P9-DTT-143

DATE DUE

Quick Table of Contents

Introductory

Medical-Surgical Nursing

Introductory Medical-Surgical Nursing

SEVENTH EDITION

Barbara K. Timby, RN,C, BSN, MS
Nursing Professor
Medical-Surgical Nursing
Glen Oaks Community College
Centreville, MI

Jeanne C. Scherer, RN, BSN, MA
Former Assistant Director and Medical-Surgical Coordinator
Sisters School of Nursing
Buffalo, NY

Nancy E. Smith, RN, MS
Chairperson
Department of Nursing
Southern Maine Technical College
South Portland, ME

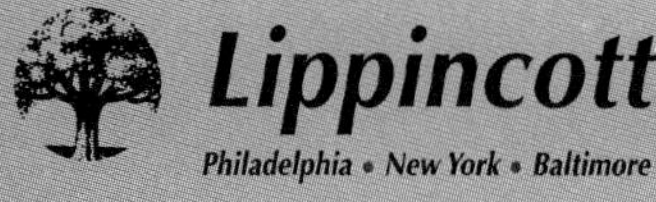
Lippincott
Philadelphia • New York • Baltimore

Acquisitions Editor: Lisa Stead
Assistant Editor: Claudia Vaughn
Senior Project Editor: Sandra Cherrey Scheinin

Senior Production Manager: Helen Ewan
Production Coordinator: Patricia McCloskey
Assistant Art Director: Doug Smock

7th Edition

9 8 7 6 5 4 3 2 1

Library of Congress Cataloging-in-Publication Data

Timby, Barbara Kuhn.
Introductory medical surgical nursing / Barbara K. Timby, Jeanne C. Scherer, Nancy E. Smith. — 7th ed.
p. cm.
Scherer's name appears first on the earlier edition.
Includes bibliographical references and index.
ISBN 0-7817-1599-7 (alk. paper)
1. Nursing. 2. Surgical nursing. I. Scherer, Jeanne C. II. Smith, Nancy E. (Nancy Ellen), 1949– . III. Title.
[DNLM: 1. Nursing Care. 2. Perioperative Nursing. WY 150T583i 1999]
RT41.S38 1999
610.73—dc21
DNLM/DC
for Library of Congress 98-30557
CIP

To Jeanne C. Scherer,
who pioneered this text and facilitated its progress
through six successful editions.
Your knowledge, enthusiasm, and friendship
will never be forgotten.

Contributors

Mary Berry, RN, BSN, MSATE
Theory and Clinical Instructor
LPN Department
School of Practical Nursing
Academy of Career and Technology
Beckley, WV

Susan G. Dudek, RD, BS
Part-Time Assistant Professor
Dietic Technology Program
Erie Community College
Williamsville, NY

Consultant Dietician
Chafee Hospital and Home
Springville, NY

Virginia Kwitkowski, MS, RN, CS, CRNP-AC
Clinical Nurse III
Nursing Department
National Institutes of Health, Warren Grant Magnuson Clinical Center
Bethesda, MD

Sharon Powell-Laney, RN, MSN, CCRN
Coordinator of Practical Nursing
Indiana County Area Vocational-Technical School
Marion Center, PA

Nancy Rayhorn, BSN, RN, BN, CGBN
Nurse Clinician
Pediatric Gastroenterology
Arizona State University
Tempe, AZ

Sally Roach, RN, MSN, CNS
Assistant Professor
University of Texas at Brownsville and Texas Southmost College
Brownsville, TX

Naomi Wilson, RN, MSN
Instructor
Department of Nursing
Southern Maine Technical College
South Portland, ME

Reviewers

James Austen, AAS, BSN
Nursing Faculty and Continuing Nursing Education Coordinator
Wetherford College
Wetherford, TX

Ann Dungan Balderee, BSN
Instructor, Vocational Nursing
Panola College
Carthage, TX

Gail Barbich, RN, MSN
Practical Nurse Teacher
James Martin School at Swenson
Philadelphia, PA

Christine Sorok Benventuti, RN, BSN
Lead Instructor Team II, LVN Program
Assistant Director of Nursing
Concorde Career Institute
Anaheim, CA

Mary Berry, RN, BSN, MSATE
Theory and Clinical Instructor
LPN Department
School of Practical Nursing
Academy of Careers and Technology
Beckley, WV

Irene Borodycia, BSN
Instructor and Coordinator
Alvernia School of Practical Nursing
Pittsburgh, PA

Jenny Burch, RN, BSN
Lead Instructor, Adult Health Nursing—Theory and Clinical
Practical Nursing Program
Spencerian College
Louisville, KY

Iva L. Burgan, BSN, MSN, RN
Coordinator of Vocational Nursing
Bee County College
Alice, TX

Marilyn F. Collins, RN, BSN, PHN
Director/Department Chairman of Health Occupations
Citrus College
Glendora, CA

Varonica Dickerson, RN, BSN
Director, Vocational Nursing
Panola College
Carthage, TX

Michelle L. Foley, RN,C, CMA
Senior Nursing Instructor
Charles E. Gregory School of Nursing
Raritan Bay Medical Center
Perth Amboy, NJ

Esther Gonzales, RN, MSN, MS, ED
Assistant Professor of Nursing
Vocational Nursing Department
Del Mar College
Corpus Christi, TX

Lois Harrion, MS, RN
Director, Vocational Nursing Program
Simi Valley Adult School and Career Institute
Simi Valley, CA

Debra Hodge, RN
Theory and Clinical Instructor
School of Practical Nursing
Academy of Careers and Technology
Beckley, WV

Kathleen A. Hutchins-Otero, ADN
LVN Instructor
San Jacinto College South
Houston, TX

Deborah Kavanagh, BSN, MS
Assistant Professor
The Union Memorial Hospital School of Nursing
Baltimore, MD

Johnnie Nichols, RN, BSN
Instructor, Vocational Nursing
Panola College
Carthage, TX

Sharon Powell-Laney, RN, MSN, CCRN
Coordinator of Practical Nursing
Indiana County Vocational Technical School of Practical Nursing
Marion Center, PA

Kathryn Sidwell, BSN
Practical Nurse Instructor
Health Occupations
Mid East Ohio Vocational School District
Zanesville, OH

Linda Snell, RN,C, DNS
Assistant Professor of Nursing
Director, Family FNP Program
D'Youville College
Buffalo, NY

Diane Vernon, MN, RN, PHN
Professor of Nursing
Department of Nursing
California State University, Los Angeles
Los Angeles, CA

Connie K. Ward, RN
Nursing Instructor
Vocational Nursing Department
Lamar University at Orange
Orange, TX

Preface

In today's changing health care environment, nurses are faced with many challenges and opportunities. The 7th edition of *Introductory Medical-Surgical Nursing* was written to help nurses meet these challenges and take advantage of expanding opportunities. The many changes to this edition reflect the changes in nursing care today. The authors have listed these changes below.

New to this Edition

Drug tables. The 7th edition includes more integration of pharmacology, with the addition of Drug Tables. In almost every chapter, a Drug Table addresses the major categories of medications prescribed for the treatment of common disorders that are discussed. The tables include categories of drugs, an example of generic and trade names, their mechanism of action, common side effects, and nursing considerations. This feature reinforces the beginning student's knowledge of drug therapy and coordinates pharmacology for students whose nursing curricula integrate this content rather than teach it as a separate course.

Additional drug information continues to appear in General Pharmacologic Considerations, a repeated feature at the end of each disorder chapter.

Nursing Guidelines. In this edition, we have presented Nursing Guidelines in special boxes separate from the text. This information reflects essential nursing information related to caring for a client with a specific disorder.

Clinical Procedures. Also new to this edition, Clinical Procedures follow a step-by-step format to help students refresh clinical skills that are commonly used when caring for clients with described disorders. The clinical procedures also include separate columns that identify nursing actions and rationales and contain illustrations, where appropriate, to further clarify the information.

Expanded discussion of psychobiologic disorders. More and more research indicates a physiologic link to conditions that were heretofore considered mental disorders. Therefore, this edition introduces students to an entire unit that focuses on the neurochemical bases for anxiety, somatoform, mood, and eating disorders. This unit also includes chapters on caring for those who are chemically dependent or who suffer from dementia and thought disorders, such as schizophrenia. This additional content provides an expanded knowledge base for students caring for clients in the community and other areas of the health care delivery system. It also prepares students for the NCLEX questions in the client needs category of Psychosocial Integrity.

Reorganization of the nursing process format. As in the 6th edition, the nursing process is emphasized extensively throughout the text. In this edition, however, the diagnosis and planning steps have been restructured into a double-column design to simulate a nursing care plan that correlates priority problems, goal statements, and nursing orders. Diagnoses from the most recent approved NANDA list are used. Collaborative problems are also included. The new arrangement assists students in the transition from their foundation in medical-surgical nursing theory to clinical practice.

Revised and Refocused Content

Emphasis on nursing management. The text continues to stress the independent and interdependent roles and responsibilities of nurses in managing the care of clients with common medical-surgical disorders. Active voice is used to direct learners toward the dynamics of nursing care.

Integrated physical assessment techniques. An overview of assessment skills is retained in Unit I. In addition, specific assessment techniques and abnormal findings are described in each Unit's introductory chapter. This separation helps students to focus on the correlation between the specific disorders presented in the text and the assessment techniques they need to use.

Strengthening of pathophysiology. After reviewing normal anatomy and physiology in each introductory unit, every disorder is accompanied by a comprehensive yet understandable discussion of the physiologic changes that occur with the disease process. The discussion builds a bridge between the disorder and the rationale for treatment measures.

More illustrations. This edition contains the addition of many new graphic art illustrations and photographs that assist visual learners to understand the concepts that are discussed.

Refocused Critical Thinking Exercises. In this edition, the Critical Thinking Exercises have been redesigned. They aim to challenge students to integrate, analyze, and apply principles discussed in each respective chapter to a representative situation. Hypothetical names of clients in the critical thinking items have been eliminated in keeping with the test development patterns established by the National Council of State Boards of Nursing and the National League for Nursing.

Identification of community and Internet resources. At the end of each chapter, students are provided with addresses, phone numbers, and web sites for organizations that provide information or client support as it relates to various disorders.

Contents

The content of the 7th edition of *Introductory Medical-Surgical Nursing* addresses the common adult disorders that are treated medically and surgically. The content has been reviewed, revised, and updated to reflect current medical and nursing practice. For example:

Unit 1, *Nursing Roles and Responsibilities*, includes chapters on Concepts and Trends in Health Care, Nursing in Various Settings, The Nursing Process, Interviewing and Physical Assessment, and Legal and Ethical Issues.

Unit 2, *Development Across the Lifespan,* contains chapters on Caring for Young Adults, Caring for Middle-Aged Adults, and Caring for Older Adults.

Unit 3, *Psychosocial Aspects of Nursing,* contains chapters on Nurse–Client Relationships and Caring for Culturally Diverse Clients.

Unit 4, *Psychobiologic Disorders,* is new to this edition. It contains chapters on Interaction of Body and Mind, Caring for Clients With Somatoform Disorders, Caring for Clients With Anxiety Disorders, Caring for Clients With Mood Disorders, Caring for Clients With Eating Disorders, Caring for Chemically Dependent Clients, and Caring for Clients With Dementia and Thought Disorders.

Unit 5, *Common Medical-Surgical Problems,* includes chapters on Caring for Clients With Infectious Disorders; Caring for Clients With Cancer; Caring for Clients With Pain; Caring for Clients With Fluid, Electrolyte, and Acid–Base Imbalances; Caring for Clients in Shock; Caring for Clients Requiring Intravenous Therapy; Caring for Perioperative Clients; and Caring for Dying Clients.

Units 6 through 17 present information on disorders according to body systems. Each unit begins with an introductory chapter that includes a general review of anatomy and physiology, a discussion of client assessment, and common diagnostic and laboratory tests that pertain to particular disorders.

Features and Learning Tools

Features and learning tools in the 7th edition of *Introductory Medical-Surgical Nursing* are easily identifiable by color highlighting, icons, or special text. They include:

Boxes. These provide quick access to vital information, summarize more detailed information found in the text, or focus the reader's attention to special concerns.

Nursing Guidelines. A new feature of this edition, these boxed displays present essential nursing information related to caring for a client with a specific disorder. Nursing Guidelines are identified with this icon.

Clinical Procedures. Also new to this edition, these step-by-step procedures reinforce skills necessary to care for clients with specific disorders discussed in the text. Clinical Procedures are identified with this icon.

Tables. These features provide additional comparative and contrasting information to assist learners in distinguishing differences in disorders and their management. Drug Tables are distinguished by this icon.

Nursing Care Plans. These are presented throughout the text to reflect the roles and responsibilities of today's nurses in planning client care.

Key Terms. These words are listed at the beginning of each chapter and are set in bold type within the text where they appear with or near their definition. Additional technical terms are italicized throughout the text.

Learning Objectives. These student-oriented objectives appear at the beginning of each chapter to serve as guidelines for acquiring specific information within each chapter.

Summary of Key Concepts. Located at the end of each chapter, the summary condenses the chapter's content and integrates information that corresponds with the learning objectives as well. The summation can be used as a preview of the chapter and a later resource for quick review.

Nutritional, Pharmacologic, and Gerontologic Considerations. Included at the end of most chapters, the content has been developed by experts in their fields. These are identified by the following icons.

Critical Thinking Exercises. These questions, which follow each chapter summary, aim to facilitate application of the material contained within the chapter, using clinical situations or rhetorical questions.

Selected Readings. These are intended to provide a guide to current literature that has been cited as references within the chapter or to encourage further independent learning about disorders discussed in the text.

Numerous illustrations and photographs. Liberally interspersed throughout the text, illustrations and photographs promote an understanding of the narrative discussions. The use of a second color calls attention to emphasized information. A section of full-color illustrations, some of which are new to this edition, aids in the assessment and identification of unique conditions. Updated photographs accurately reflect products, procedures, and client care.

Appendices. These include a guide to common medical abbreviations and laboratory tests and their normal values.

Glossary. Found at the back of the book, this is a quick reference of definitions for Key Terms and italicized words that are used throughout the text.

Detailed Table of Contents. Located at the beginning of the textbook, this provides an outline of each unit's, and chapter's subject matter.

Quick Table of Contents. Printed on the front end pages, this feature facilitates prompt location of specific chapters.

Quick Reference to NANDA-Approved Nursing Diagnoses. This list is printed on the back end page to help students become familiar with the expanding taxonomy of problems that falls within nursing's domain.

Instructor's Ancillary Package

The ancillary package includes the *Instructors Resource Manual and Testbank* with transparency acetates to accompany *Introductory Medical-Surgical Nursing,* 7th edition. Included in the Instructors' Manual are chapter overviews, chapter objectives, key terms, case study exercises, listings of multimedia and Web resources, guidelines for evaluating critical thinking exercises, and multiple-choice testbank questions on disk. Testbank questions are written and designed in accordance with the NCLEX format, and answer rationales are provided for each question, followed by identification of the specific client needs component of the nursing process. All material for critical thinking evaluations and testbank questions are derived from the textbook.

Student Study Guide

The *Study Guide to Accompany Introductory Medical-Surgical Nursing,* 7th edition, is designed for use with this text. The study guide now includes practice exercises of all question types and guidelines for students to respond to critical thinking questions, an answer key, and a student self-study disk. All questions in the study guide are also based on information in the textbook.

Acknowledgments

The authors wish to thank all those who helped in the preparation of this edition. To those at Lippincott Williams & Wilkins, especially Lisa Stead, Acquisitions Editor, and her Editorial Assistant, Claudia Vaughn, we say thank you for all your support, encouragement, and willingness to help. To Sandra Cherrey Scheinin, Senior Project Editor, we appreciate the work on the final editing process.

We are also grateful to Susan G. Dudek, RD, BS, for her contribution of the Nutritional Considerations and review of the nutritional content within the chapter. We thank Sally Roach, RN, MSN, CNS, for her contribution of the Pharmacologic and Gerontologic Considerations and review of the chapters for gerontologic and pharmacologic content. Sally also prepared most of the drug tables throughout the book as well as contributed the chapters in Unit 2, Development Across the Lifespan.

There are several contributors to whom we are grateful. They are Mary Berry, RN, BSN, MSATE; Virginia Kwitkowski, MS, RN, CS, CRNP-AC; Sharon Powell-Laney, RN, MSN, CCRN; Nancy Rayhorn, BSN, RN, BN, CGBN; and Naomi Wilson, RN, MSN.

We hope that *Introductory Medical-Surgical Nursing,* 7th edition, provides the readers with the practical knowledge and skills to manage the nursing care of clients in today's changing health care environments. We also hope that our contributions provide students with similar joys and rewards that we experience in our nursing careers.

Barbara K. Timby, RN,C, BSN, MA
Nancy Smith, RN, MS

Contents

4 Psychobiologic Disorders 97

5 Common Medical-Surgical Problems 169

10 Caring for Clients With Neurologic Disorders 541

11 Caring for Clients With Sensory Disorders 625

12 Caring for Clients With Gastrointestinal Disorders 665

13 Caring for Clients With Endocrine Problems 789

Special Features

Drug Tables

Nursing Care Plans

Clinical Procedures

Nursing Guidelines

1

Nursing Roles and Responsibilities

Chapter 1

Concepts and Trends in Health Care

KEY TERMS

Capitation
Client
Critical pathways
Diagnosis-related groups (DRGs)
Health care delivery system
Health care team
Health–illness continuum
Health maintenance
Health promotion
Health maintenance organization (HMO)
Holism
Integrated delivery system (IDS)
Managed care organization (MCO)
Preferred provider organization (PPO)
Primary care
Prospective payment systems (PPS)
Secondary care
Tertiary care

LEARNING OBJECTIVES

On completion of this chapter, the reader will:

- Explain the concepts of health and the health–illness continuum.
- Describe the role of nurses.
- Discuss the impact of economic changes on health care delivery.
- Evaluate the impact of prospective payment systems (PPS) and diagnosis-related groups (DRGs).
- Discuss the difference between capitation and fee-for-service insurance.
- Discuss methods for monitoring quality of care.
- Identify three future health care goals according to *Healthy People 2000.*
- Identify trends that will influence health care policy in the future.
- List six priorities for global health.

A career in nursing involves assisting clients to promote, maintain, and restore health, and to support clients during illness and at death. Nevertheless, the role in which nurses function in the health care system is affected by society's concept of health and changing economic policies that affect health care strategies.

Health

The constitution of the World Health Organization (WHO) defines health as "a state of complete physical, mental, and social well-being and not merely the absence of disease and infirmity." Although this definition of health is useful, it presents health and illness in absolute terms: if an individual is not functioning optimally in every way, he or she is not healthy. It also implies that the presence of an infirmity means that health is not possible.

The Health–Illness Continuum

Dunn (1961) described health as a dynamic state that ranges from high-level wellness to very poor health and death (Fig. 1–1). This definition of health allowed for many levels of health and illness. Other theorists have expanded on this idea to describe health as the ability to adapt physically, emotionally, and socially so that comfort and stability are maintained and self-expression is possible. Embedded in this definition of health is the idea that a client with chronic illness can achieve a high level of wellness if he or she can attain a high quality of life within the limits of that illness. For example, a physically disabled person would be considered healthy if he or she were physiologically stable and engaged in per-

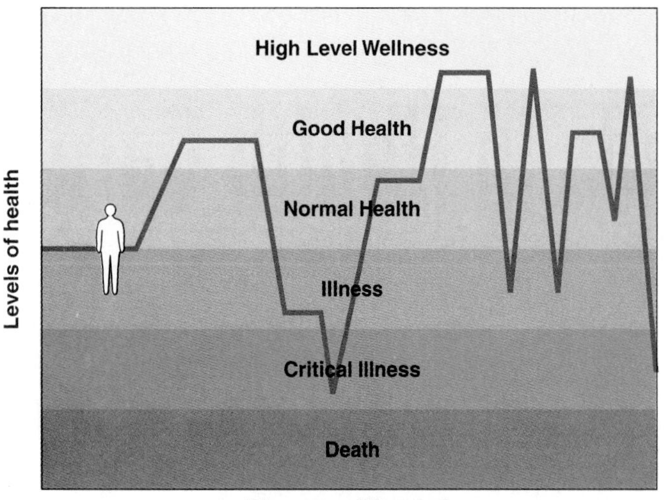

FIGURE 1-1. **The health–illness continuum** shows the different levels of health a person experiences over a lifetime.

sonal and social activities that he or she found meaningful.

Health Maintenance and Promotion

Many people now believe they have control over their well-being and are taking more responsibility for their health status. **Health maintenance** refers to protecting one's current level of health by preventing illness or deterioration, such as complying with medication regimens, being screened for diseases such as breast and colon cancer, or practicing safe sex. **Health promotion** refers to engaging in strategies to enhance health. Such strategies include eating a diet high in grains and complex carbohydrates, exercising regularly, balancing work with leisure activities, and practicing stress reduction techniques. The change in attitude from a passive role in illness to an active role in purchasing health services is reflected in this book by use of the term **client**. The client may or may not be ill, but he or she takes responsibility for meeting his or her health maintenance and promotion needs and actively participates in treatment decisions regarding health restoration.

Health Care

Although the concept of health has changed in recent decades, so too has the health care industry. Rapid advances in science and technology have contributed to the development of highly sophisticated methods for diagnosing and treating disease. At the same time, escalating health care costs have created difficult economic conditions, disparity in access to care, and brief hospital lengths of stay. The health care system has grown to include multiple outpatient, short-term, and long-term facilities with care given by a variety of providers.

Health Care Providers

The **health care team** consists of specially trained personnel who work together to help individuals meet their health care needs. The team includes physicians, nurses, psychologists, pharmacists, dietitians, social workers, respiratory and physical therapists, occupational therapists, nursing assistants, technicians, and the insurance company staff. All members of this team collaborate on client issues (medical, social, and financial) to achieve the best possible outcome. Figure 1–2 shows personnel who are part of the health care team.

THE ROLE OF THE NURSES

Nurses have multiple roles in the health care system. They collect data, diagnose human responses to

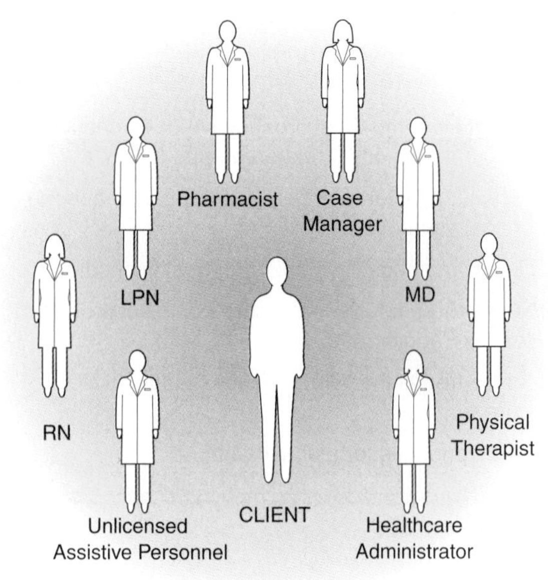

FIGURE 1-2. Members of the healthcare team.

health problems, plan, provide, and evaluate the outcomes of care in various settings according to facility policies and state nurse practice acts. They educate clients, families, and staff; manage resources; and act as advocates to help clients make informed and autonomous decisions. Nurses participate in disease prevention and health promotion activities for individuals, families, and communities and further the scientific basis for practice by participating in research. Nurses collaborate with other health care team members to provide the highest quality of care.

Nurses practice from the philosophical perspective of **holism.** Holism means that an individual and his or her health is viewed as a balance of body, mind, and spirit. Treating only the body will not necessarily restore optimum health; psychological, sociocultural, developmental, and spiritual needs must be considered as well.

The Health Care System

The **health care delivery system** refers to the full range of services that are available to individuals seeking prevention, identification, treatment, or rehabilitation of health problems. The first resource person or agency an individual contacts concerning a health need provides **primary care.** This initial contact is often with a family practitioner, an internist, or a nurse practitioner. **Secondary care** includes referrals to facilities for additional testing, consultation, and diagnosis such as cardiac catheterization. **Tertiary care** is provided in hospitals where specialists and complex technology are available. *Long-term care* or *extended care* and *rehabilitation* are provided in special facilities or units that offer prolonged health maintenance or restorative services. Examples include nursing homes, skilled nursing facilities, and rehabilitation centers. Home care is an important adjunct to inpatient care; visiting nurses and home health aides are the personnel who make earlier discharge to home possible by providing services formerly done in hospitals. Hospices and home hospice care are resources for terminally ill clients and their families.

Access to Care

As the numbers of health services expand, the health care delivery system becomes more complex, costly, and, in many cases, inaccessible. An estimated 37 million citizens in the United States do not have access to adequate health care because of the economic burden it presents. Another 25 million citizens have inadequate health care coverage. For many, health maintenance and health promotion are unaffordable luxuries. Groups most likely to be underserved are children, the elderly, ethnic minorities, and the poor. Many of these individuals delay seeking early treatment for their health problems because they cannot afford to pay for services. When the illness becomes so severe that there is no other choice but to seek medical attention, many turn to their local hospital's emergency rooms for primary care. This is an expensive alternative that usually involves long waits and no follow-up care.

Financing the Costs of Health Care

The disparities in access coupled with the high cost of health care has prompted the evaluation of spending in the entire health care industry. The 1990s has been a decade of streamlining government payment systems and finding innovative approaches from private insurers and corporate health plans. Historically, health care was paid for by private insurance, self-insurance systems, and Medicare. Under these plans there were no incentives to control costs. Hospitals and approved providers were paid what they charged; more charges meant more revenues. Not only did charges escalate at an alarming rate, but abuse and fraudulent billing escalated as well.

PROSPECTIVE PAYMENT SYSTEMS

In 1983, a **prospective payment system (PPS)** was implemented by Medicare. This system uses financial incentives to decrease total charges by reimbursing on a *fixed rate* basis. Predetermined amounts are reimbursed to hospitals for the **diagnosis-related group (DRG)** in which the client falls. The DRG system is a method of grouping clients with similar diagnoses. For example all clients receiving a hip, knee, or shoulder replacement fall into DRG 209, Total Joint Replacement, and their surgeries are reimbursed at basically the same rate. If costs are less than the reimbursed amount, the hospital makes money; if costs exceed the reimbursed amount, the hospital loses money. This reimbursement system has driven the marked decreases in hospital lengths of stay in the past 15 years.

Much of the criticism of the PPS/DRG system is related to the possible premature discharge of clients and increased responsibility for family members who may be unable to provide adequate care. Another criticism has been the shift in costs from Medicare clients to those who have private insurance. Privately insured clients were charged inflated amounts to make up for the losses in Medicare revenues. In response to this cost shifting and other economic forces, insurance companies began to challenge hospital charges aggressively, refuse payment when hospital level of care was not provided, and shift their clients into cost-containment reimbursement systems now known as managed care.

MANAGED CARE

Managed care organizations (**MCOs**) are insurers who carefully plan and closely supervise the distribution of health care services. Although it is a business venture with an emphasis on cost of services and economic use of resources, managed care focuses on prevention as the best way to manage health care costs (Box 1–1). The two most common types of managed care systems are **health maintenance organizations** (**HMOs**) and **preferred provider organizations** (**PPOs**). A third emerging MCO financing structure is called **capitation.**

Health Maintenance Organizations

HMOs are group insurance plans in which each participant pays a preset, fixed fee in exchange for health care services. This fee does not fluctuate with the type or frequency of care. The financial stability of HMOs is based on their ability to keep their members healthy and out of the hospital by periodic screening, health education, and preventive services.

The HMOs provide ambulatory, hospitalization, and home care services. Some HMOs have their own facilities; others use community agencies for services. An HMO member must receive authorization (referral) for secondary care such as second opinions with specialists or diagnostic testing. If members obtain unauthorized care, they are responsible for the entire bill. In this way, HMOs serve as the gatekeepers for health care services.

Preferred Provider Organizations

PPOs operate on the principle that costs can be controlled through competition. Acting as an agent for a health insurance company, the PPO creates a community network of providers who are willing to discount their fees for service in exchange for a steady supply of referred customers. Consumers can keep their health care costs lower if they receive care from the preferred providers. If they select providers outside the network, they pay a higher percentage of the costs.

Capitation

Capitation is a fundamentally different concept in health care financing. Instead of paying a fee for provided services as in traditional insurance plans (including HMOs and PPOs), capitation plans pay a preset fee per member per month to the health care provider, usually a hospital or hospital system. This fee covers all medical costs incurred and is paid regardless of whether or not the member requires health care services. If members do not require a lot of high-cost care, the provider makes money; if members use a lot of high-cost resources, the provider loses money. This method of financing provides the strongest incentives for limiting use of expensive services and focusing health care on health maintenance and health promotion.

BOX 1-1 Goals of Managed Care

- Use health care resources efficiently.
- Deliver high-quality care at a reasonable cost.
- Measure, monitor, and manage fiscal and client outcomes.
- Prevent illness through screening and health promotion activities.
- Provide client education to decrease risk of disease.
- Case manage clients with chronic illness to minimize number of hospitalizations.

Impact of Economic Changes on Health Care

The changes in reimbursement structures and practices have created a shift in economic and decision-making power from hospitals, nurses, and physicians to insurance companies. A great deal of criticism and concern has accompanied this shift as doctors, nurses, other providers, and consumers find themselves unable to obtain or provide care free from the economic pressuring of the insurer. Many claim that the profits posted by large insurance companies come at the expense of quality care and the jobs of health care providers. Hospitals have downsized or restructured, and sometimes closed, because of these changes. Consequently regions are left with fewer hospitals, higher nurse– client ratios, and higher client acuity levels on general medical-surgical units, skilled nursing facilities, long-term care, and home health settings.

Employment for health care workers has also been affected by changes in the health care industry. Hospitals are using unlicensed assistive personnel to perform some duties practical and registered nurses once provided and many are concerned that this will jeopardize the quality of care. Physicians' income has dropped in recent years and this trend is expected to continue.

The client's experience and satisfaction with health care may be affected as well. A single episode of illness can involve negotiating for a referral, receiving testing at a site other than the hospital, staying a short time in the hospital, transferring to a rehabilitation or skilled nursing facility (or both), and obtaining outpatient rehabilitation and home health services. Although efforts are made to coordinate care, particularly by nurse case managers (see Chap. 2), this fragmentation forces clients to build therapeutic relationships often and may leave them unsure of who is in charge.

The cost-driven changes have had positive effects as well. In an attempt to reduce redundancy of health care services and increase economic leverage, hospitals and other health care facilities are forming networks, known as **integrated delivery systems (IDS)** (Box 1–2). IDS provide a full range of health care services that should result in highly coordinated, cost-effective care. Shorter hospital stays may result in less nosocomial (acquired in the hospital) complications and quicker return to self-care. In some ways, nurses have been empowered by taking an active role in advocating for quality, nurse-provided care. New and expanded positions in the health care industry are being filled by nurses (see Chap. 2).

Additionally, the economic burden imposed on society by out-of-control health care costs had to be addressed. Another indirect positive result of the cost containment initiatives is increased attention to what constitutes quality in health care and how hospitals, practitioners, and insurance companies measure, monitor, and manage quality.

Quality of Care

Demand for evidence that hospitals and practitioners provide quality, cost-effective care comes from insurers, regulatory bodies such as the Joint Commission for Accreditation of Healthcare Organizations, and consumers. To meet this demand hospitals have formed *performance improvement committees*. These groups or hospital departments may also be called *quality improvement* or *outcomes management committees*. They assess such factors as readmission to the hospital within 30 days of discharge, average cost per case, wound infection rates, incidence of hospital-acquired pressure ulcers, and various other measures. Because insurers have so much say on the type and quantity of care provided, they too have quality improvement departments that monitor similar outcomes.

As concern for cost meets concern for quality, practitioners search for ways to ensure that all the care, teaching, and preparation are accomplished before the discharge date without overusing expensive resources. This has led to the development of protocols (also known as guidelines or standards) for managing care. One method gaining widespread use is the critical or clinical pathway. **Critical pathways** are developed by multidisciplinary teams for specific diagnoses or procedures; they standardize important aspects of care such as diagnostic workup, nursing care, education, physical therapy, and discharge planning across the estimated length of stay. By analyzing variances from the pathway (unexpected events such as delayed discharge or transfer to a more intensive level of care), clinicians can identify trends in care that are beneficial or detrimental. The team who develops the pathway can then redesign care to address the identified trend. Critical pathways are often considered a tool of case management (see Chap. 2). Figure 1–3 is an example of a critical pathway for a client with pneumonia in an emergency department.

Many other methods exist for determining the quality of care. Patient satisfaction surveys, quality of life questionnaires, functional assessment tools, number of hospital admissions per year for clients with chronic illnesses, and morbidity (complications) and mortality (deaths) rates are a few of the important measures assessed when examining quality.

BOX 1-2 Integrated Delivery Systems

Fully integrated health care delivery systems will provide:

- Wellness programs
- Preventive care
- Ambulatory care
- Outpatient diagnostic and laboratory services
- Emergency care
- General and tertiary hospital services
- Rehabilitation
- Long-term care
- Assisted living facilities
- Psychiatric care
- Home health care services
- Hospice care
- Outpatient pharmacies

Adapted from Buerhas P. (1996). Creating a new place in a competitive market: The value of nursing care. In E. Hein. *Contemporary nursing leadership: Selected readings.*

Future Trends and Goals for Health Care

The United States Public Health Service, under the direction of the Secretary of Health and Human Services, identifies national health goals. *Healthy People 2000: National Health Promotion and Disease Prevention* (1992) identified several goals that address health and access to health care:

- Increasing the span of healthy life for Americans
- Reducing health disparities among Americans
- Achieving access to preventive services for all Americans

EMERGENCY DEPARTMENT CRITICAL PATH: PNEUMONIA Exclusion Criteria: Clients with HIV, neutropenia, severe hypotension, steroid dependency > 20mg/day, those requiring mechanical ventilation, or clients on immunosuppressive or chemotherapy.

	2ND HOUR	3RD HOUR	4TH HOUR
ASSESSMENTS	REASSESSMENT/ASSESSMENT RESPONSE TO TREATMENT	REASSESSMENT/ASSESSMENT RESPONSE TO TREATMENT	REASSESSMENT/ASSESSMENT RESPONSE TO TREATMENT
CONSULTS	IF INDICATED NOTIFY ADMITTING RESIDENT		
LABS, DIAGNOSTICS PROCEDURES	1. AP/LAT CXR RESULTED 2. CBC, SMA7 3. BLOOD CULTURES X2 4. SPUTUM C + S/gmst. Y__N__ 5. ABG IF PULSE OX <92% RA 6. EKG FEMALE >55 MALE >45 OR CLINICALLY INDICATED		
INTERVENTIONS	SAFETY MEASURES AS PER STANDARD		
IV/MEDICATION	1. SALINE LOCK 2. O2 THERAPY AS PER ORDER 3. ANTIBIOTIC AS PER ALGORITHM AFTER BLOOD CULTURE AND ATTEMPT AT SPUTUM CULTURE		

Community Acquired	**Institutional**
Is the client allergic to PCN?	**Is the client allergic to PCN?**
No: **Ceftriaxone 1gm q24 •**	**No:** **Ticarcillin/Clavulanate 3.1gm q6 •**
Yes: **TMP/SMX 2amps (320mg/1600mg) IV q12 •**	**Yes:** **Ciprofloxacin 400mg IV q12 • and Clindamycin 600mg IV q8 •**
CIRCLE MEDICATION: TIME OF ADMINISTRATION _____	**CIRCLE MEDICATION: TIME OF ADMINISTRATION _____**

TEACHING	1. REASSURE AND INFORM PT/SO RE: TX PLAN AND INTERVENTIONS 2. PROVIDE CLIENT WITH PSYCHOLOGICAL SUPPORT 3. PT/FAMILY CAN VERBALIZE DISCHARGE INSTRUCTIONS? Y__N__ 4. PT/FAMILY RECEIVED WRITTEN DISCHARGE INSTRUCTIONS? Y__N__	1. REASSURE AND INFORM PT/SO RE: TX PLAN AND INTERVENTIONS 2. PROVIDE CLIENT WITH PSYCHOLOGICAL SUPPORT 3. PT/FAMILY CAN VERBALIZE DISCHARGE INSTRUCTIONS? Y__N__ 4. PT/FAMILY RECEIVED WRITTEN DISCHARGE INSTRUCTIONS? Y__N__	1. REASSURE AND INFORM PT/SO RE: TX PLAN AND INTERVENTIONS 2. PROVIDE CLIENT WITH PSYCHOLOGICAL SUPPORT 3. PT/FAMILY CAN VERBALIZE DISCHARGE INSTRUCTIONS? Y__N__ 4. PT/FAMILY RECEIVED WRITTEN DISCHARGE INSTRUCTIONS? Y__N__
D/C PLANNING AND FOLLOW-UP	DISPOSITION: 1. ADMITTED RM#____ 2. TREATED AND REFERRED 3. TX TO OTHER INSTITUTION 4. NOT EXAMINED OR TREATED 5. LEFT AMA 6. DOA/DIED IN ED TIME OF DISCHARGE________	DISPOSITION: 1. ADMITTED RM#____ 2. TREATED AND REFERRED 3. TX TO OTHER INSTITUTION 4. NOT EXAMINED OR TREATED 5. LEFT AMA 6. DOA/DIED IN ED TIME OF DISCHARGE________	DISPOSITION: 1. ADMITTED RM#____ 2. TREATED AND REFERRED 3. TX TO OTHER INSTITUTION 4. NOT EXAMINED OR TREATED 5. LEFT AMA 6. DOA/DIED IN ED TIME OF DISCHARGE________
OUTCOMES	1. CLINICALLY STABLE 2. PULSE OX > 92% (W OR W/O O2) Y__N__ 3. HR 60–135 Y__N__ 4. RR 12–35 Y__N__ 5. SBP >90 Y__N__ 6. RECEIVED FIRST DOSE OF ANTIBIOTICS Y__N__	1. CLINICALLY STABLE 2. PULSE OX > 92% (W OR W/O O2) Y__N__ 3. HR 60–135 Y__N__ 4. RR 12–35 Y__N__ 5. SBP >90 Y__N__ 6. RECEIVED FIRST DOSE OF ANTIBIOTICS Y__N__	1. CLINICALLY STABLE 2. PULSE OX > 92% (W OR W/O O2) Y__N__ 3. HR 60–135 Y__N__ 4. RR 12–35 Y__N__ 5. SBP >90 Y__N__ 6. RECEIVED FIRST DOSE OF ANTIBIOTICS Y__N__

SIGNATURE	TIME	INITIAL	SIGNATURE	TIME	INITIAL

**Shaded Area Represents MD Decision Point

FIGURE 1-3. An Emergency Department (ED) critical path for pneumonia. The first hour of care is covered by the ED's generic critical path and covers the general interventions and baseline diagnostics that lead to a working diagnosis and a specific critical path.
Abbreviations: AP/LAT CXR = Anterior, posterior and lateral chest x-rays; CBC = complete blood count; SMA7 = electrolytes, glucose; Sputum C & S/gmst = sputum culture, sensitivity and gram stain; ABG = arterial blood gas; EKG = electrocardiogram; PT/SO = patient/significant other; TX = treatment or transfer; AMA = against medical advice; DOA =dead on arrival; pulse ox = pulse oximetry; W or W/O = with or without; HR = heart rate; RR = respiratory rate; SBP =systolic blood pressure; HIV = human immunodeficiency virus.

BOX 1-3 Priorities for International Health

- Integrated, comprehensive disease control that incorporates prevention, diagnosis, treatment, and rehabilitation
- Improved training of health care professionals
- Wider use of cost-effective methods for disease prevention and management, including screening
- Intense and sustained global efforts to encourage healthy lifestyles to modify risk factors such as diet, exercise and smoking, especially among children and young adults
- Development of health-enhancing public policy including policy on financing, pricing, and taxation that will support disease prevention programs
- Alleviation of pain, reduction of suffering, and provision of palliative (comfort) care to those who cannot be cured

Adapted from World Health Organization (1997).

The Healthy People steering committee will evaluate the nation's progress in meeting these goals and identify additional health objectives in *Healthy People 2010*.

As we move into the 21st century, economics, consumer satisfaction, effectiveness of traditional medical care, alternative medicine, disease prevalence, global emergence of drug-resistant organisms, and cultural diversity are all forces that will influence the direction of health care in this nation and around the world. The WHO foresees the continued impact of infectious diseases on global health, particularly in developing nations, and an epidemic of cancer and other chronic diseases secondary to increased life expectancy combined with dramatic lifestyle changes (World Health Organization, 1997). Box 1–3 outlines the WHO priorities for international health, which can be applied to any individual nation or community. In the midst of these dramatic changes and challenges, nurses are called on to continue to provide safe, high-quality, cost-effective care to individuals, families, and communities.

SUMMARY OF KEY CONCEPTS

- Levels of health and illness exist on a continuum that ranges from high-level wellness to death.
- Individuals with chronic illness can be considered healthy if they are comfortable, stable, and able to participate in personally meaningful activity.
- Health maintenance involves activities that protect the current level of health; health promotion involves activities that enhance health.
- Health care is provided by a team of skilled clinicians who work together to achieve the best outcome. The insurer is now considered a member of the health care team.
- Nurses collect data; plan, provide, and evaluate care; educate clients and family; manage resources; and advocate on the behalf of clients.
- Holism is the philosophy that individuals are a balance of body, mind, and spirit.
- The health care delivery system is a network of services that provide help with an illness or injury, or with maintaining or improving health status.
- Health care services range from primary care by a physician or nurse practitioner for treatment and prevention services, secondary care related to diagnostic testing and consultation, to tertiary care in acute care hospitals.
- Even though Americans are more health conscious, many lack the resources to gain access to health care delivery services. Despite changes in financing health care, the cost of health care is monumental for those who are uninsured or underinsured.
- Prospective payment systems were designed by the federal government to contain Medicare costs by paying a fixed rate for specific hospital services.
- Managed care is the careful management and distribution of health care resources.
- HMOs and PPOs differ in the management of health care services in that HMOs are systems that provide a range of comprehensive health care services to their members, whereas PPOs are managed systems in which members pay lower fees for each service if done by a preferred provider.
- Capitation is a method of health care coverage that prepays the provider a set fee, regardless of the amount of care provided.
- The economic changes have had widespread impact on the health care industry including hospital downsizing, the development of multifacility networks, increased nurse–client ratios, and higher acuity-level clients in all settings.
- Positive effects of the recent changes include evaluation of the costs, efficiency, and effectiveness of health care services, less exposure to hospital environment, and increased focus on quality.
- Critical pathways are developed by a multidisciplinary team to help the client meet specific outcomes in a specified period for a particular diagnosis.
- The U.S. government has three goals for improving health care by the year 2000: (1) Americans will experience a healthier life span; (2) inequities in health care will be reduced; and (3) all Americans will have access to illness preventive services.
- Continued economic struggles, consumer satisfaction, effectiveness of traditional medical care, alternative care, cultural diversity, and global patterns of disease are all forces that will shape the distribution of health care resources in the 21st century.

CRITICAL THINKING EXERCISES

1. Interview a person who has had experience with traditional health care insurance and with managed care. Explore the advantages and disadvantages of both systems.

2. Select a health care facility where you have had student clinical experiences. Have any cost reduction measures occurred and what effect have these actions had?
3. Discuss how economic conditions affect working conditions for nurses.

Suggested Readings

American Nurses Association. (1980). *Nursing: A social policy statement.* Kansas City, MO: Author.

Dunn, H. L. (1961). *High-level wellness.* Arlington, VA: Beatty.

Flarey, D. L. (1997). Managed care: Changing the way we practice. *Journal of Nursing Administration, 27*(7/8), 16–20.

Freeman, S. R., & Chambers, K. A. (1997). Home health care: Clinical pathways and quality integration. *Nursing Management, 28*(6), 45–48.

Ireson, C. L. (1997). Critical pathways: Effectiveness in achieving patient outcomes. *Journal of Nursing Administration, 27*(6), 16–23.

Kalisch, P. A., & Kalisch, B. J. (1995). *The advance of American nursing* (3rd ed.). Philadelphia: J. B. Lippincott.

Kelly, L. Y., & Joel, L..A. (1995). *Dimensions of professional nursing* (7th ed.). New York: McGraw-Hill.

Kurzen, C. R. (1997). *Contemporary practical/vocational nursing.* Philadelphia: Lippincott-Raven.

U.S. Department of Health and Human Services. (1992). *Healthy people 2000: National health promotion and disease prevention objectives.* Boston: Jones and Barlett.

World Health Organization. (1997). *World health report 1997—Executive summary: Conquering suffering, enriching humanity.* [On-line] Available: http://www.who.ch/whr/1997/exsum97 e.htm.

Chapter 2

Nursing in Various Settings

KEY TERMS

Case management
Case method
Functional nursing
Home health care
Patient-focused care
Primary nursing
Team nursing
Total care

LEARNING OBJECTIVES

On completion of this chapter, the reader will:

- Define nursing.
- Identify and compare nursing care delivery models.
- Describe the settings in which nurses practice and discuss the type of client served in these settings.
- Identify the functions of the home health nurse.
- List services provided by home health agencies.
- Define case management and identify the nurse case manager's role.

In today's dynamic health care environment, the traditional territory, roles, and responsibilities of health care providers are being challenged. Some care that was once provided by registered nurses (RNs) in hospital intensive care units can now be managed at home by clients with the support of visiting nurses. Clients undergoing procedures that formerly required a 2-week hospital stay are now discharged in fewer than 5 days. Choice of services, treatment options, and the hospital length of stay, all traditional decisions of the attending physician, are now, in many instances, dictated by insurance companies and case managers. Throughout these changes, nursing has been called on to provide high-quality nursing care wherever it is needed and to function in both traditional and evolving roles.

Nursing Care

Definitions of Nursing

Arriving at a clear and comprehensive definition of nursing has been difficult. Florence Nightingale (1859) described the role of the nurse as putting "the patient in the best condition for nature to act upon him." Virginia Henderson (1966), a contemporary nursing theorist, envisioned the nurse's role as helping the individual (sick or well) to carry out those activities contributing to health, recovery, or a peaceful death that individuals would do for themselves if they had the necessary strength, will, or knowledge. Her definition also focused on regaining independence. The American Nurses Association (ANA) defines nursing as "the diagnosis and treatment of human responses to actual or potential health problems" (ANA, 1980, p. 9). Other definitions of nursing by selected theorists are given in Table 2–1.

Nursing is concerned with caring for the individual, family, or community and requires that nurses play a significant role in health education, prevention, and promotion. Nurses attend to client needs related to hygiene, activity, diet, the environment, medical treatment, and physical and emotional comfort. Care is provided by people with different educational levels, in diverse settings, and includes a variety of activities. The licensed practical or vocational nurse (LPN/LVN) provides care to clients under the direction of an RN or physician in a structured health care setting. LPN/LVNs care for clients with well-defined, common problems that often require a high level of technical competency and expertise. LPN/LVNs frequently work in settings in which RN supervision is available but must be sought after the LPN/LVN determines the need to do so. The RN's role is more complex, involving the management and coordination of all the care provided to a group of clients. As health care delivery models continue to change, the roles of the LPN and RN are likely to change as well.

TABLE 2-1 **Definitions of Nursing by Selected Theorists**

Theorist	Definition
Florence Nightingale (1859)	Nurses alter the environment to put the client in the best condition for nature to act.
Virginia Henderson (1966)	Nurses assist the individual to carry out those activities that the client would perform unaided if he (or she) possessed the necessary strength, will, or knowledge.
Ernestine Weidenbach (1964)	Nursing is a helping, nurturing, and caring service delivered sensitively with compassion, skill, and understanding.
Dorothea Orem (1980)	Nursing care is directed at restoring self-care abilities, which are activities that clients initiate on their own behalf in maintaining health, life, and well-being.
Imogene M. King (1981)	Nursing is the care of human beings; individuals and groups are viewed as open systems in continual interaction with the environment.

Settings and Models for Nursing Care

Hospital-Based Nursing

Nursing care is provided in a variety of settings. Although hospitals employ all level of nurses in outpatient care areas such as dialysis units, clinics, same-day surgery units, and related diagnostic departments, inpatient units have been the traditional site for much of the nursing work force. Although trends in financing suggest that less reliance on hospitals as the location for nursing care delivery will be a trend for the future, there is a great deal of interest in determining the best, most cost-effective method for providing that care. Many models for care delivery exist and can coexist within hospitals based on need.

NURSING CARE DELIVERY MODELS

Case Method

Nursing care was historically provided on a **case method** basis. One nurse provided all the services required by a particular individual. Although the nurse would accompany the client to the hospital if need be, care was provided in the home and the nurse performed many household duties as well. As times changed and care became more complex, this method became impractical and different models for the hospital-based delivery of nursing care evolved. A modern version of the case method is private duty nursing.

Functional Nursing

Functional nursing evolved during the 1930s. It is a task-oriented method in which distinct duties are assigned to specific personnel. For example, one nurse does all the vital signs, someone else makes all the beds, a third nurse does all the dressing changes, and so on. Tasks are divided and the client sees several people during the shift. Although efficient, functional nursing fragments care and is confusing for the client.

Team Nursing

Team nursing emerged in the 1950s partially in response to the fragmented care of functional nursing and to accommodate staff with varying levels of education and skill. Teams are made up of an RN team leader, other RNs, LPN/LVNs, and nursing assistants who provide care to a group of clients. The RN team leader directs the care provided by the RNs, LPNs, and aides, and works with them in various capacities. The team conference for discussion and care planning is a feature of team nursing.

Total Care

Total care refers to assignments in which a nurse assumes all the care for a small group of clients. This method focuses more on the client as whole rather than the collection of nursing tasks that need to be accomplished. Total care is often practiced in intensive care units where nurses are assigned one or two clients.

Primary Nursing

Primary nursing was initiated in the 1970s. An RN assumes 24-hour accountability for the client's care and has total responsibility for the nursing care of assigned clients during his or her shift. Secondary nurses carry out the plan of care in the primary nurse's absence. This approach is expensive because it relies entirely on RNs. However, the client is assured of having a caregiver who sees to all of his or her needs and who provides holistic and comprehensive care. There are still settings in which this model is used effectively, such as home care.

Patient-Focused Care

An updated version of primary care and team nursing called **patient-focused care** uses an RN partnered with one or more assistive personnel to care for a group of clients. The RN may work with an LPN and an assistant, or a respiratory therapist and an assistant, or a similar combination of staff. The licensed and unlicensed assistants are cross-trained to do many functions formerly done by separate departments such as drawing blood or obtaining electrocardiograms. The RN may have a role in resource management and may be held accountable for outcomes of nursing care such as skin breakdown (negative outcome) or early ambulation (positive outcome).

Community-Based Nursing

All levels of nursing care are provided in many facilities and settings besides the acute care hospital. Nursing homes, skilled nursing facilities (SNFs), rehabilitation centers, schools, single and multiple physician practices, surgicenters, industries, adult day-care centers, homes, insurance companies, and hospices are some locations in which nurses practice.

Skilled nursing facilities (SNFs) provide skilled nursing and rehabilitative care to people who have the potential to regain function but need skilled observation and nursing care during an acute illness. Clients using these facilities also require invasive procedures and therapies (eg, tube feedings, intravenous fluids, and sterile dressing changes).

Intermediate care facilities (ICFs) are nursing homes that provide custodial care for people who are unable to care for themselves because of mental or physical disabilities. These facilities do not receive reimbursement from Medicare because they are not considered medical facilities.

Rehabilitation centers provide physical and occupational therapy to clients and families to help individuals regain as much independence with activities of daily living as possible.

Hospices provide care for clients diagnosed with a terminal illness and have a life expectancy of less than 6 months. Hospice allows terminally ill clients to live as fully as possible while pain, discomfort, and other symptoms are controlled. Hospice staffs are specially trained to help families with the grief process. Many services provided by hospice are covered by Medicare.

Community health centers and local health departments provide a range of services to the districts, counties, or communities they serve. They are often funded partially or completely by federal, state, and local monies. Community mental health centers are also part of this network. Neighborhood health clinics make health care more accessible and when health facilities are more accessible, people are more likely to seek prompt treatment and reduce the need for acute care.

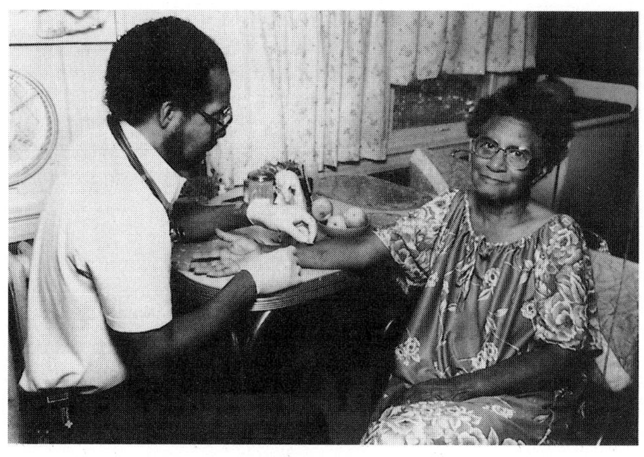

FIGURE 2-1. A home health nurse.

Home Health Nursing

The cost containment measures in the last 20 years have resulted in the expansion of **home health care** services. Home care can cover both long- or short-term health needs and provides comprehensive services. Home health nurses provide specialized care such as intravenous infusion of fluids, medications, and chemotherapy; hospice care; postcardiac surgery care; and care to ventilator-dependent clients (Fig. 2–1). The RN manages and coordinates the care the client receives and has a high level of competency in assessment, clinical skills, communication, teaching, management, and documentation abilities. The RN encourages the client and the family to develop self-care skills, with support from community resources. Box 2–1 lists other functions of the home health nurse.

BOX 2-1 Functions of the Home Health Care Nurse

- Plan, coordinate, and provide care in consultation with hospital and physician.
- Teach client and family to perform procedures, monitor symptoms, take medications, and report to physician.
- Assess client and consult with physician as needed.
- Evaluate the home environment for safety hazards, cleanliness, ability to safely store medication, family support, and adequacy of food supplies.
- Connect client and family with community resources.
- Advocate for the client when additional services are needed.
- Document care and teaching provided.
- Complete forms required for reimbursement.

TABLE 2-2 **Services Provided by Home Health Agencies**

Type of Service	Description
Physical therapy	Therapist assesses client mobility after orthopedic surgery, injury, or stroke. He or she assesses need for assistive devices. Client must meet Medicare requirements to receive physical therapy.
Speech therapy	Therapist provides rehabilitation to stroke victims and other clients with speech or swallowing disorders. Must meet Medicare requirements.
Occupational therapy	Therapist assesses need for assistive devices to aid in activities of daily living and identify issues related to fine motor movements and muscle retraining.
Social services	Social worker meets with client and family to identify difficulties with managing illness at home and provides information about financial assistance and community services.
Home health aides	Aides provide personal care such as bathing and dressing and basic skills such as taking vital signs.
Homemakers	Homemakers clean, do laundry, and shop for groceries.

Besides nursing, home health agencies provide many other services (Table 2–2).

Case Management

A new role and responsibility for nurses is in case management. **Case management** involves the careful oversight of an individual's health care so that fiscal outcomes are maximized without sacrificing quality. The person responsible for this task, usually an RN with a bachelor's or master's degree, is called the case manager (Fig. 2–2). Case managers are employed by insurers and hospitals. A hospital-based case manager may have a caseload of 15 to 25 clients depending on the acuity (degree of illness) of the clients. Not every client is aggressively case managed; those who are sickest, develop complications, or have chronic illnesses require more intensive case management. The case manager follows clients from the time admission is scheduled until the day of discharge. An insurance-based case manager often maintains contact with the client, especially one with a chronic illness, in the home. Regardless of the employer, case managers plan and coordinate the client's progress through the various phases of care so that delays, unnecessary diagnostic testing, and overuse of expensive resources are avoided. An important function of the case manager is early, thorough discharge planning. Case managers often use tools such as critical pathways (see Chap. 1), practice guidelines, and standards of care to help them plan and coordinate care. Hospitals and insurance companies may develop their own or rely on published protocols for guidance. (A cautionary note: All protocols should be developed with experts using published research.)

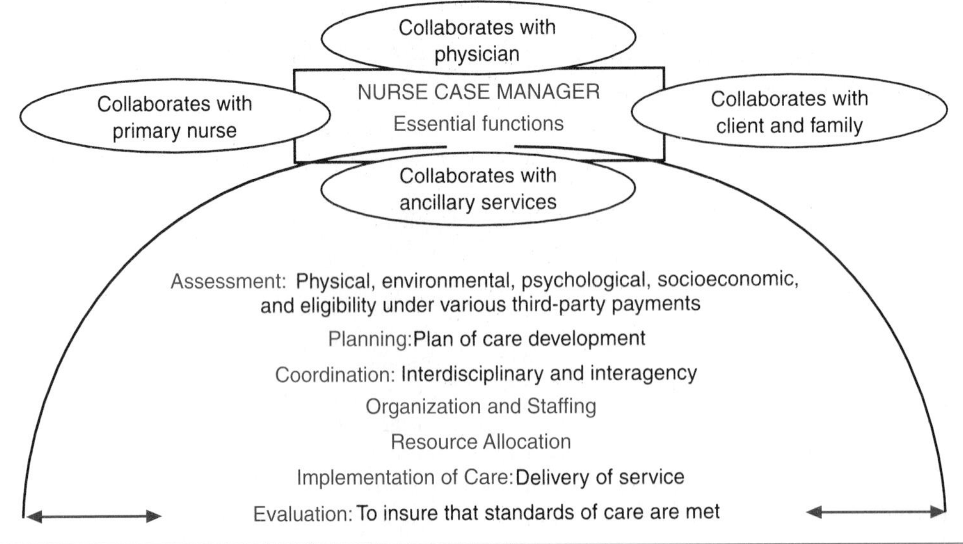
Collaborates with physician
NURSE CASE MANAGER
Essential functions
Collaborates with primary nurse
Collaborates with client and family
Collaborates with ancillary services
Assessment: Physical, environmental, psychological, socioeconomic, and eligibility under various third-party payments
Planning: Plan of care development
Coordination: Interdisciplinary and interagency
Organization and Staffing
Resource Allocation
Implementation of Care: Delivery of service
Evaluation: To insure that standards of care are met

FIGURE 2-2. Functions of the nurse case manager.

Along with the increase in responsibility, autonomy, and power, nurse case managers have increased accountability for the financial and health outcomes of care. Many employers, particularly insurance companies, measure the costs of services provided to the case manager's clients as a means of assessing his or her effectiveness. One of the complaints about case management, and its parent, managed care, is that the "bottom line" will become more important than quality. For this reason, and because they are in the best position to collect outcome data, case managers are often integral members of hospital- and insurance-based quality improvement programs.

SUMMARY OF KEY CONCEPTS

- New roles and responsibilities for nurses have grown out of economic forces in the health care industry.
- Nursing care is concerned with human responses to actual and potential health problem.
- The delivery of nursing care is usually accomplished through team nursing, primary nursing, or a combination called patient-focused care.
- Nurses practice in a variety of settings including hospitals, nursing homes, clinics, schools, and outpatient treatment centers.
- Home health services have expanded because of decreased reliance on the hospital as the setting for health care services.
- Home health nurses provide direct care, educate clients and their families to provide care, monitor health status and compliance with therapy, assess the environment for hazards, and consult with the primary care physician.
- Home health agencies provide physical therapy, speech therapy, occupational therapy, social services, home health aides, and homemakers.
- Case management is the careful monitoring and provision of services so that costs are contained without sacrificing quality.
- Nurse case managers have increased responsibility and accountability for managing financial and client health outcomes and for participating in quality improvement activities.

CRITICAL THINKING EXERCISES

1. How do you think nurses will practice in 2010?
2. What is your definition of nursing?
3. Discuss the pros and cons of case management for both the client and the nurse case manager.

Suggested Readings

American Nurses Association. (1980). *Nursing: A social policy statement.* Kansas City, MO: Author.

Ellis, J. R., & Hartley, C. L. (1995). *Managing and coordinating nursing care.* Philadelphia: J. B. Lippincott.

Ellis, J. R. & Hartley, C. L. (1997). *Nursing in today's world: Challenges, issues, and trends* (6th ed.). Philadelphia: Lippincott-Raven.

Flarey, D. L. (1995). *Redesigning nursing care delivery: Transforming our future.* Philadelphia: J. B. Lippincott.

Harrington, N., Smith, N. E., & Spratt, W. E. (1996). *LPN to RN transitions.* Philadelphia: Lippincott-Raven.

Henderson, V. (1966). *The nature and science of nursing.* New York: Macmillan.

Hunt, R., & Zurek, E. L. (1997). *Introduction to community nursing.* Philadelphia: Lippincott-Raven.

Lavin, J. & Enright, B. (1996). Charting with managed care in mind. *RN, 59*(8), 47–48.

Nightingale, F. (1859). *Notes on nursing: What it is and what it is not.* London: Harrison. Commemorative edition. (1992). Philadelphia: J. B. Lippincott.

Ostrander, F. (1996). Management and evaluation: A how-to guide for home care nurses. *American Journal of Nursing, 96*(10), 16B, 16D, 16F–G.

Schoen, M. A., & Koenig, R. J. (1997). Home health care: Past and present—Part 1. *MEDSURG Nursing, 6*(4), 230–232.

Senapartiratne, L. (1996). On the road with a home health nurse. *RN, 59*(4), 54–57.

Additional Resources

American Association of Managed Care Nurses, Inc. (AAMCN)
4435 Waterfront Drive, Suite 101
P.O. Box 4975
Glen Allen, VA 23058–4975
phone: (804) 747–9698
fax: (804) 747–5316
E-mail: sreed@aamcn.org

Chapter 3

The Nursing Process

KEY TERMS

Assessment
Client data base
Collaborative problems
Critical thinking
Evaluation
Implementation
Interventions
Long-term goals
Nursing diagnosis
Nursing process
Planning
Short-term goals

LEARNING OBJECTIVES

On completion of this chapter, the reader will:

- Describe the five steps of the nursing process.
- State the purpose of the nursing process.
- Define nursing diagnosis.
- Discuss the parts of a nursing diagnostic statement.
- Explain the five levels of human needs as identified by Maslow.
- Explain how the hierarchy of needs is used to establish nursing priorities.
- Contrast short-term and long-term goals.
- Analyze how the nurse evaluates a client's plan of care.
- Give five reasons why goals may not be accomplished.
- Define critical thinking and compare it to using the nursing process.
- List characteristics of critical thinkers.

The provision of health care is a process of problem-solving. Clients present with multiple health care needs that the caregiver must approach in an organized, systematic manner to provide efficient and effective care. The nursing process for making clinical decisions grew from problem-solving techniques and the scientific process and includes collecting information, identifying the problem, developing a goal-oriented plan, carrying out the plan, and evaluating the results. The nursing process provides the framework for nursing care in all health care settings. It is included in most states' nurse practice acts as part of the definition of nursing and is used in the organizational structure for nursing education curricula.

The Nursing Process

The **nursing process** is initiated when a client enters the health care system and consists of five steps:

- Assessment
- Diagnosis (nursing)
- Planning
- Implementation
- Evaluation

The nurse collects data (assessment), defines problems or needs (diagnosis), establishes goals and outlines actions that will help achieve the goals (planning), starts the plan (implementation), and determines the client's responses to the care provided (evaluation). Figure 3–1 depicts these five steps in a dynamic, circular model that shows that the steps are not only separate and distinct, but also interrelated and continuous.

Assessment

Assessment is the careful observation and evaluation of a client's health status. Not only is assessment the first step in the nursing process, but it also is an important, recurring nursing activity that continues as long as a need for health care exists. During assessment, the nurse methodically obtains data about the client's health and illness (Fig. 3–2). The data are documented in the medical record and contribute to the **client data base.** The data base is the result of the assessment process and includes all of the information obtained from the medical and nursing history, physical examination (see Chap. 4), and diagnostic studies. Baseline data serve as a comparison for future signs and symptoms and provide a reference for determining if a client's

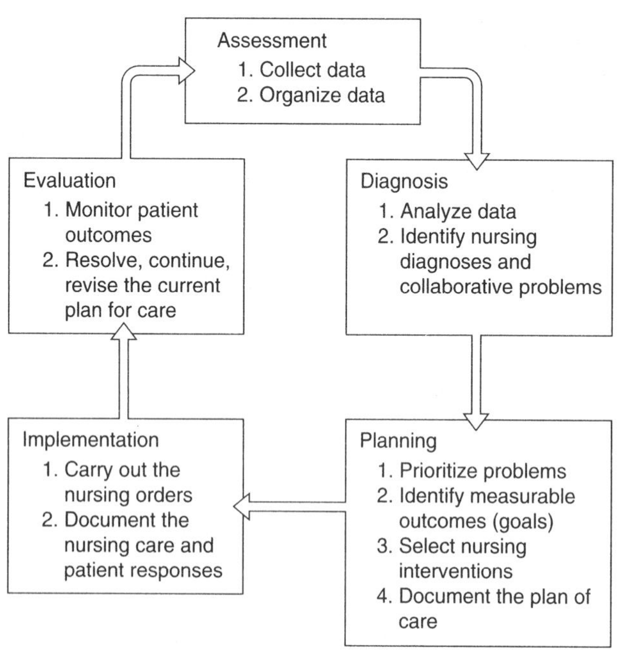

FIGURE 3-1. Steps in the nursing process.

health is improving. The importance of initial and ongoing assessment cannot be overemphasized.

Nursing Diagnosis

Once baseline information has been collected, the registered nurse (RN) examines and analyzes the client's data base to formulate the nursing diagnoses. Nursing diagnosis is analyzing data to identify and define problems. Practical nurses (LPNs) report information that suggests actual or potential health problems. Table 3–1 compares the roles of the RN and LPN in the nursing process and nursing diagnosis.

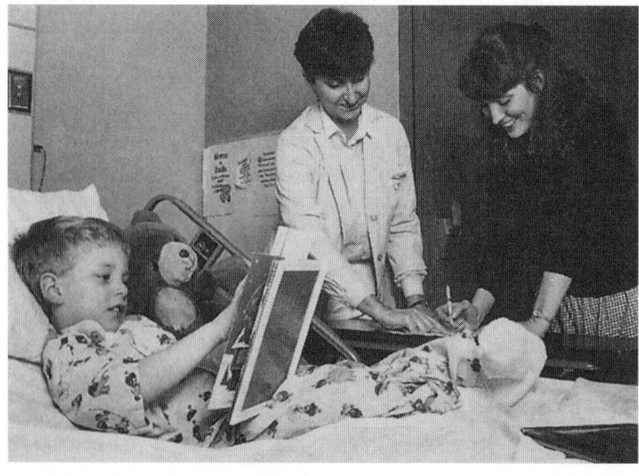

FIGURE 3-2. Nurse obtaining family history from caregiver. (Courtesy of the Department of Medical Photography, Children's Hospital, Buffalo, NY.)

A **nursing diagnosis** identifies and defines a health problem that can be solved or prevented by independent or physician-prescribed nursing actions. Table 3–2 presents different types of diagnoses. The North American Nursing Diagnosis Association (NANDA) developed the classification system for client problems and nursing diagnoses. NANDA meets every 2 years to review and update the list; a recent list is provided on the inside cover of this text. NANDA-approved nursing diagnoses should be used whenever possible. If a client's problem does not fit into any of the diagnoses approved by NANDA, the nurse can use her or his own terminology.

NURSING DIAGNOSTIC STATEMENT

A diagnostic statement includes one to three parts: (1) the name, or label, of the problem; (2) the cause of the problem; and (3) the signs and symptoms, or data, that indicate the problem. The problem portion of the statement is linked to the cause with the phrase "related to" and the data are linked to the problem and cause by the phrase "as manifested by." The following is an example of a nursing diagnostic statement:

> *Constipation* (the name of the problem) *related to* decreased fluid intake, lack of dietary fiber, and lack of exercise (causes) *as manifested by* no bowel movement for the past 3 days, abdominal cramping, and straining to pass stools (signs and symptoms).

Sometimes the cause is explained in more depth using the term "secondary to" as in "decreased fluid intake *secondary to* nausea." Different types of diagnoses also have different prefixes or stems (Table 3–3).

Potential problems are identified by the stem "risk for" as in *Risk for Impaired Skin Integrity* related to inactivity. Possible problems are identified by the stem "possible" to indicate uncertainty as in *Possible Sexual Dysfunction*. Potential and possible diagnoses do not include the third part of the statement, the data, because the data have not developed or are incomplete. Sometimes the cause may be unknown in possible diagnoses and the second part of the statement can be "related to unknown etiology." **Collaborative problems** begin with the stem "potential complication" (abbreviated PC) as in *Potential Complication: Pulmonary Embolism*. Related factors and supporting data are not used when writing collaborative problems. Wellness diagnoses begin with the stem "potential for enhanced" and do not use related factors or supporting data.

Planning

The third step of the nursing process is planning. **Planning** involves several steps: setting priorities, defining goals, and determining specific nursing in-

TABLE 3-1 **Comparison of the Role of Licensed Practical/Vocational Nurses (LPN/LVNs) and Registered Nurses (RNs) in the Nursing Process**

Nursing Process Phase	Role of LPN/LVN	Role of RN
Assessment	Gathers data, performs assessment, identifies client's strengths	Gathers more extensive biopsychosocial data, groups and analyzes data, researches additional data needed, identifies client resources
Nursing diagnosis	Not applicable	Draws conclusions, uses judgment, makes diagnosis
Planning	Contributes to development of care plans	Establishes priorities, sets short- and long-term client goals, collaborates and refers
Implementation	Provides basic therapeutic and preventive nursing measures, provides client education, records information	Manages client care (performs and delegates), provides client and family teaching, provides referrals, records and exchanges information with health care team
Evaluation	Evaluates effects of care given	Evaluates effectiveness of overall plan, analyzes new data, modifies and redesigns plan, collaborates with health team members

Adapted from Harrington, Smith, & Spratt *LPN to RN transitions*

terventions. The client and family participate in care planning as much as possible. For example, the client is consulted on specific goals and activities that are equally effective in accomplishing the goal. Respecting the right of the client to participate in her or his health care is an important ethical principle. An actively involved client is invested in carrying out the plan and reaching the goals.

ESTABLISHING PRIORITIES

The client's multiple problems are prioritized by ranking the diagnoses according to the most important, serious, or immediate needs followed by the remainder in *descending* order of importance. A framework frequently used by nurses when prioritizing client problems is the hierarchy of human needs developed by Abraham Maslow. Maslow proposed that five levels of needs motivate human behavior and he grouped them according to their significance:

- Physiologic needs (first level)
- Safety and security needs (second level)
- Love and belonging needs (third level)
- Esteem and self-esteem needs (fourth level)
- Self-actualization needs (fifth level)

The first level needs, sometimes called baseline survival needs, have the highest priority. These activities, such as eating, breathing, and drinking, sustain life. Maslow believed humans could not or would not seek to fulfill higher level needs until physiologic needs were satisfied. Any problem that poses a threat to physiologic functioning is ranked first. For example, nursing diagnoses such as *Ineffective Breathing Pattern* and *Fluid Volume Deficit* demand the nurse's attention more so than other diagnoses because the conditions may be life-threatening. Nursing diagnoses such as *Anxiety* or *High Risk for Injury* address second level needs of safety and security. *Parental Role Conflict* and *Social Isolation* are examples of nursing diagnoses that apply to the third level of love and belonging needs. Examples of nursing diagnoses that affect the fourth level of esteem and self-esteem needs are *Powerlessness* and *Ineffective Individual Coping*. *Altered Growth and Development* and *Spiritual Distress* are examples of nursing diagnoses that interfere with an individual's achieving fifth level self-actualization needs. Table 3–4

TABLE 3-2 **Types and Examples of Nursing Diagnoses**

Actual diagnosis	A problem that already exists. *Self-Care Deficit (Feeding) related to right hemiparesis as manifested by inability to grasp utensils*
Risk diagnosis	A problem that the client is at high risk for developing. *Risk for Sleep Pattern Disturbance related to changed environment (ICU)*
Possible diagnosis	A problem is suspected but more data must be collected before making a decision. *Possible Parental Role Conflict related to impending divorce*
Wellness diagnosis	No problem exists; the client desires a higher level of wellness. *Potential for Enhanced Physical Fitness*
Collaborative problem	A problem that is monitored and managed by the nurse using physician-prescribed and nursing-prescribed interventions. *Potential Complication: Phlebitis*

TABLE 3-3 **Parts of the Nursing Diagnostic Statement**

Type of Diagnosis	Stem	1. Label	2. Cause	3. Data
Actual	None	Yes	Yes	Yes
Potential	"Risk for"	Yes	Yes	No
Possible	"Possible"	Yes	Yes or No	No
Wellness	"Potential for Enhanced"	Yes	No	No
Collaborative Problem	"Potential Complication"	Yes	No	No

shows other nursing diagnoses prioritized according to Maslow's hierarchy of human needs. The entire NANDA list can be categorized in this manner.

SETTING GOALS

Developing short-term and long-term goals is an important part of the care-planning process. The client and family are included in goal setting. Goals are specific and realistic so the client can attain them and not become frustrated, and measurable so the nurse can reliably determine to what extent the client is meeting the goals. **Short-term goals** are very specific and can be met before discharge from an acute care setting. They may also be the incremental steps that need to be taken to achieve a long-term goal. An example of a short-term goal is, "The client will demonstrate safe crutch-walking before discharge." **Long-term goals** can extend beyond hospitalization. An example of a long-term goal is: "The client will accomplish activities of daily living independently."

TABLE 3-4 **Prioritizing Nursing Diagnoses According to Maslow's Hierarchy of Human Needs**

Human Need	Applicable Nursing Diagnoses
Physiologic	Impaired Swallowing Ineffective Airway Clearance Pain Urinary Retention
Safety and security	Altered Thought Processes Fear Impaired Physical Mobility Post-Trauma Response
Love and belonging	Altered Role Performance Altered Family Processes Impaired Social Interactions Risk for Loneliness
Esteem and self-esteem	Body Image Disturbance Caregiver Role Strain Chronic Low Self-Esteem Ineffective Breast-feeding
Self-actualization	Altered Growth and Development Spiritual Distress

Goals are derived from the nursing diagnosis and are stated several ways: as behavioral objectives, specific actions that the client must do; as client outcomes, meaning the desired result of treatment; or as nursing actions, used only in collaborative problems (Table 3–5). Appropriate goals indicate a time frame and can be evaluated in a measurable way.

DEFINING SPECIFIC INTERVENTIONS

The plan of care identifies interventions for achieving the goals.

Interventions are directed at relieving the cause of the problem. If the cause cannot be fixed, such as in permanent injury, interventions are directed at reducing the problem itself. For example, if a client has the nursing diagnosis of *Impaired Skin Integrity related to effects of pressure secondary to decreased mobility as manifested by a 2-cm ulcer on the right heel*, the interventions are directed at relieving pressure and its effects (decreased circulation). Such interventions would include elevating the heel off the bed to relieve pressure and having the client do ankle pumping exercises to increase blood flow to the area. If the diagnosis is *Self-Care Deficit (Feeding) related to right hemiparesis secondary to stroke as manifested by inability to grasp utensils*, interventions would be directed at working with the problem to overcome it such as providing utensils with large rubber grips.

Once interventions are determined, the RN writes the interventions in the written plan as nursing orders. Nursing orders are specific so that all health

TABLE 3-5 **Examples of Goal Statements**

Behavioral objective	By Friday 12/9, the client will demonstrate aseptic technique when changing wound dressing.
Client outcome	The client reports satisfactory pain control as measured on a scale of 1–10 within one-half hour of receiving pain medication.
Nursing action (for collaborative problems only)	The nurse will manage and minimize hypovolemia.

BOX 3-1 Characteristics of Nursing Interventions and Orders

Nursing interventions and orders are:
- Directed at preventing or minimizing the underlying causes of a problem
- Directed at minimizing problems when the cause cannot be changed
- Compatible with medical orders and other therapies
- Compatible with professional and facility standards of care
- Specific and outline what, how, when, how often, and how much
- Safe
- Individualized
- Supported by scientific rationales

team members understand exactly what to do for the client. A vague nursing order such as "encourage fluids" is likely to be interpreted differently and result in inconsistent care. If the goal is not met, determining whether the nursing measures were ineffective or whether they were carried out ineffectively would be difficult. A more appropriate nursing order would be "give the client 100 mL of juice, water, tea, or milk every hour while awake." The interventions on the nursing care plan also must be compatible with the medical orders. For instance, if the physician has prescribed complete bed rest, a nursing order to ambulate the client conflicts. Box 3–1 lists characteristics of nursing orders.

Many agencies have preprinted or computer-generated care plans that help identify nursing interventions for specific nursing or medical diagnoses. They save time by providing general suggestions for common conditions. The nurse selects appropriate interventions from the list, makes the orders specific for the individual client, and eliminates whatever is unnecessary.

Once the plan of care is drafted, it is communicated to all shifts of nursing personnel. This communication establishes a basis for continuity of care.

Implementation

The fourth step of the nursing process, **implementation** means carrying out the written plan of care, performing the interventions, monitoring the client's status, and assessing and reassessing the client before, during, and after treatments. Carrying out the plan involves the client and one or more members of the health care team. It may also include the client's family and the community.

DOCUMENTATION

Another important element of implementation is documentation. Accurate and thorough documentation in the medical record serves five functions:

- Communicates care
- Shows trends and patterns in client status
- Creates a legal document
- Supplies validation for reimbursement
- Provides a foundation for evaluation, research, and quality improvement (Alfaro-LeFevre, 1994)

By law, nursing actions, observations, and client responses must be recorded in a permanent record. This record of nursing actions should be a mirror image of the written plan. Appropriate documentation is essential in maintaining communication among members of the health care team and ensuring that the client's progress is monitored.

Evaluation

Evaluation is the fifth step of the nursing process. **Evaluation** is assessment and review of the quality and suitability of the care given and the client's responses to that care (Box 3–2). This process enables the nurse to revise goals or select alternative plans of action when goals are not met. Several possible conclusions may be reached during evaluation:

1. The goal is accomplished, the problem is solved, and the nursing orders are discontinued.
2. The goal is not met, but progress is being made and the plan of care is continued or revised with minor changes.
3. The outcome falls far short of the goal and the plan requires critical reevaluation and major revision.

Lack of progress may be due to unrealistic expectations, incorrect diagnosis of the original problem, development of additional problems, ineffective nursing measures, or a premature target date. Once the deficiency in the plan is identified, a revision can be implemented.

BOX 3-2 Evaluating Care

Evaluation includes:
- Determining if goals have been met
- Identifying the factors that interfere with achieving goals
- Deciding whether to continue, modify, or discontinue the plan

The Nursing Process and Critical Thinking

It is important to understand that the elements of the nursing process are used in many ways. These basic elements provide a framework for the **critical thinking** that must take place to provide high-quality care. The process of gathering information (assessment), defining the problem (diagnosis), developing a course of action that will resolve the problem (planning), carrying out the plan (implementation), and determining if the plan worked (evaluation) can be used over and over again with little and big problems that obstruct the effective, efficient delivery of care. For example, this process can be applied to such diverse events as a malfunctioning nasogastric drain or managing the needs of multiple clients on a busy shift.

Nurses are continually assessing the needs of their clients and are frequently confronted by situations that require multiple interventions. Developing good critical thinking skills will make nurses more efficient and effective at resolving these situations. This careful, deliberate, goal-directed thinking has predictable features that can be practiced and learned. One key feature is the ability to maintain a questioning attitude. Asking "Why is this occurring?", "Do I have all the information I need?", and "What does this mean?" are examples of questions the critical thinker asks of himself or herself (Alfaro-LeFevre, 1994). Box 3–3 outlines other characteristics of critical thinkers.

BOX 3-3 Characteristics of Critical Thinkers

Critical thinkers are:

- Aware of their strengths and capabilities (show confidence)
- Aware of their own limitations (know when to ask for help)
- Open minded (listen to new ideas and other viewpoints)
- Humble (do not have to know everything all the time)
- Creative (look for ways to improve performance)
- Proactive (anticipate problems and prevent them)
- Flexible (can modify priorities and adapt to change)
- Aware that mistakes lead to new knowledge (learn from errors)
- Willing to persevere (accept that answers may not come easily)
- Aware that the world is not ideal (realize that the best solution may not be perfect)
- Logical thinkers (establish facts, determine what is relevant, search for cause and effect, avoid jumping to conclusions)
- Able to weigh advantages and disadvantages before making decisions (foresee probable outcomes)

Adapted from Alfaro-LeFevre (1994).

SUMMARY OF KEY CONCEPTS

- The steps in the nursing process are assessment, nursing diagnosis, planning, implementation, and evaluation.
- Using the nursing process enables nurses to provide care in a systematic organized manner.
- A nursing diagnosis describes a problem that the nurse can treat independently or collaboratively.
- A nursing diagnostic statement includes one to three parts: (1) the name of the problem or label, (2) the cause, and (3)the signs and symptoms of the problem or data. A stem or prefix usually precedes the label.
- Maslow identified five levels of human needs: (1) physiologic needs, (2) safety and security needs, (3) love and belonging needs, (4) esteem and self-esteem needs, and (5) self-actualization needs.
- When planning care, nurses prioritize care by addressing the client's most important problems or needs first.
- Short-term goals are those that can be met in a very short period of time. Long-term goals are more general and may require months to accomplish.
- Goals are measurable, client centered, specific and realistic, and indicate a time frame. They must also be compatible with the medical orders. Goals for collaborative problems are nurse centered.
- Evaluation is the fifth step of the nursing process and involves comparing the outcomes of care with the stated goals.
- Several possible reasons interfere with goal accomplishment: (1) the problem was misidentified, (2) the goals were unrealistic, (3) the target date for accomplishment was premature, (4) the nursing measures were ineffective, or (5) additional problems developed.
- Nurses must develop critical thinking skills to be effective. The elements of the nursing process are a framework for critical thinking.
- Critical thinkers recognize their strengths and limitations; remain open-minded; are creative, proactive, and flexible; learn from their mistakes; persevere; recognize that the world is not ideal; think logically; and weigh advantages and disadvantages before making decisions.

CRITICAL THINKING EXERCISES

1. List several reasons why including clients in care planning is important.
2. Explain the importance of the five steps of the nursing process. Give examples of what problems might arise if steps are skipped.
3. Think of a client problem and a personal problem you encountered recently and refer to the characteristics of critical thinkers to determine which characteristics you

demonstrated. Apply the other characteristics to the problems and discuss how the outcomes might have been different.

Suggested Readings

Alfaro-LeFevre, R. (1994). *Applying nursing diagnosis and nursing process: A step-by-step guide* (3rd ed.). Philadelphia: J. B. Lippincott.

Carpenito, L. J. (1995). *Nursing care plans and documentation* (2nd ed.) Philadelphia: J. B. Lippincott.

Carpenito, L. J. (1997). *Nursing diagnosis: Application to clinical practice* (7th ed.). Philadelphia: Lippincott-Raven.

Daly, J. M., Maas, M., McCloskey, J. C., & Bulechek, G. M. (1996). A care planning tool that proves what we do. *RN, 59*(6), 26–29.

Fergy, S., Rush, S., & Wells, D. (1996). Care planning: The role of the nurse. *Nursing Times, 92*(37), 5–8.

Greenwald, D. (1996). Nursing care plans: Issues and solutions. *Nursing Management 27*(3), 33, 37–40.

Maslow, A. (1968). *Toward a psychology of being* (2nd ed.). New York: Von Nostrand.

Quackenbush, C., Damon, J., & Kramer, J. (1996). Your turn. How do you make the care plan a "living," useful document for all caregivers? *Journal of Gerontological Nursing, 22*(8), 51–52.

Scharf, L. (1997). Revising nursing documentation to meet patient outcomes. *Nursing Management, 28*(4), 38–39.

Chapter 4

Interviewing and Physical Assessment

KEY TERMS

Auscultation
Chief complaint
Closed questions
Cultural history
Focus assessment
Functional assessment
Head-to-toe method
Inspection
Objective data
Open-ended questions
Palpation
Past health history
Percussion
Physical assessment
Psychosocial history
Signs
Subjective data
Symptoms
Systems method

LEARNING OBJECTIVES

On completion of this chapter, the reader will:

- Describe the purpose of a physical assessment.
- Define subjective data, objective data, signs, and symptoms.
- List and define the components of an interview.
- Differentiate a head-to-toe method of assessment and a systems method.
- Identify four assessment techniques.

Assessment is the process of gathering information about a client's health. Through systematic assessment the nurse identifies:

- Current and past health status
- Current and past functional status
- Coping patterns
- Health beliefs and relevant cultural practices
- Risks for potential health problems
- Responses to care
- Nursing care needs
- Referral needs

Assessment is also an important standard of nursing care. The Joint Commission on Accreditation of Healthcare Organizations (JCAHO) requires that "an assessment with at least a history, physical examination, and nursing care assessment are completed within twenty-four hours of admission" (JCAHO, 1995, p. 111).

The nurse first assesses the client when he or she is admitted to the health care system. This comprehensive initial assessment establishes a data base that gives all team members relevant client information and becomes a yardstick for measuring effectiveness of care. The initial assessment consists of two parts: the interview and the physical examination. Nurses gather subjective data during the interview and objective data during the physical assessment. **Subjective data** are statements the client makes about what he or she feels. **Objective data** are facts obtained by observation, tests, and measurements. When the client tells the nurse about nausea, pain, fear, bloating, or other feelings of discomfort, he or she is providing subjective data. These feelings of discomfort are called **symptoms.** When the nurse assesses blood pressure, heart rate, or urinalysis results, he or she obtains objective data. When objective data are abnormal, they are called **signs**. Objective data often support the subjective data.

The Interview Process

The length of the interview depends on variables such as the severity of the client's condition, level of discomfort, ability to cooperate, age, and mental state. The interview process is divided into three parts: the preinterview period, the interview, and the postinterview period (Box 4–1).

The Preinterview Period

The preinterview period determines the direction of the interview process. Putting the client physically

BOX 4-1 Parts of the Interview

Preinterview Period
Establish rapport.
Explain the purpose of the interview.

Interview
Collect subjective data.
Ask open-ended questions.

Postinterview Period
Summarize what transpired during the interview.
Thank client and family for their cooperation.

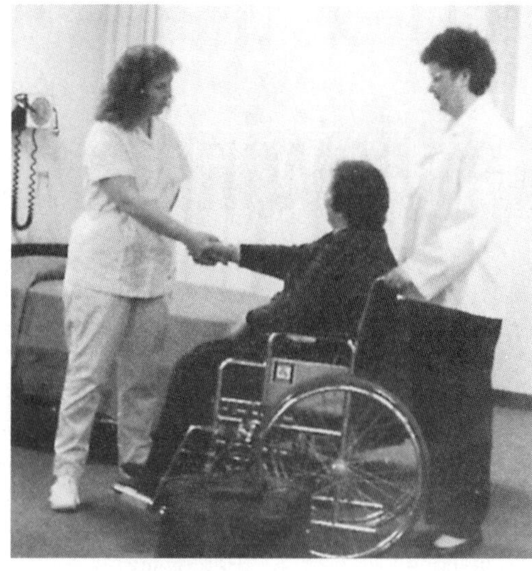

FIGURE 4-1. Greeting the client.

and emotionally at ease facilitates the exchange of information and helps to establish a bond between the client and the nurse. Start by establishing a rapport with the client and family members, and make sure the client is comfortable. Address the client by his or her surname, and introduce yourself (Fig. 4–1). Conduct the interview in a private setting to eliminate interruptions and maintain the client's confidentiality. Explain that the information obtained during the interview helps with planning care. Tell the client that all information is kept confidential, although all members of the health care team share the data.

The Interview

The components of the interview include:

1. The psychosocial and cultural history
2. Functional assessment
3. The client's chief complaint
4. A history of the present illness
5. The past health history
6. The family health history
7. A review of body systems (Box 4–2)

Following a specific pattern when conducting an interview is not necessary. The examiner can rearrange the order in which topics are discussed, digress from an established format if additional information seems pertinent, or omit areas if they are not applicable. Many institutions have assessment forms that help ensure that the data base is complete. Avoid using medical terms and ask **open-ended questions** that require discussion, rather than **closed questions** that require only a "yes" or "no" answer. Give the client ample time to answer each question and maintain frequent eye contact. Minimize reading and writing as much as possible. If the client is asked to complete the assessment form, clarify the information during the interview. Obtain biographical information, present and past health history, family history, and functional status.

PSYCHOSOCIAL AND CULTURAL HISTORY

The **psychosocial** and **cultural history** includes the client's age, occupation, religious affiliation, cultural background and health beliefs (see Chap. 10), marital status, and home and working environments. Although some of this material is found on the face sheet of the client's chart, specific aspects may need further exploration. If, for example, the client is a factory worker, the examiner would ask if the client works around hazardous chemicals or has had job-related injuries.

FUNCTIONAL ASSESSMENT

A **functional assessment** is a determination of how well the client is able to cope with activities of daily living. This is particularly important when assessing older adults or physically challenged clients of any age. Activities of daily living include self-care activities such as walking moderate distances, bathing, and toileting, and instrumental activities such as preparing meals, obtaining transportation, and dialing the telephone.

CHIEF COMPLAINT

The primary purpose of the interview is to discover what the client perceives as the health problem that needs treatment, or **chief complaint**. Recording the information in the client's own words is best. For example, "I had a terrible pain in the right side of my stomach after I ate. I never had it so bad. The doctor said maybe it's my gallbladder."

HISTORY OF PRESENT ILLNESS

Ask the client to describe all present problems including the onset, frequency, and duration of symptoms. Asking for more detailed information about one body system or problem is called a **focus assessment** because it adds depth to the original data. For example, a client may reveal that he or she has experienced abdominal pain for the past several weeks. The questioning then addresses what causes the pain, how long the pain lasts, and what makes it better or worse.

PAST HEALTH HISTORY

Obtaining the client's **past health history** is important. This includes identifying childhood diseases, previous injuries, major illnesses, prior hospitalizations, surgical procedures, drug history, and allergy history.

When discussing the client's past medical problems, ask the age at which the problem was diagnosed, the treatment prescribed, and whether it still exists. Information about past surgeries includes the type, when it was done, and whether recovery was uneventful or accompanied by complications.

Identify any current and past use of prescription and nonprescription drugs. Ask about the client's use of alcohol and tobacco because these drugs create or contribute to other health problems.

Compile a list of the client's allergies. Include sensitivities to drugs, foods, and environmental substances. If the client has a drug allergy, identify the drug and describe the client's reaction; some clients confuse a drug's side effects with an allergic response. If the client or family cannot remember the name of the drug, try to identify it from another source, such as the prescribing physician or past hospital records.

BOX 4-2 Interview Guide

The interviewer establishes a data base by asking the client questions about his or her health.

Psychosocial and Cultural History
Age; gender; marital status; number of children; occupation; highest level of education; religious affiliation; place of residence; country of origin; primary language; military service; date, location, and length of foreign travel or residence

Chief Complaint
Reason for seeking care; type, location, and severity of symptoms

Functional Assessment
Ability to walk, get in and out of bed, bathe, dress, eat and get to and from the bathroom; ability to drive, take public transportation, get groceries, or prepare meals

History of Present Illness
Chronological description of the onset, frequency, and duration of current symptoms; attempts and outcomes of self-treatment; what the client thinks caused the problem; how the illness affects the client's life at home, at work, and socially

Past Health History
Childhood diseases; physical injuries; major illnesses; previous medical or psychiatric hospitalizations; surgical procedures; drug history; use of alcohol and tobacco; allergy history

Family History
Health problems among relatives living and deceased; longevity and cause of death among deceased blood relatives

Review of Systems

General. Usual weight, recent weight change; weakness, fatigue, fever

Skin. Rashes, lumps, sores, itching, dryness, color change, changes in hair or nails

Head. Headache, head injury

Eyes. Vision, glasses or contact lenses, last eye examination, pain, redness, excessive tearing, double vision, blurred vision, spots, specks, flashing lights, glaucoma, cataracts

Ears. Hearing, tinnitus, vertigo, earaches, infection, discharge, use of hearing aids

Nose and sinuses. Frequent colds; nasal stuffiness, discharge, or itching; hay fever, nosebleeds, sinus trouble

Mouth and throat. Condition of teeth and gums, bleeding gums, dentures, if any, and how they fit, last dental examination, sore tongue, dry mouth, frequent sore throats, hoarseness

Neck. Lumps, "swollen glands," goiter, pain or stiffness in the neck

Breasts. Lumps, pain or discomfort, nipple discharge, self-examination

Respiratory. Cough, sputum (color, quantity), hemoptysis, wheezing, asthma, bronchitis, emphysema, pneumonia, tuberculosis, pleurisy; last chest x-ray film

Continued

BOX 4-2 *Continued*

Cardiac. Heart trouble, high blood pressure, rheumatic fever, heart murmurs; chest pain or discomfort, palpitations; dyspnea, orthopnea, paroxysmal nocturnal dyspnea, edema; past electrocardiogram or other heart test results

Gastrointestinal. Trouble swallowing, heartburn, appetite, nausea, vomiting, regurgitation, vomiting of blood, indigestion; frequency of bowel movements, color and size of stools, change in bowel habits, rectal bleeding or black tarry stools, hemorrhoids, constipation, diarrhea; abdominal pain, food intolerance, excessive belching or passing of gas; jaundice, liver or gallbladder trouble, hepatitis

Urinary. Frequency of urination, polyuria, nocturia, burning or pain on urination, hematuria, urgency, reduced caliber or force of the urinary stream, hesitancy, dribbling, incontinence; urinary infections, stones

Genital. Male: Hernias, discharge from or sores on the penis, testicular pain or masses, history of sexually transmitted diseases and their treatments; sexual preference, interest, function, satisfaction, and problems. *Female:* Age at menarche; regularity, frequency, and duration of periods; amount of bleeding, bleeding between periods or after intercourse, last menstrual period; dysmenorrhea, premenstrual tension; age at menopause, menopausal symptoms, postmenopausal bleeding. If the patient was born before 1971, exposure to diethylstilbestrol from maternal use during pregnancy. Discharge, itching, sores, lumps, sexually transmitted diseases and their treatments. Number of pregnancies, number of deliveries, number of abortions (spontaneous and induced); complications of pregnancy; birth control methods. Sexual preference, interest, function, satisfaction; any problems, including dyspareunia (painful intercourse)

Peripheral vascular. Intermittent claudication, leg cramps, varicose veins, past history of blood clots in the veins

Musculoskeletal. Muscle or joint pains, stiffness, arthritis, gout, backache. If present, describe location and symptoms (eg, swelling, redness, pain, tenderness, stiffness, weakness, limitation of motion or activity)

Neurologic. Fainting, blackouts, seizures, weakness, paralysis, numbness or loss of sensation, tingling or "pins and needles," tremors or other involuntary movements

Hematologic/immunologic. Anemia, easy bruising or bleeding, past transfusions and any reactions to them, status for human immunodeficiency virus infection, autoimmune disorders

Endocrine. Thyroid trouble, heat or cold intolerance, excessive sweating; diabetes; excessive thirst or hunger; polyuria

Psychobiologic. Nervousness, tension, mood; memory

Adapted from Bates, Bickley & Hockelman (1995).

FAMILY HISTORY

The family history is important because many disorders are hereditary. Ask if parents, siblings, and grandparents are living or dead. If any blood relatives in the immediate family have died, document the cause of their deaths and the ages at which they died. Identify health problems that affect other living relatives.

REVIEW OF BODY SYSTEMS

Ask general questions about each body system to trigger the client's memory of health problems that they have overlooked. For example, when reviewing the gastrointestinal system ask if the client has a history of nausea, vomiting, food intolerance, bowel irregularity, stomach ulcer, changes in the color of stool, and similar questions that suggest a current or past health problem. Asking an exhaustive number of questions for each system may not be necessary, but a few questions about each system should be included; if the client affirms that a problem exists, ask more focused questions until all data about the problem are obtained.

Postinterview Period

An effective way of ending the interview is to summarize what occurred and thank the client for cooperating. Ask the client if she or he needs more information. This provides an opportunity for the client to express concerns and ask questions.

The Physical Examination

The second part of the assessment process is the collection of objective data through a physical examination. During the **physical assessment,** the nurse examines body structures and observes the client's physical appearance, mood, mental status, behaviors, and ability to interact. The examination is conducted using one of two methods: the **systems method** of assessment or the **head-to-toe method** of assessment. The systems method approaches the examination by assessing each body system separately. The head-to-toe method approaches the examination beginning at the top of the body and progressing downward. Sometimes, parts of both methods are used. See Box 4–3 for an overview of a systems approach to a complete physical examination.

Assessment Techniques

Health care practitioners use four assessment techniques during the physical examination: inspection, palpation, percussion, and auscultation.

INSPECTION

Inspection is the systematic and intentional observation of a specific body part (Fig. 4–2*A*). Looking carefully at the skin for lesions or dryness, or examining the nail beds for cyanosis (bluish discoloration of

BOX 4-3 Components of the Physical Examination

Using inspection, palpation, percussion, and auscultation, the examiner assesses and records findings about the following attributes, body functions, and systems:

General Appraisal
Physical appearance, age, overall physical development, hygiene, grooming, posture, mobility, use of ambulatory devices, weight, height, and vital signs.

Skin and Related Structures
Color, moisture, temperature, texture, turgor, skin integrity, rash, edema (swelling caused by the collection of fluid in the tissues), warts, moles, petechiae (hemorrhagic spots on the skin), distribution of body hair, condition and shape of the fingernails and toenails

Head
Shape and size of head; texture, color, and distribution of hair

Eyes
External structures of the eyes (upper and lower lids, eyelashes, cornea, conjunctiva, sclera, iris, and pupil), pupil size and reaction to light, eye movement, anterior chambers of the eye, visual acuity

Lips and Mouth
Condition of the teeth and gums, oral cavity and mucous membranes, oral pharynx, tonsils, uvula

Ears
External ear (the earlobe, auricle, and surrounding tissues), tympanic membrane, hearing

Neck
Lymph nodes, thyroid, position of trachea, carotid arteries, neck veins

Thorax and Lungs
Shape of the chest, expansion, axilla (armpits), breathing patterns, respiratory rate and depth, use of accessory muscles, breath sounds

Breasts
Appearance, skin characteristics, nipples, presence of lumps or masses

Cardiovascular System
Radial pulse rate, apical pulse rate, heart sounds, blood pressure measurement in both arms while standing, sitting, and lying down, peripheral arteries

Abdomen
Bowel sounds, tenderness, pain, muscle resistance or rigidity, masses, scars, hernia, liver size, spleen, kidneys, abdominal aorta

Rectum
Hemorrhoids, fissures, prostate gland in male clients, stool

Genitalia
Male: Penis, scrotum, inguinal lymph nodes. *Female:* external genitalia (labia, clitoris, urethral orifice, and vaginal opening), internal structures (vaginal wall and the cervix), inguinal lymph nodes

Musculoskeletal System
Contour and size of joints, range of motion, muscle size and strength

Neurologic System
Level of consciousness, orientation, intellectual functioning, emotional state; speech patterns; short-term and long-term memory; perception of pain, heat, cold, light touch, and vibration; gait, reflexes, cranial nerves, muscle strength, movement, coordination, tendon reflexes, proprioception (or position awareness)

the skin, nail beds, or mucous membranes because of oxygen deficiency) are examples of inspection.

PALPATION

Palpation is assessing the characteristics of an organ or body part by feeling it with the hands or fingertips (Fig. 4–2*B*). The examiner palpates to assess the size of a structure and to determine general characteristics, such as firmness, tenderness, or temperature. Palpation also detects abnormal conditions, such as enlarged organs, tumors, or fluid in a cavity.

PERCUSSION

Percussion is tapping the body lightly but sharply with the fingers to elicit a sound (resonance) (Fig. 4–2*C*). Diminished resonance, a dull sound, suggests density. Dullness over the chest wall might indicate a pleural effusion (fluid in the pleural cavity). Hyperresonance, also called tympany, is a hollow sound that indicates air in a structure. A hyperresonant sound over the abdomen suggests that the bowel is distended with gas. Areas percussed are the chest and abdomen. The procedure for percussion is:

1. Place index or middle finger of the nondominant hand firmly on surface to be percussed. Only the finger should have contact with the skin surface. The other fingers and the heel of the hand should be raised off the surface.
2. Use quick, light, firm strikes with the tip of the middle finger of the dominant hand against the distal end of the nondominant finger. Use wrist motion to make the tapping movements—keep the forearm stable.
3. Deliver one to three taps, then move the nondominant finger to another area.

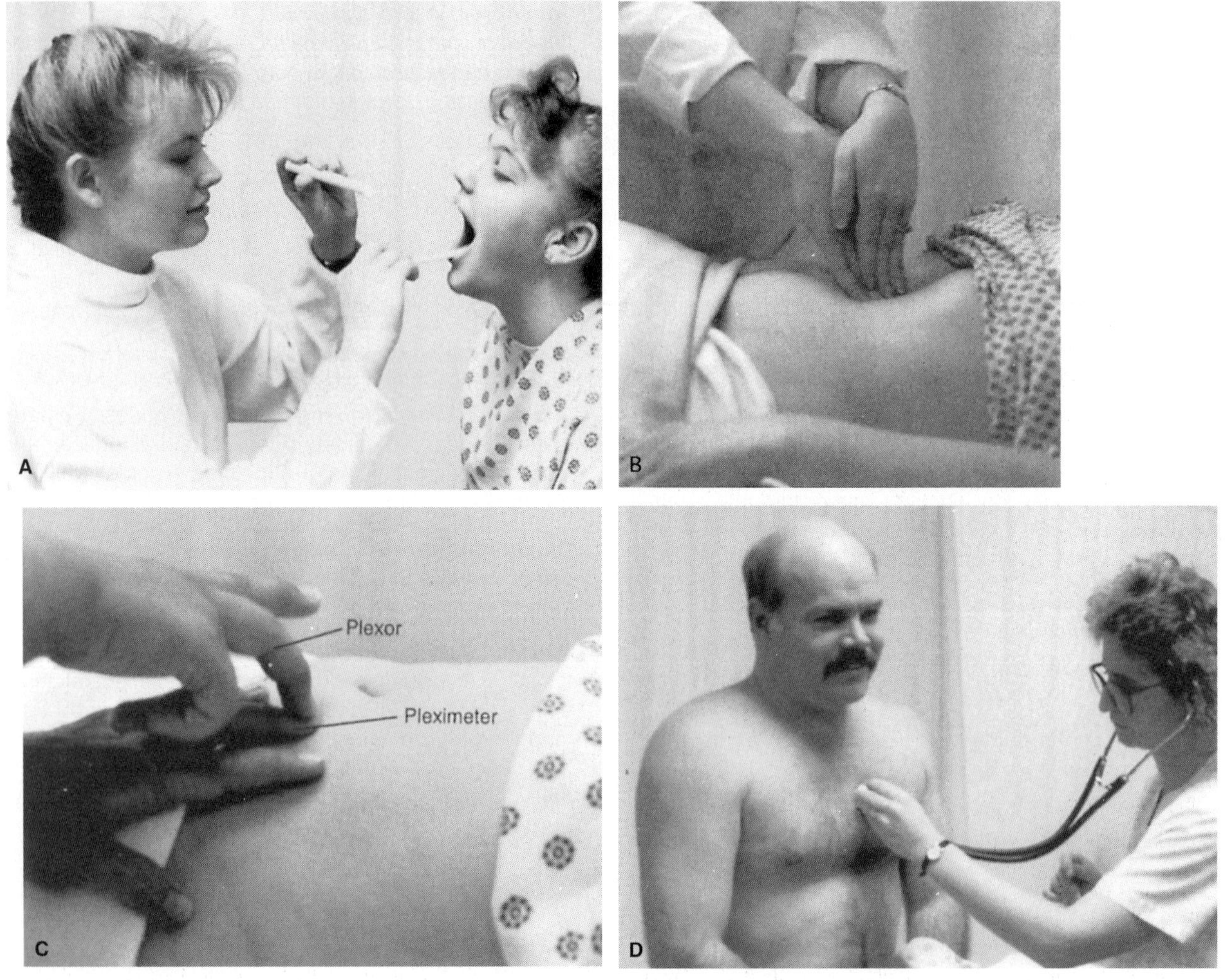

FIGURE 4-2. Assessment techniques. *(A)* Inspection, *(B)* palpation, *(C)* percussion, and *(D)* auscultation. (Courtesy of Ken Timby.)

AUSCULTATION

Auscultation means listening for normal and abnormal sounds generated by organs and structures such as the heart, lungs, intestines, and major arteries (Fig. 4–2*D*). Describe normal and abnormal sounds using descriptive terms such as high-pitched, low-pitched, harsh, blowing, crackling, loud, distant, and soft.

Performing the Examination

In-depth physical examination requires practice and skill and some components are performed by nurse practitioners or physicians. The extent of the examination performed by the licensed practical nurse or registered nurse depends on the nurse's skill, the client's condition, and facility practices. In any case, give the client an examination gown and drape and maintain the client's privacy. Provide adequate lighting in the examination area and gather all equipment, such as a penlight, stethoscope, and sphygmomanometer. Maintain Standard Precautions (see Chap. 18). Remember that clients often feel anxiety, embarrassment, and fear when undergoing a physical examination. They are concerned about the findings and the implication of those findings for their future well-being. Explaining what will happen helps the client prepare for the examination and assists in obtaining the most valid information. Avoid showing surprise or concern at any findings to prevent increasing the client's anxiety level. At the conclusion of the examination, help the client dress and get in a comfortable position, ask if he or she has any questions, and let the client and family know you will share the data with his or her physician.

SUMMARY OF KEY CONCEPTS

- An interview is done to collect subjective data and obtain information that is pertinent to the client's current health.
- Subjective data are statements made by the client about the health problem. These subjective feelings are called symptoms.
- Objective data are findings obtained through observation, tests and measurement. Abnormal objective data are called signs.
- The interview consists of the preinterview, the interview, and the postinterview phases.
- During the interview, the seven general areas covered are: psychosocial and cultural history, chief complaint, history of the present illness, past health history, family history, functional assessment, and a review of body systems.
- Maintaining privacy and a professional attitude help the client feel at ease during the interview and physical exam.
- Physical assessment can be approached by examining the client starting at the head and working down toward the toes, or by examining the client system by system.
- Inspection is looking at specific characteristics of external structures.
- Palpation is feeling parts of the body.
- Percussion is tapping parts of the body.
- Auscultation is listening to sounds with a stethoscope.

CRITICAL THINKING EXERCISES

1. How might you handle a situation in which a client's spouse offers information to the questions asked of the client? Role play a possible nurse–client scenario.
2. How might room temperature, lighting, lack of privacy, or limited time affect the assessment of a client?

Suggested Readings

Ball, R. (1997). Geriatric assessment: Special considerations of the over 65 patient. *Journal of Emergency Medical Services, 22*(3), 96–98, 100, 102.

Bates, B., Bickley, L. S., & Hoekelman, R. A. (1995). *A guide to physical examination and history taking* (6th ed.). Philadelphia: J. B. Lippincott.

Carr, K. K., & Clark, N. *Physical assessment: 7 part series.* Videocassette distributed by *American Journal of Nursing.*

Carrol, P. (1997). Only as good as the sample. *RN, 60*(9), 26–28.

Fuller, J., & Schaller-Ayers, J. (1994). *Health assessment: A nursing approach* (2nd ed.). Philadelphia: J. B. Lippincott.

Joint Commission on Accreditation of Health Care Organizations (1995). *1996 Comprehensive Accreditation Manual for Hospitals.* Illinois, JCAHO.

Weber, J. (1997). *Nurses' handbook of health assessment.* Philadelphia: Lippincott-Raven.

Williams, G. D. (1997). Preoperative assessment and health history interview. *Nursing Clinics of North America, 32*(2), 395–416.

Chapter 5

Legal and Ethical Issues

KEY TERMS

Administrative law
Advocacy
Anecdotal record
Autonomy
Beneficence
Civil law
Common law
Constitutional law
Criminal law
Deontology
Duty
Ethics
Fidelity
Good Samaritan laws
Incident report
Intentional tort
Justice
Laws
Liability
Malpractice
Negligence
Nonmaleficence
Nurse practice acts
Rights
Risk management
Statute of limitations
Statutory law
Torts
Values
Veracity
Unintentional tort
Utilitarianism

LEARNING OBJECTIVES

On completion of this chapter, the reader will:

- Discuss the differences between laws and ethics.
- Differentiate sources of U.S. law.
- Define nurse practice acts.
- Describe the function of the State Board of Nursing.
- Define negligence, malpractice, and liability.
- Discuss the elements of risk management and methods to avoid litigation.
- Identify legal issues that affect nursing practice.
- Define utilitarianism, deontology, duties, and rights.
- Discuss the characteristics of ethical values.
- Define six professional values.
- Describe factors that affect health care ethics.
- Explain an ethical decision-making model.

A system of laws and ethical beliefs provide for order and harmony within a society. **Laws** are written rules for conduct and actions. They are binding for all citizens and ensure the protection of rights. **Ethics** refers to moral principles and values that guide the behavior of honorable people. Ethical standards dictate the rightness or wrongness of human behavior. Box 5–1 highlights the differences between laws and ethics.

The health care delivery system affects and is affected by societal beliefs, values, and laws. It is accountable to society for maintaining established legal and ethical standards. Ethical and legal situations faced by nurses today involve competence, safety, optimal care, protecting clients' rights, and practicing according to professional standards of care. This chapter provides an introduction to the legal and ethical dimensions of nursing practice.

Legal Issues in Nursing Practice

Federal and state legislation directly affects the health care industry. Nurses are expected to know and understand the laws and regulations that affect their practice and the safety of their clients. Laws stem from several sources.

Sources of Law

CONSTITUTIONAL LAW

The constitution guarantees fundamental freedoms to all people in the United States. **Constitutional law** affects nurses in that it protects their basic rights, as it protects the rights of their clients. For example, freedom of speech and right to privacy are rights that nurses and clients have as citizens of the United States.

BOX 5-1 Law Versus Ethics

Laws
Rules of conduct
Guide actions and interactions within a society
Regulated by authorized organizations and law officers

Ethics
Deal with right and wrong
Consider beliefs about morals and values
Ethical guidelines do not have a formal enforcement system

Harrington, Smith & Spratt (1995)

STATUTORY LAW

Statutory law is law that any local, state, or federal legislative body enacts. These laws can have a major impact on health care providers. For example, the "DRG law" described in Chapter 1 greatly influenced health care reimbursement and length of stay. Another example of statutory law is the nurse practice act in each state.

Nurse Practice Act

Nurse practice acts define nursing practice and standards for nurses in each state. This legal statute regulates the practice of nursing to protect the health and safety of citizens. Although each state has its own nurse practice act, there are common components. A nurse practice act:

- Defines the scope of practice
- Establishes requirements for licensure and entry into practice
- Creates a board of nursing to oversee nursing practice
- Identifies legal titles for nurses, such as registered nurse and licensed practical nurse
- Determines what constitutes grounds for disciplinary action

State Board of Nursing

The responsibilities of boards of nursing include:

- Reviewing and approving nursing education programs in the state
- Forming criteria for granting licensure
- Overseeing procedures for licensure examinations
- Issuing or transferring licenses
- Implementing disciplinary procedures

COMMON LAW

Common law, also known as judicial law, is based on earlier court decisions, judgments, and decrees. These earlier decisions set precedent for interpretation of laws and evolved when courts began to present written decisions based on prior court cases. Stated another way, if one court has previously decided for a particular case and another court has a similar case, the second court will make the same decision, citing the precedent of the previous case. The court will make new rules if the precedent is outdated.

ADMINISTRATIVE LAW

Administrative law empowers federal and state agencies to create and enforce rules and regulations that concern the health, welfare, and safety of citizens. For example, the federal agency of Occupational Safety and Health Administration develops the rules and regulations that govern workplace safety. State statutory law forms nurse practice acts, but the authority to regulate that act is given to an administrative agency, often called the State Board of Nursing.

CRIMINAL LAW

Criminal law concerns offenses that violate the public's welfare. A crime is a violation of criminal law. Offenses are categorized into two types: (1) a misdemeanor, which is a minor offense, and (2) a felony, which is a serious offense. Examples of felonious crimes involving health care workers include falsification of medical records, insurance fraud, and theft of narcotics. If an individual misrepresents herself or himself as a licensed nurse, this person commits the crime of practicing without a license.

CIVIL LAW

Civil law applies to disputes that arise between individual citizens. Civil laws protect each individual's personal freedoms and property rights. Some of these include the right to be left alone, freedom from threats of injury, freedom from offensive contact, and freedom from character attacks. Plaintiff refers to the individual who brings a dispute to the court. The complaint is the formal written dispute and the restitution that the plaintiff seeks. The individual or party against whom the complaint is filed is the defendant. **Liability** means legal responsibility. If a client receives the wrong medication and is harmed as a result, the nurse is liable, or held responsible, for that harm.

Although there are various branches of civil law, tort law is most likely to affect nurses. Tort law is the body of law that governs breaches of **duty** owed by one person to another. Duties are expected actions that are based on moral or legal obligations. A **tort** is an injury that occurred because of another person's intentional or unintentional actions, or failure to act. This injury can be physical, emotional, or financial. If the defendant is found to have breached his or her duty and that breach causes harm, she or he is required to pay restitution for damages. The types of torts that involve nurses are intentional and unintentional.

Intentional Torts

An **intentional tort** is a deliberate and willful act that infringes on another person's rights or property. Examples of intentional torts include assault, battery, false imprisonment, invasion of privacy, and defamation.

ASSAULT. Assault is an act in which there is a threat or attempt to do bodily harm. This may be physical intimidation, a verbal remark, or gesture that leads the client to believe that force or injury may be forthcoming. For example, a nurse is frustrated because a client constantly turns on the call light. The nurse threatens to restrain the client's hands if this action continues. This verbal threat constitutes assault.

BATTERY. Battery is actual physical contact with another person without that person's consent. The contact can include touching a person's body, clothing, chair, or bed. A charge of battery can be made even if the contact did not cause physical harm to the individual. To protect health care workers from being charged with battery, clients sign a general permission for care and treatment at the time of admission (Fig. 5–1). Clients also sign a written consent before undergoing special tests, procedures, or surgery. A parent or guardian must provide consent if the client is a minor, mentally retarded, or mentally incompetent. In an emergency, health care providers can infer consent, meaning the law assumes that in life-threatening circumstances clients would provide consent.

Nonconsensual physical contact is sometimes justified. When mentally ill or intoxicated clients are endangering their own safety or the safety of others, health professionals may use physical force to subdue them. The nurse must clearly document that the situation required the degree of restraint used. Excessive force is never appropriate when less would have been just as effective. When recording these incidents, it is essential for the nurse to document the behavior that resulted in the use of force and the response of the client when lesser forms of restraint were tried first.

FALSE IMPRISONMENT. False imprisonment occurs when health care workers physically or chemically restrain an individual from leaving a health care institution. Mentally impaired, confused, or disoriented clients may be restrained if their safety or the safety of others is at risk. This confinement requires restraining orders, court-ordered commitments, or medical orders. A nurse cannot detain a competent client who wishes to leave the hospital before being discharged by the physician. If a client wishes to leave the hospital against medical advice, he or she signs a form (Fig. 5–2) that releases the hospital from responsibility.

The unnecessary or unprescribed application of physical or chemical restraints also creates potential liability for battery and false imprisonment. If the nurse must apply restraints and no current medical order exists, the best legal defense is to show just cause through accurate documentation. Because confined and restrained clients are unable to protect themselves or meet their own needs, charting must show that the nurse assessed the client frequently, offered fluids and nourishment, and provided an opportunity for bowel and bladder elimination. It is expected that the restraints will be discontinued when the client no longer poses a threat to himself or others.

INVASION OF PRIVACY. The right to privacy means that persons have the right to expect that they and their property will be left alone. Failure to do so is an invasion of privacy. Nonmedical torts of this nature generally include trespassing, illegal search and seizure, or wiretapping. Invasion of privacy also applies to releasing private information about a person, even if the information is true.

Medical examples of invasion of privacy include photographing an individual without consent, revealing a client's name in a public report or research paper, or allowing unauthorized persons to observe a client during treatment or care. Health professionals protect a client's privacy by:

- Obtaining a signed release for recognizable photographs for publications or presentations
- Using initials or code numbers instead of names in written reports or research papers
- Closing bedside curtains when giving personal care
- Obtaining a client's permission for a nursing student or other health care person to be present as an observer

DEFAMATION. Defamation is an act that harms a person's reputation and good name. If the character attack is uttered orally in the presence of others, it is

THREE RIVERS AREA HOSPITAL
THREE RIVERS, MICHIGAN 49093

CONSENT FOR INPATIENT, OUTPATIENT, MEDICAL AND / OR SURGICAL TREATMENT

PATIENT'S NAME: ______________________________

DATE & TIME: ______________________________

I, the undersigned, knowing that I have a condition requiring hospital and medical treatment, do hereby voluntarily consent to such routine diagnostic procedures and hospital care by Dr. ____________ ____________, his assistants or his designees, including such hospital personnel as he deems necessary.

I am aware that the practice of medicine is not an exact science and I acknowledge that no guarantees have been made to me as to the results of said outpatient care which I have hereby authorized.

If applicable, I hereby authorize Three Rivers Area Hospital to retain, preserve, and use of scientific or teaching purposes, or otherwise dispose of, at their convenience, any specimens, tissues, parts or organs taken from my (or patient's) body, as a result of the procedure or procedures authorized above.

I understand that the physician is not an employee or agent of Three Rivers Area Hospital but that as a practicing physician in the State of Michigan, he is granted the privilege to utilize the facilities of care at this hospital.

This notice is to inform you that Michigan law allows this hospital to test your blood for the presence of antibodies which may indicate you have been exposed to HIV (AIDS). This test is permitted by Michigan law and may be done without your permission if any hospital personnel are exposed to blood and body fluids in the course of care for you. This is for your protection as well as for the course of care for you. This is for your protection as well as for the protection of the physicians, nurses and other associates of this hospital.

This form has been fully explained to me and I certify that I understand its contents.

______________________________ ______________
Patient's Signature Date

______________________________ ______________
Witness Date

If patient is unable to sign or is a minor, complete the following:
Patient is a minor, ________ years of age, and/or is unable to sign because:

____

______________________________ ______________
Signature (Closest Relative or Legal Guardian) Date

______________________________ ______________
Relationship to patient Witness

FIGURE 5-1. Consent for treatment form.

called *slander*. If the damaging statement is written and read by others, it is called *libel*. Nurses must avoid offering unfounded or exaggerated negative opinions about clients, the expertise of physicians, or other coworkers. Injury occurs because the derogatory remarks may mar a person's public image or keep potential clients from seeking the services of the defamed person. If a client accuses a nurse of defamation of character, the client must prove that there was malice, misuse of privileged information, and spoken or written untruths. Nurses are at risk for defamation of character suits if they make negative comments in public areas (elevators, cafeterias) or assert opinions regarding a client's character in the medical record.

UNINTENTIONAL TORTS. An **unintentional tort** involves situations that result in injuries, although the person responsible did not mean to cause any harm. Negligence is the principal form of unintentional torts. For example, if a homeowner does not scrape the ice

THREE RIVERS HOSPITAL
THREE RIVERS, MICHIGAN 49093

Release from Responsibility for Discharge

Date: ______________________ Time: ______________ A.M.
P.M.

PATIENT: ______________________________

This is to certify that I ______________________________, a patient in the ______________________________ Hospital am being discharged against the advice of the attending physician and the hospital administration. I acknowledge that I have been informed of the risk involved and hereby release the attending physician and the hospital from all responsibility for any ill effects which may result from such discharge.

Witnesses:

____
(Signature of Patient)

____
(To be signed by the legal representative in case of a minor or of a patient who is not mentally competent, otherwise by the patient.)

FIGURE 5-2. Release form for leaving against medical advice.

or snow from a walkway and the mail carrier falls, the homeowner is liable for the injury. Although there was no harmful intent, the injury occurred because the property owner neglected to keep the path clear and dry.

NEGLIGENCE. Negligence describes the failure to act as a reasonable person would have acted in a similar situation. If harm results from the action (or failure to act), the individual can be sued for negligence. For example, a homeowner fails to repair a broken step or warn a visitor to be careful. The visitor falls and is injured. The jury decides if another reasonable, prudent person would have repaired the step or warned the visitor to be careful.

MALPRACTICE. The law defines **malpractice** as professional negligence. It refers to harm that results from a licensed person's actions or lack of action. A jury must determine if the responsible person's conduct deviated from the standard expected of others with similar education and experience. This type of tort holds health care workers to a higher standard than that used in negligence cases. Rather than being held accountable for acting as an ordinary, reasonable lay person, the court will determine if a nurse acted in a manner comparable to that of her or his peers. For example, if a client sustains a burn from warm soaks, the nurse who failed to check the water temperature could be found liable because he or she violated professional standards by not checking the temperature of the water before applying the soak to the skin. Published standards (Box 5–2), the testimony of expert witnesses, written agency policies and procedures, A Patient's Bill of Rights (Box 5–3), and standardized care plans are examples of documents that establish professional standards of care (Fig. 5–3). These help familiarize the jury with the scope of a nurse's practice.

Limiting Liability

Some measures protect nurses and other health care workers from litigation (lawsuits) or provide a foundation for legal defense. Good Samaritan laws, statutes of limitations, anecdotal records, and principles regarding assumption of risk can limit or reduce a nurse's liability.

BOX 5-2 Standards of Care

Standard I. Assessment
The nurse collects client health data.

Standard II. Diagnosis
The nurse analyzes the assessment data in determining diagnoses.

Standard III. Outcome Identification
The nurse identifies expected outcomes individualized to the client.

Standard IV. Planning
The nurse develops a plan of care that prescribes interventions to attain expected outcomes.

Standard V. Implementation
The nurse implements the interventions identified in the plan of care.

Standard VI. Evaluation
The nurse evaluates the client's progress toward attainment of outcomes.

(Reprinted with permission from Standards of Clinical Nursing Practice, © 1991, American Nurses Association, Washington, D.C.)

ASSUMPTION OF RISK

If a client is forewarned of a potential hazard to her or his safety and chooses to ignore the warning, the court may hold the client responsible. For example, if the client objects to having the side rails up or lowers the rails independently, the nurse or hospital may not be held fully accountable if an injury occurs. It is essential that the nurse document that he or she warned the client and that the client disregarded it. The same recommendation applies when clients are cautioned about ambulating only with assistance.

DOCUMENTATION

A major component in limiting liability is accurate, thorough documentation. Nurses are held responsible or liable for information that is either included or not included in reports and documentation. The work setting does not change the need for accurate and complete documentation. The medical record is a legal document and is used as evidence in court. It is essential that records be timely, objective, accurate, complete, and legible. The quality of the documentation, including neatness and spelling, can be a factor in a jury's decision. Box 5–4 provides a guide for legally safe documentation.

GOOD SAMARITAN LAWS

Good Samaritan laws have been enacted in all states. These laws provide legal immunity for rescuers who provide first aid to accident victims. The emergency is interpreted as one occurring outside of a hospital, not in an emergency department.

None of the Good Samaritan laws provide absolute exemption from prosecution in the event of an injury. Paramedics, ambulance personnel, physicians, and nurses who stop to provide assistance are still held to a higher standard of care because they have training above and beyond that of lay persons. In cases where there has been gross negligence, a total disregard for another's safety, individuals even may be charged with a criminal offense.

STATUTE OF LIMITATIONS

Each state establishes a **statute of limitations** related to civil laws. This is the designated period of time in which a person can file a lawsuit. The time is generally calculated from the time the incident occurred. However, when the injured party is a minor, the statute of limitations sometimes does not commence until the victim reaches adulthood. Once the time period expires, an injured party can no longer sue.

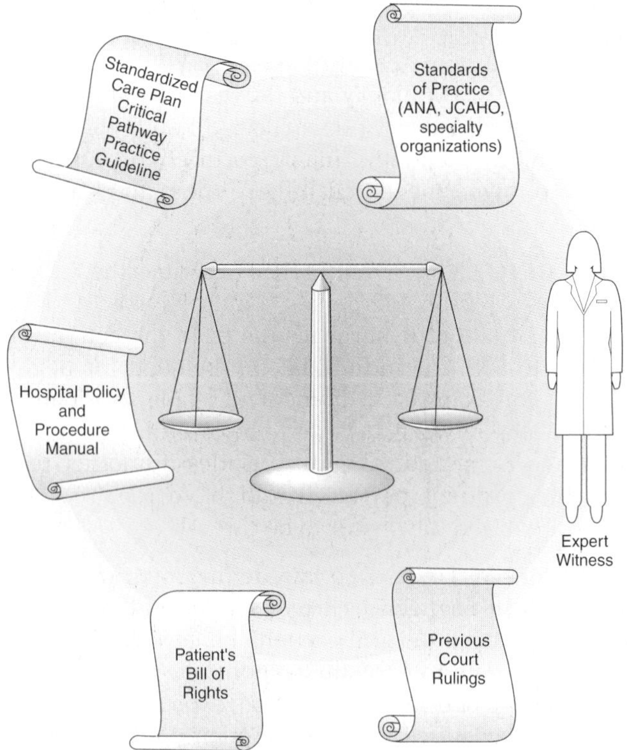

FIGURE 5-3. How the court establishes professional standards of care.

BOX 5-3 A Patient's Bill of Rights

1. The patient has the right to considerate and respectful care.
2. The patient has the right to and is encouraged to obtain from physicians and other direct caregivers relevant, current, and understandable information concerning diagnosis, treatment, and prognosis.
3. The patient has the right to make decisions about the plan of care prior to and during the course of treatment and to refuse a recommended treatment or plan of care to the extent permitted by law and hospital policy and to be informed of the medical consequences of this action.
4. The patient has the right to have an advance directive (such as a living will, health care proxy, or durable power of attorney for health care) concerning treatment or designating a surrogate decision maker with the expectation that the hospital will honor the intent of that directive to the extent permitted by law and hospital policy.
5. The patient has the right to every consideration of privacy. Case discussion, consultation, examination, and treatment should be conducted so as to protect each patient's privacy.
6. The patient has the right to expect that all communications and records pertaining to his/her care will be treated as confidential by the hospital, except in cases such as suspected abuse and public health hazards when reporting is permitted or required by law.
7. The patient has the right to review the records pertaining to his or her medical care and to have the information explained or interpreted as necessary, except when restricted by law.
8. The patient has the right to expect that, within its capacity and policies, a hospital will make reasonable response to the request of a patient for appropriate and medically indicated care and services. The hospital must provide evaluation, service, and/or referral as indicated by the urgency of the case.
9. The patient has the right to ask and be informed of the existence of business relationships among the hospital, educational institutions, other health care providers, or payers that may influence the patient's treatment and care.
10. The patient has the right to consent to or decline to participate in proposed research studies or human experimentation affecting care and treatment or requiring direct patient involvement, and to have those studies fully explained prior to consent.
11. The patient has the right to expect reasonable continuity of care when appropriate and to be informed by physicians and other caregivers of available and realistic patient care options when hospital care is no longer appropriate.
12. The patient has the right to be informed of hospital policies and practices that relate to patient care, treatment, and responsibilities.

RISK MANAGEMENT

Risk management is a concept that was developed by insurance companies. It refers to the process of identifying and then reducing the cost of anticipated losses. This term is now used by health care institutions who employ risk managers. This person has responsibility for reviewing all the problems that occur at the workplace, identifying common elements, and then developing methods to reduce the risk of their occurrence.

One of the primary tools of risk management is the **incident report** (Fig. 5–4). Hospital staff fill out incident reports when errors are made or discovered, or when an event that results in harm occurs. The incident report is not part of the medical record. It identifies the nature of the incident (who, what, where, and when), witnesses, and what actions were taken at the time. The incident report is not intended to be a punitive tool but rather a means to collect data. The incident report is factual and complete. Excuses for behaviors or actions are not included. The incident is documented in the client's record, but circumstances of the incident are not mentioned because they are not part of the client's record.

Risk management can also be applied to the individual nurse. The steps that nurses take to reduce harm to clients and avoid litigation is risk management. These steps include:

- Complying with the state's nurse practice act
- Following institutional procedures and policies
- Acknowledging personal strengths and weaknesses
- Seeking means of growth, education, and supervised experiences
- Discussing issues or problems with colleagues
- Evaluating proposed assignments and refusing to accept responsibilities for which one is not prepared
- Keeping knowledge and skills up-to-date
- Respecting client rights and developing rapport with clients
- Documenting client care accurately
- Working within the institution to develop and support management policies (Taylor, Lillis, & LeMone, 1996)

THREE RIVERS AREA HOSPITAL INCIDENT REPORT

Addressograph

Confidential - DO NOT DUPLICATE
Forward to Risk Management within 48 hours

Identification	Sex	Age	Incident Date	Time	Shift	Department
__Inpatient	__M	___	___/___/___	___:___	__1st	
__Outpatient	__F				__2nd	_________
__Visitor					__3rd	

Reason for hospitalization/presence on premises: ____________________

I. Location of Incident
__Patient Room #______
__Patient Bathroom
__Corridor
__Other ____________________

II. Type of Incident
__Fall
__Medication
__Infusion
__Lost/Found
__Burn
__Treatment/Procedure
__Equipment
__Needle/Sponge Count
__Other____________

III. Description of Incident ____________________

IV. Nature of Incident

A. Falls:

Activity Order:	Pt. Condition Prior to:	Fall Involved:	Patient/Visitor was:
__Restraints	__Weak, unsteady	__Chair, W/C	__Lying
__Bedrest only	__Alert, oriented	__Stretcher	__Standing
__BRP	__Disoriented/confused	__Tub/Shower	__Getting on/off
__Up w/asst.	__Senile	__Toilet	__Sitting
__Up AD LIB	__Unconscious	__Floor Condition(below)	__Ambulating
	__Medicated/Sedated	__Bed	__Other__________
	Med. Name _______	__Side Rails Up	__________
	Last Dose _______	__Side Rails Down	__________

B. Medications:

Incident Involved:
__Wrong Med, Tx, Procedure
__Wrong Patient
__Wrong Time
__Omission
__Incorrect Dose
__Incorrect Method of Administration
__Adverse Reaction
__Infiltration
__Other__________

Factors:
__Patient I.D. Not Checked
__Transcription
__Labeling
__Physician orders not clear
__Physician orders not checked
__Misread label/dose
__Charting
__Wrong Med from Pharmacy
__Defective equipment
__Communications
__Other______________

C. Other:
__Loss of Property
__Struck by object, equipment
__Equipment malfunction
__Anesthesia
__Patient ID
__Other______________

V. Nature of Injury (Injury sustained as a result of incident):
__Asphyxia, Strangulation, Inhalation
__Head Injury
__Contagious or infectious Disease Exposure
__Fracture or dislocation
__Viscera Injury
__Sprain or strain
__Contusion, Cut, Laceration
__Burn or Scald
__Chemical Burn
__No injury
__No apparent injury
__Other______________

VI. Action Taken:
Physician Notified __Yes __No
PT/Visitor seen by MD/T&EC __Yes __No
MD Name ______________ Time ___:___
Physician's Findings: ____________________

Other follow up: ___No __Yes - Specify____________________

____________________	__/__/__	____________________	__/__/__
Name of Person Reporting	Date	Department Director	Date
____________________	__/__/__	____________________	__/__/__
Supervisor	Date	Risk Management	Date

8311-109

FIGURE 5-4. An incident report form.

BOX 5-4 Rules for Legally Safe Charting

- Chart promptly
- Write legibly
- Chart objectively
- Chart accurately
- Chart concisely
- Use only standard abbreviations
- Do not leave vacant lines
- Sign every entry
- Keep charting free of criticism or complaints
- Make no mention of an incident report
- Do not destroy or attempt to obliterate documentation
- Record the date of a return visit, cancelled, or missed appointments
- Document all telephone conversations and follow-up instructions

ANECDOTAL RECORDS

An **anecdotal record** is a handwritten, personal account of an incident made at the time of occurrence and updated as needed. Such records are not official but are useful in refreshing the nurse's memory. Anecdotal records may be used as evidence in court particularly if there is conflicting testimony about the events that transpired.

LIABILITY INSURANCE

Today, all health care professionals need liability insurance. Liability insurance provides funds for attorneys' fees and damages awarded in malpractice lawsuits. All health care institutions carry liability insurance and some may insure their employees. However, nurses also should carry their own personal malpractice insurance so they have a separate attorney working on their sole behalf. Because the damages sought in malpractice lawsuits are so high, the attorneys hired by the hospital are sometimes more committed to defending the hospital rather than the nurse. There also have been instances in which hospitals have countersued negligent nurses for reimbursement of damages.

Ethical Practice

Nurses frequently encounter complex situations that require a decision based on determining not what is legally right or wrong, but what is morally good or bad. Ethical issues do not have absolute answers. Conflicts may arise between the desire to maintain the client's rights, and yet uphold professional values and institutional policies. For example, a mildly confused, elderly client, Mrs. S., has liver cancer but is expected to live at least several more months. She eats and drinks, but overall her intake is poor. Efforts to have her drink and eat more have failed and consent to place a feeding tube is obtained from her power of attorney. The physician asks you to assist while the tube is placed. Mrs S. resists placement and her hands must be restrained to get the feeding tube down; the restraints must be applied indefinitely to prevent her from dislodging the tube. It may be difficult in a situation like this to know what is the ethically right course of action. Mrs S. will get better nutrition this way but must endure the discomfort of the tube and wrist restraints. What are the benefits and harms of the feeding tube and the wrist restraints? Should a treatment that requires Mrs. S. to be physically restrained be provided at all? The following sections introduce theories of ethics and an ethical decision-making method that can help nurses determine their actions in perplexing situations. Box 5–5 provides definitions of terms related to ethics.

Theories of Ethics

An ethical theory is used for the purpose of determining if a particular action is good or bad. In nursing ethics, two systems or theories predominate: utilitarianism and deontology.

UTILITARIANISM

Utilitarianism, also referred to as teleologic theory, is an outcome-oriented approach for decision-making. There are two important principles: "The greatest good for the greatest number" and "the end justifies the means." When utilitarianism is used to make an ethical decision, it means that the consequences of actions must be considered and the benefits for many will outweigh the harm for a few. No action is good or bad in and of itself; the consequences of an action determine if the action was good or bad. Consequences must also be evaluated. Theorists have suggested that consequences are good if they bring pleasure and that the outcome desired by those who are affected by the act be considered above all.

An example of how utilitarianism is applied in health care can be found in the allocation of funds. If funding is being considered for vaccines for many children or organ transplants for a few, the money will go for the vaccines because a greater number will benefit (Ellis & Hartley, 1997). The advantage of using utilitarianism is that the needs of the majority are considered. The drawback of utilitarianism is that the rights of the individual are secondary.

BOX 5-5 Definitions Related to Ethics

Ethics
Decisions regarding what is right and wrong; often a system that is used to protect the rights of individuals or groups

Code of Ethics
Standards of conduct and values as defined by a profession; forms the basis for ethical decision-making by a profession

Values
The ideals and beliefs held by an individual or group; usually influenced by family, society, and religion; have a great impact on behavior

Morals
An individual's standards of right and wrong; formed in childhood; also influenced by family, society, and religion

Bioethics
Ethical questions surrounding life and death questions and concerns regarding quality of life as it relates to advanced technology

Ethical Dilemma
A situation in which an individual must choose between two alternatives that are not desirable; often involves examining rights and obligations of particular individuals; choice frequently defended

Harrington, Smith, & Spratt (1995)

DEONTOLOGY

An alternative view of ethics, **deontology,** argues that consequences are not the only important consideration in ethical dilemmas. Deontology states that duty is equally important. Duties are part of our understanding of the situations and relationships in which we find ourselves. We know intuitively that we must keep promises, return borrowed items, or help an injured person (Quinn & Smith, 1987). We have an obligation to perform or avoid some actions, regardless of the consequences, because of our duties to others. For example, the deontologist would say that lying is never acceptable because it disregards one's duty to tell the truth, and abortion is unethical because it violates the duty to respect and preserve life (Zerwekh & Claborn, 1994).

Implied in the concept of duties is the idea of **rights.** Another individual is entitled to what we have a duty to provide. For example, a person has a right to have his or her belongings returned or to have promises kept. This is a particularly important concept in nursing practice. Nurses have a professional duty to their clients, and those clients have a right to expect that the nurse will perform his or her duties (see Box 5–3).

One advantage of using the deontologic approach is that the rights of each person are considered. A second advantage is that the obligation to duty and moral thinking is foremost, and thus the decisions for similar situations are the same. However, it may be difficult to apply the deontologic method when the consequence of the decision can be harmful to an individual. For example, the decision to maintain life for all infants regardless of the outcome may be difficult when the infant is severely deformed and will require many invasive and expensive procedures to survive in a vegetative state.

Factors That Influence Ethical Decision-Making

Selecting a system for ethical decision-making should simplify the process. However, most nurses do not necessarily use one system or another; they also are influenced by a number of factors and not just by knowledge of ethical theory.

PROFESSIONAL VALUES

Values are the beliefs that individuals find most meaningful. People value many different ideas and not all ideas are ethical. Ethical values are rules or principles a person uses to make decisions about right and wrong and have four characteristics:

1. Ethical values are consistent.
2. Ethical values take priority over other values.
3. Ethical values concern the treatment of others.
4. Ethical values are well thought out (Quinn & Smith, 1987).

Professional values are principles intended to support the ethical conduct of the profession. Some of those values do not differ from personal values, whereas some may come from a person's professional education. Several values guide the decisions that nurses make.

Beneficence

Beneficence is the duty to do good for the clients assigned to the nurse's care. This "good" includes technical competence and a humanistic, holistic approach. Stated another way, a nurse ought to prevent or remove harm, and promote or do good (Edge and Groves, 1994). The nurse has a duty to remove wrist restraints whenever possible (removing a harm) and to help the client regain independence (promoting and doing good). The principle of beneficence directly supports the nurse's role of client advocacy. **Advocacy** is the safeguarding of clients' rights and the support of their interests. For example, if a client is being discharged before mastering a complicated dressing change, the nurse advocates for an additional day in the hospital or home health visits.

Nonmaleficence

Nonmaleficence is the duty to do no harm to the client. If a nurse fails to check an order for an unusually high dose of insulin and administers it, he or she has violated the principle of nonmaleficence. Sometimes it is difficult to reconcile nonmaleficence with medical care because the choice of treatment may initially cause harm, even though the outcome is potentially good. For example, a client with colon cancer has a resection with a colostomy and endures the pain of surgery. In addition, the client undergoes unpleasant chemotherapy and radiation treatments. Although harmed in many ways, the ultimate goal is for the client to be free of cancer. In these cases, the treatment is still ethically right because the intended effect is good and outweighs the bad effect. If the outcome is likely to be poor despite the treatment, what is ethically right may be difficult to determine.

Autonomy

Autonomy refers to a client's right to self-determination or freedom to make choices without opposition. Nurses respect the client's right of autonomy even if the decision conflicts with the nurse's values. Through their advocacy role, nurses support clients' autonomy.

Justice

Justice is the duty to be fair to all people regardless of age, gender, race, or other factors. The American Nurses Association Code of Ethics (Box 5–6) has the principle of justice as its first statement. A conflict can occur if there are limited health care resources or when fairness to one means discrimination to another.

Fidelity

Fidelity is the duty to maintain commitments of professional obligations and responsibilities. This is generally defined by nurse practice acts.

Veracity

Veracity is the duty to tell the truth. The nurse is obligated to provide factual information to the client so that he or she may exercise autonomy. There are potential conflicts if the family or physician withholds information from the client. The issues of beneficence and nonmaleficence can enter into this ethical conflict.

LEGISLATIVE AND JUDICIAL INFLUENCES

Society's struggles with ethical issues result in legislative and judicial decisions that affect ethical decisions. For example, the issue of declaring death and removing life support has become more difficult with

BOX 5-6 Code for Nurses

1. The nurse provides services with respect for human dignity and the uniqueness of the client, unrestricted by considerations of social or economic status, personal attributes, or the nature of health problems.
2. The nurse safeguards the client's right to privacy by judiciously protecting information of a confidential nature.
3. The nurse acts to safeguard the client and the public when health care and safety are affected by incompetent, unethical, or illegal practice by any person.
4. The nurse assumes responsibility and accountability for individual nursing judgments and actions.
5. The nurse maintains competence in nursing.
6. The nurse exercises informed judgment and uses individual competency and qualifications as criteria in seeking consultation, accepting responsibilities, and delegating nursing activities.
7. The nurse participates in activities that contribute to the ongoing development of the profession's body of knowledge.
8. The nurse participates in the profession's efforts to implement and improve standards of nursing.
9. The nurse participates in the profession's efforts to establish and maintain conditions of employment conducive to high-quality nursing care.
10. The nurse participates in the profession's effort to protect the public from misinformation and misrepresentation and to maintain the integrity of nursing.
11. The nurse collaborates with members of the health professions and other citizens in promoting community and national efforts to meet the health needs of the public.

Reprinted with permission from Code for Nurses With Interpretive Statements. Kansas City, American Nurses Association, 1985.

advances in technology. Formerly, the loss of cardiac and respiratory function was the deciding factor in determining death. However, with greater abilities to maintain cardiac and respiratory function, society has had to redefine death. Brain criteria, including lack of movements or breathing, absence of reflexes, a flat electroencephalogram, and unresponsiveness are now included in definitions of death. These are widely accepted by most states. The ethical issues for many nurses are related to their own beliefs about the dignity of life, the harvesting of donor organs from an individual who is brain dead, and supporting the family members who may be asked to make decisions. The legality of brain death has removed some of the uncertainties for nurses regarding ethical issues.

Another topic engendering much debate is physician-assisted suicide and euthanasia. Many people fear a prolonged and painful death. This has given rise to a movement for a legally sanctioned, medically assisted, peaceful death as an option for clients of sound mind with terminal illnesses.

THE IMPACT OF TECHNOLOGY

The developments of science and technology have created ethical issues that were unheard of even 10 years ago. Some examples include the successful impregnation of a woman past menopause that has caused some governments to consider age limitations for such procedures, genetic engineering that has the potential to harm humans or lead to discrimination, and cloning that raises difficult questions about the creation of life and individuality. These advances, once in the realm of science fiction, now pose serious ethical dilemmas. Nurses will be involved with these issues and will have particular problems if the duty to the client is obscured by the need to promote science and progress.

HEALTH CARE REFORM

Cost control, shorter hospital stays, increased client acuity, and interest in alternative health care are factors that will have an impact on ethical decision-making. The discharge of clients to their homes when they are sicker and more vulnerable is of great concern. Issues related to the allocation of health care dollars to those who need it the most or who have the greatest potential to have a positive outcome also are ethically challenging. Nurses will continually face questions that make them examine their own values as they relate to providing quality care to clients and their families.

Ethical Decision-Making

Nurses use a problem-solving method (the nursing process) to provide care to clients. Health care providers use a similar problem-solving approach for ethical dilemmas. The following steps can be used when making ethical decisions:

1. Obtain as much information as possible to understand the situation. Identify the problem and describe it. Determine what values are involved and who will be affected by the decision. A statement of the dilemma (after looking at all the data) helps to see the issue as clearly as possible.
2. List all the possible options for solving the dilemma; this is referred to as brainstorming. Do not determine the consequences at this point.
3. Examine the pros and cons of each option, foreseeing possible consequences from both a utilitarian and a deontologic approach. Consider the effects on the individual.
4. Make the decision and follow through on it.
5. Evaluate the decision in terms of effects and results.

Ethics Committees

Hospitals and other health care institutions often have ethics committees to help resolve ethical dilemmas and make decisions on a per case basis. Ethics committees are composed of individuals with diverse backgrounds. They often include physicians, nurses, clergy, social workers, and community members. Ethics committees establish guidelines and policies before an ethical dilemma develops. However, they may also be called on to act as an advocate for clients who are no longer mentally capable of making their own decisions. Having a resource for reviewing difficult cases by a committee of individuals with different perspectives often helps to ensure that a careful and unbiased decision is made.

SUMMARY OF KEY CONCEPTS

- Laws are written rules of conduct approved by an authorized body. Ethics are moral principles and values that guide a person's actions.
- Nurse practice acts protect the public from unqualified practitioners and are enforced by each respective state's board of nursing.
- Criminal laws affect the public's welfare. Conviction results in a fine, jail term, or both.

- The State Board of Nursing is responsible for reviewing and approving nursing education programs, granting licensure, overseeing licensure examinations, and implementing disciplinary procedures.
- Civil laws protect individual citizens' rights and freedoms; the injured citizen sues the accused. If guilty, the defendant pays legal fees and restitution for damages.
- Intentional torts are civil infractions in which a person deliberately acted aggressively toward another (eg, an assault or battery). Unintentional torts are those in which the accused did not purposely cause harm to another. Negligence and malpractice are unintentional torts.
- Legal issues that may affect nurses include working outside the scope of practice as defined in the nurse practice act, falsifying medical records, committing insurance fraud, stealing narcotics, or engaging in an intentional or unintentional tort.
- Negligence is determined by comparing the accused person's actions with the reasonableness with which others would have acted. Malpractice is determined by examining how closely the accused person's actions deviated from the accepted standard for a similarly licensed individual with comparable education and experience.
- Nurses can avoid being sued by following agency policies and procedures, strengthening clinical weaknesses, finding acceptable alternatives when unprepared for an assignment, accurately documenting information, and respecting clients' rights.
- Immunity from prosecution may occur under the provisions of a Good Samaritan law or through expiration of the statute of limitations.
- The medical record is a legal document. All information entered in the record must be accurate and complete, dated and timed, legible, objectively written, and signed.
- All nurses should have personal liability insurance separate from their employer to ensure that the lawyer who represents the nurse will act in the nurse's best interests.
- Utilitarianism is a consequence-oriented theory of ethics.
- Deontologic theory is duty based.
- Duties are moral or legal obligations.
- Rights are those freedoms or actions to which one has a just moral and or legal claim.
- Ethical values are consistent, take priority over other concerns, involve the welfare of others, and are well considered and thoughtfully examined.
- Professional values include beneficence, nonmaleficence, autonomy, justice, fidelity, and veracity.
- Ethical issues in health care are influenced by professional values, judicial and legislative acts, technology, and industry-wide economic conditions.
- An ethical decision-making model uses a problem-solving approach for ethical dilemmas, and includes obtaining information, exploring options, making a decision, and evaluating the decision.

CRITICAL THINKING EXERCISES

1. A confused client has attempted to get out of bed by climbing over the side rails. What actions would you take to protect yourself from being sued?
2. A liver becomes available for transplant. The tissue matches an adolescent and a middle-aged client who both are in need of the organ. If you were responsible for deciding which client receives the organ transplant, what criteria would you use?
3. Consider the case of Mrs. S. (see p. 41) Discuss the ethical issues involved from the standpoint of values. Assess the situation from a utilitarian and a deontologic viewpoint using the ethical decision-making model. Decide if you think inserting the feeding tube and using wrist restraints was ethically good.

Suggested Readings

Davis, A. J. (1997). Selected ethical issues in planned social change and primary health care. *Nursing Ethics: An International Journal for Health Care Professionals, 4*(3),239–240.

Edge, R. S., & Groves, J. R. (1994). *The ethics of health care: A guide for clinical practice.* Albany, Delmar Publishers, Inc.

Ellis, J. R., & Hartley, C. L. (1997). *Nursing in today's world: Challenges, issues and trends* (6th ed.). Philadelphia. J. B. Lippincott-Raven.

Giuliano, K. K. (1997). Organ transplants. Tackling the tough ethical questions. *Nursing, 27*(5), 34–40.

Haddad, A. (1997). Acute care decisions. Ethics in action...assisted suicide. *RN, 60*(3), 17–18, 20, 69.

Harrington, N., Smith, N. E. & Spratt, W. E. (1996). *LPN to RN transitions.* Philadelphia. Lippincott-Raven.

Kopf, R. (1993). Are your medical records a legal asset or liability? Legal documentation guideline. *Journal of Nursing Law, 1*(1), 5–13.

Laudebache, P. (1995, September-October). Limiting liability to avoid malpractice litigation. *American Journal of Maternal Child Nursing, 20*, 243–248.

Moniz, D. M. (1996). When things go wrong...malpractice lawsuits. *Nursing, 26*(2), 45.

Quinn, C. A., & Smith, M. D. (1987). *The professional commitment: Issues and ethics in nursing.* Philadelphia: Saunders.

Scanlon, C., & Rushton, C. H. (1996). Assisted suicide: Clinical realities and ethical challenges. *American Journal of Critical Care, 5*(6), 397–405.

Simpson, R. L. (1996). Ethics and privacy in a technologically driven health care network. *Nursing Administration Quarterly, 21*(1), 81–84.

Spinstead, K. (1996). Cost versus quality: Making ethical decisions in home care today. *Caring, 15*(10), 38, 40, 44.

Taylor, C., Lillis, C., & LeMone, P.(1996). *Fundamentals of nursing: The art and science of nursing care* (3rd ed.). Philadelphia: Lippincott-Raven.

Terry, P., & Rushton, C. H. (1996). Allocation and scarce resources: Ethical challenges, clinical realities. *American Journal of Critical Care, 5*(5), 326–330.

Zerwekh, J., & Claborn, J. C. (1994). *Nursing today: Transitions and trends.* Philadelphia: Saunders.

2

Development Across the Life Span

Chapter 6

Caring for Young Adults

KEY TERMS

Autonomy
Developmental stage
Developmental tasks
Development
Doubt
Growth
Guilt
Industry
Inferiority
Initiative
Intimacy
Isolation
Mistrust
Psychosexual stages
Psychosocial stages
Role confusion
Shame
Trust

LEARNING OBJECTIVES

On completion of this chapter, the reader will:

- Differentiate growth from development.
- Explain the terms developmental stage and developmental task.
- Name Erikson's eight psychosocial stages of development.
- Describe the attributes associated with each stage of psychosocial development.
- List at least six characteristics of maturity.
- Describe the physical, social, and emotional characteristics of young adults.
- Discuss at least three areas for health teaching when caring for young adults.

Nurses provide care to all individuals from birth to old age. It is important to prepare clients for the physical changes and common life experiences that occur at various stages throughout life. To do this, nurses must be knowledgeable about how aging affects health and familiar with social changes that are characteristic of each period in the life cycle. The first part of this chapter is a discussion on growth and development followed by a review of the developmental life stages, tasks, and crises commonly encountered in each. Following the overview of the developmental phases, the chapter focuses on the physical and psychosocial development of the young adult, the stage roughly between the ages of 18 to 35.

Growth and Development

Growth refers to an increase in body size and is measured by changes in height and weight. **Development** refers to the ability to perform physical, intellectual, social, and psychological tasks. Development is measured by evaluating a person's physical coordination, language skills, and ability to solve problems, establish and maintain relationships, and cope during crises. Although development depends heavily on physical growth and maturation, social relationships and life experiences also affect development.

At one time, it was commonly believed that growth and development ceased after adolescence. Now development is considered a lifelong process of transitions during which people change according to their unique age-related experiences.

Developmental Stages

A **developmental stage** is a period of life during which there are unique physical and behavioral changes. The human life span is a continuous series of developmental stages. Each stage is separate and distinct from the previous stage and from the stage that follows. All individuals develop in the same cycle and pattern of progression. During each stage, individuals are challenged to complete specific **developmental tasks,** activities unique to a particular stage. Accomplishing the tasks within each stage is critical to future development. Handling a task out of sequence, either prematurely or belatedly, can cause frustration and emotional crises. Consider the impact of trying to toilet train a child too soon, or of having a first child close to menopause, or of being forced to retire early due to health changes. These situations create psychic stress when the tasks occur during atypical periods of life.

Finally, one's degree of success in accomplishing the developmental tasks of each stage influences the outcome of each successive stage. Failure to complete the developmental tasks in a timely manner makes eventual achievement difficult. Mastery of the tasks empowers one to succeed in future challenges.

Erik Erikson divided developmental stages into eight periods that span the life cycle. Erikson suggested that each stage is influenced by social relationships and coined the term **psychosocial stages.** He proposed that a person acquires one of two opposing attributes at each developmental stage (Fig. 6–1). He maintained that either a positive or negative outcome results, depending on an individual's success or failure in accomplishing the developmental tasks. The following is a brief overview of the psychosocial stages up to and including young adulthood. The stages of middle and late adulthood are discussed in subsequent chapters.

Early Psychosocial Stages

INFANCY AND TRUST VS. MISTRUST

During infancy, birth to approximately 18 months of age, a baby's developmental task is to communicate and satisfy basic needs. Infants indicate they are hungry, cold, hot, wet, or tired primarily through crying, pointing, and other body language. When the parents or caretakers consistently respond to their needs, infants develop a sense of **trust** or reliance on others. When physical and emotional needs are ignored, the infants acquire a general **mistrust** of others. If trust is not acquired, it handicaps the individual during future developmental stages.

EARLY CHILDHOOD AND AUTONOMY VS. SHAME AND DOUBT

Erikson observed that a major developmental task during the toddler years, ages 18 months to 3 years, is eliminating urine and feces in a socially acceptable manner. The emotional consequences, as Erikson saw it, depended on the approval or disapproval of significant persons, usually the parents. Erikson proposed that when toddlers learn to suppress immediate gratification, such as delaying urinating or defecating until an appropriate time, they are praised and accepted. The approval results in **autonomy,** a sense of pride in self. When toddlers are met with impatience or criticism for toileting accidents, **shame** or **doubt** develop: shame, for having disappointed parents, or doubt in one's ability to live up to parental expectations. Autonomy lays a positive foundation for the next developmental stage.

THE PRESCHOOLER AND INITIATIVE VS. GUILT

During ages 3 to 6 years, the child seeks to perform tasks modeled by parents and identifies with the same-sex parent. Little girls imitate their mothers by helping to cook or wash dishes; little boys use tools or carry a briefcase like their fathers. **Initiative**, the positive result of this stage, develops when children feel that the work they do is appreciated and encouraged.

Constant, unwarranted, or harsh discipline in the absence of praise can create overwhelming feelings of **guilt** and low self-esteem.

Development is enhanced during this stage when parents or caregivers supervise the child in appropriate activities and praise the child's accomplishments. Giving the preschool child opportunities to complete tasks within his or her ability helps to promote industry, a characteristic of the next developmental stage.

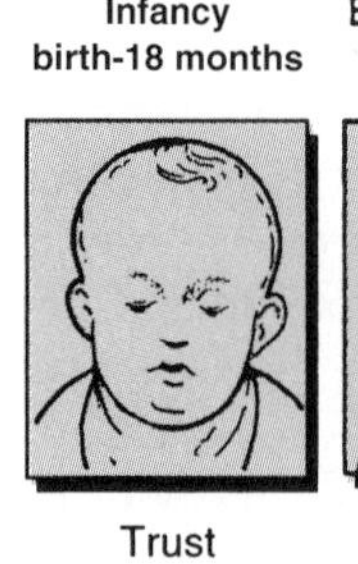

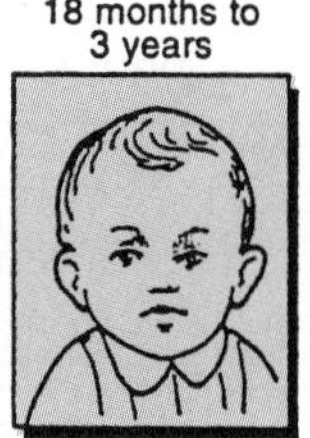
Early childhood
18 months to
3 years
Autonomy
vs. Shame,
Doubt

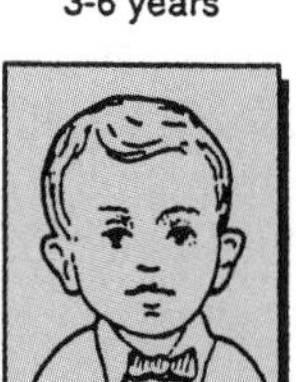
Pre-school age
3-6 years
Initiative
vs.
Guilt

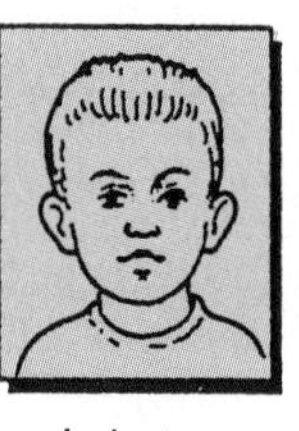
School age
6-12 years
Industry
vs.
Inferiority

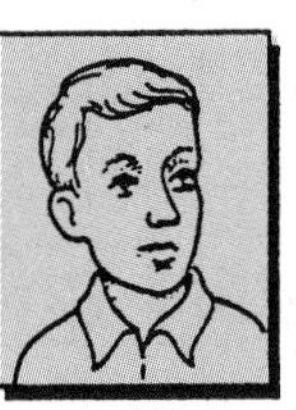
Adolescence
12-18 years
Identity
vs. Role
Confusion

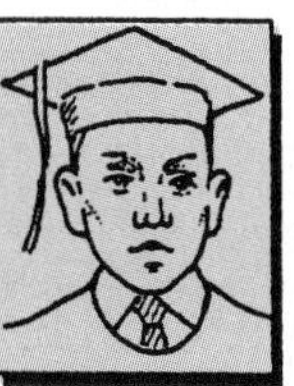
Young adult
18-35 years
Intimacy
vs.
Isolation

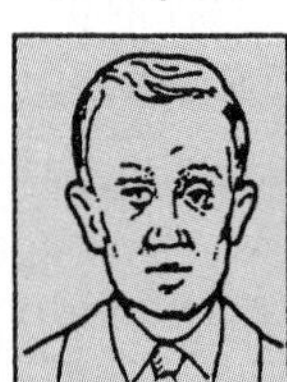
Middle-aged adult
35-65 years
Generativity
vs.
Stagnation

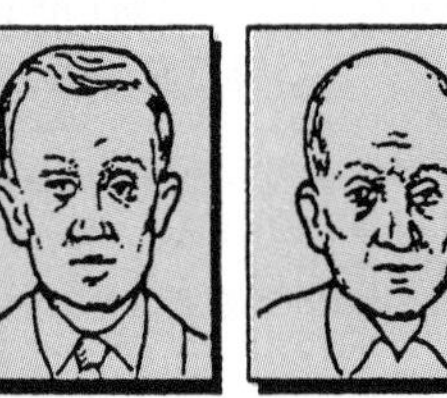
Older adult
65+ years
Ego
Integrity vs.
Despair

FIGURE 6-1. Erikson's psychosocial stages of development.

THE SCHOOL-AGE CHILD AND INDUSTRY VS. INFERIORITY

The tasks during early school age, 6 to 12 years, include paying attention, following directions, cooperating with others, and completing work in a timely and acceptable manner. If the child developed the negative attributes of mistrust, shame or doubt, and guilt in the previous stages, his or her self-confidence is diminished. This child appears withdrawn, feels inadequate, and experiences failure, all of which contribute to a sense of **inferiority** at this stage. Contrast the child who has acquired the positive attributes of trust, autonomy, and initiative during previous stages. This child enjoys new challenges and is eager to engage in efforts to produce work of high quality—examples of **industry.**

ADOLESCENCE AND EGO IDENTITY VS. ROLE CONFUSION

In adolescence, ages 12 to 18, the child strives to establish self-identity, or **ego identity.** Before adolescence, children identify themselves primarily in terms of their position in the family, such as son or daughter, brother or sister. During adolescence, the healthy child explores alternative value systems, develops a sense of self beyond the family, and eventually adopts values that are compatible with his or her personal beliefs. Adolescents must perceive that they are valuable parts of society and find satisfactory roles within it.

In contrast, some adolescents are reluctant to oppose or question parental or adult views. This leads to **role confusion** because these adolescents never develop true self-identity, and they attempt to fulfill the dreams and expectations of others. Some adolescents consider suicide as an escape from hopelessness and depression. Suicide is the third leading cause of death among adolescents. Confusion over role identity, substance abuse, and family stress are factors that contribute to suicidal behaviors.

YOUNG ADULTHOOD AND INTIMACY VS. ISOLATION

Erikson observed that the developmental tasks during young adulthood, ages 18 to 35, involve leaving the home, forming lasting relationships with nonrelatives, and committing to a career (Fig. 6–2). If the young adult forms friendships with others and has a significant, intimate relationship with one individual, a basis for closeness with others results. The young adult then acquires the positive attribute of **intimacy,** the ability of a person to enter into personal relationships that reaffirm one's own identity. Acquiring intimacy during this period enhances one's capability to become a productive and happy member of society. The inability to form a close relationship with another results in loneliness and **isolation.**

The Young Adult

The young adult stage is a period of life like no other. Young persons are establishing independence from their parents, developing their own lifestyle, forming new relationships with friends, coworkers, and a spouse, and taking on increasing responsibilities, such as working full time and raising children. Developing the qualities that transform adolescents into mature adults is a gradual process. Characteristics of maturity are listed in Box 6–1.

Social Characteristics

The young adult's social network undergoes major changes: relationships with former classmates dwindle after high school graduation; peer conformity loses its importance; and new acquaintances met at college, work, or in the community replace the formerly close friendships. Young adults eventually leave their parents' home. Education after high school and employment offer the opportunity for greater independence.

Many young adults establish credit and acquire debts for the first time in their lives. Financial independence requires a budget and money management. Marriage and starting a family increase the financial responsibilities of this age group.

Sexuality is at its peak at this stage. It is not unusual for young adults to have several romantic relationships and become sexually active. This age group has access to contraception and safer sex practices but often still risks unprotected sex. Unsafe sex practices among nonmonogamous heterosexuals contributes to the rising incidence of young adults infected with acquired immunodeficiency syndrome (AIDS).

Emotional Characteristics

Young adulthood can be both physically and psychologically stressful. Frequently, young adults face a variety of crises: rejection within a relationship or divorce; the possibility or actuality of contracting AIDS and dealing with a life-threatening illness; and job insecurity and financial obligations. Young adults who have not developed effective coping strategies resort

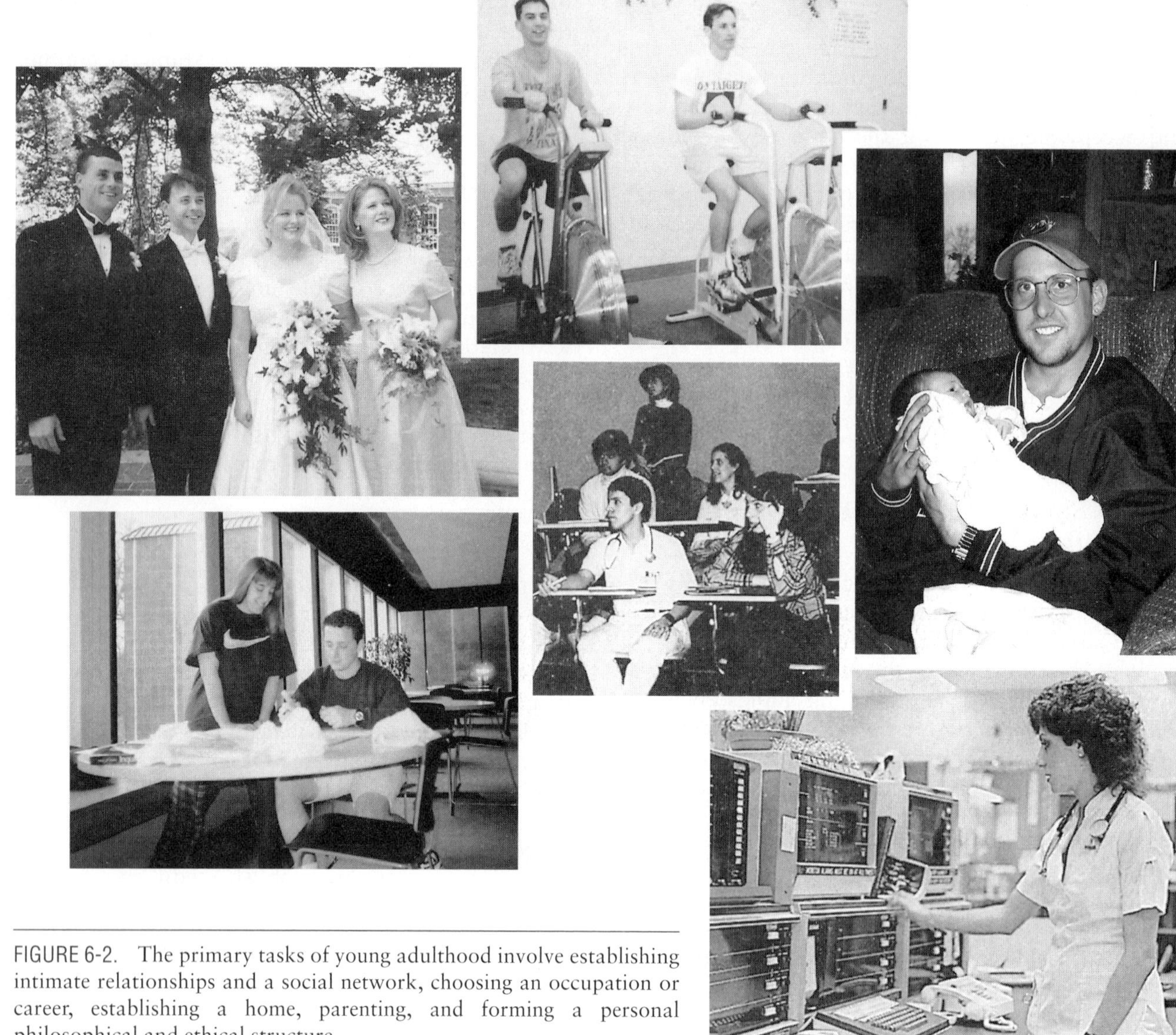

FIGURE 6-2. The primary tasks of young adulthood involve establishing intimate relationships and a social network, choosing an occupation or career, establishing a home, parenting, and forming a personal philosophical and ethical structure.

to maladaptive measures such as alcohol or drug abuse. Substance abuse impairs judgment and physical reaction time, thereby increasing the incidence of accidents, homicide, and suicide among young adults.

Marriage contributes to a stable lifestyle, whereas the birth of a first child can be emotionally unsettling. Some young parents doubt their ability to care for a child. The stress becomes more anxiety provoking if the baby has special needs or becomes sick. Parenthood can become extremely stressful if financial and emotional crises are not resolved.

Physical Characteristics

Most people are healthiest and attain peak physical performance as young adults. Injury from automobile accidents, homicide, or other accidents is a greater cause of health problems than physical illness. The following is a brief overview of the physical characteristics of the young adult.

MUSCULOSKELETAL SYSTEM

Young adults are generally physically strong and resilient. They enjoy remarkable agility and stamina because the musculoskeletal system is functioning optimally. Proprioception, the ability to sense and coordinate body movements, and the speed of reaction time reach their peak between ages 20 and 30. By about age 20, changes in general appearance no longer occur at such a rapid rate as during adolescence. Growth for nonpregnant females and most

BOX 6-1 Characteristics of Adult Maturity

- Developing personal self-reliance
- Learning from past experiences
- Communicating feelings
- Respecting others
- Coping with stressors
- Restraining impulses
- Being accountable
- Accepting consequences of decisions

males is complete. Some men grow a few more inches between the ages of 18 and 20.

COGNITION AND SENSORY-PERCEPTION

The brain in a young adult is totally developed and, therefore, cognitive ability is complete. The ability to problem solve continues to be refined as the young adult goes through the process of life experiences. Sensory organs undergo slight changes. Hearing, which is most acute at about age 14, gradually declines. Significant hearing loss, if identified at this time, is more likely associated with a history of childhood middle ear infections or exposure to loud music during adolescence.

THE INTEGUMENT

Skin blemishes, a problem during puberty and adolescence, tend to resolve. Facial hair for young men is more widely distributed and requires daily shaving. Wisdom teeth or third molars, if present, erupt during early young adulthood. For men who inherit male pattern baldness, early thinning or loss of hair at the hairline may be noted.

THE CARDIOVASCULAR SYSTEM

Minor changes occur in the heart and vascular system. There is a 1% loss of myocardial strength for each subsequent year of age. Early narrowing of the coronary arteries and other vascular changes begin occurring as well. A diet high in saturated fat contributes to the building of plaque on the walls of the coronary arteries beginning the pathologic process of atherosclerosis. Effects of this process are not evident for many years.

CHANGES RELATED TO PREGNANCY

Pregnancy causes unique physical changes: the breasts and uterus enlarge; there is an increase in circulatory volume; skin pigmentation changes occur, the most obvious of which is the darkening about the nipples and a brown line, called linea nigra, in the midline of the pregnant abdomen. Some women develop a dark area across the cheeks and forehead, called chloasma or "mask of pregnancy." The thyroid gland may increase in size due to metabolic changes. Posture and gait compensate for the shift in the center of gravity caused by the enlarging fetus. The lumbar curve is accentuated to resemble lordosis to accommodate the increasing abdominal girth.

Nursing Implications

When caring for young adults, nurses must be aware of common patterns of behavior that affect the health and well-being of individuals within this age group. Because they are seeking health care for the first time as an adult, young adults have minimal knowledge of community health care resources. In addition, nurses are likely to find that young adults tend to seek health care only when they experience an acute emergency. In many cases, young adults delay seeking medical care due to an inability to pay for treatment.

Health Promotion

Nurses should understand that young adults perceive themselves as perpetually healthy and invincible. Consequently, many disregard early warning signs of diseases. They often do not consider preventive health measures a priority and disregard healthy behaviors such as obtaining early prenatal care, performing breast or testicular self-examinations, or scheduling regular health and dental examinations.

Nutrition

Having reached maximum growth, young adults require fewer calories as during adolescence. Failure to modify previous eating habits leads to an increase in body fat, although body weight may remain stable.

Physical attractiveness is extremely important to young adults. It is not uncommon for young adults to become compulsive about exercising or to follow unhealthy fad diets. Some develop eating disorders (see Chap. 15). Overeating and subsequent obesity sometimes occur as a result of using food to cope with unhappiness.

Illness and Hospitalization

Young adults continue to adjust to their physical characteristics and to work through feelings about sexuality. They are apt to develop great anxiety when faced with a medical examination or need for surgery. It is essential to carefully explain necessary procedures and to provide privacy. Such measures convey to young adults that the nurse is concerned about their welfare, understands their feelings, and respects their right to privacy. The nurse often finds during data base interviews that young adult clients have no knowledge about their family's health history nor their personal history of childhood diseases. For this reason, nurses need to collaborate with a family member or rely on past medical records to obtain a comprehensive health history.

During hospitalization, young adults are as frightened as younger clients but show their fear in less obvious ways. It is important for the nurse to realize that young adults also require reassurance, even though they tend to conceal their need for it. The nurse is especially supportive of young adults by allowing them to express ideas and ask questions about matters that interest or concern them, and by conveying respect for them as individuals. The nurse also helps young adults cope with their illness, whether temporary or permanent, and teaches them preventive health care measures.

Human Immunodeficiency Virus (HIV)

Nurses who work in public health agencies, acute care settings, and long-term health care facilities are likely to see an increase in young adults diagnosed with HIV. The total reported HIV infected cases in adults under 25 years old as of July 1997 was 12,673; the total number of adult cases in July 1997 was 85,386. Individuals infected with HIV can remain asymptomatic for as long as 10 years, yet they are capable of transmitting the virus to others. This information indicates a need for nurses to educate teenagers and adults about the advantages of sexual abstinence, maintaining monogamous relationships with an uninfected partner, or using other safer sex practices. Unfortunately, when HIV becomes active, infected adults succumb to and need treatment for opportunistic infections and eventually require terminal care (see Chap. 42). As of 1997, AIDS is the leading cause of death among men aged 25 to 44 and the third cause of death among women in this same age group. Overall, AIDS is the eighth leading cause of all adult deaths in the United States. AIDS remains a major threat to this age group.

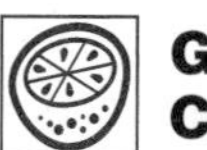

General Nutritional Considerations

Lean body mass and basal metabolic rate peak in early adulthood then gradually decline each successive decade. If calorie intake is not adjusted downward or physical activity decreases, gradual weight gain occurs.

Because peak bone mass is not attained until 30 to 35 years of age, it is important for young adults to consume adequate calcium to maximize bone density. The Recommended Daily Allowance (RDA) for calcium and other bone-building nutrients was replaced in the fall of 1997 with new Dietary Reference Intakes (DRIs). For young adults the recommendation for calcium intake increased to 1000 mg daily or at least three servings from the Milk Group.

Irregular eating habits, reliance on fast food, and frequent fad dieting may be "outgrown" as young adults mature and adopt a more stable lifestyle.

Despite counseling for wellness promotion, young adults may not recognize the long-term value of a healthful diet.

Vitamin supplements are widely used, though only a few groups actually need them: people on very low-calorie diets, strict vegetarians, pregnant and lactating women, people with malabsorption disorders and certain other chronic diseases, and people who use specific medications that interfere with vitamin absorption or metabolism.

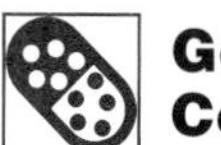

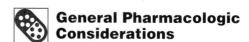

General Pharmacologic Considerations

All clients who take medication after discharge from the hospital should be cautioned about combining the use of prescription drugs with nonprescription drugs unless approved by the physician. Interactions of various drugs can cause serious adverse effects.

Although the incidence of acne declines in the young adult, some cases persist. Young women prescribed isotretinoin (Accutane) for severe acne must be warned that this drug has been associated with birth defects and under no circumstances should pregnancy occur while this drug is being taken. Effective contraception is essential during administration of this drug and for 1 month after discontinuing the drug. If pregnancy is suspected, stop the medication and notify the health care provider immediately.

Caution all young adults about mixing medications (both over-the-counter and prescription) with alcohol. The action of many drugs is potentiated when used with alcohol.

If pregnant, women must not take any drug, legal or illegal, prescription or nonprescription, unless the use of the drug is prescribed or recommended by the health care provider.

SUMMARY OF KEY CONCEPTS

- Growth refers to increases in body size, whereas development refers to the ability to perform physical, intellectual, social, and psychological tasks.

- Developmental stages are periods in life during which there are unique physical and behavioral changes. A developmental task is a process of socialization that is best accomplished at a particular time in life.
- Erikson proposed eight developmental stages that extend over the entire life span from birth to old age.
- From birth through young adulthood, individuals acquire one from each of the following pairs of attributes: during infancy, trust or mistrust; during early childhood, autonomy, shame or doubt; as preschoolers, initiative or guilt; in the early school years, industry or inferiority; as adolescents, ego identity or role confusion; and as young adults, intimacy or isolation; middle-aged adults acquire generativity or stagnation; and older adults develop ego integrity or despair.
- The characteristics that differentiate the maturity of adulthood from the immaturity of childhood and adolescence include developing personal self-reliance, learning from past experiences, communicating feelings, respecting others, restraining impulses, being accountable, and accepting the consequences of decisions.
- Young adults are physically strong and focused on their physical attractiveness. Pregnancy and childbearing occurs predominantly at this time. The numbers of friendships decrease but the quality with the few who remain is increased. Many experience emotional highs and lows because of their economic instability and active lifestyles.
- Nurses who care for young adults must teach methods for health promotion and disease prevention, especially in areas such as reducing risks for HIV, receiving early prenatal and illness care, and scheduling periodic health and dental examinations.

CRITICAL THINKING EXERCISES

1. Discuss the ways adults can promote the acquisition of positive characteristics among children from birth through adolescence.
2. Describe the typical physical, emotional, and social characteristics of young adults.
3. When planning a health promotion program for a group of young adults, what topics are most important to include?

Suggested Readings

Bailey, D. S., & Bailey, D. R. (1997). *Therapeutic approaches in mental health/psychiatric nursing* (4th ed.). Philadelphia: Davis.

Doornbos, M. M. (1997). The problems and coping methods of caregivers of young adults with mental illness. *Journal of Psychosocial Nursing and Mental Health Services, 35*(9), 22–26, 41–42.

Graves, K. L. (1995). Risky sexual behavior and alcohol use among young adults: Results from a national survey. *American Journal of Health Promotion, 10*(1), 27–36.

Kerr, D. L., & Gascoigne, J. L. (1996). Getting to know generation X: Health education for the thirteenth generation. *Journal of Health Education, 27*(5), 268–276.

MacKinnon, D. P., Williams-Avery, R. M., & Pentz, M. A. (1995) Youth beliefs and knowledge about the risks of drinking while pregnant. *Public Health Reports, 110*(6), 754–763.

Nettina, S. M. (1996). *The Lippincott manual of nursing practice* (6th ed.). Philadelphia: Lippincott-Raven.

Roye, C. F., & Coonan, P. R. (1997). Emergency! Adolescent rape. *American Journal of Nursing, 97*(4), 45.

Saltonstall, R. (1993). Healthy bodies, social bodies: Men's and women's concepts and practices of health in everyday life. *Social Science and Medicine, 36*(1), 7–14.

Scherer, J., & Roach, S. (1996). *Introductory clinical pharmacology* (5th ed.). Philadelphia: Lippincott-Raven.

Seymour, M., Hoerr, S. L., & Huang, Y. (1997). Inappropriate dieting behaviors and related lifestyle factors in young adults: Are college students different? *Journal of Nutrition Education, 29*(1), 21–26.

Steptoe, A., Wardle, J., Vinck, J., et al. (1994). Personality and attitudinal correlates of healthy and unhealthy lifestyles in young adults. *Psychology and Health, 9*(5), 331–343.

Stiffman, A. R., Dore, P., Cunningham, E. F. (1995). Person and environment in HIV risk behavior change between adolescence and young adulthood. *Health Education Quarterly, 22*(2), 211–226.

Ziff, M. A., Conrad, P., & Lachman, M. E. (1995). The relative effects of perceived control and responsibility on health and health-related behaviors in young and middle-aged adults. *Health Education Quarterly, 22*(1), 127–142.

Chapter 7

Caring for Middle-Aged Adults

KEY TERMS

Generativity
Keratotic lesion
Menopause
Mid-life crisis
Osteoporosis
Presbycusis
Presbyopia
Sandwich generation
Stagnation

LEARNING OBJECTIVES

On completion of this chapter, the reader will:

- List the developmental tasks associated with middle age.
- Name and discuss the two characteristics associated with the tasks of middle-age development.
- Describe the physical, social, and emotional characteristics of middle-aged adults.
- Discuss at least three unique problems the nurse deals with when caring for middle-aged adults.

Middle age, from age 35 to 65, is characterized as the established years. During this period, the individual has a chance to actualize the earlier struggles to establish a home and career. Middle-aged adults have the opportunity to analyze their assets and channel their energies into accomplishing life goals that are unfulfilled.

The Adult in Middle Life

The middle years are characterized by the pursuit of activities that provide self-satisfaction and community responsibility. These adults are often described as being the **sandwich generation** because they are raising their children and assuming more responsibility for their aging parents. Consequently, they are sandwiched between two generations. Some also must care for their grandchildren. Such added responsibilities can thwart the middle-aged adult's independence and create a crisis. The well adjusted middle-aged adult views the added responsibilities of aging parents and children as part of life.

Middle Adulthood and Generativity vs. Stagnation

Triggered by the realization that life is rapidly advancing, the middle years are the time when adults take inventory of their lives. The young adult years were focused on making goals; middle-aged adults evaluate if, and how well, their goals are being achieved.

Middle-aged adults are more likely to philosophically ponder the purpose for and value of their existence. With the knowledge that their remaining years are limited, middle-aged adults want to survey their achievements and pursue opportunities for self-fulfillment, a characteristic referred to as **generativity.** Middle-aged adults become more caring, giving, and productive. Many middle-aged adults spend time comforting, advising, and listening to younger family members or close friends and volunteering in civic activities to contribute to the community (Fig. 7–1).

On self-examination, however, some middle-aged adults are disappointed to find that their energies have not been invested wisely. The feeling that nothing of true significance has been accomplished along with a lack of commitment to future endeavors is referred to as **stagnation.** The major developmental tasks of the middle-aged adult are summarized in Box 7–1.

Social Characteristics

During middle age, adults remain socially involved with a variety of relatives and friends. As children marry, their social network expands to include sons-

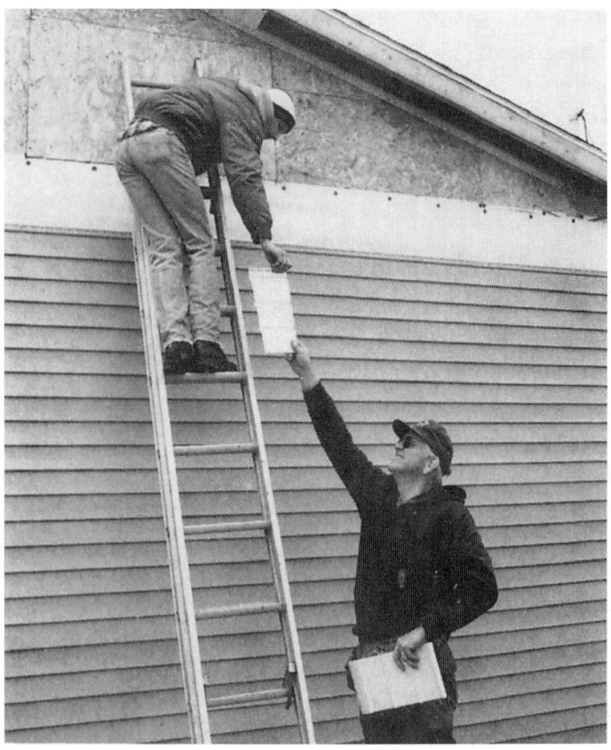

FIGURE 7-1. The middle-aged adult often becomes involved in community activities. These Habitat for Humanity volunteers make it possible for the organization to renovate or build affordable homes that are sold to low-income people at no interest.

and daughters-in-law. When children leave home, middle-aged couples have more time to spend with each other. For many, this strengthens the relationship. Others find that the relationship has changed since the years of childrearing, causing them to feel distant and estranged from one another. Irreconcilable differences lead to separation or divorce. Couples who remain together tend to be more financially secure than they were during early adulthood and many start to focus on ensuring that their savings will be adequate during their retirement years.

BOX 7-1 Major Developmental Tasks of the Middle-Aged Adult

- Reassessing life accomplishments and goals
- Adjusting to role changes
- Accepting physical, emotional, and social changes associated with middle-age
- Planning for retirement
- Strengthening relationships with spouse, family, friends, or companions
- Adjusting to responsibilities of aging parents
- Developing skills, hobbies, or activities that provide satisfaction

Emotional Characteristics

Personality is viewed as a variety of dynamic traits that continue to develop and change throughout adulthood. New events and challenges influence personality in many adults. Aging tends to be emotionally difficult in the American culture. Americans value youth and their energy more than the experience and wisdom of middle-aged and older adults. As a consequence of feeling unfulfilled and unappreciated, some middle-aged individuals develop a **mid-life crisis**. These middle-aged adults often view themselves as less likely to accomplish the goals of their youth. Even those who have accomplished their goals and seem successful have feelings of dissatisfaction. To relieve their feelings of insecurity and unhappiness over the loss of their youth, some have cosmetic surgery, wear clothing styles more characteristic of younger adults, have extramarital affairs, or abandon their current lifestyle to seek a more meaningful existence. Fortunately, most middle-age adults adapt to the changes and challenges of mid-life.

Financial insecurity also continues to stress middle-aged adults. Unemployment jeopardizes pension plans, retirement packages, and health insurance benefits. Without insurance coverage, serious illness or injury can mean financial ruin. Another financial burden includes caring for elderly parents, formerly the pillars of security and support, now dependent on their middle-aged children. Some middle-aged adults struggle with guilt for being unable to assume the care that aging parents require and worry about finding an adequate caregiver or nursing home.

Physical Characteristics

The middle years are productive years, yet there is a subtle change in the pace of living. Evidence of declining physical abilities becomes apparent. Early signs of aging appear. These changes can be traumatic, especially in the American culture that emphasizes youth and glamour.

MUSCULOSKELETAL SYSTEM

Height remains constant until the late stages of middle adulthood when there is a slight decline. Muscle mass is gradually replaced by adipose and connective tissue, which compromises strength. Range of joint motion diminishes due to a sedentary lifestyle or from damage to joints from hard work.

Bone mass becomes increasingly porous, particularly in women after menopause, leading to **osteoporosis.** For some, these debilitating processes can go unnoticed until a simple injury occurs with serious consequences, such as a fracture or delayed healing.

SENSORY-PERCEPTION

There is a gradual decline in visual accommodation, the ability to focus an image on the retina. Around ages 40 to 50 many individuals notice difficulty in reading small print or performing other tasks that require close vision. This condition, called **presbyopia,** is caused by a loss of elasticity in the lens of the eyes. Because the lens tends to be more rigid, it requires longer time to adjust to rapid changes in light and darkness. Changes in the lens such as thickening, loss of flexibility, and an increase in opacity cause glare sensitivity.

Presbycusis is the loss of hearing associated with aging. High-pitched sounds diminish first. Some people, particularly those in later middle years, find that the decrease interferes with hearing and communicating with others.

THE INTEGUMENT

Subcutaneous fat disappears toward the end of the middle-age period creating a bony appearance to the face. Age lines or wrinkles are evident at the forehead, corners of the eyes, and mouth. The skin appears wrinkled and dry due to chronic exposure to the sun. **Keratotic lesions,** elevated, darkly pigmented skin plaques, appear as moles on the scalp, face, neck, or trunk. The hair loses texture and color. Baldness becomes more evident among men. Change in the balance of estrogen and testosterone causes facial hair or hair growth about the nipples and chest area in postmenopausal women. Many adults lose one or more permanent teeth.

THE CARDIOVASCULAR SYSTEM

Cardiovascular disease is the leading killer of adults today. Genetics and lifestyle play important roles. Men are at higher risk in comparison to premenopausal women; however, the risks equalize for men and women after menopause. Arteries continue to fill with deposits of fat while calcium infiltrates the fatty plaque making the arteries hard and inelastic. Mild hypertension (high blood pressure) is a common sign of early heart disease.

THE URINARY SYSTEM

Men over the age of 50 begin to notice slight changes in urinary patterns, such as hesitancy, reduced force of urinary stream, or feeling of fullness in the bladder, which are indicators of prostatic hypertrophy (see Chap. 60). Women who have had several children often experience stress incontinence due to a relaxation of the pelvic floor muscles. Coughing, sneezing, or laughing causes a leakage of urine.

BOX 7-2 Secondary Sex Changes With Decreased Estrogen

- Breasts begin to droop and sag.
- Mucous membrane of the vagina becomes dry and easily irritated.
- Pubic hair becomes sparse and gray.
- Vaginal lubrication decreases.
- Mood swings are common.
- Hot flashes and headaches occur.
- Bones become more brittle due to a loss of calcium.
- Vascular changes are accelerated.

REPRODUCTIVE CHANGES

Although sexuality continues throughout the life span, the frequency and vigor of intercourse is likely to decrease. Couples have a variety of contraceptive measures available to limit family size during their reproductive years. The use of oral contraceptives, however, especially among middle-aged women who smoke, increases the risk for blood clot formation. Women between the ages of 40 and 55 develop a dramatic physiologic change in the reproductive system known as **menopause** (see Chap. 58). Ovulation becomes irregular toward late mid-life and eventually ceases. Reduction in estrogen also causes changes in secondary sex characteristics (Box 7–2). As men age, the ability to achieve and sustain an erection is slightly diminished and the prostate gland enlarges. Male fertility extends long past that of women.

Nursing Implications

Health Promotion

Many middle-aged clients become concerned about their physical condition after the illness or death of a friend. They recognize the negative effects of neglecting their health and seek to reform poor health habits. It is important for the nurse to identify health risks and teach clients ways to modify or refrain from behaviors that contribute to preventable diseases. Health teaching includes smoking cessation, refraining from excessive alcohol, eating a low-fat diet, exercising regularly, and obtaining regular screening for colorectal, prostate, breast, and cervical cancer. Breast self-examination on a monthly basis is important for women in this age group to aid in early detection of breast cancer.

Nutrition

Weight tends to increase in middle age. Approximately 30% of all middle-aged adults are overweight and 60% of adults aged 50 to 59 are considered obese. Weight gain is a combination of consuming excessive calories, decreasing metabolic rate, and decreasing activity. The diet should include all nutrients needed to maintain and repair body tissue, with a decrease in caloric intake to compensate for decreased activity levels and a decreased metabolism. Because calcium in the bone is constantly being broken down and replenished, calcium requirements remain high. A regular exercise program helps to prevent weight gain, maintains bone mass, and compensates for lowered metabolism.

As adults age, poor dentition affects the ability to chew food. If the diet is deficient in whole grains, fresh fruits, and uncooked vegetables to compensate for the inability to chew, stool volume and moisture are reduced, which contributes to a pattern of bowel irregularity and constipation.

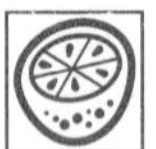

General Nutritional Considerations

Food preferences and eating habits are well established, making it difficult for some clients to accept special diets or dietary restrictions. Some clients view a "diet" as punishment or not worthwhile.

Promoting a healthful diet during the mid-life years, before evidence of chronic disease is apparent, may help reduce the risk of a variety of disorders. From a psychological standpoint, modifying eating habits to prevent disease may be easier than doing so to treat disease. Urge clients to eat more fruits and vegetables, choose foods lower in fat and higher in fiber, and avoid overeating. Maintaining an active lifestyle, with both aerobic activity and weight training, helps promote weight management.

Because aging causes everyone to lose bone mass, new calcium requirements for all adults over age 50 are increased to 1,200 mg/day, or about four servings from the milk group.

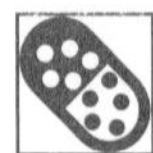

General Pharmacologic Considerations

- Clients must thoroughly understand drug use: quantity of the drug (number of capsules or tablets, amount of liquid); the time it is to be taken (eg, 10 AM and 2 PM); and any instruction relating to a specific drug.
- Noncompliance is a problem with adults who perceive themselves as healthy. Appropriate and thorough client teaching helps diminish noncompliance.
- Menopausal women face a decision concerning estrogen replacement therapy (ERT). The nurse provides up-to-date information on the risks and benefits of ERT to assist the client in making an informed choice.
- To diminish the possibility of osteoporosis in postmenopausal women who do not elect ERT, a bone resorption inhibitor such as alendronate (Fosamax) is often prescribed. Women taking alendronate are instructed to ingest the drug in the morning with 6 to 8 ounces of water and to remain upright for 30 minutes after ingestion.
- Men with prostate hypertrophy should be cautioned that some medications can exacerbate urinary retention. These men should be instructed to check with the primary care provider before taking over-the-counter or prescription medications.

SUMMARY OF KEY CONCEPTS

- Middle age is the period when adults evaluate their progress in reaching goals, plan for and use their remaining opportunities in life wisely, and cope with the changes associated with aging.
- Middle-aged adults acquire either generativity or stagnation on completion of this stage of development. Generativity is a feeling of satisfaction with personal life accomplishments and a reinvestment of time and energy in self-fulfilling activities. Stagnation involves feelings of remorse and lack of commitment toward remaining opportunities for future achievements.
- Middle age marks the start of physical decline. Strength and muscle tone decrease, weight increases, bones become more brittle and fragile, especially in women, and teeth are weak or diseased if dental care is neglected. Vision and hearing often diminish. The skin tends to becomes dry and wrinkled and shows pigment changes. Vascular disease continues to progress. There is loss of fertility in women and a decline in sexual performance for both sexes.
- Middle-aged adults have usually acquired more emotional and financial stability than at any other time in their lives. They are often faced with the care of dependent children, aging parents, and grandchildren. Some find this time richly satisfying, whereas others feel overwhelmed by responsibilities and disappointed by their lack of accomplishments.
- Nursing approaches directed toward the needs of middle-aged adults include helping them cope with the onset of chronic diseases, sustaining their independence, promot-

ing adequate nutrition, and supporting their role within their family.

CRITICAL THINKING EXERCISES

1. A middle-aged client is admitted for observation following an incidence of chest pain. Based on what you know about the physical, emotional, and social characteristics of an individual in this age group, what assessments are important to make and why?
2. A 72-year-old male's health is generally good, but he needs assistance with activities of daily living because he is blind in one eye and has only partial vision in the other. He lives with his 51-year-old son and daughter-in-law who are also responsible for their 3-year-old granddaughter. Explain how this situation represents the "sandwich generation." What are some potential problems in this situation? What would be the 51-year-old son's greatest stressor? What suggestions would you offer the son who feels his life is disrupted by the responsibility of his grandchild and elderly father?

Suggested Readings

Burman, M. E. (1996). Daily symptoms and responses in adults: A review. *Public Health Nursing, 13*(4), 294–301.

DeLaune, S. C., & Ladner, P. K. (1998). *Fundamentals of nursing: Standards and practice.* Albany, NY: Delmar.

Edelman, C. L., & Mandle, C. L. (1994). *Health promotion throughout the lifespan* (3rd ed.). St. Louis: Mosby–Year Book.

Eschleman, M. M. (1996). *Introductory nutrition and nutrition therapy* (3rd ed.). Philadelphia: Lippincott-Raven.

Rosdahl, C. B. (1995). *Textbook of basic nursing* (6th ed.). Philadelphia: J. B. Lippincott.

Schuster, A. (1992). *The process of human development: A holistic life-span approach* (3rd ed.). Philadelphia: J. B. Lippincott.

Ziff, M. A., Conrad, P., & Lachman, M. E. (1995). The relative effects of perceived personal control and responsibility on health and health-related behaviors in young and middle-aged adults. *Health Education Quarterly, 22*(1), 127–142.

Additional Resources

American Association of Retired Persons
http://www.aarp.org/
601 E. St. NW
Washington, DC 20049
800–424–3410

Children of Aging Parents
Suite 302-A
1609 Woodbourne Road
Levittown, PA 19057
(215) 945–6900
(800) 227–7294

Volunteers of America
Suite 400
3939 North Causeway Boulevard
Metairie, LA 70002
(504) 837–2652

Chapter 8

Caring for Older Adults

KEY TERMS

Ageism
Antioxidants
Autophagocytosis
Despair
Ego integrity
Elder abuse
Free radicals
Gerontology
Kyphosis
Life review
Pet therapy
Reality orientation
Reminiscence therapy
Senescence
Validation therapy

LEARNING OBJECTIVES

On completion of this chapter, the reader will:

- List five trends for which society should prepare in view of the growing population of aging adults.
- Define gerontology.
- Discuss three theories of aging.
- Define ageism and how it affects older adults.
- Identify developmental tasks for the older adult.
- Contrast the developmental characteristics of ego integrity and despair.
- Discuss physical characteristics that are unique to the adult older than age 65.
- Identify social characteristics of older adults.
- Discuss factors that affect the emotional health of older adults.
- Discuss ways that a nurse's attitude concerning the aged can affect their care.
- List approaches the nurse can use when teaching older adults.
- Identify nursing care measures that are especially important when providing physical care for an older adult.
- Describe pet therapy, reality orientation, and reminiscence therapy.

Older adults play a vital role in society, the home, the workplace, and the community. They offer others with less maturity the wisdom of life experiences. Health care workers play an important role in helping older adults maintain their independence, health, and productivity.

The Older Adult

Senescence is the last stage in the life cycle. During senescence there is a gradual degeneration of body processes. Diet, exercise, stress reduction, and health promotion activities play a role in slowing the rate of senescence. This developmental period is subdivided into three categories: the young-old, ages 65 to 74, who are still active and vibrant; the middle-old, ages 75 to 84; and the old-old, over age of 85, who are physically frail (Fig. 8–1).

According to the United States Bureau of the Census, the number of people over age 65 is increasing rapidly. Life expectancy has been extended in both sexes to nearly 75 years (U.S. Department of Health and Human Services, 1992). The number of people aged 85 and older will be seven times greater in the middle of the next century (U.S. Senate Special Committee on Aging, 1991). The federal government has identified 10 major trends (Box 8–1) that society should prepare for in response to the growing population of older adults. *Centenarians* (those age 100 and over) are also increasing in number. By the year 2080 some estimate that there will be approximately 1 million centenarians living in the United States (Rybash, Roodin, & Hoyer, 1995).

Gerontology

Gerontology is the study of aging, including physiologic, psychological, and social aspects. Scientists are conducting much research to determine the actual

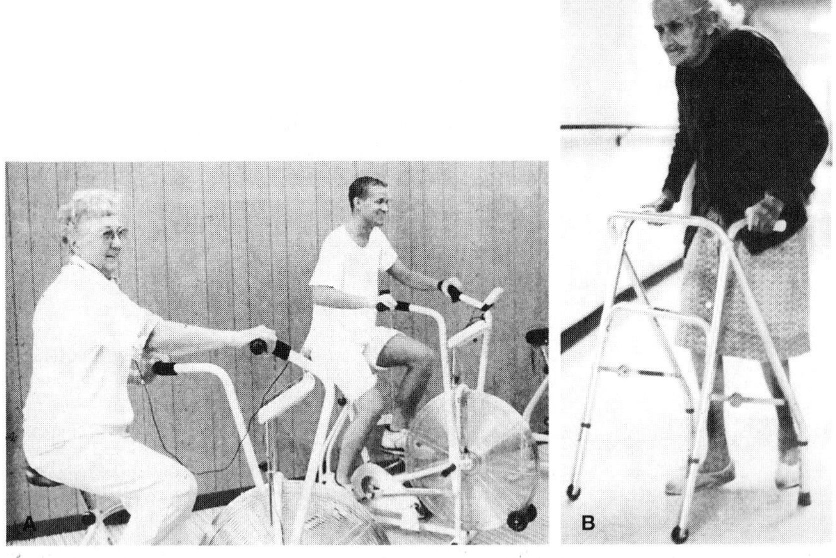

FIGURE 8-1. *(A)* This woman is representative of many healthy, active, youthful, older adults. *(B)* Others, like this woman, fall at the opposite end of the spectrum and show multiple signs of physical decline.

causes of the aging processes. The goal of this extensive research is to find ways to extend both the quantity and the quality of life.

Theories of Aging

It is an established fact that physical characteristics change throughout the life cycle. As one ages, the hair turns gray, skin becomes wrinkled, bones demineralize, and blood vessels become hard and inelastic. What biologic mechanism triggers these changes remains a mystery. Some theories that attempt to explain the aging process include autophagocytosis, the stress response, impairment of the immune response, alterations in DNA replication, and cellular damage by free radicals. No one theory fully explains the aging process and it is likely that aging is a combination of physiologic phenomena.

Autophagocytosis

Autophagocytosis literally means "to eat self." This does not mean total consumption of the cell, but portions of it are consumed to reduce its size. This process is used when the cell senses that adverse conditions exist. A smaller cell results in a temporary decrease in energy needs, and increases the potential for survival. During this process, a brown-colored residue called *lipofuscin* is formed. Scientists have noted that this cellular pigment accumulates in increasing amounts as in-

BOX 8-1 Ten Trends in the Older Adult Population in the United States

1. There are more elderly than ever before in history.
2. The elderly are an increasing proportion of our population.
3. Growth of the elderly will be steady but undramatic until 2011 when the baby boomers begin to reach age 65.
4. Elderly women outnumber elderly men.
5. More persons will survive to the oldest ages.
6. As more survive, more also face chronic illness and disabilities.
7. Issues surrounding the care of the frail elderly will become more prevalent. At the same time, the young-old have become pacesetters in new ways to spend the retirement years.
8. The elderly population will be more diverse in terms of racial composition and Hispanic origin in the coming decades.
9. The educational attainment of the elderly population will increase significantly in the coming years because younger cohorts were more likely to have completed high school and attended college than is true for the elderly of today.
10. Some elderly are economically secure. Others, especially many of the oldest old, those living alone, African Americans, American Indians, some Asian groups, and Hispanics have relatively high rates of poverty.

(Source: Taeuber CM. U.S. Bureau of the Census, Sixty-five plus in America, Current Population Reports, P 23-178. Washington, DC: U.S. Government Printing Office, 1992.)

dividuals age. Cell shrinkage caused by autophagocytosis contributes to the decrease in weight and height of older adults and to the atrophy of tissues and organs.

Stress Response

Hans Selye, a gifted physician of the early 20th century, pioneered a theory concerning stress and its effects on the body. He proposed that physical, psychological, and social changes produce biologic stress. Regardless of the stress-producing stimulus, Selye maintained that the physiologic response, which he called the *general adaptation syndrome*, is always the same (see Chap. 11). Gerontologists hypothesize that the defense mechanisms associated with the stress response eventually weaken, leading to death.

Decline of the Immune System

One of the most important mechanisms for preserving health is the immune system. Scientists have discovered that as individuals age, the immune system becomes impaired and the body's defenses are weakened and vulnerable to overwhelming infection and cancer. An increased incidence of each is associated with advancing age. Others theorize that as the immune system declines, the body misidentifies normal cells as foreign. The autoimmune theory of aging is that the body's defenses attack the healthy cells, advancing the aging process.

Faulty DNA Replication

The deoxyribonucleic acid (DNA) molecule present in each cell programs cellular reproduction. DNA is susceptible to damaging agents such as free radicals (see later discussion). A damaging agent locked onto the DNA molecule has the potential for scrambling the genetic code. The dysfunctional DNA is then unable to program the continued, orderly synthesis of proteins. When this happens repeatedly, fewer cells are capable of replication. In the young, cells resist agents that damage DNA or repair the damage efficiently. Because billions of cells are damaged in the aging process, tissue disorganization occurs and leads to organ failure.

Free Radicals

Free radicals are unstable atoms with excessive energy capable of damaging DNA molecules. It is possible that free radicals are responsible for changes associated with aging. Chronic exposure to substances such as radiation and environmental toxins damage DNA, causing cellular changes. Healthy cells resist the damaging effects of free radicals using chemicals called **antioxidants** that block the chemical reactions that cause free radicals. Scientists are investigating the antioxidant properties of vitamins C and E, and provitamin A, known as beta-carotene and found in the pigments of deep yellow and dark green fruits and vegetables.

Ageism

Ageism describes behaviors and beliefs that depict older adults in a negative, inaccurate, or stereotypical manner. Ageism results in the older adult being characterized as a sick, feeble, rigid, disagreeable, opinionated, or demented individual who lives in the past. According to information compiled by the U.S. Senate Special Committee on Aging (1991), the American Association of Retired Persons, the Federal Council on Aging, and the U.S. Administration on Aging, older adults are remarkably healthy and productive until the extremes of old age. Some Americans believe that the significant part of life is over after middle-age. This view undermines the dignity of older people who sense that they are not expected to remain physically or mentally healthy (Fig. 8–2). Ageism can prevent older adults from obtaining new jobs or force them into early retirement. In some situations older adults are avoided, treated disrespectfully, or ignored.

Late Adulthood

Late adulthood is the period beginning at the age of 65 and continuing until death. During late adulthood there are developmental tasks to complete (Box 8–2). Older adults must discover activities to fill the time previously spent at work and raising families. It is important that these activities sustain a sense of usefulness and self-worth. In addition, older adults must adjust to many losses such as the loss of friends or a spouse, loss of income, loss of health and agility, and loss of independence. Aging adults must face their own death.

Ego Integrity vs. Despair

As aging adults deal with life's remaining challenges, they acknowledge the permanency of past decisions

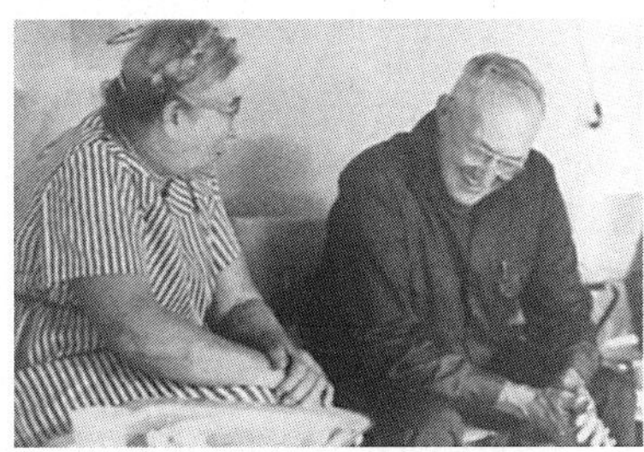
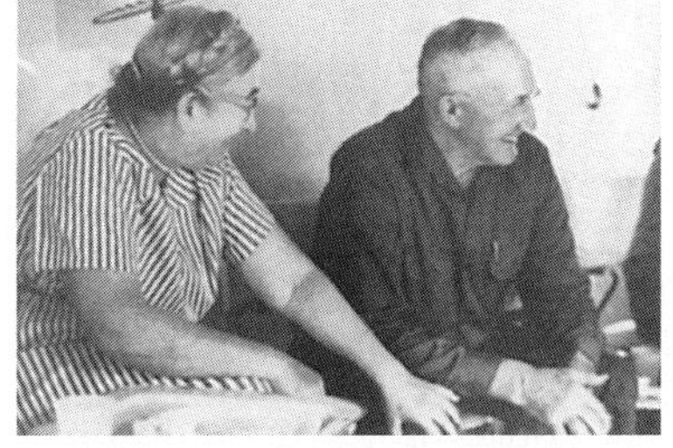
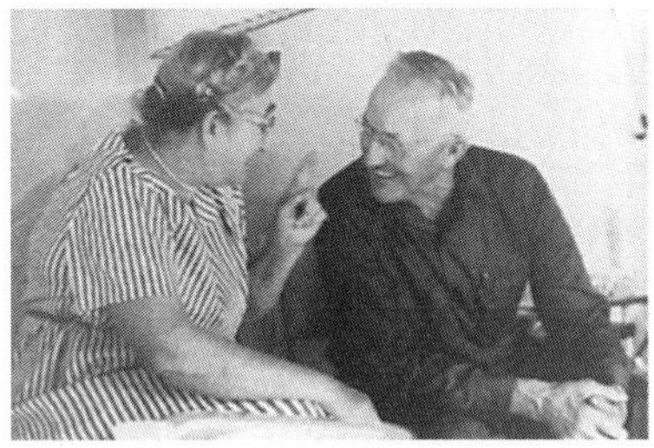
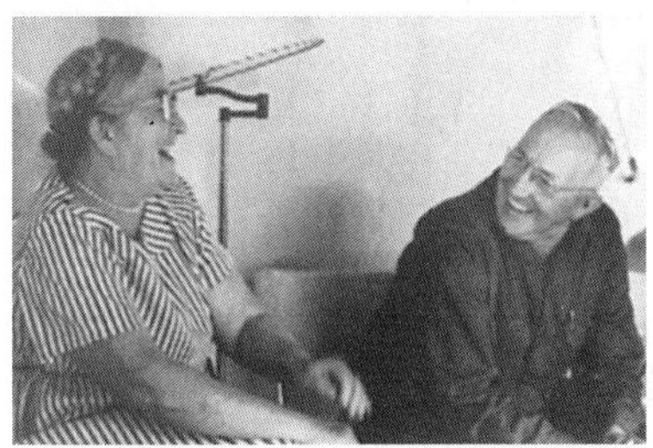

FIGURE 8-2. This older couple is enjoying social interaction. (Photos by Karen Baldwin.)

and actions. They develop either a sense of **ego integrity** or *despair* as they reflect on their lives. Ego integrity is a feeling of personal satisfaction that life has been happy and fulfilling. **Despair,** on the other hand, results when an individual views life as disappointing and unfulfilling and anguishes over what might have been. Most older adults engage in **life review.** This is looking back at one's life and reviewing decisions, choices, conflicts, and resolutions. For integrity to emerge in the older adult, a life review results in the belief that life has been meaningful and well spent. Despair is the predominate feeling if, after a life review, the older adult feels that life has been ineffective, decisions were poor, and life has been filled with unresolved conflict.

BOX 8-2 Developmental Tasks of the Older Adult

- Adjust to the physical limitations brought about by aging.
- Find satisfaction in retirement.
- Secure acceptable living arrangements.
- Develop meaningful social relationships.
- Adjust to losses accompanying aging (eg, loss of friends, family, or spouse through death, reduced income, functional loss, etc.).
- Recognize meaning in one's life.
- Accept and prepare for one's own death.

Social Characteristics

Working and raising a family previously provided many social contacts for the older adult. Some older adults feel bored and lonely when they retire, with a loss of self-esteem because their former activities and contacts are curtailed.

DEPENDENCE

Approximately 9 million Americans aged 65 or older were living alone in 1989 (U.S. Senate, 1991). The other two-thirds lived with a companion or in supervised living arrangements, such as an extended care facility or a nursing home. Many older adults find dependence on others difficult to accept, even though they recognize the need for it. Some deny that they need assisted living and insist on remaining at home even when it jeopardizes their safety.

HOUSING

Finding safe and affordable living accommodations is difficult for many older people. Retirement communities combine smaller residences with conveniences such as an infirmary, shopping services, and recreational facilities. The older adult must part with treasured objects to accommodate a smaller dwelling. Familiar objects and mementos are extremely comforting to the older adult because they are reminders of past accomplishments and relationships.

ECONOMIC CONCERNS

Older adults face economic concerns related to decreased income. Compulsory retirement or serious and chronic illnesses are major factors contributing to financial worries. Although studies show that older workers tend to be conscientious, careful, accurate, and dependable, many employers are reluctant to hire them. There is a significant growth in the number of older adults engaged in part-time employment and employers may be recognizing the value of older adults because trends suggest that more retired people are re-entering the work force.

Medical expenses increase for older adults, adding to economic concerns. The enactment of Medicare, federal legislation providing health benefits to the aged, has been an important advance in helping older adults meet health care costs.

Older adults also need to employ others to carry out tasks they can no longer perform, such as caring for the lawn, painting, and cleaning. Most older adults rely on Social Security, a fixed income that does not increase at the same rate as the cost of living. Consequently, as older adults live longer, their money does not stretch as far. They are less able to buy material goods as costs continue to rise.

Emotional Characteristics

Although personality continues to evolve throughout life, basic temperament is stable into old age. Thus, if an individual's temperament was cheerful and optimistic during youth, that is usually the demeanor in old age. A bitter, complaining young person will often carry that attitude into old age. The ability to cope with the crises of diminished health, dependence, leisure time, fixed income, and alternative housing depends on the coping skills established much earlier in life.

LONELINESS

All people have emotional needs for love, companionship, and acceptance. Hobbies or other special interests and social contacts help older adults cope. Some become involved in community volunteer work or take advantage of activities and meeting places specifically for older adults.

The problem of loneliness is acute for many older people. Besides being faced with a lack of contact with former coworkers, the older adult also is faced with separation from family and friends and the death of a spouse. Community meal sites and senior centers try to meet the older adult's need for companionship by providing opportunities for socialization.

Pets also fill the void (Fig. 8–3). For older adults living alone, pets serve as family substitutes, provide comfort, and decrease feelings of loneliness. Many extended care facilities are using **pet therapy** and have a resident cat or dog. The activity and playfulness of the animal stimulate aged persons who are uncommunicative. Pets can decrease anxiety and depression and provide the older adult with the feeling of being needed and loved.

DEPRESSION AND SUICIDE

Many older adults experience depression. Symptoms such as fatigue, irritability, loss of interest in surroundings, decreased ability to concentrate, or feelings of worthlessness are often viewed as natural consequences of aging, and many older adults with depression receive no treatment. This is unfortunate because older adults respond well to antidepressants such as amitriptyline (Elavil), nortriptyline (Aventyl, Pamelor), trazodone (Desyrel, Trazon), and fluoxetine (Prozac).

Although older adults represent only 13% of the population, they account for 20% of all suicide attempts. More suicide attempts occur in individuals

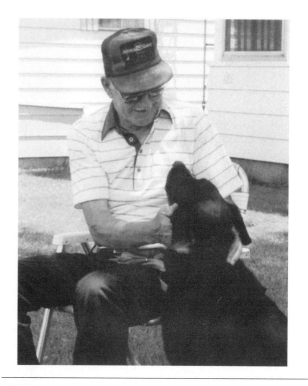

FIGURE 8-3. Pets provide companionship to many older adults.

age 65 or older than in any age group. The risk for suicide is greater in those who live alone, have health problems, or abuse alcohol. Men are more likely to actually commit suicide, but more women attempt it. Death of a spouse is also associated with an increased risk of suicide. The nurse or health care provider investigates any expressions of hopelessness or helplessness. It is appropriate to ask older adults who seem depressed if they have considered harming themselves or ending their life.

FEAR FOR SAFETY

Many older adults who live alone, particularly those living in urban settings, are vulnerable to crimes against their property and person. Some cope with these fears by becoming isolated prisoners in their own homes. Older adults are also the victims of fraud or con games.

Older adults may become victims of **elder abuse** when they depend on others for care and support. Abuse may be physical, in the form of beatings; psychological, in the form of threats; social, in the form of abandonment or unreasonable confinement; and material, in the form of theft or mismanagement of money. The abuser is often a caretaker or family member. Older adults at risk for abuse are frail, dependent, and cognitively or physically impaired. Adult Protective Services, a division of each state's Department of Social Services, investigates and safeguards older adults who are suspected victims of abuse.

Physical Characteristics

The nurse can expect to see a functional decline in the absence of any specific illness in the older adult. In caring for the gerontologic client, it is essential to recognize the normal physiologic variations that occur with aging. In addition, older adults often manifest diseases with milder or atypical symptoms. Many of the physical changes seen in the older adult are a progression of the changes that occur during middle age.

MUSCULOSKELETAL SYSTEM

The older adult continues to experience a decrease in height due to compression of the disks between the vertebrae. This, combined with a weakening of the chest muscles, causes the spine to take on an obvious thoracic curve known as **kyphosis** or humpback. With a change in the center of gravity, the older adult assumes a wider stance when standing and walking. The hips and the knees tend to be flexed at all times. There may be stiffness in the weight-bearing joints and limitation in their range of motion. Muscles atrophy, yet they are more clearly defined because of the loss of subcutaneous fat. There is a general, progressive loss of muscle fibers causing flabby thin muscles particularly of the arms and legs.

The physical limitations seen in the elderly are the result of inactivity, not degenerative changes. Remaining as active a possible helps slow the loss of physical ability. Arthritis is the leading chronic condition that affects the musculoskeletal system among people over the age of 65. Arthritis results in joint stiffness, limitation of movement, and deformity. Osteoporosis causes a loss of bone mass, particularly in older women, and places the older adult at increased risk for spontaneous fractures.

COGNITION

The incidence of serious cognitive deficits, like Alzheimer's disease (see Chap. 17), increases with age. Most older adults have better long-term memory than short-term memory. The older adult does not respond quickly to questions in an interview. One should not assume, however, that the individual is cognitively impaired. Diminished hearing or anxiety slows a client's responses. Clinical depression, common among older adults, is often mistaken for dementia.

SENSORY-PERCEPTION

Most older adults wear glasses. The *presbyopia* (age-related loss of visual acuity for near vision) that began in the middle years becomes more pronounced. Visual acuity declines at an accelerated rate as structures of the eye degenerate. Most people over age 70 have some degree of cataract formation. Many avoid driving at night because of the difficulty in adjusting to the glare of oncoming headlights.

Hearing loss also becomes more pronounced. *Presbycusis* (age-related hearing loss) that began in the middle years progresses. Presbycusis is gradual with initial loss of ability to hear high-pitched sound, followed by a decreased ability to hear middle- and low-pitched sounds. The nurse must look for signs of hearing loss because older adults do not always report hearing difficulties. Signs of hearing loss include:

- Cupping the hand behind the ear
- Asking the person to repeat what was said
- Agreeing without waiting for the completion of the sentence
- Speaking in an excessively loud or quiet voice or acting indifferent

Position sense and reaction time decline gradually until about age 70, when the rate of decline becomes rapid. The deterioration of these two faculties, together with diminished vision, is a common cause of accidents. Consequently, many older adults are injured in falls.

THE INTEGUMENT

Gradual changes in the skin and in the body's ability to adjust to heat and cold occur with age. The skin is drier, is prone to wrinkling, and becomes thin, flaky, and susceptible to irritation. Small brown pigmented freckles called *lentigines*, or liver spots, appear about the hands, arms, and face or other areas exposed to sun and weather. Older adults bruise easily due to capillary fragility. Diabetes and vascular disease predispose older adults to poor healing.

Facial features change as the result of loss of subcutaneous tissue. Wrinkles appear and the face seems to sag. The hair becomes drier, thinner, and gray. Nails, particularly toenails, often thicken and become brittle from poor circulation to the extremities. Teeth are lost due to neglected oral hygiene. The gums recede and teeth loosen as the bones in the jaw shrink in size.

The body gradually loses its ability to adjust to extremes of temperature. It is harder for older people to keep warm because their metabolism is lower. In hot weather, they do not lose heat as well as younger people because the blood vessels in their skin dilate slowly and their sweating mechanism does not function as effectively.

THE CARDIOVASCULAR SYSTEM

Important cardiovascular changes occur with aging, including a decrease in cardiac output (volume of blood pumped by the heart) and in vital capacity (the amount of air exhaled after taking a deep breath). The aorta and arteries stiffen and become less flexible with age, and the circulatory system responds less efficiently to the demands of activity and exercise. Common changes in vital signs include increased blood pressure, irregular pulse, and shortness of breath on exertion. Older adults also experience postural hypotension (rapid drop in blood pressure when rising or standing from a lying or sitting position).

Impaired arterial circulation makes the skin feel cool and causes the feet to appear purplish or bluish when in a sitting or standing position. Varicose veins (bulging, twisted veins in the legs) cause the lower extremities to swell and fatigue easily.

REPRODUCTIVE CHANGES

The breasts of older women lose their suppleness and hang flat against the chest wall. Men appear to have more prominent breasts due to a slight decrease in testosterone. Both genders remain sexually active, but both require more stimulation to become aroused. The penis and testes decrease in size, whereas the prostate gland enlarges. Erections are more brief. In women, the vagina becomes shorter and narrower. Discomfort and bleeding may occur during intercourse due to diminished lubrication and thinning of the epithelium.

THE URINARY SYSTEM

Both men and women develop urinary problems as they age. The bladder capacity decreases in both sexes. Men awaken at night to void because the enlarged prostate gland blocks complete emptying of urine. It becomes necessary to urinate more frequently. For women, ligaments and muscles stretched during pregnancy fail to keep the bladder suspended. As elastic tissue and pelvic floor muscles weaken, stress incontinence, leakage of urine with increased abdominal pressure during coughing, sneezing, laughing, or lifting, occurs. Another type of chronic incontinence is urge incontinence, leakage of urine because of an inability to delay voiding.

THE GASTROINTESTINAL SYSTEM

Older adults have many gastrointestinal problems such as constipation, indigestion, or increased flatulence (gas). Virtually every area of the gastrointestinal tract is affected by age. In the oral cavity, taste buds decrease in number and saliva production diminishes. The older adult is at increased risk for aspiration because food remains in the esophagus for a longer period of time and the gag reflex is weaker. The cells of the colon atrophy and peristalsis slows, resulting in constipation and flatulence.

Implications for Nursing

Nurses will care for greater numbers of older adults in a variety of health care settings as this population continues to increase. The plan of care includes early discharge planning and appropriate use of community resources.

Teaching the Older Adult

Older adults retain the ability to learn new information but require more time during the teaching process. Proceed slowly to allow time to think about and respond to new ideas. Speak slowly and distinctly if the client has a hearing deficit and ensure that the older client is wearing glasses (if necessary) and that the lighting is adequate. Provide ample opportunity for questions to clarify misunderstood information. If visual aides such as graphs, pictures, or printed material are used, use materials that are clear, uncluttered, and large enough to be seen. If a hearing aid is worn make certain that the client is wearing it and that it is working properly. If possible include another person who will assist the client after discharge. Ask questions about past experiences and relate the new information to these past experiences. The older client has a vast fund of knowledge and helping him or her draw on this knowledge facilitates learning new information.

Depression and Suicide

It is extremely important for nurses to be aware of the high incidence of depression and the potential for suicide in the older adult. This is true both in the home setting and in the extended care facility. Assess the older adult for signs of increased alcohol consumption, decreased interest in friends and social activities, complaints of fatigue, anger, and feelings of hopelessness. Ask depressed clients about suicidal thoughts or intentions. If an older adult confides suicidal thoughts, report those intentions immediately to the nursing supervisor and primary care physician. Immediately remove any potential articles that could be used to commit suicide from the environment such as guns, razors, knives, scissors, and medications (both prescription and nonprescription). Have someone stay with the person. The number of suicides in the older population can be decreased significantly by recognizing and treating depression in the elderly in appropriate and effective ways. (See Chap. 14 for more information on depression and suicide.)

Nutrition and Dietary Modifications

Nutritional deficiencies are a serious problem for the older adult. Dietary insufficiencies are related to loss of or changes in teeth, boredom at eating alone, fatigue, or lack of money. The diet of older adults tends to be high in carbohydrates, which are more affordable on a fixed income. In addition, because many shop irregularly, they may depend on a stockpile of processed foods that have an extended shelf life. Older adults benefit from a diet lower in calories but high in nutrients because absorption of the nutrients is diminished.

Some older clients require a soft diet and foods that are easy to digest. Chewing is difficult for some because of diminished production of saliva or improperly fitted dentures. Many benefit from supplemental vitamins and minerals or nourishing between-meal snacks. Tracking body weight is a good assessment tool for evaluating the nutritional status of older adults. Weight gain or loss of 5% in a 4-week period is reported to the health care provider for analysis.

Physical Care

The nurse helps older adults maintain their dignity and self-respect by promoting hygiene and grooming. Clients feel better about themselves when their hair is neatly arranged, their skin is clean and healthy, and they are dressed attractively.

Older adults must learn to adjust to their increasing physical limitations, but self-care is always encouraged. Older adults quickly lose their ability to care for themselves when someone does it for them. If the nurse performs activities of daily living for clients when they are capable of performing these activities without help, they may think they are no longer considered capable of managing such tasks. Surrendering self-care functions that help maintain their independence and contact with reality leads to unnecessary dependence on others, as well as a loss of self-esteem.

SKIN AND NAIL CARE

Decreased circulation to the extremities results in prolonged healing time for injuries or infections. If the skin on the legs and feet is very dry, cream or lotion is necessary after bathing. Thickened, brittle toenails are carefully trimmed after soaking the feet in water. If the older adult has very thick nails, diabetes, or a peripheral vascular disease, professional nail care is indicated.

BATHING AND HYGIENE

A daily partial bath and a biweekly tub bath are adequate because frequent bathing dries the skin. The older client *must* be helped getting in and out of a tub. A stall shower is desirable because it avoids the need to step over an elevated edge and lower oneself into the tub. A shower chair is ideal for the weak and unsteady client. The shower offers the most thorough rinsing of soap from the skin, thus helping to minimize skin irritations. Whatever method of bathing is used, care is taken to ensure privacy.

Some older women have a vaginal discharge or urinary incontinence. The vaginal mucous membrane becomes thin and subject to infection. If the nurse or family member detects this problem, consult the physician regarding use of a cleansing douche or oral medication. The client is kept clean and comfortable with good perineal care and the use of disposable pads.

ELIMINATION

Bowel and urinary elimination may pose problems for older adults. Frequency of urination is common. Care is taken to prevent falls when the client gets up during the night to use the toilet. The call button is nearby so that the client can obtain assistance. For those who are unable to wait for assistance, a commode, bedpan, or urinal is left within easy reach. Constipation is more likely to occur in those who are immobile, who fail to drink sufficient fluids, or whose diet lacks sufficient bulk. Helping the client maintain adequate fiber and fluid intake and to have a regular time for evacuation helps restore regularity. Enemas, mild laxatives, or stool softeners are ordered by the physician if other methods of relieving constipation are ineffective.

MOBILITY

Confinement in bed causes adverse effects among older people. Because older adults expand their chests less fully, confinement in bed, which accentuates this problem, often leads to the development of hypostatic pneumonia (pneumonia that occurs as a result of shallow breathing).

Pressure ulcers (bedsores) are common among older adults because they have diminished subcutaneous fat. Frequent position changes and pressure-relieving devices are necessary for clients who are inactive. Muscle tone is readily lost during prolonged bed rest; extreme weakness results and is difficult to overcome. To combat these complications, alternative activity such as active or passive exercises must be promoted.

PHYSICAL COORDINATION

Some older adults are slower in their movements and responses. Attempts to make them hurry result in confusion, anxiety, and accidents. The thoughtful nurse prepares everything clients need for self-care and then lets them proceed at their own pace to complete those aspects of care that they can perform.

SAFETY

The nurse ensures that the environment is safe for the older client. Beds that are left in a high position are a potential danger because older adults can misjudge the distance to the floor and fall when getting out of bed. The bed is left in the low position except when direct nursing care is administered. A dim night light helps the older person become oriented to the surroundings and prevents falling or tripping over objects when the client gets out of bed. The call button is placed within reach.

Nighttime agitation and confusion are common among older adults, particularly when they are moved from familiar surroundings to a hospital or nursing home. Unfortunately, this problem is commonly mismanaged. Physical restraints are too quickly applied before alternative measures are tried. Restraints increase the individual's frustration and distress. The nurse tries to determine the cause of the client's confusion and then attempts to reduce or eliminate it. Causes of agitation include the need to urinate, the discomfort of constipation, being too hot or cold, fatigue, pain, fear, or loneliness. Meeting physical or emotional needs is often all that is needed to quiet a restless client.

SLEEP

Older adults usually require less sleep than younger adults. Keeping older clients awake and active during the day facilitates sleep at night. Sedatives and hypnotics, even when administered in low doses, can result in wakefulness, excitement, and confusion. The nurse can provide a warm, caffeine-free beverage, an extra blanket, or soft music to promote restful sleep.

ORIENTATION

Measures to help older clients maintain contact with reality can prevent episodes of confusion. The older adult benefits from **reality orientation** (Nursing Guidelines 8–1). Reality orientation involves using various techniques that reinforce the client's awareness of the date, time, place, names or roles of individuals involved in their care, and current events.

COMMUNICATION

An important aspect of encouraging communication involves stimulating older adults to talk about past experiences and events. This is referred to as

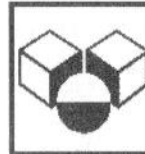

Nursing Guidelines 8-1

Reality Orientation

- Prominently display the date.
- Identify yourself and address the client by name each time there is interaction.
- Reinforce the time of day during routine activities ("Mrs. Green, it's 2 PM and time for your pill.")
- Give the client a few pages of the newspaper to read.
- Discuss current events.
- Compare events from day to day.
- Routinely tune in radio or television news programs.
- Encourage social interaction with other clients.

reminiscence therapy and is a good technique for reinforcing self-esteem. Older adults have a need to talk about past events, achievements, and losses. Asking them to recall their personal history encourages communication between the older adult, health care personnel, and the family.

Validation therapy, developed by Naomi Feil, is a method of communicating with the elderly who are confused, disoriented, and act out in inappropriate ways because of a permanent and progressive loss of cognitive ability. Feil believes these individuals are seeking to communicate feelings through their behavior. In validation therapy the nurse seeks to reassure the client and gain understanding of the client's behavior or words spoken. For example, the woman who cares for and nurtures a doll may need validation of her role as a mother or the assurance of the love of her children. In this case the nurse says, "I know you love your children" or "You are such a good mother." To say "That is not a baby, but a doll," is presenting reality, but would cause emotional pain or agitation in many older adults. By seeking to validate feelings, the nurse provides comfort and affirming feelings.

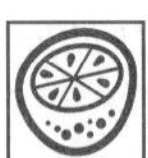

General Nutritional Considerations

The eating habits of older adults are affected by such factors as limited income, inadequate cooking facilities, social isolation, and poor dentition. Older adults, particularly those living alone, are at risk for nutritional deficiencies. Nutritional care of the older adult is client centered and based on the person's physical and psychosocial status. Rigid dietary restrictions are bypassed in favor of quality of life and independent functioning.

Calcium balance, energy balance, bowel elimination, and sense of well-being may all be improved with physical activity. Encourage the client to be as active as possible.

Increasing fiber and fluid intake may help alleviate constipation. Clients with altered dentition who cannot chew fresh fruits and vegetables may find using wheat bran and whole grain breads and cereals the most practical method of increasing fiber intake. A soft, ground, or pureed diet may be necessary if chewing or swallowing is impaired.

Thirst is not a reliable indicator of need in the elderly. Encourage ample fluid intake of 6 to 8 glasses daily to maintain hydration and normal urine and fecal output.

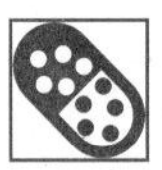

General Pharmacologic Considerations

Because drugs are excreted more slowly by older clients, lower doses of many pharmacologic agents, particularly narcotics, sedatives, hypnotics, and other central nervous system depressants, are indicated. In some instances, toxicity results when normal doses are administered.

Many medications cause confusion in the elderly. When an older adult experiences sudden confusion, an evaluation of the medication regimen is necessary to identify the drug or drugs that cause or contribute to the confusion. All older adults need a periodic review of their medication regimen. In some situations polypharmacy is practiced (the taking of a large number of prescription and nonprescription drugs). Some of these drugs could be inappropriate and cause needless adverse reactions.

Some medications cause depression in the elderly. Antipsychotics, hypnotics, some antihypertensives and cardiovascular drugs, and the narcotic analgesics are drugs associated with the development of depression in the elderly. Careful monitoring of the older client who takes these drugs is essential. Antidepressants need to be taken up to 8 weeks before a therapeutic effect is observed. Warn family members and caregivers to take precautions against suicide until a therapeutic effect is achieved.

General Gerontologic Considerations

Older clients with arthritis or other conditions that cause loss of strength or coordination may request that prescriptions be filled without using childproof caps.

Nurses caring for gerontologic clients must dispel stereotypical thinking and view the older adult as an individual with unique qualities and characteristics.

SUMMARY OF KEY CONCEPTS

- Because more adults in America are living longer, society must prepare for a larger population of people who will enjoy a longer period of retirement, need alternative living arrangements, be dependent on limited incomes, have more chronic diseases, be at risk for injury, and require more assistance with their physical care.

- Gerontology is the study of aging. This specialty focuses on determining what causes aging and possible measures to delay its onset and progress.
- Several theories have been proposed to explain aging: autophagocytosis occurs; stressors wear out the body's resources; the immune system becomes dysfunctional; and DNA replication is altered by environmental toxins or other dangerous substances like free radicals.
- Ageism is prejudice against older people. Negative stereotypes are extremely damaging to the self-image of older adults and perpetuate a myth that they cannot live vital and productive lives and make contributions to society.
- During the period of late adulthood, older adults must deal with multiple physical, emotional, and social losses; manage time; engage in useful projects; and begin to prepare for death.
- Late adulthood is a time during which adults gain a sense of ego integrity, being content and satisfied during later years, or experience despair if disappointed and regretful over lost opportunities.
- Older adults are at increased risk for depression and suicide. Symptoms of depression are often attributed to other disorders or disregarded as a part of normal aging.
- Depression can be successfully treated in the older adult, but careful monitoring is required for up to 8 weeks after treatment with the antidepressant is started or until a therapeutic effect is noted.
- Older adults tend to lose height, experience problems with weight gain or loss, lose short-term memory, have a worsening of visual and hearing deficits, develop gray hair and dry skin, have impaired circulation in their extremities, and experience urinary incontinence or retention.
- Social problems among older adults include loneliness and isolation from living a distance from their children, losing a spouse and friends through death, living alone, becoming economically impoverished, and being unable to afford increased health care costs.
- Older adults are affected emotionally by their loneliness and fear for personal safety.
- When teaching older clients, the most important principles to keep in mind are to convey a feeling of confidence that they are able to learn and to relate new concepts to something the person already knows. Other techniques include presenting information in small amounts; using a clear, distinct voice, allowing time for questions; and using pictures and large print aides for those who are visually impaired.
- Skin care is modified to include less frequent bathing and to use creams to keep the skin lubricated and intact. Showers are safer than bathtubs because they present less risk of falling. Dentures are cleaned regularly. The diet is modified to accommodate the client's ability to chew and alterations in digestion. A record of elimination patterns helps identify bowel and bladder needs.
- In health care agencies, beds are kept in low position and the signal light is within reach at all times. Floor lights help maintain orientation. Restraints, sedatives, and hypnotics are avoided unless absolutely necessary because they tend to agitate older adults.
- Pet therapy is being used to promote social interaction and communication. Reminiscence writing and oral storytelling help maintain memory and reinforce individuality. To maintain reality orientation, nurses use interventions such as placing large printed words on doors or using large numbered calendars and clocks that can be easily seen.
- Reminiscence therapy, life review, reality orientation, and validation therapy are all methods to help the older adult adjust to aging and develop increased feelings of self-esteem.

CRITICAL THINKING EXERCISES

1. An 82-year-old client sits alone all day in the nursing home. He spends his time staring at the television with no obvious interest. When the nursing staff try to involve him in various activities, he becomes irritated or says that he is too tired. What are some possible reasons for the client's behavior? What actions(s) could you take to help him?
2. The nursing home asks you to help organize a reality orientation program for the older adults in the facility. Many of the nursing assistants are unaware of the intervention. How would you explain reality orientation to the nurse assistants? What are some suggestions you could make to reinforce reality for the elderly clients in the nursing home?

Suggested Readings

Birchenall, J. M., & Streight, M. E. (1993). *Care of the older adult* (3rd ed.). Philadelphia: J. B. Lippincott.

Dudek, S. G. (1993). *Nutrition handbook for nursing practice* (2nd ed.). Philadelphia: J. B. Lippincott.

Eliopoulos, C. (1996). *Gerontological nursing* (4th ed.). Philadelphia: Lippincott-Raven.

Feil, N. (1992). *Validation: The Feil method.* Cleveland, OH: Edward Feil Productions.

Lueckenotte, A. G. (1994). *Pocket guide to gerontologic assessment* (3rd ed.). St. Louis: Mosby.

Matteson, M. A., & McConnell, E. S. (1996). *Gerontological nursing: Concepts and practice* (2nd ed.). Philadelphia: Saunders.

Rybash, J. M., Roodin, P. A., & Hoyer, W. J. (1995). *Adult development and aging* (3rd ed.). Dubuque, IA: Brown Communication.

Stabb, A. S., & Hodges, L. C. (1996). *Essentials of gerontological nursing: Adaptation to the aging process.* Philadelphia: Lippincott-Raven.

Taeuber, C. M. (1992). *Sixty-five plus in America.* Washington, DC: U.S. Department of Commerce.

U.S. Department of Health and Human Services. (1992). *Healthy people 2000: National health promotion and disease prevention objectives.* Boston: Jones and Bartlett.

U.S. Senate Special Committee on Aging, American Association of Retired Persons, Federal Council on the Aging, U.S. Administration on Aging. (1991). *Aging America: Trends and projections.* Washington, DC: U.S. Department of Health and Human Services.

Additional Resources

Administration on Aging
U.S. Department of Health and Human Services
330 Independence Avenue, SW
Washington, DC 20201
(202) 619–0724
http://www.aoa.dhhs.gov

National Aging Information Center
330 Independence Ave., SW
Room 4656
Washington, DC 20201
(202) 619–7501
http://aoa.dhhs.gov/naic/

Alliance for Aging Research
Suite 305
2021 K Street, NW
Washington, DC 20006
(202) 785–8574

Gerontological Society of America
Suite 350
1275 K Street, NW
Washington, DC 20006
(202) 842–1275
httpd://www.geron.org

National Association of Area Agencies on Aging
Suite 100
11122 16th Street, NW
Washington, DC 20006
(202) 296–8130

3

Psychosocial Aspects of Nursing

Chapter 9

Nurse–Client Relationships

KEY TERMS

Affective learner
Affective touch
Cognitive learner
Comfort zone
Formal teaching
Hearing
Informal teaching
Intimate space
Introductory phase
Kinesics
Learning capacity
Learning needs
Learning readiness
Learning style
Listening
Motivation
Nonverbal communication
Nurse–client relationship
Paralanguage
Personal space
Proxemics
Psychomotor learner
Public space
Social space
Task-oriented touch
Teaching plan
Terminating phase
Therapeutic communication
Verbal communication
Working phase

LEARNING OBJECTIVES

On completion of this chapter, the reader will:

- Name three phases in a nurse–client relationship.
- Differentiate between verbal, nonverbal, and therapeutic communication.
- Give at least two examples of therapeutic and nontherapeutic communication techniques.
- List and explain five components of nonverbal communication.
- Give the names of four proxemic zones and explain what is meant by a client's "comfort zone."
- Differentiate between task-oriented and affective touch.
- Explain the learning styles of cognitive, affective, and psychomotor learners.
- Name three variables that affect learning.
- Compare informal with formal learning.
- Discuss at least five nursing guidelines for teaching adult clients.

The word *relationship* refers to an association between two people. In this case, the relationship is the one between nurses and the people for whom they care. Communicating therapeutically, listening empathetically, sharing information, and providing client education are among the most important processes that occur within the context of the nurse–client relationship.

The Nurse–Client Relationship

The **nurse–client relationship** exists during the period of time when the nurse interacts with clients, sick or well, to promote or restore their health, cope with their illness, or die with dignity. As in any effective relationship, both parties have unique responsibilities to the other (Table 9–1).

Phases of the Nurse–Client Relationship

The nurse–client relationship progresses through three phases: the introductory phase, the working phase, and the terminating phase. Box 9–1 shows an example of the activities that occur in each of the three phases.

INTRODUCTORY PHASE

The **introductory phase** starts when the nurse and the client get acquainted and the client identifies one or more health problems for which care is sought. Both bring preconceived ideas about the other to the initial interaction and these assumptions are eventually confirmed or dismissed. The nurse demonstrates courtesy, active listening, empathy, competency, and appropriate communication skills to convey to the

TABLE 9-1 **Nurse–Client Responsibilities**

Nursing Responsibilities	Client Responsibilities
Possess current knowledge.	Identify current problem.
Be aware of unique age-related differences.	Describe desired outcomes.
Perform technical skills safely.	Answer questions honestly.
Be committed to the client's care.	Provide accurate historic and subjective data.
Be available and courteous.	Participate to the fullest extent possible.
Allow client to participate in decisions.	Be open and flexible to alternatives.
Remain nonjudgmental.	Comply with the therapeutic regimen.
Advocate on the client's behalf.	Keep follow-up appointments.
Provide explanations in language that is easily understood.	
Promote independence.	

client that he or she is valued. Partnership and advocacy in the client's health care is demonstrated by:

- Treating each client as a unique person
- Respecting the client's feelings
- Striving to promote the client's physical, emotional, social, and spiritual well-being
- Encouraging the client to participate in problem-solving and decision-making
- Accepting that a client has the potential for growth and change
- Communicating in terms and language that the client understands
- Using the nursing process to individualize the client's care
- Involving those persons to whom the client turns for support, such as family and friends, when providing care
- Implementing health care techniques that are compatible with the client's value system and cultural heritage

BOX 9-1 Examples of Phase-Related Activities

Client	Nurse
INTRODUCTORY PHASE	
Seeks help in managing diabetes	Determines what the client needs to learn
WORKING PHASE	
Practices skills and returns the demonstrations to the nurse	Develops and implements a teaching plan that includes monitoring blood sugar and insulin administration
TERMINATION PHASE	
Demonstrates desired competencies	Refers client to diabetic clinic for future follow-up

WORKING PHASE

The **working phase** involves mutually planning the client's care and putting the plan into action. Both the nurse and the client participate. Each shares in performing those tasks that will lead to the desired outcomes identified by the client. During the working phase, the nurse supports the client's independence. Doing too much is as harmful as doing too little.

TERMINATING PHASE

The **terminating phase** occurs when there is mutual agreement that the client's immediate health problems have improved and the nurse's services are no longer necessary. The nurse uses compassion and a caring attitude when facilitating the client's transition to other health care services or back to independent living.

Communication

Communication is an exchange of information. It involves both sending and receiving messages between two or more individuals. It is followed by feedback indicating that the information is understood or needs further clarification (Fig. 9–1).

Therapeutic Communication

Communication occurs on a social or therapeutic level. **Therapeutic communication** refers to using words and gestures to promote a person's physical and emotional well-being. Techniques that are helpful are identified in Table 9–2.

In situations where clients are quiet and noncommunicative, the nurse must avoid assuming that the client has no problems or understands everything.

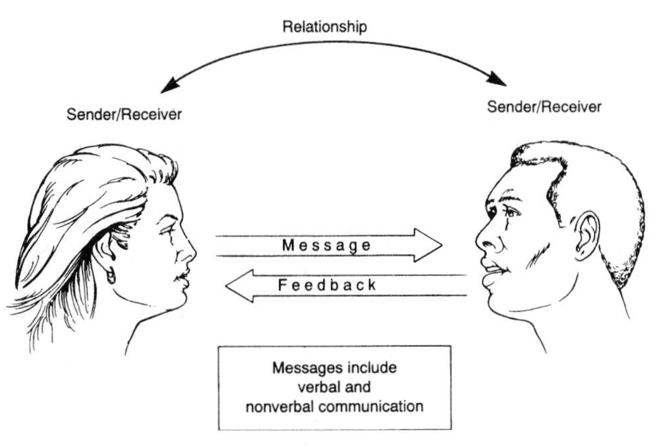

FIGURE 9-1. Communication is a two-way process.

On the other hand, it is never appropriate to probe and press an unwilling client to communicate. It is advantageous to wait because it is not unusual for reticent clients to share their feelings and concerns after they feel that the nurse is sincere and trustworthy.

The response of the nurse to a vocal and emotional client must also be handled delicately. For instance, when clients are angry or cry, the best nursing approach is to allow them to express their emotions without fear of retaliation or censure.

Although nurses have the best intentions of interacting therapeutically with clients, some fall into traps that block or hinder therapeutic communication. Table 9–3 lists common examples of nontherapeutic communication.

Verbal Communication

Verbal communication is communication that uses words. It includes speaking, reading, and writing. Verbal communication is affected by:

- Attention and concentration
- Language compatibility
- Verbal skills
- Hearing and visual acuity
- Motor functions involving the throat, tongue, and teeth
- Noise and distracting activity
- Interpersonal attitudes
- Literacy
- Cultural similarities

Listening

Listening is as important during communication as speaking. In contrast to **hearing,** which is perceiving sounds, **listening** is an activity that includes attending to and becoming fully involved in what the client

TABLE 9-2 **Therapeutic Communication Techniques**

Technique	Use	Example
Broad openings	Relieves tension before getting to the real purpose of the interaction	"Wonderful weather we're having."
Giving information	Provides facts	"Your surgery is scheduled at noon."
Direct questioning	Acquires specific information	"Do you have any allergies?"
Open-ended questioning	Encourages the client to elaborate	"How are you feeling?"
Reflecting	Confirms that the conversation is being followed	Client: "I haven't been sleeping well." Nurse: "You haven't been sleeping well."
Paraphrasing	Restates what the client has said to demonstrate listening	Client: "After every meal, I feel like I will throw up." Nurse: "Eating makes you nauseous, but you don't actually vomit."
Verbalizing what has been implied	Shares how a statement has been interpreted	Client: "All the nurses are so busy." Nurse: "You're feeling that you shouldn't ask for help."
Structuring	Defines a purpose and sets limits	"I have 15 minutes. If your pain is relieved, I could go over how your test will be done."
Giving general leads	Encourages the client to continue	"Uh, huh," or "Go on."
Sharing perceptions	Shows empathy for how the client is feeling	"You seem depressed."
Clarifying	Avoids misinterpretation	"I'm afraid I don't quite understand what you're asking."
Confronting	Calls attention to manipulation, inconsistencies, or lack of responsibility	"You're concerned about your weight loss, but you didn't eat any breakfast."
Summarizing	Reviews information that has been discussed	"You've asked me to check on increasing your pain medication and getting your diet changed."
Silence	Allows time for considering how to proceed; or, arouses the client's anxiety to the point that it stimulates more verbalization	

TABLE 9-3 **Nontherapeutic Communication Techniques**

Technique and Consequence	Example	Improvement
Giving False Reassurance		
Trivializes the unique feelings of the client and discourages further discussion	"You've got nothing to worry about. Everything will work out just fine."	"Tell me about your specific concerns."
Using Clichés		
Provides worthless advice and curtails exploring alternatives	"Keep a stiff upper lip."	"It must be difficult for you right now."
Giving Approval or Disapproval		
Holds the client to a rigid standard; implies that future deviation may lead to subsequent rejection or disfavor	"I'm glad you're exercising so regularly." "You should be testing your blood sugar each morning."	"Are you having any difficulty fitting regular exercise into your schedule?" "Let's explore some ways that will help you test your blood sugar each morning."
Agreeing		
Does not allow the client flexibility to change his or her mind	"You're right about needing surgery immediately."	"Having surgery immediately is one possibility. What others have you considered?"
Disagreeing		
Intimidates the client; makes the person feel foolish or inadequate	"That's not true! Where did you get an idea like that?"	"Maybe I can help clarify that for you."
Demanding an Explanation		
Puts the client on the defensive; the client may be tempted to make up an excuse rather than risk disapproval for an honest answer	"Why didn't you keep your appointment last week?"	"I see you couldn't keep your appointment last week."
Giving Advice		
Discourages independent problem-solving and decision-making; provides a biased view that may prejudice the client's choice	"If I were you, I'd try drug therapy before having surgery."	"Share with me the advantages and disadvantages of your options as you see them."
Defending		
Indicates such a strong allegiance that any disagreement to the contrary is not acceptable	"Ms. Johnson is my best nursing assistant. She wouldn't have let your light go unanswered that long."	"I'm sorry you had to wait so long."
Belittling		
Disregards how the client is responding as an individual	"Lots of people learn to give themselves insulin."	"You're finding it especially difficult to stick yourself with a needle."
Patronizing		
Treats the client in a condescending manner as less than capable of making an independent decision	"Are *we* ready for *our* bath yet?"	"Would you like your bath now, or should I check with you later?"
Changing the Subject		
Alters the direction of the discussion to a topic that is safer or more comfortable	Client: "I'm so scared that a mammogram will show I have cancer." Nurse: "Tell me more about your family."	"It is a serious disease. What concerns you the most?"

says. Empathic listening implies that the nurse attempts to perceive the emotions and meanings of the client. When the nurse conveys this quality to clients, it helps them to feel both understood and valued (Oermann, 1991). How empathetically one listens is often demonstrated through nonverbal means.

When communicating with most American clients, it is best to position oneself at the client's level and make frequent eye contact (see cultural exceptions in Chap. 10). Nodding and encouraging the client to continue with comments, such as "Yes, I see," conveys interest in what is being said. The nurse guards against sending messages that indicate boredom such as looking out a window or interrupting a comment.

Nonverbal Communication

Nonverbal communication is the exchange of information without using words. It is what is *not* said. Nonverbal communication consists of components such as kinesics, paralanguage, proxemics, touch, and silence.

KINESICS

Kinesics refers to body language, or those collective nonverbal techniques such as facial expressions, posture, gestures, and body movements. Even clothing style and accessories (eg, jewelry) can affect the context of communication.

PARALANGUAGE

Paralanguage is vocal sounds, not actually words, that communicate a message. Some examples include drawing in a deep breath to indicate surprise, clucking the tongue to show disappointment, and whistling to get someone's attention. Crying, laughing, and moaning are additional forms of paralanguage. Vocal inflections, volume, pitch, and rate of speech add yet another dimension to communication.

PROXEMICS

Proxemics refers to the use of space when communicating. In general, four proxemic zones are common when Americans communicate. They include an **intimate space, personal space, social space,** and **public space** (Table 9–4).

Most Americans tolerate strangers up to a 2- to 3-foot area. Determining the circumference of a person's **comfort zone,** the area which when intruded, does not create anxiety, is important because physical closeness is common during nursing care. Approaches that relieve a client's anxiety about being close include explaining beforehand how a nursing procedure will be performed and ensuring that the client is properly draped.

TOUCH

Touch is a tactile stimulus produced by personal contact with another person or object. In the context of nursing, touch is either task-oriented, affective, or both (Brady & Nesbitt, 1991). **Task-oriented touch** involves the personal contact that is required when performing nursing procedures (Fig. 9–2). **Affective touch** is used to demonstrate concern or affection (Fig. 9–3). Most people respond positively to being touched. However, even though its intention is to communicate caring and support, affective touching should be used cautiously because there is a great deal of variation among individuals. In general, affective touch is used therapeutically when a client is:

- Lonesome
- Uncomfortable

TABLE 9-4 **Proxemic Zones**

Zone	Distance	Purpose
Intimate space	Within 6 inches	• Lovemaking • Confiding secrets • Sharing confidential information
Personal space	6 inches to 4 feet	• Interviewing • Physical assessment • Therapeutic interventions involving touch • Private conversations • Teaching one-on-one
Social space	4–12 feet	• Group interactions • Lecturing • Conversations that are not intended to be private
Public space	12 or more feet	• Giving speeches • Gatherings of strangers

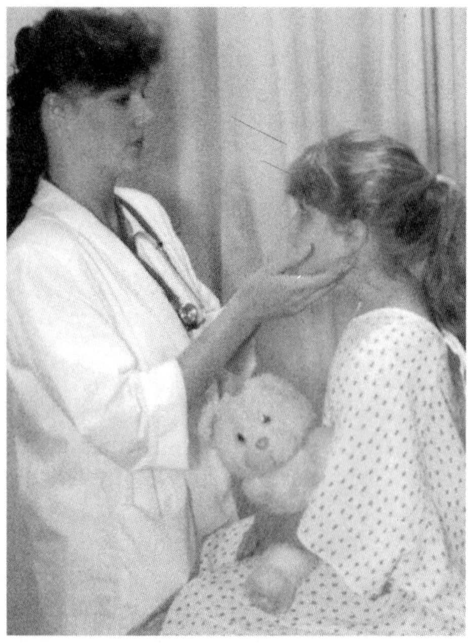

FIGURE 9-2. Task-oriented touch. (Courtesy of Ken Timby.)

- Near death
- Anxious, insecure, or frightened
- Disoriented
- Disfigured
- Semiconscious or comatose
- Visually impaired
- Sensory deprived

SILENCE

Silence is the art of remaining quiet. One of its therapeutic uses is to encourage a client's verbal communication; others include using silence to provide a personal presence and a brief period of time during which clients can process information or respond to a question.

Client Teaching

Sharing information and performing *client teaching* are essential nursing activities that promote a person's ability to understand the hospital environment and independently meet his or her own health needs. Limited hospitalization time demands that nurses begin teaching clients as soon as possible after admission. Teaching is either formal or informal and the most efficient teaching occurs when the nurse presents information compatible with the client's learning style.

Learning Styles

A **learning style** is the manner in which a person best comprehends new information. Usually people fall into one of three categories: cognitive, affective, or psychomotor (Table 9–5). The **cognitive learner** processes information best by listening to or reading facts and descriptions. The **affective learner** is more attuned to learning when presented with information that appeals to his or her feelings, beliefs, and values. A **psychomotor learner** likes to learn by doing (Fig. 9–4).

Learner Assessment

One way to determine a client's learning style is to ask, "When you learned to add fractions, what helped you most: listening to the teacher's explanation, recognizing the value of fractions in cooking or carpentry, or actually working sample problems?" Although most favor one style of learning, learning tends to be optimized by presenting information through a combination of the three styles.

Besides determining the style of learning a client prefers, the nurse assesses the learning needs of the client, his or her learning capacity, motivation for learning, and learning readiness.

LEARNING NEEDS

Client education begins with an assessment of **learning needs**. Learning needs are those concepts and skills that the client and family must acquire to restore, maintain, or promote health. For example, the diabetic client needs to learn to self-administer insulin, a skill, and to understand how diabetes affects

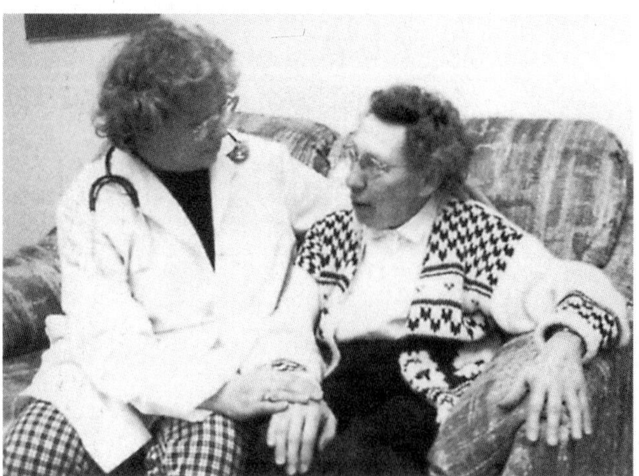

FIGURE 9-3. Affective touch. (Courtesy of Ken Timby.)

TABLE 9-5 **Activities That Promote Learning According to Styles**

Cognitive Learners	Affective Learners	Psychomotor Learners
Listing	Advocating	Assembling
Identifying	Supporting	Changing
Naming	Accepting	Emptying
Describing	Promoting	Filling
Summarizing	Internalizing	Adding
Selecting	Valuing	Removing

circulation, a concept. Distinguishing the important skills and concepts a client must learn and then assessing what the client already knows helps in identifying goals, tailoring the teaching plan to the individual, and evaluating outcomes.

LEARNING CAPACITY

Learning capacity refers to a person's intellectual ability to understand, remember, and apply new information. Illiteracy, sensory deficits, and a shortened attention span require special adaptations when implementing client teaching.

MOTIVATION

Motivation is the desire to acquire new information. Learning occurs at an accelerated rate when a person has a purpose or reason for mastering it. Some motivating forces include restoring independence, preventing complications, facilitating discharge, and returning to the comfort of home.

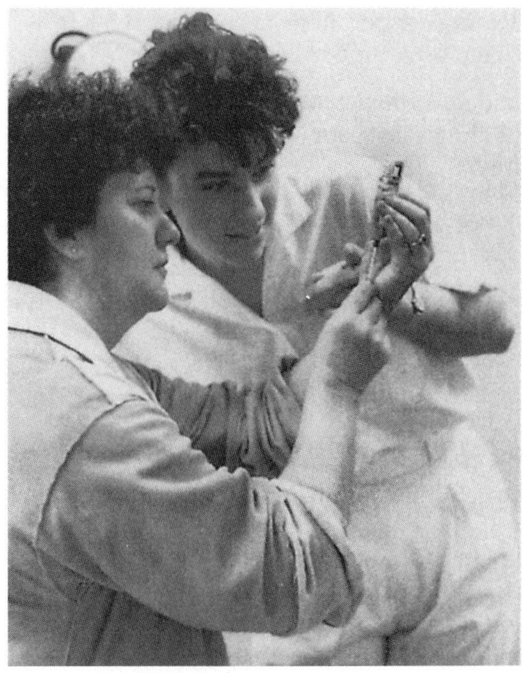

FIGURE 9-4. A nurse implements teaching for a client who is a psychomotor learner. (Courtesy of Ken Timby.)

LEARNING READINESS

Learning readiness pertains to the optimal time for learning. Ideally, it occurs when a client is in a state of physical and psychological well-being. For example, a client who is in pain, uncomfortably warm or cold, anxious or depressed is not in the best condition for learning. In these situations, it is best to restore comfort and then attend to teaching.

Informal and Formal Teaching

Informal teaching is unplanned. It occurs spontaneously, usually at the client's bedside. **Formal teaching** requires a plan to avoid being haphazard. A **teaching plan** is the organized arrangement of content in a specific time frame. It facilitates reaching goals, providing essential information, and ensuring the client's comprehension before being discharged. Developing a plan and implementing it gradually and sequentially avoids overwhelming the client with new information or learning skills that are difficult to perform. The suggestions in Nursing Guidelines 9–1 on the next page are useful when teaching adult clients.

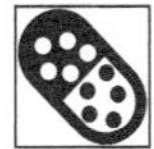

General Pharmacologic Considerations

Some medications dull mental ability and make concentration more difficult. This can affect the client's ability to learn new material and to remember specific details taught during a teaching session.

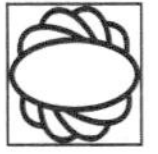

General Gerontologic Considerations

Older adults tend to lose the ability to hear at high-pitched ranges. Therefore, it is best to lower the voice pitch during communication and avoid using letters that are

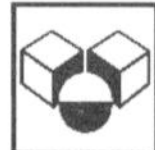

Nursing Guidelines 9-1

Teaching Adult Clients

- Identify the value or purpose for learning new information.
- Determine if the client is comfortable at the moment.
- Make sure the adult is wearing glasses or using a hearing aid, if one or the other is needed.
- Reduce noise and distractions in the environment.
- Sit at eye level unless doing group teaching and face the client(s).
- Use short sentences of 10 words or less.
- Avoid speaking rapidly.
- Keep technical terms and medical jargon to a minimum; define words whenever necessary.
- Use words that a seventh to ninth grader would understand.
- Present one, but no more than three new ideas at each teaching session.
- Review frequently.
- Use the active form of the verb rather than passive (eg, "Wipe straight down the center of the incision," rather than "The incision is wiped down the center.").
- Use examples with which the learner can identify.
- Relate new information to prior learning.
- Build in a learner performance evaluation, such as asking the client to repeat or paraphrase prior information, demonstrate a skill, or apply the information to a hypothetical situation, such as "What would you do if. . . ."
- Terminate teaching if the client cannot remain attentive.

formed with high-pitched sounds like "f," "s," "k," and "sh."

Communicate with hearing-impaired adults by inserting a stethoscope into the client's ears and speaking into the bell or using a magic slate, chalkboard, flash cards, or writing tablets.

Older adults have a lifetime of past experiences that are useful as a foundation for new learning.

When teaching older adults, choose printed materials that feature persons of similar age in a positive manner.

Avoid using printed materials that are cluttered with extensive amounts of information.

Booklets, pamphlets, and brochures that are printed in black on white matte paper improve visual clarity.

Healthy older adults do not have a significant decrease in cognitive ability and are able to learn new information. They do, however, learn more efficiently when they are allowed to progress at their own pace.

Learning motor skills may be more difficult for older adults due to physiologic changes. More time may be needed to learn new activities.

An appreciation of the older adult as an individual with unique needs and concerns is the foundation of a positive nurse–client relationship with the older adult.

When the older adult constantly tells the same story or asks the same question, make an effort to see if there is a hidden or unspoken message of fear or concern that the older adult is too apprehensive to discuss.

During the introductory phase of the nurse–client relationship, take time to actively listen to the older adult. Allow ample time for a response to questions. Remember the health history of an older adult may span over 80 years.

Clarify any questionable information with a family member or the primary caregiver. Older adults may have short-term memory impairment, even though long-term memory remains intact.

SUMMARY OF KEY CONCEPTS

- The nurse–client relationship progresses through three phases: the introductory, working, and terminating phases.
- Therapeutic communication, empathic listening, sharing information, and providing client teaching are important components of communication and the nurse–client relationship.
- Verbal communication uses words; nonverbal communication is an exchange of information without using words; therapeutic communication uses words and gestures to promote a person's physical and emotional well-being.
- Examples of therapeutic communication techniques are paraphrasing and verbalizing what has been implied; examples of nontherapeutic communication include giving false reassurance and using clichés.
- Components of nonverbal communication include the use of kinesics, which is a term for body language; paralanguage, which is vocal sound; proxemics referring to space, touch or personal contact; and silence, the art of remaining quiet.
- The four proxemic zones include a person's intimate, personal, social, and public space. A person's comfort zone is the area, which when intruded, does not stimulate anxiety.
- Nursing care involves two types of touch. Task-oriented touch occurs when assessing clients and performing physical care; affective touch occurs when demonstrating concern or emotional feelings.
- Communication is essential during teaching, and teaching is most efficient when it is compatible with a client's learning style.
- There are three basic categories of learning styles. Cognitive learners prefer processing information by listening or reading; affective learners grasp information better when it appeals to their feelings, beliefs, or values; psychomotor learners retain information better by performing hands-on tasks.
- Client education, whether formal or informal, begins with an assessment of learning needs.
- Regardless of a person's learning style and learning needs, three variables affect the teaching-learning process. They include a person's capacity to learn, motivation to learn, and learning readiness.
- Teaching can occur informally during a spontaneous moment or formally when it is planned according to sequenced content and time.
- Some nursing guidelines that are appropriate to follow when teaching adults include: presenting one, but no

more than three new ideas at a time, keeping technical terms to a minimum, reviewing frequently, relating new information to prior learning, and building in some type of learner performance evaluation.

CRITICAL THINKING EXERCISES

1. Role play a nurse–client interaction and analyze the types of verbal and nonverbal communication that occur.
2. Create a nurse–client scenario that demonstrates nontherapeutic communication and then revise it to demonstrate a more therapeutic version.
3. Explain how you would teach a cognitive, affective, and psychomotor learner how to follow a low-calorie diet or other health-related concept.

Suggested Readings

Brady, B. A., & Nesbitt, S. N. (1991). Using the right touch. *Nursing, 21*, 46–47.

Marken, S. (1997). Learning to listen. *American Journal of Nursing, 97*(4), 16D, 16F.

Oermann, M. H. (1991). *Professional nursing practice, a conceptual approach.* Philadelphia: J. B. Lippincott.

Rankin, S. H., & Stallings, K. D. (1996). *Patient education: Issues, principles, practices.* Philadelphia: Lippincott-Raven.

Rega, M. D. (1993). A model approach for patient education. *MED-SURG Nursing, 2*, 477–479, 495.

Chapter 10

Caring for Culturally Diverse Clients

KEY TERMS

Biologic variation
Culture
Ethnicity
Ethnocentrism
Generalization
Health beliefs
Health practices
Race
Stereotype
Subculture
Transcultural nursing

LEARNING OBJECTIVES

On completion of this chapter, the reader will:

- Differentiate between the terms culture, race, and ethnicity.
- Explain why the American culture is described as being Anglicized.
- Define the term subculture and list four major subcultures in the United States.
- Discuss two factors that can lead to bigotry or discrimination against members of minority subcultures.
- Explain the difference between generalizing and stereotyping.
- List five ways in which people from subcultural groups may differ from Anglo-Americans.
- Explain the meaning of the term "transcultural nursing."
- Give three characteristics of transcultural nursing.
- List at least five ways of demonstrating culturally sensitive nursing care.

Despite the fact that people vary in many ways, such as their age, gender, country of origin, language, education, and religion, the tendency among some nurses has been to interact with clients as if differences did not exist. Although this may seem politically correct, many nurses now believe that ignoring what is unique about a person's personal and cultural heritage is actually detrimental. Consequently, there is a movement toward identifying what is distinct about clients as cultural groups and what is unique about clients as individuals within those groups.

Culture

Culture refers to the "set of traditions that are transmitted from generation to generation" (Andrews & Boyle, 1995, p. 9). One's cultural heritage is often the foundation for language, communication style, rituals, customs, religion, health beliefs, and health practices. Individuals from particular cultures also tend to share biologic and physiologic characteristics.

The United States has been described as a "melting pot" in which culturally diverse groups have become assimilated; however, that is not the case. Individuals from various cultural groups have settled, lived, and worked in the United States (Box 10–1), while sustaining their particular ethnicity.

Ethnicity

Ethnicity is the bond or kinship people feel with their country of birth or place of ancestral origin. Ethnicity can exist regardless of whether a person has ever lived outside the United States. Pride in one's ethnic heritage is demonstrated by valuing certain physical characteristics, giving one's children ethnic names, wearing unique items of clothing (Fig. 10–1), appreciating folk music and dance, and eating native food.

When two or more cultural groups mix, their differences become more obvious. Consequently, some cultural groups have been victimized as a result of bigotry, which is based on stereotypical assumptions and ethnocentrism.

BOX 10-1 Culturally Diverse Groups Within the United States

City or Region	Cultural Group
New England	Irish
Detroit, Buffalo, Chicago	Polish
Upper Midwest (Minnesota, North Dakota)	Scandanavians
Ohio and Pennsylvania	Amish (Pennsylvania Dutch)
New York (Spanish Harlem)	Puerto Rican
Miami (Little Cuba)	Cuban
San Francisco (Chinatown)	Chinese
Manhattan (Little Italy)	Italian
Louisiana	Cajun (French/Indian)
Southwest	Latin American/Native American
Hawaiian Islands	Japanese/Chinese

Race

The term **race** is often confused with ethnicity and culture. Race refers to **biologic variation** and was originally made up of three divisions: Mongoloid, Negroid, and Caucasoid. The divisions are based primarily on differences in obvious physical features such as eye shape, skin color, and hair texture. Racial mixing has blurred the distinctions among races. However, race is still used as a label to identify extremely large subgroups of humankind that share certain physical, and in some instances, physiologic characteristics.

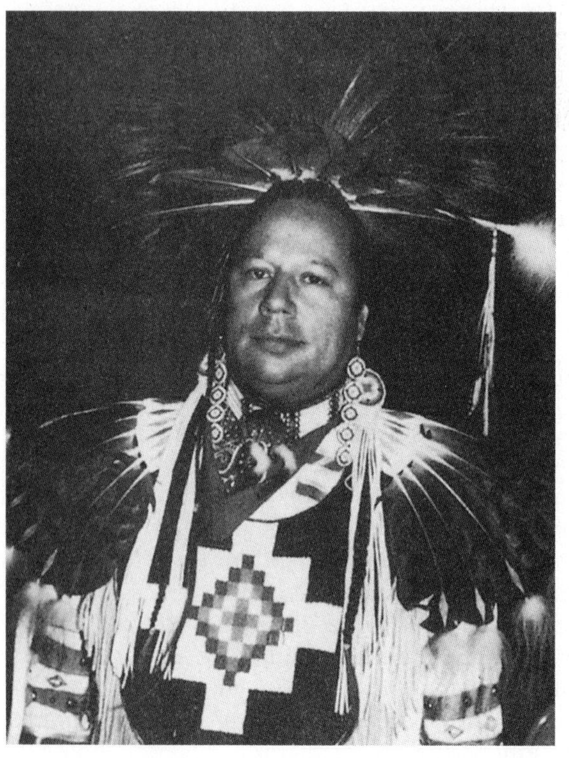

FIGURE 10-1. A Native American in Tribal dress. (Courtesy of Ken Timby.)

Still, physical differences, particularly skin color, are mistakenly associated with culture. Therefore, it is essential that nurses not equate skin color or other physical feature with culture. To do so leads to two possible erroneous assumptions: (1) that all people with certain physical attributes share essentially the same culture, and (2) that all people with physical similarities have cultural values, beliefs, and practices different from those of Anglo-Americans.

Stereotyping

A **stereotype** is a fixed attitude about *all people* who share a common characteristic, such as age, gender, race, religion, or country of origin.

Because stereotypes are preconceived ideas that are usually unsupported by facts, they tend to be neither real nor accurate. In fact, they can be dangerous because they are dehumanizing and interfere with accepting others as unique individuals.

Ethnocentrism

Ethnocentrism is the belief that one's own ethnic heritage is the norm and superior to others. The danger in ethnocentrism is that those who are different may be considered deviant and undesirable. Ethnocentrism was the basis for the Holocaust, the planned extinction of an entire ethnic group—European Jews, and plays a role in the racist attitudes against African Americans in this country.

Anglo-American Culture

The American culture is described as *Anglicized*, or English-based, because it evolved primarily from the culture of British settlers. It is foolish, however, to suggest that all people who live in America necessarily embrace the whole of Anglo-American culture.

American Subcultures

The term **subculture** refers to a unique cultural group that coexists within a dominant culture. Major American subcultures based on ethnic background include

TABLE 10-1 **American Subcultural Groups***

Subculture	Countries	Percent of American Population
African American	Africa, Haiti, Jamaica, West Indian Islands, Dominican Republic	12.1%
Latino	Mexico, Puerto Rico, Cuba, South and Central America	9%
Asian American	China, Japan, Korea, Philippines, Thailand, Indochina, Vietnam, Pacific Islands	2.9%
Native Americans	North American Indian nation and tribes including Eskimos and Aleuts	0.8%

*As reported by the U.S. Census Bureau in 1990.

African Americans, Latinos, Asian Americans, and Native Americans (Table 10–1) (Fig. 10–2). Subcultures form because of other shared characteristics as well, such as occupation (astronauts, miners, nurses), religion (Catholics, Jehovah's Witnesses), age (senior citizens, teenagers), or geographic location (New Englanders, Midwesterners, Southerners). One must remember that subcultures can be further subdivided to provide more meaningful cultural information; for example, there are over 500 Native American tribes and several Asian American subgroups such as Korean, Japanese, and Chinese.

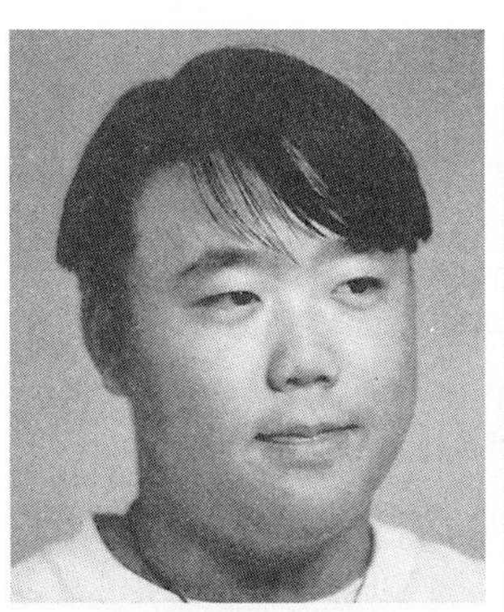
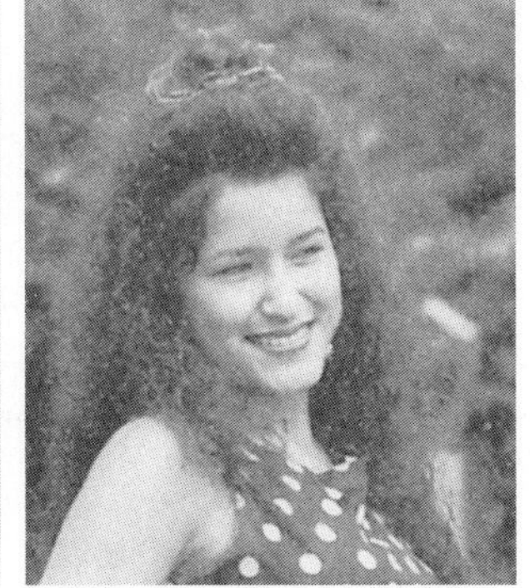
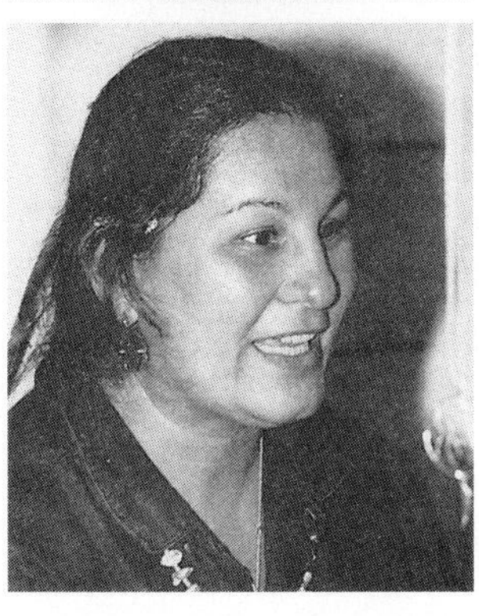
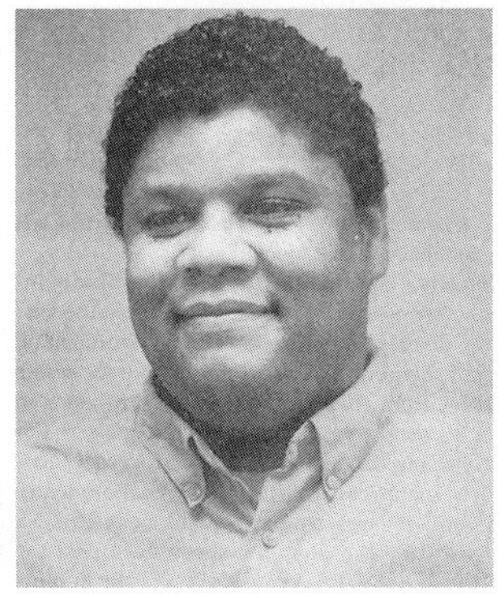

FIGURE 10-2. Individuals representative of major American subcultures; upper left, Asian American; upper right, Latino; lower left, Native American; lower right, African American.

Although Anglo-American culture still predominates in the United States, those who trace their ancestry to western European countries are gradually becoming the minority. The Bureau of the Census predicts that by the middle of the 21st century, the majority of American citizens will be of African, Asian, Hispanic, or Arabic descent (Kavanaugh, 1993).

Disease Prevalence

There are several diseases, such as sickle cell anemia, hypertension, diabetes, and stroke, that occur with much greater frequency among ethnic subcultures than in the general population. The incidence of some chronic diseases and their complications is the result, in part, of socioeconomic status. Minority cultural groups tend to be less affluent and their access to expensive health care is often limited. Without preventive health care, early detection, and treatment, higher death rates are bound to occur. The United States has committed itself to reducing the disparity in health care among all Americans by the year 2000 (U.S. Department of Health and Human Services, 1992). As the richly varied population in America today becomes even more culturally diverse, nurses will need to acquire the skills and knowledge necessary to practice transcultural nursing.

Transcultural Nursing

Transcultural nursing, a term coined by Madeline Leininger in the 1970s, refers to nursing care that is provided within the context of another's culture. Transcultural nursing is culturally sensitive and characterized by:

- Accepting each client as an individual
- Possessing knowledge of health problems that affect particular cultural groups

- Planning care compatible with the client's health belief system

To provide culturally sensitive care, nurses must become skilled at managing language differences, understanding biologic and physiologic variations, promoting health teaching that will reduce prevalent diseases, and respecting alternative health beliefs or health practices.

Diversity and Nursing Care

It is important to understand the distinction between generalizations and stereotypes because cultural information can be misused and nurses may inadvertently fall into the trap of stereotyping. Stereotyping refers to assuming that a person possesses certain characteristics without ascertaining if that assumption is true. It tends to reduce individuals and groups to caricatures. **Generalization** also starts with an assumption about a person's cultural traits but recognizes that each individual lives within the context of his or her culture in unique ways. General knowledge leads the nurse to *specific questions* about how the client is similar to or different from others in their cultural group (Lipson, Dibble, & Minarik, 1996). *It is always wrong to assume that all people who affiliate themselves with a particular group behave or believe exactly alike.* There is, of course, diversity within cultural groups.

LANGUAGE

Differences in language can be a significant barrier when providing nursing care. Among all of the different cultural groups living in the United States, many do not speak English or have learned it as their second language and do not speak it well. In addition, most individuals prefer to speak in their native tongue especially when they are under stress. A translator should be used when neither the nurse nor the client speak the same language. Care should be taken when asking family members to interpret; embarrassment and lack of medical knowledge can result in miscommunication. Refer to Nursing Guidelines 10–1 for additional communication techniques.

COMMUNICATION STYLES

When the nurse from one culture and the client from another speak the same language, the *manner* in which they do so may result in miscommunication. What is an accepted pattern during verbal interactions for one may be unusual, rude, or offensive to another. Understanding that unique cultural characteristics involving verbal and nonverbal communication exist can facilitate the transition to culturally sensitive care.

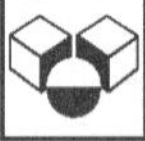

Nursing Guidelines 10-1

Communicating With Non-English-Speaking Clients

When Clients Speak No English

- Learn a second language, especially one spoken by a large ethnic population serviced by the health agency.
- Speak words or phrases in the client's language, even if it is not possible to carry on a conversation.
- Refer to an English/foreign language dictionary for bilingual vocabulary words; *Taber's Cyclopedic Medical Dictionary* contains medical words and phrases in Spanish, Italian, French, and German.
- Construct a loose-leaf folder or file cards with words in one or more languages spoken by clients in the community.
- Develop a list of employees or individuals to contact in the community who speak a second language and are willing to act as translators; in an extreme emergency, international telephone operators may be able to provide assistance.
- Select a translator who is the same gender as the client and approximately the same age, if possible.
- Look at the client, not the translator, when asking questions and listening to the client's response.

When English is a Second Language

- Determine if the client speaks or reads English, or both.
- Speak slowly, not loudly, using simple words and short sentences.
- Avoid using technical terms, slang, or phrases with a double or colloquial meaning like "Do you have to use the john?"
- Ask questions that can be answered by a "yes" or "no."
- Repeat the question without changing the words, if the client appears confused.
- Give the client sufficient time to process the question from English to the native language, and respond back in English.
- Rely heavily on nonverbal communication, and pantomime if necessary.
- Avoid displaying impatience.
- Ask the client to "read this line," to determine the client's ability to follow written instructions, which are provided in English.

Verbal Differences

There are general communication patterns found among the major American subcultures. The nurse is advised to carefully observe or tactfully question the client about communication preferences and to tailor the interview accordingly.

Native Americans are rather private people and may be hesitant to share much personal information with a stranger. They may also fear an encounter with non-Indian health care providers because of the long history of careless treatment of Native Americans. They may interpret questioning as prying or meddling. Be patient when awaiting an answer and listen carefully; listening is a valued skill and impatience is seen as disrespectful (Lipson et al., 1996). Some may be skeptical of Anglo-American nurses who write down what they say because Native Americans preserved their history through the oral tradition rather than written records; it may be useful to write notes after the interview instead of during it, if possible. Navajos, currently the largest tribe of Native Americans, feel that no person has the right to speak for another, and they may refuse to comment on a family member's health problems.

African Americans have in the past been victimized by the health care system as unknowing research subjects; consequently, they may be distrustful. Show professionalism by addressing clients by their last names and introducing yourself. Follow-up thoroughly with requests; respect the client's privacy and ask open-ended rather than direct questions until trust has been established. Because of their experiences as victims of Anglo-American discrimination, African Americans may be hesitant to give any more information than what is asked.

Latinos are characteristically more comfortable sitting close to the interviewer and letting the interaction slowly unfold. Many Latinos may speak English, but still can have difficulty with medical terminology. They may be embarrassed to ask the interviewer to speak slowly, so be sure to provide information and ask questions carefully without displaying impatience. If an interpreter is required, have someone of the same gender translate. Latino men generally are protective and authoritarian when it comes to women and children. Men expect to be consulted in decision-making when a family member is the primary client.

Asian Americans feel more comfortable positioned more than an arm's length from the interviewer. They tend to respond with brief, factual answers with little elaboration, perhaps because they value simplicity, meditation, and introspection. Asian Americans may not openly disagree with authoritarian figures, like physicians and nurses, because of their respect for harmony. Their reticence can conceal a potential for noncompliance when a particular therapeutic regimen is unacceptable from their perspective.

Nonverbal Differences

Personal space, touch, eye contact, and the use of silence are all communication factors that are culturally determined. Although it may be natural for Anglo-Americans to look directly at a person while speaking, eye contact may offend Asian Americans, Native Americans, and other cultural groups who feel that lingering eye contact is an invasion of privacy. Others avoid eye contact with authority figures as a sign of respect. Even the Anglo-American custom of a strong handshake can be interpreted as offensive by some Native Americans, who may be more comfortable with just a light passing of the hands.

Anglo-Americans, in general, are open to providing personal health information and expressing their positive and negative feelings. Asian Americans, however, tend to control demonstrating emotion or revealing that they are physically uncomfortable (Zborowski, 1952, 1969), especially when among people with whom they are unfamiliar. Similarly, Latino men may not show feelings or readily discuss their symptoms because it may be interpreted as less than manly (Andrews & Boyle, 1995). The male Latino behavior can be attributed to *machismo*, their belief that virile men are physically strong and must deal with their emotions in private.

Cultural Assessment

ASSESSING CULTURAL HERITAGE

Cultural ignorance can have a profound effect on an individual's or group's access to quality health care. It provides the motivation for expanding the knowledge base about people from different cultures. Additionally, it is important to recognize all the areas in which cultural differences subtly manifest themselves. These areas include:

- Communication patterns
- Hygiene practices, including feelings about modesty and accepting the help of others
- The use of special clothing or amulets
- Food preferences
- Management of symptoms such as pain, constipation and depression
- Rituals surrounding birth and death
- Spiritual or religious orientation, especially as it relates to health care
- Family relationships including expectations of elders and children
- Patterns of interacting with health care providers (Lipson et al., 1996)

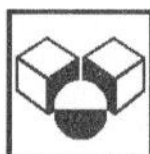

Nursing Guidelines 10-2

Performing a Cultural Assessment

Ask about or observe for the following cultural elements:

- Where was the client born? How long has the client lived in this country?
- What is the client's ethnic background? Does the client identify strongly with others from the same cultural background? Does the client live in a neighborhood with others of the same ethnic or cultural background?
- To whom does the client turn for support? Who is the head of the family and is he or she involved in decision-making about the client?
- What is the client's primary language and literacy level?
- What is the client's religion and is it important in his or her daily life? Are there religious rituals related to sickness, death or health that the client observes?
- Has the client sought the advice of traditional healers?
- What are the client's communication styles? Does the client avoid eye contact and maintain physical distance? Is the client open and verbal about symptoms?
- What are the client's food preferences or restrictions?
- Does the client participate in cultural activities such as dressing in traditional clothing and observing traditional holidays and festivals?

Adapted from Lipson, J. G., Dibble, S. L., & Minarik, P. A. (1996). Culture and nursing care: A pocket guide. *San Francisco: UCSF Nursing Press.*

An assessment of cultural characteristics should be included in any initial assessment (Nursing Guidelines 10–2), along with an assessment of health practices and beliefs.

ASSESSING HEALTH BELIEFS AND PRACTICES

Health beliefs and **health practices,** ideas about what causes illness, the role of the sick person, what must occur for health to be restored, and how one stays healthy, exist and are perpetuated under the influence of strong cultural affiliations (Table 10–2). To discover the health beliefs and practices of an individual, it is useful to ask specific questions that elicit this information (Nursing Guidelines 10–3). Assessment of these factors helps the nurse to:

- Identify the client's beliefs about his or her health or illness.
- Recognize health-seeking behaviors on which to capitalize to promote health.
- View the situation from the client's perspective.
- Distinguish behaviors that do not contribute to health restoration, maintenance, or promotion.
- Perceive issues that can compromise the treatment plan.
- Establish a mutually agreed on plan of care (McSweeney, Allan, & Mayo, 1996).

Developing Transcultural Sensitivity

Increasing one's awareness of America as a multicultural nation is a beginning step toward transcultural nursing. Examining personal beliefs, communication habits, and health care practices is another step toward transcultural practice and enabling the elimination of barriers to cross-cultural care. The following recommendations are offered for developing

TABLE 10-2 **Traditional Health Beliefs and Practices**

Cultural Group	Health Belief	Health Practices
Anglo-Americans	Illness is caused by infectious microorganisms, organ degeneration, and unhealthy lifestyles.	Physicians are consulted for diagnosis and treatment; nurses provide physical care.
African Americans	Supernatural forces can cause disease and influence recovery.	Individual and group prayer is used to speed recovery.
Asian Americans	Health is the result of a balance between *yin* and *yang* energy; illness results when equilibrium is disturbed.	Acupuncture, acupressure, food, and herbs are used to restore balance.
Latinos	Illness and misfortune occur as a punishment from God, referred to as *castigo de Dios,* or they are caused by an imbalance of "hot" or "cold" forces within the body.	Prayer and penance are performed to receive forgiveness; the services of lay practitioners who are believed to possess spiritual healing power are used; foods that are "hot" or "cold" are consumed to restore balance.
Native Americans	Illness occurs when the harmony of nature (Mother Earth) is disturbed.	A *shaman,* or medicine man, who has both spiritual and healing power, is consulted to restore harmony.

*As reported by the U.S. Census Bureau in 1990.

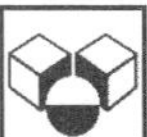

Nursing Guidelines 10-3

Assessing Health Beliefs and Practices

Initial assessment of the client should include the following questions:

- What have you done in the past and what do you do now to maintain health?
- How do these activities help you maintain your health?
- What practices could you add to help promote health?
- What is your definition of good health?
- Do you have any difficulties with performing activities that will restore, maintain, or promote health?
- What do you call your health problem?
- What do you think has caused this problem?
- Why do you think it started when it did?
- What does this problem do to you?
- What are the difficulties that this health problem has caused you, personally, in your family, or at work?
- What do you fear most about this health problem?
- What kind of treatment do you think will help? What are the most important results you hope to get from this treatment?

Adapted from McSweeney, J. C., Allan, J. D., & Mayo, K. (1997). Exploring the use of explanatory models in nursing research and practice. Image: Journal of Nursing Scholarship, *29(2), 243–248.*

a growing expertise in culturally sensitive nursing care:

- Learn to speak a second language.
- Use techniques for facilitating interactions, like sitting within the client's comfort zone and making appropriate eye contact.
- Become familiar with physical differences among ethnic groups.
- Perform physical assessments, especially of the skin, using techniques that will provide accurate data.
- Perform cultural and health beliefs assessment and plan care accordingly.
- Consult the client on ways to solve health problems.
- Never ridicule a cultural belief or practice, verbally or nonverbally.
- Integrate cultural practices that are helpful or harmless within the plan of care.
- Modify or gradually change unsafe practices.
- Avoid removing religious medals or clothing that hold symbolic meaning for the client; but, if this must be done, keep them safe and replace them as soon as possible.
- Provide food that is customarily eaten.
- Advocate that clients be routinely screened for diseases to which they are genetically or culturally prone.
- Facilitate rituals by whomever the client identifies as a healer within his or her belief system.
- Apologize if cultural traditions or beliefs are violated.

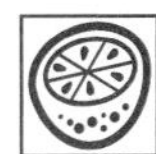

General Nutritional Considerations

Culture defines what food is; how food is obtained, stored, prepared and served; when food is eaten; differences in food habits based on age, gender and status; and the meaning of food. Within any cultural or ethnic group, individual food habits can vary greatly. Generalizations about usual dietary practices are intended only as a guide.

African Americans are at higher risk for hyptertension, stroke, diabetes and obesity. Limiting fat, sodium and excess calories may help prevent or treat these disorders. Because lactose intolerance is common, calcium intake may be inadequate if milk is avoided. In the South, "soul food" refers to both the cooking style (usually barbecued or fried) and particular foods consumed (eg, pork, corn products, greens).

Throughout Latin America, traditional food practices are influenced by Indian and Spanish cultures and local food availability. Obesity is common among Latino Americans and the prevalence of diabetes is high. Calcium intake may be adequate because milk intake is often low.

Rice is the staple food in most Asian cultures; starch intake is therefore high among Asian Americans and fat intake is low. Meat is used more as a condiment than as a main entree in traditional cooking, and preparing food usually takes more time than cooking the food. Lactose intolerance is common. Because of extensive use of soy sauce, limiting sodium intake is difficult.

Traditional food habits of Native Americans stem from cultural and religious beliefs and are influenced by geography and food availability. Although staple foods vary among tribes, corn, squash, and beans are used extensively in most traditional cooking. Many plant foods are also used in traditional medicinal practices. Obesity, diabetes, and lactose intolerance are common health problems among Native Americans.

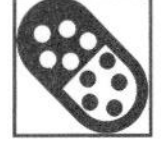

General Pharmacologic Considerations

Almost all cultures and ethnic groups have traditional folk remedies that are used as medicine within that group. These preparations have pharmacologic actions that can affect physiology and cause drug interactions.

Folk healing beliefs and practices are important aspects of healing and methods should be found to combine these practices with the medically prescribed treatment. Noncompliance with the pharmaceutical regimen may be a problem with those who use folk remedies unless at least some of these remedies can be incorporated into the treatment regimen.

When a drug is prescribed, the nurse asks the client if any herbal medicines or teas have been or are presently being used and informs the physician of the client's use of these products.

Biologic and physiologic variations may play a role in the way a drug is absorbed and metabolized. The nurse must be alert to any idiosyncrasies from the norm in drug action or the appearance of unusual adverse drug reactions, which may or may not be due to the person's inherited characteristics.

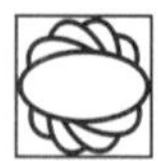

General Gerontologic Considerations

A grandmother or an older aunt is often considered the matriarch (female head or leader) in an African American family.

The advise of spiritual healers and the use of folk medicines are more often used by the older generation. For example, some Hispanics, especially older Hispanics, use a traditional folk healer, the "curandero" for managing health problems. If used exclusively for health care needs, problems can arise that need a more conventional medical approach.

Aging Asians tend to be cared for and live with one of their children. It is considered rude to suggest that an aging parent be placed in a nursing home.

Older Asian women are very modest and often prefer not to be examined or cared for by men. Rather than be touched during a physical assessment, they prefer to point to a model to indicate where they are experiencing symptoms (Giger & Davidhizar, 1995). Latino women also are frequently uncomfortable being cared for by male nurses.

An aging male Latino's self-image and security may be threatened by illness, especially those that cause obvious physical changes or dependence on a woman for care.

Nurses must take the time to listen to the older adult in a nonjudgmental manner. If the nurse is not culturally sensitive to the older adult's beliefs regarding health issues, communication is blocked and health care needs may not be identified.

SUMMARY OF KEY CONCEPTS

- Culture is the traditions that are transmitted from generation to generation; ethnicity is the bond or kinship people feel with their country of birth or place of ancestral origin; race is a term that refers to a large group of people who share similar physical characteristics.
- The culture in America as a whole is referred to as being Anglicized because its traditions have been largely influenced by early settlers from Great Britain.
- A subculture is a unique cultural group that coexists within a dominant culture. There are four major subcultures within the United States: African Americans, Latinos, Asian Americans, and Native Americans.
- Members of minority subcultures are often the victims of bigotry and discrimination because of stereotyping, fixed and often false attitudes about those who share common characteristics, and ethnocentrism, the belief that the dominant culture's ethnic heritage is the norm and, therefore, superior to others.
- Generalizations about other cultures leads the nurse to perform a cultural assessment to determine in what ways the individual subscribes to or deviates from his or her cultural background.
- Subcultural groups differ from Anglo-Americans in one or more of the following ways: language, communication style, biologic and physiologic variations, prevalence of diseases, and health beliefs and practices.
- Transcultural nursing refers to nursing care that is provided within the context of another's culture. It is distinguished by (1) accepting each client as an individual, (2) possessing knowledge of health problems that affect particular cultural groups, (3) assessing the client's cultural background and health beliefs and practices, and (4) planning care within the client's health belief system to achieve the best health outcomes.
- Some ways that nurses can demonstrate culturally sensitive nursing include: learning a second language, performing physical assessments and care according to the client's unique biologic variations, consulting with each client as to his or her cultural preferences, advocating for modifications in diet and dress according to the client's customs, respecting cultural health beliefs, and allowing clients to continue cultural health practices that are not harmful.

CRITICAL THINKING EXERCISES

1. How might a culturally sensitive nurse prepare for the home care of a non–English-speaking client from Pakistan or some other foreign country?
2. Discuss how a culturally sensitive nurse might handle the fact that a pregnant woman wears a chicken bone about her neck, which she believes will protect her unborn child from birth defects.
3. Answer the first five questions in Nursing Guidelines 10–2 to gain insight into your own health beliefs and practices. Consider the variables discussed in Nursing Guidelines 10–3 and discuss ways in which these cultural values are frequently ignored in the health care setting and how this might affect outcomes and the client's experience with health care.

Suggested Readings

Andrews, M. M., & Boyle, J. S. (1995). *Transcultural concepts in nursing care* (2nd ed.). Philadelphia: J. B. Lippincott.

Giger, J. N., & Davidhizar, R. E. (1995). *Transcultural nursing: Assessment and intervention* (2nd ed.). St. Louis: Mosby.

Kavanaugh, K. H. (1993, Summer). Transcultural nursing: Facing the challenges of advocacy and diversity/universality. *Journal of Transcultural Nursing, 5*, 4–13.

Leininger, M. (1996). Major directions for transcultural nursing: A journey into the 21st century. *Journal of Transcultural Nursing, 7*(2), 28–31.

Lipson, J. G., Dibble, S. L., & Minarik, P. A. (1996). *Culture and nursing care: A pocket guide*. San Francisco: UCSF Nursing Press.
McSweeney, J. C., Allan, J. D., & Mayo, K. (1997). Exploring the use of explanatory models in nursing research and practice. *IMAGE: Journal of Nursing Scholarship, 29*(2), 243–248.
Spector, R. E. (1996). *Cultural diversity in health and illness* (4th ed.). East Norwalk, CT: Appleton & Lange.
U.S. Bureau of the Census. (1990). *General population characteristics*. Washington, DC: U.S. Government Printing Office.
U.S. Department of Health and Human Services. (1992). *Healthy people 2000: National health promotion and disease prevention objectives*. Boston: Jones and Bartlett.
Zborowski, M. (1952). Cultural components in response to pain. *Journal of Social Issues, 8*, 16–30.
Zborowski, M. (1969). *People in pain*. San Francisco: Jossey Bass.

Additional Resources

Alliance of Genetic Support Groups
4301 Continental Ave., NW
Suite 404
Washington, DC 20008-2304
(800) 336-GENE
http://medhlp.netusa.net/www/agsg.htm

Alternative Medicine Homepage
http://www.pitt.edu/~cbw/altm.html
or write: Charles B. Wessel, MLS
Falk Library of the Health Sciences
University of Pittsburgh
Pittsburgh, PA 15261
e-mail: cbw@med.pitt.edu

CultureNurse.org
340 Commerce Ave., SW
Grand Rapids, MI 49503-4129
e-mail: webmaster@culturenurse.org
http://nursing.simplenet.com/main/mainindex.html

Department of Health and Human Services
Health Resources and Services Administration
Office of Minority Health
200 Independence Ave., SW
Washington, DC 20201
(202) 619-0257
http://www.os.dhhs.gov/

Families USA
1334 G St, NW
Washington, DC 20005
(202) 628-3030
http://familiesusa.org

4

Psychobiologic Disorders

Chapter 11

Interaction of Body and Mind

KEY TERMS

Biofeedback
Brain mapping
Coping mechanisms
Distress
Eustress
General adaptation syndrome
Hardiness
Humor
Imagery
Immunopeptides
Limbic system
Mental status examination
Neuropeptides
Neurotransmitters
Placebo effect
Psyche
Psychobiologic disorders
Psychoneuroendocrinology
Psychoneuroimmunology
Psychosomatic diseases
Receptor
Soma
Stress-related disorders
Stress
Stress management

LEARNING OBJECTIVES

On completion of this chapter, the reader will:

- Explain why mental illnesses are now considered psychobiologic disorders.
- Name two chemical substances transmitted between neurons and give examples of each.
- Discuss two new areas of neuroscience that are being studied to learn more about psychobiologic disorders.
- Name three psychodynamic factors that affect behavior.
- List four examples of techniques used for assessing clients with psychobiologic disorders.
- Distinguish between stress, eustress, and distress.
- Describe the general adaptation syndrome and name the three stages it includes.
- Explain the purpose of coping mechanisms and the outcomes that may result from their use.
- List the defining features of hardiness.
- Discuss techniques the nurse can suggest for helping clients cope with stressors.
- Discuss the rationale for a mind–immune system connection.
- Discuss four explanations for the development of psychosomatic diseases.
- Discuss interventions nurses use to foster effective coping skills.
- Name four psychobiologic interventions that can be used therapeutically.

Once thought to be completely separate structures, the mind, the central nervous system (CNS), and the body are now viewed as a single communicating entity. Recent research has uncovered anatomic and chemical links between the body and the mind and new fields of science have emerged to research these linkages and their impact on health. *Psychobiology* is the study of the biochemical basis of thought, behavior, affect, and mood. **Psychobiologic disorders** are those in which evidence exists of a link between biologic abnormalities in the brain and altered cognition, perception, emotion, behavior, and socialization. **Psychoneuroendocrinology** is the study of how fluctuations in pituitary, adrenal, thyroid, and reproductive hormones alter cognition, perception, behavior, and mood. **Psychoneuroimmunology** studies the connections among the emotions, the CNS, the neuroendocrine system, and the immunologic system. Although a new and not completely developed science, psychoneuroimmunology is the focus of a great deal of interest. Research in this field studies how stress predisposes to infection, autoimmune disorders (see Chap. 41), and cancer. All these overlapping fields study the anatomy, physiology, and pathology of the brain.

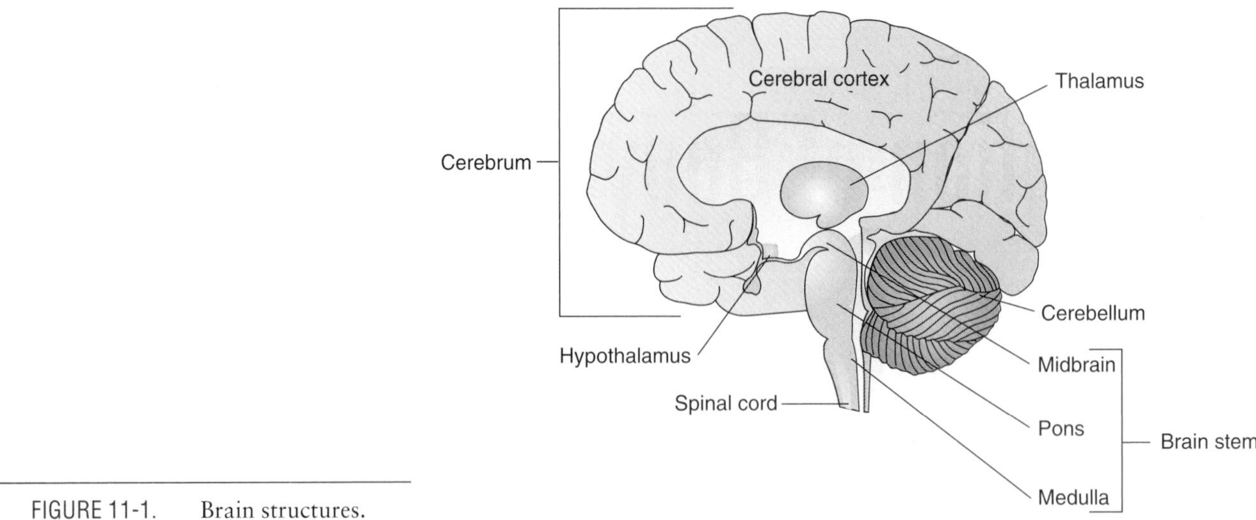

FIGURE 11-1. Brain structures.

The Brain and Psychobiologic Function

The brain is a complex organ made up of the cerebrum, brain stem, and cerebellum (Fig. 11–1). The *cerebrum* is the largest component of the brain. It is the basis for sensory perception, voluntary movement, personality, intelligence, language, thoughts, judgment, emotions, memory, creativity, and motivation. The outer layer of the cerebrum, the *cerebral cortex*, is the major pathway of physiologic intercommunication. The cortex receives, processes, integrates, and relays information to appropriate functional areas of the brain. The **limbic system** is a network within the brain that contains structures involved in emotions and related physiologic functions. It includes the *thalamus*, which connects many brain centers and modulates movement, sensation, behavior, and emotions. The limbic system also includes the *hypothalamus*, which controls the autonomic nervous system and coordinates the endocrine and immune systems via pituitary-adrenocortical connections (Porth, 1998). Because of its neuroendocrine and neuroimmunologic roles, the limbic system affects and determines many psychobiologic activities.

Neurotransmitters and Receptors

RECEPTORS

Receptors are structures found on the surface of cells throughout the body and brain. Each cell has mil-

TABLE 11-1 **Selected Neurotransmitters**

Neurotransmitters	Abbreviation	Examples of Functions
Serotonin (5-hydroxytryptamine)	5-HT	Stabilizes mood Induces sleep Regulates temperature Controls appetite
Dopamine	DA	Integrates thoughts Promotes movement in concert with ACH Stimulates hypothalamic endocrine activity Enhances judgment
Norepinephrine	NE	Affects attention and concentration Raises energy level Heightens arousal
Acetylcholine	ACH	Assists memory storage Promotes movement in concert with DA Prepares for action
Gamma-Aminobutyric Acid	GABA	Reduces arousal and aggression Inhibits excitatory neurotransmitters like NE and DA Decreases seizure potential

lions of different receptors. These receptors sense and pick up chemical messages that arrive in the extracellular fluid. The chemical messenger may be thought of as a specific key that fits into a specific receptor and binds to it. Only those messengers that have molecules in exactly the right shape can bind with specific receptors. For example, opiate receptors can bind with only chemicals in the opiate group such as heroin, morphine, or endorphins. Once binding occurs, the message is received and the cell begins to respond. Chemical messengers may be natural or man made and the message may cause the cell to perform any number of activities. Neurotransmitters and neuropeptides are the messengers that play a significant role in regulating all physical, emotional, and mental processes.

NEUROTRANSMITTERS

Neurotransmitters (Table 11–1) are chemical messengers. They communicate information that affects thinking, behavior, or bodily functions across the synaptic cleft between neurons (Fig. 11–2). The chemicals, which are synthesized in the neuron and then stored in vesicles in the axon, are released and attach themselves (bind) momentarily to the receptors on postsynaptic neurons. After the chemicals have transmitted their information, they are:

- Broken down into inactive substances by enzymes like monoamine oxidase
- Recaptured by the releasing neuron for later use, a process called reuptake
- Weakened by becoming diluted in intercellular fluid

Neurons are classified by the type of neurotransmitter they release; for example, cholinergic neurons release acetylcholine, and dopaminergic neurons release dopamine.

Neuropeptides are a separate type of neurotransmitter. They include chemicals such as:

- Substance P, which transmits the sensation of pain
- Endorphins and enkephalins, morphine-like neuropeptides that interrupt transmission of substance P and promote a feeling of well-being
- Neurohormones released by interactions between the hypothalamus, pituitary, and the endocrine glands they stimulate

Different areas of the brain contain different types of neurons with specific neurotransmitters. Each neurotransmitter has a different stimulating or inhibiting effect on neurons. All brain function including thoughts, emotions, or sending messages to organs and muscles, is dependent on these neurotransmitters (Barry, 1996).

Receptors for neurotransmitters and neuropeptides are found not only throughout the CNS, but in the endocrine and the immune systems as well. This suggests that these systems communicate with each other through chemical messages. This concept has tremendous implications for how the mind and emotions can affect physical well-being and how physical status can affect the mind (Barry, 1996; Goleman & Gurin, 1993; Pert, 1997).

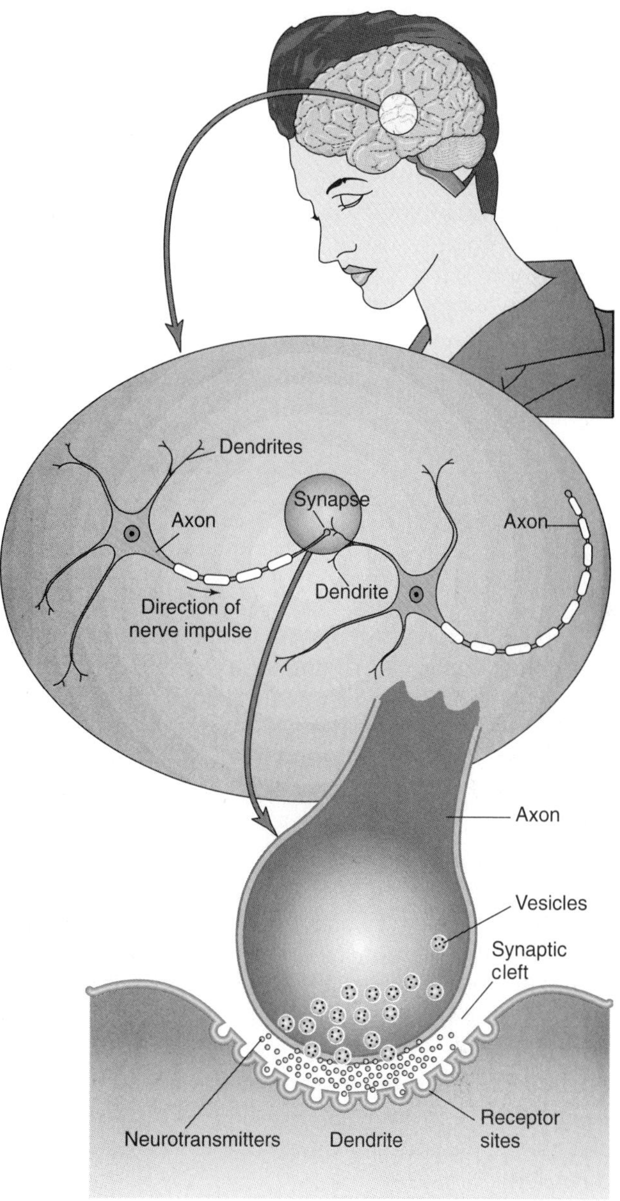

FIGURE 11-2. Neurotransmitter anatomy.

Psychobiologic Illness

Historically, many believed mental illness to be the result of character defects, evidence of demonic possession, or punishment by God. These myths persist, which explains why individuals with mental illness are sometimes feared and stigmatized. The study of brain structure, chemistry, and genetics has begun to replace ignorance and misinformation about mental illness with facts. Brain pathology is now seen as the major factor contributing to mental illnesses, now called psychobiologic disorders. Three major types of psychobiologic disorders are somatoform and anxiety disorders (see Chaps. 12 and 13), mood disorders (see Chap. 14), and thought disorders (see Chap. 17). Other conditions with a biologic basis include eating disorders (see Chap. 15) and chemical dependency (see Chap. 16).

Etiology and Pathophysiology

BIOLOGIC FACTORS

The neurotransmitters dopamine, norepinephrine, epinephrine, serotonin, and acetylcholine are often implicated in the psychobiology of mental illness (Hayes, 1995). Because the neurotransmitters are concentrated in different areas of the brain, disruption of a neurotransmitter system results in the specific symptoms associated with that area of the brain. For example, dopamine influences movement, memory, thoughts, and judgment and the disorganized thought patterns and bizarre behavior of schizophrenia have been correlated with excess levels of dopamine; low levels of dopamine cause the impaired balance and uncontrolled tremors of Parkinson's disease. Serotonin is found in areas that regulate sleep, appetite, sexual behavior, and mood. Imbalances in serotonin are thought to be responsible for depression, eating disorders, sleep disturbances, and obsessive-compulsive disorder.

Other insights into brain physiology came from observing the effects of medications on behavior and symptoms (psychopharmacology). The theory that depression results from decreased levels of norepinephrine and serotonin was first postulated when the monoamine oxidase inhibitors, which block the inactivation of norepinephrine and serotonin (see Chap. 14), were found to alleviate depression. Similarly, antianxiety medications like the benzodiazepines (see Chap. 13) activate gamma-aminobutyric acid receptors that inhibit arousal, excitement and aggression.

PSYCHODYNAMIC FACTORS

Psychodynamic factors (forces that shape behavior) also influence psychological equilibrium and may be tied to brain chemistry as well. Some researchers postulate that emotion, memory, and learned behavior are linked by the neurotransmitter network (Pert, 1997). These psychodynamic factors have long been components of psychiatric theory and include intrapersonal development, interpersonal interactions, and learning.

Intrapersonal Development

Sigmund Freud proposed that disordered behavior is the result of intrapersonal (within oneself) conflicts that arise during a particular stage of development during infancy through adolescence. Freud placed great emphasis on sexual aspects of behaviors between an infant and mother, conflicts surrounding toilet training, awareness of gender differences and genital pleasure, rivalry with the same-gender parent, investment of energy in intellectual pursuits, and efforts to establish relationships with members of the opposite sex.

Interpersonal Interaction

Other theorists, like Erik Erikson (see Chap. 6) and Harry Stack Sullivan, proposed that mental health or illness is a consequence of social relationships and interpersonal interactions. Some go further to suggest that one's mental stability is affected not only by significant others, but also by social systems, such as one's neighborhood, city, and country. The more positive the social system, the better the chances are that a person will be mentally healthy and well adjusted.

Learning

The theory that adaptive and maladaptive behavior is learned and repeated because of rewarding reinforcement was proposed by psychologist B. F. Skinner. This theoretical perspective is applied in a variety of circumstances such as when young children are offered candy to induce toilet training or when privileges are withdrawn to extinguish unacceptable behaviors.

Assessment Findings

SIGNS AND SYMPTOMS

Brain dysfunction can cause a mix of psychobiologic signs and symptoms. Symptoms for each specific mental disorder have been established by the American Psychiatric Association (1994) in the *Diagnostic and Statistical Manual of Mental Disorders*, a book that classifies psychiatric disorders. Commonly seen symptoms include anxiety, mood changes, abnormal eating patterns, chemical dependence, or thought disturbances. Ultimately, the client's signs and symptoms affect relationships with others and interfere with age-related role responsibilities.

Besides a comprehensive personal and family medical history, clients undergo a mental status examination and laboratory, diagnostic, and psychological testing.

MENTAL STATUS EXAMINATION

A **mental status examination** is one component of a thorough neurologic examination. It is an array of observations and questions that elicit information about a person's cognitive and mental state. The components of an extensive mental status examination include obtaining data about the client's:

- Physical appearance
- Orientation
- Attention and concentration
- Short- and long-term memory
- Movement and coordination
- Speech patterns
- Mood
- Intellectual performance
- Perception
- Insight
- Judgment
- Thought content

Nurses regularly conduct mini mental status examinations (Box 11–1). Changes in the total score are used to evaluate changes in the client's condition.

PSYCHOLOGICAL TESTS

Psychological tests are administered to detect personality characteristics, interpersonal conflicts, and self-concepts. Examples of various psychological tests are described in Table 11–2.

LABORATORY AND DIAGNOSTIC TESTS

Measuring levels of neurotransmitters and neuropeptides is difficult, expensive, and sometimes impossible. Unfortunately, a definitive diagnosis for many psychobiologic disorders occurs more often by ruling out other diseases that manifest similar symptoms. The reader is referred to Chapter 44 for a description of tests such as electroencephalography (EEG), computed tomography, magnetic resonance imaging, and positron emission tomography, which clients may undergo.

One of the newest diagnostic tools, brain mapping, suggests that diagnosing psychobiologic disorders more efficiently in the future will be possible. **Brain mapping** is a technique for comparing a client's brain activity patterns from an EEG or other electronic image with a computerized data base of electrophysiologic abnormalities. A growing data base of distinctive patterns for seizure disorders, schizophrenia, depression, dementia, anxiety disorders, attention deficit disorder, and others now exists for comparison.

Medical and Nursing Management

Treatment of psychobiologic disorders is dependent on the specific diagnosis and includes psychotherapy, cognitive therapy, behavior modification, or drug therapy (refer to Chaps. 12 through 17). Drug therapy is aimed at correcting the underlying biochemical abnormality and is particularly useful in mood disorders (see Chap. 14), anxiety (see Chaps. 12 and 13), and schizophrenia (see Chap. 17). The goals of psychotherapy, cognitive therapy, and behavior modification are to uncover repressed thoughts and emotions and identify healthier coping mechanisms. Nurses play an active role in all aspects of treatment including administering and monitoring response to drug therapy, implementing behavior modification plans, and providing individual and group counseling.

The Brain and Psychosomatic Function

In addition to the study of the biologic basis of mental illness, brain chemistry and its impact on physical health are currently being widely researched as well. Emotions, which originate in brain structures and chemicals, can have a powerful influence on an individual's health and sense of well-being. Stress has been implicated in the development or exacerbation of autoimmune diseases, anorexia nervosa, obsessive-compulsive disorder, panic attacks, thyroid conditions, heart disease, functional and inflammatory disorders of the gastrointestinal tract, chronic pain conditions, and diabetes.

Stress

According to Selye's theory (1956), **stress** is a physiologic response to biologic stressors like surgical trauma

BOX 11-1 Mini-Mental State Examination

Orientation

(Score 1 point for correct response)

1. What is the year?
2. What is the season?
3. What is the date?
4. What is the day of the week?
5. What is the month?
6. Where are we? building or hospital?
7. Where are we? floor?
8. Where are we? town or city?
9. Where are we? county?
10. Where are we? state?

Registration

(Score 1 point for each object identified correctly, maximum is 3 points)

11. Name three objects at about one each second. Ask the patient to repeat them. If the patient misses an object, repeat them until all three are learned.

Attention and Calculation

(Score 1 point for each correct answer up to maximum of 5 points)

12. Subtract 7's from 100 until 65 (or, as an alternative, spell "world" backward).

Recall

(Score 1 point for each correct answer, maximum of 3)

13. Ask for names of three objects learned in question 11.

Language

14. Point to a pencil and a watch. Ask the patient to name each object. Score 1 point for each correct answer, maximum of 2 points.
15. Have the patient repeat "No ifs, ands, or buts." Score one point if correct.
16. Have the patient follow a three-stage command: "(1) Take the paper in your right hand. (2) Fold the paper in half. (3) Put the paper on the floor." Score 1 point for each command done correctly, maximum of 3 points.
17. Write the following in large letters: "CLOSE YOUR EYES." Ask the patient to read the command and perform the task. Score 1 point if correct.
18. Ask the patient to write a sentence of his or her own choice. Score 1 point if the sentence has a subject, an object, and a verb.
19. Draw the design printed below. Ask the patient to copy the design. Score 1 point if all sides and angles are preserved and if the intersecting sides form a quadrangle.

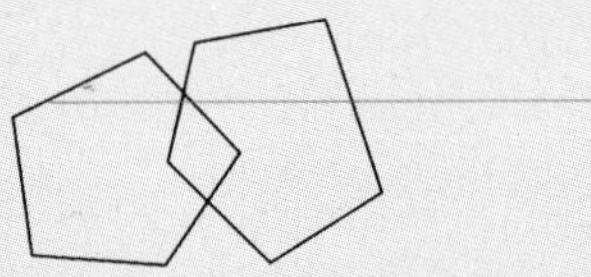

From Folstein, M. E., Folstein, S. E., McHugh, P. R. Mini-mental state: A practical method for grading the cognitive state of patients for the clinician. *Journal of Psychiatric Research, 12*(189), 1975. Used with permission.

TABLE 11-2 **Psychological Tests**

Test	Description
Minnesota Multiphasic Personality Inventory (MMPI)	True and false test of 550 questions; used to analyze which ones of nine clinical personality traits are manifested by the client's responses.
Beck Depression Inventory	Client rates self according to statements that concern mood.
Draw-a-Person (tree, house, family) Test	Client's drawing is analyzed for symbolism about his or her self-perception or other emotional data.
Word Association Test	Client is asked to quickly provide a response to words, such as "mother . . . work . . .", etc. Responses are analyzed for psychological significance.
Thematic Apperception Test (TAT)	Client is asked to look at pictures and then tell a story about them. Recurring themes in the stories suggest the underlying basis of emotional problems.
Rorschach Test	The client is asked to indicate what is seen in each of 10 separate inkblots.

or infection, psychological stressors such as worry and fear, or sociologic stressors including a new job or increased family responsibilities.

Stress is not an entirely negative concept. Just the right amount of stress, called **eustress,** is what maintains a healthy balance in life. Some amount of stress helps individuals to pursue goals, learn to solve problems, or manage life's predictable and unpredictable crises. Excessive, ill-timed, or unrelieved stress is called **distress.** It triggers the **general adaptation syndrome**, a nonspecific physiologic response (Box 11–2). This response, which can cycle many times through the alarm and resistance stages before reaching the exhaustion stage, occurs through the neuroendocrine and autonomic nervous systems.

PHYSIOLOGIC STRESS RESPONSE

The autonomic nervous system consists of the sympathetic and the parasympathetic divisions. The most common pathway for the stress response is through the sympathetic division. The sympathetic division stimulates body systems, arousal, and anxiety in response to stress using acetylcholine and norepinephrine. This response overrides the parasympathetic nervous system's control, which causes many metabolic processes to slow and is the automatic regulator of all body systems. A few individuals respond to stressors through the parasympathetic pathway.

PSYCHOLOGICAL STRESS RESPONSE

Just as the physical body responds to stressors, the **psyche,** or mind, also reacts to stress. **Coping mechanisms** are unconscious tactics to protect the self from feeling inadequate or threatened (Table 11–3). These mechanisms function like psychological first-aid by helping temporarily to avoid the emotional impact of a stressful situation. When used appropriately and in moderation, coping mechanisms allow maintenance of psychological equilibrium and lead to psychological growth. However, if coping mechanisms are overused they become dysfunctional. In addition, some individuals develop maladaptive coping mechanisms such as abusing alcohol or other substances.

Some people have developed a particularly effective coping style called **hardiness** (Kobasa, 1979). Hardiness is characterized by:

- A commitment to something meaningful versus alienation
- A sense of having control over the sources of stress versus a feeling of helplessness
- The perception of life events as a challenge rather than a threat

Refer to Nursing Guidelines 11–1 for interventions that can foster effective coping skills.

BOX 11-2 General Adaptation Syndrome

Stressor
↓
ALARM
↓
Autonomic Nervous System
↓ ↓

Sympathetic Division (norepinephrine)	Parasympathetic Division (acetylcholine)
↓	↓
• Increased heart rate	• Decreased gastric motility
• Increased force of heart contraction	• Increased intestinal peristalsis
• Increased rate and depth of respirations	• Contraction of urinary bladder muscles
• Vasoconstriction	
• Increased blood pressure	
• Increased muscle tension	

RESISTANCE
↓
Hypothalamus/Pituitary/Adrenal Axis
↓
Adrenocorticotropic Hormone (ACTH)
↓
Adrenal Cortex
Glucocorticoids (cortisol)
–Increased blood sugar
–Altered fat and protein metabolism
–Decreased capillary permeability
–Decreased inflammatory response
Mineralcorticoids (aldosterone)
–Conservation of sodium
–Excretion of potassium
–Reduced urine output
↓
EXHAUSTION
↓
Cardiac Failure
Renal Failure
Inadequate Immune Response

TABLE 11-3 **Coping Mechanisms**

Mechanism	Description and Example
Repression	Forgetting about situations that produced stress *Example:* Wiping from memory the experience of being sexually abused
Suppression	Purposely avoiding thinking about an issue *Example:* A person indicates that he or she will sleep on a problem or has turned the problem over to God.
Denial	Rejecting information *Example:* Refusing to accept a life-threatening diagnosis
Rationalization	Relieving personal accountability by attributing responsibility to someone or something else *Example:* Blaming failure on a test to the manner in which the test was constructed
Displacement	Taking anger out on something or someone else who is less likely to retaliate *Example:* Kicking the wastebasket after being reprimanded by the boss
Regression	Behaving in a manner characteristic of a much younger period of life *Example:* A child who is toilet-trained begins to wet and soil himself when a new sibling is born
Projection	Attributing that which is unacceptable in oneself on to another *Example:* A racially biased individual accuses a person of another race of being prejudiced.
Somatization	Manifesting emotional stress with physical symptoms *Example:* A person who dreads an appointment, develops diarrhea or a severe headache, which may provide an excuse for missing the appointment.
Compensation	Excelling at something to make up for a weakness of another kind. *Example:* A physically disadvantaged person becomes a motivational speaker.
Sublimation	Channeling one's energies into an acceptable alternative *Example:* A nonathletic person becomes a sports writer.
Reaction/Formation	Acting just the opposite to one's feelings *Example:* Being extremely nice to someone who is disliked
Identification	Taking on the characteristics of another to meet unconscious needs *Example:* In an effort to feel accepted, an adolescent dresses like others in the same age range.

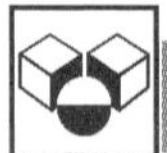

Nursing Guidelines 11-1

Fostering Effective Coping Skills

- Explore the coping strategies the client has found helpful in the past and encourage their continued use.
- Encourage clients to re-establish priorities and to strike a healthy balance between work and play.
- Suggest cultivating relationships with family and friends who are supportive.
- Teach the client assertiveness skills by role playing how to (1) clearly state feelings, and (2) say "no" to unreasonable requests.
- Discuss time management techniques like (1) getting up earlier, (2) avoiding procrastination, (3) performing stressful tasks when there is maximum energy, and (4) eliminating or delegating unwanted tasks.
- Recommend a daily exercise program to reduce stimulating neurotransmitters and release endorphins and enkephalins such as (1) beginning with a 5- to 10-minute workout, (2) increasing the duration by 5 minutes each day, and (3) building up to a 30- to 45-minute period of exercise.
- Tell the client to avoid using alcohol or other nonprescribed sedative drugs as forms of self-treatment.
- Suggest writing about feelings in a diary if verbalizing traumatic or angry thoughts is difficult.
- Suggest stress management education and joining a support group.

Psychosomatic Illnesses

Psyche refers to the mind, and **soma,** the body. The term *psychosomatic* means pertaining to the mind–body relationship and *psychosomatic illness* refers to illnesses influenced by the mind; the term is often used interchangeably with stress-related. In the past, psychosomatic had a negative connotation suggesting that a client's illness was not legitimate. However, psychoneuroimmunologic research in the last two decades has given the term a much more holistic meaning, reflecting the concept that the mind and the body are not separate. **Psychosomatic diseases** (Box 11–3) are bona fide medical conditions associated with or aggravated by stress. Many health care providers now believe that all illnesses, if not psychosomatic in origin, have a psychosomatic component.

Etiology and Pathophysiology

BIOLOGIC FACTORS

In addition to the known effects of stress on the autonomic nervous system, studies show that stressful events such as preparing for exams or undergoing job strain also can affect the immune system. The purpose

BOX 11-3 Stress-Related Diseases and Disorders

Allergic and hypersensitivity disorders
Anovulation
Bronchial asthma
Bruxism
Cancer
Cardiac dysrhythmias
Connective tissue disorders
Eczema
Hair loss
Herpes simplex infection
Hypertension
Infertility
Irritable bowel syndrome
Low back pain
Multiple sclerosis
Nervous tics
Psoriasis
Rheumatoid arthritis
Temporo-mandibular joint disorder
Tension headaches
Ulcerative colitis

of the immune system is to defend the body from cancer and invading microorganisms. Stress can lower the numbers of white blood cells, the immune system's disease fighters. Research also shows that chronic stress, or very intense stress such as the death of a spouse, has more of an impact on health than temporary stressors. This seems to be particularly true when there is a lack of supporting relationships. Several studies have shown a connection between poorer immune function and loneliness; other studies have shown improved immune function when emotions are shared with others (Kiecolt-Glaser & Glaser, 1993).

Support for a biologic connection between the mind and the immune system is found in research that demonstrates that the immune system and the brain communicate with each other through the chemical messenger system using neurotransmitters and immunopeptides. **Immunopeptides** (or immunotransmitters) are called *cytokines* and function in the same way as neurotransmitters; they relay messages throughout the immune system and to the brain (Pert, 1997). Immune cells can also secrete small quantities of neurochemicals. In addition, nerve cells connecting the organs of the immune system (thymus, spleen, and lymph nodes) to the brain have been identified. This ability to communicate through chemicals implies that the immune system can make the brain aware of processes going on at distant sites in the body and that the brain can send messages directing the immune system's actions. The powerful actions of neurotransmitters, especially in states of excess or depletion, suggest that the psychological state can have a significant impact on immune function.

Many psychosomatic or stress-related diseases involve allergic, inflammatory, or altered immune responses (see Chap. 41). They are characterized by physical symptoms that cycle through periods of *remission*, or absence, and *exacerbation*, or recurrence with the symptomatic episodes often occurring when the client is under stress. The brain–immune connection suggests that changes in body chemistry during periods of stress trigger an autoimmune (self-attacking) response or result in immunosuppression. However, invasion of the body by disease-causing microorganisms, including cancer cells, is not sufficient cause for disease; disease occurs when defenses are compromised or unable to recognize foreign material. This is why psychological variables that influence immunity have the potential to influence the onset and progression of immune system-mediated diseases (Cohen & Herbert, 1996, p. 127).

PSYCHODYNAMIC FACTORS

Psychological characteristics and an increased incidence of illness have been observed for centuries. Research suggests that there may be a generic, disease-prone personality with character traits that include anger and hostility, depression, anxiety, and other personality features (Pelletier, 1993). The type of disease that develops is related to an individual's health habits, environmental exposure, family history, and other socioeconomic factors.

Anger

Although anger is a normal emotion, many people fail to express it, perhaps feeling threatened by possible retaliation. They expend vast amounts of energy maintaining a facade of being happy and well adjusted. However, the effect of chronically suppressing anger and the neurochemical changes that accompany it may be the triggering mechanism for a dysfunctional immune response.

Conversely, evidence suggests that the excess expression of hostility and anger is correlated with an increased incidence of heart attacks and may be the result of low levels of serotonin. The frequent activation of the sympathetic nervous system in persons prone to anger and hostility is another factor implicated in the development of heart disease.

Dependence

Others propose that unmet dependency needs and fears of rejection or abandonment provoke feelings of insecurity among some individuals with psychosomatic disorders (Townsend, 1993; Johnson, 1996). Helplessness is related to dependence and numerous studies have shown that people who feel powerless in their lives have more illnesses than those who have a sense of control.

Ambivalence

Ambivalence means feeling or acting in two opposing ways at the same time. For example, an individual may feel hostility toward the persons from whom they most want love and approval, or he or she may act independently and yet desire dependence. These unresolved conflicts may affect neurotransmitter and immune functioning and be another key to the development of physical disorders.

Life Events

Additional insight into emotions and the risk for developing stress-related diseases is based on the Social Readjustment Rating Scale that rates life events according to how stressful they are (Box 11–4). The potential for a stress-related disease increases with the sum that a person scores. Particularly important is the sense of control a person has over these events; a recent history of uncontrollable life events puts a person at increased risk for disease.

BOX 11-4 Social Readjustment Rating Scale

Rank	Life Event	LCU Value
1	Death of spouse	100
2	Divorce	73
3	Marital separation	65
4	Jail term	63
5	Death of close family member	63
6	Personal injury or illness	53
7	Marriage	50
8	Fired at work	47
9	Marital reconciliation	45
10	Retirement	45
11	Change in health of family member	44
12	Pregnancy	40
13	Sex difficulties	39
14	Gain of new family member	39
15	Business readjustment	39
16	Change in financial state	38
17	Death of close friend	37
18	Change to different line of work	36
19	Change in number of arguments with spouse	35
20	Mortgage over $10,000	31
21	Foreclosure of mortgage or loan	30
22	Change in responsibilities at work	29
23	Son or daughter leaving home	29
24	Trouble with in-laws	29
25	Outstanding personal achievement	28
26	Wife begins or stops work	26
27	Begin or end school	26
28	Change in living conditions	25
29	Revision of personal habits	24
30	Trouble with boss	23
31	Change in work hours or conditions	20
32	Change in residence	20
33	Change in schools	20
34	Change in recreation	19
35	Change in church activities	19
36	Change in social activities	18
37	Mortgage or loan less than $10,000	17
38	Change in sleeping habits	16
39	Change in number of family get-togethers	15
40	Change in eating habits	15
41	Vacation	13
42	Christmas	12
43	Minor violations of the law	11

Social events are ranked from most stressful to least stressful. Each event is assigned a life change unit (LCU), which correlates with the severity of stress that is associated with it. The client is instructed to circle those events that have occurred in the last 6 months. The sum of LCUs for the marked items is then calculated to predict the individual's potential for developing a stress-related illness. A score of less than 150 LCUs is considered low risk; a score between 150 and 199 is an indicator of mild risk; moderate risk is associated with a score between 200 and 299; and a score over 300 places the individual at major risk. (Holmes TH, Rahe RH. The social adjustment rating scale. J Psychosom Res August 1967; 11:216. Copyright © 1967, Pergamon Press, Ltd.)

Assessment Findings

SIGNS AND SYMPTOMS

Many stress-prone individuals seek medical attention when they experience symptoms in one or more organs affected by the sympathetic nervous system. Clients may present with heart palpitations, pounding headaches, breathlessness, tightness in the chest, chest pain, chronic pain, irritability, epigastric pain, abdominal discomfort and bloating, or constipation alternating with diarrhea. Many other illnesses, including cancer and cardiovascular disease, are not so obviously related to stress but are thought to have a psychosomatic component. The biopsychosocial effects of stress and mental state should be considered in the evaluation and treatment of all illnesses.

LABORATORY AND DIAGNOSTIC FINDINGS

Diagnostic tests are done to determine the extent of the disease and all physical causes for the client's symptoms. Because other conditions such as excessive intake of caffeine, cocaine use, mitral valve prolapse, hyperthyroidism, hypoglycemia, and lactose intolerance, to name a few, can mimic the signs and symptoms of some stress-related diseases, it is important to conduct tests before assuming that the disorder is only stress induced.

Medical and Nursing Management

Treatment involves standard medical care pertinent to the diagnosis, control of the physical symptoms, and implementation of methods effective in managing stress and supporting the immune system. Nurses have an important role in participating in the treatment and education of clients regarding these methods. At one time dismissed by the medical community, stress management and other techniques have gained acceptance based on studies that suggest psychological factors can reduce the effects of stress on the immune system and facilitate healing.

PSYCHOBIOLOGIC INTERVENTIONS

The Placebo Effect

The **placebo effect** refers to the power for healing that can arise simply from the individual's belief that a treatment will be effective. The placebo effect was first observed during drug research. In most drug trials half the research volunteers receive the drug being studied while the other half receive an inactive substance known as a *placebo*. None of the volunteers or the researchers know which drug the subjects are receiving. When the results of the studies are analyzed, researchers find that 30% or more of the individuals who received the placebo experienced improvement. This is thought to show how a person's belief system positively influences health and that a purely psychological basis for recovery exists. In other words, when clients believe in the prescribed plan for treatment, it potentiates a positive outcome. Harnessing the psychological forces that create a "placebo effect" by communicating caring, optimism about treatment, and the belief that the client has the ability to recover can have a significant impact on wellness.

Other methods that have a positive psychobiologic effect include stress management techniques, biofeedback, imagery, and humor therapy. Many of these techniques are helpful even when illness is purely biologic in origin such as recovering from hip replacement surgery.

Stress Management

Stress management programs are particularly useful for clients who wish to prevent stress-related illnesses and for those with chronic disorders. These programs offer instruction in relaxation techniques and effective coping strategies including assertiveness training and developing a network of social support.

Biofeedback

Biofeedback is a technique in which an individual voluntarily controls one or more physiologic functions, such as body temperature, heart rate, blood pressure, and brain waves. Initially, clients are attached to a machine that transforms a physiologic activity, like heart rate, into a pulsating waveform, digital numbers, or audible sound. While receiving feedback from the machine, clients try to alter a particular function, such as decrease the heart rate. If the machine's signal changes, it helps them determine if they are successful. Eventually, clients do not need to rely on the response from the device; they can alter their physiology at will. Biofeedback is currently being used in the United States to reduce hypertension and rapid heart rates, manage pain, abort seizures, relieve migraine headaches, and produce dilation of peripheral blood vessels in individuals with vascular disorders.

Imagery

Imagery is a psychobiologic technique in which the mind is used to visualize a positive physiologic effect. When using imagery, clients conjure up mental images of their body waging and winning a battle with the disease process. For example, clients might visualize their white blood cells being produced in large numbers. They then imagine the white cells destroying cancer cells. Lab values of white cell counts taken before and after such imagery sessions often show that the numbers of white blood cells have dramatically increased.

Humor

Humor can be used therapeutically. Laughter stimulates the immune system by increasing the number of white blood cells and lowering cortisol, which suppresses immune function (Wooten, 1996). Laughter can cause the release of the neuropeptides, endorphins and enkephalins. Norman Cousins (1979) shared his own pain-relieving and healing experiences using humor in his book, *Anatomy of an Illness*.

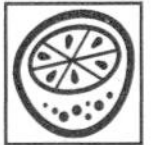

General Nutritional Considerations

Some people overeat in response to stress while others deny normal hunger. Assess for changes in appetite, eating patterns, and weight. Encourage clients to eat at regular intervals to avoid both overeating and undereating.

Dietary interventions for some psychosomatic diseases may be necessary only during times of exacerbation, such as avoiding lactose during acute ulcerative colitis. For other psychosomatic diseases, such as irritable bowel syndrome, dietary interventions are recommended whether or not symptoms are present.

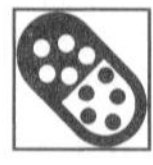

General Pharmacologic Considerations

A complete current medication history is obtained for each client, including nonprescription drugs. Some people who experience stress take over-the-counter drugs, stimulants, and tranquilizers that they may not mention unless asked.

Anti-inflammatory drugs and corticosteroids are often given to treat the symptoms of various psychosomatic diseases. Drug treatment is considered symptomatic rather than curative.

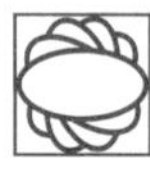

General Gerontologic Considerations

The function of the immune system diminishes with age resulting in an increase in the incidence of infection, cancer and autoimmune disease.

Elderly clients who have developed positive coping skills continue to cope well as they age.

Some older adults feel helpless and unable to cope when released from a health care facility without adequate discharge planning.

Emotional distress and impaired self-care abilities have been identified as major factors to rehospitalization of older adults.

Loss of a network for support increases an older adult's vulnerability and reaction to stressors.

Adults who have chronic psychosomatic diseases are likely to manifest debilitating effects in late adulthood.

SUMMARY OF KEY CONCEPTS

- Mental illnesses are those disorders that historically were considered the result of maladaptive psychological responses; these same diseases are now more correctly referred to as psychobiologic disorders because evidence indicates that brain pathology causes alterations in cognition, thinking, perception, emotion, behavior, and socialization.
- Malfunctions within the cerebrum and the structures found within it are associated with psychobiologic disorders.
- The cerebral cortex, the outer layer of the cerebrum, receives, processes, integrates, and relays information to appropriate functional areas of the brain.
- The limbic system contains many structures involved in emotional expression.
- Normal brain function depends on an elaborate network of neurons that transmit information biochemically with neurotransmitters. Neurotransmitters, like serotonin, dopamine, norepinephrine, acetylcholine, and γ-aminobutyric acid, are chemical messengers. Neuropeptides, a type of neurotransmitter, include substance P, endorphins, and enkephalins, and a variety of neurohormones.
- Two new areas of neuroscience are psychoneuroendocrinology that studies how fluctuations in pituitary, adrenal, thyroid, and reproductive hormones alter cognition, perception, behavior, and mood and psychoneuroimmunology, the study of how stress predisposes to infection, autoimmune disorders (antibodies attacking healthy cells), and cancer.
- Besides brain pathology, other psychodynamic factors that effect behavior include intrapersonal development, interpersonal interactions, and learning.
- Some signs and symptoms of psychobiologic disorders include anxiety, physical changes such as altered bowel elimination, mood changes, and thought disturbances.
- Techniques used to assess clients with psychobiologic disorders include a mental status examination, standard neurologic tests, psychological tests, and perhaps brain mapping.
- Stress-related diseases occur partially or wholly because of excessive stimulation of either the sympathetic or parasympathetic divisions of the autonomic nervous system, and decreased resistance to disease. Some examples of stress-related diseases are hypertension, skin disorders such as eczema and psoriasis, and irritable bowel syndrome.
- Stress is a physiologic response to biologic, psychological, and social stressors. There are two types of stress: eustress and distress. Eustress is just the right amount of stress to maintain a healthy balance in life. Distress is stress that is excessive, ill-timed, or unrelieved.
- The general adaptation syndrome is a nonspecific physiologic stress response consisting of three stages: alarm, resistance, and exhaustion.
- Coping mechanisms are unconscious tactics that protect the self-concept, or ego, from feeling inadequate. When used appropriately and in moderation, coping mechanisms allow individuals to maintain their psychological equilibrium.
- Hardiness is characterized by a sense of commitment to something, a feeling of control over stressful events, and a perception that stressors are a challenge rather than a threat.
- Nurses help clients cope with stressors by exploring positive coping strategies, reestablishing priorities, encouraging the cultivation of supportive relationships, implementing time management techniques, promoting daily exercise, and avoiding alcohol and drug abuse.
- Psychosomatic diseases are medical conditions associated with or aggravated by stress.
- Psychosomatic diseases generally have three common characteristics: (1) they usually involve allergic, inflammatory, or altered immune responses; (2) they cycle through periods of remissions and exacerbations; and (3) symptomatic episodes coincide with periods of stress.

- Some examples of psychosomatic diseases include bronchial asthma, multiple sclerosis, irritable bowel syndrome, ulcerative colitis, rheumatoid arthritis, and various skin disorders (eg, eczema and psoriasis).
- Several explanations have been proposed for why psychosomatic diseases develop. They may be a consequence of biochemical changes in the stress response that go awry, or pathologic consequences of suppressed anger, stress from unmet dependency needs, or conflict over ambivalent feelings.
- Psychosomatic diseases are treated medically by treating symptoms, reducing or eliminating the inflammatory or altered immune responses, and offering stress management techniques.
- To help clients express anger, nurses can encourage them to ventilate their feelings without the threat of retaliation, to role play communicating feelings they find difficult to express to others, or to write about their feelings in a diary.
- Five psychobiologic interventions that are used therapeutically include fostering a placebo effect, stress management techniques, imagery, biofeedback, and humor.

CRITICAL THINKING EXERCISES

1. Discuss situations in which the mind influences physiologic functions.
2. What would you say to someone who characterizes mental illness as the manifestation of a poor character?
3. Discuss how psychobiologic interventions can be integrated into nursing care.
4. What behaviors are therapeutic for avoiding the development of psychosomatic diseases?

Suggested Readings

American Psychiatric Association. (1994). *Diagnostic and statistical manual of mental disorders* (4th ed.). Washington, DC: Author.

Barry, P. (1996). *Psychosocial nursing: Care of physically ill patients and their families* (3rd ed.) Philadelphia: Lippincott-Raven.

Bartol, G. M., & Eakes, G. G. (1995). A study of the meanings assigned to the term psychosomatic among health professionals. *Perspectives in Psychiatric Care, 31*(1), 24–29.

Cohen, S., & Herbert, T. (1996). Health psychology: Psychological factors and physical disease from the perspective of human psychoneuroimmunology. *Annual Review of Psychology, 47*, 113–142.

Courts, N. F., & Bartol, G. M. (1996). Psychosomatic: Connotations for people who are neither nurses nor physicians. *Clinical Research, 5*(3), 283–293.

Cousins, N. (1979). *Anatomy of an illness.* New York: Norton.

Giedt, J. F. (1997). Guided imagery: A psychoneuroimmunological intervention in holistic nursing practice. *Journal of Holistic Nursing 15*(2), 112–127.

Goleman, D., & Gurin, J. (1993). What is mind/body medicine? In D. Goleman & J. Gurin (Eds.), *Mind/body medicine: How to use your mind for Better Health* (pp. 3–18). Yonkers, NY: Consumer Reports Books.

Hayes, A. (1995). Psychiatric nursing: What does biology have to do with it? *Archives of Psychiatric Nursing, IX*(4), 216–224.

Johnson, B. S. (1996). *Psychiatric mental health nursing: adaptation and growth,* 4th ed. Philadelphia: Lippincott.

Kiecolt-Glaser, J., & Glaser, R. (1993). Mind and immunity. In D. Goleman & J. Gurin (Eds.), *Mind/body medicine: How to use your mind for better health* (pp. 39–64). Yonkers, NY: Consumer Reports Books.

Kobasa, S. (1979). Stressful life events, personality and health: an inquiry into hardiness. *Journal of Personality and Social Psychology, 42*(1), 1–11.

Lazar, J. (1996). Mind-body medicine in primary care. *Primary Care, 23*(1), 169–182.

Pelletier, K. (1977). *Mind as healer, mind as slayer.* New York: Dell.

Pelletier, K. (1993). Between mind and body: Stress, emotions, and Health. In D. Goleman & J. Gurin (Eds.), *Mind/body medicine: How to use your mind for better health* (pp. 19–38). Yonkers, NY: Consumer Reports Books.

Pert, C. (1997). *Molecules of emotions: Why you feel the way you feel.* New York: Scribner.

Richman, J. (1995). The life-saving function of humor with the depressed and suicidal elderly. *Gerontologist, 35*(2), 271–273.

Schleifer, S. J., Keller, S. E., Camerino, M., et al. (1983). Suppression of lymphocyte function following bereavement. *Journal of the American Medical Association, 250*, 374–377.

Selye, H. (1956). *The stress of life.* New York: McGraw-Hill.

Townsend, M. C. (1993). *Psychiatric mental health nursing: concepts of care.* Philadelphia: FA Davis.

Wooten, P. (1996). Humor: An antidote for stress. *Holistic Nursing Practice, 10*(2), 49–56.

Additional Resources

Society for Traumatic Stress Studies
60 Revere Drive, Suite 500
Northbrook, IL 60062
(708) 480–9080

The Mind/Body Medical Institute
Division of Behavioral Medicine
New England Deaconess Hospital
185 Pilgrim Road
Boston, MA 02215
(617) 732–9530

Stress Reduction Clinic
University of Massachusetts Medical Center
Worcester, MA 01655
(508) 856–1616

The Academy for Guided Imagery
P.O. Box 2070
Mill Valley, CA 94942
(800) 726–2070

The American Self-Help Clearinghouse
St. Clares-Riverside Medical Center
25 Pocono Road
Denville, NJ 07834
(201) 625–7101

Chapter 12

Caring for Clients With Somatoform Disorders

KEY TERMS

Histrionic
Insight-oriented therapy
La belle indifference
Malingering
Secondary gain
Somatization
Somatoform disorders

LEARNING OBJECTIVES

On completion of this chapter, the reader will:

- Describe the coping mechanism referred to as somatization.
- Explain why malingering is not a somatoform disorder.
- Name at least three somatoform disorders.
- Discuss three explanations for the development of somatoform disorders.
- Describe the characteristics of somatoform disorders.
- Explain the meaning of insight-oriented therapy.
- Name three nursing diagnoses that are common to clients with somatoform disorders.

The care of clients who suffer from somatoform disorders is challenging because the symptoms, which are very real and distressing, are not due to any specific pathology. By understanding the psychological origins of these disorders, nurses can provide better care for clients who suffer physically from underlying emotional factors.

Somatoform Disorders

Somatoform disorders are conditions that have their basis in the coping mechanism of somatization. **Somatization** is the manifestation of unconscious emotional distress through physical symptoms. Although many people have physical illnesses worsened by stress and emotional conflict (see Chap. 11), somatizers (people with somatoform disorders) have no physiologic basis for their symptoms and often go from doctor to doctor seeking relief. Somatoform disorders are not to be confused with **malingering,** which is the deliberate faking of an illness to acquire financial compensation, obtain drugs, or be relieved of responsibilities from work or school. The psychological origin of the somatizer's symptoms is unknown to them and their illnesses seem very real. Types of somatoform disorders are listed in Table 12–1.

Etiology and Pathophysiology

Several theories exist to explain somatoform disorders. One belief is that the chronic release of neurotransmitters and neuroendocrine hormones in response to stress negatively affects regions in the brain that facilitate adaptation and coping behaviors. Another theory suggests that physical symptoms provide relief from psychological tension when it cannot be dealt with on a conscious level. Converting emotional pain into a physical disorder may be a justifiable way to obtain attention and compassion from others—an outcome referred to as **secondary gain**. Still other theories suggest that parental failure to respond to an infant's needs or inadvertent reward during times of routine childhood illnesses lay the groundwork for somatization.

TABLE 12-1 **Somatoform Disorders**

Disorder	Description
Somatization disorder	Clients experience multiple and chronic physical symptoms in a variety of organ systems.
Hypochondriasis	Clients are preoccupied with minor symptoms and develop an exaggerated belief that they have signs of major or life-threatening diseases.
Conversion disorder	Clients have a sudden loss of sensory or motor function usually following an emotionally traumatic experience, yet appear indifferent to the consequences of the impairment (**la belle indifference**).
Somatic pain disorder	Clients experience significant pain in the absence of any medical or traumatic condition.
Body dysmorphic disorder	Clients are overly concerned about a physical characteristic (shape or length of nose, size of hips, etc.), which by most standards are normal.

Regardless of the cause, clients with somatoform disorders experience physical distress that interferes with the quality of their lives. In some cases, it impairs social interactions and affects their ability to perform activities of daily living and role responsibilities.

Assessment Findings

SIGNS AND SYMPTOMS

Clients seek diagnosis and treatment for symptoms that generally involve the gastrointestinal, cardiopulmonary, genitourinary, and neurosensory systems. Some may have illnesses that are highly symbolic in nature, for example, imagined heart ailments after termination of a romance. Some somatizers appear **histrionic,** a term that comes from the word hysteria, when describing their symptoms. They are animated, dramatic, and prone to exaggeration. Others, like those with conversion disorder, appear apathetic. They often have multiple symptoms and many provide a history of extensive medical consultations, diagnostic procedures, and surgical interventions. Despite this, the symptoms persist or are replaced by others. The physical examination usually reveals symptoms that do not fit with known patterns of disease or injury. Often, these symptoms become more distressing during emotional crises, although most somatizers do not acknowledge that a relationship exists. The symptoms often provide some secondary gain: they distract from dealing with emotional problems, they provide a means for gaining attention, or they relieve the client from performing unwanted responsibilities.

DIAGNOSTIC FINDINGS

Despite comprehensive laboratory and diagnostic tests, no etiology or pathology is identified. In some cases, all current medications are temporarily discontinued to determine if a drug–drug interaction may explain the client's symptoms. When all investigative approaches prove negative, it is presumed that the symptoms are the consequence of a psychobiolgic process.

Medical Management

Differentiating the somatizer from a client with an actual illness is important. The physician, of course, attempts to discover the basis for symptoms when they occur; however, repeated diagnostic testing can reinforce the client's belief that something really is physically wrong. Although many clients with somatoform disorders resist it, they are eventually referred to psychiatrists or psychologists for insight-oriented psychotherapy.

Insight-oriented psychotherapy helps clients understand the cause and relationship between their emotional distress and physical symptoms. Goals of treatment include avoiding further unnecessary procedures and diagnostic testing, minimizing disability, and helping the client find other coping mechanisms that will prevent translating emotional stress into bodily symptoms. Therapy may be brief and can be followed by one or two sessions as needed if extreme stress results in a recurrence. Antianxiety medications are avoided or only prescribed for a brief period because of their potential for abuse and addiction among clients with chronic symptoms.

Nursing Management

The nurse supports the client emotionally. Above all the nurse avoids conveying to the client that the symptoms are unreal or that they can be consciously controlled. If psychological counseling becomes a part of the medical treatment plan, the nurse reinforces the idea that the mind influences the body and that both may need treatment from time to time.

The nurse's role in caring for clients with somatoform disorders includes, but is not limited to the following:

Nursing Diagnoses and Collaborative Problems	Nursing Interventions
Altered Comfort related to maladaptive coping Goal: The client's discomfort will be reduced.	Assess physical complaints matter of factly without emphasizing undue concern, yet avoiding dismissing them altogether. Show empathy for the client's distress. Implement prescribed medical treatment measures when they are appropriate. Use distraction, deep-breathing, muscle relaxation, and imagery to relieve discomfort.
Ineffective Individual Coping related to mismanagement of unconscious stressors Goals: The client will identify a connection between stress and physical symptoms. The client will use coping strategies, other than somatizing, for managing stressors.	Express a caring attitude. Accept the client's need to use somatizing as a coping mechanism until alternative coping strategies are acquired. Give the client permission to ventilate feelings and provide positive feedback when the client talks about emotional issues. Offer the suggestion that a link may exist between underlying emotional conflict and how the client feels physically. Explore the rewards the client's symptoms provide. Reinforce the client's developing awareness. Encourage the client to use previously successful coping strategies.

General Pharmacologic Considerations

Numerous drugs may be prescribed for somatoform disorders. The course of treatment is usually of short duration due to adverse reactions or lack of therapeutic effect.

Psychotropic medications and prescription analgesics are usually avoided in clients with somatoform disorders.

When medications are prescribed for clients with somatoform disorders, careful monitoring is necessary since these clients may overuse or abuse drugs.

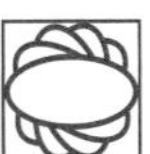

General Gerontologic Considerations

Loss of a network for support increases an older adult's vulnerability and reaction to stressors.

Older adults who are socially isolated may focus on themselves and become preoccupied with bodily illness.

By focusing on somatoform disorders, older adults may obtain more attention and care from family members than they would otherwise.

SUMMARY OF KEY CONCEPTS

- Somatization is an unconscious coping mechanism in which people express emotional distress through physical symptoms.
- Somatoform disorders are those in which clients experience physical symptoms, but no identifiable pathology is found.
- Malingering, the conscious faking of an illness or injury, is not considered a somatoform disorder because clients who malinger do not experience any physical symptoms although they may try to convince people otherwise.
- Examples of somatoform disorders include somatization disorder, hypochondriasis, conversion disorder, somatic pain disorder, and body dysmorphic disorder.
- Somatoform disorders may develop because a chronic stress response negatively affects regions in the brain that facilitate adaptation and coping behaviors, because physical symptoms provide relief from psychological tension when it cannot be dealt with on a conscious level, or because they are a learned means of dealing with stressors. Some somatizers may derive secondary gain from being physically ill.
- Somatoform disorders generally have some common characteristics such as the symptoms affect the gastrointestinal, cardiopulmonary, sexual/reproductive, or neurosensory systems; the symptoms become more distressing during emotional crises, although most do not acknowledge that a relationship exists; and the symptoms often provide some underlying reward.
- Clients with somatoform disorders may improve with insight-oriented therapy, a form of psychotherapy in which clients are helped to understand the cause and relationship between their emotional problems and physical symptoms.
- When caring for clients with somatoform disorders, the nurse may implement interventions for managing their altered comfort and ineffective coping.

CRITICAL THINKING EXERCISES

1. Discuss the physical, emotional, social, and financial implications that can result from having a somatoform disorder.
2. What behaviors might be therapeutic to avoid the development of somatoform disorders?

Suggested Readings

Harrison, S., Watson, M., & Feinmann, C. (1997). Does short-term group therapy affect unexplained medical symptoms? *Journal of Psychosomatic Research, 43*(4), 399–404.

Johnson, B. S. (1996). *Psychiatric-mental health nursing: Adaptation and growth* (4th ed.). Philadelphia: Lippincott-Raven.

Townsend, M. C. (1993). *Psychiatric mental health nursing: Concepts of care.* Philadelphia: Davis.

Additional Resources

National Mental Health Consumers' Self-Help Clearinghouse
1211 Chestnut Street
Philadelphia, PA 19107
(800) 553–4539

The American Self-Help Clearinghouse
St. Clares-Riverside Medical Center
25 Pocono Road
Denville, NJ 07834
(201) 625–7101

Chapter 13

Caring for Clients With Anxiety Disorders

KEY TERMS

Anxiety
Anxiety disorders
Behavioral therapy
Cognitive therapy
Desensitization
Fear

LEARNING OBJECTIVES

On completion of this chapter, the reader will:

- Differentiate anxiety from fear.
- Name four levels of anxiety and explain how each differs from the others.
- Give six areas of nursing management that apply to the care of anxious clients.
- Give three examples of anxiety disorders.
- List categories of drugs used to treat anxiety disorders.
- Name and discuss two types of psychotherapy used in the treatment of anxiety disorders.
- List six nursing interventions that are helpful for reducing anxiety.
- Discuss areas of teaching for clients with anxiety disorders.

Questions remain whether anxiety disorders are strictly biologic, learned, the result of unconscious emotional conflicts, or a combination of all three. Probably, physical and psychological factors have a dual role. A person is first genetically predisposed to an anxiety disorder and then manifests a disorder when exposed to situational triggers. Although anxiety and fear are normal human responses, anxiety disorders are not.

Anxiety and Fear

Anxiety is different from fear, but these terms are often used interchangeably. **Anxiety** is a vague uneasy feeling the cause of which is not readily identifiable. It is evoked when anticipating nonspecific danger. **Fear** is a feeling of terror in response to someone or something specific perceived as dangerous or threatening. Because it is usual for clients to be anxious in an environment that is unfamiliar, or to be fearful of pain, suffering, or death, both reactions are common in hospitals or health care agencies.

Because many medical and surgical clients temporarily feel vulnerable, they are prime candidates for experiencing anxiety. Recognizing the signs of escalating anxiety, understanding the consequences, and intervening appropriately is important.

Levels of Anxiety

Anxiety can range from mild, which is constructive, to moderate, severe, and panic levels (Table 13–1). Mild anxiety prepares individuals to take action in situations where it is appropriate. For example, mild anxiety before a test causes most to study. Other levels of anxiety tend to be destructive; they provoke responses that interfere with physical and emotional well-being.

Nursing Management

BUILDING TRUST

Building trust is especially critical to developing a therapeutic relationship with an anxious client. Being available and attentive to the client's needs accomplishes this. Do not leave an anxious client alone, especially during a new or potentially frightening experience.

TABLE 13-1 **Levels of Anxiety**

Level	Behavioral Manifestations	Physical Manifestations
Mild	Heightened attention Expanded sensory perception Focused on stimuli Reality remains intact Accurate processing of information Feels in control	Increased muscle tone Slight increase in heart rate, blood pressure, breathing Noticeable perspiration
Moderate	More easily distracted Slight impairment of concentration Able to redirect attention Learning takes more effort Perception narrows Difficulty problem-solving Irritability Feels inadequate	Tense muscles and slight hand or leg tremors Nonpurposeful activity occurs Change in rate, pitch, and volume of speech Respiratory depth and vital signs increase Disturbed sleep
Severe	Short attention span Unable to concentrate Cannot remain focused Perception reduced Impaired ability to learn May process information inaccurately or incompletely Aware of extreme discomfort Takes effort to control emotions Feels incompetent	Hyperventilation and dizziness Tachycardia and heart palpitations Hypertension Impaired fine motor movement Limited communication
Panic	Exaggerates details Perception is distorted Learning disabled Fragmented thoughts Unable to control emotions Feels helpless	Incoherent speech Haphazard movement usually in an effort to escape Dyspnea Fainting Tremors Diaphoresis

RESTORING COMFORT

The nurse's interventions are guided by what will bring relief to a particular person. Ask the client to suggest methods that may be personally comforting. Some find it helpful for the nurse to give support in nonverbal ways, like remaining with them without talking, holding a hand, or stroking the skin. Others prefer to talk about how they feel, but are more relaxed if the nurse remains physically distant (Fig. 13–1).

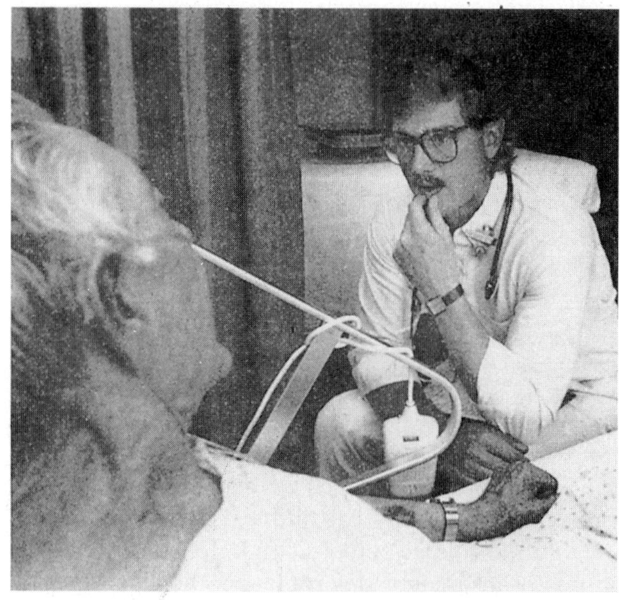

FIGURE 13-1. A nurse listens to an anxious client. (Courtesy of Suzanne Weaver, Bay Health Systems.)

MODIFYING COMMUNICATION

Avoid interrupting anxious clients when they talk. Although verbalizing does not relieve anxiety, it can be beneficial. Talking helps in processing information and exploring methods for dealing with problems. Some clients prefer not to discuss their anxiety and fears with the nurse. When this occurs, the nurse respects the client's right to privacy. However, offering a referral to a health professional like a psychiatrist or medical social worker with counseling expertise is appropriate.

ADJUSTING TEACHING

Because an anxious client's attention and concentration are limited, directions or explanations are simple, brief, and repeated frequently. To determine a client's level of comprehension, it is helpful to ask the person to paraphrase what has been taught.

The client also benefits from reducing sensory stimulation such as dimming the lights and eliminating as much noise as possible. Avoid expecting a great deal of self-reliance or independence until the client feels more in control.

HELPING PROBLEM-SOLVE

Problem-solving ability is impaired when clients are anxious and they may look to the nurse for advice in decision-making. However, nurses avoid influencing their clients' choices. Instead, nurses help clients follow a step-by-step process in formulating decisions. The problem-solving process includes:

1. Identifying problems
2. Determining their causes
3. Exploring possible solutions
4. Examining the pros and cons of each option
5. Selecting the choice that is most compatible with personal values

Once the client arrives at a decision, the nurse advocates on the client's behalf for its implementation—even if it is not one the nurse would personally choose. The nurse also respects the client's right to change his or her mind at any time.

ENSURING SAFETY

Persons experiencing panic-level anxiety can act impulsively and endanger their safety, for example, by jumping out of a window or running into the street. The nurse remains calm to help the panicky individual reduce the anxiety to a more manageable level. Having only one nurse interact with the client is usually best because responding to multiple sources of stimulation adds to a client's agitation. If the client is extremely unstable, it is wise to avoid touching the person or getting physically close. Intruding within the client's personal space is likely to trigger an increase in anxiety.

Anxiety Disorders

Anxiety disorders are a group of psychobiologic illnesses that result from activation of the sympathetic division of the autonomic nervous system. They tend to be chronic and sometimes appear without any logical explanation. Some examples of anxiety disorders include generalized anxiety disorder, panic disorder, phobic disorders, post-traumatic stress disorder, and obsessive-compulsive disorder (Table 13–2).

Etiology and Pathophysiology

Genetic studies suggest that many anxiety disorders have a familial pattern. This can imply an inherited faulty physiology, maladaptive learning, or acquisition of personality traits modeled after those displayed by significant others.

The symptoms are manifested because the neurotransmitter norepinephrine floods the limbic system

TABLE 13-2 **Anxiety Disorders**

Disorder	Manifestations
Generalized anxiety disorder (GAD)	Tension and worrying out of proportion to the reality of everyday living; signs and symptoms of moderate anxiety.
Panic disorder	Abrupt but recurring symptoms of severe anxiety that arise suddenly and quickly mount to panic level before spontaneously subsiding.
Phobic disorders	Exaggerated fears that cause avoidance of the phobic stimulus. Those with *agoraphobia*, fear of losing control in a public place, may become homebound.
Post-traumatic stress disorder (PTSD)	Psychic reexperience of traumatic event like rape, murder, war tragedies, and natural disasters in nightmares or conscious flashbacks. Many cope by becoming emotionally numb and detaching themselves from social interactions.
Obsessive-compulsive disorder (OCD)	Recurring thoughts that provoke anxiety are temporarily relieved by repeatedly performing some act like checking, counting, cleaning, or washing. Most realize that their actions are illogical.

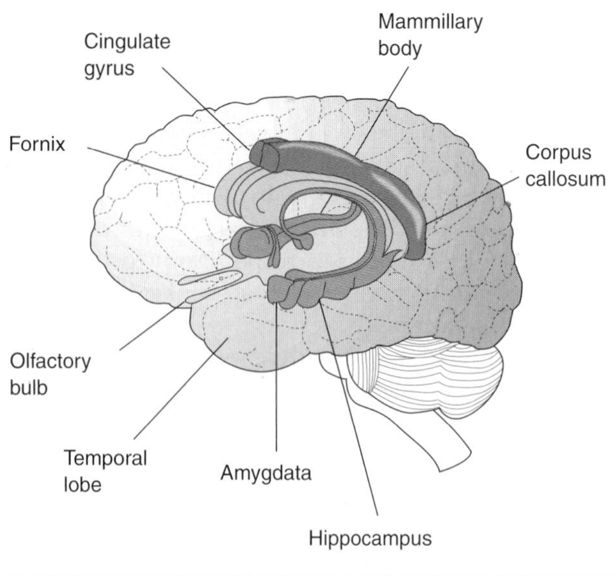

FIGURE 13-2. The limbic system

(Fig. 13–2). The limbic system, which surrounds the brain stem, is a ring of structures made up of lobes of the cortex, the thalamus, the hypothalamus, and others. This complex of neural tissue is a physiologic network for emotions, survival and behavioral responses, motivation, and learning. The biochemical changes brought on by norepinephrine trigger physical arousal in the cortex and the neuroendocrine pathways involving the hypothalamus, pituitary, and adrenal glands.

Other biochemical mechanisms also may contribute to the development of anxiety disorders. A dysregulation of gamma-aminobutyric acid (GABA), a neurotransmitter that should buffer or extinguish the activity of norepinephrine, is one possibility. The second possibility is that serotonin (5-HT) becomes depleted. This would explain why some who have anxiety disorders develop depression or improve when antidepressant drugs are given (see Chap. 14).

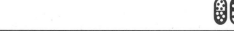

TABLE 13-3 **Drugs Used to Treat Anxiety**

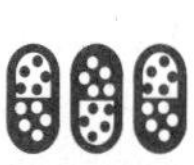

Category of Drug/Example/ Mechanism of Action	Side Effects	Nursing Considerations
Benzodiazepine		
alprazolam (Xanax) Exact mechanism of action is not understood but is thought to increase the inhibitory effects of GABA, making the cells less responsive to norepinephrine	Transient mild drowsiness, sedation, fatigue, lethargy, disorientation, lightheadedness, constipation, diarrhea, nausea, dry mouth, drug dependence	Instruct client to avoid alcohol and other CNS depressants. Warn that effect is increased with cimetidine, disulfiram, omeprazole, valproic acid, and oral contraceptives. Avoid operating machinery or driving. Tell client to report all side effects and to avoid stopping the drug abruptly.
Nonbenzodiazepine axiolytics		
buspirone (BuSpar) Exact mechanism unknown but does bind with serotonin and dopamine receptors	Dizziness; nervousness; insomnia, headache; lightheadedness; dry mouth; abdominal distress; vomiting; palpitations; chest pain; hyperventilation	Instruct client to avoid alcohol and other CNS depressants. Avoid operating machinery or driving. Report side effects. Inform client that frequent small meals and sucking on ice chips will alleviate gastrointestinal disturbances and dry mouth.
Beta-adrenergic blockers		
propranolol hydrochloride (Inderal) Decreases the impact of the sympathetic nervous system by reducing CNS sympathetic outflow and blocking beta adrenergic receptors.	Fatigue, nausea, vomiting, diarrhea, flatulence, constipation, bradycardia, congestive heart failure, arrhythmias, impotence, decreased libido, decreased activity tolerance	Monitor heart rate, blood pressure and postural changes. Avoid alcohol. Review all medication as propranolol can interact with many other drugs. Warn client not to discontinue drug abruptly. Administer with food. Tell client to report all side effects. Warn diabetics that signs and symptoms of hypoglycemia may be obscured by propranolol and to manage blood sugars carefully.
Centrally acting sympatholytics		
clonidine hydrochloride (Catapres) Decreases sympathetic outflow from the CNS and inhibits sympathetic nervous system effects	Drowsiness, sedation, dizziness, constipation, dry mouth, anorexia, impotence, weight gain, weakness; nightmares	Monitor blood pressure and postural changes. Avoid alcohol. Inform client to take as prescribed and not to miss doses or abruptly discontinue. Tell client to report any side effects and that side effects will disappear once drug is discontinued.

CNS, central nervous system; GABA, gamma-aminobutyric acid

Assessment Findings

SIGNS AND SYMPTOMS

Clients seek treatment for symptoms they interpret as cardiovascular, respiratory, or neurologic. Many are concerned about heart palpitations, breathlessness, chronic fatigue, tension headaches, and sleep disturbances. Blood pressure is often elevated and the heart rate is increased. Some acknowledge having unrealistic worries or fears, exaggerated startle reactions, flashbacks of previously traumatic events, avoiding situations that provoke symptoms, and performing ritualistic behaviors.

DIAGNOSTIC FINDINGS

Laboratory blood tests and diagnostic tests like electrocardiography are essentially normal. Positron emission tomography and computed tomography scans have shown abnormal brain utilization of glucose. Magnetic resonance imaging has demonstrated atrophy in some areas of the brain in selected anxiety disorders. However, most clients with anxiety disorders are diagnosed on their symptomatology and history.

Medical Management

The medical management of anxiety disorders includes drug therapy combined with cognitive and behavioral psychotherapy.

DRUG THERAPY

Symptoms of anxiety are relieved by benzodiazepines, such as alprazolam (Xanax); nonbenzodiazepine anxiolytic drugs, such as buspirone (BuSpar); beta-adrenergic blockers, such as propranolol (Inderal); and centrally acting adrenergic inhibitors, such as clonidine (Catapres) (Table 13–3). Certain anxiety disorders such as obsessive-compulsive disorder and agoraphobia seem to improve more readily when treated with antidepressants (see Chap. 14) such as clomipramine (Anafranil), fluvoxamine (Luvox), and paroxetine (Paxil).

The benzodiazepines are sedating and have the potential to be addicting and are generally reserved for short-term therapy. The dosage or frequency of administration is gradually decreased to avoid withdrawal symptoms.

PSYCHOTHERAPY

Psychotherapy involves talking with a psychiatrist, psychologist, or mental health counselor. Some clients respond better when therapy sessions are conducted one on one; others, such as those with post-traumatic stress disorder, respond better to group interactions.

Cognitive Therapy

One type of psychotherapy useful in treating clients with anxiety disorders is cognitive therapy. **Cognitive therapy** is a type of psychotherapy in which the therapist helps clients alter their irrational thinking, correct their faulty belief systems, and replace negative self-statements with positive ones. This therapy is based on the theory that it is not events that provoke anxiety, but the person's interpretation of events. By reshaping a person's viewpoint, the disorder can be minimized or eliminated.

Behavioral Therapy

Behavioral therapy attempts to extinguish undesirable responses by learning other adaptive techniques. One example that is sometimes used with clients who have phobic disorders or obsessive-compulsive disorder is desensitization. **Desensitization** involves providing emotional support while gradually exposing a person to whatever it is that provokes anxiety. If anxiety escalates, the therapist coaches the client to perform relaxation or breathing exercises to overcome symptoms. Eventually, the client can tolerate the anxiety-provoking experience independently by learning methods for eliminating physical and emotional discomfort.

NURSING PROCESS
The Client With Anxiety

Assessment

Observe for evidence of various levels of anxiety: pacing, talking excessively, complaining, crying, being withdrawn, trying to run away. Encourage the client to express anxiety by asking open-ended questions such as "How are you feeling now?" Ask the client to rate his or her anxiety level using a scale from 0 to 10, and to indicate the level at which anxiety is tolerable. Ask the client if he or she has an effective method for controlling anxiety. Assess the client's use of and knowledge about antianxiety medication.

Diagnosis and Planning

Nursing care of the client with anxiety includes but is not limited to the following:

Nursing Diagnoses and Collaborative Problems	Nursing Interventions
Anxiety related to faulty perception of danger **Goal:** The client's anxiety will return to a tolerable level.	Instruct and help the client with mild to moderate anxiety to perform one or more of the following anxiety-reducing measures and to continue tech-

niques until anxiety level is tolerable:

- Counting backward from 100 in groups of three
- Breathing slowly and deeply in through the nose and out the mouth
- Progressively relaxing groups of muscles from the toes up to the head
- Repeating positive statements such as "I am in control," "I am safe," "I am relaxed,"
- Visualizing a pleasant, relaxing place
- Listening to a relaxation audiotape or soothing music

Powerlessness related to feeling helpless in managing symptoms

Goal: The client will affirm the ability to self-control anxiety symptoms.

Suggest the client keep a diary documenting the numbers of times anxiety interferes with activities, techniques used to restore equilibrium, and the length of time symptoms lasted.

Have client review diary to identify techniques that reduce frequency or duration of anxiety.

Recommend that the client say, "Stop," when thoughts of losing control occur.

Reinforce when the client implements anxiety-reducing techniques successfully or independently.

Risk for Ineffective Management of Therapeutic Regimen related to knowledge deficit of drug and dietary modifications

Goal: The client will safely manage his or her own self-care.

Explain the routine for self-administering prescribed drugs.

Emphasize that alcohol and other sedating drugs must be avoided when taking benzodiazepines.

Emphasize compliance with drug therapy although it may take a week or more to feel a beneficial effect.

Advise the client to discuss discontinuing drug therapy with the prescribing physician because abrupt withdrawal may exacerbate anxiety.

Tell the client to avoid caffeine, nicotine, or stimulating drugs such as nonprescription diet pills and some allergy or cold tablets.

Provide information on anxiety self-help groups.

Evaluation and Expected Outcomes

- The client's anxiety level has diminished to a tolerable level on a scale of 0 to 10.
- The client has developed a specific coping technique that works well for him or her.
- The client knows of resources that can provide support or therapy.
- The client is knowledgeable about the therapeutic and adverse effects of antianxiety medication.

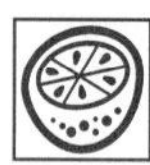

General Nutritional Considerations

Clients with anxiety should avoid caffeine.

Although some clients lose their appetite, others may react to stress by overeating. Assess current weight status and recent weight fluctuations.

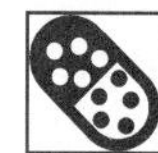

General Pharmacologic Considerations

A complete current medication history is obtained for each client, including nonprescription drugs. Many people who experience anxiety take over-the-counter drugs, stimulants, and tranquilizers that they may not mention unless asked.

Antianxiety drugs such as alprazolam or diazepam are used in the short-term treatment of anxiety. Long-term treatment is not recommended because prolonged use can result in drug dependence.

Antianxiety drugs may cause drowsiness or blurred vision. The client is advised to use caution while driving or performing tasks requiring mental alertness.

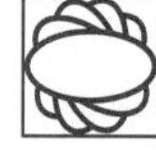

General Gerontologic Considerations

Anxiety in the older adult is caused by feelings of vulnerability and limitations associated with age.

Because most antianxiety agents are excreted by the kidney, older adults with impaired kidney function are at increased risk for toxicity.

Anxiety may be manifested in the older adult as confusion, behavior changes, or withdrawal.

Many older adults on fixed incomes experience financial problems related to housing and medical expenses that can produce anxiety.

Antianxiety drugs may cause short periods of memory impairment that can aggravate an already existing cognitive disorder.

SUMMARY OF KEY CONCEPTS

- Anxiety is a vague uneasy feeling the cause of which is not readily identifiable. Fear is a feeling of terror in response to someone or something specific perceived as dangerous or threatening.
- The four levels of anxiety are mild, moderate, severe, and panic. Mild anxiety is constructive; the other three are destructive. Each level is distinguished by increased intensity in behavioral and physical symptoms.
- When nurses care for anxious clients they focus on building trust, restoring comfort, modifying verbal communication, adjusting teaching strategies, helping with the problem-solving process, and ensuring safety.
- Although experiencing anxiety is normal, some individuals develop pathologic conditions called anxiety disorders. Anxiety disorders are conditions that result from activation of the sympathetic division of the autonomic nervous system. Some examples include generalized anxiety disorder, panic disorder, phobic disorders, post-traumatic stress disorder, and obsessive-compulsive disorder.
- Anxiety disorders are usually treated with drugs that block the effects of norepinephrine. Some of these include anxiolytics from the benzodiazepine and nonbenzodiazepine families, beta-adrenergic blockers, and centrally acting antiadrenergics. However, some anxiety disorders (eg, obsessive-compulsive disorder) respond well to antidepressant drug therapy.
- Drug therapy is combined with psychotherapy when treating clients with anxiety disorders. Two commonly used techniques are cognitive therapy and behavioral therapy. The former helps clients alter their irrational thinking, correct their faulty belief systems, and replace negative with positive self-statements. The latter helps extinguish undesirable anxiety responses by learning other adaptive techniques.
- Nurses can help clients reduce anxiety by using distraction, deep breathing exercises, progressive muscle relaxation, positive self-statements, visualization, and music.
- Clients taking antianxiety medication are taught to take drugs as prescribed and to avoid using alcohol or other nonprescribed sedative drugs.
- Nurses teach clients to eliminate stimulating chemicals in food, beverages, tobacco products, and over-the-counter drugs.
- The nurse suggests joining a self-help group.

CRITICAL THINKING EXERCISES

1. Discuss nursing interventions that would be appropriate when a client tells you that she feels anxious about her upcoming surgery.
2. Explain how you would approach teaching an anxious client about his or her discharge instructions.

Suggested Readings

Armstrong, M. A., & Rose, P. (1997). Group therapy for partners of combat veterans with post-traumatic stress disorder. *Perspectives on Psychiatric Care, 33*(4), 14–18.

Benham, E. (1995). Coping strategies: A psychoeducational approach to post-traumatic symptomatology. *Journal of Psychosocial Nursing and Mental Health Services, 33*(6), 30–35.

Blair, D. T., & Ramones, V. A. (1996). The undertreatment of anxiety: Overcoming the confusion and stigma. *Journal of Psychosocial Nursing and Mental Health Services, 34*(6), 9–18.

Cadieux, R. J. (1996). Recognizing and treating persistent anxiety in a stressful world. *Women's Health Digest, 2*(4), 272–275.

Chez, N. (1994). Helping the victim of domestic violence. *American Journal of Nursing, 94*(7), 32–37.

Clark, C. C. (1997). Post-traumatic stress disorder: How to support healing. *American Journal of Nursing, 97*(8), 26–32.

Dossey, B. (1996). Help your patient break free from anxiety. *Nursing, 26*(10), 52–54.

Roye, C. F., & Coonan, P. R. (1997). Emergency! Adolescent rape. *American Journal of Nursing, 97*(4), 45.

Valent, S. M. (1996). Diagnosis and treatment of panic disorder and generalized anxiety in primary care. *Nurse Practitioner: American Journal of Primary Health Care, 21*(8), 26, 32–34, 37–38.

Vallone, D. C. (1997). Antidepressants and antiolytics. *RN, 60*(7), 27–32.

Additional Resources

Anxiety Disorders Association of America
6000 Executive Boulevard
Suite 513
Rockville, MD 20852
(301) 231–9350
E-mail: anxdis@aol.com

Council on Anxiety Disorders
Route 1, Box 1364
Clarkesville, GA 30523
(910) 722–7760
E-mail: xjrg06@aol.com

Phobics Anonymous
P.O. Box 1180
Palm Springs, CA 92263
(619) 322-COPE

Panic Disorder Information Line
National Institute of Mental Health
5600 Fishers Lane
Room 7C-02
Rockville, MD 20857
(800) 647–2642

Mental Health Net
http://www.cmhc.com/

Internet Mental Health
http://www.mentalhealth.com/p1.html

Recovery, Inc.
802 Dearborn Street
Chicago, IL 60610
(312) 337–5661

Chapter 14

Caring for Clients With Mood Disorders

KEY TERMS

- Affect
- Bipolar disorder
- Cyclothymia
- Dysthmia
- Electroconvulsive therapy
- Euthymia
- Major (unipolar) depression
- Mania
- Monoamine hypothesis
- Mood
- Neurobiologic theory
- Norepinephrine
- Reactive (secondary) depression
- Serotonin

LEARNING OBJECTIVES

On completion of this chapter, the reader will:

- Discuss the signs and symptoms of mood disorders.
- Explain the neurobiologic theory as it applies to mood disorders.
- Name three neurotransmitters that, when imbalanced, affect mood.
- Identify types of drugs that are used to treat mood disorders and nursing considerations that apply to their administration.
- Give three criteria that are characteristics of a high risk for suicide.
- Discuss nursing measures that are useful in preventing suicide.
- Discuss the nursing management of clients with common mood disorders.

The term **mood** refers to a person's overall feeling state and may be thought of as a continuum with extremes of emotion existing at either end or pole (Fig. 14–1). Mood is displayed in a person's **affect,** the verbal and nonverbal behavior that communicates feelings (Box 14–1).

People with normal moods are referred to as **euthymic;** they are capable of experiencing a variety of feelings, all of which are situationally appropriate. Individuals with *mood disorders* experience a persistent, extreme mood or severe, unpredictable mood swings that interfere with social relationships. The primary mood disturbances include major (unipolar) depression and bipolar disorder, formerly called manic-depressive syndrome. **Dysthymia,** a feeling of unremitting sadness, is similar to major depression but is less severe. **Cyclothymia,** a swing back and forth in sad and elated moods, resembles bipolar disorder, but the extremes of mood are not as pronounced. **Mania** refers to the frenzied state of euphoria exhibited by persons during the manic phase of bipolar disorder. *Seasonal affective disorder* (SAD) is a mood disorder characterized by depressive feelings that develop during darker winter months and then disappear in the spring.

Brain function, and consequently, mood depends on the dynamic interplay of neurotransmitters (see Chap. 11). The **neurobiologic theory** postulates that biochemical dysregulation alters the brain's physiology and causes mood disorders and neurologic problems. Decreased or excessive amounts of neurotransmitters, receptor sensitivity, or impaired regulation of neurotransmitters are all thought to play a role in mood disorders (Abrams, 1995). Drug therapy is aimed at either enhancing or inhibiting these processes.

While research continues to investigate what causes the imbalance in neurotransmitters, other possible factors in mood disorders include genetic predisposition, electrolyte imbalance, loss of significant others, habitual negative thought patterns, environmental stressors, and endocrine imbalances involving the hypothalamus, pituitary, adrenal cortex, and thyroid.

Major Depression

Everyone experiences depression at some time in his or her life. In the majority of cases, transient depression is a normal reaction to loss, such as the death of a loved one; disappointment, such as being fired from a job; or

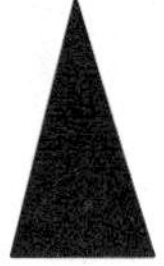

FIGURE 14-1. Mood continuum.

overwhelming events, like being heavily in debt. When feeling sad can be directly attributed to a situation or cause, it is referred to as **reactive** or **secondary depression.** Generally, reactive depression is self-limiting; when circumstances change or there is help from supportive others, depression is relieved. Nevertheless, many people experience **major** or **unipolar depression**, a sad mood for which there is no obvious relationship to situational events. Over 8 million Americans experience unexplained feelings of depression.

Etiology and Pathophysiology

The most widely accepted neurobiologic theory for depression is the **monoamine hypothesis,** which postulates that depression is the result of a deficiency of one or more of the monoamine neurotransmitters—**serotonin, norepinephrine,** and dopamine. Other theories suggest that infantile rejection or neglect, learned feelings of helplessness, chronic exposure to discrimination, or distorted or false perceptions about oneself are implicated in the development of depression.

BOX 14-1 Examples of Mood and Affect

Mood	Affect
happy	smile brisk walk attentive to appearance positive attitude cooperative creative gregarious
depressed	gloomy inactive neglectful of appearance empty feeling no initiative insensitive to others' feelings isolative

Assessment Findings

SIGNS AND SYMPTOMS

The predominant feature of major depression is a persistent sad mood accompanied by multiple physiologic and cognitive (thought) changes represented by the acronym SAD IMAGES (Box 14–2). Because the manifestations of depression may be similar to those of other conditions (Box 14–3), the diagnosis is made while simultaneously investigating and eliminating alternative reasons for the clinical findings.

DIAGNOSTIC FINDINGS

Studies that identify metabolites of serotonin and norepinephrine in urine and cerebrospinal fluid are financially prohibitive. A dexamethasone suppression test (DST), which theoretically indicates major depression when there is failure to suppress the release of cortisol after an oral dose of dexamethasone, may be ordered, although its usefulness is controversial. Laboratory tests such as thyroid function analysis and drug screening may be done to detect underlying conditions.

Medical Management

Two of the most commonly used treatments for depression are drug therapy and, in severe cases, electroconvulsive therapy (ECT).

BOX 14-2 Signs and Symptoms of Major Depression

S ad mood
A ppetite change; increased or decreased
D isturbed sleep; insomnia or hypersomnia

I nability to concentrate
M arked decrease in pleasure
A pathy, including disinterest in sex
G uilty feelings
E nergy changes; restlessness or inactivity
S uicidal thoughts

BOX 14-3 Conditions That Mimic Depression

- Hypothyroidism
- Brain tumor
- Alcohol or sedative abuse
- Stimulant withdrawal
- Chronic hypoxia
- Side effects of drug therapy such as corticosteroids, antihypertensives such as reserpine (Reserfia), methyldopa (Aldomet), propranolol (Inderal)

ANTIDEPRESSANT DRUG THERAPY

The three main categories of drugs that relieve the symptoms of depression are tricyclic antidepressants (TCAs), monoamine oxidase inhibitors (MAOIs), and selective serotonin reuptake inhibitors (SSRIs) (Table 14–1). All antidepressants, regardless of the category, increase or potentiate serotonin. Some TCAs and all MAOIs also increase levels of norepinephrine. Because norepinephrine is a stimulant, increasing it is often desirable for depressed clients who lack energy and tend to sleep a lot.

Pharmacotherapy is not without its concerns, however. Therapeutic levels and, therefore, symptom relief, may not be evident for 2 weeks with SSRIs and may take as long as 6 weeks with TCAs. Paradoxically, suicide risk increases just as antidepressants begin to take effect because the still-depressed client may now have the energy to carry out his or her plan. MAOIs can produce a potentially fatal hypertensive crisis when combined with certain foods and drugs (Box 14–4) and careful client education must occur.

TABLE 14-1 **Antidepressant Drug Therapy**

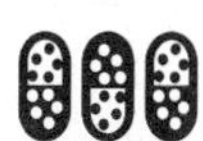

Drug Category and Mechanism of Action	Side Effects	Nursing Considerations
Tricyclic Antidepressants		
amitriptyline (Elavil) nortriptyline (Pamelor) imipramine (Tofranil) Block the reuptake of serotonin and norepinephrine	Orthostatic hypotension, sedation, dry mouth, blurred vision, weight gain, constipation, urinary retention	Inform client that symptomatic relief may not occur for 2–6 weeks. Caution to rise slowly from a lying or sitting position. Inform client that blurred vision and dry mouth will decrease over time. Discuss the increased potential for suicide as energy increases before depression resolves. Discontinue gradually.
Monoamine Oxidase Inhibitors		
phenelzine (Nardil) tranylcypromine (Parnate) Block the enzyme that breaks down monoamines	Headache, insomnia, severe hypertension with certain foods and drugs, orthostatic hypotension, transient impotence, constipation or diarrhea, dry mouth, blurred vision	Provide information on diet and drug restrictions to avoid hypertensive crisis. Advise wearing a Medic-Alert bracelet. Educate client about lethal interaction with demerol. Explain that there may be a 2–6 week delay before symptoms improve. Take last dose before bedtime to avoid sleep disturbances. Allow at least a 14-day interval between discontinuing TCA and initiating an MAOI.
Selective Serotonin Reuptake Inhibitors		
fluoxetine (Prozac) sertraline (Zoloft) paroxetine (Paxil) Block the reuptake of serotonin but not norepinephrine	Weight loss, insomnia, tremor, nervousness, headache, decreased libido, impotence, interference with liver enzymes that potentiates the risk for altered metabolism of other drugs	Instruct to avoid caffeine and other foods or drugs that are cardiac stimulants. Monitor blood pressure and heart rate. Allow at least 14 days before switching to an MAOI. Monitor for central serotonin syndrome (confusion, agitation, sweating, increased reflexes, shivering incoordination, fever) which can result from a drug-drug interaction.

BOX 14-4 MAOI Food, Beverage, and Drug Restrictions

Food and Beverages to Avoid

Aged, hard cheese	Pepperoni, sausage
Chocolate	Sour cream
Pickled herring	Broad beans (fava beans)
Overripe bananas	Monosodium glutamate
Chicken liver	Beer
Dried fish	Soy sauce
Fermented meat (salami)	Red wine
Yogurt	Meat tenderizer

Drugs to Avoid

Cold and allergy medications	Meperidine (Demerol)
Appetite suppressants	Antidepressants in other categories
Antiasthmatics	Local anesthetics with epinephrine
Antihypertensives	

Signs and symptoms of hypertensive crisis include:

- Headache
- Nausea
- Vomiting
- Sweating
- Palpitations
- Visual changes
- Neck stiffness
- Sensitivity to light
- Tachycardia

Antidepressant selection is based on the client's symptoms and the drug's potential side effects. The SSRIs are becoming more popular because they are not as lethal as the TCAs if the client overdoses, produce fewer side effects, and do not require dietary and drug restrictions like the MAOIs. Antidepressants with different mechanisms of action may be combined to achieve a greater therapeutic effect and it is not unusual for some clients to respond better to a drug in one category rather than another, or to another drug in the same category. Lithium, a mood-stabilizing drug (discussed later), or a thyroid hormone may be added. If the client's mood has not improved after a reasonable trial of 6 weeks on a particular regimen, a different one may be prescribed.

ELECTROCONVULSIVE THERAPY

Electroconvulsive therapy (ECT) uses the application of an electric stimulus to the temporal region of the head to produce a brief, generalized seizure. Although the exact mechanism of action is unknown, the belief is that ECT achieves its effect by either increasing circulating levels of monoamine neurotransmitters or by improving transmission to the receptor site.

Electroconvulsive therapy is generally reserved for depressed clients who:

- Have not responded to drug therapy
- Are intolerant to the side effects of antidepressant medications
- Are so seriously suicidal that their safety is jeopardized by waiting for antidepressants to become effective

Except for clients who are extremely suicidal, ECT can be administered on an ambulatory, outpatient basis (Nursing Guidelines 14–1). Many clients experience af-

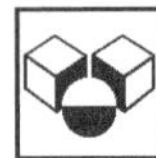

Nursing Guidelines 14-1

Managing the Care of a Client Undergoing Electroconvulsive Therapy (ECT)

Pretreatment Responsibilities

- Keep the client in a fasting state for 8 to 12 hours before ECT.
- Check that the client has signed a consent form for ECT.
- Confirm that anticonvulsant drugs have been discontinued so as to ensure a therapeutic seizure.
- Give the client an opportunity to verbalize fears or questions.
- Collaborate with those responsible for performing a venipuncture to initiate the administration of intravenous fluid and provide access for intravenous medications.
- Complete the presurgical checklist (see Chap. 24).
- Administer pretreatment medications such as atropine sulfate or glycopyrrolate (Robinul).

Post-ECT Care

- Monitor vital signs at frequent regular intervals.
- Position the client laterally to prevent aspiration.
- Keep the client oxygenated per mask or nasal cannula.
- Suction the airway if necessary.
- Orient the client to person, place, and time.
- Administer prescribed analgesia for headache or muscle aches.
- Reorient and repeat information at intervals to compensate for the temporary memory loss and confusion.
- Acknowledge the client's frustration with memory loss, and explain that the deficit is usually temporary.
- Offer food and fluids as the client is able to tolerate them.
- Discontinue fluid therapy as ordered or flush medication lock to ensure future use.
- Keep environmental stimuli to a minimum until the client is capable of processing information accurately.

tereffects including headache, soreness of skeletal muscles, temporary confusion, short-term patchy memory loss, and brief learning disability. ECT is usually contraindicated for clients with cardiac or neurovascular pathologies.

Nursing Management

Nursing responsibilities when caring for a depressed client include ensuring the safety of suicidal clients, assisting clients who neglect their basic needs, administering antidepressant therapy, preparing and recovering clients who receive ECT, and teaching clients skills and strategies that will promote their safe self-care after discharge.

SUICIDE PREVENTION

If a client is depressed, assume that he or she may also be suicidal. One of the most reliable suicide assessment techniques is to bluntly ask, "Do you feel like killing yourself?" Unfortunately, some depressed clients conceal their suicidal thoughts, provide only vague verbal or behavior clues (Box 14–5), or assume that others are aware of their despair but have chosen to ignore it.

If a client admits to being suicidal, determine whether or not he or she has a plan. Having a plan increases the seriousness of the risk. Assess if the plan is feasible and whether it is one that is considered of high or low lethality. *High lethality methods* are those from which the possibility of rescue is remote. Some examples include shooting oneself, hanging, jumping from a bridge or building, throwing oneself in front of a train or truck, driving into a tree, wall, or off a cliff. *Low lethality methods* are those that allow a window of time in which the suicidal person may be found and rescued. Low lethality methods include overdosing on medications, cutting the wrists, or inhaling carbon monoxide.

In almost all cases, people who are suicidal are ambivalent—they would choose life rather than death if they held some hope for the future. Despite conscientious efforts to prevent suicide, some individuals cannot be stopped.

Nursing care of the suicidal client includes, but is not limited to, the following:

Nursing Diagnoses and Collaborative Problems	Nursing Interventions
Risk for Self-Directed Violence related to feelings of hopelessness **Goal:** The client will not harm self; the client will identify a reason for living.	Move the client close to the nursing station. If the client is not hospitalized, encourage the person to not remain alone, or talk to the client as long as possible on the phone while contacting a 911 operator. Make a verbal or written contract with the client that he or she will not attempt suicide. Clients often honor their commitment. Confiscate any objects that may be used for self-harm, such as belts, shoelaces, safety razors, sharp combs or keys, knives, etc. Observe the client's whereabouts at least every 15 minutes, and spend time interacting with the client. Keep the client busy and involved in activities.
Ineffective Individual Coping related to feelings of helplessness and worthlessness **Goal:** The client will identify one or more alternatives to suicide.	Acknowledge the client's feeling of despair and indicate that you want to help but do not make promises you cannot keep. Emphasize hope and previous positive experiences and outcomes. Explore other courses of action rather than suicide to appeal to the desire to live. Discuss previous coping strategies and encourage using some that were effective in the past.

BOX 14-5 Clues of Suicidal Intentions

Clear Verbal Clues

"I'm planning to kill myself."
"I wish I were dead."

Vague Verbal Clues

"I just can't stand it any longer."
"Nobody needs me anymore."
"Life has lost its meaning for me."
"You won't be seeing me anymore."
"I'm getting out."
"Everybody would be better off without me."

Behavioral Clues

Giving away a valued possession
Donating large sums of money to charity
Putting personal affairs in order
Writing poetry with morbid themes
Composing a suicide note
Making funeral arrangements
Buying a gun; stockpiling pills
Lifting of depressed mood (may indicate a plan and energy to carry it out)

	Develop a plan for maintaining safety in the future such as talking with a trusted friend or calling a crisis hotline.

BASIC NEEDS

Depressed clients may not eat, bathe, shave, shampoo or style their hair. In some cases, self-care is neglected due to lack of energy. Cleanliness and grooming also may be ignored because depressed clients have low self-esteem and little concern for social acceptance.

Nursing management of depressed clients includes, but is not limited to, the following:

Nursing Diagnoses and Collaborative Problems	Nursing Interventions
Self-Care Deficit: Bathing/Hygiene/Grooming related to lack of motivation	Break hygiene into small tasks that may be completed a few at a time.
Goal: The client will bathe, perform oral hygiene, and care for hair independently.	Collaborate on a deadline for completing bathing, hygiene, and grooming.
	Acknowledge accomplishments when the client meets a goal; efforts that are positively reinforced are more likely to be repeated.
	Assist the client when deadlines expire, but do so without commenting on the client's inaction. Criticism reinforces low self-esteem.
Altered Nutrition: Less than Body Requirements related to anorexia	Monitor food intake at each meal.
Goal: The client's weight will be maintained within ±2 lb.	Provide nutritional supplements such as Ensure, Enrich, or Sustecal between meals and at bedtime.
	Develop a list of preferred foods and arrange to have a variety from which the client can snack.
Sleep Pattern Disturbance related to depression	Keep the client busy during the day and discourage from napping or going to bed early.
Goal: The client will sleep a maximum of 8 hours, but only at night.	Include forms of active exercise during the day, but not before bedtime.

CLIENT AND FAMILY TEACHING

Before being discharged, the nurse teaches the client about common side effects of medication and how to manage or minimize them, provides information on drug–drug and drug–food interactions, and describes the signs and symptoms of hypertensive crisis. The nurse emphasizes avoiding alcohol, not only because it increases sedation but even more so because alcohol interferes with judgment and may contribute to acting on suicidal ideas. If periodic laboratory tests are necessary, the nurse informs the client when and where to schedule them. The nurse also provides the client with resources for postdischarge care such as an appointment with a psychiatrist or mental health counselor, referral to support groups, or a telephone number where emergency psychiatric assistance is available at any time. Finally, the nurse teaches family members to take the following steps:

- Keep the lines of communication open.
- Support the client in his or her coping strategies.
- Monitor and report the return of severely depressed symptoms.
- Eliminate potential means for suicide such as a household gun.

Bipolar Disorder

Bipolar disorder is characterized by cycling between depression, euthymia, and euphoria. Some individuals experience a mild manic phase, referred to as *hypomania*; others, known as rapid cyclers, experience at least four episodes of mania and depression a year.

Etiology and Pathophysiology

Extremes in levels of norepinephrine—excessive in mania and inadequate during depression—seem to be responsible for the symptoms of bipolar disorder. In severe cases, excess dopamine may cause distorted thinking and hallucinations. Genetic predisposition is also implicated in the development of bipolar disorder.

Assessment Findings

SIGNS AND SYMPTOMS

Signs and symptoms of the depressive phase of bipolar disorder are the same as those for major depression. During the manic phase, clients are hyperactive and often display an exaggerated sense of their own importance. They can quickly become angry and aggressive with those who attempt to restrain their burst of energy and wild ideas. Because judgment is impaired—another characteristic of the disorder—reckless and impulsive behavior like sexual promiscuity, criminal activity, spending sprees, gambling, and risky business transactions can occur. The surge of norepinephrine allows manic-phase bipolars to go without sleep for long periods of time, and causes rapid thinking that is displayed by racing speech. When extremely ill, some individuals experience psychotic features such as hallucinations. Combined with their *delusions*, which are illogically false beliefs, the client with bipolar disorder can be homicidal or suicidal.

DIAGNOSTIC FINDINGS

It may eventually be possible to predict who will develop bipolar disorder with the use of gene mapping. However, at the present time there are no objective tests and the diagnosis is made on the basis of the client's history. The key indicator is the client's description of a pattern of emotional "highs" and "lows." A family member with bipolar disorder is a risk factor as is a history of substance abuse, because undiagnosed individuals naively attempt to self-medicate to relieve the depressive episodes.

Medical Management

Bipolar disorder is managed by the administration of one or more mood-stabilizing medications (Table 14–2). Lithium (Eskalith, Lithane, Lithobid), a chemical element, is usually the initial drug of choice. However, lithium:

- May be ineffective for some
- Has a delay of 5 to 14 days in achieving therapeutic benefits
- Has a narrow range of safety between a therapeutic serum level (0.8–1.2 mEq) and toxic level (1.5 mEq),

TABLE 14-2 **Mood-Stabilizing Medications** 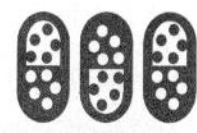

Drug Example and Mechanism of Action	Side Effects	Nursing Considerations
Lithium carbonate (Eskalith, Lithane, Lithobid) Alters sodium transport in nerve and muscle cells, increases intraneural stores and inhibits release of norepinephrine and dopamine	Hand tremors, nausea, vomiting, diarrhea, thirst, polyuria, sedation, thyroid dysfunction, wrist and ankle edema at therapeutic level	Administer with meals. Withhold if serum level is > 1.5 mEq. Female clients should use contraception and avoid breast-feeding.
valproic acid (Depakote) May increase levels of gamma-aminobutyric acid	Drowsiness, mild tremor, ataxia, nausea, vomiting, diarrhea, blood dyscrasias, liver toxicity	Administer with meals. Caution to avoid activities that require alertness and coordination. Monitor blood for therapeutic level.
carbamazepine (Tegretol) Decreases rate of neuronal impulse transmission	Dizziness, drowsiness, unsteady gait, nausea, vomiting, fluid retention, edema, blood dyscrasias, skin rash, liver toxicity	Administer with meals. Caution to avoid activities that require alertness and coordination. Increased risk of central nervous system toxicity when given with lithium. Increased risk of liver toxicity when given with monoamine oxidase inhibitor. Monitor blood for therapeutic levels. Female clients should use contraceptives at all times.
clonazapam (Klonopin) May increase brain levels of GABA	Drowsiness, dizziness, unsteady gait, nausea, vomitting, constipation, blood dyscrasias, dry mouth, liver toxicity	Collaborate with the physician on baseline bood tests before initiating therapy. Administer drug with food or milk. Drowsiness may be potentiated if combined with alcohol or other sedative drugs. Monitor lab findings during therapy and withhold drug if there is bone marrow suppression or serious elevation in liver enzymes. Advise sucking on hard candy or more frequent oral hygiene to relieve dry mouth. Advise females that there is an increased incidence of birth defects if taken during pregnancy, and to use a reliable contraceptive while taking this drug. Never discontinue the drug abruptly.

- May be nontherapeutic or dangerously elevated when taken in combination with other drugs (Box 14–6)
- Causes side effects that challenge compliance
- Requires periodic laboratory tests to monitor serum blood levels

The American Psychiatric Association's Practice Guideline for the Treatment of Bipolar Disorder (1994) now recommends the use of anticonvulsants such as valproic acid derivatives (Depakote, Depakene, Valproate), and others such as carbamazepine (Tegretol), alone or in combination with lithium, for controlling mood swings. Antipsychotics such as haloperidol (Haldol) (see Chap. 17) may also be prescribed for a brief period to induce sedation and control hallucinations and delusional thinking.

Nursing Management

During an acute manic phase, the nurse keeps the client and others safe, assists the client to process information accurately, and ensures that the client's basic needs are met (Nursing Care Plan 14–1).

Before mood-stabilizing drugs are administered, the nurse obtains medical orders for baseline laboratory tests and initiates those referrals. Once drug therapy commences, the nurse administers medications as prescribed, observes for and collaborates with the physician in relieving side effects, and monitors drug levels as reported by laboratory analysis.

CLIENT AND FAMILY TEACHING

Before being discharged, the client and his or her significant others are educated on these aspects:

- The disease process
- How prescribed drugs help in symptom management
- Drug effects and side effects
- Signs of drug toxicity and actions to take
- Frequency of blood tests
- The advantages of wearing a Medic-Alert bracelet

In addition to arranging outpatient therapy, the nurse informs the client and others of support groups that can continue the educational and therapeutic processes. Both the client and those who live in the same environment need to understand the signs of relapse, such as an inability to sleep for several days in a row or increasingly impulsive behavior such as making unnecessary purchases. The nurse also reviews the signs of cycling into a depressed mood so that indications for reinitiating medical care are clear.

BOX 14-6 Drugs Affecting Serum Lithium Levels

Increase Serum Lithium Level	Decrease Serum Lithium Level
tetracycline	theophylline
thiazide diuretics	aminophylline
nonsteroidal anti-inflammatory drugs (NSAIDs)	carbamazepine
haloperidol	sodium bicarbonate
	osmotic diuretics

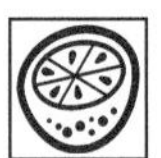

General Nutritional Considerations

Tryptophan, tyrosine, and phenylalanine are known as aromatic amino acids. Tryptophan is a precursor of the neurotransmitter serotonin; tyrosine and phenylalanine are nutritional building blocks of the neurotransmitters dopamine and norepinephrine. Food intake can increase brain levels of tryptophan and tyrosine and the speed with which they are converted to neurotransmitters.

Some studies indicate that a high-carbohydrate, low-protein meal or snack alters neurotransmitter levels in the brain and thus affects mood. Insulin secreted by the pancreas in response to eating causes most amino acids to leave the blood and enter muscle cells. Tryptophan is the exception; with the decrease in blood concentration of other competitive amino acids, tryptophan is readily transported across the blood–brain barrier and floods the brain, which converts it to serotonin. Carbohydrate-generated serotonin may promote calmness, fatigue, or sleepiness. However, in depressed people, a high carbohydrate load may elevate mood. (Starchy meals or snacks that contain significant amounts of protein provide enough competing amino acids to inhibit the brain's uptake of tryptophan and the subsequent production of serotonin.)

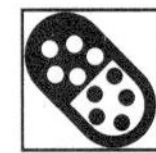

General Pharmacologic Considerations

Pregnant women should always consult with their obstetrician before taking any medication. Lithium and the MAOIs are especially hazardous to the fetus.

Lithium is excreted in breast milk as well as other body fluids. Therefore, there is a potential for lithium toxicity in breast-fed infants whose mothers take lithium.

Dietary and drug restrictions must be continued for 2 weeks after the discontinuation of an MAOI to avoid a hypertensive episode.

The nurse must monitor for signs and symptoms of lithium toxicity: diarrhea, vomiting, nausea, drowsiness, muscular weakness, twitching, and lack of coordination.

NURSING CARE PLAN 14-1

Managing the Care of a Client with Bipolar Disorder/Acute Manic Phase

Potential Problems and Nursing Diagnoses	Nursing Management	Outcome Criteria
Altered Thought Processes related to excessive levels of norepinephrine and dopamine	Orient client to person, place, time, and events. Provide information in small amounts using brief sentences. Reduce distracting stimuli such as noise and activity. Present reality when client is delusional; do not press the issue if it causes agitation. Monitor whereabouts to ensure that the client does not wander from the unit or health care agency.	Is oriented and has an accurate perception of circumstances surrounding admission
Risk for Violence Self-Directed or Directed at Others related to impulsivity and diminished ability to process information accurately	Take client to room or other secluded area when there are signs of aggression. Set firm limits for behavioral expectations using a modulated and controlled tone of voice. Offer the client a large muscle activity like playing basketball to reduce anger and excess energy. Administer prescribed short-acting sedative if aggressive behavior escalates and others are endangered. Obtain a medical order to seclude or restrain if the client becomes violent. Initiate suicidal precautions if data suggests vulnerability for self-harm.	No injuries to self or others
Risk for Altered Nutrition: Less than Body Requirements related to increased activity and distraction from eating	Consult dietitian about increasing calories at meal times. Offer liquid nutritional supplements three times a day. Provide finger foods that may be consumed throughout the day.	Maintains admission weight
Risk for Fluid Volume Deficit related to polyuria secondary to lithium therapy and inattention to thirst	Monitor intake and output. Offer at least 2.5 to 3 quarts of liquid per day. Observe for dry oral mucosa. Monitor electrolyte values.	Well hydrated as evidenced by moist mucous membranes.
Sleep Pattern Disturbance related to hyperaroused state	Administer mood-stabilizing drug therapy, which may induce drowsiness. Schedule rest periods each hour even if the client does not sleep. Direct to bed at acceptable hour for sleep at night. Do not disturb sleep once it occurs.	Sleeps at least 6 hours within a 24-hour period
Self-Care Deficit: Bathing, Hygiene, Grooming related to decreased attention and concentration	Prepare necessities for bathing, grooming and hygiene for the client. Supervise hygiene and provide assistance if needed. Spread uncompleted tasks throughout the remainder of the day. Help client to dress appropriately and remain dressed.	Is clean and groomed on a daily basis

Polyuria can occur with administration of lithium. Unless contraindicated due to disease condition, an increase in fluids up to 3,000 mL/d may be required to maintain fluid balance.

Some antidepressants, particularly TCAs, may trigger a manic phase in individuals with bipolar disorder.

Complaints of a headache (especially an occipital headache) may indicate a hypertensive crisis in those receiving MAOIs and should be reported to the health care provider immediately.

Drugs used to treat depression require 3 to 4 weeks before a therapeutic effect is seen. Therefore, it is critical to monitor the client closely for the first month of therapy, especially if the client has suicidal tendencies.

Caution the patient to avoid alcohol and other central nervous system depressants while taking any of the psychotropic drugs.

The patient taking valproic acid (Depakote, depakene) must be monitored closely for hepatotoxicity periodically during therapy. Frequent liver function tests and serum ammonia concentrations may be ordered.

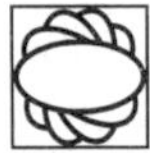

General Gerontologic Considerations

Impaired regulation of neurotransmitters in the elderly suggests that older adults may be biologically predisposed to depression and thought disorders.

Cognitive impairment in the depressed older adult can be easily confused with dementia. It is important to distinguish between the two because depression in the elderly can usually be treated successfully.

When lithium is used to treat bipolar disorder in the elderly, it must be carefully monitored. Because the drug is eliminated by the kidney, age-related changes in the elderly may reduce renal clearance, predisposing these clients to lithium toxicity.

In older adults psychotropic drugs are prescribed at the lowest possible drug dosage that will produce a therapeutic effect due to the potential for increased adverse reactions and possible toxicity.

There is an increased risk of orthostatic hypotension in the elderly from psychotropic drugs because of a decrease in function of the blood pressure-regulating mechanism in the older adult.

Older adults may require longer (up to 8 weeks) to obtain a therapeutic effect when taking antidepressants for depression.

Antidepressants must be used cautiously in older adults with cardiovascular disease. Older men with prostatic enlargement may be more susceptible to urinary retention.

Older adults who seek treatment for subacute physical symptoms, such as loss of appetite, trouble sleeping, lack of energy, and weight loss, may actually be depressed.

The losses that accompany aging and chronic or terminal illness may trigger feelings of hopelessness, which increase the risk for suicide.

The rate of suicide is highest among older adults; it is 50% higher than in other age groups (Klebanoff & Smith, 1997). Older adults who are depressed often use a lethal means to ensure successful suicide.

As individuals with bipolar disorder age, their depressive episodes may increase in frequency and last longer.

SUMMARY OF KEY CONCEPTS

- Individuals with major depression experience a predominant mood of sadness.
- Individuals with bipolar depression experience both depressive and manic episodes.
- It is now thought that mood disorders develop when there is an imbalance of neurotransmitters known as monoamines.
- The major monoamines that are associated with mood disorders are serotonin and norepinephrine, and to a lesser extent dopamine.
- Mood disorders are diagnosed primarily on the basis of signs and symptoms, family history, and elimination of other diseases and disorders.
- The symptoms of mood disorders can be relieved with antidepressant agents and mood-stabilizing drugs or electroconvulsive therapy (ECT), which theoretically affects levels of neurotransmitters.
- The three primary categories of antidepressants are tricyclics (TCAs), monoamine oxidase inhibitors (MAOIs), and selective serotonin reuptake inhibitors (SSRIs).
- Achieving the therapeutic effect from antidepressants may take from 2 to 6 weeks once treatment is begun.
- Clients who take MAOIs must adhere to dietary and drug restrictions to avoid a hypertensive crisis.
- The therapeutic range of lithium is very close to toxic range.
- Electroconvulsive therapy is useful for relieving the depression of extremely suicidal clients, those who do not respond to antidepressants, and those who cannot tolerate antidepressant side effects.
- People with mood disorders are often suicidal.
- Suicide, in most, but not all cases, is preventable.
- Suicidal clients tend to give verbal and behavioral clues of their intentions; however, some of these clues may be quite subtle.
- The best method for assessing suicide potential is to ask the client directly.
- The potential for suicide increases when a person has a plan, when the plan includes a highly lethal method, and when it is feasible that the client could carry out the plan.
- The risk for suicide increases when antidepressant drugs begin to produce therapeutic effects; at that time, depressed clients may have the energy to act on their suicidal ideas.
- Nurses plan measures for ensuring that clients with mood disorders and those in the immediate environment are protected from self-destructive and violent acts.

- One of the chief nursing responsibilities when managing the care of clients with mood disorders is to provide health teaching about the disease and, in most cases, the need for life-long drug therapy.

CRITICAL THINKING EXERCISES

1. There are two depressed clients. One feels suicidal, but has no plan for carrying it out. The other indicates that he would kill himself with a gun, but has none. Describe the similarities and differences in their nursing care.
2. What physical consequences might occur for the client in a manic episode?
3. What problems might family members experience as a result of living with a person with a mood disorder?

Suggested Readings

Abrams, A. C. (1995). *Clinical drug therapy* (4th ed.). Philadelphia: J. B. Lippincott.

American Psychiatric Association. (1994). Practice guideline for the treatment of patients with bipolar disorder. *American Journal of Psychiatry, 151*(12s), iii–36.

Badger, J. (1995). Reaching out to the suicidal patient. *American Journal of Nursing*, 95(3), 24–31.

Cerrato, P. (1992). Pasta: The perfect pick-me-up? *RN, 55*(5), 79–82.

Fernstrom, J. (1994). Dietary amino acids and brain function. *Journal of American Dietetic Association, 94*(1), 71–77.

Klebanoff, N. A., & Smith, N. M. (1998). *Behavior management in home care.* Philadelphia: Lippincott-Raven.

Lippincott's nursing drug guide. (1998). Philadelphia: Lippincott-Raven. 94(12), 18-25.

Valente, S. M. (1994). Recognizing depression in elderly patients. *American Journal of Nursing, 94*(12) 19–25.

Additional Resources

Mental Health Infosearch
http://www.mhsource.com

Mental Health Net
http://www.cmhc.com/

National Institute of Mental Health (NIMH)
Information Resources and Inquiries Branch
Office of Scientific Information, Room 15C
5600 Fishers Lane
Rockville, MD 20857
(301) 443–4513

National Mental Health Association
1021 Prince Street
Alexandria, VA 22314–2971
(800) 969-NMHA

Friends and Advocates of the Mentally Ill
432 Park Ave. South
New York, NY 10016
(212) 684-FAMI

Society for Light Treatment and Biological Rhythms
P.O. Box 478
Wilsonville, OR 97070
(503) 694–2404

National Depressive and Manic Depressive Association
730 North Franklin, Suite 501
Chicago, IL 60610
(800) 82-NDMDA
(312) 642–0049

National Foundation for Depressive Illness
P.O. Box 2257
New York, NY 10116
(212) 370–7190

National Committee on Youth Suicide Prevention
666 Fifth Ave.
New York, NY 10103
(212) 957–9292

Chapter 15

Caring for Clients With Eating Disorders

KEY TERMS

Anorexia nervosa
Behavioral therapy
Binge eating disorder
Body mass index
Bulimarexia
Bulimia nervosa
Compulsive overeating
Eating disorders
Family counseling
Food binges
Group psychotherapy
Individual psychotherapy
Normal eating
Nutritional therapy
Purge
Satiety

LEARNING OBJECTIVES

On completion of this chapter, the reader will:

- Differentiate normal eating from the characteristics of an eating disorder.
- Name four types of eating disorders.
- Describe two forms of anorexia nervosa.
- Name two neurotransmitters that affect the appetite and satiety center in the brain.
- Discuss two reasons why most anorectics induce self-starvation.
- Identify the tool used to evaluate a person's size in relation to norms within the adult population.
- Give the healthy range for body mass index.
- List four components of treatment for clients with anorexia nervosa.
- Name at least two problems that are the focus of nursing when managing the care of clients with anorexia nervosa.
- Discuss the nurse's role for managing the nutrition of a client hospitalized with anorexia nervosa.
- Give two examples of how bulimics compensate for binging.
- Name a biochemical that research indicates may play a role in bulimia nervosa.
- Name two problems, besides nutrition, that are the nursing focus when caring for clients with bulimia nervosa.
- Differentiate between binge eating disorder and compulsive overeating.
- Name four biochemicals, besides norepinephrine and serotonin, that may play a role in overeating syndromes.
- Discuss at least three psychosocial problems that may accompany overeating syndromes.
- Name a support group that individuals with overeating syndromes find particularly helpful.

A rich variety of foods, sufficient for energy needs, growth and repair of cells, and maintenance of weight, is required to preserve health. Depending on such variables as gender, age, physical condition, activity level, and height, normal eating involves consuming approximately 1,500 to 2,500 calories per day, usually spread over three meals and two to three snacks. **Normal eating** occurs in response to hunger and ceases when **satiety** (a feeling of comfortable fullness) is attained.

Eating Disorders

Collectively, eating disorders are those in which eating

- Is outside the range of normal
- Is accompanied by anxiety and guilt
- Results in physiologic imbalances

Eating disorders affect half a million people at any given time and are more prevalent among middle to upper middle class young women between the ages of 12 and 25. Often, clients with eating disorders strive to keep their illness secret; family and friends may only become aware of their problem when emotional and behavioral symptoms are repeatedly noted (Table 15–1) or when serious health consequences ensue (Table 15–2). Box 15–1 is a self-test that can assist individuals in determining if their eating pattern is abnormal.

Anorexia nervosa, bulimia nervosa, binge eating, and compulsive overeating are eating disorders. Obe-

TABLE 15-1 **Signs and Symptoms of Eating Disorders**

Eating Disorder	Physical	Emotional	Behavioral
Anorexia nervosa	Decrease of 25% in body weight; weight is 85% or less of normal; lanugo; alopecia; cold intolerance; amenorrhea; constipation; abdominal pain	Distorted body image; hatred of a particular body part; low self-esteem; depression; isolation; perfectionism	Restriction of food choices and intake; ritualistic handling of food (cutting into tiny pieces, arranging food a certain way, using certain plates and utensils only); weighing oneself frequently; denial of hunger
Bulimia nervosa	Inability to accurately interpret hunger and fullness signals; swelling of parotid glands (chipmunk cheeks); frequent weight fluctuations; irregular menses	Feeling unable to control eating; depressive mood and frequent mood swings; black and white thinking; exaggerated concern about weight	Excessive exercise, use of diuretics, and laxatives; secret eating of high-calorie, high-carbohydrate foods; alternately binging and fasting
Binge eating and compulsive overeating	Obesity; discomfort after eating	Preoccupation with weight, eating, and dieting; attributes professional and social success and failure to weight; feels disgust or guilt after eating; feels lack of control over eating	Frequent dieting, restricts activities due to embarrassment about weight; eating when not hungry; rapid eating; eating alone

sity is a consequence of overeating; therefore, some clients who are obese also have an eating disorder.

Anorexia Nervosa

Anorexia nervosa is an eating disorder characterized by an obsession for thinness that is achieved through self-starvation. It occurs more often in women. Among girls who are 12 to 18 years of age, 1 of 200 develops anorexia nervosa.

There are two subtypes of anorectics: those who lose weight by exclusively restricting their intake of calories, and those who manifest **bulimarexia,** a pattern of both food restriction and purging to avoid absorbing the food that is consumed.

Etiology and Pathophysiology

The cause of anorexia nervosa is unknown. Many authorities believe that anorexia and all the other eating

TABLE 15-2 **Complications of Eating Disorders**

Disorder	Potential Complications
Anorexia nervosa	Amenorrhea Anemia Arrhythmias Bradycardia Cardiac arrest Constipation Dehydration Edema Electrolyte imbalance Fatigue Heart failure Internal organ shrinkage Kidney failure Osteoporosis, fractures Peripheral neuropathy
Bulimia nervosa	Anemia Arrhythmias Cardiac arrest Cardiomyopathy Cathartic colon (from laxative abuse) Chronic sore throat Constipation Dehydration Diarrhea Electrolyte imbalance Erosion of tooth enamel Esophagitis Esophageal tears Gastric dilatation and rupture Heart failure Kidney and liver damage Mitral valve prolapse Pancreatitis Parotid gland enlargement Peptic ulcer
Binge eating and compulsive overeating	Arthritis Coronary artery disease Embolism Fatigue Gastric dilatation Hiatal hernia High blood pressure Obesity Shortness of breath Toxemia of pregnancy

BOX 15-1 Eating Behavior Self-Test

______Even though people tell me I'm thin I feel fat.
______I get anxious if I can't exercise.
______My menstrual periods are irregular or absent (female).
______My sex drive is not as strong as it used to be (male).
______I worry about what I will eat.
______If I gain weight, I get anxious or depressed.
______I would rather eat by myself than with family or friends.
______Other people talk about the way I eat.
______I get anxious when people urge me to eat.
______I don't talk much about my fear of being fat because no one understands how I feel.
______I enjoy cooking for others, but I don't usually eat what I've cooked.
______I have a secret stash of food.
______When I eat I'm afraid I won't be able to stop.
______I lie about what I eat.
______I don't like to be bothered or interrupted when I'm eating.
______If I were thinner I would like myself better.
______I have missed work or school because of my weight or eating habits.
______I tend to be depressed and irritable.
______I feel guilty when I eat.
______I avoid some people because they bug me about the way I eat.
______My eating habits and fear of food interfere with friendships or romantic relationships.
______I cut my food into tiny pieces, eat it on special plates, make patterns on my plate with it, or spit it out before swallowing it.
______I am hardly ever satisfied with myself.
______I have taken laxatives to control my weight.
______I have vomited to control my weight.
______I want to be thinner than my friends.
______I have said or thought, "I would rather die than be fat."
______I have fasted to lose weight.
______In romantic moments I cannot let myself go because I am worried about my fat and flab.

If you answer yes to any of these questions; discuss your eating habits with your physician.

Adapted from Anorexia Nervosa and Eating Disorders, Inc.

disorders result from a combination of physiologic and psychodynamic factors. Evidence suggests that neurotransmitters influence eating by binding with receptors in the appetite center of the hypothalamus. Anorectics may experience a down-regulation or insensitivity to *norepinephrine* and may also have increased *serotonin* levels that fool the brain into believing satiety has occurred (Kaye & Weltzin, 1991). Individuals with this disorder are often perfectionists, have low self-esteem, and possess an intense desire to please others. Refusal to eat is also thought to be a form of self-control used to cope with life experiences or dysfunctional family relationships. Whatever the cause, failure to consume adequate nourishment eventually deprives all body systems of the nutritional elements required for homeostasis, growth, and cellular repair. Starvation can lead to serious medical conditions and death from cardiac failure or arrhythmia.

Assessment Findings

SIGNS AND SYMPTOMS

Despite the use of the term "anorexia," persons with this disorder do experience hunger, but they control the urge to eat because of a morbid fear of becoming fat. It is not uncommon to find that the anorectic consumes an average of 600 to 900 calories per day and often less. Eventually anorectics weigh 85% or less of others of similar build, age, and height and consider themselves obese despite appearing emaciated.

When confronted with the fact that they are in jeopardy of dying, clients deny the seriousness of everyone's concern. Clients may appear skeleton-like and develop a growth of fine body hair called *lanugo* that, in the absence of subcutaneous fat, helps to maintain body temperature by preventing heat loss. Anorectics tend to be hypotensive and may have irregular, low pulse rates. Severe malnutrition causes anorectics to be constipated, feel cold most of the time, have frequent infections, and cease menstruating. Many conceal their starvation by hiding or disposing of food and dressing in bulky clothing.

DIAGNOSTIC FINDINGS

Body mass index (BMI), a mathematical computation based on height and weight (Box 15–2), is used to evaluate a person's size in relation to norms within the adult population. In anorectics, the BMI is typically 16 or less. Anemia is usually present and electrolyte levels, especially potassium and sometimes sodium, are often dangerously low. Deficiencies in serum proteins are reflected in low albumin, transferrin, and ferritin levels. Cardiac irregularities are identified by electrocardiography.

Medical Management

Treatment involves four aspects: nutritional therapy, drug therapy, psychotherapy, and family counseling.

BOX 15-2 Body Mass Index Formula, Calculation, and Interpretation

Formula $BMI = \frac{\text{weight in kg}}{\text{height } m^2}$

Calculation

1. Divide pounds by 2.2 = kilograms
2. Divide height by 39.4 = meters
3. Square the answer in step 2 by multiplying the number times itself.
4. Divide weight in kg by m^2

Interpretation

Anorectic	BMI = ≤16
Underweight	BMI = 16–19
Healthy	BMI = 19–25
Mild to moderately obese	BMI = 25–35
Severely obese	BMI = ≥35

Nutritional therapy includes providing nourishing meals, supplemental vitamins and minerals, intravenous fluids and electrolytes, tube feedings, or total parenteral nutrition. Once the client's weight improves or stabilizes, outpatient treatment begins.

To promote compliance with the weight gain regimen, **behavioral therapy** is instituted. By eating, the client earns privileges for having visitors and participating in social and physical activities. The privileges are rewards used to reinforce desired behavior.

Antidepressant medications such as amitriptyline (Elavil) are administered (see Chap. 14). Bulimarexic clients have responded to drug therapy with the antihistamine cyproheptadine (Periactin), which seems to have antiseritonergic activity.

Individual and **group psychotherapy** are used to help clients gain insight into their distorted perceptions of thinness and the motivations for persisting in weight-loss behaviors. Counseling and involvement in self-help groups for several years are often indicated. **Family counseling** is aimed at relieving the power struggle between those who try to convince the client to eat and the anorectic who refuses. It also focuses on learning skills for undoing *enmeshment*, the habit of being so involved with one another that a loss of personal identity and exclusion of others occurs.

Nursing Management

The nurse performs a physical assessment, maintains caloric and fluid intake flow sheets, and implements the plan for behavioral and nutritional therapy. The role of the nurse in caring for clients with anorexia nervosa includes, but is not limited to the following:

Nursing Diagnoses and Collaborative Problems	Nursing Interventions
Alteration in Nutrition: Less than Body Requirements related to fear of gaining weight	Consistently assign the same few nurses to the client's care to promote a therapeutic alliance, maintain consistency, and avoid manipulation.
Goal: The client will gain 2 to 5 lb/week by a mutually agreed on target deadline. The client will attain and maintain a BMI of at least 20.	Establish a contract for expected weight restoration and target date. Include the rewards for reaching goals and consequences for failures.
	Weigh the client regularly, but randomly to avoid **water loading,** a technique in which anorectic clients attempt to demonstrate weight gain by consuming a large volume of water and avoiding urination before being weighed.
	Work with the dietitian to provide at least 6 to 8 meals each day with a total caloric value between 1,500 and 2,000 calories; then gradually increase the total calories to between 2,500 to 4,000/day.
	Allow the client at least 30 minutes to consume the meal.
	Observe the client during mealtime to prevent the client from hiding rather than eating food.
	Remove dietary tray after 30 minutes without commenting on food that has not been eaten.
	Record the percentages of food consumed so the dietitian can analyze the caloric intake.
	Restrict the client's use of the bathroom for 2 hours after meals or accompany the client to the bathroom to prevent purging.
	Give the client a liquid nutritional supplement for the uneaten calories at meals.
	Implement behavioral rewards or consequences consistently and fairly.
	Administer prescribed drug therapy and ensure that clients attend group and individual psychotherapy.
Body Image Disturbance related to unresolved psychosocial conflicts	Encourage the client to talk about perceptions of body image, but avoid opposing the client's views.

Goal: The client will develop a realistic perception of self and the motivation for thinness.	Offer the observation that investing energy in weight control acts as a distraction from dealing with psychosocial issues of more substance. Help the client to clarify issues underlying controlling weight gain and promoting weight loss. Suggest that perfection is not possible and that no goal is worth dying for.

FAMILY TEACHING

Counsel and educate family members by offering the following suggestions:

- Focus on the person rather than the eating disorder.
- Provide unconditional love.
- Avoid inflicting guilt for the family distress that the disorder causes in daily living.
- Give the anorectic individual the power to make decisions and facilitate changes in matters other than eating.

Prepare the family for potential hospitalization should the client become medically unstable or relapse, and explain that clients with anorexia often resist hospitalization and attempt to discredit the staff, agency, and treatment approaches to facilitate being discharged. If that happens, it is especially important to avoid manipulation and to demonstrate united support for each other and the plan for treatment.

Bulimia Nervosa

Bulimia nervosa is characterized by two episodes of secret **food binges** (rapid consumption of a large number of calories) per week that are followed by behaviors intended to prevent weight gain. The abnormal eating pattern persists at least 6 months. There are two types of bulimics: (1) those who **purge** (eliminate nutrients) afterward with self-induced vomiting, laxatives, enemas, or diuretics, and (2) those who do not purge, but who compensate by fasting, using diet pills, or engaging in excessive exercise.

Etiology and Pathophysiology

Research suggests that bulimic individuals have a biochemically induced compulsion to eat created by increased sensitivity to norepinephrine in the appetite center of the hypothalamus and reduced levels of serotonin, which disguises the point of satiety. *Endorphins*, morphine-like chemicals synthesized in the brain, and opioid peptides are lower in bulimic persons and create cravings for sweet and high-fat foods (Brewerton, et al., 1992; Drewnowski, et al., 1992). Additionally, bulimic persons may purge in an effort to be thin, which is a standard for attractiveness in American society.

Bulimia nervosa has been linked to a seizure disorder. Once the binge begins, it is difficult to control. Eating is terminated by

- abdominal pain
- interruption (discovery by others) or
- sleeping

After the eating frenzy, bulimics feel so guilty that they purge, fast (abstain from food for a longer than usual time—not days on end like someone with bulimarexia), or exercise.

Episodic binging and purging between periods of controlled eating cause the weight to fluctuate widely. Self-induced vomiting and use of emetics like ipecac damage teeth; abuse of laxatives and enemas contributes to constipation. The nonprescribed use of diuretics and diet pills predisposes to cardiac problems.

Assessment Findings

SIGNS AND SYMPTOMS

During a binge, 3,500 to 11,500 calories of food is consumed in 2 hours or less. Self-induced vomiting results in hoarseness, inflammation of the esophagus and oral pharynx, calluses on the back of the hand and fingers from repeatedly stimulating the gag reflex, erosion of tooth enamel, and swollen parotid glands. Bulimic clients tend to be of normal weight or slightly overweight; however, their weight can fluctuate as much as 10 lb in a week.

DIAGNOSTIC FINDINGS

Diagnosis is based on the clinical findings and a history of persistent binging and purging. Serum electrolytes may be altered depending on the time that has elapsed since the last purge and the blood draw. A radiograph of the upper gastrointestinal tract shows an overstretched or stenotic esophagus from frequent regurgitation and inflammation followed by scarring.

Medical Management

Treatment of bulimia includes drug therapy with antidepressants or anticonvulsants, individual and group therapy, and behavior modification techniques.

Nursing Management

The nurse collects the history and current health information, explains the medical therapy regimen, refers the client to the dietitian for a safe weight loss program, and provides emotional support.

Some of the nurse's interventions include but are not limited to the following:

Nursing Diagnoses and Collaborative Problems	Nursing Interventions
Risk for Altered Nutrition: More than Body Requirements related to poor impulse control **Goal:** The client will consume 2,000 to 3,000 calories per day divided among three meals plus or minus snacks.	Help client identify feelings, situations, or foods that trigger binging episodes. Explore alternative coping mechanisms for dealing with triggering stimuli. Explain that starving leads to binging; therefore, eating regularly is better than periods of fasting to lose weight. Discuss alternatives for aborting or interrupting the eating binges, such as calling a friend, leaving the binging location, and stocking low-calorie food. Adulterate the binge food making it unpalatable, like dropping it in dirt or soaking it in vinegar if all else fails.
Ineffective Individual Coping related to managing guilty feelings by binging and purging **Goal:** The client will implement effective coping mechanisms for dealing with guilt and stressors.	Encourage the client to forgive herself or himself for binging and purging. Reinforce the data that suggest the disorder has a biochemical component that she or he cannot totally control. Formulate a contract with the client to seek out the nurse or another support person when feeling the urge to purge. Suggest that the client discard all purging paraphernalia such as medications and enema equipment. Discuss alternative coping strategies for reducing or eliminating guilt, such a referring to a diary to reinforce that the binging and purging are being reduced, substituting some other positive behavior like meditating or writing about a pleasurable experience.
Low Self-Esteem related to poor impulse control and ineffective methods to control weight **Goal:** The client will report increased self-esteem.	Have clients write down or verbally list their positive attributes. Help dispel the faulty perception that losing control in reference to binging and purging means the client is a total failure. Offer praise for reducing the frequency or duration of binging and elimination of compensating behaviors.

CLIENT TEACHING

Some important areas to reinforce during health teaching include:

- Following a dietary plan that is compatible with the food pyramid (Fig. 15–1)
- Eating at a slow pace
- Eating only in the presence of others

Binge Eating Disorder and Compulsive Overeating

Binge eating disorder is characterized as the inability to control overeating, feeling guilty, but not engaging in compensating behaviors to prevent weight gain. **Compulsive overeating** is characterized as eating when not hungry or regardless of feeling full. Some

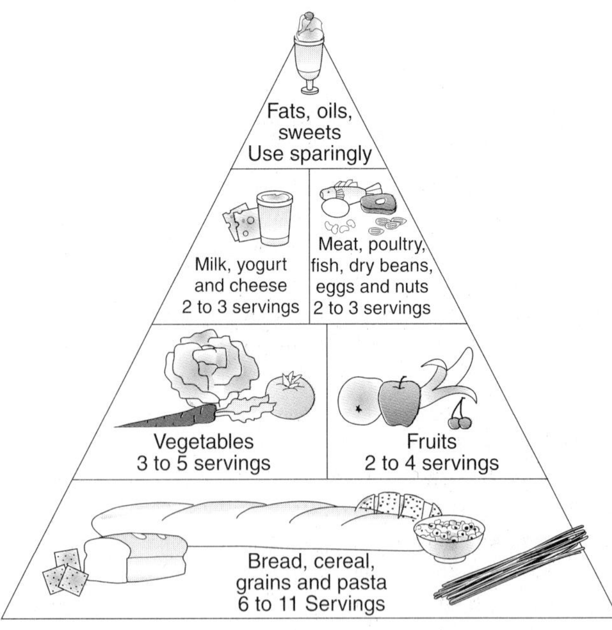

FIGURE 15-1. The food pyramid.

individuals have both problems simultaneously. Either may result in obesity.

Etiology and Pathophysiology

The cause of overeating syndromes is still unknown. Because people with eating disorders suffer from anxiety, depression, and compulsive behavior, there is speculation that a biochemical factor is involved in binge eating and compulsive overeating. The imbalance of neurotransmitters is thought to involve norepinephrine and serotonin, which affect the appetite center in the brain. There may be more extensive neuroendocrine disequilibrium involving *cortisol,* a hormone released by the adrenal cortex in response to stress (see Chap. 11); *cholecystokinin,* a hormone secreted by the mucosa of the upper small intestine that causes laboratory animals to stop eating when feeling full; and imbalances in *neuropeptide Y* and *peptide YY,* psychoactive chemicals that stimulate eating behavior in research animals. Also, many overeaters state they use food as a way of coping with stress.

Ultimately, overeating leads to many physical and emotional problems. As a consequence of obesity, many individuals develop hyperlipidemia, (elevated blood fat levels), hypertension, type II diabetes, degenerative arthritis, and sleep apnea. There is a higher risk for gallbladder disease, heart disease, and some types of cancer. Many feel unhappy, ashamed, and disgusted with themselves. They tend to become socially isolated to avoid being noticed and possibly rejected.

Assessment Findings

SIGNS AND SYMPTOMS

Overeaters are typically overweight and have a history of unsuccessful attempts at dieting. Clients tend to eat in the absence of hunger. They have preferences for high-sugar and high-fat foods that they may nibble over several hours or gorge on until they feel uncomfortably full. Some report that they overeat or binge when they are angry, sad, bored, or anxious. They often have a history of other compulsive behaviors such as alcohol or drug abuse. Some reveal that they have considered suicide or have performed *self-mutilation,* such as cutting and burning themselves, pulling their hair, and interfering with wound healing to cope with their intense feelings, to punish themselves, or to experience physical pain to counteract the consequences of feeling emotionally numb.

DIAGNOSTIC FINDINGS

People with overeating syndromes generally have a BMI that is 30 or above. Other laboratory and diagnostic tests reflect secondary complications from obesity such as elevated blood sugar, cholesterol, and serum lipid levels.

Medical Management

A comprehensive approach to treating overeating syndromes involves weight reduction, psychotherapy, and self-help support groups. The first step is a sensible weight loss regimen that is prescribed by a dietitian. Strict dieting is discouraged because it tends to worsen binge eating. To help clients lose weight and remain compliant, short-term drug therapy may be used. Prescribed medications include antidepressants such as selective serotonin reuptake inhibitors, for example; fluoxetine (Prozac), that seem to promote weight loss.

Support groups, like Overeaters Anonymous (see Additional Resources), or group therapy in eating disorder clinics are helpful adjuncts to individual psychotherapy. In some cases, surgery is an option for severely obese clients with medical complications (see Chap. 53).

Nursing Management

The nurse interviews the client with sensitivity to the individual's self-consciousness about weight and emotional problems. A comprehensive physical assessment is performed. Privacy is provided when measuring weight and height.

The nurse's role in caring for clients with overeating syndromes includes, but is not limited to the following:

Nursing Diagnoses and Collaborative Problems	Nursing Interventions
Alteration in Nutrition: More than Body Requirements related to insensitivity to satiety **Goal:** The client will consume only the prescribed number of calories per day.	Follow the meal plan for three meals and three snacks each day that has been developed by a dietitian in conjunction with nutritional counseling. Emphasize that the client not deviate from the plan. Recommend using a scale and measuring utensils to comply with portion sizes. Stick to a prepared shopping list and buy only the size or amount that is needed.

	Schedule the day with planned activities preferably involving others to prevent opportunities for secretive binging.
Risk for Loneliness related to self-consciousness concerning appearance and eating behaviors **Goal:** The client will participate in social relationships.	Accept the client for herself or himself. Seek the client out for verbal interactions. Encourage contacting friends or support persons or joining social or self-help groups. Cultivate leisure activities that can be shared with others.

CLIENT TEACHING

The nurse counsels clients with overeating syndromes to:

- Obtain and persist with treatment from professionals who are experienced in treating eating disorders.
- Follow the label directions for taking prescribed medications; report any untoward effects.
- Avoid popular nonprescription diet pills. These generally contain phenylpropanolamine and caffeine, which are central nervous system stimulants. They can increase heart rate and blood pressure and cause dizziness, irritability, insomnia, and dry mouth.
- Strict dieting or fasting is the leading cause of binging.
- Exercising with the advice of a physician can reduce the appetite and increase weight loss.
- Nutritional and weight loss centers are generally ineffective in the long run because they do not offer the comprehensive services most clients need to keep from gaining weight once the target weight is reached.
- Labels that say "sugar free" or "contains no cholesterol" do not mean that the ingredients are calorie free or even low calorie.
- Talk to a close friend or support person about your feelings.
- Overeaters Anonymous is a free self-help group that is modeled after the 12-step program of Alcoholics Anonymous.
- Remember that recovery is a day-by-day process; it is self-defeating to dwell on the lack of previous success or relapses that may occur.

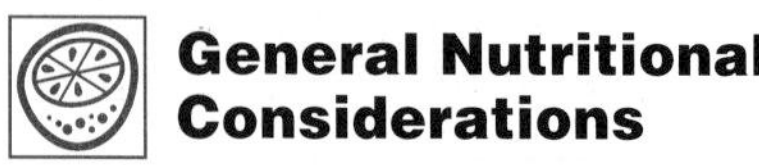

General Nutritional Considerations

The focus of treatment for anorexia nervosa is the resumption of normal eating behaviors, not simply restoring body weight. Initially, as few as 1,500 calories may be prescribed because large amounts of food, as well as high-fat foods and gassy vegetables may cause gastrointestinal discomfort after constipation. No foods are restricted, but "diet" foods (artificially sweetened beverages, fat-free foods) should be avoided. Ongoing nutritional counseling may be needed throughout the maintenance period.

Like anorectic individuals, clients with bulimia nervosa need to resume normal eating behaviors and avoid restrictive practices. They may also need to accept a body weight higher than they would like. Fears and misconceptions about food and weight should be identified and corrected; clients who are persuaded to occasionally eat small amounts of a high-calorie food are less likely to binge later. Clients are advised not to skip meals or snacks, to use appropriate utensils, to not pick at food, and to not feel guilty about occasional planned indulgences.

Rather than produce long-term weight management, restrictive low-calorie diets increase preoccupation with food and weight, and increase the risk of binge eating. It is estimated that 95% of people who lose weight regain it within 5 years, and some dieters gain back more than they originally lost. The newer approaches to weight management stress that all foods are acceptable and teach clients to recognize and differentiate between physiologic and psychological hunger.

Clients with binge eating need to establish a regular, balanced, healthy eating pattern that includes three daily meals, planned snacks, and decreased avoidance of "trigger" foods. Eating is nonrestrained but is self-regulated as clients respond to their internal cues. Discussion of weight control treatment is not appropriate until binge eating is eliminated. Because it produces favorable health benefits and is more likely to be maintained, a weight loss goal of 10% to 20%, rather than attaining an "ideal" weight, should be encouraged.

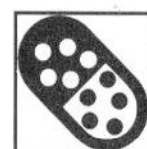

General Pharmacologic Considerations

Adolescent girls with insulin-dependent diabetes sometimes reduce their dose of insulin to promote weight loss. The practice is unsafe for obvious medical reasons.

Constipation in anorexia nervosa may be treated with a stool softener (eg, docusate sodium [Colace, Regutol]), but harsh laxatives should never be administered. Constipation is usually relieved when the anoretic client begins to eat normally.

There is no drug therapy that is universally given for those with an eating disorder. However, some clients with certain types of anorexia nervosa gain weight on the drug cyproheptadine (Periactin). If this drug is given to increase weight, monitor for the following adverse reactions: dry mouth, dry eyes, sedation, photosensitivity, lethargy, and constipation.

If chlorpromazine (Thorazine) is given, the severely emaciated client is at increased risk for hypotension and hypothermia.

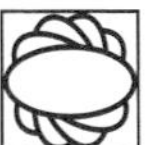

General Gerontologic Considerations

Older adults may experience severe weight loss as the result of major depression, but it is extremely rare for older adults to have an excessive fear of gaining weight or an excessive desire for weight loss. Any adult with a significant weight loss should be assessed for depression.

At times, older adults may simply refuse to eat, resulting in self-starvation. Self-starvation over the loss of health, the diagnosis of a terminal disease, or inability to cope with life's losses is related to major depression or faulty coping skills and is not classified as an eating disorder.

SUMMARY OF KEY CONCEPTS

- Normal eating occurs in response to hunger and ceases when satiety is attained.
- There are four types of eating disorders. They are anorexia nervosa, bulimia nervosa, and two overeating syndromes, binge eating disorder and compulsive overeating.
- Anorexia nervosa, characterized by an obsession for thinness and self-starvation, is manifested in two ways: totally restricting food intake or combining food restriction with purging by vomiting, laxative abuse, enemas, diuretics, and exercise.
- Two neurotransmitters that affect the appetite and satiety centers in the brain are norepinephrine and serotonin. Either or both may be imbalanced in eating disorders.
- Most anorectic individuals practice self-starvation because of a morbid fear of becoming fat or an obsession for thinness.
- Calculating BMI is a tool that is used to evaluate a person's size in relation to norms within the adult population. A BMI between 19 and 25 is considered healthy.
- Recovery from anorexia nervosa increases if it includes nutritional therapy, drug therapy, psychotherapy, and family counseling.
- Although only severely malnourished clients with anorexia nervosa are hospitalized, when they are, the nurse is concerned with promoting the intake of nourishing food and helping the client deal with disturbance in body image.
- When managing the anorectic client's nutritional problem, the nurse contracts with the client on the amount of weight gain and target date, identifies rewards and loss of privileges for not meeting goals, guards against techniques that clients use to disguise their failure to gain weight, collects data to monitor caloric intake, prevents discarding or purging food, administers drugs to correct imbalances of neurotransmitters, and ensures that clients participate in psychotherapy.
- Bulimic clients compensate for binging either by purging afterward with self-induced vomiting, laxatives and enemas, or diuretics, or they compensate by fasting, using diet pills, or participating in excessive exercise.
- Researchers have detected a link between low levels of beta-endorphin, an opioid peptide, and bulimic behaviors.
- Besides the nutritional aspects of care, nursing management of clients with bulimia nervosa includes helping them find more effective ways of coping with their guilt over binging and purging and improving their self-esteem.
- There are two overeating syndromes—binge eating disorder, characterized by episodic overeating without compensating behaviors to prevent weight gain, and compulsive overeating, characterized by eating when not hungry or regardless of feeling full.
- Besides an imbalance of norepinephrine and serotonin, overeating syndromes may also be influenced by other neurochemicals such as cortisol, cholecystokinin, neuropeptide Y, and peptide YY.
- Clients with binge eating disorder and compulsive overeating suffer from anxiety, depression, other compulsive behaviors, such as alcoholism and drug abuse, suicidal ideation, and self-mutilation.
- Overeaters Anonymous, a free self-help group that is modeled after the 12-step program of Alcoholics Anonymous, has been helpful to many individuals who are obese or have overeating syndromes.

CRITICAL THINKING EXERCISES

1. Based on the food pyramid, explain what a healthy diet consists of on a daily basis.
2. Calculate the BMI of a person who is 63 inches tall and weighs 175 pounds. What conclusion is appropriate based on your calculation?
3. What weight loss strategies are appropriate to recommend and discourage for an obese client who is a compulsive overeater?

Suggested Readings

Amara, A., & Cerrato, P. L. (1996). Eating disorders–still a threat. *RN, 59*(6), 30–35.

Brewerton, T. D., Lydiard, R. B., Laraia, M. T., et al. (1992). Beta-endorphin and dynorphin in bulimia nervosa. *American Journal of Psychiatry, 149*(8), 1086–1090.

Bruce B., & Wilfley, D. (1996). Binge eating among the overweight population: A serious and prevalent problem. *Journal of the American Dietetic Association, 96*, 58–61.

Drewnowski, A., Krahn, D. D., Demitrack, M. A., et al. (1992). Taste responses and preferences for sweet high fat foods: Evidence for opioid involvement. *Physiology and Behavior, 51*(2), 371–379.

Katrina, K., King, N., & Hayes. D. (1996). *Moving away from diets.* Lake Dallas, TX: Helm Seminars Publishing.

Kaye, W. H., & Weltzin, T. E. (1991). Serotonin activity in anorexia and bulimia nervosa: Relationship to the modulation of feeding and mood. *Journal of Clinical Psychiatry, 52*: 41–48.

Polivy, J. (1996). Psychological consequences of food restriction. *Journal of the American Dietetic Association, 96*, 589–592.

Ponto, M. (1995). The relationship between obesity, dieting and eating disorders. *Professional Nurse, 10*(7), 422–425.

Additional Resources

American Anorexia Nervosa Association, Inc.
133 Cedar Lane
Teaneck, NJ 07666

National Anorexic Aid Society, Inc. (NAAS)
P.O. Box 29461
Columbus, OH 43229

Anorexia Nervosa and Associated Disorders (ANAS)
550 Frontage Road, Suite 2020
Northfield, IL 60093

Bulimic Anorexic Self-Help, Inc.
6125 Clayton Avenue, Suite 215
St. Louis, MO 63139
(800) 227–4785, (314) 567–4080

Center for the Study of Anorexia and Bulimia
1 West 91st Street
New York, NY 10024
(212) 595–3449

Overeaters Anonymous
6075 Zenith Court, NE
Rio Rancho, NM 87124
(505) 891–2664
http://www.overeatersanonymous.org/

Binge Eating Program
Western Psychiatric Institute and Clinic
3811 O'Hara Street
Pittsburgh, PA 15213
(412) 624–2823

Chapter 16

Caring for Chemically Dependent Clients

KEY TERMS

Addiction
Alcoholism
Aversion therapy
Blackouts
Cross-tolerance
Detoxification
Gateway substances
Methadone maintenance therapy
Opiate dependence
Physical dependence
Polydrug abuse
Psychological dependence
Relapse
Rule of One Hundreds
Substance abuse
Tolerance
Withdrawal

LEARNING OBJECTIVES

On completion of this chapter, the reader will:

- Discuss the health and social consequences of substance abuse.
- List four steps in the progression toward chemical dependence.
- Explain tolerance and give two mechanisms by which it occurs.
- Discuss the meaning of withdrawal.
- Name four addictive substances that are commonly abused and at least three other categories of abused drugs.
- List two physiologic explanations and two psychosocial factors for the development of chemical dependency.
- Explain two ways abused drugs produce their effects.
- Define alcoholism and list three symptoms.
- Name four components of treatment for alcoholism.
- Discuss the nursing management of alcoholic clients.
- List five potential health consequences of tobacco use.
- Discuss the components of a successful smoking cessation program.
- Discuss elements of recovery programs.

Chemical dependency and substance abuse are serious public health and social problems. They contribute significantly to the morbidity (incidence of disease) and mortality (deaths) from liver damage, cardiopulmonary disease, and infectious diseases such as hepatitis and acquired immunodeficiency syndrome (AIDS). Alcohol and drug abuse also are major factors in domestic and child abuse, crime, traffic and boating fatalities, assaults, and murders.

Substance Abuse

Substance abuse is the use of a drug in a manner that differs from its accepted purpose. Generally, it is the consequences of inappropriately taking drugs—primarily mind and mood altering substances—that is of major concern.

Commonly abused drugs include alcohol, cocaine, heroin, hallucinogens, amphetamines, marijuana, barbiturates, volatile hydrocarbons such as those found in glue, and nicotine. From the standpoint of morbidity and mortality, alcohol and nicotine are the most harmful substances. Tobacco use has been so widely accepted and its psychoactive properties so subtle that the negative effects on social and occupational obligations seem minor. Yet tobacco is an addictive substance that contributes annually to the deaths of 450,000 people, as many as are caused by alcohol, cocaine, heroin, suicide, homicide, motor vehicle accidents, fire, and AIDS combined (Munzer, 1997).

Chemical Dependence

Chemical dependence occurs when a person must take a drug to avoid withdrawal symptoms. **Addiction** is sometimes used interchangeably with depen-

BOX 16-1 Signs of Alcohol or Drug Addiction

Regularly drinking or taking more than was originally planned
Unsuccessful attempts to reduce or regulate use
Spending excessive amounts of time obtaining, consuming, or recovering from the effects of the drug
Continued use despite negative consequences
Drinking or consuming drugs alone
Failure to fulfill major role obligations at work school or home
Tolerance to alcohol and sedative drugs
Withdrawal symptoms when drug is not consumed

dence but more accurately refers to the drug-seeking behaviors that interfere with work, relationships, and normal activities (Box 16–1). **Withdrawal** refers to the physical symptoms and craving that occur when an abused substance is abruptly stopped (Table 16–1). **Tolerance** refers to the reduction in a drug's effect after persistent use, and occurs because the body becomes more efficient at inactivating the drug. As a consequence of tolerance, increasing amounts of the substance are taken to obtain the desired effect.

Etiology and Pathophysiology

The causes of chemical dependence are complex and involve many psychobiologic factors. Substance abuse often begins with curious experimentation, and progresses to habituation, to **psychological** and **physical dependence**, to addiction (Table 16–2). One factor that explains drug abuse is the self-reinforcing pleasurable effects these drugs produce in the limbic system of the brain. Stimulant drugs such as cocaine and amphetamines affect norepinephrine, dopamine, and acetylcholine. Depressant drugs such as alcohol, heroin, and barbiturates cause effects similar to those of gamma-aminobutyric acid (GABA), endorphins, and enkephalins. These drugs either mimic the neurotransmitters by attaching to their receptor sites or block their reuptake (see Chap. 11).

In alcoholism, accumulating evidence suggests a genetic component that results in an altered metabolism of alcohol (Box 16–2) (Olms, 1983). Instead of converting acetaldehyde to acetic acid, some acetaldehyde combines with dopamine to form an addictive substance called *tetrahydroisoquinoline* (TIQ). TIQ is only formed in the brains of alcoholics, not those who drink socially. Other researchers have identified a variant gene for dopamine among alcoholics that

TABLE 16-1 **Commonly Abused Substances**

Drug	Effects	Signs and Symptoms of Toxicity	Signs and Symptoms of Withdrawal
Alcohol	Central nervous system depressant • Lethargy • Slurred speech • Slowed motor reaction • Impaired judgment • Decreased social inhibition	Nausea and vomiting, loss of coordination, belligerence, stupor, coma	Anxiety, agitation, elevated vital signs, hyperactive reflexes, tremors, diaphoresis, insomnia, hallucinations, seizures
Cocaine	Central nervous system stimulant • Tachycardia • Hypertension • Increased energy • Feeling of well-being • Insensitivity to pain and fatigue • Weight loss	Restlessness, paranoia, irritability, auditory hallucinations, convulsions, respiratory or cardiac arrest	Depressed mood, lethargy, impaired concentration, craving for drug
Heroin	Central nervous system depressant • Initial brief rush of euphoria • Sedating • Reduces motivation, attention, and concentration • Alters sensitivity to stressors • Relieves pain • Lowers vital signs, especially respiratory rate • Slows peristalsis • Constricts pupils • Decreases interest in sex	Respiratory depression, hypothermia, pin-point pupils, coma	Yawning, runny nose, perspiration, goose bumps, anorexia, vomiting, diarrhea, dilated pupils, insomnia, elevated vital signs, drug craving

TABLE 16-2 **Patterns of Substance Abuse**

Experimentation	Habituation	Dependence	Addiction
Initial use Low dose Finds experience pleasurable No discomfort from abstinence	Repeated use Uniform doses Seeks to re-experience pleasure No discomfort from abstinence	Frequent use Doses increase Craves ongoing pleasure from drug Experiences minor physical discomfort if drug is not used	Unremitting use High doses Needs drug to feel "normal" Experiences severe withdrawal symptoms if drug is not used

locks onto receptors, triggering sensations of pleasure and reward (Noble, 1996).

Psychosocial dynamics are also a component in substance use and abuse. Observing family members, peers, and role models who use alcohol, tobacco, and other drugs, influences impressionable teenagers and youngsters. The promotion of alcohol in American culture fosters its use and abuse also. Many people abuse drugs in a dysfunctional effort to cope with psychosocial stressors.

Treatment

Initiating treatment is one of the most difficult hurdles in treating chemical dependency. Clients deny their addiction, rationalize drug use, or blame life situations for their drug and drinking habits. Often, dependent individuals must "hit bottom" before they seek help. Once treatment is sought and withdrawal is managed, recovering individuals must learn new methods to cope with the stressors of life, repair relationships damaged by addiction, and develop new interests and activities to fill the time once devoted to using drugs or alcohol.

Although some individuals quit taking the abused substance unassisted, most people benefit from a treatment plan that involves abstinence, counseling, and support of peers through a 12-step program. Twelve-step programs are free and provide specific guidelines (steps) for becoming and staying drug and/or alcohol free. Frequent attendance at meetings is encouraged (daily, if necessary) where members share their experiences and discuss the 12 steps and other topics related to recovery.

BOX 16-2 Normal and Alcoholic Metabolism of Alcohol

Ethyl alcohol
↓
Acetaldehyde + dopamine → Tetrahydroisoquinoline (TIQ)
↓
Acetic acid (vinegar)
↓
Carbon dioxide + water

Altered alcohol metabolism shown in red

Alcohol Dependence

Alcoholism is a chronic, progressive multisystem disease characterized by an inability to control the consumption of alcohol. Unchecked, the disease is fatal. Because women generally weigh less than men they are affected sooner and more seriously.

Assessment Findings

SIGNS AND SYMPTOMS

Although the client may emphatically deny problem drinking, he or she typically has a history of increasing alcohol consumption. Many manifest a great tolerance for alcohol and a **cross-tolerance,** reduced effect for other sedative-hypnotic drugs. **Blackouts,** periods of amnesia for events and activities that happen while drinking, occur even in the early stages of drinking. Family and friends note alcoholic behaviors, and social or legal repercussions occur. A history of marital, financial, and occupational problems reflects the individual's inability to control drinking despite negative consequences. Many have been arrested for driving under the influence of liquor (DUIL).

A host of alcohol-related physical symptoms can occur with persistent drinking. Esophagitis, gastritis, enlarged liver, esophageal and rectal bleeding, and pancreatitis are common. Memory is impaired and clients may experience sexual dysfunction such as impotence or decreased libido. Studies also implicate alcohol in liver cancer, stroke, metabolic deficiencies, aspiration pneumonia, cardiomyopathy, blood dyscrasias, and neurologic disorders.

Acutely intoxicated alcoholics may enter the tertiary care hospital with altered mental status, acute gastric bleeding, or as victims of trauma or violence. When this occurs, management of alcohol withdrawal is as important as management of the related conditions.

DIAGNOSTIC FINDINGS

A *blood alcohol level* (BAL) measures the percentage of alcohol in the blood, indicating the extent of alcohol toxicity (Table 16–3). Elevated glutamyltransferase (GTT), aspartate transferase (AST), and alanine transferase (ALT) levels reflect alcohol-induced liver disease. Levels of pancreatic enzymes (amylase and lipase) may also be elevated.

Medical Management and Rehabilitation

To break the progression of alcoholism, clients undergo detoxification, nutritional therapy, psychotherapy, drug therapy, and are encouraged to continue rehabilitation by joining a support group such as Alcoholics Anonymous.

DETOXIFICATION

Alcohol withdrawal is a potentially fatal condition. **Detoxification** (detox) is the process of stabilizing the client with a sedative drug while the alcohol is metabolized from his or her system and withdrawal symptoms subside. Drugs used in detoxification are lorazepam (Ativan), chlordiazepoxide (Librium), and diazepam (Valium) (Table 16–4). Initially, these medications are administered frequently and in high doses to compensate for the client's cross-tolerance; they are then tapered and discontinued. A beta-adrenergic blocker such as propranolol (Inderal) is given to reduce the dangerously elevated heart rate and blood pressure that can occur. Intravenous hydration with glucose and added vitamins support the client metabolically until the condition stabilizes.

NUTRITIONAL THERAPY

Alcoholics often are undernourished and suffer from deficiencies of B vitamins. Injections of thiamine for 3 days followed by oral administration and folic acid supplements are often prescribed. Vitamin therapy prevents neurologic complications known as *Wernicke's encephalopathy* and *Korsakoff's psychosis*.

PSYCHOTHERAPY

Individual or group psychotherapy helps the client to gain greater insight into the emotional problems that have led to or resulted from alcohol dependence.

SUPPORT GROUPS

Alcoholics Anonymous (AA) was the first 12-step self-help program. Founded in 1926 by an alcoholic physician, AA is composed of and run by recovering alcoholics to help people who are dependent on alcohol get sober and stay sober. It emphasizes personal accountability, spirituality, and powerlessness over alcohol. Family members are encouraged to attend meetings of *Al Anon*, *Alateen*, or *Adult Children of Alcoholics* (ACOA) to learn more about how they have been affected by alcoholism.

DRUG THERAPY

Disulfiram (Antabuse) is a drug given to recovering alcoholics who cannot control the compulsion to drink. It is a form of **aversion therapy** because it deters drinking by causing unpleasant physical reactions when alcohol is consumed or absorbed through the skin (see Table 16–4). Life-threatening cardiopulmonary complications and even death can occur. Naltrexone (Trexan, Re Via), a narcotic antagonist, is also used as an adjunct for recovering alcoholics. It decreases the effects

TABLE 16-3 **Blood Alcohol Level and Associated Impairment**

Blood Alcohol Level	Percentage of Blood Alcohol	Physical and Behavioral Effects
50 mg/dL	0.05%	Mood changes, loosening of inhibition, decreased judgment, slight euphoria
80–100 mg/dL	0.08–0.1%	Reduced muscle coordination, decreased reaction time, impaired vision
200 mg/dL	0.2%	Staggering, poor control of emotions, easily angered
300 mg/dL	0.3%	Mental confusion, stupor
400 mg/dL	0.4%	Coma
500 mg/dL	0.5%	Respiratory depression, death

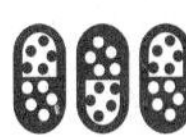

TABLE 16-4 **Drugs Used in the Recovery From Chemical Dependence**

Drug Category and Use	Side Effects	Nursing Considerations
Benzodiazepine		
chlordiazepoxide hydrochloride (Librium)—management of acute alcohol withdrawal	Sedation, confusion, restlessness, bradycardia, tachycardia, urinary retention or incontinence, drug dependence	If giving intravenously, use a large vein and monitor vital signs carefully. Intramuscular injection can be quite painful; reconstitute with special diluent only, monitor injection sites, administer slowly. Observe client for excessive sedation and use cautiously in clients with impaired kidney or liver function.
Antialcoholic Agent		
disulfiram (Antabuse)—blocks oxidation of alcohol resulting in the accumulation of acetaldehyde	*If alcohol is used:* flushing, throbbing headaches, dyspnea, vomiting, tachycardia, hypotension, blurred vision; severe reactions can result in convulsions, myocardial infarction, death. *Disulfiram* alone: drowsiness, headache, dermatitis	Do not administer until at least 12 hours has elapsed since last exposure to alcohol. Inform client that all sources of alcohol must be avoided and to wear a medical identification bracelet. Arrange for follow-up liver and blood studies. Inform client of potential side effects and to report them to a health care provider.
Smoking Deterrent		
nicotine transdermal (Nicotrol)—binds to nicotinic receptors in central and peripheral nervous system	Headache, insomnia, diarrhea, constipation, pharyngitis, burning and itching at site, backache, chest pain, dysmenorrhea	Explain application, site rotation, and disposal of used patches so that pets or children do not come in contact with product. Inform client of side effects and to report any that occur.
Narcotic Antagonist		
naltrexone hydrochloride (Trexan, ReVia)—blocks the effects of opioids and aids in the abstinence from alcohol	Insomnia, anxiety, nervousness, low energy, abdominal pain, nausea, vomiting, decreased potency, delayed ejaculation, rash, joint and muscle pain, increased thirst	Induces sudden withdrawal so do not use until 7 to 14 days has elapsed since last exposure to opioids. Inform client that small doses of opioids will have no effect. Larger doses may overcome the inhibiting effect but coma or death may occur. Tell the client to report any side effects.
Narcotic Agonist Analgesic		
methadone (Dolophine)—binds with opioid receptors in the central nervous system and produces euphoria, analgesia, and sedation	Light-headedness, dizziness, sedation, nausea, vomiting, respiratory depression, circulatory depression, shock, cardiac arrest	A single liquid oral dose is used for maintenance. Constipation may be severe, ensure that client is taking a stool softener. Use with caution in clients receiving sedatives, hypnotics, tranquilizers, tricyclic antidepressants and monoamine oxidase inhibitors—respiratory depression, hypotension and coma can occur.

of alcohol should the person **relapse** (return to drinking).

Nursing Management

The nurse includes questions about the use of alcohol when establishing the client's data base. The *CAGE Screening Test* is helpful in detecting alcoholic behaviors (Box 16–3). If the client admits to consuming alcohol, the nurse determines the type, how much, and when the last drink was consumed. The latter information is important because withdrawal symptoms occur within 3 to 72 hours after a client's last drink. A

BOX 16-3 CAGE Questionnaire for Alcoholism

1. Have you ever felt that you ought to **C**ut down on your drinking?
2. Have people **A**nnoyed you by criticizing your drinking?
3. Have you ever felt **G**uilty about your drinking?
4. Have you ever had a drink first thing in the morning to steady your nerves or get rid of a hangover (**E**ye-opener)?

From Ewing, J. A. (1984). Detecting alcoholism: The CAGE questionnaire. *Journal of the American Medical Association, 252,* 1905–1907.

history of seizures or other severe symptoms in previous withdrawals merits close observation for a similar reaction.

The nurse monitors the client for signs and symptoms of withdrawal. Nurses often use the **Rule of One Hundreds** as an indicator of escalating withdrawal. It refers to a body temperature ≥100°F. pulse rate ≥100 beats/min, or diastolic blood pressure of ≥100 mm Hg. The rise in any one of these three vital signs suggests the need for sedative medication as the physiologic consequences of withdrawal may be extremely difficult to counteract once they have begun.

NURSING PROCESS
The Client With Alcohol Dependence

Assessment

Use the CAGE questionnaire to determine if the client has a drinking problem. Determine usual daily amount consumed and time of last drink. Ask if client has experienced withdrawal symptoms and, if so, describe. Assess client's use of all prescribed and nonprescribed drugs. Assess vital signs.

Diagnosis and Planning

Nursing Diagnoses and Collaborative Problems	Nursing Interventions
Potential Complication: Alcohol withdrawal **Goal:** The nurse will manage and minimize alcohol withdrawal.	Assess and consult with physician regarding need for sedative to manage symptoms of withdrawal. Monitor for therapeutic effect of sedative. Assess vital signs every 2 hours and monitor for onset of symptoms such as low grade fever, tremors, anxiety, insomnia, disorientation, tachycardia, and elevated diastolic blood pressure. Monitor for seizure activity, hallucinations, extreme tremors, agitation, diaphoresis, and other signs of severe withdrawal.
Altered Nutrition: Less than Body Requirements related to inadequate consumption of nutrients **Goal:** The client's nutrition will improve as evidenced by consuming at least 75% of food that is served.	Obtain a baseline weight. Determine the client's food preferences. Collaborate with the dietary department to provide six small meals each day and an ample variety of snacks. Monitor dietary intake and record data in the medical record.
Sleep Pattern Disturbance related to sympathetic nervous system stimulation secondary to withdrawal **Goal:** The client will sleep for at least 6 hours.	Eliminate any sources of caffeine. Reduce environmental stimuli. Suggest relaxation techniques such as a warm bath, soothing music, or light reading before bedtime. Offer a back massage if sleeplessness persists.
Anticipatory Grieving related to loss of alcohol use, social activities, and contacts **Goal:** Client will accept the loss of alcohol and the activities and contacts associated with it.	Let the client ventilate feelings concerning potential losses. Explore alternatives that may substitute for potential losses. Encourage the family or significant others to support one another. Promote sharing of experiences between the client and others who are further ahead in their recovery.
Health Seeking Behavior related to a desire to abstain from alcohol **Goal:** The client will proceed with a plan for attaining sobriety.	Provide the locations where AA meetings are held and explain that a sponsor may be selected who will provide social and emotional support. Recommend that the client begin reading the "Big Book" of Alcoholics Anonymous that describes the 12 steps to recovery. Prepare the client for possible relapse by role playing situations that may entice drinking.

Evaluation and Expected Outcomes

- Vital signs are stable.
- Symptoms of withdrawal are controlled.
- The client is eating a well balanced diet.
- The client sleeps an adequate number of hours per night.
- The client demonstrates a willingness to cope with losses associated with overcoming dependence on alcohol.

CLIENT TEACHING

Teach the client taking disulfiram to avoid alcohol even in its most obscure forms (Box 16–4), that mild reactions can occur at a blood level as low as 0.05%, and that a reaction can occur within 5 to 10 minutes of absorbing alcohol. Reactions are possible for up to 2 weeks after discontinuation.

Nicotine Dependence

Nicotine, the stimulant drug in tobacco, is the most heavily used addictive substance in the United States. The drug is absorbed by inhaling cigarettes, cigars,

BOX 16-4 Obscure Sources of Alcohol

- Liquid cough and cold medications
- Liquid sleep medications
- Flavoring extracts
- Mouthwash
- Rubbing alcohol
- Aftershave lotions
- Fruitcake with alcohol

and pipe tobacco; or it is absorbed through the mucous membranes of the mouth from loose tobacco.

Although nicotine causes disease and dysfunction throughout the body, American society condones and even endorses tobacco use. Smoking is responsible for 90% of deaths due to lung cancer, 90% of deaths due to chronic obstructive lung disease, 35% of all cancer deaths, and 21% of all deaths from coronary artery disease (Munzer, 1997). Tobacco contains more than 40 carcinogenic chemicals. It is the major cause of oropharyngeal cancers and contributes to cerebrovascular disease, peripheral vascular disease, and cancers of the urinary tract, esophagus, and pancreas.

Smokeless tobacco (chewing tobacco) exposes the oral cavity to carcinogens, inhaled tobacco targets the lungs and distant organs, and cigars or pipes repeatedly expose the oral cavity and esophagus to harmful substances. Smoking raises carbon monoxide levels in the blood and causes constriction of peripheral blood vessels. It disrupts the structure of alveoli, causing them to become overstretched and inelastic, and is implicated in the development and recurrence of gastric ulcers. Although smoking and tobacco use has decreased in recent decades, approximately 25% of adults use tobacco and medical costs are estimated at $53 billion annually. Passive absorption of smoke also causes disease in nonsmokers.

Nicotine is an addictive, mood-altering substance that produces tolerance resulting in increased use over years and withdrawal symptoms when its use is discontinued. Users light up or chew to maintain blood and brain levels; nicotine is then distributed throughout the body, metabolized in the liver, and excreted by the kidneys. Frequency of tobacco use is also governed by conditioned, learned responses meaning that the habit of smoking is reinforced by past patterns of use. This is important in that smoking cessation strategies must target both the physical dependence and the conditioned behaviors.

Medical Management

All smokers and tobacco users are advised to quit and provided with materials that inform them of methods for doing so. Various levels of intervention are available and include minimal approaches such as brief counseling and follow-up, or more intense intervention such as enrollment in behavior modification programs. These programs help the client in managing temptation, extinguishing preconditioned cues to smoke, and providing rewards for goal achievement. Pharmacologic therapy using nicotine substitutes (gum, patch, inhaler) (see Table 16–4), which are gradually tapered and stopped, helps the client avoid withdrawal symptoms and is an adjunct to other interventions.

Relapse is common and only 10% to 15% of smokers who quit remain tobacco free for a year. However, attempts to quit are a predictor for eventual success; 60% of those who try and fail do ultimately succeed.

Nursing Management

Nurses help clients who smoke by counseling them to quit and providing them with information on various programs. Nurturing the client's belief that he or she can be successful is an important supportive measure. Because many clients fear gaining weight, the nurse informs them that typical weight gain in the year after cessation is 9 to 10 lb. The nurse then helps the client plan strategies to offset the tendency for weight gain such as beginning a walking program or substituting fruits for high-calorie desserts and reducing fat in the diet. If the client is unwilling to contemplate quitting, the nurse informs him or her of the dangers of passive smoke to others and encourages them to abstain from smoking in the presence of nonsmokers, especially children. The nurse also takes an active role in promoting individual and community health by learning smoking cessation techniques and providing seminars to the public.

Cocaine Dependence

Cocaine, obtained from the leaves of the coca plant, is a central nervous system (CNS) stimulant. The powder form of cocaine is snorted (inhaled through the nose) or dissolved and injected intravenously. *Crack*, a purified form of cocaine with a crystalline or rocklike appearance, is smoked either by placing it in a pipe or by sprinkling it onto or mixing it with tobacco or marijuana. Cocaine may be freebased, which reduces it to its purest form. It is then smoked by sprinkling it onto a cigarette or inhaling it through a pipe. Freebasing cocaine provides an intense physical experience as the drug is absorbed, more so than when it is taken by other routes. It also produces an increased risk of toxic effects and overdose reactions.

Assessment Findings

SIGNS AND SYMPTOMS

Signs and symptoms of the drug's effect may be brief (see Table 16–1) because cocaine is fully metabolized in several minutes. There are signs that correlate with its route of administration and consequences of chronic use.

Ulceration of the nasal mucosa and perforation of the nasal septum are found in those who snort cocaine. Needle marks are found along the pathways of veins in those who inject cocaine intravenously. Those who smoke or freebase may have burns on their faces, fingertips, or eyebrows from using or leaning over a lighted pipe. Long-term abusers of cocaine experience anorexia, weight loss, memory impairment, personality and behavioral changes, psychosis, and hallucinations. Those who smoke or inhale cocaine may have a chronic cough and pulmonary congestion.

Cocaine addicts often have a problem with **polydrug abuse,** abuse of more than one substance. It is common for them also to take sedative drugs such as alcohol, minor tranquilizers, barbiturates, and marijuana to offset their agitation and irritability.

DIAGNOSTIC FINDINGS

Drug toxicology tests are done on blood and urine. Metabolites of cocaine can be found in urine up to 36 hours after its use. Other abused substances are also identified.

Medical Management and Rehabilitation

Cocaine toxicity (see Table 16–1) requires immediate treatment because the condition is life-threatening. Referral to Cocaine Anonymous, which is based on AA, provides a source of ongoing support for the cocaine addict. Participation in individual and group psychotherapy and Cocaine Anonymous are encouraged to help the client in eliminating all forms of drug abuse. The recreational use of other drugs can lead to relapse.

To help the cocaine addict with recovery, medications like bromocriptine (Parlodel) and amantadine (Symmetrel) are used temporarily. They increase or mimic the effects of dopamine, the neurotransmitter that is most likely responsible for the reward and reinforcing effect of cocaine. Antidepressants are prescribed to relieve the *dysphoria* (depression) that occurs during withdrawal. Amino acid precursors such as phenylalanine and tyrosine, the substances from which the neurotransmitters norepinephrine and dopamine are made, are included in drug therapy to replace levels depleted by chronic use. Research is currently underway to develop a drug that can neutralize cocaine in the blood thus reducing the amount available for brain uptake.

Nursing Management

The nurse assesses the client's history of drug use, current physical condition, and signs of toxicity and withdrawal. The nurse implements medical treatment during a life-threatening emergency. Later, the effects of drug abuse and risks for continuing drug-taking behaviors are explained. The nurse monitors the client for suicidal ideation (see Chap. 14) and administers medications that provide support during withdrawal.

Opiate Dependence

Opiate dependence is an addiction to CNS depressant drugs, narcotics, that are either derived from opium or are chemically similar. Opioid is a term for synthetic narcotics. Some examples of opiate drugs include heroin (diacetylmorphine), codeine, morphine, meperidine (Demerol), methadone, hydromorphone (Dilaudid), oxycodone, and opium as in tincture of paregoric. Opiates produce a state of sedation after an initial phase of euphoria. The rate at which tolerance and chemical dependency occurs is related to the drug, the dose, and frequency of use. Sharing needles during the intravenous administration of any abused substance can lead to AIDS, hepatitis, and septicemia.

Assessment Findings

SIGNS AND SYMPTOMS

Refer to heroin in Table 16–1 for the effects of opiates. Chronic use is evidenced by anorexia, weight loss, constipation, malnutrition, needle marks, and scarring (tracks) along the paths of veins.

DIAGNOSTIC FINDINGS

A urine drug screen reveals evidence of opiate use. Rapid recovery (within 2–5 minutes) from lethargy, hypotension, and respiratory depression after the intravenous administration of a narcotic antagonist such as naloxone (Narcan) supports the diagnosis of narcotic overdose.

Medical Management and Rehabilitation

Withdrawal symptoms are treated with the alpha-adrenergic blocker clonidine (Catapres) to inhibit the release of norepinephrine. Methadone (Dolophine), another narcotic, may be used to eliminate or control withdrawal symptoms.

One method for helping the heroin addict stay off drugs is methadone maintenance therapy. **Methadone maintenance therapy** involves substituting one addicting drug for another. The advantage is that because methadone is a synthetic drug prepared by a pharmaceutical company, the drug is untainted and the dose is reliable. The rationale behind methadone maintenance therapy is that it forestalls withdrawal, avoids a toxic overdose, and theoretically reduces crime because the drug is provided legally. Another drug used for opiate addiction is naltrexone (Trexan, Re Via), which is a nonaddicting, long-acting narcotic antagonist that blocks the effects of opiates. If clients return to opiate abuse while taking naltrexone, they do not experience the previous level of opiate effects.

Psychotherapy is an important aspect of rehabilitation. It involves treating the complex web of social problems that accompanies the addiction. Clients also are referred to Narcotics Anonymous, a self-help organization modeled after AA.

Nursing Management

The nurse's role is similar to that discussed for other types of chemical dependence with a few exceptions that apply to administering drug therapy. If naltrexone is prescribed, the client must be opiate free for at least 7 days. The nurse advises the client who takes methadone to tell health care providers or wear a Medic Alert tag in case there is a time when the client needs a narcotic, tranquilizer, or barbiturate. Because methadone is a narcotic, lower doses of other sedative drugs are necessary because the combination can potentiate their depressant action.

Other Abused Substances

A variety of other substances are abused and addictive. Some examples include hallucinogens, amphetamines, marijuana, barbiturates, tranquilizers, and volatile hydrocarbons. Signs and symptoms follow the same pattern as with previously discussed substances: experimental use progresses through stages of increased use until dependence and addiction occur; there is failure to meet social, familial, or occupational obligations with an increase in defensive mechanisms to explain behavior; disturbances in mood and physical function occur as the result of drug abuse. Treatment and recovery include withdrawal, abstinence, and ongoing enrollment in a support group.

General Nutritional Considerations

Nutritional interventions for alcoholism include correcting nutrient deficiencies and modifying the diet as needed for complications. Parenteral nutrition may be indicated for clients with acute pancreatitis; a low-fat diet may improve symptoms of chronic pancreatitis. Protein intake is adjusted for clients with acute and chronic liver disease.

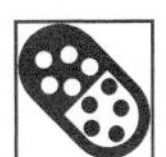

General Pharmacologic Considerations

A reaction to disulfiram can occur up to 2 weeks after the drug is discontinued. Inform the client to avoid all forms of alcohol (cough syrups, elixirs, etc.) for at least 2 weeks after discontinuing the drug.

Used nicotine patches contain enough nicotine to cause serious adverse reactions in children. Nicotine gum should be stored out of the reach of children.

A careful drug history is obtained from chemically dependent clients because these individuals tend to abuse multiple substances.

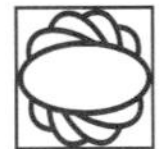

General Gerontologic Considerations

Alcoholism may be difficult to identify in the older adult because symptoms such as tremors or memory loss mimic changes associated with aging.

Alcohol abuse diminishes significantly after age 70.

Older adults who drink alcohol exhibit greater impairment than younger adults and recover more slowly.

Prolonged use of alcohol over the years can result in neurologic deficits such as confusion, ataxia, and loss of cognitive ability.

Older adults may abuse over-the-counter and prescription drugs rather than illicit drugs.

SUMMARY OF KEY CONCEPTS

- Substance abuse follows a natural progression from curious experimentation, to habituation, psychological and physical dependence, and addiction.
- Tolerance refers to the reduction in a drug's effect after a period of persistent use. It occurs because the body develops mechanisms for using the drug more effectively or inactivating the substance more efficiently.

- Withdrawal refers to the physical symptoms and craving that occur when an abused substance is abruptly stopped.
- Four addictive substances that are commonly abused are alcohol, cocaine, heroin, and nicotine, the most heavily used addictive drug in the United States.
- Two physiologic explanations for the mechanism of chemical dependency are (1) drugs produce pleasurable effects in the limbic system of the brain and (2) dependency is a result of a genetic predisposition.
- Psychosocial factors contributing to substance abuse include (1) peer pressure, (2) observing role models who take drugs, and (3) learned maladaptive coping behaviors.
- Abused drugs produce their effects by mimicking neurotransmitters or blocking their reuptake.
- Alcoholism is a chronic, progressive multisystem disease characterized by inability to control alcohol consumption, increased tolerance, and blackouts.
- To break the progress of alcoholism, clients undergo detoxification, nutritional support, and individual and group psychotherapy. They are encouraged to continue rehabilitation by joining a support group such as Alcoholics Anonymous (AA).
- The nursing management of alcohol- or drug-dependent clients includes collecting data about patterns of use, last drink or drug taken, and past symptoms of withdrawal. During detoxification, the nurse monitors for signs of withdrawal, administers sedative medications as needed, implements measures to improve the client's nutrition, promotes undisturbed sleep, and assists with anticipatory grieving.
- Tobacco use is the single most common preventable cause of death in the United States. Tobacco use causes cancer and chronic obstructive pulmonary disease and contributes to coronary artery and peripheral vascular disease.
- Smoking cessation can be accomplished without specific intervention by just quitting, enrolling in a behavior modification program, and using decreasing doses of nicotine substitutes. Few people are successful with their first attempt, but many succeed eventually.
- Persons who abuse cocaine may also abuse sedative drugs such as alcohol, minor tranquilizers, barbiturates, and marijuana to offset their agitation and irritability.
- Methadone maintenance therapy used in the rehabilitation of opiate addicts forestalls withdrawal, avoids a toxic overdose, and reduces crimes because the drug is provided legally.
- Medications help in withdrawal and abstinence. Some alcoholic clients benefit from receiving disulfiram (Antabuse); both alcoholics and opiate-dependent clients have a decrease in relapse when receiving naltrexone (Trexan); smokers may use nicotine substitutes; bromocriptine (Parlodel) and amantadine (Symmetrel) assist the cocaine addict in withdrawing from cocaine use.

CRITICAL THINKING EXERCISES

1. Compare chemical dependency on a CNS depressant with that of a CNS stimulant.
2. Discuss the type of chemical dependence you believe is most detrimental (physically, socially, and so on) and support your belief with several reasons.
3. Discuss the drugs used to promote recovery from chemical dependence. Include the addiction for which each is used, side effects, and nursing implications.
4. What topics can you discuss with a client who expresses a desire to quit smoking but does not know how to start?

Suggested Readings

Alexander, D. E., & Gwyther, R. E. (1995). Alcoholism in adolescents and their families: Family focused assessment and management. *Pediatric Clinics of North America, 42*(1), 217–234.

Blank-Reid, C. (1996). How to have a stroke at an early age: The effects of crack, cocaine and other illicit drugs. *Journal of Neuroscience Nursing, 28*(1), 19–27.

Brent, M. J. (1997). Unexpected alcohol withdrawal. *American Journal of Nursing, 97*(6), 52–53.

Kending, S. (1995). Women at risk for infection: The woman who is chemically dependent. *Journal of Obstetric, Gynecologic, and Neonatal Nursing, 24*(8), 776–781.

MacKinnon, D. P., Williams-Avery, R. M., & Pentz, M. A. (1995). Youth beliefs and knowledge about the risks of drinking while pregnant. *Public Health Reports, 110*(6), 754–763.

Marcus, M. T., Gerace, L. M., & Sullivan, E. J. (1996). Enhancing nursing competence and substancing abusing clients. *Journal of Nursing Education, 35*(8), 361–366.

Noble, E. P. (1996). The gene that rewards alcoholism. *Scientific American Science & Medicine, 3*(2), 52–61.

Munzer, A. (1997). Smoking and smoking cessations. In Kelley, W. (ed.). *Textbook of internal medicine.* Philadelphia: Lippincott-Raven.

Olms, D. (1983). *The disease concept of alcoholism.* Bellville: Gary Whiteaker Company.

Ryan, L. A. (1997). Alcohol withdrawal? This protocol works. *RN, 60*(8), 17–20.

Additional Resources

National Institute on Drug Abuse
5600 Fishers Lane
Rockville, MD 20857
http://www.nida.nih.gov.NIDAHome.html

Alcoholics Anonymous
475 Riverside Drive
New York, NY 10163
(212) 870–3400

Al Anon and AlaTeen
P.O. Box 862
Midtown Station
New York, NY 10018
(212) 302–7240

Adult Children of Alcoholics
1225 East 11 Mile Road
Royal Oak, MI 48067
(810) 541–4013

Narcotics Anonymous
P.O. Box 9999
Van Nuys, CA 91409
(818) 780–3951

Mothers Against Drunk Driving (MADD)
669 Airport Freeway
Suite 310
Hurst, TX 76053
(817) 268–6233

National Council on Alcoholism
12 West 21st Street
New York, NY 10010
(212) 206–6770

Action on Smoking and Health (ASH)
2013 H Street, NW
Washington, DC 20006
(202) 659–4310

Chapter 17

Caring for Clients With Dementia and Thought Disorders

KEY TERMS

Acalculia
Agnosia
Agraphia
Alexia
Alzheimer's disease
Aphasia
Apraxia
Ataxia
Delirium
Delusions
Dementia
Depot injections
Extrapyramidal side effects
Hallucinations
Mentation
Negative symptoms
Neuritic plaques
Neurofibrillary tangles
Positive symptoms
Respite care
Schizophrenia

LEARNING OBJECTIVES

On completion of this chapter, the reader will:

- Differentiate between delirium and dementia, and give one example of a condition that causes each.
- List five etiologic factors linked to Alzheimer's disease.
- Name four pathologic changes associated with Alzheimer's disease.
- Give the characteristic of stages 1 through 7 on the Global Deterioration Scale.
- Name the first symptom of Alzheimer's disease.
- Identify two methods for diagnosing Alzheimer's disease.
- Explain the mechanism of drug therapy in Alzheimer's disease.
- Describe the focus of nursing management when caring for clients with Alzheimer's disease.
- List six nursing diagnoses common to clients with Alzheimer's disease.
- Give three characteristics of schizophrenia.
- Name two psychobiologic explanations for schizophrenia.
- Differentiate between positive and negative symptoms, and give two examples of each.
- Discuss how most people with schizophrenia are managed medically.
- Name three examples of antipsychotic drugs and their mechanisms of action.
- Explain the term extrapyramidal side effects, and list four examples.
- Describe a technique to prevent schizophrenic clients' noncompliance with drug therapy.
- Summarize the nursing management of clients with schizophrenia.
- List five nursing diagnoses common to clients with schizophrenia.

Changes in **mentation,** mental activity, can occur anytime during the life cycle. *Cognitive functions,* such as short-term memory and learning ability, change gradually as people get older, but many acute, chronic, reversible, and irreversible conditions that impair thinking processes can occur at any age.

Delirium

Delirium is a sudden, transient state of confusion. Delirium can be the result of high fever, head trauma, brain tumor, drug intoxication or withdrawal, metabolic disorders (eg, liver or renal failure), and inflammatory disorders of the central nervous system (CNS) such as meningitis or encephalitis. Treating the underlying medical condition usually restores mental functions.

TABLE 17-1 **Comparison of Dementia and Delirium**

Dementia	Delirium
Onset	
Gradual	Sudden
Presentation	
Alert	Blunted
Attentive	Inattentive
Course	
Stable	Unstable
Progressive deterioration	Fluctuations in function
Extended	Brief
Duration	
Permanent	Temporary
Treatment	
Symptomatic or supportive	Specific
Outcome	
Incurable	Curable

Dementia

Dementia refers to conditions in which a gradual, irreversible loss of intellectual abilities occurs. Although clients with dementia display signs and symptoms similar to those of delirium, several differences exist (Table 17–1). The most common cause for dementia in adults is Alzheimer's disease.

Alzheimer's Disease

Alzheimer's disease is a progressive, deteriorating brain disorder. Two types exist: early onset (after age 40) and late onset (after age 70) with late onset being most common.

Etiology and Pathophysiology

Genetic abnormalities on chromosomes 14, 19, and 21 have been associated with Alzheimer's disease. One theory suggests a defective gene (ApoE4) causes weakness in the neuronal cell membranes. This stimulates a response by the immune system that results in excess beta amyloid, a starchy component that accumulates in the brains of Alzheimer's victims. Beta amyloid causes injury to neurons in the area of the brain responsible for producing acetylcholine, the neurotransmitter that is critical for memory and cognition (Lombard & Germano, 1997). Other theories include aluminum toxicity, zinc deficiency or excess, previous head injury, and viral *sequela* (aftereffects).

Four pathologic changes occur in the brain:

1. Decreased size of the cortex
2. Deficiency of the neurotransmitter acetylcholine, especially in the cortex and hippocampus
3. Presence of **neuritic plaques,** deposits of beta amyloid and degenerating nerve cells
4. **Neurofibrillary tangles**, twisted bundles of nerve fibers (Fig. 17–1)

The decrease in the size of the cerebral cortex along with acetylcholine deficiency explains the cognitive deficits and alterations in emotions that accompany the disease. The degree to which plaque and tangles are present is directly related to the severity of disease manifestations.

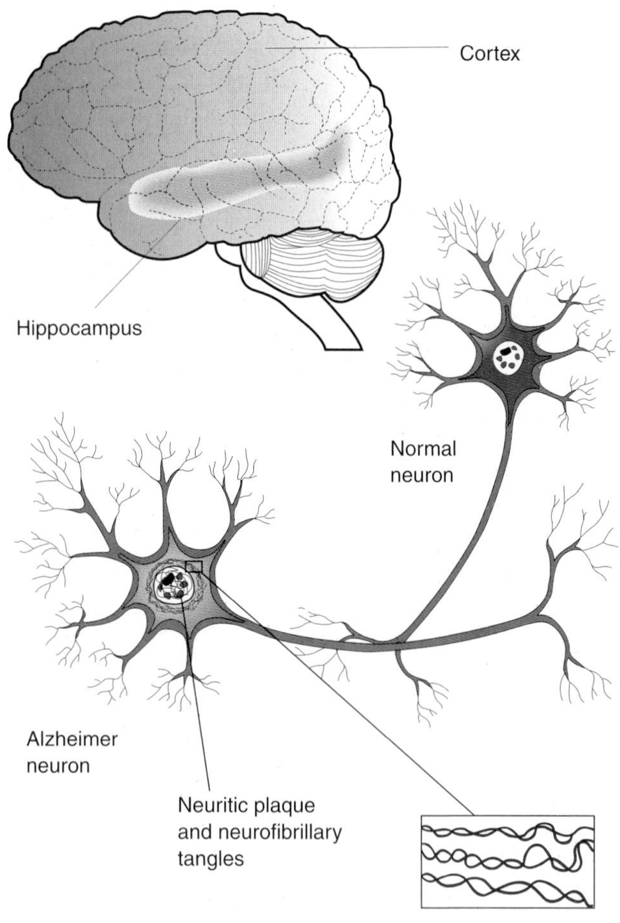

FIGURE 17-1. Neurofibrillary tangling and neuritic plaques in Alzheimer's disease.

Assessment Findings

SIGNS AND SYMPTOMS

The onset is usually insidious and symptoms may develop slowly over years. Memory loss, the classic symptom, is confined at first to recent information, but eventually long-term memory and the ability to make appropriate judgments and problem solve becomes impaired as well. Alzheimer's disease progresses through seven distinct stages that correspond with those identified in the Global Deterioration Scale (Table 17–2).

TABLE17-2 **Global Deterioration Scale**

Stage	Characteristic	Manifestations
1	Normal mentation	None
2	Forgetfulness	Concern for self-identified memory changes such as forgetting location of items, forgetting familiar names. No objective demonstration of memory deficit. No social consequences for minor memory loss.
3	Early confusion	One or more of the following: getting lost in an unfamiliar location others notice a decline in work performance deficit in word and name finding little retention of what has been read difficulty remembering names of new acquaintances loss or misplacement of valuable objects impaired ability to concentrate Objective demonstration of memory deficit Denies memory and cognitive deficits Mild to moderate anxiety
4	Late confusion	Deficits in the following areas: current and recent events personal history counting backward in series of numbers traveling and handling finances Inability to perform complex tasks such as preparing dinner for guests Strongly denies impairment Affect becomes blunted Retreats from challenges
5	Early dementia	Needs assistance of others Memory loss for important information like address and telephone number Some disorientation to time or place Difficulty counting backward by 4s or 2s May have difficulty choosing proper clothing
6	Middle dementia	May forget name of spouse or others who are significant Unaware of recent events and experiences Memory of past sketchy Unaware of date and surroundings Difficulty counting backward and sometimes forward in 10s Requires assistance with activities of daily living May be incontinent Needs assistance to travel Confuses day and night Personality and emotional changes such as: delusional thinking repetition of cleaning anxiety, agitation, violence cannot keep a thought long enough to carry it out
7	Late dementia	Loss of verbal ability Grunting may be evident Incontinent; requires help with toileting and feeding Loss of motor skills for walking, sitting, head control, and smiling

Adapted from Reisberg, B., Ferris, S. H., Leon, J. J., & Crook, T. (1982). The global deterioration scale (GDS): An instrument for the assessment of primary degenerative dementia. *American Journal of Psychiatry, 139,* 1136–1139.

Disturbances in behavior, personality changes, and depression also occur. As the disease advances, memory, cognition, awareness, and the ability to care for self deteriorates markedly. Clients may wander away and become lost. Periodic incidences of violent behavior may occur. Problems with speaking (**aphasia**), reading (**alexia**), writing (**agraphia**), and calculating (**acalculia**) develop. Inability to recognize objects and sounds (*visual*, *tactile*, and *auditory* **agnosia**), difficulty walking (**ataxia**), and tremors occur. In the final stage of the disease, an inability to accomplish activities of daily living (ADL; **apraxia**), such as grooming, toileting, and eating, despite intact motor function, makes the client totally dependent on others.

DIAGNOSTIC FINDINGS

The diagnosis is usually made by excluding other causes for the client's symptoms. A computed tomography (CT) scan shows shrinking of the cerebral cortex, but this is not apparent in the early stages of the disease. Photon emission tomography (PET) and magnetic resonance imaging (MRI) provide structural and metabolic information about the brain. Slower than normal brain waves are detected by electroencephalography (EEG). None of these diagnostic tests are specific for Alzheimer's disease, which until recently could only be confirmed by examining the brain during a postmortem examination. A new diagnostic test called Nymox AD7C detects evidence of beta amyloid protein in cerebrospinal fluid. By ruling out Alzheimer's disease, it may save many clients emotional agony, time, and money spent on nonspecific tests.

Medical Management

No cure exists for Alzheimer's disease; treatment is mainly supportive. A cholinesterase inhibitor drug that increases acetylcholine by inhibiting the enzyme that degrades it may be prescribed to improve cognitive function. Examples include tacrine (Cognex) and donepezil (Aricept) (Table 17–3). Antidepressants or tranquilizers may help the agitated or depressed client.

Nursing Management

The major focus of nursing management is to help the client and caregiver in maintaining the highest possible quality of life by supporting mental and physical functions and ensuring safety. Most clients are initially cared for in their homes and a home health nurse can instruct the family about physical care, the disease process, and treatment. He or she also will provide emotional support and intervene if the caregiver becomes overburdened. *Risk for Caregiver Role Strain* is related to being overwhelmed by responsibilities, fatigue, and depression. The goal of nursing intervention is to have the caregiver feel comfortable and knowledgeable about implementing plans that will provide needed relief. To accomplish this, the nurse can:

- Assess the caregiver's strengths, limitations, and ability to manage caretaking activities.
- Suggest scheduling **respite care**, brief relief from caretaking responsibilities, with family and friends on a regular rotating basis.
- Provide a list of agencies that offer social services such as the county's commission on aging and Social Security and Medicare agencies.

TABLE 17-3 **Drug Therapy for Alzheimer's Disease**

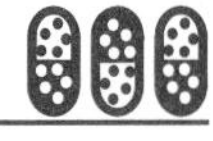

Drug Category/Mechanism of Action	Side Effects	Nursing Considerations
Cholinesterase Inhibitor		
tacrine (Cognex) Provides for increased levels of acetylcholine in the cortex by inhibiting cholinesterase, the enzyme that breaks down acetylcholine	Headache, fatigue, confusion, dizziness, nausea, vomiting, diarrhea, gastrointestinal upset, abdominal pain, loss of appetite, skin rashes, hepatotoxicity	Administer on an empty stomach on an around-the-clock schedule. Do not abruptly discontinue. Arrange for regular blood tests to determine transaminase levels. Inform client and family of side effects and to report any that occur. Tell client to exercise caution if performing tasks that require alertness.
donepezil (Aricept) Inhibits the breakdown of acetylcholine	Nausea, vomiting, diarrhea, bradycardia, possibly worsens asthma and chronic obstructive pulmonary disease	Tell client that frequent small meals may minimize gastrointestinal upset. Monitor heart rate and report bradycardia (heart rate <60).

- Develop a list of people who may be contacted in an emergency, including a 24-hour hotline for the home health nursing agency.
- Recommend that the caregiver and client take care of legal matters such as wills, transferring titles, and preparing an advanced directive (see Chap. 25).
- Suggest establishing *durable power of attorney* designating who may make decisions regarding finances or health care when the client becomes *incompetent*, the legal term for the inability to understand the risks or benefits of decisions.
- Advise the caregiver to obtain *guardianship* or *conservatorship*, court-appointed responsibility, for managing the client's care and assets if the client is already incompetent.
- Encourage the caregiver to place the client in a long-term nursing facility while taking a well deserved vacation.

The nurse should routinely evaluate the caregiver's use of respite care. He or she should seek relief at least 1 or 2 days a week.

NURSING PROCESS
The Client With Alzheimer's Disease

Assessment

The nurse interviews both the client and the family because the client may be unable to give a complete history. Assessment includes a neurologic examination to assess muscular strength, balance, and gait. The nurse does a mini mental state examination (see Chap. 11) and evaluates the client's behavior, emotional status, cognitive and motor skills, ability to carry out ADLs, and level of orientation.

Diagnosis and Planning

When it becomes necessary to transfer the client from his or her home, the nurse meets the client's physical needs on a full-time basis and helps the family cope during the client's deterioration. When caring for clients with Alzheimer's disease, the nurse's attends to, but is not limited to the following:

Nursing Diagnoses and Collaborative Problems	Nursing Interventions
Altered Thought Processes related to global cognitive deficits	Orient the client frequently to person, place, and time.
Goal: The client will be reoriented and participate in life experiences to his or her potential.	Assign consistent caregivers.
	Get the client's attention by using the name preferred.
	Keep explanations or directions short and simple.
	Give gentle reminders or model the action desired.
	Involve the client in one idea or task at a time.
	Maintain a structured daily routine.
	Reduce stimuli that decrease the client's attention and concentration, like noise and activity.
	Promote interactions that tap into the client's long-term memory such as reminiscing; offer the client cues such as, "I understand you were . . . (a school teacher)."
	Give the client plenty of time to respond to questions. Try to understand what the client wants to convey.
	Include the client in group activities, even if there is little or no socialization. Change activities or distract the client if he or she becomes angry, hostile, or uncooperative.
	Make sure that the client is wearing an identification bracelet with an address and telephone number in case he or she wanders away. Photograph the client in case a search is necessary.
	Install alarms on exit doors and respond immediately when one sounds.
Impaired Physical Mobility and Risk for Injury related to ataxia	Help the client don supportive walking shoes.
Goal: The client will move about freely and safely.	Provide assistance with ambulation.
	Remove hazards, such as footstools, small tables, or liquid spills, from the ambulatory area.
	Keep the environment well-lighted.
	Maintain the bed in low position. Use **restraint alternatives,** protective or adaptive devices for fall protection and postural support; always use the least restrictive intervention.
	Place a bed monitor under the client's mattress to call attention to times when the client gets out of bed without signaling for assistance.

Self-Care Deficit (specify bathing/hygiene, feeding, dressing/grooming, toileting) related to apraxia and agnosia **Goal:** The client will manage self-care or needs will be met for the client when he or she is unable to do so.	Encourage the client to continue doing whatever self-care is possible. Open food containers and cut food into bite-size pieces. Seat the client across from others at meal times so he or she can mimic how to eat. Offer the client water, beverages, and snacks at frequent intervals to maintain nutrition and fluid volume; tell the client to "swallow" if he or she forgets. Toilet the client at scheduled intervals and keep a record of bowel elimination. Hand the client a utensil, comb, brush, electric razor, or other self-care item and show the client how to use it. Modify clothing with Velcro or suspenders so that they are easily donned and removed. Help the client or dress the client in clothing that is appropriate for the occasion and temperature.
Sleep Pattern Disturbance related to confusion between day and night **Goal:** The client will obtain at least 6 hours of uninterrupted sleep or return to sleep after awakening.	Keep the client active during daytime hours, but avoid excess fatigue. Restrict the consumption of beverages that contain stimulants such as coffee, tea, cola. Make sure the room is comfortably warm or cool, that the client has urinated, and satisfied his or her thirst just before bedtime. Dim the lights and reduce unnecessary noise. Provide a lighted clock at the bedside if the client can interpret the information. Redirect the client gently but firmly to return to bed if night time wandering occurs.
Risk for Altered Family Processes related to guilt over placing the client in a care facility. **Goal:** The family will remain united and supportive over the decision to transfer the client's care to others.	Acknowledge and empathize with the family's ambivalent feelings. Emphasize the skills and services provided at the facility. Let the family participate in developing or revising the plan of care. Keep the family informed of the client's progress or lack thereof. Encourage the family to visit and participate in the client's care to whatever level they want. Allow the family privacy when they interact and make an area available to them for special occasions like birthdays and anniversaries. Keep a current list of family phone numbers, their relationship to the client, and indications for which they prefer to be called. Prepare the family ahead of time for the deterioration that will most likely occur.

evaluation and expected outcomes

- The client participates in ADLs.
- The client interacts with family and staff.
- Agitation and confusion are reduced.
- The client takes adequate foods and fluids.
- The client sleeps 6 to 8 hours each night.
- Family displays effective coping skills.

Schizophrenia

Schizophrenia is a thought disorder characterized by deterioration in mental functioning, altered sensory perception, and changes in *affect* (emotion). Schizophrenic clients improve with drug therapy but, unfortunately, never fully recover. Because the condition is lifelong and appears in young adulthood, it causes considerable anguish among families who must deal with both the burden of health care costs and the responsibility for caring for a loved one with this illness.

Etiology and Pathophysiology

Schizophrenia, historically attributed to emotional dysfunction, is now categorized as a psychobiologic disease because of recent findings in brain and neurotransmitter chemistry. Many neurotransmitter imbalances are involved in schizophrenia. Dopamine excess is believed to be the major cause of the symptoms, with imbalances of norepinephrine, serotonin (5-HT), and gamma-aminobutyric acid (GABA) (see Chap. 11) also playing a role. The disease is known to have a familial or genetic component. Other theories suggest that the anatomic and physiologic changes associated with schizophrenia are the result of a viral infection experienced by the mother during pregnancy. The neurochemical imbalance produces a variety of manifestations characterized by disturbed thinking, with themes that may include suspiciousness, persecution, being controlled, grandiosity (belief in one's importance), religious fixation, preoccupation with sex, a love interest, illness, or a body part—or no ideas at all.

Assessment Findings

SIGNS AND SYMPTOMS

The onset of symptoms is generally late adolescence to early adulthood. Clients manifest a range of symptoms categorized as positive or negative. **Positive symptoms** include **delusions**, **hallucinations**, and fluent but disorganized speech. **Negative symptoms**, sometimes called defect symptoms, are marked by impoverished speech and an inability to enjoy relationships or express emotions (Box 17–1). Positive symptoms are more easily managed than negative symptoms. Classic symptoms are inexplainable sensory experiences such as hearing voices or seeing apparitions of people who are not really there. These occur in combination with peculiar patterns of speaking and odd motor behaviors. The client also tends to abandon relationships and interactions with others, and loses motivation for working, going to school, or other goal-driven behaviors. Hygiene and appearance tend to lose the importance they once had.

DIAGNOSTIC FINDINGS

The diagnosis is made primarily on the symptomatology and by ruling out other possible causes. CT and PET scans, MRIs, and brain mapping (see Chap. 11) may show decreased brain size and activity especially in the frontal and temporal lobes.

Medical Management

Schizophrenic clients are referred to the care of psychiatrists. Once the client is within the mental health system, every effort is made to avoid institutionalization. The exception is when the client is dangerous to himself or others. Generally, community mental health services are selected that meet the client's needs for psychotherapy, drug administration, and social needs; such as housing, job assistance, and money management; in an outpatient setting.

DRUG THERAPY

Antipsychotic drugs are the mainstay of treatment. These drugs, also called major tranquilizers or neuroleptics, belong to several different chemical families but all block receptors for dopamine. Some examples of antipsychotic drugs are haloperidol (Haldol), fluphenazine (Prolixin), risperidone (Risperdal), clozapine (Clozaril), and olanzapine (Zyprexa) (Table 17–4).

Risperdal, clozapine, and olanzapine, newer drugs called atypical antipsychotics, produce their effects with less incidence of **extrapyramidal side effects** (EPS), movement disorders associated with traditional drugs (Box 17–2). But clozapine has the potential adverse effect of dangerously depressing bone

BOX 17-1 Positive and Negative Symptoms of Schizophrenia

Positive	Negative
Delusions, false beliefs that cannot be changed by logical reasoning	*Concrete thinking*, an inability to explain abstract ideas
Hallucinations, sensory experiences that others do not perceive, like auditory, visual, tactile, olfactory, or gustatory (involving taste)	*Thought blocking*, inability to recall information for a period of time
Loose associations, a sequence of ideas that are slightly connected	*Symbolism*, attaching significance to an insignificant object or idea
Inappropriate affect, a display of emotional feeling inconsistent for the situation	*Blunted* or *flat affect*, little or no display of feeling
Peculiarities in speech like *echolalia*, repeating what others say; rhyming, using unrelated words in a sentence (*word salad*), or inventing new words (*neologisms*)	*Anhedonia*, inability to experience pleasure
Bizarre behavior such as *stereotopy*, repetitious movement; and *echopraxia*, mimicking the movement of others	*Catatonia*, immobility
	Posturing, assuming statuesque positions
	Autism, social withdrawal
	Self-neglect of hygiene, eating, work, finances, etc
	Poverty of thought, lacking any opinions or ideas

TABLE 17-4 **Drugs Used in the Treatment of Schizophrenia**

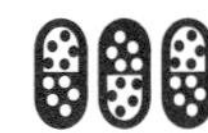

Drug Category/Mechanism of Action	Side Effects	Nursing Considerations
Antipsychotics		
haloperidol (Haldol) Blocks postsynaptic dopamine receptors	Drowsiness, pseudoparkinsonism, dystonia, akathisia, neuroleptic malignant syndrome, arrhythmias, suppression of cough reflex, anaphylactoid reactions, anemia, dry mouth, constipation, urinary retention	Monitor older clients for dehydration and aspiration potential. Withdraw drug gradually. Tell client to avoid driving. Instruct client to drink fluids and report any side effects.
fluphenazine (Prolixin) blocks postsynaptic dopamine receptors	Drowsiness, extrapyramidal syndromes, arrhythmias, suppression of cough reflex, dry mouth, constipation, urinary retention.	Tell client to avoid alcohol. Do not mix oral concentrate with caffeine-containing beverages, teas, or apple juice. Monitor older clients for signs of dehydration. Tell client to drink plenty of fluids and to report any side effects.
risperidone (Risperdal) blocks dopamine and serotonin receptors in the brain	Insomnia, agitation, headache, anxiety, drowsiness, nausea, vomiting, constipation, tardive dyskinesias, neuroleptic malignant syndrome, seizures	Monitor for seizures when initiating therapy or increasing dose. Increase dose gradually until therapeutic effect is achieved. Tell client not to stop taking drug abruptly or to make up missed doses, but to contact the health care provider. Instruct client that drug may not be taken during pregnancy and to report any side effects.
olazapine (Zyprexa) blocks dopamine and serotonin receptors	Dizziness, drowsiness, headache, weight gain, orthostatic hypotension, extrapyramidal symptoms	Instruct clients in measures to offset orthostatic hypotension, such as rising slowly and doing ankle pumps before standing. Monitor for extrapyramidal symptoms, initiate anticholinergic drugs, decrease, discontinue or switch medications as directed.

marrow function and clients who take clozapine must have a weekly blood count. If the white blood cell count drops too low, the drug is discontinued. Anticholinergic drugs such as trihexyphenidyl (Artane) and benztropine (Cogentin) are given to prevent or relieve EPS. Antipsychotics are sometimes combined with anticonvulsant drugs such as clonazepam (Klonopin) and carbamazepine (Tegretol).

Noncompliance with drug therapy is the leading cause for the return of disease symptoms and the need for short-term hospitalization. For this reason, some nonhospitalized clients are given **depot injections**, intramuscular injections of antipsychotic drugs in an oil suspension that are gradually absorbed over 2 to 4 weeks.

BOX 17-2 **Extrapyramidal Side Effects (EPS)**

Movement Disorder	Explanation
Akinesia (pseudoparkinsonism)	The client appears to have symptoms of Parkinson's disease (see Chap. 44) such as hand tremors, stooped posture, stiff shuffling gait
Akathisia	Inability to sit or stand still
Dystonia	Sudden severe muscle spasm usually in the neck, tongue, or the eyes
Tardive dyskinesia	Involuntary muscle movement usually in the face such as tongue thrusting, continuous chewing, grimacing, lip smacking, blinking; irreversible once manifested

NURSING PROCESS
The Client With Schizophrenia

Assessment

When caring for clients in acute care or community mental health settings, perform a mini mental status examination (see Chap. 11) during the initial contact and periodically thereafter to monitor for changes.

Assess client for positive and negative symptoms of schizophrenia including presence of delusions, bizarre speech patterns, hallucinations, agitation, stupor, and social withdrawal. Assess physical status including hygiene and nutritional condition.

Diagnosis and Planning

Nursing care includes, but is not limited to the following:

Nursing Diagnoses and Collaborative Problems	Nursing Interventions
Altered Thought Processes related to brain changes as manifested by illogical beliefs **Goal:** The client's thoughts will be reality based as evidenced by a decrease or absence of delusions.	Administer antipsychotic drugs as prescribed. Do not argue about the validity of the client's delusions or try to convince him or her otherwise, but reinforce that you do not share the belief. Shift the client's focus to what is real in the "here and now" when he or she dwells on the delusion. Direct the client to a quiet place when he or she becomes agitated to help restore calm and prevent loss of control.
Altered Sensory Perception (Specify: auditory, visual, olfactory, tactile, gustatory) related to brain changes as manifested by hallucinations **Goal:** The client will acknowledge that the hallucinations are not real or will minimize their importance.	Intervene when it appears that the client is experiencing a hallucination such as assuming a listening pose, or laughing or talking when others are absent or uninvolved in interaction. State that you do not hear or see anyone, but acknowledge that the experience must seem real and frightening to the client. Stay with the client throughout the hallucination. Avoid touching the client without prior warning because the client may respond violently to what he or she perceives as a threat. Call auditory hallucinations "the voices" rather than using a personal pronoun like "they," which suggests the words are coming from real people. Ask the client to share the content of the hallucination to obtain data for determining if the client's safety or that of others is in jeopardy. Distract the client from attending to the hallucination. Teach the client the technique of voice dismissal, which refers to saying "stop" or "be gone" to halt the hallucination.
Impaired Verbal Communication related to disordered thinking as manifested by neologisms and other speech oddities **Goal:** The client will communicate effectively with staff and others.	Never imply that the client's illogical communication is understood; ask the client, "What do you mean by . . . ?", or "I'm sorry I do not understand what you mean . . ."
Self-Care Deficit (Specify type) related to lack of motivation, illogical fears, emotional withdrawal **Goal:** The client will perform activities of daily living.	Explain where hygiene is done and how to obtain soap, shampoo, toothpaste, etc. Direct client to care for self at an appropriate time. Assist if the client is unable to initiate or complete self-care. Praise any accomplishments that are deserved. Monitor food and fluid intake and toileting patterns. Provide nutritious snacks if the client eats insufficiently.
Impaired Social Interactions related to autism as evidenced by absence from group meetings, reluctance to participate in group activities **Goal:** The client will interact independently with one person initially and more than one as comfort level improves.	Accompany client to group meetings and activities. Sit by the client, but do not manipulate the client into participating. Share some time after the group experience and use open-ended questions to explore the outcome with the client. Verbally compliment the client when possible for speaking voluntarily with others or acting appropriately in a social situation. Suggest ways the client can improve interactions with others.

Evaluation and Expected Outcomes

- The client shows improved concentration and level of orientation.
- The client reports a decrease in delusions and hallucinations.
- Communication is coherent and understandable.
- The client manages self care.
- Socialization and participation in group activities are enhanced.

FAMILY TEACHING

The nurse helps the family cope by teaching them about the client's illness, the treatment plan, and prognosis. It is also important to encourage the family to be supportive and involved, while allowing the client to remain as independent as possible. Give the family a referral to a social worker and crisis telephone numbers. Direct the family to local community mental health associations and support groups.

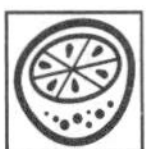

General Nutritional Considerations

Alzheimer's disease can have a devastating impact on nutritional status. Forgetfulness, alterations in smell and taste, and decreasing ability to self-feed impair intake.

Increased agitation significantly increases calorie requirements. Nutritionally dense foods that are easy to consume, such as liquid supplements, help maximize intake.

Clients in the later stages of Alzheimer's disease may not only be incapable of feeding themselves, they also may not know what to do when food is placed in their mouths.

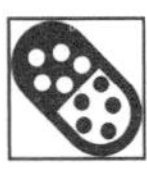

General Pharmacologic Considerations

Tacrine therapy in clients with Alzheimer's is not curative and will become ineffective with time. Achieving maximum benefits with Tacrine takes up to 2 months of continuous treatment.

Antipsychotic drugs do not cure mental illness, but they calm the unmanageable client and make some more responsive to other forms of therapy.

Monitor the client taking an antipsychotic drug for symptoms of neuroleptic malignant syndrome and notify the primary health care provider immediately if fever, dyspnea, tachycardia, hypertension, severe muscle stiffness, or loss of bladder control occurs.

Advise clients to take all antipsychotic drugs as directed and to avoid double dosing if a dose is missed.

Advise clients not to stop antipsychotic drugs abruptly; nausea, vomiting, sweating, tachycardia, headache, and insomnia can occur.

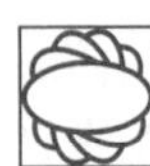

General Gerontologic Considerations

Alzheimer's disease affects approximately 45% of individuals over age 85.

Tacrine can be dissolved in orange juice or other liquid if the older adult has difficulty swallowing.

Geriatric clients require lower dosages of antipsychotic drugs.

The older adult taking haloperidol (Haldol) is at risk for dehydration. Report lethargy, decreased thirst, weakness, and dry mucous membranes.

Older adults are particularly susceptible to tardive dyskinesia. Report symptoms immediately because the drug must be discontinued.

SUMMARY OF KEY CONCEPTS

- Delirium refers to a sudden, transient state of confusion. It can be the result of high fever, trauma, infection, drug reactions, or metabolic disorders. Dementia refers to a gradual, irreversible loss of intellectual abilities.
- The cause of Alzheimer's disease is unknown, but there are five possible links to its development: (1) a genetic predisposition, (2) aluminum toxicity, (3) autoimmune pathology, (4) earlier head injury, and (5) viral sequela.
- Four pathologic changes are associated with Alzheimer's disease: decreased size of the cortex, deficiency of the neurotransmitter acetylcholine, presence of neuritic plaques, and neurofibrillary tangles.
- The Global Deterioration Scale describes mental state and deterioration from normal to forgetfulness, early confusion, late confusion, and early, middle, and late dementia.
- Short-term memory loss is the first symptom of Alzheimer's disease.
- Alzheimer's disease is definitively diagnosed by examining the brain of a person after death or by detecting beta amyloid protein in the cerebrospinal fluid.
- Drugs used in managing the care of those with Alzheimer's disease may improve cognitive functioning by inhibiting the enzyme that degrades acetylcholine.
- The major focus of nursing management when caring for a client with Alzheimer's disease is to maintain the client and caregiver's quality of life, sustain the client's physical and mental functions, ensure safety, and assist and support the family in home care and decision-making concerning extended care.
- Alzheimer's disease can severely affect nutritional status.
- Nursing diagnoses that are common when planning care for a client with Alzheimer's disease include *Altered Thought Processes*, *Impaired Physical Mobility*, *Self-Care Deficit*, and *Sleep Pattern Disturbance*. The nurse may also diagnose *Risk for Caregiver Role Strain* and *Risk for Altered Family Processes*.
- Schizophrenia is characterized by deterioration in mental functioning, altered sensory perception, and changes in affect.
- Signs and symptoms associated with schizophrenia are believed to be the result of excess dopamine and possible imbalances of norepinephrine, serotonin, and gamma-aminobutyric acid.
- Clients with schizophrenia manifest positive symptoms such as delusional thinking and hallucinations, and negative symptoms such as concrete thinking and blunted affect.
- Every effort is made to keep from institutionalizing schizophrenic clients by stabilizing them with drug therapy and providing a variety of community mental health services.
- Clients with schizophrenia are treated with antipsychotic drugs. Three examples include haloperidol (Haldol), fluphenazine (Prolixin), and clozapine (Clozaril), which are believed to achieve their therapeutic effect by blocking receptor sites for dopamine.

- Antipsychotic drugs can cause extrapyramidal side effects such as pseudoparkinsonism, akathisia, dystonia, and tardive dyskinesia.
- Some schizophrenic clients are given depot injections, intramuscular administration of antipsychotic drugs in an oil suspension that are gradually absorbed over 2 to 4 weeks, to prevent noncompliance with drug therapy.
- The nursing management of clients with schizophrenia includes making periodic mental status assessments, administering medications, observing for drug side effects, teaching the client and family about the disease and its treatment, and directing them to community mental health services and support groups.
- Nurses may diagnose and design interventions for *Altered Thought Processes, Altered Sensory Perception, Impaired Verbal Communication, Self-Care Deficit,* and *Impaired Social Interactions.*

CRITICAL THINKING EXERCISES

1. Discuss the similarities and differences between Alzheimer's disease and schizophrenia.
2. In what ways are the interventions for the nursing diagnosis of *Altered Thought Processes* different for a client with Alzheimer's disease and schizophrenia?
3. Discuss nursing interventions that are appropriate when a client with schizophrenia expresses a delusional belief or experiences a hallucination.

Suggested Readings

Baily, K. P. (1996). Pharmacologic agents for the treatment of schizophrenia: Similarities and differences. *Journal of the American Psychiatric Nurses Association, 22*(5), 181–185.

Castle, L. N. (1997). Beyond medication: What else does the patient with schizophrenia need to reintegrate into the community? *Journal of Psychosocial Nursing and Mental Health Services, 35*(9), 18–21, 41–42.

Everitt, J. (1995). Schizophrenia and family support: Interventions to reduce relapse rate. *Mental Health Nursing, 15*(5), 12–15.

Hall, G. R., & Wakefield, B. (1996). Acute confusion in the elderly. *Nursing, 26*(7), 32–37.

Holmberg, S. K., & Kane, C. F. (1995). Severe psychiatric disorder and physical health risk. *Clinical Nurse Specialist, 9*(6), 287–292, 298.

Kovach, C., Weisman, G., Chaudhury, H., et al. (1997). Impact of a therapeutic environment for dementia care. *American Journal of Alzheimer's Disease, 12*(3), 99–110.

Lombard, J., & Germano, C. (1997). *The brain wellness plan: Breakthrough medical, nutritional, and immune-boosting therapies.* New York: Kensington.

McDougall, G. J. (1996). Predictors of the use of memory improvement strategies by older adults. *Rehabilitation Nursing, 21*(4), 202–209.

Nihart, M. A. (1996). The neurobiology of schizophrenia. *Journal of the American Psychiatric Nurses Association, 2*(5), 181–185.

Whitlatch, C. J., Feinberg, L. F., & Sebesta, D. S. (1997). Depression and health in family caregivers: Adaptation over time. *Journal of Aging and Health, 9*(2), 222–243.

Additional Resources

Alzheimer's Association
919 North Michigan Avenue
Suite 1000
Chicago, IL 60611–1676
(800) 272–3900

Alzheimer's Disease Education and Referral (ADEAR) Center
P.O. Box 8252
Silver Spring, MD 20907–8252
(800) 438–4380

Eldercare Locator
1112 16th Street, NW
Washington, DC 20036
(800) 677–1116

Children of Aging Parents (CAPs)
1609 Woodbourne Road
Suite 302A
Levitown, PA 19057
(800) 227–7294

National Institute on Aging
Public Information Office
Federal Building
Room 5C27, Building 31
9000 Rockville Place
Bethesda, MD 20892
(301) 496–1752

National Alliance for the Mentally Ill
200 North Glebe Road
Suite 1015
Arlington, VA 22203–3754
(800) 950–6264

Schizophrenics Anonymous
15920 West Twelve Mile
Southfield, MI 48076
(313) 477–1983

American Schizophrenic Association Hotline
(800) 847–3802

5

Common Medical-Surgical Problems

Chapter 18

Caring for Clients With Infectious Disorders

KEY TERMS

Community-acquired infections
Culture
Generalized infections
Host
Immunizations
Infectious disorders
Infectious process cycle
Leukocytosis
Localized infections
Microorganisms
Mode of transmission
Multidrug resistance
Nonpathogens
Nosocomial Infections
Opportunistic infections
Pathogens
Phagocytosis
Portal of entry
Portal of exit
Reservoir
Sensitivity
Sepsis
Septicemia
Standard precautions
Susceptibility
Transmission-based precautions
Virulence

LEARNING OBJECTIVES

On completion of this chapter, the reader will:

- Explain the meaning of infectious disorders.
- Describe microorganisms and list at least three examples.
- List three factors that influence whether an infection develops.
- Differentiate between pathogens and nonpathogens.
- List at least five factors that increase susceptibility to infection.
- Name six components of the infectious process cycle.
- Explain the difference between mechanical and chemical defense mechanisms.
- Differentiate between localized and generalized infections.
- Describe the events that occur during the inflammatory process.
- Name at least three diagnostic tests ordered for clients suspected of having an infectious disorder.
- Discuss the medical management of clients with infectious disorders.
- Name three nursing interventions that prevent or control infectious disorders.
- List three reasons why clients in health care agencies are at increased risk for infection.
- Explain the role of an infection control committee.
- List at least four measures that have reduced community-acquired infections.
- Provide at least three health teaching recommendations that help reduce the incidence of infectious disorders.
- Discuss measures to take if a needle stick injury occurs.

Microorganisms and Infectious Disorders

Infectious disorders are conditions caused by microorganisms. **Microorganisms**, commonly called "germs," are living plants and animals that are so small they can only be seen with a microscope.

Once microorganisms invade, one of three events occurs: (1) the body's immune defense mechanisms eliminate them (see Chap. 41), (2) they reside in the body without causing disease, or (3) they cause an infection or infectious disease. Factors that influence whether an infection develops are the type of microorganism, its characteristics, and susceptibility of the **host**, the person on or in whom the microorganism resides.

Types of Microorganisms

Microorganisms that infect living tissue include bacteria, viruses, fungi, rickettsiae, protozoans, mycoplasmas, and helminths. Some cause *communicable* or *contagious diseases*, infectious diseases that are transmissible to other people. Examples of communicable diseases are measles, streptococcal sore throat, sexually transmitted diseases, and tuberculosis.

BACTERIA

Bacteria are single-celled microorganisms. They appear in a variety of shapes: round (cocci), rod-shaped (bacilli), or spiral (spirochetes) (Fig. 18–1). *Aerobic bacteria* require oxygen for growth and multiplication, whereas *anaerobic bacteria* grow and multiply in an atmosphere that lacks oxygen. A growing number of bacteria such as *Staphylococcus aureus*, *Streptococcus pneumoniae*, and the enterococcus (intestinal bacteria) *Escherichia coli*, are developing **multidrug resistance**, the ability to remain unaffected by antimicrobial drugs such as antibiotics (Box 18–1).

BOX 18-1 Causes of Antibiotic Resistance

- Bacterial mutations that interfere with the mechanism of antibiotic action
- Inappropriate prescription of antibiotics for viral infections
- Less than full compliance when taking prescribed antibiotics
- Prophylactic (preventive) administration of antibiotics in the absence of an infection
- Environmental dispersal of antibiotic solutions that intermingle with microorganisms such as when partially empty intravenous bags are deposited in waste containers, and droplets are released when purging IV tubing or removing air from syringes used to inject antibiotics
- Administration of antibiotics to livestock, leaving traces of drug residue after slaughter

VIRUSES

Viruses are the smallest agents known to cause disease and can only be seen with high-powered magnification using an electron microscope. They are also filterable, meaning they pass through very small barriers. Viruses are divided into two types: (1) those whose nucleic acid composition consists of deoxyribonucleic acid (DNA), or (2) those whose nucleic acid consists of ribonucleic acid (RNA). Viruses use the metabolic and reproductive materials of living cells or tissues to multiply. Some viral infections, such as the common cold, are minor and *self-limiting*; that is, they terminate with or without medical treatment. Others, such as rabies, poliomyelitis, and viral hepatitis, are more serious and may be fatal. On occasion, viruses may be dormant in a living host, reactivate from time to time, and cause the infection to recur. An example of this phenomenon is the herpes simplex virus, which causes cold sores (fever blisters) (see Chap. 68).

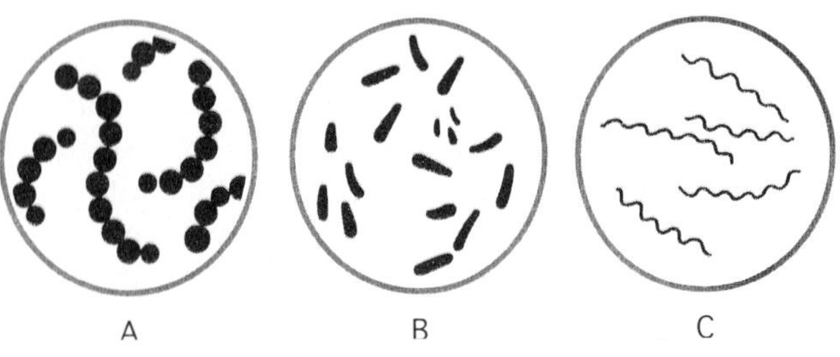

FIGURE 18-1. Classification of bacteria according to shape: (A) cocci, (B) bacillis, (C) spirochetes.

FUNGI

Fungi are divided into two basic groups: *yeasts* and *molds*. Only a small number of fungi appear to produce disease in humans. There are three types of fungus (mycotic) infections: superficial (dermatophytoses), that effect the skin, hair, and nails; intermediate, that chiefly affect subcutaneous tissues; and deep (systemic), that affect deep tissues and organs.

RICKETTSIAE

Rickettsiae are microorganisms that resemble but are different from bacteria. Like viruses, they invade living cells and cannot survive outside a living organism or a host. Rickettsial diseases are transmitted by arthropods (invertebrate animals with a segmented body, an external skeleton, and jointed, paired appendages), such as the flea, tick, louse, or mite.

PROTOZOANS

Protozoans are single-celled animals that are classified according to their motility (ability to move). Some protozoans possess *amoeboid motion*; they extend their cell walls and their intracellular contents flow forward. Others move by means of *cilia*, hairlike projections, or *flagella*, whiplike appendages. Still others have little or no movement.

MYCOPLASMAS

Mycoplasmas are single-celled microorganisms that lack a cell wall and, therefore, are pleomorphic (assume many shapes). They are similar but not related to bacteria. Mycoplasmas primarily infect the surface linings of the respiratory, genitourinary, and gastrointestinal tracts.

HELMINTHS

Helminths are infectious worms, some of which are microscopic. They are divided into three major groups: nematodes, or roundworms; cestodes, or tapeworms; and trematodes, or flukes. Some helminths enter the body in the egg stage, whereas others spend the larval stage in an intermediate host, then enter the human host. The organisms mate and reproduce in the definitive host and then are excreted, and the cycle begins again.

Characteristics of Microorganisms

Not all microorganisms are dangerous. Some are **nonpathogens** because they are generally harmless to healthy humans. For example, the normal microbial *flora* (microscopic plants) present in the intestine help synthesize vitamin B_{12}, biotin, vitamin K, and folic acid. **Pathogens**, on the other hand, have a high potential for causing infectious diseases. The ability of a microorganism to cause infection depends on a number of factors: its ability to move or be moved from one place to another, its **virulence** (power to produce disease), the number present, the duration of exposure, its ability to invade the host, and the **susceptibility** (prone to disease) of the host.

Given the right set of circumstances, both pathogens and nonpathogens can produce an infection. Unless and until the supporting host becomes weakened, normal flora remain in check. However, even benign microorganisms can produce **opportunistic infections**, those in which nonpathogenic or remotely pathogenic microorganisms take advantage of favorable situations and overwhelm the host (Box 18–2). More often than not, however, infections are caused by common pathogens.

BOX 18-2 Factors That Increase Susceptibility to Infection

- Inadequate nutrition
- Poor hygiene
- Suppressed immune system
- Chronic illness
- Insufficient white blood cells
- Prematurity
- Aging
- Compromised skin integrity
- Weakened cough reflex
- Diminished blood circulation
- Disregard for immunizations
- Overcrowding and homelessness

Infection Transmission

Like the links in a chain, components in the **infectious process cycle** must be present to transmit an infectious disease from one human or animal to a susceptible host (Fig. 18–2). Besides the infectious agent and host, an appropriate reservoir, exit route, mode of transmission, and portal of entry are necessary.

RESERVOIR

A **reservoir** is the environment in which the infectious agent is able to survive and reproduce. The reservoir may be human, animal, or nonliving, such as contaminated food and water. A human or animal that harbors (or is the reservoir of) an infectious microorganism but does not show active evidence of the infectious disease is a *carrier*. Nonliving reservoirs are *fomites*.

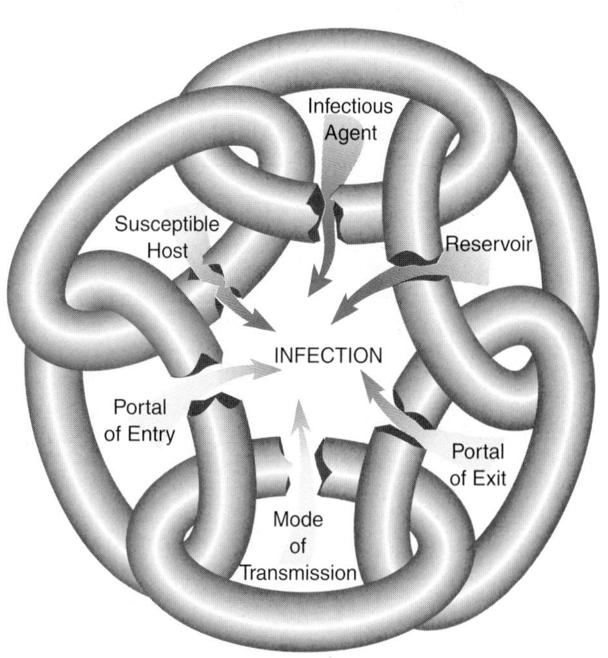

FIGURE 18-2. The infectious process cycle.

PORTAL OF EXIT

The **portal of exit** is the route by which the infectious agent escapes from the reservoir such as through the respiratory, gastrointestinal, or genitourinary tract, from the skin and mucous membranes, and blood and other body fluids.

MODE OF TRANSMISSION

A microorganism's **mode of transmission** refers to the manner in which it is transferred or moved from its reservoir to the susceptible host. There are five potential modes of transmission: contact, droplet, airborne, vehicle, and vector transmission (Table 18–1).

PORTAL OF ENTRY

An infectious agent gains entrance into a susceptible host through a **portal of entry**. Some infectious agents may have only one portal of entry; others may use several. Staphylococci, for example, can cause disease by entering through the respiratory tract (pneumonia), skin (boils), blood (internal abscesses), or gastrointestinal tract (food poisoning).

Although many microorganisms are present in reservoirs, they may be prevented from producing an infection because of human defense mechanisms.

Defense Mechanisms

Humans and other animal species have developed both mechanical and chemical defense mechanisms. *Mechanical defense mechanisms* are those that act as a physical barrier for preventing microorganisms from gaining entry or those designed to expel microorganisms before they multiply. Examples of mechanical defenses are the skin and mucous membranes, physiologic reflexes (eg, sneezing, coughing, and vomiting), and macrophages.

Chemical defense mechanisms destroy or incapacitate microorganisms with naturally produced biologic substances. Examples of chemical defense mechanisms include enzymes, secretions, and antibody substances.

SKIN AND MUCOUS MEMBRANES

The first line of defense against invading microorganisms is unbroken skin and mucous membranes. They separate underlying body tissues from microorganisms in the environment. The normal flora (eg, microorganisms) found on the skin compete with pathogenic microorganisms for nutrients, thereby retarding the growth of pathogens in these areas. In addition, the skin, which is acidic (because of the acetic acid in perspiration), creates an undesirable medium for the multiplication of pathogenic microorganisms.

Mucus, a sticky substance secreted from mucous membranes, traps microorganisms and debris on its surface. For example, mucous membrane secretions of the vagina favor the growth of nonpathogenic acid-producing bacteria, known as Doederlein's bacilli. The acid environment is unfavorable for multiplication of pathogenic bacteria and fungi. However, a change in vaginal pH or destruction of the normal flora can favor the development of a vaginal infection (see Chap. 61).

PHYSIOLOGIC REFLEXES

If microorganisms gain entry, they can be forcefully expelled by sneezing, coughing, and vomiting. Coughing is promoted by the action of *cilia*, hairlike projections in the upper respiratory tract, that beat in an upward direction.

TABLE 18-1 **Common Modes of Transmission**

Route of Transmission	Description	Example
Contact		
Direct	Infected to susceptible person	Sexual intercourse
Indirect	Contaminated substance to susceptible person	Handling a contaminated paper tissue
Droplet	Spray of moist particles within a 3-ft radius of infected person	Sneezing, coughing, talking
Airborne	Suspension and transport on air currents beyond 3 ft	Inhalation of microorganisms attached to dust particles
Vehicle	On or in contaminated food, water, objects, equipment	Eating or drinking tainted products
Vector	Infected animal or insect to susceptible person	Transfer from bites of mosquitoes, bats, ticks, etc

TABLE 18-2 **Types of Infections**

Type	Description	Common Signs and Symptoms/Examples
Localized	Confined to a small area	Pain, redness, warmth, and swelling, collection of fluid that may be purulent, swollen lymph nodes, and leukocytosis
Generalized	Systemic or widespread in one or more organs	Fever, chills, shivering, rapid pulse and respirations, hypotension (see septic shock in Chap. 22), headache, fatigue, anorexia, marked leukocytosis
Opportunistic	Infections that occur among immunocompromised hosts	Common infections include yeast infections in the mouth, bladder infections, gastroenteritis, and a type of pneumonia caused by the protozoan *Pneumocystis carinii* (see Chap. 42)
Community-acquired	Transmitted from one infected species to another	Same as generalized plus organ or disease specific manifestations (eg, a rash with chickenpox, diarrhea with dysentery)
Nosocomial	Acquired in a health care agency and not present prior to admission	Same as localized and generalized plus additional manifestations depending on the tissue that is infected
Acute	Sudden onset with serious and sometimes life-threatening manifestations	Appendicitis, an inflammation of the appendix secondary to a localized infection (see Chap. 51)
Chronic or subacute	An extended infection that resists treatment	Bacterial endocarditis, an inflammation of the inner muscle layer of the heart (see Chap. 30)
Secondary	A complication of some other disease process that occurred first	Infection in a person who has experienced severe burns

MACROPHAGES

Macrophages are specialized cells that make up the mononuclear phagocyte system, formerly known as the reticuloendothelial system (see Chap. 40). These cells are located throughout tissues of the body, in the liver (*Kupffer's cells*), the spleen, and lymphoid tissue (eg, the tonsils). Their primary function is to ingest dead cells and foreign material including microorganisms.

BIOLOGIC SUBSTANCES

Lysozyme (muramidase), an enzyme capable of splitting (lysing) the cell wall of some gram-positive bacteria, is present in tears, saliva, mucus, skin secretions, and some internal body fluids such as gastric juices. This enzyme is *bactericidal* (destroys bacteria) and thus acts as a defense against some pathogenic bacteria.

Antibodies, complex proteins also referred to as *immunoglobulins*, are formed when macrophages consume microorganisms and display their distinct cellular markers from their surface. Antibodies work with other white blood cells (WBCs) by rendering microorganisms more easily ingested, or phagocytized, in one of several ways: by *lysing* (dissolving or reducing the size of the foreign invader), by *neutralizing* their *toxins* (poisons released by some microorganisms), by *opsonizing* (coating) them, by *agglutinating* (clumping) them together, or by *precipitating* (solidifying) them.

Interferon, another chemical protein, is produced by the WBCs and other body cells in response to viral infections and other factors. Interferon appears to trigger infected cells to manufacture an antiviral protein. Because interferon also appears to inhibit cell reproduction, it is being used in the adjunct treatment of some cancers and viral disorders with positive results.

Despite all the various defense mechanisms, humans continue to succumb to infections of one type or another (Table 18–2). Regardless of the infectious process, all infections share some common pathophysiologic characteristics.

Pathophysiology

Localized Infections

The initial localized reaction to an invading microorganism activates the *inflammatory process* (Fig 18–3)—the first event is a cellular response that results in leakage of fluid, colloids, and ions from the capillaries into the tissues between the cells, producing swelling. It is followed by a vascular response that produces redness and heat, and a chemical response that causes pain. WBCs—neutrophils, macrophages, monocytes, and lymphocytes—move to the injury site to destroy the toxins produced by the pathogens and to remove debris from the area. More WBCs are manufactured as they are needed, a process referred to as **leukocytosis**.

To prevent the spread of pathogenic microorganisms to adjacent tissues, a fibrin barrier forms around the injured area. Inside the barrier, a thick, white exu-

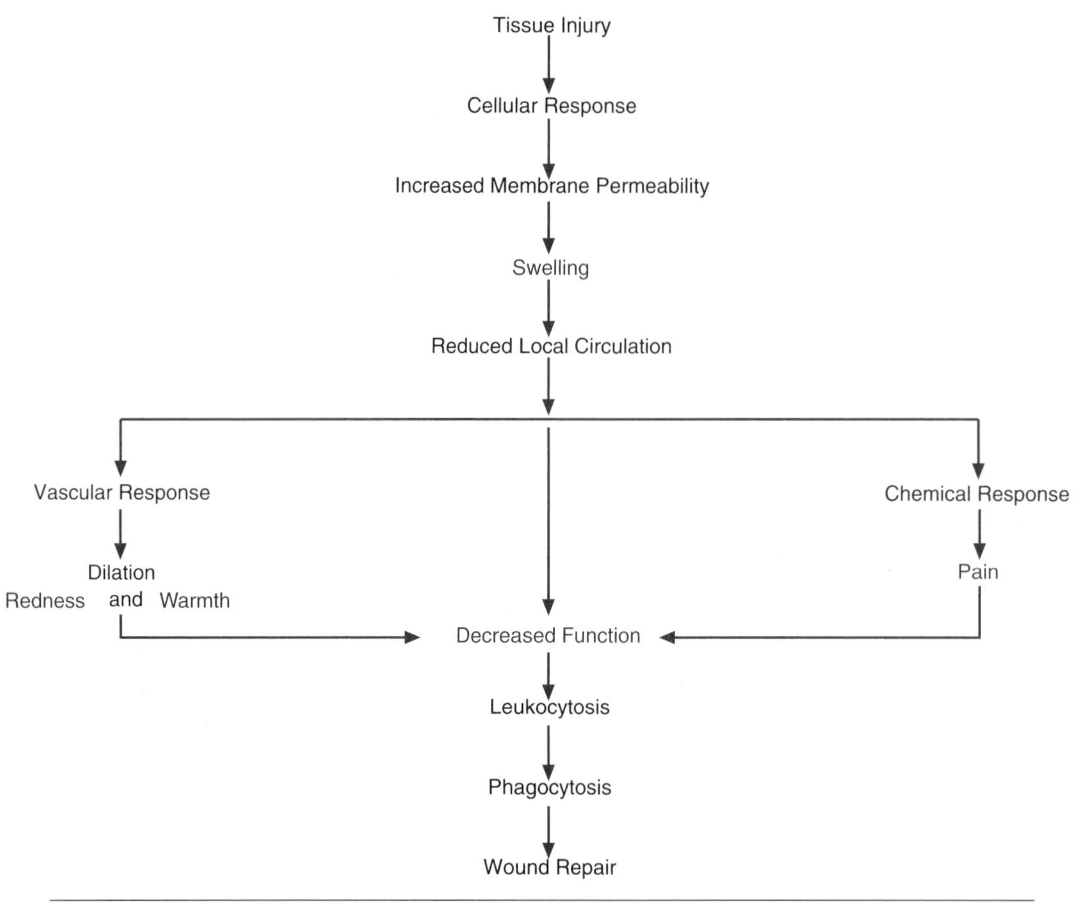

FIGURE 18-3. The inflammatory process.

date (pus) accumulates. This collection of pus is called an *abscess*. The abscess may break through the skin and drain, or continue to enlarge internally.

If the lymph nodes in the area become involved, they become enlarged and tender, an inflammatory condition referred to as *lymphadenitis*. If this defense mechanism is unable to contain the infection, the microorganisms begin to travel from node to node (see Chap. 39). Because the lymphatic system drains into the venous system, the microorganisms may eventually reach the bloodstream causing a condition called **septicemia** or **sepsis**, which leads to a generalized infection.

Generalized Infections

The pathophysiology of a **generalized infection** varies depending on the virulence of the pathogen and condition of the host. During the early stages, some persons have few symptoms, whereas others are acutely ill. Fever, which is the body's attempt to destroy the pathogen with heat, occurs and rises as the infection worsens. The person feels chilled despite the fever because surface blood vessels constrict to prevent loss of body heat. Muscles may contract to produce additional heat, causing uncontrollable shivering. Sweating stops as circulation is diverted to blood vessels deep within the body. The pulse and respiratory rates rise in proportion to the fever. Some clients experience a drop in blood pressure. If hypotension becomes severe, *septic shock*, *bacteremic shock*, or *toxic shock* (see Chap. 22) may ensue.

One of the major ways to limit an infection is early diagnosis and specific treatment.

Diagnostic Tests

A physical examination and thorough history are essential for the diagnosis of an infectious disease or process. Diagnosing some infectious diseases, however, requires additional tests and laboratory examinations to identify the microorganism.

White Blood Cell Count and Differential

An elevation in the number and type of WBCs (leukocytes), whose main function is **phagocytosis** (consuming pathogens, dead cells, and cellular debris), is indicative of an inflammatory and possibly infectious process. Although a total WBC count provides important information, a differential—one that indicates the percentage of WBC subtypes—is even more valuable. An elevation of neutrophils, the largest subtype of leukocytes, is an indication that the body is in the early stages of responding to an invading pathogen. As their numbers become depleted, bone marrow produces additional cells called "band cells" (bands) that eventually mature and take their place. An elevation of monocytes, the largest sized subtype of WBCs, is the body's second line of defense.

Culture and Sensitivity Test

A **culture** is used to identify bacteria within a specimen taken from a person with symptoms of an infection. The source of the specimen may be body fluids or wastes, such as blood, sputum, urine, or feces, or the *purulent exudate,* collection of pus, from an open wound (Clinical Procedure 18–1). The specimen is cultured. This involves placing a small amount of the specimen in or on a special growth medium. The specimen is incubated for a specific time period (usually 48–72 hours), then examined microscopically. To facilitate examination, the specimen is stained or dyed (colored). One stain is the Gram stain. Those bacteria that absorb the color are classified as *gram-positive;* those that do not, are *gram-negative.* The microorganisms may also be tested for pathogenicity or virulence with a coagulase test. When a culture is reported as *coagulase-positive,* it is more virulent than a culture of the same microorganism that produces a negative (*coagulase-negative*) response.

Sensitivity studies are done to determine which antibiotic inhibits the growth of a nonviral microorganism and will be most effective in treating the infection.

Examination for Ova and Parasites

Most ova (eggs) and parasites (those that live at the expense of the host) are intestinal worms. Therefore, the stool is examined for evidence of any forms within the infecting microorganism's life cycle. Generally, three random stools are collected from a bedpan, not the toilet. Urine and toilet paper may alter the specimen and therefore must be disposed of separately. Clients suspected of having intestinal ova and parasites are advised to perform scrupulous handwashing to avoid reinfecting themselves and others.

Skin Tests

Skin testing determines the presence of a specific active or inactive infection. Diseases for which skin testing may be done include histoplasmosis, mumps, tuberculosis, diphtheria, and coccidioidomycosis. The material for skin testing is injected intradermally (Fig. 18–4). The reaction is read after a specified time period (usually 48–72 hours). The size of the *induration* (hard elevated tissue), not including the surrounding area of *erythema* (redness) is measured in millimeters (mm). The measurement determines whether the reaction is significant. For example, a tuberculin skin test is considered positive if the induration is 15 mm or greater in persons with no known risk factors for tuberculosis; smaller measurements are significant in certain risk groups, such as those who are immunocompromised.

Immunologic Tests

Immunologic tests may be used to determine the presence of antigen (substances that stimulate an immune response) and antibody reactions (see Chap. 40). Examples include *agglutination tests,* for example the cold agglutinins test, which may reveal the presence of high antibody titers confirming immunity to rubella (measles); *precipitation tests,* for example the C-reactive protein test and erythrocyte sedimentation rate, which are elevated in some inflammatory diseases; *complement-fixation tests,* which, when elevated, indicate an inflammatory process; and *immunofluorescence tests,* which identify immunoglobulins, antibodies formed by the immune system.

Other Tests

Depending on the disease, other diagnostic tests may be used. Radiography (plain films or contrast studies), computed tomography scanning, and magnetic resonance imaging may be used to locate abscesses, identify displacement of organs or structures that may indicate abscess formation, and detect changes in tissues in areas such as the bones or the lung.

Medical Management

In some cases, supportive therapy such as rest, fluids, adequate nutrition, and antipyretics such as aspirin or acetaminophen (Tylenol) for a significantly elevated fever, may be advised while the infectious disease runs its course (Table 18–3). If the etiology is amenable

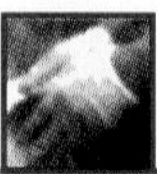

Clinical Procedure 18-1
Collection of a Wound Specimen for Culture

PURPOSE	EQUIPMENT
• To identify the pathogen infecting a wound	• Clean gloves • Culturette, a tube containing a swab and transport medium • Plastic zip-lock bag • Laboratory request slip • Paper bag for soiled dressing, if there is one • Sterile dressing materials and tape for reapplication

Nursing Action	Rationale
ASSESSMENT	
Check the medical orders.	Collaborates nursing activities with the medical plan for care
PLANNING	
Obtain the necessary equipment.	Prevents unnecessary delays in the plan of care
IMPLEMENTATION	
Check the client's identification.	Prevents errors
Wash your hands and don clean gloves.	Reduces the transmission of microorganisms
Remove the current dressing and discard it in a paper bag.	Confines vehicle that may transmit pathogens
Open the culturette and remove the swab from the tube taking care to avoid touching anything other than the wound with the tip.	Facilitates collecting a specimen without superimposing microorganisms from other sources.
Swab the wet drainage and saturate a large portion of the cotton tip, if possible.	Ensures collecting an adequate and reliable specimen
Avoid contact with the skin surrounding the wound.	Prevents collecting insignificant microorganisms
Insert the swab directly into the center of the culturette tube.	Prevents transferring pathogens to the outer surface where they may be transmitted to others.
Seal the culturette tube.	Prevents evaporation of the wet specimen
Crush the ampule of transport medium while holding the sealed end of the tube up.	Saturates the swab and maintains the concentration of microorganisms
Make sure that the swab is in contact with the transport medium.	Ensures that the specimen will not become degraded.
Place the sealed culturette inside the zip-lock plastic bag.	Confines potential sources of pathogen transmission
Remove gloves and wash your hands.	Removes microorganisms
Redress the wound.	Covers the wound so that drainage is wicked away from the local tissue
Complete the information that is requested on the laboratory slip.	Promotes accurate identification of the specimen and test results
Deliver the specimen to the laboratory immediately.	Facilitates prompt examination or measures that will ensure microbial growth and reproduction
Document the collection of the specimen, appearance of the wound and exudate, and reapplication of wound dressing.	Records implemented care and assessment findings

to drug therapy, antimicrobials such as antibiotics, sulfonamides, and antiviral drugs are prescribed.

Infected wounds may be *debrided*, a process of removing dead and damaged tissue. Wound irrigations, hydrotherapy (whirlpool), and the application of wet-to-dry dressings may accomplish the same objective.

With secondary infections, treatment of the primary condition may relieve the infectious process.

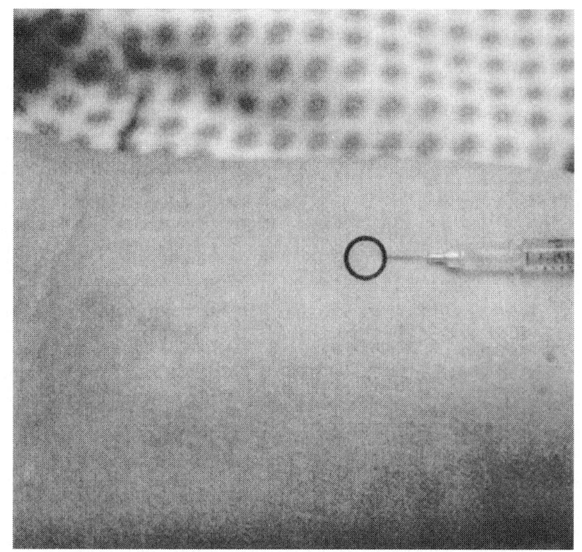

FIGURE 18-4. Forming a wheal. (Courtesy of Ken Timby.)

Bone marrow transplantation or administration of drugs that boost WBC production such as filgrastim (Neupogen) may help immunosuppressed clients.

Nursing Management

The nurse obtains a client's history, gathers subjective and objective data paying particular attention to manifestations of an inflammatory response, evidence of unusual drainage, and generalized data like a fever, lassitude (feeling tired), and loss of appetite. The nurse also prepares the client for diagnostic tests and collects specimens that will be cultured.

Handwashing remains the single most important measure for preventing the spread of infection. It is essential that everyone in a health care agency conscientiously follows handwashing guidelines (Box 18–3). Four elements are necessary to reduce the number of microorganisms on the hands: a cleansing agent, friction, running water, and time. The hands are washed with a cleansing agent such as soap. Friction and the lather from the cleansing agent lift the microorganisms from the skin's surface. Running water removes the cleansing agent and many of the microorganisms. To be effective, time is essential: 30 to 60 seconds of washing is recommended for hands not grossly contaminated.

BOX 18-3 Handwashing Guidelines

Handwashing should be performed:

- When arriving and leaving work
- Before and after contact with each client
- Before and after equipment is handled
- Before and after gloving
- Before and after specimens are collected
- Before preparing medications
- Before serving trays or feeding clients
- Before eating
- After toileting, hair combing, or other hygiene
- After cleaning a work area

Follow standard precautions, formerly called universal precautions, during the care of all clients. **Standard Precautions** (Box 18–4) are techniques that are used to prevent the potential for transmitting pathogens in blood or other body fluids when a person's infectious status is unknown (Fig. 18–5). When, and if, a client is diagnosed with an infectious condition, **transmission-based precautions** (Table 18–4), those that interfere with the manner in which a particular pathogen is spread, are implemented.

The nurse administers drug therapy and observes for evidence of the client's improvement such as a reduction in temperature, heart rate, and WBC count. Perform wound care regularly; keep dressings dry and intact. The nurse also implements measures that promote the client's comfort such as reducing fever

TABLE 18-3 **The Course of Infectious Diseases**

Stage	Characteristic
Incubation period	Infectious agent reproduces, but there are no recognizable symptoms. The infectious agent may, however, exit the host at this time and infect others.
Prodromal stage	Initial symptoms appear, which may be vague and nonspecific. They may include mild fever, headache, and loss of usual energy.
Acute stage	Symptoms become severe and specific to the tissue or organ that is affected. For example, tuberculosis is manifested by respiratory symptoms.
Convalescent stage	The symptoms subside as the host overcomes the infectious agent.
Resolution	The pathogen is destroyed. Health improves or is restored.

BOX 18-4 Standard Precautions

- Wear clean gloves when touching:
  - blood, body fluids, secretions and excretions, and items containing these body substances
  - mucous membranes
  - nonintact skin
- Perform handwashing immediately
  - when there is direct contact with blood, body fluids, secretions and excretions, and contaminated items
  - after removing gloves
  - between client contacts
- Wear a mask, eye protection, face shield during procedures and client care activities that are likely to generate splashes or sprays of blood, body fluids, secretions, and excretions
- Wear a cover gown during procedures and client care activities that are likely to generate splashes or sprays of blood, body fluids, secretions or excretions or cause soiling of clothing
- Remove soiled protective items promptly when the potential for contact with reservoirs of pathogens is no longer present.
- Clean and reprocess all equipment before reuse by another client.
- Discard all single-use items promptly in appropriate containers that prevent contact with blood, body fluids, and secretions and excretions, contamination of clothing, and transfer of microorganisms to other clients and the environment.
- Handle, transport, and process linen soiled with blood, body fluids, and secretions and excretions in such a way as to prevent skin and mucous membrane exposures, contamination of clothing, or transfer to other clients and the environment.
- Prevent injuries with used needles, scalpels, and other sharp devices by
  - never removing, recapping, bending, or breaking used needles
  - never pointing the needle toward a body part
  - using a one-handed "scoop" method, special syringes with a retractable protective guard or shield for enclosing a needle, or blunt-point needles
  - depositing disposable and reusable syringes and needles in puncture-resistant containers
- Use a private room or consult with an infection control professional for the care of clients who contaminate the environment, or who cannot or do not assist with appropriate hygiene or environmental cleanliness measures.

and measures that prevent or restore impaired skin integrity and improve nutrition and fluid intake.

Methods for preventing or controlling nosocomial infections and infectious communicable diseases, also known as community-acquired infections, are especially important. Nurses have valuable skills to contribute in these two aspects of health care.

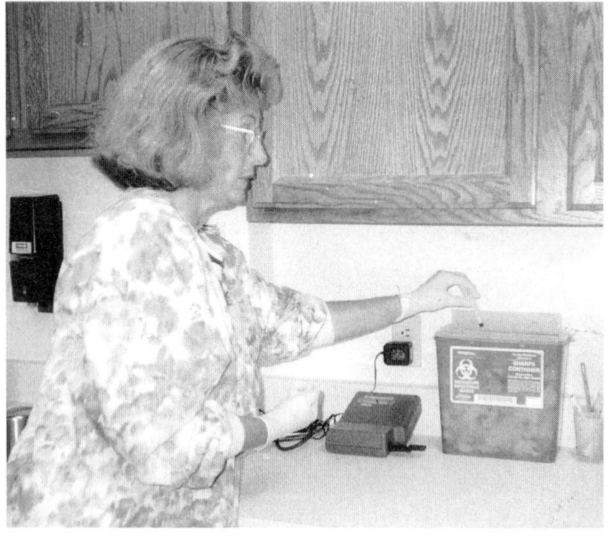

FIGURE 18-5. A nurse deposits an uncapped syringe in a biowaste container after it's used.

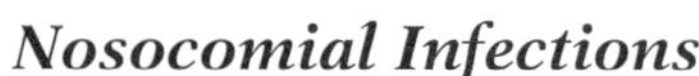

Nosocomial Infections

Nosocomial infections are those acquired while being cared for in a health care agency and the infection was not present, as either an active, incubatory, or chronic infection, at the time of admission. There are many reasons why nosocomial infections occur. Hospitalized clients are more susceptible to infections than well people, because they are exposed to pathogenic microorganisms in the hospital's environment, may have incisions or invasive equipment such as intravenous lines that compromise skin integrity, or may be immunosuppressed due to poor nutrition, their disease process, or its treatment. Also, because hospital personnel are in frequent and direct contact with many clients, there is a high risk for transmitting pathogenic microorganisms between and among clients. Visitors also carry a potential for introducing pathogens into the hospital environment as might equipment (eg, wheelchairs) and facilities used in common with others (eg, shared bathrooms).

TABLE 18-4 **Transmission-Based Precautions**

Type of Precaution	Location	Protection	Examples of Diseases
Airborne	Private room Negative air pressure* Discharge of room air to environment or filtered before being circulated	Follow Standard Precautions. Wear a mask for airborne pathogens or particulate air filter respirator in the case of tuberculosis. Place a mask on the client if transport is required.	Tuberculosis Measles Chickenpox
Droplet	Private room, or in a room with a similarly infected client(s) or one in which there is at least 3 feet between other client(s) and visitors	Follow Standard Precautions. Wear a mask when entering the room, but especially when within 3 feet of the infected client. Place a mask on the client if a transport is required.	Influenza Rubella Streptococcal pneumonia Meningococcal meningitis
Contact	Private room, or in a room with similarly infected client(s), or Consult with an infection control professional if the above options are not available.	Follow Standard Precautions. Don gloves before entering the room. Remove gloves before leaving the room. Change gloves after contact with infective material. Perform handwashing with an antimicrobial agent immediately after removing gloves. Wear a gown when entering the room if there is the possibility that your clothing will touch the client or items in the room, or if the client is incontinent, has diarrhea, an ileostomy, a colostomy, or wound drainage not contained by a dressing. Avoid transporting the client, but, if required, use precautions that minimize transmission. Clean bedside equipment and client care items daily. Use items such as a stethoscope, sphygmomanometer and other assessment tools exclusively for the infected client and terminally disinfect them when precautions are no longer necessary.	Gastrointestinal, respiratory, skin, or wound infections that are drug resistant Acute diarrhea Draining abscess

*Negative air pressure pulls air from the hall into the room when the door is opened, as opposed to positive air pressure, which pulls room air into the hall.

Source: Centers for Disease Control and Prevention. Draft guideline for isolation precautions in hospitals; notice. Federal Register November 7, 1994, 59:55552–55570.

PREVENTION AND CONTROL

To help prevent and control nosocomial infections, nurses apply principles of medical and surgical asepsis whenever they care for clients. They are further guided by recommendations from the health care agency's infection control committee, which is usually composed of representatives from various areas and departments of the hospital, such as medical staff, nursing service, clinical laboratories, pathology, operating room, housekeeping, and dietary service. The responsibilities of the infection control committee include surveillance, the process of detecting, reporting, and recording nosocomial infections; educating hospital personnel about methods for reducing nosocomial infections; providing guidelines for the prevention of infectious diseases, and investigating and following up outbreaks of nosocomial infections. Infection control guidelines generally establish policies for pre- and postemployment health examinations, sterilization procedures and methods, disposal of garbage and biologic wastes, and housekeeping techniques; designate precautions to be followed for a specific infection; and define the procedures for managing contaminated materials such as linen, equipment, and supplies used in the care of infectious clients (Fig. 18–6).

Many **community-acquired** (communicable, contagious) **infections** have been contained or eliminated because of advances in the prevention and treatment of infectious diseases. These advances include the discovery and use of antibiotics, the development of immunizing agents, guidelines for the proper disposal of human wastes, legislation controlling the preparation and sale of foods, immunization programs, and public education.

To help prevent and control community-acquired infections, nurses encourage childhood **immunizations** (Table 18–5), vaccines that stimulate the body to produce antibodies against a specific disease organism, to reduce the incidence of some infectious diseases. However, parental apathy or the inability to afford health care can pose a potential problem in

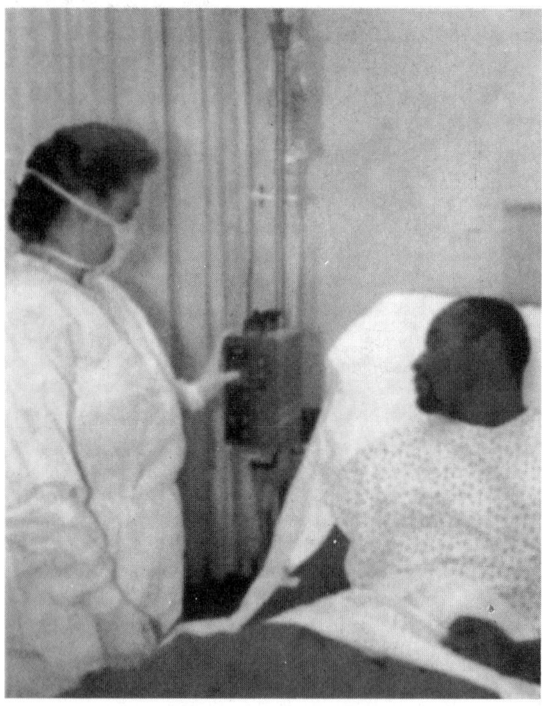

FIGURE 18-6. Gowns, masks, and gloves are worn if there is close client contact or handling of infected materials.

children obtaining immunizations. The immunization of children protects *all* people—children as well as adults who may not have developed sufficient immunity. Local, state, and federal public health agencies and the World Health Organization cooperate in the detection and control of communicable diseases. Because of their combined efforts, the incidence of many infectious diseases has been reduced and some (eg, smallpox) have been virtually eliminated.

The most personal avenue for preventing and controlling infectious diseases is education. Ideally, education about general health measures begins early in life. Parents must instruct their children in proper handwashing and in personal cleanliness and grooming and model similar behaviors.

Client and Family Teaching

To reduce the potential for infection, the nurse teaches the client and family members to:

- Perform frequent handwashing, especially before eating, after using the toilet, and after contact with nasal secretions.
- Bathe daily and perform other forms of personal hygiene such as oral care.
- Keep the home environment clean; household bleach diluted 1:10 or 1:100 is an excellent disinfectant.
- Keep immunizations current. Tetanus vaccine is recommended every 10 years; the influenza vaccine is repeated yearly; and one dose of pneumococcal pneumonia vaccine lasts a lifetime.
- Investigate the need for vaccinations, water purification techniques, and foods to avoid when traveling outside the United States.
- Practice a healthy lifestyle such as eating the recommended servings from the food pyramid (see Chap. 15) and using safe food handling practices.
- Use and immediately discard disposable paper tissues rather than reuse a cloth handkerchief.
- Avoid sharing personal care items such as washcloths and drinking cups.
- Use safe sex practices.
- Stay home from work or school when ill rather than expose others to infectious pathogens.
- Avoid crowds and public places when there are local outbreaks of influenza.
- Follow posted infection control instructions when visiting hospitalized family members and friends.
- Understand that antibiotic therapy is not always appropriate for every infectious disease, but when it is, take the full dose for the prescribed period of time.

Needle Stick Injuries

One of the greatest threats to health care workers is the potential for acquiring blood-borne infectious diseases such as hepatitis B (HBV) and acquired immunodeficiency syndrome (AIDS). Following Standard Precautions (see Box 18–3) reduces this potential. However, gloves are not impervious to penetration by sharp objects such as needles that may contain blood. Despite following policies and precautions for avoiding blood-borne pathogens and using new needleless access devices on intravenous lines, needle stick injuries continue to occur. Should an accidental injury occur, health care workers are advised to follow postexposure recommendations, which include:

- Reporting the injury to one's supervisor immediately
- Documenting the injury in writing
- Identifying the person or source of blood, if possible
- Obtaining the human immunodeficiency virus (HIV) and hepatitis B status, if it is legal to do so. Unless the client gives permission, testing and revealing HIV status is prohibited.
- Obtaining counseling on the potential for infection

TABLE 18-5 **Recommended Childhood Immunization Schedule**

Vaccine	Doses	Acceptable Age Range for Immunization
Hepatitis B (HBV)	1st dose 2nd dose 3rd dose	birth–2 months 1–4 months 6–18 months or 11–12 years if not immunized earlier
Diphtheria, Tetanus, Pertussis (DTaP or DTP)	1st dose 2nd dose 3rd dose booster booster Td booster	2 months 4 months 6 months 15–18 months 4–6 years 11–16 years; repeat T every 10 years
Haemophilus influenzae B (HiB)	1st dose 2nd dose 3rd dose booster	2 months 4 months 6 months 12–15 months
Poliomyelitis (OPV or IPV)	1st dose 2nd dose 3rd dose booster	2 months 4 months 12–18 months 4–6 years
Measles, Mumps, Rubella (MMR)	1st dose 2nd dose	12–15 months 4–6 years or 11–12 years
Varicella (Var) (chickenpox)	one dose	12–18 months; 11–12 years if not immunized earlier or never acquired the disease

DTaP, diphtheria, tetanus, acellular pertussis; IPV, inactivated (injected) polio vaccine; OPV, oral polio vaccine; Td, full dose of tetanus, reduced dose of diphtheria.

Recommendations are based on those approved by the Advisory Committee on Immunization Practices, the American Academy of Pediatrics, and the American Academy of Family Physicians (January–December 1997)

- Receiving the most appropriate postexposure prophylaxis
- Being tested for the presence of disease antibodies at appropriate intervals
- Receiving instructions on monitoring potential symptoms and medical follow-up

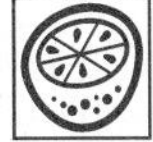

General Nutritional Considerations

Infection causes changes in body metabolism including an increase metabolic rate and an increase in the breakdown of glycogen, fat, and protein tissue.

Fever is a major determinant of caloric needs during infection. Basal metabolic rate (BMR) increases by 7% for each degree of Fahrenheit of temperature above normal. For instance, the BMR for a person with a temperature of 103.6° is increased by 35% (5° above normal × 7%/degree = 35% increase). This translates into an extra 350 to 700 calories per day, based on an average BMR range of 1,000 to 2,000 calories per day.

Protein needs can increase to 1.5 to 2.5 g/kg body weight for severe infections (normal protein requirement is 0.8 g/kg). Milk, milk drinks, and commercial supplements may be used to add significant amounts of proteins and calories.

Fluid needs depend on the severity of the fever and the presence of complicating factors such as diarrhea, vomiting, and excessive sweating. Encourage the intake of ice water, broth, fruit juices, milk, popsicles, and gelatin. Tea, coffee, and carbonated beverages containing caffeine promote diuresis and should be avoided.

Clients who are acutely ill may accept and tolerate a full liquid diet with in-between-meal supplements better than solid food. Advance the diet as tolerated to maximize intake.

For clients on transmission-based precautions, meals are served on disposable dinnerware. The tray is made as attractive as possible to encourage eating. Uneaten food is disposed in the toilet and plastic containers deposited in sealed bags before removal from the room.

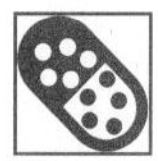

General Pharmacologic Considerations

Antibiotics can cause an overgrowth of microorganisms not affected by the antibiotic. This overgrowth can cause a superinfection leading to a potentially serious and life-threatening diarrhea called pseudomembranous colitis. Report fever, abdominal cramps, and severe diarrhea immediately.

Antipyretic drugs (eg, aspirin and acetaminophen) usually are ordered for an elevated temperature.

When an antipyretic drug is administered rectally, the suppository is inserted high in the rectum. The client is checked in 30 minutes to ensure that the suppository has not been expelled.

Antibiotics are administered *on time* and at regular intervals around-the-clock to maintain therapeutic blood levels.

When antibiotics are administered, observe the client for adverse drug effects. Nausea, vomiting, anorexia, diarrhea, and rash are adverse effects of some antibiotics but also are symptoms associated with some infectious diseases. An accurate history and physical examination at the time of admission and ongoing documentation of the client's symptoms, help distinguish between symptoms related to the infectious disease and those possibly caused by antibiotic therapy.

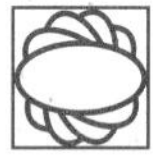

General Gerontologic Considerations

Chronic diseases and inadequate nutrition predispose older adults to infections and infectious diseases.

Infection in older adults is more serious because their defense mechanisms are less efficient.

Symptoms of infectious disease are subtle, atypical or blunted in the elderly. For example temperature is less elevated with pneumonia or urinary tract infection. Confusion and changes in behavior are often signs of infection among older adults.

Residents in nursing homes tend to acquire infections involving the urinary tract, skin, and respiratory tract.

Pneumonia and influenza are the fifth leading cause of death in people older than age 65. Morbidity and mortality can be reduced by immunizing for pneumococcal pneumonia and influenza.

Visitors with respiratory infections are tactfully advised to avoid visiting older adults until their symptoms are relieved, or they are provided with a mask.

When transmission-based precautions are necessary, older adults may become confused because of decreased social contact and the lack of environmental stimulation from television, radio, windows, reading materials, and so on.

Some older adults who had tuberculosis as children can experience a reactivation of the disease if they become seriously ill.

SUMMARY OF KEY CONCEPTS

- Infectious disorders are conditions caused by microorganisms.
- Microorganisms are living plants and animals that are so small they cannot be seen except with a microscope. Examples include bacteria, viruses, fungi, rickettsiae, protozoans, mycoplasmas, and helminths.
- Three factors that influence whether an infection develops are the type of microorganism, its characteristics, and susceptibility of the host.
- Nonpathogens are microorganisms that are generally harmless to healthy humans. Pathogens are microorganisms that have a high potential for causing infectious diseases.
- Factors that increase a person's susceptibility to infection include inadequate nutrition, poor hygiene, suppressed immune system, chronic illness, and insufficient leukocytes.
- For an infection to develop, six components—collectively referred to as the infectious process cycle—must be present: an infectious microorganism, reservoir, portal for exit, mode for transmission, portal of entry, and susceptible host.
- Mechanical and chemical defense mechanisms prevent many infectious disorders from occurring. Mechanical defenses, like the skin, or reflexes that expel microorganisms, like coughing, act as a physical barrier to microorganisms. Chemical defenses destroy or incapacitate microorganisms with naturally produced biologic substances like enzymes and antibodies.
- Whenever tissue is infected or injured, the inflammatory response occurs. It proceeds from a cellular response that causes swelling and reduced circulation, to a vascular response that produces redness and warmth, and a chemical response that produces pain. Collectively the physiologic responses result in decreased function. Afterward leukocytosis and phagocytosis occur to facilitate cellular repair.
- Examples of diagnostic tests that may be ordered for clients suspected of having an infectious disorder include a WBC count and differential, a culture and sensitivity, and skin tests.
- Medically, clients with infectious disorders are given general supportive treatment as the infectious disorder follows its natural course or antimicrobial therapy is administered. Some immunocompromised clients may undergo a bone marrow transplant or receive a drug that boosts production of WBCs.
- Examples of nursing techniques useful for preventing or controlling infections include conscientious handwashing and following standard and transmission-based precautions.
- Clients cared for in health care agencies are at greater risk for infection because they are exposed to microorganisms that are different than those in their home environment, they often have equipment or procedures that impair their skin integrity, and they are cared for by health care workers who may transfer microorganisms from one client to another during the course of care.

- Infection control committees develop policies and guidelines for preventing infections within the health care agency.
- Handwashing is the best technique for limiting infections. To be effective, it must include a cleansing agent, friction, running water, and sufficient time.
- Community-acquired infections have been reduced because of the discovery and use of antibiotics, the development of immunizing agents, proper disposal of human wastes, sanitary control of the sale and preparation of foods, mandatory immunization programs, and public education.
- Important information to teach clients to prevent infections includes maintain personal hygiene, keep the home environment clean, obtain appropriate immunizations, avoid contact with individuals who have infectious diseases, and follow the advice of the physician in regard to antibiotic therapy.
- Nurses and other health care workers are at risk for infection from blood-borne microorganisms. Therefore, if a penetrating injury occurs, such as a needle stick, it is important to report and document the incident, be tested for evidence of the disease, receive counseling regarding infection risks and possible postexposure treatment, and comply with long-term medical follow-up.

CRITICAL THINKING EXERCISES

1. Use the *Infectious Process Cycle* illustrated in Figure 18–2 to trace the viral transmission of a common cold from one person to another.
2. List specific examples of ways that pathogens are spread among clients and health care workers; then identify techniques for preventing their transmission.
3. Select any infectious disease and identify the type of microorganism that causes it, its usual reservoir, exit route, mode of transmission, and port of entry.

Suggested Readings

Borton, D. (1996). Gloves on or off? *Nursing, 26*(5), 57.

Borton, D. (1997). Isolation precautions: Clearing up the confusion. *Nursing, 27*(1), 49–51.

Calianno, C. (1996). Nosocomial pneumonia: Repelling a deadly invader. *Nursing, 26*(5), 34–39.

Garner, J. (1996). Guideline for isolation precautions in hospitals. *Infection Control and Hospital Epidemiology, 17*(1), 53–80.

Removing protective garb. (1996). *Nursing, 26*(11), 62–64.

Ruth-Sahd, L., & Pirrung, M. (1997). The infection that eats patients alive. *RN, 60*(3), 28–31, 33–34.

Shoevin, J., & Young, M. S. (1992). MRSA: Pandora's box for hospitals...methicillin resistant *Staphylococcus aureus*. *American Journal of Nursing, 92*, 48–52.

Additional Resources

Centers for Disease Control and Prevention
1600 Clifton Road, NE
Atlanta, GA 30333
http://www.cdc.gov@cdcl/diseases.html

Center for Food Safety and Applied Nutrition
200 C Street, SW
Washington, DC 20204
http://vm.cfsan.fda.gov/list.html

National Institute of Allergy and Infectious Disease (gopher server)
gopher://odie.niaid.nih.gov

Pan American Health Organization
Regional Office of the World Health Organization
525 23rd Street, NW
Washington, DC 20037
http://www.paho.org
(202) 974–3000

Outbreak (information on emerging diseases)
http://www.objarts.com/cgi-outbreak-unreg/dynaserve.exe/index.html

Chapter 19

Caring for Clients With Cancer

KEY TERMS

Alopecia
Antineoplastic
Benign
Biotherapy
Brachytherapy
Cancer
Carcinogens
Chemotherapy
Extravasation
Gene Therapy
Leukopenia
Malignant
Metastasis
Neoplasms
Radiation Therapy
Stomatitis
Thrombocytopenia
Vesicants

LEARNING OBJECTIVES

On completion of this chapter, the reader will:

- Discuss the pathology and etiology of cancer.
- Differentiate between benign and malignant tumors.
- Name factors that contribute to the development of cancer.
- Identify the warning signs of cancer.
- Describe ways to reduce the risks of cancer.
- Discuss methods for diagnosing cancer.
- Describe systems for staging and grading malignant tumors.
- Differentiate various treatments and methods for managing cancer.
- Discuss various adverse effects that occur with cancer treatments and methods used to treat those effects.
- Discuss the emotional impact associated with the diagnosis of cancer.
- Use the nursing process as a framework for caring for clients with cancer.

Cancer is characterized by abnormal, unrestricted cell proliferation. Malignant tumors invade healthy tissues and compete with normal cells for oxygen, nutrients, and physical space. The nursing specialty related to caring for clients with cancer is called oncology nursing. The diagnosis of cancer is frightening for most people, although reactions of clients depend on the particular diagnosis, location, stage, treatment, effects on bodily functions, and prognosis.

Pathophysiology

The cell is the basic structural unit in plant and animal life forms. Differentiated cells work together to perform specific functions. Cell regeneration occurs through cell division and reproduction. Abnormal changes in cells can occur for many reasons. These abnormal cells reproduce in the same way, but they do not have the regulatory mechanisms to control growth. As a result, the abnormal cell growth proliferates in an uncontrolled and unrestricted way.

New growths of abnormal tissue are called **neoplasms** or tumors. They are classified according to their cell of origin and whether their manner of growth is **benign**, not invasive or spreading, or **malignant,** invasive and capable of spreading. Table 19–1 classifies tumor cells. The first part of the name indicates the particular cell or tissue (Bullock, 1996). The suffix *-oma* indicates it is a tumor. Four main classifications of tumors according to tissue type are:

- Carcinomas (cancers originating from epithelial cells)
- Lymphomas (cancers originating from organs that fight infection)
- Leukemias (cancers originating from organs that form blood)
- Sarcomas (cancers originating from connective tissue, such as bone or muscle)

TABLE 19-1 **Classification of Tumor Cells**

Origin	Malignant	Benign
Skin	Basal cell carcinoma	
	Squamous cell carcinoma	Papilloma
	Malignant melanoma	Nevus (mole)
Epithelium	Adenocarcinoma	Adenoma
Muscle	Myosarcoma	Myoma
Connective tissue		
Fibrous tissue	Fibrosarcoma	Fibroma
Adipose (fatty) tissue	Liposarcoma	Lipoma
Cartilage	Chondrosarcoma	Chondroma
Bone	Osteosarcoma	Osteoma
Nerve tissue	Neurogenic sarcoma	Neuroma
	Neuroblastoma	Ganglioneuroma
	Glioblastoma	Glioma
Bone marrow	Multiple myeloma	
	Leukemia	

The major differences between benign and malignant (cancerous) neoplasms are shown in Table 19–2.

Cancer can spread (**metastasis**) by direct extension to adjacent tissues, extension from lymph vessels into the tissues adjacent to lymphatic vessels, transportation by blood or lymph systems, and diffusion within a body cavity. The area in which malignant cells first form is the *primary site*. The regions to which cancer cells spread are *secondary* or metastatic sites. Metastasis is one of the most discouraging characteristics of cancer because even one malignant cell can give rise to a metastatic lesion in a distant part of the body. Metastatic tumors are treated aggressively whenever possible to improve the quality of life and to lengthen survival time. When a malignant tumor is removed, generally a lymph node dissection is also done, along with a wide excision of the tumor (Fig. 19–1).

Benign tumors remain at the original site of their development. They may grow large, but their rate of growth is slower than that of malignant tumors. Benign tumors usually do not cause death unless their location impairs the function of a vital organ, such as the brain. On the other hand, malignant tumors grow rapidly, and, unless completely removed before metastasis has occurred, they are likely to spread.

Etiology

Certain factors and agents appear to be related to the development of many cancers. Factors believed to cause cancer are called **carcinogens**. These include chemical agents, environmental factors, dietary substances, viruses, defective genes, and hormones.

Chemical agents in the environment are believed to account for 85% of all cancers. Effects of tobacco smoke and nicotine are related to cancers of the lung, mouth, throat, neck, esophagus, pancreas, cervix, and bladder. Prolonged exposure to certain chemicals such as asbestos and coal dust is associated with some cancers. Chemical substances in the workplace can cause cancer. Organs most affected are the lungs, liver, and kidneys because they are involved with biotransformation and excretion of chemicals.

Environmental factors include prolonged exposures to sunlight, radiation, pollutants, and possibly electromagnetic fields from microwaves, power lines, and cellular phones.

Diet is a risk factor in cancer development. What a person does not consume is as important as what he or she consumes. Food high in fat, smoked foods, foods preserved with salts or alcohol, and foods with nitrates are associated with an increased risk for cancer. Foods believed to reduce the risk of cancer are

TABLE 19-2 **Characteristics of Benign and Malignant Tumors**

Benign Tumors	Malignant Tumors
Usually slow steady rate of growth	Generally rapid rate of growth; can be unpredictable
Growth remains localized	Invades surrounding tissue and metastasizes to other tissues
Generally remain encapsulated	Rarely encapsulated
When palpated, the tumor is smooth, easily defined, and movable.	When palpated, the tumor has irregular borders and is immobile.
Less profuse blood supply	Greater than normal blood supply
Cells resemble the cells of the tissue of origin.	Cells cannot be readily identified as to tissue of origin.
Only destroy normal tissue by compression or obstruction of normal tissue	Invade normal tissue and compete with normal cells for oxygen and nutrients; also destroy by compression and destruction
When removed, recurrence is rare.	When removed, recurrence is more common.
Rarely fatal	Fatal if not treated

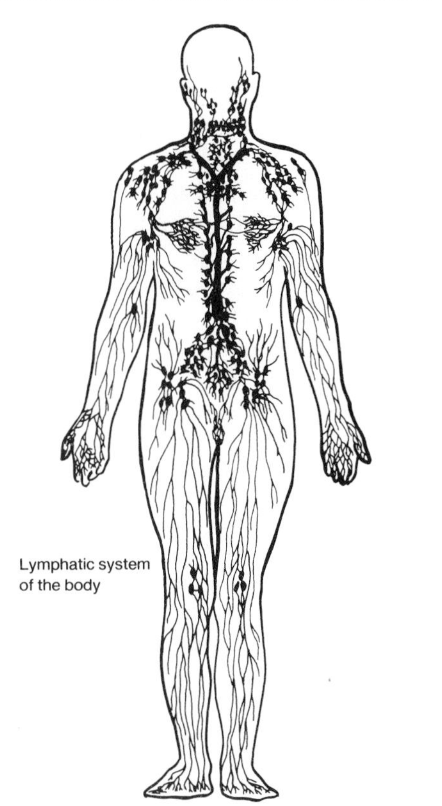

FIGURE 19-1. One route by which malignant cells can spread to other areas of the body is the lymphatic system. Cancer cells also can be carried by the blood.

high in fiber, cruciferous, (cabbage, broccoli), and high in carotene (winter squash, carrots, cantaloupe). Vitamins A, C, and E also seem to have anticancer value. Table 19–3 provides guidelines for dietary modifications that are believed to reduce the risk of cancer.

Viruses are implicated in many cancers. The cell changes incorporated into the genetic information by the virus may result in the formation of cancerous cells. An example is Kaposi's sarcoma associated with human immunodeficiency virus (HIV) (Bullock, 1996).

Defective genes are responsible for diverse cancers. Some types of leukemia, retinoblastoma (eye tumor in children), and skin cancers are associated with genetic factors. Breast, prostate, and colorectal cancers are also associated with defective genes.

Medically prescribed interventions such as immunosuppressive drugs, hormone replacements, and anticancer drugs have been associated with increased incidence of cancer in individuals or their offspring when exposed in utero.

TABLE 19-3 **Diet Modifications for Reducing the Risk of Cancer**

- Decrease the intake of red meat.
- Increase the number of servings of cruciferous vegetables such as broccoli, cabbage, and cauliflower.
- Reduce the intake of processed meats that contain nitrites and nitrates as preservatives.
- Increase fiber intake.
- Decrease fat intake to 20–30% of total daily calories.
- Increase intake of food rich in vitamins A and C, such as fruits and yellow and leafy green vegetables.
- Reduce alcohol intake to no more than one drink per day.

Assessment Signs and Symptoms

Cancer is an insidious disease. It initially may not cause any symptoms or the signs may be vague. This underscores the importance of educating the public about prevention and self-examination so that cancer can be diagnosed in its earliest stages. Seven warning signals of cancer (CAUTION) published by the American Cancer Society are:

Change in bowel or bladder habits
A sore that does not heal
Unusual bleeding or discharge
Thickening or lump in breast or elsewhere
Indigestion or difficulty in swallowing
Obvious change in wart or mole
Nagging cough or hoarseness

Better education has produced an awareness of the warning signals and factors that influence the development of cancer. Public education stresses the importance of periodic physical examinations and cancer screening programs. Self-examination of the breasts, testicles, and skin is emphasized and taught. Avoidance of factors that predispose a person to cancer and early detection increase the chances of curing the disease. Table 19–4 lists healthy habits that reduce the risk of cancer.

TABLE 19-4 **Healthy Lifestyle Habits that Reduce the Risk of Cancer**

- Learn and practice self-examination techniques on a regular basis.
- See physician or nurse practitioner on a regular basis.
- Include periodic colon exams, mammograms, Pap smears, testicular exams, and prostate-specific antigen testing as indicated.
- Eat a healthy diet (see Table 19-3).
- Abstain from smoking or using tobacco products.
- Avoid overexposure to the sun; use sunscreen with SPF of 15 or greater.
- Maintain weight within suggested limits.
- Exercise regularly.
- Practice safety in the workplace to avoid exposure to chemicals and radiation.
- Limit alcohol intake.

Diagnosis

Cancer is diagnosed by history, physical examination, and diagnostic studies. In some cases the physical examination is unremarkable, but the client's history is suspicious for cancer. In addition, the client is evaluated for risk factors.

Many diagnostic studies are used to establish a diagnosis of cancer. The physician, using information obtained during the history and physical examination, selects tests that help establish a diagnosis.

Laboratory Tests

The chemical composition of blood and other body fluids is altered by the presence of specific cancers. Specialized tests have been developed for *tumor markers,* which are specific proteins, antigens, hormones, genes, or enzymes released by cancer cells. These include:

- *Acid phosphatase*: indicates that prostate cancer has metastasized to other parts of the body if blood levels of this enzyme are elevated.
- *CA-19–9*: detects an antigen that indicates pancreatic cancer.
- *CA-125*: measures the antigen that is diagnostic for ovarian cancer.
- *Prostate specific antigen (PSA)*: detects prostate cancer when levels are elevated; this test is more specific than acid phosphatase.

Other laboratory tests may be useful in establishing a diagnosis. Although abnormal values do not directly indicate a malignant process, they may help in formulating a total clinical picture. For example, a complete blood count may detect anemia in a client with possible colon cancer. Occult blood in the stool may indicate colorectal cancer.

Radiologic Tests

- *X-ray studies*: These studies, such as plain films or radiographs using contrast media or specialized equipment, detect tumors in specific organs. A contrast medium is a substance that highlights, outlines, or provides more detail than shown in a plain film. A barium enema is an example of a study done with contrast medium.
- *Computed tomography (CT)*: The CT scan provides three-dimensional cross-sectional views of tissues to determine tumor density, size, and location.
- *Magnetic resonance imaging (MRI)*: Similar to a CT scan, the MRI uses magnetic fields for sectional images. It helps visualize tumors hidden by bones.
- *Radioisotope studies*: These studies use radioactive materials (given orally or intravenously) to help diagnose various malignancies. A scanner then identifies areas of increased, decreased, or normal distribution.
- *Ultrasound*: Ultrasound uses high frequency sound waves to detect abnormal variations of a body organ or structure. The sound wave reflections are projected on a screen and may be recorded on film. These studies help differentiate solid and cystic tumors of the abdomen, breasts, pelvis, and heart.

Other Studies

- *Biopsy*: Tissue samples excised from the body are directly examined microscopically for malignant or premalignant processes. Tissue samples may be obtained during a surgical procedure, through insertion of a biopsy needle under local anesthesia, or during endoscopic procedures. A biopsy provides the most definitive method for diagnosing cancer.
- *Frozen section*: During some surgeries, when a tumor or node is removed, it is taken to the pathologist for immediate examination. The specimen is quickly frozen and then sliced into very thin pieces so that it may be examined under a microscope. Once the preliminary findings are known, the surgeon makes a decision regarding the type of surgery needed. The client is made aware of the possibilities before surgery.
- *Endoscopy*: Fiberoptic instruments are flexible tubes that contain optic fibers that enable light to travel in a straight line or at various angles and illuminate the area being examined. Specific areas of the body are examined with endoscopy: gastroscopy, bronchoscopy, and colonoscopy. Tissue biopsies are done if a malignancy is suspected.
- *Cytology*: Microscopic examination of cells from various areas of the body are used to diagnose malignant or premalignant disorders. Cells are obtained via needle aspiration, scraping, brushing, or sputum. An example of a cytologic test is the Papanicolaou's (Pap) smear used in diagnosing changes in the endometrium, cervix, and vagina (see Chap. 58).

Staging of Tumors

Before a client is treated for cancer, the tumor is staged and graded based on the manner in which tumors tend to grow and the cell type of the tumor. The American Joint Commission on Cancer developed a grading system referred to as the TNM classification system: *T* indicates the size of the tumor; *N* stands for the involvement of regional lymph nodes; and *M* refers to the presence of metastasis. Table 19–5 gives a more detailed description of the TNM classification system.

A second classification system also stages tumors according to size, evidence of metastasis, and the presence or absence of lymph node involvement:

- *Stage I*: malignant cells are confined to the tissue of origin, no signs of metastasis
- *Stage II*: limited spread of cancer in the local area, generally to area lymph nodes
- *Stage III*: tumor larger or probably has invaded surrounding tissues or both
- *Stage IV*: cancer has invaded or metastasized to other parts of the body

Grading of tumors involves the differentiation of the malignant cells. Basically there are two classifications: differentiated and undifferentiated. Cancer cells are evaluated in comparison to normal cells. *Well differentiated* cells are those that most closely resemble the tissue of origin. *Undifferentiated cells* bear little resemblance to the tissue of origin. Cell differentiation is classified on a grade of I to IV. The higher the number, the less differentiated the cell type. Tumors with poorly differentiated cells are graded IV. These tumors are very aggressive and unpredictable and the prognosis usually poor.

Medical Management of Cancer

Three basic methods are used in the treatment of cancer: (1) surgery, (2) radiation therapy, and (3) chemotherapy. Another method, bone marrow transplantation, is also used for treating selected cancers. Biotherapy, gene therapy, and other alternative therapies may also be used. Cancer frequently is treated with a combination of therapies using established protocols.

TABLE 19-5 **TNM Staging System and Classification**

Symbol	Meaning
T	Primary tumor
TO	No evidence of primary tumor
Tis	Carcinoma in situ
T1, T2, T3, T4	Progressively larger tumor size and extension
N	Regional lymph nodes
NO	No regional lymph node involvement
N1, N2, N3	Increasing regional lymph node involvement
M	Distant metastasis
MO	No distant metastasis
M1	Presence of distant metastasis
Example: T2, N1, MO	Indicates that the primary tumor has grown and spread to regional lymph nodes but has not metastasized

Surgery

Surgery may range from excision of the tumor alone to extensive excision, including removal of the tumor and adjacent structures such as bone, muscle, and lymph nodes. The type and extent of the surgery depends on the extent of disease, actual pathology, age and physical condition of the client, and anticipated results. When tumors are confined and have not invaded vital organs, the surgery is more likely to be curative. Surgery that helps to relieve uncomfortable symptoms or prolong life is considered palliative. Reconstructive or plastic surgery may be done after extensive surgery to correct defects caused by the original surgery. Some surgeries are disfiguring or are so profound that the client may have difficulty adjusting to body changes and disfigurement. In these cases, radiation therapy may be a better option. Preoperative and postoperative care is discussed in Chapter 24. Specific surgeries are addressed in separate chapters.

Radiation Therapy

Radiation therapy uses high-energy ionizing radiation, such as high-energy x-rays, gamma rays, and radioactive particles (alpha and beta particles, neutrons, and protons), to destroy cancer cells. Cell destruction occurs as a result of disruption of cell function and division and alteration of DNA molecules. Cell death can occur immediately or when the cell is unable to reproduce. The goal of radiation therapy is to destroy malignant, rapidly dividing cells without permanently damaging the surrounding healthy tissues. Normal and malignant cells can both be destroyed. However, the more rapidly reproducing malignant cells are more sensitive to radiation because radiation affects cells undergoing mitosis (cancer cells) more than cells in slower growth cycles (normal tissue). Radiation therapy is applied externally or internally, both with curative and palliative intent. Nearly 60% of all clients with cancer will receive some form of radiation for their treatment and about 60% of those are cured of their disease (Washington & Leaver, 1997).

EXTERNAL RADIATION THERAPY

External radiation therapy makes use of high-energy x-rays aimed at a specific location in the body. A treatment plan, using beams from multiple directions, is developed and customized for each client. Clients usually have external radiation done on an outpatient basis. Their skin is marked with a marker or tattoo to identify the reference points for the treatment plan. Clients are instructed not to wash these markings off until the therapy is complete.

Expected side effects occur as a result of the destruction of normal cells in the area being irradiated and are specific to the anatomic site treated. These include: **alopecia** (hair loss); erythema (local redness and inflammation of the skin); desquamation (shedding of epidermis; can be dry or moist); alterations in oral mucosa including **stomatitis** (inflammation of the mouth); xerostomia (dryness of the mouth); change or loss in taste, and decreased salivation; anorexia (loss of appetite); nausea; vomiting; diarrhea; cystitis (inflammation of the bladder); pneumonitis (inflammation of the lungs); fatigue; and bone marrow suppression if marrow-producing sites are irradiated, resulting in anemia (decreased red blood cells, decreased hemoglobin or volume of packed red blood cells), **leukopenia** (decreased white blood cell count), or **thrombocytopenia** (decreased platelet count).

Effects of radiation are cumulative and often the client experiences chronic or long-term side effects after therapy is completed. Many times these effects are the result of decreased blood supply and normal tissue destruction. The changes are irreversible. Effects that can occur include: fibrosis (abnormal formation of scar tissue) in the small intestine, lungs, and bladder; cataracts; disturbances in blood cell formation; sterility; and formation of new cancers.

INTERNAL RADIATION THERAPY

Internal radiation therapy **(brachytherapy)** involves the direct application of radioisotopes within the body (sealed sources). Radioisotopes such as iridium, cesium, and iodine 125 in a sealed applicator are inserted into body cavities. Cancers treated in this way are those affecting the mouth, tongue, breast, vagina, cervix, endometrium, bladder, rectum, and brain. Sealed radioisotopes can also be in containers such as tubes, wires, needles, seeds, or capsules. Internal radiation therapy has the advantage of delivering a higher dose within the tumor while at the same time sparing more normal surrounding tissue. Unsealed sources of radiation (radiation in a suspension or solution), such as iodine 131 or strontium 90, may be administered orally, intravenously, or topically using various kinds of applicators.

A client must be hospitalized when receiving internal radiation therapy because radiation is emitted from the client during therapy. Specific orders for treatment and precautions to be taken, as well as the type and dosage of the radioactive substance, time and area of insertion, type of applicator used, and when the material is to be removed are noted in the client's chart. If any orders are unclear, the nurse should contact the radiation oncologist or radiation safety officer. Table 19–6 lists safety measures to be followed when a client is receiving radiation therapy. Everyone involved in the client's care must recognize the necessity for limitations to radiation exposure. The degree of possible hazard depends on the type and amount of radioactive material used. Generally, no special precautions are required when a small amount of a radioactive substance is used for diagnostic studies. If necessary, precautions are specified by the radiation oncologist, personnel informed, and a radiation sign posted (Fig. 19–2).

When radioisotopes are used in the treatment of cancer, three safety principles must always be kept in mind: time, distance, and shielding (where applicable).

Time

Time refers to the length of exposure. The less time spent in the vicinity of a radioactive substance, the less radiation received. Nurses must plan carefully and work quickly and efficiently so minimal time is spent at the bedside. Careful psychological preparation helps the client accept the limited amount of nursing time.

Distance

Distance refers to the length in feet between the person entering the room and the radioactive source (the client). The inverse square law applies to radiation exposure. The rate of exposure varies inversely to the square of the distance from the source (client). For example, nurses standing 4 feet away from the source of radiation receive 25% of the radiation they

TABLE 19-6 **Safety Measures for Protecting Health Care Personnel and Visitors From Excessive Exposure to Radiation**

Client is placed in private room; some rooms have walls that are lined with lead.

Standardized sign (see Fig. 19-2) is placed on door to designate the room as a radiation room.

Anyone entering the room must have knowledge of the precautions required. Children under age 18 and pregnant women are never permitted in the room.

Health care personnel limit time spent in the room and limit distance from source of radiation by working as far away from the source of radiation as possible.

The physician and radiation safety personnel are notified if the sealed sources become dislodged.

When the client has unsealed sources, gloves must be worn at all times. Policies regarding disposal of body fluids and contaminated articles such as dressings must be adhered to.

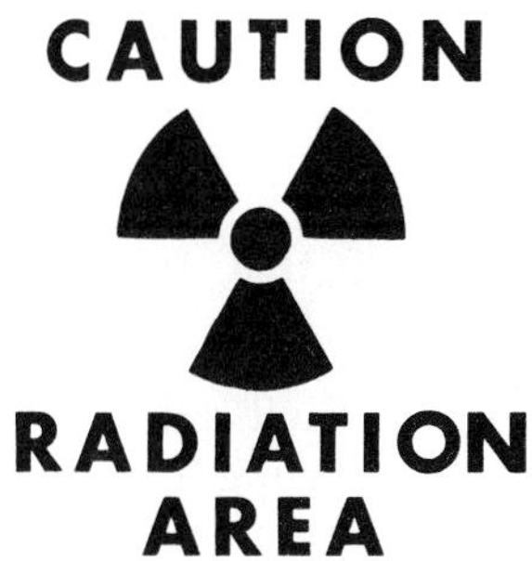

FIGURE 19-2. International radiation symbol.

would receive if they were standing 2 feet away from the source (Fig. 19–3).

Shielding

Shielding is the use of any type of material to lessen the amount of radiation that reaches an area. The material usually used is lead, such as lead-lined gloves and lead aprons. Other materials, such as concrete walls, have the capability of shielding.

The National Committee on Radiation Protection publishes guides for radiation safety. The effects of long and short exposures must be considered. The latent period between the exposure and the accumulated biologic effect is often long, and great care is taken to protect occupationally exposed workers from radiation injury that can accumulate over the years. Pregnant women should avoid exposure to radioactive substances. Nursing Guidelines 19–1 lists standard interventions for clients receiving radiation therapy. When providing information, clients need to know: the type and duration of treatment; what is required of the client; possible side effects; skin and mouth care; nutritional and dietary concerns; and precautions needed.

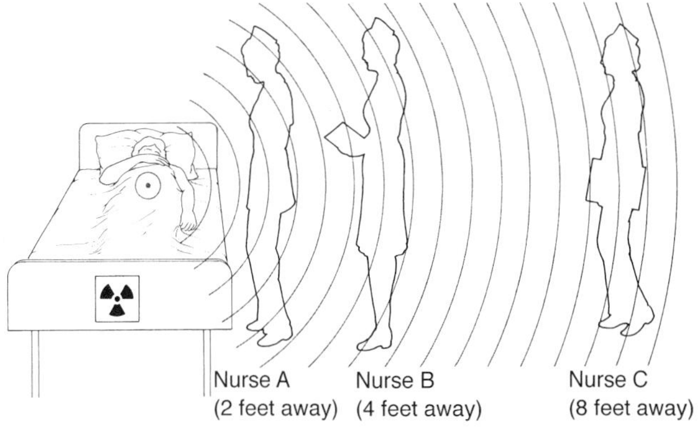

FIGURE 19-3. Examples of distance. Nurse B receives about 25% of the radiation received by Nurse A, and Nurse C receives about 25% of the radiation received by Nurse B.

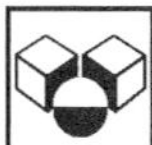

Nursing Guidelines 19-1

Managing Clients Receiving Radiation Therapy

- Provide information regarding the safety of radiation: effects on others, effects on tumor, and side effects related to radiation.
  - Teach client about the actual procedure of external or internal radiation therapy.
  - Explain to client the need for optimal nutritional intake.
- Protect the skin from irritation
  - Assess client's skin and mucous membranes for changes, particularly the areas being treated.
  - Advise client that the effects of radiation on skin include redness, tanning, peeling, itching, hair loss, and decreased perspiration.
  - Cleanse with mild soap (be careful not to wash radiation marks)
  - Use tepid water
  - Use electric razors
  - Moisturize with mild water-based lubricant lotions
  - Wear loose cotton clothing
  - Protect skin from sun exposure, chlorine, and wind
  - Avoid heat lamps and heating pads
  - Report any blistering (use prescribed creams or ointments)
- Maintain intact oral mucous membranes.
  - Teach client to:
  - Report oral burning, pain, open lesions, or problems with swallowing; use nonalcoholic mouthwash
  - Brush with soft toothbrush and avoid electric toothbrushes
  - Floss gently; use WaterPik cautiously
  - Keep lips moist with lip balm
  - Avoid alcoholic beverages, very hot drinks and foods, highly seasoned foods, acidic foods, and tobacco products
  - Assess lesions—culture as necessary
  - Monitor client for signs of bone marrow suppression: decreased leukocyte, erythrocyte, and platelet counts.
  - Assess client for signs of bleeding; assess lesions and culture as necessary.
  - Monitor client for signs and symptoms related to area of irradiation: cerebral edema, malabsorption, pleural effusion, pneumonitis, esophagitis, cystitis, and urethritis.
  - Encourage client to share fears and anxieties related to radiation therapy.
  - Inform client that fatigue is a common effect of radiation therapy.

CLIENT AND FAMILY TEACHING

For clients who will receive radiation therapy on an outpatient basis, it is important for the nurse to instruct the client to:

- Avoid the use of ointments or creams on the area receiving radiation therapy unless their use has been prescribed or recommended by a physician or radiation therapist.
- Avoid extremes of heat or cold; heating pads; ultraviolet light; diathermy; whirlpool, sauna, or steam baths; direct sunlight. If receiving radiation to the head or scalp, avoid shampooing with harsh shampoos (baby or mild shampoo is okay), tinting, permanent waving, hair dryers, curling irons, and hair products or treatments of any kind unless approved by the physician or radiation therapist.
- Bathe carefully. Avoid using soap and friction over the area being radiated. Skin markings must *not* be washed off because they are used as guides for setting and adjusting the treatment machine over the area to be radiated.
- Wear loose clothing to avoid irritation of the irradiated areas.

Chemotherapy

Chemotherapy uses **antineoplastic** drugs to destroy tumor cells, usually by interfering with cellular function and reproduction. Antineoplastic drugs are classified according to their relationship to cell division and reproduction.

CELL CYCLE-SPECIFIC DRUGS

Antineoplastic drugs are most effective when cell division is occurring. Cell cycle-specific drugs are used to treat rapidly growing tumors because they attack cancer cells when they enter a specific phase of cell reproduction. They are administered in multiple repeated doses to produce a greater cell kill and to halt the growth of tumor cells. Examples of cell cycle-specific agents are antimetabolites and Vinca alkaloids.

CELL CYCLE-NONSPECIFIC DRUGS

Cell cycle-nonspecific drugs are effective during any phase of the cell cycle, whether reproducing or resting. These drugs are used for larger tumors that are not as fast growing. The amount of drug given is more important than the frequency it is given. Examples of cell cycle-nonspecific agents are alkylating agents, antitumor antibiotics, nitrosureas and hormones.

Many drugs are given in combination with or following radiation therapy. Table 19–7 provides examples of various antineoplastic agents.

TABLE 19-7 **Antineoplastic Drugs**

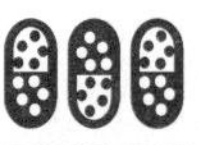

Category	Mechanism of Action	Common Drugs
Cell Cycle Specific		
Antimetabolites	Interfere with the biosynthesis of metabolities/nucleic acids necessary for RNA and DNA synthesis	cytarabine, 5-fluorouracil, FUDR, methotrexate (MTX), hydroxyurea, 6-mercaptopurine, 6-thioguanine, 5-azacytadine, pentostatin, leustatin, edatrexate
Plant alkaloids/natural products (Vinca alkaloids)	Cause metaphase arrest by inhibiting mitotic tubular formation; inhibit DNA and protein synthesis	vincristine (VCR), vinblastine, vindesine, VP-16, VM-26, taxol
Cell Cycle Nonspecific		
Alkylating agents	Alter DNA structure by misreading of DNA code, breaks in DNA molecule, cross-linking of DNA strands	amsacrine, nitrogen mustard, cyclophosphamide, ifosfamide, melphalan, chlorambucil, thiotepa, carboplatin, cisplatin, busulfan
Nitrosoureas	Similar to alkylating agents; cross blood–brain barrier	carmustine (BCNU), lomustine (CCNU), semustine (methylCCNU), streptozocin
Antitumor antibiotics	Interfere with DNA synthesis by binding DNA; prevent RNA synthesis	dactinomycin, bleomycin, daunorubicin, idarubicin, plicamycin, mitomycin, mitoxantrone, doxorubicin
Hormonal agents	Bind to hormone receptor sites that alter cellular growth; block binding of estrogens to receptor sites (antiestrogens); inhibit RNA synthesis	androgens, estrogens, antiestrogens, progesterone, steroids
Miscellaneous agents	Unknown: too complex to categorize	asparaginase, procarbazine, M-AMSA, hexamethylmelamine, dacarbazine (DTIC), mitoxantrone, methyl-GAG

Adapted from Smeltzer, S. C., & Bare B. G. (1996). *Brunner and Suddarth's textbook of medical-surgical nursing* (8th ed., pp. 282–283). Philadelphia: Lippincott-Raven.

TABLE 19-8 **Treatment of Extravasation**

General Measures	Specific Measures	
Stop administration of drug.	Vesicant:	
Leave needle in place.	Doxorubicin	Elevate and rest extremity.
Gently aspirate residual drug and blood into tubing or needle.		Apply topical cooling for 24 h. Give hydrocortisone as ordered.
Give antidote as ordered.	Nitrogen mustard	Apply cold compresses. Give thiosulfate as ordered.
	Vinca alkaloids (vinblastine, vincristine, vendesine)	Apply warm compresses. Do not apply ice—increases skin toxicity. Give hyaluronidase as ordered.
	Mitimycin	Apply ice. Give dimethyl sulfoxide (DMSO) as ordered.

Adapted from Carpenito, L. J. (1995). *Nursing care plans and documentation: Nursing diagnoses and collaborative problems.* Philadelphia: J. B. Lippincott.

ROUTES AND DEVICES FOR ADMINISTRATION OF CHEMOTHERAPY

Chemotherapeutic drugs are administered by a number of routes. The most common are the oral and intravenous (IV) routes, but they are also given intramuscularly, intraperitoneally, intra-arterially, intrapleurally, topically, intrathecally, or directly into a cavity.

Intravenous administration is monitored closely to prevent leakage of the drug into the surrounding tissues. This is referred to as **extravasation.** Most agents have the potential to be very irritating. Blistering and tissue necrosis are possible effects of extravasation. If a client complains of burning or pain during the chemotherapy infusion, the drug must be discontinued. Vesicant neoplastics are particularly damaging. If **vesicants** are being administered, there are protocols for treating the extravasation (Table 19–8).

Various vascular devices are used to administer chemotherapy. These devices are particularly beneficial for long-term chemotherapy. The client does not have to endure repeated venipunctures. In addition, they are advantageous when a client has poor veins. Peripheral vascular access devices are special catheters inserted into a peripheral or central vein so that the catheter tip is located in the superior vena cava or right atrium. Examples include peripheral indwelling catheters (PIC lines), peripherally inserted central catheters (PICC lines), and tunneled central catheters (Hickman catheters, Broviac catheters).

Central vascular access devices include the implantable vascular access device (IVAC), also referred to as a port. A metal or plastic port encloses a self-sealing silicone rubber septum. The port is surgically implanted subcutaneously. A silicone catheter attached to the port is threaded subcutaneously to the right atrium. The port is accessed by inserting a needle in the septum of the port.

Chemotherapy infusion pumps are used for some cancers. These devices provide constant infusion of an antineoplastic drug directly into the cancerous organ. A small pump (similar in size to a hockey puck) is surgically implanted subcutaneously in the abdomen or applied externally. Vascular access devices are particularly beneficial for long term chemotherapy. The client does not have to endure repeated venipunctures. In addition, they are advantageous when a client has poor veins, especially from damage caused by antineoplastics.

ADVERSE EFFECTS OF CHEMOTHERAPY

Nursing management of the client receiving chemotherapy varies depending on the drug, dose administered, and route used. Nursing Guidelines 19–2 provides standard care for managing clients receiving chemotherapy. Some clients experience little discomfort or have few adverse effects. Others have a wide range of symptoms. The tissues most susceptible to the chemotherapy are those with rapidly growing cells, such as epithelial tissue, hair follicles, and bone marrow. Adverse effects associated with chemotherapy include:

- Nausea and vomiting are the most common adverse effects to occur during the first 24 hours after chemotherapy administration; use of concurrent antiemetics helps to reduce the incidence and severity.
- Stomatitis (inflammation of the mouth) and mouth soreness or ulceration: may occur as a result of destruction to the epithelial layer.

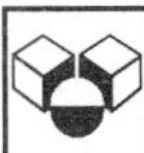

Nursing Guidelines 19-2

Managing Clients Receiving Chemotherapy

- Monitor client for symptoms of anaphylactic reaction:
  - Urticaria (hives)
  - Pruritus (itching)
  - Sensation of lump in throat
  - Shortness of breath and/or wheezing
- Assess client for electrolyte imbalances (see Chap. 21).
- Teach the client and family to report the following:
  - Excessive fluid loss or gain
  - Change in level of consciousness
  - Increased weakness or ataxia (lack of muscle coordination)
  - Paresthesia (numbness, prickling, or tingling)
  - Seizures
  - Persistent headache
  - Muscle cramps or twitching
  - Nausea and vomiting
  - Diarrhea
- Prevent extravasation of vesicant drugs.
- Implement measures to treat extravasation of vesicant medications if it occurs (see Table 19-8).
- Teach client to increase fluid intake to 2,500 to 3,000 mL/day unless contraindicated.
- Assess client for signs of bone marrow depression—decreased WBC, RBC, granulocytes, and platelet count.
- Assess for signs of bleeding.
- Assess for signs of infection.
- Monitor for signs of renal insufficiency:
  - Elevated urine specific gravity
  - Abnormal electrolyte values
  - Insufficient urine output (<30 mL/hour)
  - Elevated blood pressure
  - Elevated BUN (blood urea nitrogen)
  - Elevated serum creatinine
- Inform client about the reasons for nausea and vomiting.
- Administer antiemetic medications before and during administration of chemotherapy, or as indicated.
- Encourage the following dietary modifications:
  - Eat small, frequent meals
  - Eat slowly
  - Eat cool, bland foods and liquids
  - Suck on hard candy during chemotherapy if taste alterations occur
  - Avoid:
    - Hot or very cold liquids
    - Food with fat and fiber
    - Spicy foods
    - Caffeine
- Assess oral mucosa for dryness, redness, swelling, lesions, ulcerations, viscous (sticky) saliva, or white patches.

(Continued)

- Instruct client to:
  - Maintain regular and meticulous oral hygiene
  - Avoid mouthwashes with alcohol or lemon
  - Use soft toothbrush
  - Floss gently—omit if excessive bleeding occurs
  - Avoid smoking
  - For viscous secretions, use rinses that assist in loosening the mucus (1/4 strength hydrogen peroxide and warm water. Do not use for long periods of time)
- Tell client to report any difficulty swallowing.
- Administer oral pain medications and antimicrobials as indicated.
- Encourage client to share fears and anxieties related to chemotherapy.
- Provide client with information and explanations related to chemotherapy.

- Alopecia (loss of hair): occurs when rapidly growing cells of the hair follicles are affected by the chemotherapy.
- Bone marrow depression: inhibits the manufacture of red and white blood cells and platelets. Severe anemia, bleeding tendencies, leukopenia (abnormal decrease in white blood cell count), and thrombocytopenia (abnormal decrease in the number of platelets) may occur if bone marrow depression is profound. Blood transfusions may be necessary, as well as protection of the client from infections.
- Fatigue: results from the above effects and from chemotherapy and the increased metabolic rate that occurs with cell destruction.

CLIENT AND FAMILY TEACHING

For clients who will be receiving chemotherapy on an outpatient basis, it is important for the nurse to instruct the client to:

- Keep all appointments for chemotherapy treatments.
- Follow recommendations of the physician or health care personnel regarding diet, oral fluids, and what adverse effects to report.
- Purchase a wig, cap, or scarf before therapy begins, if hair loss is anticipated. Regrowth of hair usually occurs within 4 to 6 months after therapy; new growth of hair may be a slightly different color and texture.
- Have periodic evaluations and examinations as recommended.

Bone Marrow Transplantation

Cancers that are very sensitive to high doses of chemotherapy and radiation therapy may be treated with bone marrow transplantation (BMT). The survival rate following BMT for malignant disease is approximately 40% to 50% (Smeltzer & Bare, 1996). There are three possible sources for BMT: autologous (client receives BMT from self); allogenic (BMT is from a compatible donor); and syngeneic (BMT is from an identical twin).

AUTOLOGOUS BONE MARROW TRANSPLANTATION

An *autologous BMT* involves harvesting the client's own bone marrow and storing it in a frozen state. The client then receives intensive chemotherapy (also referred to as *ablative chemotherapy*) and radiation therapy to eliminate any remaining tumor. The client's own bone marrow is then reinfused. The harvested bone marrow may also be treated with chemotherapy to kill any malignant cells present. Until the bone marrow is reinfused, the client is at high risk for infections and bleeding. This type of transplant is done for clients who have cancer affecting the bone marrow but do not have a matched donor or for clients who have aggressive cancer that has not affected the bone marrow (Smeltzer & Bare, 1996).

ALLOGENIC BONE MARROW TRANSPLANTATION

An *allogeneic BMT* is usually done for the client who has cancer affecting the bone marrow. Bone marrow is obtained from a compatible donor. The client receives ablative chemotherapy and total body irradiation to destroy the cancer cells and bone marrow and then receives the donor bone marrow IV. It takes 2 to 4 weeks for the transplanted marrow to establish itself and to begin producing blood cells. Clients receive immunosuppressant drugs to prevent rejection of the bone marrow. The first 3 months following transplantation are the most critical for the client in terms of rejection, infection, hemorrhage, nausea, vomiting, and fatigue.

SYNGENEIC BONE MARROW TRANSPLANTATION

Syngeneic BMT requires that the client have an identical twin. The process is the same as for allogeneic BMTs. Because the donor is an identical tissue match, immunosuppressant drugs are not needed as there is no issue with bone marrow rejection (Smeltzer & Bare, 1996).

NURSING MANAGEMENT

Nursing management for the client receiving a BMT is crucial. Before receiving a BMT, the client is thoroughly evaluated in terms of physical condition, organ function, nutritional status, complete blood studies including assessment for past antigen exposure such as hepatitis or cytomegalovirus, and psychosocial status.

When clients are ready to receive a BMT, they undergo intensive chemotherapy or whole body radiation. Because a large amount of tissue is treated, nausea, vomiting, diarrhea, and stomatitis often occur. In addition, until the transplanted bone marrow begins to produce blood cells, these clients have no physiologic means to fight infection, which makes them very prone to infection. It is imperative that nurses monitor clients closely and ensure measures are taken to prevent infection. Clients are also at risk for bleeding, renal complications, and liver damage.

After the BMT, clients are closely monitored for at least 3 months because complications related to the transplant can still occur. Infections are common, as is graft versus host disease (GVHD), which occurs as a result of a reaction between the recipient and donor tissue. The client's immune system is deficient because of the chemotherapy and radiation therapy. Throughout the entire BMT procedure, clients are also assessed in terms of their psychological status. Clients experience many mood swings and need support and assistance throughout this process. Their families and significant others also require support. Nursing Guidelines 19–3 describes standard management of clients receiving a bone marrow transplant.

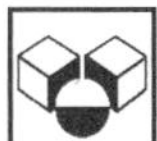

Nursing Guidelines 19-3

Managing Clients Receiving a Bone Marrow Transplant

- Assess client's nutritional status.
- Monitor client for signs and symptoms of infection.
- Monitor client for signs of renal insufficiency (see guidelines for clients receiving chemotherapy).
- Assess clients for signs and symptoms of graft-versus-host disease (GVHD): irritability, pulmonary infiltration, hepatitis, enlarged spleen, enlarged lymph nodes, anemia, sepsis, diarrhea, maculopapular rash, and skin desquamation.
- Implement Standard Precautions and use protective isolation as needed.
- Assist client with thorough hygiene.
- Review information related to prevention of infection, signs of rejection, importance of adherence to medical regimens and follow-up, medication instructions, and dietary needs.
- Encourage client to discuss anxieties and fears.
- Provide ongoing information about recovery phase and status of recuperation.

Biotherapy

Biotherapy (also called immunotherapy) uses biologic response modifiers (BRMs) to stimulate the body's natural immune system to restrict and destroy cancer cells. This treatment is fairly new and still in trial phases. Recent research has demonstrated that the body's natural immunity is a defense against cancer. Natural immunity is a process of surveillance, recognition, and attacking foreign cells (Rosdahl, 1995). Use of BRMs attempts to manipulate the natural immune response by restoring, modifying, stimulating, or augmenting the natural defenses (Smeltzer & Bare, 1996).

The results of biotherapy vary. Some clients respond well, others have little or no response. Generally, biotherapy is not instituted until other treatments such as surgery, radiation therapy, and chemotherapy have been used.

There are three categories of biotherapy: nonspecific, monoclonal antibodies, and cytokines.

NONSPECIFIC BIOTHERAPY

Nonspecific biotherapy uses nonspecific agents such as bacille Calmette-Guerin (BCG) or *Corynebacterium parvum* to act as antigens to stimulate an immune response. When these antigens are injected into a client, the goal is for the stimulated immune system to destroy malignant growths. These agents are useful in treating melanoma, colorectal cancer, and localized bladder cancer (Smeltzer & Bare, 1996).

MONOCLONAL ANTIBODY BIOTHERAPY

Monoclonal antibody biotherapy uses monoclonal antibodies, a form of BRM. Specific tumor cells are injected into mice. Antibodies produced by the immune system in the mice are harvested and infused into the client. The goal is for the antibodies to overwhelm and destroy the tumor cells. Clinical trials have been used for solid tumors and cancers affecting the blood with limited success. There is a high incidence of allergic reactions, headaches, wheezing, tachycardia, nausea and vomiting, rash, fever, and chills.

CYTOKINES

Cytokines are substances that the cells of the immune system produce to enhance the immune system. There are four categories of cytokines: interferons, interleukin-2, colony-stimulating factors, and tumor necrosis factor. Table 19–9 describes the action of cytokines. In general, they stimulate the immune system or assist in inhibiting tumor growth. Side effects include flulike symptoms, gastrointestinal disturbances, alopecia, and low blood counts.

Gene Therapy

It is theorized that many cancers occur as a result of gene alterations. Treatment strategies include replacing altered genes with correct genes, inhibiting defective genes, and introducing substances that cause genes or cancer cells to be destroyed (Smeltzer &

TABLE 19-9 **Cytokines**

Cytokines are substances produced by the cells of the immune system that promote the activities of the immune system and may have antiviral, antibacterial, and antitumor effects.

Interferons	• Naturally occurring protein molecules produced in response to viral infections • Inhibit growth of tumor cells • Used in the treatment of hairy cell leukemia and AIDS-related Kaposi's sarcoma
Interleukin-2	• Produced by lymphocytes • Stimulates production of T-cell lymphocytes; known to enhance production of other cytokines • Used in trial treatments of melanoma, sarcoma, non-Hodgkin's lymphoma, and renal cancer
Colony-stimulating factors	• Hormone-like substances produced by the immune system • Stimulate production of blood cells: neutrophils, lymphocytes, platelets, erythrocytes, monocytes, and macrophages • Do not treat cancers, but used to treat negative effects of treatments that affect bone marrow • Higher doses of chemotherapy can be given with less suppression of bone marrow function.
Tumor necrosis factor	• Naturally produced by macrophages • Exact mechanism of action not understood; stimulates other cells in the immune response and directly kills tumor cells. • Research being done with melanoma and renal and lung cancers

TABLE 19-10 **Alternative Methods of Cancer Treatment**

Method	Description
Imagery, relaxation techniques, and stress reduction exercises	Used to reduce pain, promote relaxation, and enhance conventional treatment methods. Approach based on beliefs that there is a link between the immune system and cancer and that these methods boost the immune system's ability to fight the cancer cells.
Medicinal agents	Many "cures" for cancer have been concocted from plants, herbs, flowers, and fluids of humans and animals. Although a few merit scientific investigation, many are considered quackery. The use of vitamins, minerals, proteins, and other ingredients is advocated for treatment of many cancers and prevention of treatment side effects.
Special diets	Many diet regimens are advocated as treatment for certain cancers or as adjuncts to treatment. Examples include organic foods, macrobiotic diets, and particular foods that reportedly kill cancer cells.
Spiritual methods	These methods are derived from powers of faith that individuals believe will help them to overcome cancer. Examples include faith healing, laying on of hands, and prayer.

Bare, 1996). **Gene therapy** is being investigated in the treatment of brain tumors; melanoma; and renal, breast, and colon cancers, usually when other therapies have failed.

Alternative Treatments and Therapies

Alternative treatment and therapies include imagery, medicinal therapy, special diets, and spiritual approaches. Table 19–10 describes various methods used in the treatment of cancer. It is difficult for health care professionals to condone unconventional therapies because many of the methods do not have a scientific foundation. There are also legal and ethical implications if health care personnel participate in unaccepted methods of treatment. Information provided to clients must be factual and understandable. Although some alternative methods have successfully augmented conventional treatments, many methods have no positive effects, and indeed some are actually harmful.

Psychological Support

The diagnosis of cancer is frightening and frequently overwhelming. Psychological support for the client is as important as the medical treatments and physical care. Clients have many reactions ranging from anxiety, fear, and depression to feelings of guilt related to viewing cancer as a punishment for past actions or failure to practice a healthy lifestyle. They also may express anger related to the diagnosis and their inability to be in control. Clients have the right to know their diagnosis, treatment plan, and prognosis. In this way they can make informed decisions. A client's acceptance of the diagnosis of cancer may never happen. However, when clients are provided with adequate information and supported psychologically, they are more likely to face their diagnosis and be involved with their care and treatment. Families and significant others also require support to assist their loved one.

NURSING PROCESS
The Client With Cancer

Assessment

Assess the client's level of understanding about the diagnosis, treatment plan, and follow-up care. Determine the client's strengths, coping mechanisms, response to the diagnosis, and emotional and physical support systems. Assess the family's response to illness. Ascertain the client's overall physical condition, energy and pain levels, and nutritional and fluid status.

Diagnosis and Planning

The following plan of care is intended as a guide and should not be limited to this information.

Nursing Diagnoses and Collaborative Problems	Nursing Interventions
Anxiety or Fear related to diagnosis of cancer, change in health status, hospitalization and medical or surgical interventions, and possibility of death	Encourage client to share thoughts and feelings; maintain frequent contact with client.
	Provide accurate and sufficient information. Answer questions, explain procedures, and provide alternatives.
Goal: The client will express feelings and demonstrate effective coping mechanisms.	

Nursing Diagnosis	Nursing Interventions
	Allow client to express anger, despair, and fear without judgment. Promote a sense of hope. Explore coping strategies; recommend participation in a cancer support group.
Body Image Disturbance related to changes in appearance **Goals:** The client will verbalize understanding of changes in appearance. The client will demonstrate coping methods and adaptation to changes client is experiencing.	Encourage client to verbalize how changes are affecting him or her. Openly discuss sadness or depression as normal responses. Suggest techniques minimizing changed physical appearance (prostheses, wigs, reconstructive surgeries). Assess client for maladaptive responses such as denial, isolating oneself, or reluctance to participate in care. Refer client to support group or counseling.
Grieving related to anticipated loss and altered role status **Goals:** The client will identify and verbalize feelings. The client will continue to make future-oriented plans, even if one day at a time. The client will verbalize understanding of the dying process.	Encourage client to express feelings of loss. Discuss coping strategies that the client has used successfully in the past. Reduce environmental stressors. Provide privacy when grief is overwhelming. Stay with client, if he or she desires, and convey acceptance of emotions. Focus on the present and support the client's self-esteem.
Pain related to disease and effects of surgery, radiation therapy, chemotherapy, and other treatments **Goals:** The client will report pain relief. The client will use relaxation methods and other alternatives for reducing pain and discomfort.	Refer to Nursing Guidelines 20-1 in Chapter 20 for implementing an effective pain management program. Develop the pain management plan with the client, physician, and other health care professionals.
Fatigue related to disease, treatments, and physical and psychological stresses **Goals:** The client will participate in daily care as much as possible. The client will identify measures to conserve energy and to improve energy levels	Identify energy level by asking client to evaluate it on a scale of 0 to 10 (0, not tired; 10, total exhaustion). Plan care around energy level and allow for rest periods. Assist client in identifying energy pattern by recording levels on an hourly basis for 2 to 3 days to detect trends. Encourage discussion about effect of fatigue on self-care and role function. Identify which activities are most difficult and assist client as needed while encouraging as much self-care as possible. Suggest relaxation therapy and guided imagery to enhance energy level (Carpenito, 1997). Promote adequate nutritional intake.
Impaired Skin Integrity and Altered Mucous Membranes related to the disease, effects of radiation and chemotherapy, immobilization, decreased immunity, or poor nutrition **Goal:** The client will demonstrate measures to prevent skin or tissue impairment complications or to promote tissue or skin healing.	Explain the necessity for regular and meticulous oral hygiene. Instruct client on appropriate oral hygiene measures. Implement nursing measures for skin care (see guidelines for managing clients receiving radiation therapy and chemotherapy).
Risk for Fluid Volume Deficit related to excessive loss from vomiting, diarrhea, or bleeding, or as a result of inadequate fluid intake. **Goal:** The client will achieve adequate fluid balance.	Monitor intake and output, weight, and vital signs. Assess client for decreased urine output, decreased skin turgor, dry mucous membranes. Encourage adequate fluid intake. Monitor complete blood count, electrolytes, and serum albumin.
Infection, Risk for related to immunosuppression, malnutrition, and invasive procedures **Goal:** The client will demonstrate interventions that prevent or reduce infections.	Implement standard precautions. Assess client continually for signs of infection (Table 19–11). Stress the necessity of thorough hygiene, including oral hygiene. Monitor CBC and differential. Obtain cultures as needed. Administer antibiotics as ordered.
Altered Nutrition: Less than Body Requirements related to the disease, results of surgery, chemotherapy, radiation therapy, other therapies, fatigue, or emotional distress **Goals:** The client will increase dietary intake. The client will demonstrate knowledge of necessity for adequate intake of nutrients and fluids.	Monitor daily food intake. Encourage the intake of sufficient calories, nutrients, and fluids. (See guidelines for managing clients receiving radiation therapy and chemotherapy.) Administer antiemetics, vitamins, and supplements as ordered or recommended. Review laboratory studies to monitor for signs of dehydration, biochemical imbalances, and malnutrition.

Evaluation

- The client and family share anxieties about diagnosis and care.
- The client adopts methods for coping with body changes.
- The client's pain is controlled.
- The client is able to participate in care without becoming exhausted.
- The client's skin and mucous membranes are intact.
- The client maintains adequate nutritional and fluid intake.

Client and Family Teaching

Clients and their families or significant others require much support and education to understand the diagnostic procedures, make treatment choices, participate in prevention of complications, and recognize side effects and other adverse signs. Teaching is focused on:

- Information about medications, treatments, and procedures
- Adverse effects associated with treatment
- Possible changes in body image or function that can occur
- Resources for support
- Follow-up needed after discharge from the hospital

When developing a plan for client and family teaching, it is important to consider facts such as the type of malignancy, treatment given, proposed treatments, condition of the client, and effectiveness of the family support system. These facts will determine the areas to discuss in more detail. The nurse should be aware of any explanations or information given to the client and family by other health care providers. It is important to allow time for clients to express their feelings or discuss their home care. This also helps to identify issues the client or family does not understand.

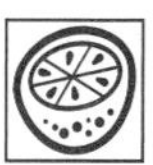

General Nutritional Considerations

Improving the client's nutritional status not only improves quality of life, but may make cancer cells more susceptible to treatment. Good nutrition also promotes better rehabilitation, may lessen the adverse effects of treatment, and may increase the chance of survival. Conversely, poor nutritional status may potentiate the toxicity of cancer treatments.

Malnutrition is not an inevitable consequence of cancer, yet, once established, it can be difficult to reverse. To prevent malnutrition, it is usually more effective to increase the nutrient density of foods consumed rather than expecting a client to eat more food. Fortifying casseroles, bev-

TABLE 19-11 **Factors That Predispose Clients With Cancer to Infection**

Factors	Underlying Pathology
Impaired skin and mucous membrane integrity	Loss of first line of defense against microorganisms.
Chemotherapy	Bone marrow suppression leads to decreased leukocyte production. Skin and mucous membrane integrity is impaired. Organ damage can predispose clients to infection.
Radiation therapy	Bone marrow suppression leads to decreased leukocyte production. Skin and mucous membrane integrity is impaired
Biologic response modifiers	May cause bone marrow suppression and organ dysfunction
Malignancy	Malignant cells can infiltrate bone marrow and interfere with leukocyte and lymphocyte production.
Malnutrition	Interferes with immune response May contribute to impaired skin and mucous membrane integrity
Medications	Antibiotics disturb the balance of normal flora, which may lead to a pathogenic process (most common in gastrointestinal tract).
Catheters (intravenous, urinary, other) and invasive procedures	Creates port of entry for microorganisms Impairs skin integrity
Contaminated equipment	Harbor microorganisms (ie, stagnant water in oxygen equipment, old suctioning tubing)
Age	Organ immaturity or declining organ function Immature immune system or decreased production and function of the immune system
Chronic illness	Associated with impaired organ function and altered immune responses
Prolonged hospitalization	Increased incidence of nosocomial (hospital-acquired) infections

Adapted from Smeltzer, S. C., & Bare, B. G. (1996). *Brunner and Suddarth's textbook of medical-surgical nursing* (8th ed., p. 291). Philadelphia: Lippincott-Raven.

erages, cereals, and other foods with skim milk powder, whole milk, cheese, cream cheese, peanut butter, eggs, butter, and honey increases density without increasing volume. Small frequent feedings are also beneficial.

Side effects of cancer and cancer therapies can have a devastating impact on the client's ability to eat, which may change from day tp day or meal to meal. Clients with nausea fare better with low-fat foods and "dry" meals (liquids are taken between meals). Clients receiving chemotherapy should avoid eating or drinking for 1 to 2 hours after treatment to avoid nausea.

Clients with anorexia should consume small, frequent meals. Encourage clients to view eating as part of therapy, not as a voluntary activity.

Clients with vomiting need to replenish fluids by taking water or flat beverages every 10 to 15 minutes.

Clients who develop taste alterations from chemotherapy often complain that meats taste "bad" or "rotten." Offer cold protein alternatives such as cheese, cottage cheese, protein beverages, and sandwiches. Assure the client that it is not necessary to eat meat to consume adequate protein intake.

Sucking on hard candy during chemotherapy infusion may help clients avoid a bitter or metallic taste.

Clients with fatigue should rest before meals and avoid items that require a lot of chewing.

Clients with difficulty swallowing should use gravies and sauces liberally. Semisolid foods may be better tolerated than liquids. Avoid extremely hot foods.

A high fluid intake is necessary to promote excretion of chemotherapeutic drugs. Water, milk, fruit juices, and high-protein beverages are all good choices; beverages containing caffeine should be avoided and empty calorie soft drinks should be limited.

Clients with a sore mouth should avoid highly seasoned foods, acidic juices, salty items, and coarse breads and cereals. Cold food and beverages may be better tolerated than warm items.

Force feeding, weighing the client, and using nutritional support are contraindicated for palliative care.

General Pharmacologic Considerations

The client taking an antineoplastic agent must be monitored for symptoms of gout, which include increased uric acid levels, joint pain, and edema. Allopurinol may be prescribed to decrease the uric acid level. The client is encouraged to increase fluid intake (up to 2,000 mL/day) if condition permits.

Anemia may occur as an adverse reaction to the antineoplastic agents. Fatigue, dyspnea, or orthostatic hypotension are reported immediately.

Most antineoplastic agents are teratogenic. The female client must use birth control measures throughout therapy. If pregnancy is suspected, the primary health care provider is notified immediately.

Because antineoplastic drugs can depress the immune system, advise clients to avoid crowds (eg, shopping malls, movie theaters) and individuals with colds, flu, or other infectious diseases.

If stomatitis occurs the primary health care provider may prescribe topical agents to make eating easier. If stomatitis pain is severe, an analgesic may be prescribed.

Antineoplastic drugs used in the treatment of cancer are potentially toxic agents. Nurses must be thoroughly familiar with adverse effects and toxicity of these agents. The dose or length of treatment depends, in some cases, on the client's response to therapy.

Many antineoplastic drugs have a profound effect on the bone marrow. Clients are observed for signs of bone marrow depression (fever, sore throat, chills), infection, and bleeding (oozing from venipuncture or parenteral injection sites, bleeding from gums, or signs of blood in urine or stools).

Intravenous or intra-arterial administration of antineoplastic agents may lead to thrombophlebitis. Sites are inspected daily for tenderness, pain, swelling, or induration above or below site of use.

Nausea, vomiting, and diarrhea may occur from therapy. These adverse effects must be reported immediately because dehydration and electrolyte imbalance often occur rapidly. Antiemetic or antidiarrheal drugs or IV fluid and electrolyte replacement may be needed.

Allopurinol (Zyloprim) may be prescribed when uric acid levels rise during chemotherapy.

Drugs may be ordered for other adverse effects that may occur during radiation therapy: acetaminophen for fever, antibiotics for infection, and various ointments and creams (applied exactly as prescribed) for skin irritation.

General Gerontologic Considerations

Older adults with cancer may have additional problems with nutrition, adequate fluid intake, skin care, and complications related to inactivity.

Older adults often have decreased resistance to infection, which may pose problems if they receive antineoplastic agents that have a depressant effect on the bone marrow.

Because of concurrent disease and the effect of the aging process on the body's tissues and organs, older adults may not receive the same treatments for cancer that a younger client does.

Older adults, faced with long and sometimes rigorous cancer treatment, may refuse treatment.

Older adults who have undergone extensive surgery for cancer require detailed home care planning before discharge from the hospital.

Arthritis, as well as general muscular stiffness, may make lying supine on an x-ray table difficult for older adults. It may be necessary to pad bony prominences and provide support to the back or legs during radiation therapy.

The skin of older adults is often dry. Intense itching and dryness may be experienced during and after radiation therapy; therefore, additional treatment of skin problems may be necessary. The skin is inspected frequently for signs of breakdown, evidence of excessive scratching, and infection.

Older adults are often more prone to electrolyte imbalance. Excessive vomiting during or after treatments may result in a serious electrolyte imbalance.

Older adults who receive internal radiation therapy may experience difficulty in lying still until the end of the treatment. These clients are checked more frequently for displacement of the applicator.

SUMMARY OF KEY CONCEPTS

- Cancer is characterized by abnormal, unrestricted cell proliferation. Malignant tumors invade healthy tissues and compete with normal cells for oxygen, nutrients, and physical space.
- Cancer cells metastasize by invading surrounding tissues, via lymph and blood systems, or through diffusion into a body cavity.
- Factors that cause cancer are called carcinogens. Chemical agents, environmental factors, dietary issues, viruses, genetic and familial factors, and hormonal influences are all potential carcinogens.
- Research has increased public awareness of risk factors. Education efforts are directed at teaching people ways to prevent or decrease the risks of cancer.
- Many specific diagnostic tests are used to diagnose cancer. Specialized tests are referred to as tumor markers, in that the tests identify specific proteins, antigens, hormones, genes, or enzymes released by cancer cells.
- Tumors are staged according to the ways in which tumors tend to grow and the particular cell types. The TNM classification system and other classification systems are used to determine treatment methods.
- Three basic methods are used (alone or in combination) in the treatment of cancer: surgery, radiation therapy, and chemotherapy. Bone marrow transplantation is also used in treating some types of cancer. Biotherapy, gene therapy, and other alternative therapies are also being used.
- Adverse effects of radiation therapy, chemotherapy, bone marrow transplantations, and other therapies can be problematic. Careful assessment is essential in preventing or reducing these effects. Treatments of adverse effects have decreased some of the problems, but these effects still produce great anxiety and fear in clients and their families.
- The role of the nurse is significant in the care of clients with cancer. The nursing process provides a framework for planning and implementing care.

CRITICAL THINKING EXERCISES

1. A client with endometrial cancer has been told that she will be treated with internal radiation therapy. Discuss what information needs to be included in a teaching plan for this client.
2. A client with leukemia is scheduled for an allogeneic bone marrow transplant. Discuss the information the client should know before this procedure is performed.

Suggested Readings

Bullock, B. L. (1996). *Pathophysiology: Adaptations and alterations in function* (4th ed.) Philadelphia: Lippincott-Raven.

Carpenito, L. J. (1995). *Nursing care plans and documentation: Nursing diagnoses and collaborative problems* (2nd ed.). Philadelphia: J. B. Lippincott.

Carpenito, L. J. (1997). *Nursing diagnosis: Application to clinical practice* (7th ed.). Philadelphia: Lippincott-Raven.

Dearborn, P., De-Muth, JS., Requarth, AB., and Ward, SE (1997). Nurse and patient satisfaction with three types of venous access devices. *Oncology Nursing Forum, 24*(1):Suppl, 34–40.

Coleridge-Smith, E. (1996). Achieving good cancer pain control at home. *Community Nurse, 2*(1), 18, 20.

Koopmeiners, L., Post-White, J., Gutknecht, S., Ceronsky, C., Nickelson, K., Drew, D., Mackey, K. W., & Kreitzer, M. J. (1997). How healthcare professionals contribute to hope in patients with cancer. *Oncology Nursing Forum, 24*(9), 1507–1513.

Macklin, D. (1997). How to manage PICCs. *AJN 97*(9), 26–33.

Martsoff, D. S. (1997). Cultural aspects of spirituality in cancer care. *Seminars in Oncology Nursing, 13*(4), 231–236.

Masoorli, S. (1997). Managing complications of central venous access devices. *Nursing 97, 27*(8), 59–64.

Riddell, A., & Fitch, M. I. (1997). Patients' knowledge and attitudes toward the management of cancer pain. *Oncology Nursing Forum, 24*(10), 1775–1784.

Rosdahl, C. B. (1995). *Textbook of basic nursing* (6th ed.). Philadelphia: J. B. Lippincott.

Smeltzer, S. C., & Bare, B. G. (1996). *Brunner and Suddarth's textbook of medical-surgical nursing* (8th ed.). Philadelphia: Lippincott-Raven.

Washington, C. M., & Leaver, D. T. (1997). *Principle and practice of radiation therapy: Practical applications*. St. Louis: Mosby.

Wilby, M. L. (1998). Improving the health profile: Decreasing risk for cancer through primary prevention. *Holistic Nursing Practice, 12*(2), 52–61.

Additional Resources

Cancer Pain Education for Patients and Families
http://coninfo.nursing.uiowa.edu/CancerPain/

OncoLink University of Pennsylvania Cancer Center
http://cancer.med.upenn.edu/psychosocial/

International Cancer Alliance
http://www2/ari/net/icare/

Cancer Guide
http://cancerguide.org/

Chemotherapy and You
http://cancernet.nci.nih.gov

American Cancer Society
http://www.cancer.org

Home Care Guide for Advanced Cancer
http://www.acponline.org

Chapter 20

Caring for Clients With Pain

KEY TERMS

Acute pain
Analgesic
Chronic pain
Cutaneous pain
Equianalgesic dose
Gate-closing mechanisms
Gate control theory
Intractable pain
Neuropathic pain
Pain
Pain management
Pain perception
Pain threshold
Pain tolerance
Patterning theory
Referred pain
Somatic pain
Specificity theory
Substance P
Visceral pain

LEARNING OBJECTIVES

On completion of this chapter, the reader will:

- Define the term pain.
- Explain how the sensation of pain is transmitted to the brain.
- Name two chemical substances that block pain transmission.
- List three pain transmission theories.
- Name four types of pain classified according to their location, two types classified according to duration, and one type that has atypical characteristics.
- Give three characteristics distinguishing acute from chronic pain.
- Differentiate between pain perception, pain threshold, and pain tolerance.
- Explain why it is difficult to assess pain and list seven essential components of pain assessment.
- Name four tools for assessing the intensity of pain.
- Identify at least five occasions when it is important to assess a client's pain.
- Explain pain management and list four techniques commonly used.
- Name two categories of analgesic drugs.
- Identify two surgical procedures performed on clients with intractable pain.
- Discuss the nursing management of clients with pain.
- List at least three nursing diagnoses, besides *Pain*, that are common among clients with pain.
- Discuss information pertinent to teach clients and family about pain management.

Pain is a privately experienced, unpleasant sensation usually associated with disease or injury that also has an emotional component referred to as *suffering*. Pain is a complex phenomena not yet fully understood. Various theories have been proposed to explain how pain is received by higher centers of the brain and dissipated before it arrives there.

Pain Theories

Pain theories include the specificity theory, the pattern theory, and the gate control theory. No one theory is all-encompassing.

Specificity Theory

The **specificity theory** states that pain is a separate sensation transmitted by specific pain receptors to higher centers of the brain. The transmission of pain begins with some type of cellular disruption that signals *nociceptors*, specialized pain receptors (Fig. 20–1). The nociceptors then transmit the pain message to the brain via the spinal cord using various neurotransmitters, one of which is called **substance P.** Pain transmission can be blocked or reduced with naturally produced morphine-like chemicals, *endorphins* and *enkephalins* (see Chap. 11), that bind to the nociceptor's membrane and interfere with the transmission of substance.

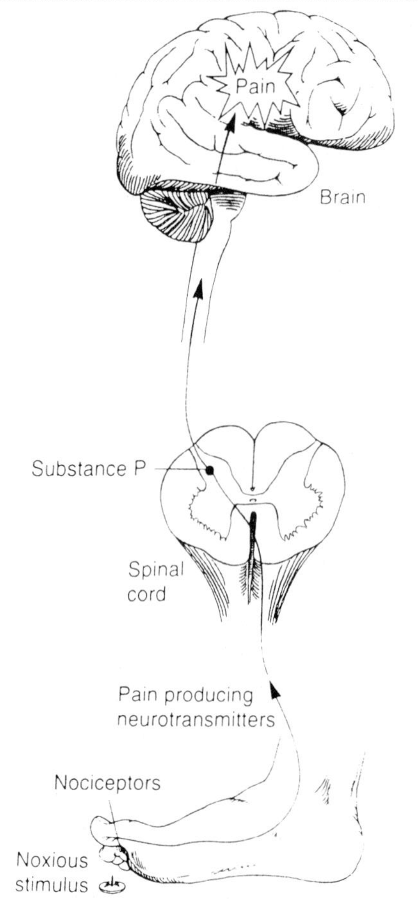

FIGURE 20-1. Pain transmission pathway.

Patterning Theory

The **pattern theory** proposes that pain and nonpainful sensations are transmitted by nonspecific receptors over a common pathway to higher centers of the brain; different patterns of activity determine whether the sensation is interpreted as painful or not painful.

Gate Control Theory

The **gate control theory** is a modification of the other two theories. It suggests that "gates" in the spinal cord control the transmission of pain sensations to higher levels of the brain. This theory helps to explain why interventions, such as massage and others examples that are discussed later, achieve their **analgesic** (pain-relieving) effect.

The gate control theory only partially explains the complex phenomenon of pain. Many other important factors, such as endogenous opioids, learned behaviors, and culture, influence the experience of pain.

Types of Pain

Several types of pain have been described according to their source (cutaneous, somatic, visceral, referred, or neuropathic) and duration (acute or chronic).

CUTANEOUS AND SOMATIC PAIN

Cutaneous pain originates at the skin level, and the depth of the trauma determines the type of sensation that is experienced. According to Bullock and Rosendahl (1992), damage confined to the epidermis produces sensations of itching and burning. At the dermis level, pain is localized and superficial; subcutaneous tissue injury produces an aching, throbbing pain. **Somatic pain** is generated from deeper connective tissue structures such as muscles, tendons, and joints.

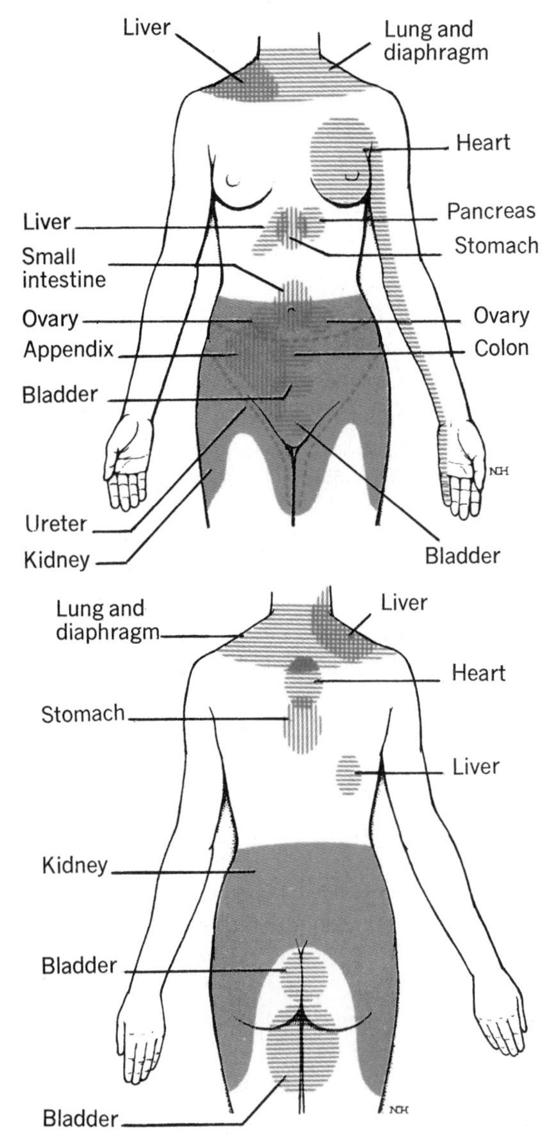

FIGURE 20-2. Common areas of referred pain.

TABLE 20-1 **Characteristics of Acute and Chronic Pain**

Acute Pain	Chronic Pain
Recent onset	Remote onset
Symptomatic of primary injury of disease	Uncharacteristic of primary injury or disease
Specific and localized	Nonspecific and generalized
Severity associated with the acuity of the injury or disease process	Severity out of proportion to the stage of the injury or disease
Favorable response to drug therapy	Poor response to drug therapy
Requires less and less drug therapy	Requires more and more drug therapy
Diminishes with healing	Persists beyond healing stage
Suffering decreases	Suffering intensifies
Associated with sympathetic nervous system responses such as hypertension, tachycardia, restlessness, anxiety	Absence of autonomic nervous system responses; manifests depression and irritability

VISCERAL AND REFERRED PAIN

Visceral pain arises from internal organs that are diseased or injured and tends to be referred or poorly localized. **Referred pain** describes discomfort that is perceived in a general area of the body, but not in the exact site where an organ is anatomically located (Fig. 20–2). Visceral pain is usually accompanied by other autonomic nervous system symptoms such as nausea, vomiting, pallor, hypotension, and sweating.

Neuropathic pain, also called functional or psychogenic pain, is pain with atypical characteristics. It is often experienced days, weeks, or even months after the source of the pain has been treated and resolved (Copstead, 1995). This leads some to speculate that there is a dysfunctional chemical message that is being transmitted to the brain. One example of neuropathic pain is *phantom limb pain* and *phantom limb sensation* in which individuals with amputated limbs perceive that the limb still exists and that sensations such as burning, itching, and deep pain are located in tissues that have been surgically removed.

ACUTE AND CHRONIC PAIN

Pain varies according to its duration. **Acute pain** has a short duration, whereas **chronic pain** lasts longer than 6 months. Either type may be intermittent—meaning there are periods of relief. Other characteristics differentiate acute from chronic pain (Table 20–1).

Pain Perception, Threshold, and Tolerance

Pain perception, the conscious experience of discomfort, occurs when the pain threshold is reached. The **pain threshold** is the point at which the pain-transmitting neurochemicals reach the brain causing conscious awareness. Pain thresholds tend to be the same among healthy persons. However, people tolerate or bear the sensation of pain differently. **Pain tolerance** is the amount of pain a person endures once the threshold has been reached. Pain tolerance is often influenced by learned behaviors that are gender, age, and culture specific.

Pain Assessment

There is no perfect way for determining if pain exists and how severe it is. McCaffery, a nursing expert on pain states, "Pain is whatever the person says it is, and exists whenever the person says it does" (McCaffery & Beebe, 1989.).

Unfortunately, there are several groups of clients from whom assessment data cannot always be validly obtained (Box 20–1). Because machines or laboratory tests cannot measure pain, nurses rely on subjective information that clients supply and suggestive signs that may indicate pain and discomfort (Box 20–2). A full pain assessment includes the client's description of its onset, quality, intensity, location, and duration (Table 20–2). In addition, nurses assess for accompanying symptoms such as nausea or dizziness, and what makes the pain better or worse.

BOX 20-1 Underassessed and Undertreated Clients

- Infants
- Children under age 7
- Culturally diverse clients
- Mentally challenged (retarded) clients
- Clients with dementia (diminished brain function)
- Hearing or speech impaired clients
- Psychologically disturbed clients

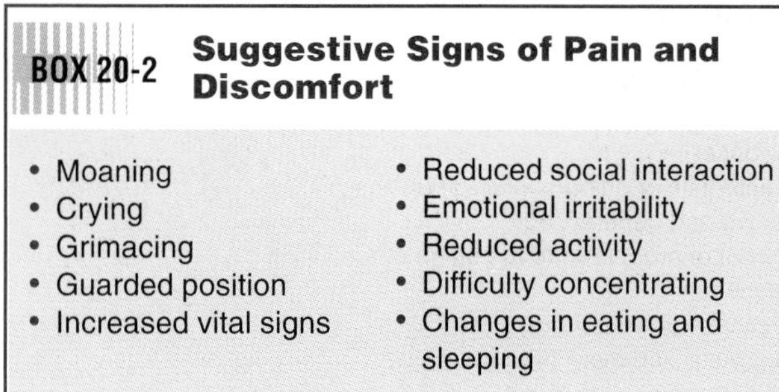

BOX 20-2 Suggestive Signs of Pain and Discomfort

- Moaning
- Crying
- Grimacing
- Guarded position
- Increased vital signs
- Reduced social interaction
- Emotional irritability
- Reduced activity
- Difficulty concentrating
- Changes in eating and sleeping

Assessment Tools

Four assessment tools for quantifying pain intensity include a numeric scale, a word scale, a linear scale, and a picture scale (Fig. 20–3). Clients identify how their pain compares with the choices on the scale. One scale is not better than another. A numeric scale is commonly used when assessing adults. The picture scale is usually best for pediatric, culturally diverse, and mentally challenged clients.

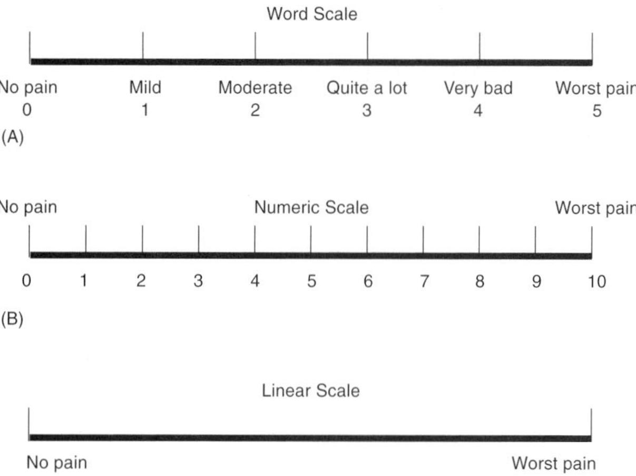

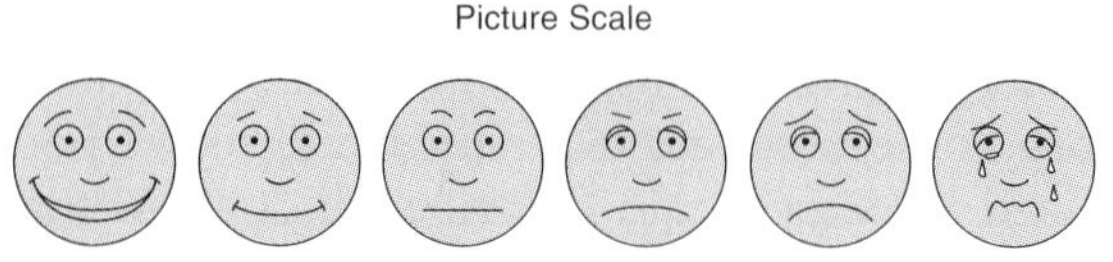

FIGURE 20-3. Pain assessment tools: (A) Word scale, (B) numeric scale, (C) linear scale (D) picture scale.

Assessment Standards

To improve pain control, Donovan and Miaskowski (1992) recommend pain assessment at any time the nurse considers it appropriate and routinely in the following circumstances:

- When the client is admitted
- At least once per shift when pain is an actual or potential problem
- When the client with pain is at rest, and when involved in a nursing activity
- After each potentially painful procedure or treatment
- Before implementing a pain management intervention, such as administering an analgesic drug, and again 30 minutes after its implementation

Pain assessment findings are documented in the medical record.

Pain Management

Pain management refers to the techniques used to prevent, reduce, or relieve pain. The Joint Commission on Accreditation of Healthcare Organizations (JCAHO) requires evidence that the pain of terminally ill clients is being adequately treated (Donovan & Miaskowski, 1992). As of 1992, the American Pain Society, working with the *Agency for Health Care Policy and Research (AHCPR)*, a division of the U.S. Department of Health and Human Services, developed *Stan-*

TABLE 20-2 **Components of a Pain Assessment**

Characteristic	Description	Examples
Onset	Time or circumstances under which the pain became apparent	After eating, while shoveling snow, during the night
Quality	Sensory experiences and degree of suffering	Throbbing, crushing, agonizing, annoying
Intensity	Magnitude of the pain, like moderate, severe; or a quantifying scale, such as from 0 to 10	None, slight, mild, a level of "7"
Location	Anatomic site	Chest, abdomen, jaw
Duration	Time span of the pain	Continuous, intermittent, hours, weeks, months

BOX 20-3 Standards for the Relief of Acute Pain and Cancer Pain

Standard I
Acute pain and cancer pain are recognized and effectively treated.

Standard II
Information about analgesics is readily available.

Standard III
Patients (clients) are informed on admission, both orally and in writing, that effective pain relief is an important part of their treatment, that their communication of unrelieved pain is essential, and that health professionals will respond quickly to their reports of pain.

Standard IV
Explicit policies for use of advanced analgesic technologies are defined.

Standard V
Adherence to standards is monitored by an interdisciplinary committee.

*Reprinted with permission from American Pain Society, Skokie, Illinois.

dards for the Relief of Acute Pain and Cancer Pain (Box 20–3) in an effort to improve the manner in which pain is assessed and controlled.

Pain Management Techniques

Four general techniques for achieving pain management include:

1. Blocking brain perception
2. Interrupting pain-transmitting chemicals at the site of injury
3. Using gate-closing mechanisms
4. Altering pain transmission at the level of the spinal cord

Any one or a combination of these techniques may be used.

DRUG THERAPY

Drug therapy is the cornerstone for managing pain. The World Health Organization recommends following a three-tiered approach according to the client's pain intensity and response to selected drug therapy (Fig. 20–4).

Opioid and Nonopioid Analgesics

Opioid and opiate analgesics such as morphine and meperidine (Demerol) are controlled substances referred to as narcotics. They interfere with pain perception centrally (at the brain). Nonopioids are not narcotics; they relieve pain by altering neurotransmission at the peripheral level (site of injury) (Table 20–3). Antidepressants are prescribed in some circumstances because they increase the amount of available serotonin, which blocks pain transmission.

Analgesic drugs are administered by oral, rectal, transdermal, or parenteral (injected) routes, including a continuous infusion that may be instilled into the spinal canal or self-administered intravenously by clients. When changing from a parenteral to an oral route, it is best to administer an **equianalgesic dose** (an oral dose that provides the same level of pain relief as when the drug is given by a parenteral route) (Table 20–4).

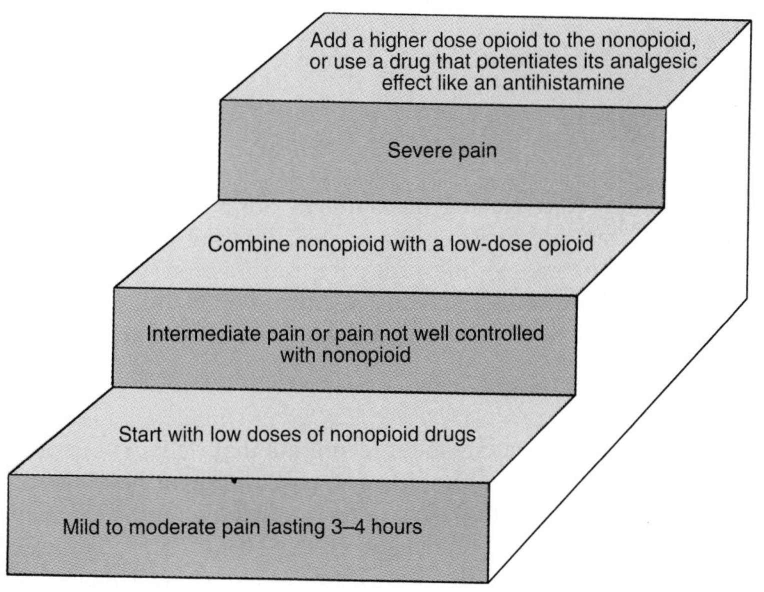
Add a higher dose opioid to the nonopioid, or use a drug that potentiates its analgesic effect like an antihistamine
Severe pain
Combine nonopioid with a low-dose opioid
Intermediate pain or pain not well controlled with nonopioid
Start with low doses of nonopioid drugs
Mild to moderate pain lasting 3–4 hours

FIGURE 20-4. World Health Organization (WHO) analgesic ladder.

TABLE 20-3 **Analgesic Drug Therapy**

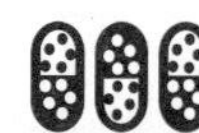

Drug Category/Example and Mechanism of Action	Side Effects	Nursing Considerations
Opioids		
Morphine sulfate, oxycodone (Roxicodone), hydromorphone (Dilaudid), meperidine (Demerol) Binds with opiate receptors in the central nervous system.	Sedation, euphoria, nausea, vomiting, constipation, paralytic ileus, respiratory depression, urinary retention, physical dependence, hypotension	Do not administer if respirations are < 12/min. Encourage clients to cough and deep breathe to avoid atelectasis. Monitor for excessive sedation. Monitor bowel activity. Maintain safety precautions such as keeping side rails up and call bell within reach. Instruct client to call for assistance before ambulating. Administer before pain is severe to increase effectiveness.
Nonopioids		
Nonsteroidal anti-inflammatory drugs (NSAIDs): ibuprofen (Motrin), aspirin Inhibits the production of prostaglandins that increase sensitivity to pain.	Headache, dizziness, nausea, gastritis and ulcers, constipation, increased bleeding time, bone marrow depression, tinnitus, dyspnea, anaphylactoid reactions, renal impairment, rash	Administer with food. Inform client of potential side effects and instruct client to take only as prescribed. Caution clients not to take more than one NSAID at a time.
	Nausea, gastritis, dizziness, tinnitus, occult bleeding, increased clotting time	Give with food. Report any side effects, including bleeding gums or bruising easily.
Antidepressants		
Tricyclic antidepressant amitriptyline (Elavil) Blocks the reuptake of serotonin.	Sedation, confusion, dry mouth, constipation, nausea, orthostatic hypotension, urinary retention, tachycardia, palpitations, bone marrow depression	Give at bedtime if sedation is a problem. Avoid alcohol. Report any side effects. Do not stop drug abruptly.

Patient-Controlled Analgesia

Patient-controlled analgesia (PCA) allows clients to self-administer their own narcotic analgesic by means of an intravenous pump system (Fig. 20–5). The drug is infused when the client presses a hand-held button. The dose and time interval between doses is programmed into the device to prevent accidental overdosage.

Intraspinal Analgesia

In *intraspinal analgesia,* a narcotic or local anesthetic is infused into the subarachnoid or epidural space of the spinal cord by means of a catheter inserted by a physician. The intraspinal analgesic is administered several times per day or as a continuous low-dose infusion. This method of analgesia relieves pain with minimal systemic drug effects. When used for clients who require long-term analgesia, there is less chance of affecting the subcutaneous tissues with repeated injections that may eventually lessen drug absorption.

TABLE 20-4 **Examples of Adult Equianalgesic Doses**

Drug	Parenteral Dose	Oral Dose
morphine sulfate	10 mg q 3–4 h	30 mg q 3–4 h
meperidine (Demerol)	100 mg q 3 h	300 mg q 2–3 h
hydromorphone (Dilaudid)	1.5 mg q 3–4 h	7.5 mg q 3–4 h
pentazocine (Talwin)	60 mg q 3–4 h	150 mg q 3–4 h

Adapted from Carr, C. B., Jacox, A. K., Chapman, C. R., et al. (1992, February). *Acute pain management: Operative or medical procedures and trauma. Clinical Practice Guideline No. 1.* (AHCPR Pub. 92-0032). Rockville, MD: Agency for Health Care Policy and Research.

GATE-CLOSING MECHANISMS

Gate-closing mechanisms are nondrug techniques that produce a sensation, usually through the skin (cutaneous), to interrupt pain transmission. Examples include transcutaneous electrical nerve stimulation, application of heat or cold, acupuncture, and acupressure.

Transcutaneous Electrical Stimulation

Transcutaneous electrical nerve stimulation (TENS) is a pain management technique that delivers bursts of electricity to the skin and underlying nerves. It is safe for managing acute and chronic pain, and it does not produce systemic side effects or addiction. The electricity is delivered from a battery-operated unit through electrode patches that are placed at appro-

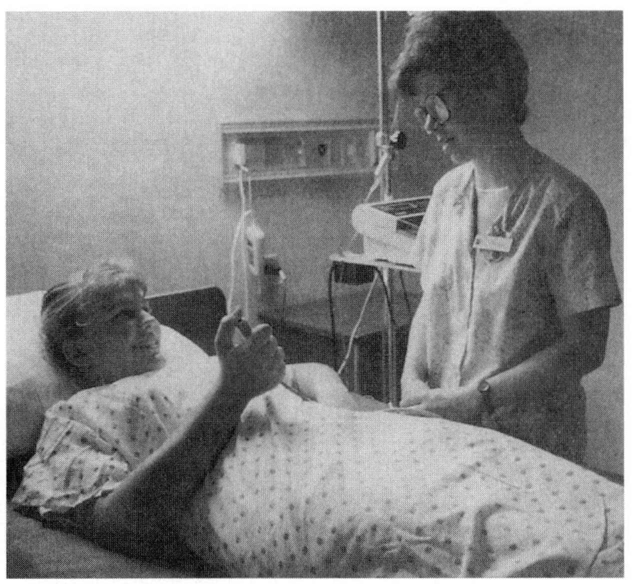

FIGURE 20-5. Patient-controlled analgesia.

priate sites, such as directly over the affected area, at areas along a nerve pathway, or at points distal to the painful area (Fig. 20–6). The electrical stimulus is perceived as a pleasant tapping, tingling, vibrating, or buzzing sensation. Placement sites, intensity of electrical current, rate of electrical bursts, and duration can be changed according to the client's response.

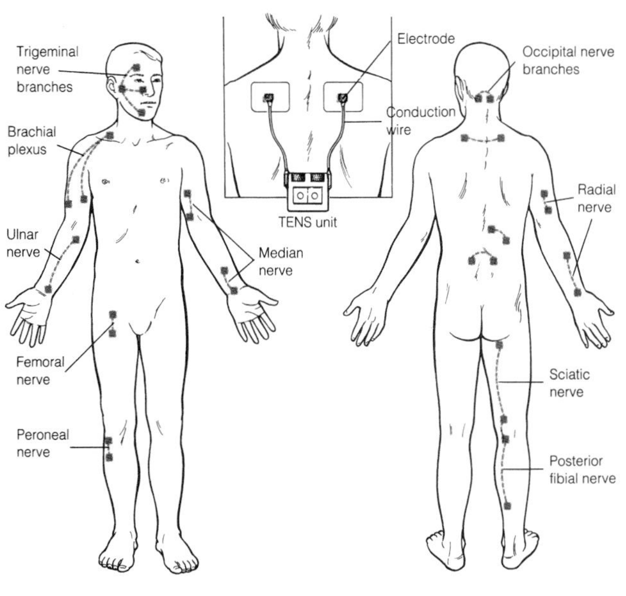

FIGURE 20-6. Transcutaneous electric nerve stimulation (TENS) unit may be placed close to source of pain to activate various sensory nerves. The purpose is to flood the gates in the spinal cord and block the perception of pain. Various sites are used depending on the location of the painful stimulus. (Bullock BL, Rosendahl PP. Pathophysiology: adaptations and alterations in function. 3rd ed. Philadelphia, JB Lippincott, 1992: 1025)

Heat and Cold

Applications of heat using a heating pad, hydrotherapy, or moist hot packs may provide relief of chronic pain or minor or moderate pain, such as that caused by arthritis, muscle strain or sprain, and soft tissue injury. In addition to controlling bleeding and swelling resulting from minor injuries, application of cold may be used for minor or moderate pain.

Acupuncture and Acupressure

Acupuncture is a pain management technique in which long, thin needles are inserted into the skin. *Acupressure* uses tissue compression, rather than needles, to reduce pain. The location for needle placement and pressure is based on 2,000-year-old traditions practiced in Chinese medicine. Relief of pain, especially chronic pain, is not permanent and repeated treatments are almost always necessary.

Although both techniques have been demonstrated to prevent or relieve pain, their exact mechanism is not completely understood. Some speculate the twisting, vibration, or pressure are forms of cutaneous stimuli that close the gates to pain-transmitting neurochemicals. Another theory is that acupuncture and acupressure stimulate the body to release endorphins and enkephalins.

SPINAL SURGERY TECHNIQUES

Intractable pain, pain that does not respond to analgesic medications, noninvasive measures, or nursing management, requires more drastic measures. Neurosurgical procedures that provide pain relief include rhizotomy and cordotomy.

Rhizotomy

A *rhizotomy* is a surgical procedure on the spine that involves a laminectomy (see Chap. 47) followed by sectioning of the posterior (sensory) nerve root just before it enters the spinal cord. Sectioning a spinal nerve prevents sensory impulses from entering the spinal cord and going to the brain. This results in a permanent loss of sensation in the area supplied by the sectioned nerve. More than one nerve may need to be sectioned to produce the desired results. A chemical rhizotomy (using chemicals such as alcohol or phenol to destroy the nerve) or a percutaneous rhizotomy (use of radio frequency waves to destroy pain fibers) are alternatives that may provide the same result. This procedure usually is reserved for terminally ill clients.

Cordotomy

A *cordotomy* is an interruption of pain pathways in the spinal cord. A laminectomy is performed and sensory nerve tracts in the vertebral column are destroyed, thus preventing sensory nerve impulses from going to the brain. Loss of sensation is permanent. A *percutaneous cervical cordotomy* is basically the same procedure as a cordotomy but is performed under local anesthesia. It carries less risk and usually is better tolerated by terminally ill clients. Guided by fluoroscopy, the surgeon inserts a needle through the skin (percutaneous) in the neck (cervical) near the mastoid process. Pain pathways are interrupted by movement of the needle.

OTHER NONINVASIVE TECHNIQUES

Various other techniques are used singly or as adjuncts to more traditional pain management techniques. Some include imagery, biofeedback, humor, breathing exercises and progressive relaxation, and distraction. Refer to Chapters 11 and 12 for a review of these techniques. In addition, in some situations, for example clients with severe burns, hypnosis is used. *Hypnosis* is a technique in which a person assumes a trancelike state during which perceptions are altered. During hypnosis, a suggestion is made that a person's pain will be eliminated or the sensation will be experienced in a more pleasant way.

NURSING PROCESS
The Client With Acute Pain

Assessment

Assess the source of the client's pain and related factors such as what makes the pain better or worse. Use a pain assessment scale to determine severity. Ask client at what level would pain be tolerable. Assess vital signs. Assess subjective interpretation of pain.

Diagnosis and Planning

The nurse works collaboratively with the client and physician to implement the best approaches for managing and reducing pain (Nursing Guidelines 20-1). Other interventions for the client in pain include but are not limited to the following:

Nursing Diagnoses and Collaborative Problems	Nursing Interventions
Pain related to release to cellular injury or disease **Goal:** The client will rate his or her pain at a lower level (specify) 30 minutes after implementing a pain management technique.	Implement Nursing Guidelines 20-1: Managing Pain
Anxiety or **Fear** related to concerns about the significance and seriousness of pain. **Goal:** The client will report feeling more relaxed and less fearful of what the pain represents.	Share with client the usual pattern of pain for clients with similar conditions; clarify any unrealistic ideas. Take time to be an attentive and concerned listener when the client talks about his or her pain. Offer to stay with the client or have someone else do so when anxiety or fears are at a heightened level. Implement techniques that promote distraction such as engaging in conversation or watching television.
Self-Care Deficit (specify type) and **Activity Intolerance** related to reduced endurance secondary to the drain of energy used to cope with pain. **Goal:** The client will demonstrate an increased tolerance for activity and independence in managing activities of daily living.	Place the call light within easy reach. Distribute required self-care activities between periods of rest. Assist client when he or she becomes fatigued or unable to continue with activity or self-care.

When narcotic analgesics are administered, the nurse monitors for and implements measures for managing side effects. Problems that may develop with opioid and opiate therapy include *Risk for Impaired Gas Exchange* related to respiratory depression, *Constipation* related to slowed peristalsis, *Risk for Injury* related to drowsiness and unsteady gait, *Risk for Altered Nutrition: Less than Body Requirements* related to anorexia and nausea, *Risk for Fluid Volume Deficit* related to reduced oral intake, and Sleep Pattern Disturbance (excessive or interrupted sleep) related to depression of the central nervous system.

Evaluation

- The client reports that pain is gone or at a tolerable level.
- The client perceives the pain experience realistically and copes effectively.
- The client is able to participate in self-care activities without undue pain.

Client and Family Teaching

The nurse encourages the client and family to:

- Discuss with the physician what to expect from the disorder, injury, or its treatment.
- Talk with the physician about any concerns that relate to drug therapy.
- Share information about what drugs or pain-relieving techniques have been helpful, and those that have not, during previous episodes.
- Identify drug allergies to avoid adverse effects.

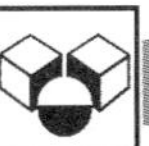

Nursing Guidelines 20-1

Managing Pain

- Assess, monitor, and document characteristics of the client's pain and possible related factors at appropriate intervals.
- Never doubt or minimize the client's description of pain or need for relief.
- Assess accompanying aspects of the pain experience such as disturbed sleep, impaired physical mobility, anorexia, depressed mood, and interference with relationships and role performance.
- Determine results of pain management techniques already attempted.
- Develop a written plan for managing pain. Collaborate with the client on setting realistic goals with specific outcome criteria.
- Modify or eliminate factors that contribute to pain such as emptying the bladder or bowel, changing body positions, limiting movement or activity, altering environmental temperature, and decreasing social isolation.
- Let the client choose from available options for controlling pain. Explain the goal or mechanism for each technique implemented.
- Consult with the physician on the best analgesic, including dose, schedule, and route of administration and follow the written medical orders. Advocate for the client if the drug or prescription is not adequately controlling the pain. Obtain the best equianalgesic dose when switching from a parenteral to oral route.
- Administer pain medication before an activity that produces or intensifies pain.
- Monitor for side effects of opioid drug therapy such as respiratory depression, decreased levels of consciousness, nausea, vomiting, and constipation.
- Use nondrug nursing interventions such as distraction, breathing exercises, imagery, progressive relaxation, and massage if the client is open to their use.
- Evaluate the outcomes of interventions, document results objectively. Revise the pain management plan if goals are unmet.

- Inform the physician about other medications being taken to avoid drug–drug interactions.
- Take prescribed drugs exactly as directed and report untoward effects.
- Avoid taking over-the-counter drugs unless the physician has been consulted; follow label directions for administration.
- Avoid alcohol and sedative drugs if the analgesic causes sedation.
- Keep analgesic drugs out of the reach of children; request childproof caps.
- Never share medications with others or take someone else's medications for pain.

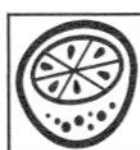

General Nutritional Considerations

Painful procedures are performed at times least likely to interfere with meals.

Pain medications administered 30 to 45 minutes before meals may enable the client to consume an adequate intake.

Small, frequent meals may help maximize intake in clients with drug- or pain-related anorexia. Solicit food preferences.

A high-fiber diet (ie, whole grain breads and cereals, fresh fruits and vegetables) along with increased fluids may help clients with constipation related to narcotic analgesics.

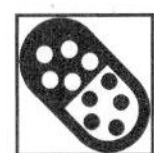

General Pharmacologic Considerations

Analgesic administration is timed to permit maximum client cooperation in care.

Some nonnarcotic analgesics, when used daily over an extended period, can cause undesirable side effects, such as gastrointestinal bleeding and hemorrhagic disorders.

Transdermal fentanyl (Duragesic) may be used to manage chronic pain in clients requiring opioid analgesic therapy. This drug is released into the systemic circulation over a period of 72 hours.

The primary health care provider or dentist should be informed before any procedure when pain medications, especially salicylates or nonsteroidal anti-inflammatory agents, are used on a regular basis.

An over-the-counter analgesic agent such as aspirin, ibuprofen, or acetaminophen, should not be used consistently to treat chronic pain without first consulting a physician.

General Gerontologic Considerations

Pain perception may be diminished in older adults causing some acute conditions to go unreported to medical personnel.

Older adults experience a higher peak effect and longer duration of pain relief from an opioid.

Older adults taking nonsteroidal anti-inflammatory drugs are at increased risk for renal toxicity and gastrointestinal problems.

Confused older adults may not be able to report pain, but may exhibit other signs such as agitation, behavior changes, or irritability.

A reduced dose of analgesics, especially opioid analgesics, may be prescribed for the older adult initially. The nurse carefully assesses the older client for pain relief.

SUMMARY OF KEY CONCEPTS

- Pain is an privately experienced, unpleasant sensation usually associated with disease or injury; it also has an emotional component referred to as suffering.
- The transmission of pain begins with some type of cellular disruption that signals nociceptors, specialized pain receptors. The nociceptors transmit the pain message to the brain via the spinal cord using various neurotransmitters, one of which is called substance P.
- Pain transmission can be blocked or reduced with two naturally produced morphine-like chemicals, endorphins and enkephalins.
- The three theories concerning pain transmission are the specificity theory, the pattern theory, and the gate control theory.
- Pain is classified in several ways. Types of pain include cutaneous, somatic, visceral, referred, and neuropathic pain, and acute and chronic pain.
- Pain perception is the conscious experience of discomfort. Pain threshold is the point at which the pain-transmitting neurochemicals reach the brain causing conscious awareness. Pain tolerance is the amount of pain a person endures once the threshold has been reached.
- Pain is difficult to assess because machines and laboratory tests cannot measure it. Nurses are limited to subjective information clients supply and suggestive signs that may indicate discomfort.
- A pain assessment includes the client's description of its onset, quality, intensity, location, and duration, symptoms that accompany pain, and what, if anything, makes it better or worse.
- Four assessment tools for quantifying pain intensity include a numeric scale, word scale, linear scale, and picture scale.
- Pain assessment is essential: when the client is admitted, at least once per shift when pain is an actual or potential problem, when the client in pain is at rest or involved in a nursing activity, after each potentially painful procedure or treatment, and before and 30 minutes after a pain management intervention.
- Pain management refers to the techniques used to prevent, reduce, or relieve pain. Four general techniques for achieving pain management are blocking brain perception, interrupting pain-transmitting chemicals at the site of injury, using gate-closing mechanisms, and altering pain transmission at the level of the spinal cord.
- Opioid and nonopioid analgesics are the cornerstones of pain management.
- Gate-closing mechanisms are nondrug techniques that produce a sensory experience, usually through the skin to interrupt pain transmission. Examples include transcutaneous electrical nerve stimulation, application of heat and cold, acupuncture, and acupressure.
- Two surgical procedures used to relieve intractable pain are rhizotomy and cordotomy.
- Nurses may independently use noninvasive pain management techniques such as imagery, humor, breathing exercises, progressive relaxation, and distraction.
- Nursing management of clients with pain includes working collaboratively with the client and physician to implement the best approaches for reducing pain, implementing nursing interventions for pain management, monitoring and managing drug side effects, teaching clients information important to communicate to health care workers, and teaching clients how to self-administer analgesics.
- Three nursing diagnoses, besides *Pain*, common among clients with pain include *Anxiety* or *Fear*, *Self-Care Deficit*, and *Activity Intolerance*.
- Pertinent information to teach clients includes to identify drug allergies and problems that have been encountered with previously prescribed analgesics, to take the prescribed drug according to directions, and to never share medications.

CRITICAL THINKING EXERCISES

1. What questions should the nurse ask when a client states he or she has pain?
2. Discuss how acute pain after surgery is different from that experienced by a client with chronic back pain.
3. Discuss nursing interventions that are appropriate if a client does not experience adequate pain relief from a prescribed analgesic.

Suggested Readings

Allcock, N. (1996). Factors affecting the assessment of pain: A literature review. *Journal of Advanced Nursing, 24*(6), 1144–1151.

Berkowitz, C. M. (1997). Epidural pain control–your job, too. *RN, 60*(8), 22–27.

Bullock, B. L., & Rosendahl, P. P. (1992). *Pathophysiology, adaptations and alterations in function* (3rd ed.). Philadelphia: J. B. Lippincott.

Brooks, K. (1997). Reducing epidural catheter infections. *Nursing, 27*(5), 15.

Carr, E. C. J., & Thomas, V. J. (1997). Anticipating and experiencing postoperative pain: The patients' perspective. *Journal of Clinical Nursing, 6*(3), 191–201.

Caudill, M. A., Holman, G. H., & Turk, D. (1996). Effective ways to manage chronic pain. *Patient Care, 30*(11), 154–155, 159–162, 164–167.

Cerrato, P. (1996). Acupuncture: Where East meets West. *RN, 59*(10), 55–57.

Copstead, L. C. (1995). *Perspectives on pathophysiology.* Philadelphia: Saunders.

Donovan, M. I., & Miaskowski, C. (1992). Striving for a standard of pain relief. *American Journal of Nursing, 92*, 106–107.

McCaffery, M. (1997). Pain management handbook. *Nursing, 27*(4), 42–45.

McCaffery, M., & Beebe, A. (1989) *Pain: Clinical manual for nursing practice.* St. Louis: Mosby.

Reed, J., Lesiuk, N., & MacQuarrie, V. Focus on quality: managing postoperative gas pain. *Canadian Nurse, 93*(8), 43, 45.

Additional Resources

American Pain Society
4700 West Lake Avenue
Glenview, IL 60025
http://www.ampainsoc.org

American Chronic Pain Association
P.O. Box 850
Rocklin, CA 95677
(916) 632–0922

American Society of Pain Management Nurses
2755 Bristol Street, Suite 110
Costa Mesa, CA 92628
(714) 545–1305

Agency for Health Care Policy and Research
Executive Office Center
Suite 501
2101 East Jefferson St.
Rockville, MD 20852
http://www.ahcpr.gov/

World Health Organization
1211 Geneva 27, Switzerland
http://www.who.dk/

National Commission for the Certification of Acupuncturists
1424 16th Street, NW
Suite 601
Washington, DC 200036

Chapter 21

Caring for Clients With Fluid, Electrolyte, and Acid–Base Imbalances

KEY TERMS

Acidosis
Acids
Active transport
Alkalosis
Anions
Anion gap
Bases
Bicarbonate-carbonic acid buffer system
Cations
Chvostek's sign
Circulatory overload
Compensation
Dehydration
Dependent edema
Electrolytes
Extracellular
Facilitated diffusion
Filtration
Generalized edema
Hemoconcentration
Hemodilution
Hypervolemia
Hypovolemia
Interstitial fluid
Intracellular fluid
Intravascular fluid
Ions
Osmosis
Passive diffusion
Pitting edema
Third-spacing
Trousseau's sign

LEARNING OBJECTIVES

On completion of this chapter, the reader will:

- Name two main fluid locations in the human body and two subdivisions.
- List three chemical substances that are components of body fluid.
- Identify five processes by which water and dissolved chemicals are relocated.
- List two types of fluid imbalance.
- Explain the difference between hypovolemia and dehydration.
- Explain what hemoconcentration and hemodilution means.
- Give the average fluid intake per day for adults.
- List four ways in which fluid is normally lost from the body.
- Identify at least five assessments characteristic of hypovolemia.
- Discuss nursing interventions for fluid volume deficit.
- Identify assessment data pertinent to hypervolemia.
- Explain the potential consequence of hypervolemia.
- List and identify the differences in three types of edema.
- Explain how edema is graded.
- Discuss nursing interventions for managing hypervolemia.
- Name two nursing diagnoses, besides fluid volume excess, that are common among clients with hypervolemia.
- Explain third-spacing and medical techniques for relocating this fluid.
- List at least three factors each that contribute to electrolyte loss and excess.
- Name four electrolyte imbalances that pose a major threat to well-being.
- Discuss the nursing management of clients with electrolyte imbalances.
- Discuss the role of acids and bases in body fluid.
- Explain pH and identify the normal range of plasma pH.
- Identify two chemicals and two organs that play major roles in regulating acid–base balance.
- Give the names of two major acid–base imbalances and subdivisions of each.
- Discuss the significance of maintaining acid–base balance.
- List three components of arterial blood gas findings that are used to determine the status of acid–base imbalance.
- Discuss the nursing management of clients with acid–base imbalances.

About 60% of the adult human body is water. Put another way, for every 100 lb of body weight, approximately 60 lb is water. The majority of the body's water is located within cells (**intracellular fluid**), with the rest in **extracellular** (outside the cells) locations such as between cells (**interstitial fluid**) and the plasma, or serum, portion of blood (**intravascular fluid**) (Fig. 21–1). The volume of fluid in each location varies with age and gender (Table 21–1).

There is a continuous translocation (movement back and forth) of fluid and an exchange of chemicals within and among all the areas where water is located. Some of the chemicals involved are **electrolytes**, substances that when dissolved in fluid carry an electrical charge; **acids**, substances that release hydrogen into fluid; and **bases**, substances that bind with hydrogen. The delicate balance of fluid, electrolytes, acids, and bases is ensured by an adequate intake of water and nutrients, mechanisms for regulating fluid volume, and by various physiologic processes.

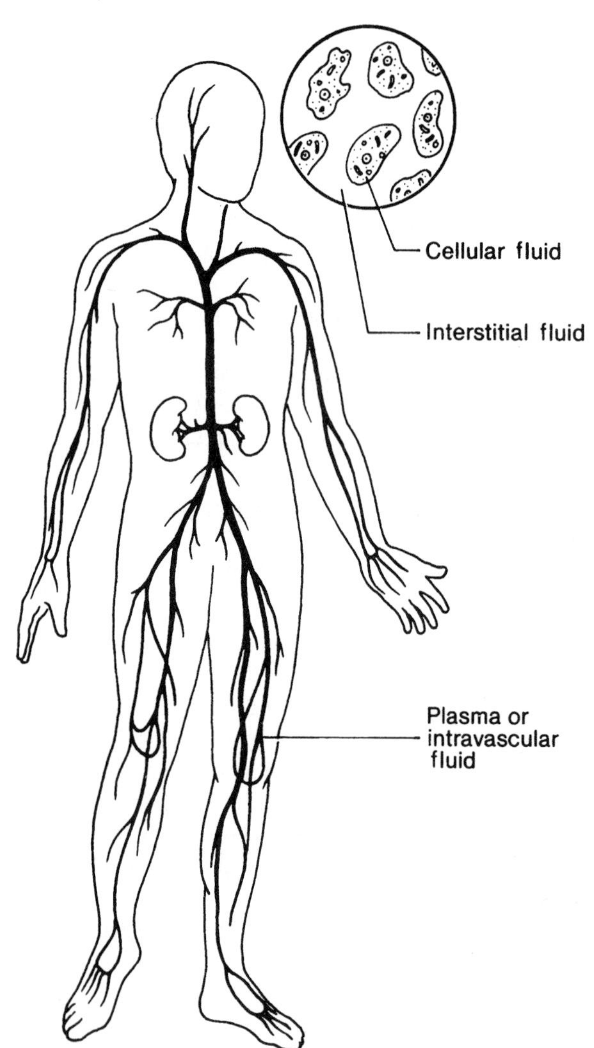

FIGURE 21-1. Normal distribution of body fluid.

Fluid Regulation

In healthy adults, oral fluid intake averages about 2,500 mL/day. However, it can range between 1,800 to 3,000 mL/day with a similar volume of fluid loss (Table 21–2). Under normal conditions, several mechanisms maintain equivalents between fluid intake and loss. For example, as body fluid becomes concentrated, the brain triggers the sensation of thirst, which then stimulates a person to drink fluid. As fluid volume increases, fluid is lost, primarily through urination, in a proportionate volume to maintain or restore equilibrium. Other mechanisms for fluid loss include bowel elimination, perspiration, and breathing. Losses from the skin in areas other than where sweat glands are located and from the vapor in exhaled air are referred to as *insensible losses* because they are, for practical purposes, unnoticeable and unmeasurable.

Fluid and Chemical Distribution

Once water and chemical substances are absorbed, their movement and relocation at the cellular level are governed by physiologic processes such as osmosis, filtration, passive diffusion, facilitated diffusion, and active transport.

OSMOSIS

Osmosis is the movement of water through a *semipermeable membrane*, one that allows some but not all substances in a solution to pass through, from a dilute (*hypotonic*) to more concentrated (*hypertonic*) area. *Tonicity* refers, in this case, to the quantity (concentration) of substances dissolved in the water. The power to draw water in the direction of greater concentration is referred to as *osmotic pressure*. *Colloids*, large-sized substances such as serum proteins (eg, albumin, globulin, and fibrinogen) and blood cells, do not readily pass through cell and tissue membranes. Their presence contributes to fluid concentration and acts as a force for attracting water—a property referred to as *colloidal osmotic pressure*.

Fluid distribution via osmosis occurs in the following ways: if the concentration is higher within the cell, water is drawn through the membrane into the cell from the interstitial space. The process continues until the concentration is the same (*isotonic*) on both

TABLE 21-1 **Percentages of Body Fluid According to Age and Gender**

Fluid Compartment	Infants	Male Adults	Female Adults	Older Adults
Intravascular	4%	4%	5%	5%
Interstitial	25%	11%	10%	15%
Intracellular	48%	45%	35%	25%
Total	77%	60%	50%	45%

sides of the membrane. The reverse is true as well: if the concentration is higher in the interstitial space, water is pulled from the cell (Fig. 21–2).

Filtration is a process that promotes movement of fluid and some dissolved substances through a semipermeable membrane according to pressure differences. Filtration relocates water and chemicals from an area of high pressure to an area with lower pressure. For example, at the arterial end of a capillaries, fluid is under higher pressure than at the venous end. Filtration causes the fluid and some dissolved substances such as oxygen to move to the interstitial space. The majority of water is then reabsorbed at the venous end of capillaries by colloidal osmotic pressure (Fig. 21–3).

Filtration also affects the manner in which the kidneys excrete fluid and wastes and then selectively reabsorb water and other chemicals that need to be conserved. The kidneys filter about 180 liters of fluid from blood each day. All but 1 to 1.5 liters is reabsorbed.

Passive diffusion is a physiologic process in which dissolved substances such as electrolytes move from an area of high concentration to an area of lower concentration through a semipermeable membrane. Passive diffusion, like osmosis, remains fairly static (unchanged) once equilibrium occurs.

Facilitated diffusion is a process in which certain dissolved substances require the assistance of a carrier molecule to pass through a semipermeable membrane. For example, the distribution of glucose molecules is facilitated inside cells with the help of the carrier substance, insulin.

Active transport requires an energy source, a substance called *adenosine triphosphate* (ATP), to drive dissolved chemicals from an area of low concentration to one that is higher—just the opposite of passive diffusion. An example of active transport is the *sodium–potassium pump system*. Its function is to move potassium from lower concentrations in the extracellular fluid into cells where it is highly concentrated. It also moves sodium, which is in lower amounts within the cells, to extracellular fluid, where it is more abundant.

Metabolic disorders that diminish ATP seriously affect normal cellular functions by impairing the distribution of chemicals within intracellular and extracellular fluid. The normal functioning of the body can be disrupted whenever there is a significant change in fluid volume or its distribution.

Fluid Imbalances

Fluid imbalance is a general term describing any of several conditions in which the body's water is not in the proper volume or location within the body. Common fluid imbalances include hypovolemia, hypervolemia, and third-spacing.

Hypovolemia

Hypovolemia (fluid volume deficit) refers to a low volume of extracellular fluid. Generally there is a similar

TABLE 21-2 **Daily Fluid Intake and Losses**

Sources of Fluid		Mechanisms of Fluid Loss	
Oral liquids	1,200–1,500 mL/day	Urine	1,200–1,700 mL/day
Food	700–1,000 mL/day	Feces	100–250 mL/day
Metabolism	200–400 mL/day	Perspiration	100–150 mL/day
		Insensible losses	
		Skin	350–400 mL/day
		Lungs	350–400 mL/day
Total	2,100–2,900 mL/day	**Total**	2,100–2,900 mL/day
Median amount	2,500 mL/day	**Median amount**	2,500 mL/day

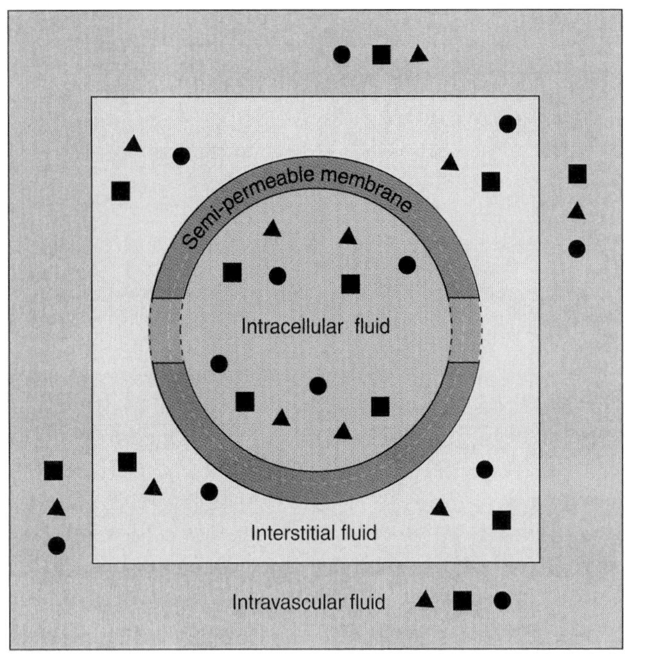

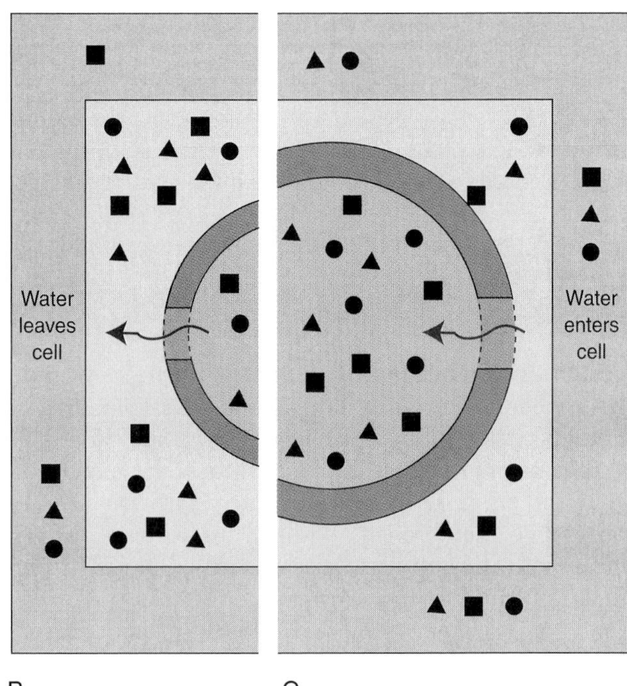

FIGURE 21-2. Movement of intracellular and extracellular fluid by osmosis. (A) Equal translocation of water due to similar concentrations on both sides of the semipermeable membrane. (B) Fluid leaves in greater proportions from the cell to dilute the area of concentration; the cell shrinks. (C) Greater proportions of water move inside the concentrated cellular fluid; the cell enlarges.

depletion in dissolved chemical substances, such as electrolytes, as well. **Dehydration** results when the volume of body fluid is significantly reduced in both extracellular and intracellular compartments (Fig. 21–4).

ETIOLOGY AND PATHOPHYSIOLOGY

Factors that contribute to hypovolemia or fluid volume deficits include inadequate fluid intake; fluid loss in excess of fluid intake such as with hemorrhage, prolonged vomiting or diarrhea, wound loss as in the case of a burn injury, or profuse urination or perspiration; and translocation of fluid to compartments where it is trapped, such as the abdominal cavity or interstitial spaces (eg, third-spacing). When there is a decrease in circulatory volume, the heart compensates by increasing the heart rate to maintain an adequate cardiac output (see Chap. 30). Blood pressure falls with postural changes or it may become

FIGURE 21-3. Dynamics of capillary fluid filtration.

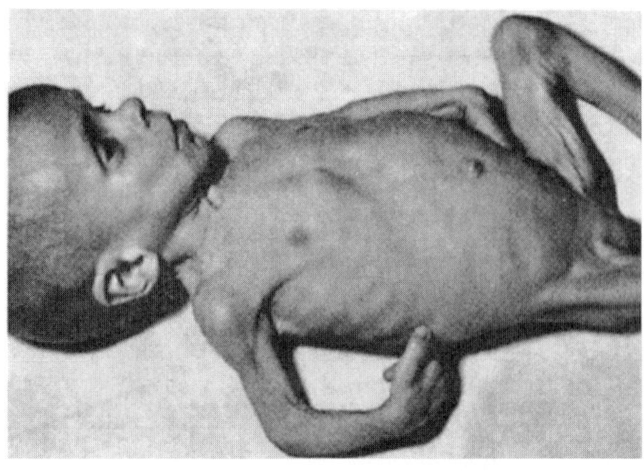

FIGURE 21-4. A severe case of dehydration.

severely lowered when there is a rapid loss of blood. **Hemoconcentration**, high ratio of blood components in relation to watery plasma, increases the potential for forming blood clots and urinary stones and compromises the kidney's ability to excrete nitrogen wastes. Hypovolemia eventually depletes intracellular fluid, which can affect cellular functions. One example is the change in mentation that usually occurs.

ASSESSMENT FINDINGS

Signs and Symptoms

One of the earliest symptoms of hypovolemia is thirst. Other signs and symptoms are listed in Table 21–3.

Diagnostic Findings

Evidence of hemoconcentration is reflected in an elevated hematocrit and blood cell counts, a consequence of water deficiency. Urine specific gravity is high. Serum electrolytes tend to remain normal because they are depleted in proportion to the water loss (Bullock, 1996). The central venous pressure (CVP) (see Chap. 29) is below 4 cm H_20.

MEDICAL MANAGEMENT

Fluid deficit is restored by treating its etiology, increasing the volume of oral intake, prescribing intravenous fluid replacement (see Chap. 23), controlling fluid losses, or a combination of these.

NURSING MANAGEMENT

Gather assessment data that provide evidence of the client's fluid status (Nursing Guidelines 21–1). Identify the nursing diagnosis *Fluid Volume Deficit* and its etiology such as fluid loss in excess of intake. Implement nursing measures and medical orders to restore the fluid intake to at least 2000 mL/day and a urine output that is ±500 mL of intake. Refer to Nursing Guidelines 21–1 for specific methods for restoring fluid balance. Monitor and document the client's response.

Client and Family Teaching

The nurse teaches clients who have a potential for hypovolemia to:

- Respond to thirst because it is an early indication that fluid volume is reduced
- Consume at least 8 to 10 glasses of fluid each day and more during hot, humid weather
- Drink water as an inexpensive means for meeting fluid requirements
- Include a moderate amount of table salt or foods containing sodium each day
- Rise slowly from a sitting or lying position to avoid dizziness and potential injury

Hypervolemia

Hypervolemia (fluid volume excess) means there is a high volume of water in the intravascular fluid compartment.

ETIOLOGY AND PATHOPHYSIOLOGY

It is caused by fluid intake that exceeds fluid loss, such as from excessive oral intake or rapid infusion of intravenous fluid. Hypervolemia is also a consequence of heart failure (see Chap. 35) when the heart cannot adequately distribute fluid to the kidney for

TABLE 21-3 **Signs and Symptoms of Fluid Volume Deficit and Excess**

Assessment	Fluid Deficit	Fluid Excess
Weight	Weight loss ≥ 2 lb/24 h	Weight gain ≥ 2 lb/24 h
Blood pressure	Low	High
Temperature	Elevated	Normal
Pulse	Rapid, weak, thready	Full, bounding
Respirations	Rapid, shallow	Moist, labored
Urine	Scant, dark yellow	Light yellow
Stool	Dry, small volume	Bulky
Skin	Warm, flushed, dry	Cool, pale, moist
	Poor skin turgor	Pitting edema
Mucous membranes	Dry, sticky	Moist
Eyes	Sunken	Swollen
Lungs	Clear	Crackles, gurgles
Breathing	Effortless	Dyspnea, orthopnea
Energy	Weak	Fatigues easily
Jugular neck veins	Flat	Distended
Cognition	Reduced	Reduced
Consciousness	Sleepy	Anxious

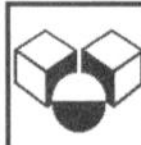

Nursing Guidelines - 21-1

Assessing and Managing Fluid Volume Deficit

- Weigh every client on admission. Weigh clients at risk for fluid volume deficit daily, at the same time of day, on the same scale, and dressed similarly. Record weight in the medical record. Report a loss of 2 lb (1 kg) or more in 24 hours; a 2-lb loss is the equivalent of 1 liter of fluid.
- Keep a daily record of fluid intake and output volumes.
- Measure urine output hourly or every shift depending on the client's acuity level. Report a trend in which the hourly urine output is less than 50 mL or the 24-hour output is less than 500 mL.
- Observe urine for dark yellow color, strong odor, and specific gravity 1.022 or greater.
- Monitor laboratory blood tests for evidence of *hemoconcentration* such as an elevated hematocrit and blood cell count.
- Record vital signs every 5 to 15 minutes or at 1-, 2-, or 4-hour intervals depending on the client's acuity level.
- Assess *skin turgor* (elasticity) by lifting the skin over the sternum, inner thigh, or forehead each shift. *Skin tenting,* a quality in which the skin remains elevated and is slow to return to the underlying tissue, is an indication of dehydration.
- Observe the tongue for furrowing (linear channels) and dry oral mucous membranes.
- Inform the client about the need to increase consumption of oral fluids. Set a target goal for oral intake per hour, per shift, and per 24-hour period; a goal of 3,000 to 4,000 mL is not excessive for clients who are dehydrated. Schedule the bulk of fluid intake during times when the client is awake (eg, more intake during daytime hours than throughout the night).
- Obtain a list of fluids the client prefers; include gelatin, popsicles, ice cream, and sherbet as alternatives to liquid beverages if they are allowed.
- Provide a variety of liquids at the bedside for the client to drink; replace with a fresh supply periodically. Ensure that fluids are at an appropriate temperature.
- Offer small volumes frequently, rather than expecting the client to consume a large volume at any one time.
- Relieve nausea, vomiting, mouth discomfort, and other problems that interfere with consuming oral liquids.
- Evaluate goals by recollecting assessment data and analyzing trends especially in intake and output totals. Report results to the physician, especially if collaborative efforts with the client fall short of goals.

filtration. It can also result from inadequate fluid elimination as may occur with kidney disease (see Chap. 62). Fluid retention (reduced fluid loss) also can occur secondarily to an excessive intake of salt (sodium chloride), adrenal gland dysfunction (see Cushing's disease, Chap. 55), or the administration of corticosteroid drugs such as prednisolone (Delta-Cortef).

Hypervolemia can lead to **circulatory overload**, a volume that exceeds what is normal for the intravascular space, and has the potential for compromising cardiopulmonary function if it remains unresolved. The excess volume raises blood pressure and causes the heart to increase the force of its contractions. As the excess volume is distributed to the interstitial space **pitting edema**, indentations in the skin following compression, may be noted (Fig. 21–5). However, edema does not generally occur until there is a 3-liter excess in the intravascular volume (Monahan, Drake, & Neighbors, 1994).

ASSESSMENT FINDINGS

Signs and Symptoms

Early signs of hypervolemia are weight gain, elevated blood pressure, and more effort to breathe. There may be evidence of **dependent edema** (body areas most affected by gravity), such as the feet and ankles, or sacrum in clients who are confined to bed. Rings, shoes, and stockings may leave marks in the skin. The jugular neck veins may appear prominent when the client is in a sitting position. Eventually there are moist breath sounds caused by fluid congestion in the lungs. See Table 21–3 for a listing of signs and symptoms of hypervolemia.

Diagnostic Findings

The blood cell counts and hematocrit are low due to **hemodilution**, reduced ratio of blood components to watery plasma. Urine specific gravity is also low reflecting the larger proportion of water. CVP is above 10 cm H_2O.

MEDICAL MANAGEMENT

The condition causing the fluid excess is treated. Oral and parenteral fluid intake is restricted. *Diuret-*

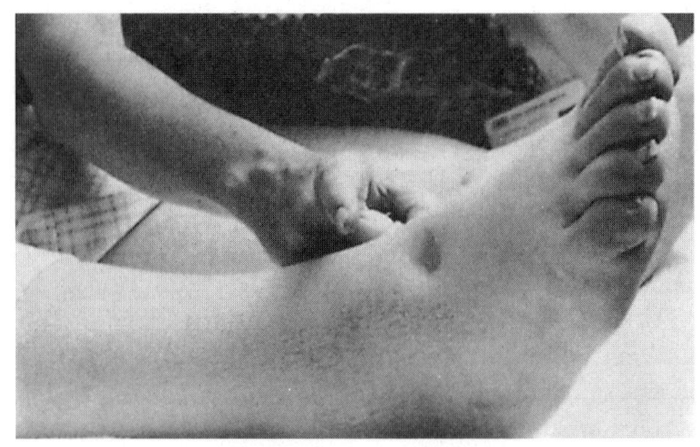

FIGURE 21-5. Pitting edema.

ics, drugs that promote urinary excretion, are prescribed. Salt and sodium intake is limited.

NURSING PROCESS
The Client With Fluid Volume Excess

Assessment

Obtain a baseline weight and weigh the client daily thereafter on the same scale and at the same time each morning before breakfast. A 2-lb weight gain in 24 hours is indicative of retaining a liter of fluid. Maintain accurate intake and output records and report significant differences. Auscultate the lungs for abnormal breath sounds, assess neck veins for distention, and record the blood pressure, heart rate, and respiratory rate. Observe the client's activity tolerance. Assess for pitting edema by gently pressing the skin over a bony area, such as the tibia or dorsum of the foot for up to 5 seconds and observe the results (Fig. 21–6). Inspect the edematous skin for cracks and breakdown.

Diagnosis and Planning

Care of a client with hypervolemia includes, but is not limited to, the following:

Nursing Diagnoses and Collaborative Problems	Nursing Interventions
Fluid Volume Excess related to intake that exceeds fluid loss (or reduced fluid loss in relation to intake) **Goal:** The client's fluid status will return to normal as evidenced by a loss of weight, reduction in edema, blood pressure within normal limits, and urine output at least 2000 mL/day.	Assess the following on a regular basis or as often as necessary: vital signs, daily weight, intake and output, breath sounds, location and extent of edema. Use guidelines established by the physician for restricting oral fluid. Work out a plan with the client for distributing the allotted oral volume over a 24-hour period. Ration fluid so the client has an opportunity to consume some at times other than meals. Collaborate with the dietitian on modifying the diet to meet salt/sodium restrictions and to avoid foods that are sweet or dry to control thirst.
Altered Comfort: Dry Mouth and Thirst related to restriction of oral fluid **Goal:** The client's mouth will be moist despite fluid restrictions.	Provide frequent oral hygiene. Let the client rinse the mouth with water and expectorate it rather than swallow it. Substitute ice chips for liquids to give the appearance and sensation of consuming a larger volume of fluid. Provide a measured volume of fluid in a squeeze bottle or spray atomizer to extend the volume of allotted fluid.
Risk for Impaired Skin Integrity related to poor circulation secondary to edema **Goal:** The client's skin will remain intact.	Change the client's position every 2 hours and keep the legs elevated higher than the heart. Use pressure-relieving devices around bony prominences. Teach the inactive client to contract and relax leg muscles every 2 hours while awake to promote venous circulation.

Evaluation and Expected Outcomes

- Lungs are clear and the client's respirations are unlabored.
- The client loses 1 lb/day.
- Edema decreases.
- Electrolyte values are within normal limits.
- The skin is intact.
- Elevations in blood pressure or heart rate resolve.

Client and Family Teaching

The nurse educates the client by:

- Showing the client common containers and indicating the volume each holds
- Identifying foods that are high in salt or sodium (Box 21–1).
- Informing the client or family how to read food labels and look for the words salt, sodium, and other sources of sodium such as baking soda or powder
- Providing information concerning diuretic drug therapy
- Listing ways to determine if fluid excess is reoccurring or has resolved

Third-Spacing

Third-spacing describes the translocation of fluid to tissue compartments, where it becomes trapped and useless. It is associated with the loss of colloids as may occur with *albuminemia,* a low level of albumin in the blood, or conditions such as burns and severe allergic reactions in which capillary and cellular membrane permeability is altered. Fluid translocation follows the shift in osmotic pressure to other locations. If the translocation depletes fluid volume in the intravascular area, it can lead to hypotension, shock, and circulatory failure (see Chap. 22).

ASSESSMENT FINDINGS

Signs and Symptoms

The client manifests signs and symptoms of hypovolemia with the exception of weight loss. The fluid

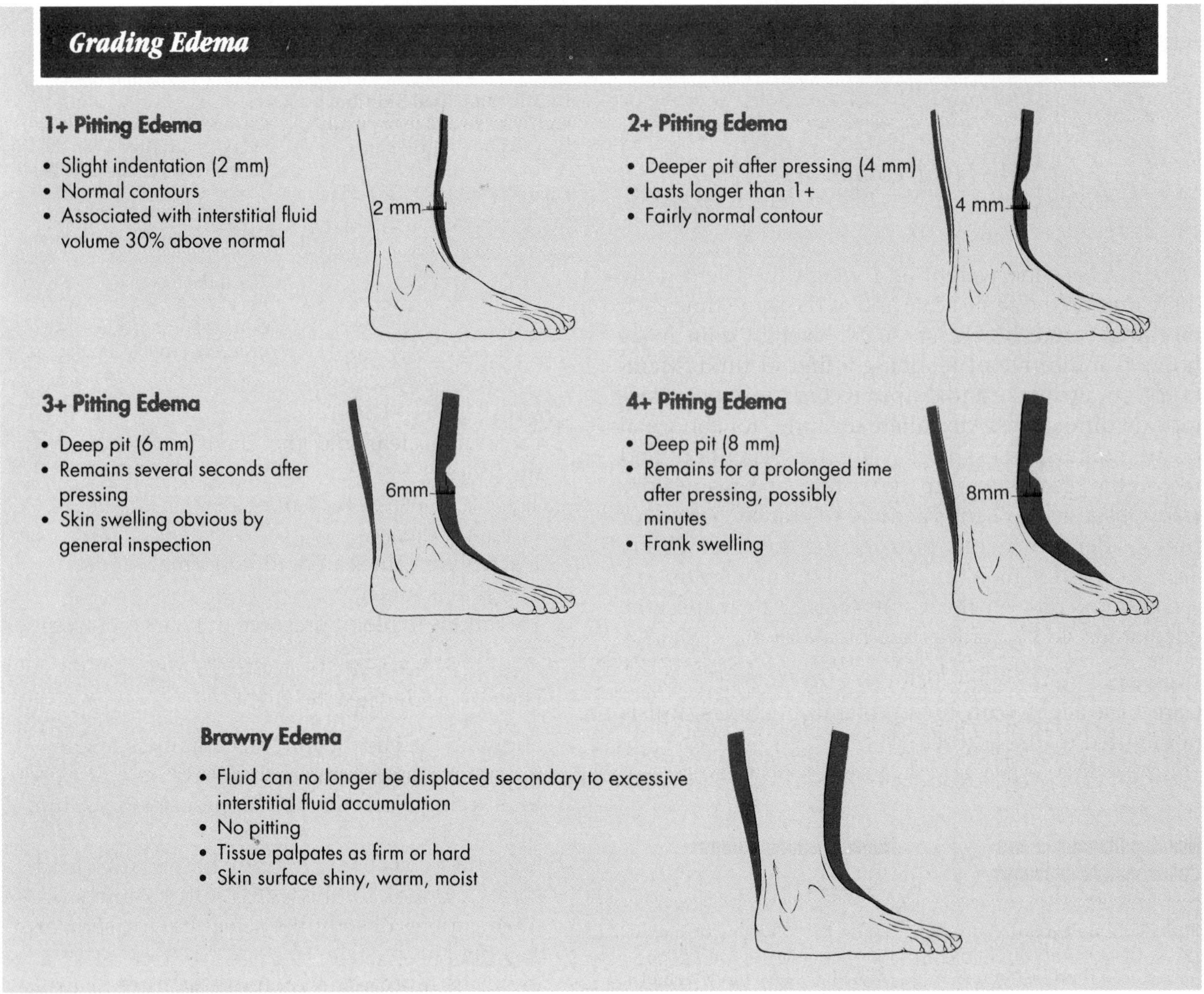

Grading Edema

1+ Pitting Edema

- Slight indentation (2 mm)
- Normal contours
- Associated with interstitial fluid volume 30% above normal

2+ Pitting Edema

- Deeper pit after pressing (4 mm)
- Lasts longer than 1+
- Fairly normal contour

3+ Pitting Edema

- Deep pit (6 mm)
- Remains several seconds after pressing
- Skin swelling obvious by general inspection

4+ Pitting Edema

- Deep pit (8 mm)
- Remains for a prolonged time after pressing, possibly minutes
- Frank swelling

Brawny Edema

- Fluid can no longer be displaced secondary to excessive interstitial fluid accumulation
- No pitting
- Tissue palpates as firm or hard
- Skin surface shiny, warm, moist

FIGURE 21-6. Grading edema is somewhat subjective and therefore assessment findings may vary depening on the clinician. These criteria are offered to assist in documentation.

BOX 21-1 Foods High in Salt (Sodium)

- Processed meats—hot dogs and cold cuts
- Salted and smoked fish
- Cheeses, especially processed varieties
- Peanut butter
- Powdered cocoa or hot chocolate mixes
- Canned vegetables
- Foods preserved in brine—pickles, olives, sauerkraut
- Tomato and tomato-vegetable juices
- Canned soup and instant soups or bouillon
- Boxed casserole mixes
- Salted snack foods
- Seasonings—catsup, gravy mixes, soy sauce, monosodium glutamate (MSG), pickle relish, tartar sauce, mustard, horseradish, barbecue sauce, steak sauce

volume remains relatively unchanged, but the percentages in various locations are altered. There may be signs of localized enlargement of organ cavities like the abdomen if it fills with fluid, a condition referred to as *ascites* (see Chap. 54). There may be **generalized edema** in all the interstitial spaces, which is sometimes called *brawny edema* or *anasarca*.

Diagnostic Findings

Laboratory blood tests and urine specific gravity are borderline normal or reveal evidence of hemoconcentration. CVP is lower than normal, as are other hemodynamic measurements (pressure as it relates to intravascular volume, see Chap. 29).

MEDICAL MANAGEMENT

The medical priority is to restore circulatory volume in hypotensive clients and eliminate the trapped fluid. This is done by administering intravenous solutions–sometimes at rapid rates–and blood products, like albumin, to restore colloidal osmotic pressure. The administration of albumin pulls the trapped fluid back into the intravascular space. When this occurs, clients who were previously hypovolemic, can suddenly become hypervolemic. An intravenous diuretic may be ordered to reduce the potential for circulatory overload.

NURSING MANAGEMENT

Nursing care of clients with third-spacing combines the assessment techniques for detecting both hypo- and hypervolemia. Policies and practices vary concerning how much responsibility practical/vocational nurses may assume with regard to intravenous fluid therapy and the administration of intravenous medications.

Electrolytes

Electrolytes are in both intracellular and extracellular water. They include **ions**, positively and negatively charged substances, such as potassium, magnesium, sodium, phosphate, sulfate, calcium, chloride, bicarbonate, protein, and organic acids. Sodium, calcium, and chloride ion concentrations are higher in extracellular fluid whereas potassium, magnesium, and phosphate concentrations are higher within the cell. These differences are responsible for electrical potentials that develop across the cell membrane and perhaps also for the degree of permeability of the membrane.

Electrolyte Imbalances

Electrolyte imbalances occur when there is a deficit, excess, or translocation of electrolytes to any one or more fluid compartments. A loss or gain in fluid is generally accompanied by a similar change in electrolytes. Electrolyte imbalances are identified primarily by measuring their levels in the serum (watery portion of blood).

Etiology and Pathophysiology

Electrolyte deficits occur as a result of inadequate dietary intake of food that is their natural source. Other causes include administering intravenous solutions that contain none, or only some, of the needed electrolytes, and by conditions that deplete water and substances dissolved therein, such as vomiting and diarrhea. Administration of certain medications (eg, diuretics) also depletes electrolytes.

Factors that contribute to an excess of electrolytes include an overabundance of orally consumed or parenterally administered electrolytes, kidney failure, and endocrine (glandular) dysfunction, especially the pituitary gland and adrenal cortex. Sodium, potassium, calcium, and magnesium deficits or excesses are of particular concern.

Sodium Imbalances

Sodium (Na^+), the chief **cation** (positive charged electrolyte) in extracellular fluid, is essential for the maintenance of normal nerve and muscle activity, the regulation of osmotic pressure, and preservation of acid–base balance. The principal role of sodium is the regulation and distribution of fluid volume in the body. Normal sodium concentration ranges from 135 to 145 mEq/L. A lower than normal serum sodium level is *hyponatremia; hypernatremia* occurs with higher than normal serum sodium levels.

HYPONATREMIA

Causes of hyponatremia include profuse diaphoresis along with excessive ingestion of plain water or administration of nonelectrolyte intravenous fluids, profuse diuresis, loss of gastrointestinal secretions (eg, in prolonged vomiting, gastrointestinal suctioning, or draining fistulas), or Addison's disease (see Chap. 56).

Assessment Findings

Hyponatremia is manifested by mental confusion, muscular weakness, anorexia, restlessness, elevated body temperature, tachycardia, nausea, vomiting, and personality changes. If the deficit is severe, symptoms are more intense and convulsions or coma can occur. The serum sodium level is below 135 mEq/L.

Medical Management

When possible, the underlying cause is corrected. If the deficit is mild, treatment includes oral administration of sodium (foods high in sodium, water to which salt has been added, and salt tablets). Administration of intravenous solutions containing sodium chloride (see Chap. 23) are prescribed if the deficit is severe.

HYPERNATREMIA

Hypernatremia is an excess of sodium in the blood. Causes include profuse watery diarrhea, excessive intake of salt without sufficient ingestion of water, high fever, decreased water intake (eg, in elderly, debilitated, unconscious, or retarded clients), excessive administration of solutions that contain sodium, excessive water loss without an accompanying loss of sodium, and severe burns.

Assessment Findings

Hypernatremia results in thirst; dry, sticky mucous membranes; decreased urine output; fever; a rough, dry tongue; and lethargy, which can progress to coma if the excess is severe. The serum sodium level is above 145 mEq/L.

Medical Management

Treatment depends on the cause of the imbalance and includes the oral administration of plain water or intravenous administration of a hypotonic solution, such as 0.45% sodium chloride or 5% dextrose (see Chap. 23). In mild cases of hypernatremia, sodium intake may be restricted until laboratory test results are normal.

Nursing Management for Sodium Imbalances

Nursing management includes early detection of a sodium imbalance especially in those at risk for developing hypo- or hypernatremia. The nurse apportions oral fluids according to target volumes, maintains accurate intake and output measurements, assesses vital signs every 1 to 4 hours, and closely monitors the infusion of intravenous fluids. Prescribed dietary restrictions or supplements are implemented. The nurse gathers data that indicate an increase or decrease of symptoms and notifies the physician if symptoms become worse or laboratory values show a significant change.

Potassium Imbalances

The potassium cation (K^+) is the chief electrolyte found in intracellular fluid. Potassium has the same functions intracellularly as sodium has extracellularly. A deficit of potassium in the blood is called *hypokalemia*; an excess is *hyperkalemia*.

HYPOKALEMIA

Potassium-wasting diuretics (eg, furosemide [Lasix], ethacrynic acid [Edecrin], and hydrochlorothiazide [HydroDiuril]) contribute to hypokalemia. Loss of fluid from the gastrointestinal tract (eg, in severe vomiting or diarrhea, draining intestinal fistulas, or prolonged suctioning) also causes potassium loss. Taking large doses of corticosteroids, intravenous administration of insulin and glucose, and prolonged administration of nonelectrolyte parenteral fluids can deplete potassium.

Assessment Findings

Hypokalemia causes fatigue, weakness, anorexia, nausea, vomiting, cardiac arrhythmias (abnormal heart rate or rhythm, especially in people receiving cardiac glycosides such as digitalis preparations), leg cramps, muscle weakness, and paresthesias (abnormal sensations). Severe hypokalemia results in hypotension, flaccid paralysis, and even death from cardiac or respiratory arrest. Hypokalemia produces characteristic changes in the electrocardiogram (ECG) waveform (Fig. 21–7). The serum potassium level is below 3.5 mEq/L. Symptoms may not be apparent until the serum potassium level is below 3.0 mEq/L.

Medical Management

Treatment includes (when possible) elimination of the cause. Mild hypokalemia is treated by increasing oral intake of potassium-rich foods or using a prescribed potassium oral replacement such as K-Lor, K-Lyte, and Klorvess. Severe hypokalemia is treated with intravenous administration of a potassium salt, such as potassium chloride.

HYPERKALEMIA

Hyperkalemia can occur with severe renal failure when the kidneys are unable to excrete potassium; severe burns; the administration of potassium-sparing diuretics; overuse of potassium supplements, salt substitutes (which contain potassium instead of sodium), or potassium-rich foods; crushing injuries;

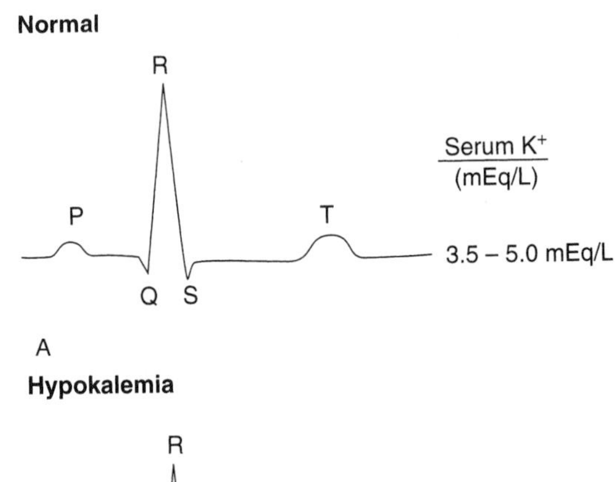

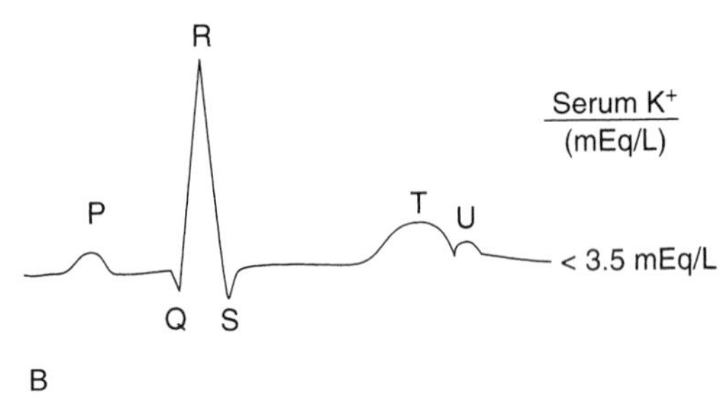

FIGURE 21-7. (A) Normal ECG waveforms. (B) The appearance of a U wave suggests hypokalemia.

Addison's disease; and rapid administration of parenteral potassium salts.

Assessment Findings

Hyperkalemia results in diarrhea, nausea, muscle weakness, paresthesias, and cardiac arrhythmias. The serum potassium level is above 5.5 mEq/L. Hyperkalemia also causes unique changes in ECG waveforms (Fig. 21–8) that can forewarn of a potential for sudden cardiac death.

Medical Management

Treatment depends on the cause and severity of the excess. Mild hyperkalemia is treated by decreasing the intake of potassium-rich foods or discontinuing oral potassium replacement until laboratory values are normal. Severe hyperkalemia is treated with the administration of a cation-exchange resin such as Kayexalate (see renal failure, Chap. 63) or a combination of regular insulin and glucose administered intravenously. Peritoneal dialysis or hemodialysis, techniques for removing toxic substances from the blood, also may be used (see Chap. 63).

Nursing Management for Potassium Imbalances

The nurse assesses clients for conditions that have the potential for causing potassium imbalances, identifies signs and symptoms associated with potassium imbalances, monitors the laboratory findings measuring serum potassium, administers medications that restore potassium balance, and evaluates the client's response to medical therapy. The nurse consults with the physician when a client is receiving prolonged intravenous fluid therapy without the addition of potassium. If intravenous potassium is ordered, *it must be diluted in an intravenous solution* and *administered at a rate not to exceed 10 mEq/h*. The infusion is observed frequently to verify that it is being administered at the appropriate rate.

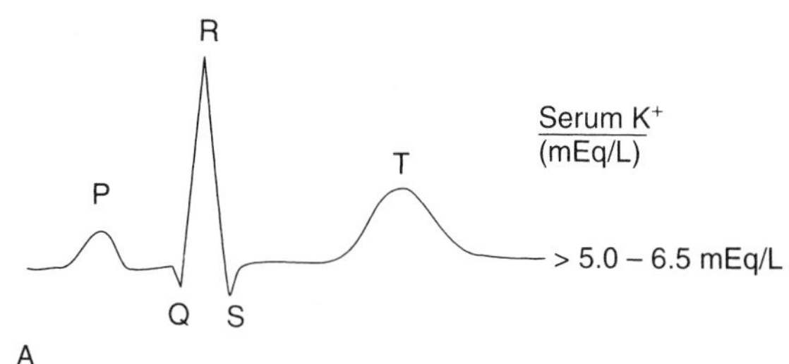

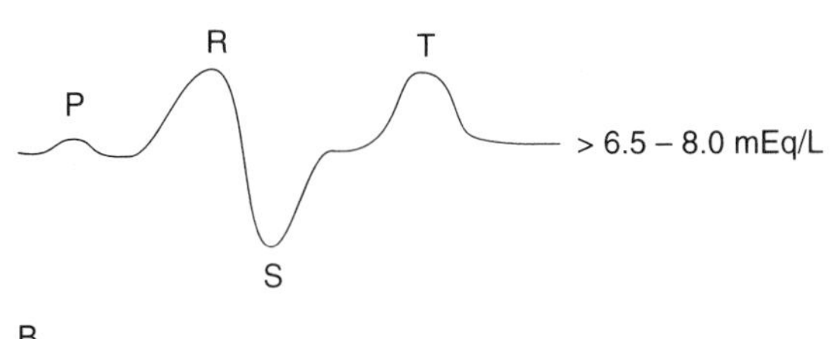

FIGURE 21-8. (A) A tall or peaked T wave is indicative of hyperkalemia, as well as (B) a widened QRS complex.

Client and Family Teaching

Clients who are at risk for potassium imbalances, are informed about:

- Medications that cause urinary excretion of potassium, such as diuretics.
- Foods that are sources of potassium—abundant in vegetables, dried peas and beans, wheat bran, and fruits. Rich sources include bananas, oranges, orange juice, melon, prune juice, potatoes, and milk.
- Taking oral potassium supplements shortly after meals or with food to avoid gastrointestinal distress. Effervescent tablets or liquids are taken with a full glass of water.

Calcium Imbalances

Most of the body's calcium (Ca^{++}) is found in bones and teeth. A small percentage (about 1% of total body calcium) is in the blood. The level of calcium in the blood is regulated by the parathyroid glands. Calcium is necessary for the clotting of blood; smooth, skeletal, and cardiac muscle function; and the transmission of nerve impulses. Vitamin D is necessary for the absorption of calcium in the intestine. *Hypocalcemia* occurs when there is a lower than normal serum calcium level; *hypercalcemia* when there is an above normal level.

HYPOCALCEMIA

Causes of hypocalcemia include vitamin D deficiency, hypoparathyroidism, severe burns, acute pancreatitis, certain drugs, administration of multiple units of blood that contain an anticalcium additive over a short period of time, intestinal malabsorption disorders, and accidental surgical removal of the parathyroid glands.

Assessment Findings

Hypocalcemia is evidenced by tingling in the extremities and the area around the mouth (circumoral paresthesia), muscle and abdominal cramping, carpopedal spasms referred to as **Trousseau's sign** (Fig. 21–9), mental changes, positive **Chvostek's sign** (spasms of the facial muscles when the facial nerve is tapped) (Fig. 21–10), laryngeal spasms with airway obstruction, tetany (muscle twitching), seizures,

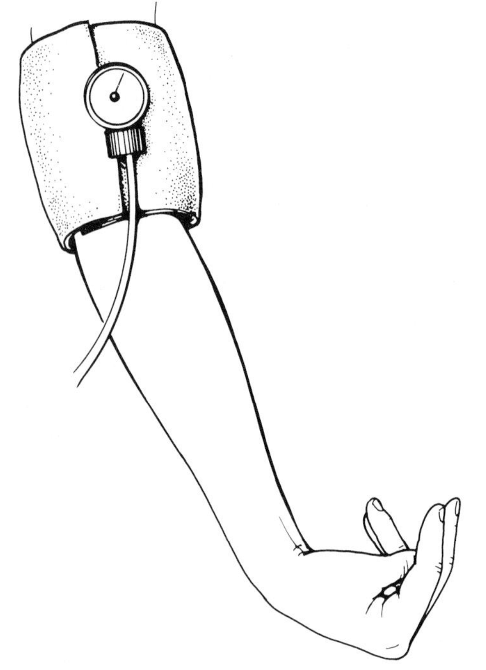

FIGURE 21-9. Trousseau's sign, a characteristic of hypocalcemia, is evidenced by a carpopedal spasm when circulation of blood is occluded in the arm for 3 minutes.

bleeding, and cardiac arrhythmias. Hypocalcemia is present if the total serum calcium level is below 8.8 mg/dL (normal range, 9–11 mg/dL) or the ionized calcium level is below 4.4 mg/dL (normal, 4.4–5.4 mg/dL).

Medical Management

Treatment includes administration of oral calcium and vitamin D for mild deficits and intravenous administration of a calcium salt, such as calcium gluconate, for severe hypocalcemia.

HYPERCALCEMIA

Hypercalcemia is associated with parathyroid gland tumors, multiple fractures, Paget's disease, hyperparathyroidism, excessive doses of vitamin D, prolonged immobilization, some chemotherapeutic agents, and certain malignant diseases, such as multiple myeloma, acute leukemia, and lymphomas.

Assessment Findings

Hypercalcemia causes deep bone pain, constipation, anorexia, nausea, vomiting, polyuria, thirst, pathologic fractures, and mental changes (usually decreased memory and attention span). Chronic hypercalcemia can promote the formation of kidney stones. The total serum calcium level is above 10.0 mg/dL and the ionized calcium level is above 5.4 mg/dL.

Medical Management

Treatment includes determining and correcting the cause when possible. Mild hypercalcemia is treated by increasing oral fluid intake and limiting calcium consumption until laboratory studies are normal. Acute hypercalcemia is treated by the administration of one or more of the following: intravenous sodium chloride solution (0.45% or 0.9%) and a diuretic such as furosemide (Lasix) to increase calcium excretion in the urine, oral phosphates, or calcitonin (Cibacalcin), a synthetic hormone for regulating calcium levels. Hypercalcemia associated with cancer or chemotherapy is treated on an individual basis. A decrease in drug dosage or the discontinuation of therapy may be necessary. Corticosteroids or plicamycin (Mithracin), an antineoplastic agent, may also be used to treat hypercalcemia of malignant diseases that do not respond to other forms of therapy.

Nursing Management for Calcium Imbalances

The hypocalcemic client is closely monitored for neurologic manifestations (tetany, seizures, and spasms), cardiac arrhythmias, and airway obstruction because emergency interventions may be necessary. If the deficit is severe, seizure precautions are instituted. Clients with severe muscle cramping are maintained on bed rest for comfort and to avoid accidental falls. Because a low calcium level interferes with clotting, the client is routinely checked for signs of bruising or bleeding. The client with mild hypercalcemia is encouraged to drink a large quantity of oral fluids. The nurse collaborates with the dietitian

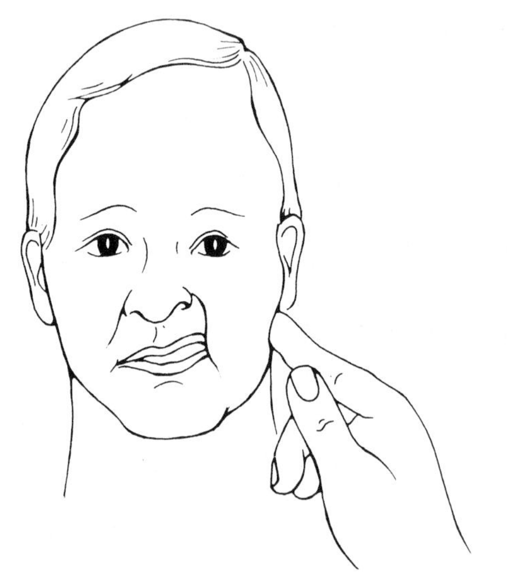

FIGURE 21-10. Chvostek's sign, unilateral spasm of facial muscles, is elicited in hypocalcemic clients by tapping over the facial nerve which lies approximately 2 cm anterior to the earlobe.

when calcium is restricted from the diet. The client is encouraged to ambulate as tolerated. Assistance is provided and the client is instructed to wear shoes to avoid falls that may result in pathologic fractures.

Client and Family Teaching

A teaching plan includes:

- Follow the physician's recommendations regarding the addition or restriction of calcium in the diet. Milk and dairy products are rich sources of dietary calcium. Nondairy sources are turnip and mustard greens, collards, kale, broccoli, canned fish with bones, and calcium-enriched orange juice.
- Lactose-free milk and nonprescription lactase enzyme are available for those who have an intolerance to lactose.
- Take prescribed drugs or those recommended by the physician as directed; do not exceed or omit a dose.

Magnesium Imbalances

Magnesium (Mg^{++}) is found in bone cells and in specialized cells of the heart, liver, and skeletal muscles. Only a small percentage of the total magnesium found in the body is present in extracellular fluid. Magnesium is involved in the transmission of nerve impulses, plays a role in muscle excitability, and is an activator for a number of enzyme systems, including the functioning of B vitamins and the use of potassium and calcium. A lower than normal serum level of magnesium is *hypomagnesemia;* a higher than normal serum level is *hypermagnesemia.*

HYPOMAGNESEMIA

Conditions that can be accompanied by hypomagnesemia include chronic alcoholism, diabetic ketoacidosis, severe renal disease, severe burns, severe malnutrition, toxemia of pregnancy (eclampsia), intestinal malabsorption syndromes, excessive diuresis (drug induced), hyperaldosteronism (see Chap. 56), and prolonged gastric suction.

Assessment Findings

Signs and symptoms of hypomagnesemia include tachycardia and other cardiac arrhythmias, neuromuscular irritability, paresthesias of the extremities, leg and foot cramps, hypertension, mental changes, positive Chvostek's sign and Trousseau's sign (see hypocalcemia), dysphagia (difficulty swallowing), and convulsions. The serum magnesium level is below 1.3 mEq/L (normal range, 1.3–2.1 mEq/L).

Medical Management

Treatment includes administration of oral magnesium salts or the addition of magnesium-rich foods to the diet (see General Nutritional Considerations at the end of this chapter). A severe magnesium deficit is treated with intravenous administration of magnesium sulfate.

HYPERMAGNESEMIA

Hypermagnesemia can occur as a consequence of renal failure, Addison's disease, excessive use of antacids or laxatives that contain magnesium, and hyperparathyroidism.

Assessment Findings

Clients with hypermagnesemia experience flushing and a feeling of warmth, hypotension, lethargy, drowsiness, bradycardia (slow heart rate), muscle weakness, depressed respirations, and coma. The serum magnesium level is above 2.1 mEq/L.

Medical Management

Treatment includes decreasing the oral magnesium intake or discontinuing the administration of parenteral replacement. In severe hypermagnesemia, hemodialysis may be necessary. If respiratory failure occurs, mechanical ventilation is essential.

Nursing Management for Magnesium Imbalances

Clients with hypomagnesemia are closely observed for arrhythmias and early signs of neuromuscular irritability, which are reported to the physician immediately. If intravenous magnesium sulfate is administered, the blood pressure is checked frequently to detect hypotension because its administration can produce vasodilation. Calcium gluconate is kept available as an antidote in the event there is an adverse reaction during the administration of magnesium sulfate. If dysphagia occurs, the nurse consults with the physician and dietitian on alternatives or modifications in dietary management.

When caring for clients with hypermagnesemia or its potential, vital signs are closely monitored. The nurse notifies the physician immediately if there are significant changes, especially in respiratory rate, rhythm, or depth.

Client and Family Teaching

A teaching plan for clients with magnesium imbalances includes:

- Check with the physician, pharmacist, or nurse concerning antacids or laxatives that contain magnesium.
- If use of an antacid or laxative is allowed, follow the physician's recommendations regarding the frequency of use.

Acid–Base Balance

Besides water and electrolytes, body fluid also contains acids and bases. One of the chief acids is carbonic acid (H_2CO_3). An example of a base, sometimes referred to as an alkaline substance, which neutralizes acids is bicarbonate (HCO_3). Acid and base content influence the pH of body fluid.

The symbol *pH* refers to the amount of hydrogen ions in a solution; pH can range from 1, which is highly acid, to 14, which is highly basic. A pH of 7.0 is considered neutral. The more hydrogen ions in a solution, the more acidic it is. Acidity is indicated by a pH of less than 7. The degree of alkalinity is identified by a pH greater than 7. Normal plasma pH is 7.35 to 7.45, or slightly alkaline. The body maintains the normal plasma pH by two mechanisms: chemical regulation and organ regulation.

Chemical Regulation

Chemical regulation occurs through one or more buffering systems in which hydrogen ions are either added or eliminated. Adding hydrogen ions increases acidity; removing hydrogen ions promotes alkalinity. The major chemical regulator of plasma pH is the **bicarbonate-carbonic acid buffer system**. Maintaining a ratio of 20 parts bicarbonate to 1 part carbonic acid results in a normal plasma pH.

Oxygen Regulation

The ratio of bicarbonate to carbonic acid is facilitated by the lungs and kidneys. Carbon dioxide is one of the components of carbonic acid:

CO_2 (carbon dioxide) + H_2O (water) = H_2CO_3 (carbonic acid).

The lungs regulate carbonic acid levels by releasing or conserving carbon dioxide by increasing or decreasing the respiratory rate, volume, or both. The kidneys assist in acid–base balance by retaining or excreting bicarbonate ions. If an imbalance in acids or bases occur, these regulatory processes are accelerated and referred to as **compensation**.

Acid–Base Imbalances

An imbalance in acids or bases is life-threatening. Death occurs quickly if plasma pH is outside the range of 6.8 to 8.0 (Sherwood, 1995). Arterial blood gas (ABG) results are the main tool for measuring blood pH, carbon dioxide content ($PaCO_2$), and bicarbonate. An acid–base imbalance may accompany a fluid and electrolyte imbalance.

There are essentially two types of acid–base imbalances: acidosis or alkalosis. **Acidosis** occurs when there is an excessive accumulation of acids or an excessive loss of bicarbonate in body fluids; **alkalosis** occurs when there is an excessive accumulation of base or a loss of acid in body fluids (Fig. 21–11). Either can occur as a result of metabolic or respiratory alterations resulting in four subtypes: metabolic acidosis, metabolic alkalosis, respiratory acidosis, and respiratory alkalosis.

Metabolic Acidosis

Metabolic acidosis is a condition that results in a reduction in plasma pH due to an increase in organic acids (acids other than carbonic acid) or a decrease in bicarbonate. Organic acids increase during periods of anaerobic metabolism when cells attempt to produce ATP for energy without oxygen. Anaerobic metabolism is much less efficient than aerobic (with oxygen) metabolism, and produces by-products such as lactic acid. Anaerobic metabolism occurs during shock and cardiac arrest. Acids also accumulate in starvation and diabetic ketoacidosis (see Chap. 57) when fatty acids accumulate due to an inability to use glucose for energy. It may also be a consequence of renal failure because the kidney cannot reabsorb bicarbonate for the purpose of buffering the blood. Acids also accumulate with aspirin (acetylsalicylic acid) overdosage, and during periods of profuse diarrhea. Or it may occur with loss of intestinal fluid via wound drainage when bicarbonate can be lost in disproportionate amounts.

ASSESSMENT FINDINGS

Signs and Symptoms

Metabolic acidosis is accompanied by deep and rapid breathing (*Kussmaul's breathing*), a compensatory mechanism for ridding the body of carbon dioxide so as to avoid forming carbonic acid. The client may experience anorexia, nausea, vomiting, headache, confusion, flushing, lethargy, malaise, drowsiness, abdominal pain or discomfort, and weakness. Dangerous cardiac arrhythmias can develop and the force of cardiac contractions can be weakened. In severe stages, stupor and coma occur, which may be shortly followed by death.

Diagnostic Findings

The ABG values generally show a decrease in pH and plasma bicarbonate (HCO_3). Initially, the $PaCO_2$

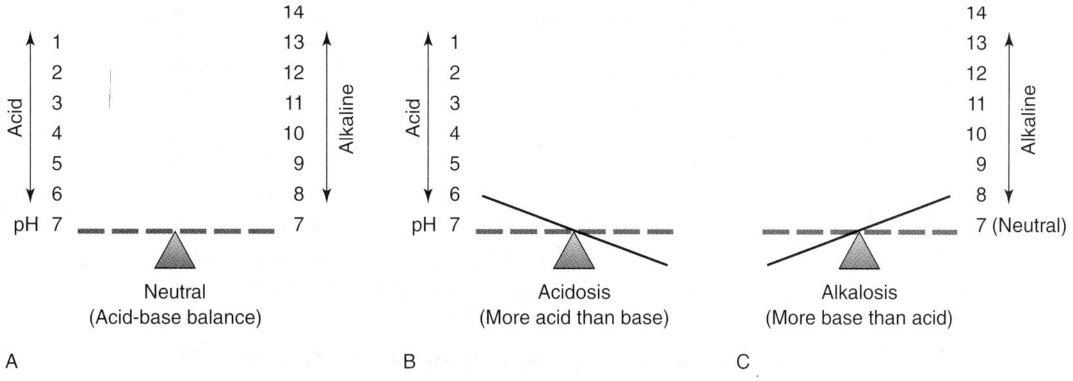

FIGURE 21-11. Acid–base balance; appropriate ratio of acids and bases to maintain pH in neutral zone. (B) pH is less than 7 when acids are in excess proportion. (C) pH is greater than 7 when bases are in excess proportion.

is normal, a condition referred to as an *uncompensated state*. As the rapid and deep breathing becomes effective, $PaCO_2$ decreases. Until the pH returns to normal, it is referred to as a *partially compensated state*. When the pH returns to normal, it is referred to as a *fully compensated state*, even though the HCO_3 and $PaCO_2$ are abnormal (Table 21–4). In a fully compensated state, regardless of the initial imbalance and current abnormal values, the client is out of danger.

Some laboratories also report the anion gap with the ABG findings. The **anion gap** (or R factor), the difference between sodium and potassium cation (positive ions) concentrations and the sum of chloride and bicarbonate **anions** (negative ions) in extracellular fluid, reflects the remaining anion content from substances like lactic acid, ketones (by-products of fat metabolism), and others. Determining the anion gap helps differentiate whether metabolic acidosis is caused by a loss of base or accumulation of acid. *Normal anion gap acidosis* (12 ± 4 mEq/L) results from a loss of bicarbonate; *high anion gap acidosis* results from an accumulation of metabolic acids.

MEDICAL MANAGEMENT

Treatment includes elimination of the cause and replacement of fluids and electrolytes that may have been lost as a consequence of the accompanying etiology. Intravenous bicarbonate is administered for severe metabolic acidosis.

TABLE 21-4 **Arterial Blood Gas Trends in Acid–Base Imbalances**

Condition	pH	HCO_3	$PaCO_2$
Acid–Base Balance	7.35–7.45	22–26 mEq/L	35–45 mmHg
Metabolic Acidosis			
Uncompensated	<7.35	<22 mEq/L	normal
Partially compensated	<7.35	<22 mEq/L	<35 mmHg
Fully compensated	7.35–7.45	<22 mEq/L	<35 mmHg
Metabolic Alkalosis			
Uncompensated	>7.45	>26 mEq/L	normal
Partially compensated	>7.45	>26 mEq/L	>45 mmHg
Fully compensated	7.35–7.45	>22 mEq/L	>45 mmHg
Respiratory Acidosis			
Uncompensated	<7.35	normal	>45 mmHg
Partially compensated	<7.35	>26 mEq/L	>45 mmHg
Fully compensated	7.35–7.45	>26 mEq/L	>45 mmHg
Respiratory Alkalosis			
Uncompensated	7.45	normal	<35 mmHg
Partially compensated	7.45	<22 mEq/L	<35 mmHg
Fully compensated	7.35–7.45	<22 mEq/L	<35 mmHg

Metabolic Alkalosis

Metabolic alkalosis is a condition that results in an increase in plasma pH due to an accumulation of base bicarbonate or a decrease in hydrogen ion concentration. Factors that promote an increase in base bicarbonate include excessive oral or parenteral use of bicarbonate-containing drugs or other alkaline salts, a rapid decrease in extracellular fluid volume (eg, in diuretic therapy), and when there is a loss of hydrogen and chloride ions (eg, in vomiting, prolonged gastric suctioning, hypokalemia, or hyperaldosteronism) resulting in retention of sodium bicarbonate and an increase in base bicarbonate.

ASSESSMENT FINDINGS

Signs and Symptoms

Clients in metabolic acidosis can manifest anorexia, nausea, vomiting, circumoral paresthesias, confusion, carpopedal spasm, hypertonic reflexes, and tetany. The respiratory rate and volume decrease in a compensatory effort to produce more carbonic acid to increase and restore the acidic level in the blood.

Diagnostic Findings

Initially, ABGs show an increase in pH and HCO_3 and normal $PaCO_2$ levels (see Table 21–4). As compensatory respiratory mechanisms result in slower and more shallow breathing, there is an elevation in $PaCO_2$; eventually, the pH may return to normal.

MEDICAL MANAGEMENT

Treatment involves eliminating the cause. It may include prescribing potassium (as a potassium salt) if hypokalemia is present or sodium chloride solutions to correct volume depletion when there has been a rapid decrease in extracellular fluid volume.

Respiratory Acidosis

Respiratory acidosis, which may be either acute or chronic, is caused by carbonic acid excess, which causes the pH to drop below 7.35. Conditions that predispose to acute respiratory acidosis include pneumothorax, hemothorax, pulmonary edema, acute bronchial asthma, atelectasis, hyaline membrane disease or other forms of respiratory distress in the newborn, pneumonia (see Chap. 28), some drug overdoses, and head injuries. Chronic respiratory acidosis is associated with chronic respiratory disorders (see Chap. 28) such as emphysema, bronchiectasis, bronchial asthma, and cystic fibrosis.

ASSESSMENT FINDINGS

Signs and Symptoms

Acute respiratory acidosis is associated with extreme respiratory insufficiency. The client may make frantic efforts to breathe, breathe slowly or irregularly, or stop breathing. Expiratory volumes are decreased. Lung sounds my be moist or absent in some lobes. Tachycardia is usually present, and cardiac arrhythmias can develop. Cyanosis, a dusky appearance to the skin, may be evident. The accumulation of carbon dioxide leads to behavioral changes (mental cloudiness, confusion, disorientation, hallucinations), tremors, muscle twitching, flushed skin, headache, weakness, stupor, and coma. Responses to chronic respiratory acidosis are less prominent and can include an increased breathing effort, lack of energy, reduced activity, dull headache, and weakness.

Diagnostic Findings

The ABG values show a decrease in pH and an increase in the $PaCO_2$. As the kidney attempts to compensate, which may take 2 to 3 days, the HCO_3 rises, followed by a return to normal pH if full compensation occurs (see Table 21–4).

MEDICAL MANAGEMENT

Treatment is individualized, depending on the cause of the imbalance and whether the condition is acute or chronic. Mechanical ventilation may be necessary to support respiratory function. Intravenous sodium bicarbonate is administered when ventilation efforts do not adequately restore a balanced pH. Heart rate and rhythm are monitored to detect sudden cardiac changes. In less acute situations, treatment may include the administration of pharmacologic agents, such as bronchodilators and antibiotics to improve breathing. Suctioning of the airway may be necessary if the client is too weak to cough secretions.

Respiratory Alkalosis

Respiratory alkalosis is due to a carbonic acid deficit that occurs because rapid breathing releases more carbon dioxide than necessary with expired air. *Tachypnea* (rapid breathing) may be the result of acute anxiety, high fever, thyrotoxicosis (overactive thyroid), early salicylate (aspirin) poisoning, hypoxemia (low oxygen in the blood), and mechanical ventilation.

Assessment Findings

Signs and Symptoms

The most obvious manifestation is an increase in respiratory rate. It is accompanied by light-headedness, numbness and tingling of the fingers and toes, circumoral paresthesias, sweating, panic, dry mouth, and, in severe cases, convulsions.

Diagnostic Findings

The ABG values indicate a pH above 7.45 and a $PaCO_2$ below 35 mm Hg. If the kidney compensates by excreting bicarbonate ions, the HCO_3 falls below 22 mEq to restore pH (see Table 21–4).

Medical Management

Treatment aims to correct the cause of the rapid breathing. Having the client breathe into a paper bag that is held over the nose and mouth and rebreathe expired air may be useful temporarily. Sedation may be necessary, when the tachypnea is caused by extreme anxiety.

Nursing Management for Acid–Base Imbalances

The nurse carefully documents all presenting signs and symptoms to provide accurate baseline data. The nurse monitors the laboratory findings; compares ABG findings with previous results, if there are any; and reports current results to the physician as soon as they are obtained. The same applies to abnormal electrolyte levels. Accurate intake and output records are maintained to monitor the client's fluid status. The nurse implements prescribed medical therapy, such as administering fluid and electrolyte replacements, suctioning the airway, maintaining mechanical ventilation, and monitoring the cardiac rate and rhythm (see Chap. 29). The nurse administers cardiopulmonary resuscitation at any time it becomes necessary.

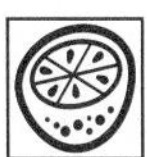

General Nutritional Considerations

Because salt and sodium compounds are used extensively in food processing and manufacturing, it is estimated that processed and convenience foods account for 75% of the sodium in the average American diet. Naturally occurring sources such as milk, meats, and certain vegetables provide 10% of the sodium consumed. The remaining 15% comes from salt added during cooking and at the table.

The daily value for sodium that appears on the Nutrition Facts food label is 2,400 mg/day, far more than the estimated minimum requirement for healthy adults, yet considerably less than most Americans consume. Under normal circumstances, the body maintains sodium balance over a wide range of intakes by regulating urinary sodium excretion.

Magnesium is found in cocoa, chocolate, nuts, soybeans, dried peas and beans, green leafy vegetables, and whole grains, especially wheat germ and bran. The need for magnesium may be increased by physical stress and by high intakes of calcium, protein, vitamin D, or alcohol.

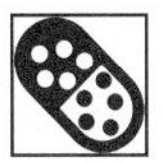

General Pharmacologic Considerations

The dosage of electrolytes is carefully measured and given only as directed by the physician because these agents are potentially dangerous.

Sodium and calcium products are given cautiously to clients with edema, congestive heart failure, or renal dysfunction.

Calcium replacement is given cautiously to clients with kidney stones because high levels of calcium in the kidney tubules may contribute to additional stone formation.

Sodium chloride and potassium chloride may be given to help correct metabolic alkalosis.

Clients may experience burning along the vein with intravenous infusion of potassium. The discomfort is in proportion to its concentration. If the client can tolerate the fluid, it may be helpful to consult with the physician on the possibility of diluting the potassium in a larger volume of intravenous solution.

Clients receiving a digitalis preparation are closely monitored for digitalis toxicity, which can be precipitated by potassium and magnesium deficits.

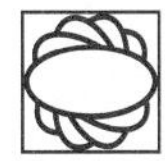

General Gerontologic Considerations

The skin loses elasticity during the process of aging. Therefore, assessing skin turgor may be an ineffective technique for detecting fluid volume deficit. If skin turgor is assessed use the skin of the forehead.

Older adults may deplete fluid volume if they take a diuretic, yet be unaware of the problem because a reduced sensation of thirst often occurs with aging.

A common electrolyte imbalance in the older adult is hypernatremia; it may be manifested as a change in mental status.

A decrease in renal function in the older adult can cause an inability to concentrate urine and is associated with fluid and electrolyte imbalance.

Older adults have a tendency to drink less water and, therefore, may incur chronic fluid volume deficit and other electrolyte imbalances.

A poor appetite, erratic meal patterns, the inability to prepare nutritious meals, or financial circumstances may influence nutritional status, resulting in electrolyte imbalance.

Aging often is accompanied by chronic disorders, such as cardiac and renal disease, which may be treated by drug therapy. The effect of certain drugs (eg, digitalis) may be modified in the presence of some electrolyte imbalances.

Poor respiratory exchange caused by chronic lung disease, inactivity, or thoracic skeletal changes may lead to chronic respiratory acidosis.

Overuse of sodium bicarbonate (baking soda), an inexpensive substitute for commercial antacids, may lead to metabolic alkalosis.

SUMMARY OF KEY CONCEPTS

In the human body, water is located in two major areas: inside the cell (intracellular fluid) and outside the cell (extracellular fluid). Extracellular fluid is subdivided into that which is located between cells (interstitial fluid) and within the blood (intravascular fluid).

Three chemicals within body fluid include electrolytes, acids, and bases.

- Five physiologic processes by which water and chemicals are relocated include osmosis, filtration, passive diffusion, facilitated diffusion, and active transport.
- Two types of fluid imbalances are hypovolemia or hypervolemia. Dehydration is different from hypovolemia, a reduction in intravascular water; dehydration is a reduction in intracellular and extracellular fluid volume.
- Intravascular fluid imbalances are demonstrated by hemoconcentration, a high ratio of blood components in relation to watery plasma, or hemodilution, a reduced ratio of blood components to watery plasma.
- Most adults consume approximately 2,500 mL of fluid per day, but the amount can range between 1,800 to 3,000 mL without significant consequences. Water is lost from the body in four ways: urination, losses in stool, perspiration, and from the surface of skin and exhaled vapor. Fluid loss approximates fluid intake in healthy individuals.
- A deficit in fluid volume is reflected by a loss of at least 2 lb of weight in 24 hours, fluid intake that is well below fluid losses, dark urine that has a high specific gravity, poor skin turgor, dry oral mucous membranes, furrowed tongue, and elevated hematocrit and blood cell counts in the absence of blood disease.
- When caring for a client with actual or potential fluid volume deficit, the nurse collects and records appropriate data, provides oral fluid replacement after developing a plan and target goals with the client, and consults with the physician if interventions to promote fluid balance fall short of goals.
- Assessments for determining hypervolemia are similar to those for detecting hypovolemia except the findings are opposite. Additional assessments include listening for abnormal lung sounds and checking for signs of edema. Nursing management of clients with excess fluid volume include limiting fluid intake and implementing medical therapy that may include the administration of drugs that promote urinary excretion.
- Two nursing diagnoses, besides *Fluid Volume Excess*, that may develop among clients who manifest edema or who must limit their oral intake include: *Risk for Impaired Skin Integrity* and *Risk for Altered Oral Mucous Membranes*.
- Third-spacing describes a unique fluid imbalance in which fluid moves into tissue compartments where it becomes trapped and useless. To redistribute the fluid, intravenous solutions that may include blood or albumin may be administered.
- Electrolyte deficits occur as a result of inadequate oral intake of food, prolonged administration of nonelectrolyte intravenous solutions, excessive fluid loss, and potent response to diuretic therapy. Electrolyte excesses occur with excessive intake of electrolyte sources without their comparable excretion, which may happen in certain endocrine or kidney diseases.
- Four electrolytes that have serious consequences when imbalanced include sodium, potassium, calcium, and magnesium.
- Nursing management of clients with actual or potential electrolyte imbalances includes early detection of electrolyte imbalances, ensuring adequate nutrition, maintaining oral fluid intake, implementing prescribed drug and fluid therapy, monitoring the client's response, and keeping the physician informed of the client's progress, or lack of it.
- Acid and base content influences the pH, or hydrogen ion concentration, of body fluid, which must be maintained within a range of 7.35 to 7.45. An imbalance in acids or bases is life-threatening.
- Acid–base balance is regulated by maintaining an adequate ratio of bicarbonate to carbonic acid ions. The ratio is regulated primarily via the lungs and kidney.
- Two major acid–base imbalances are acidosis or alkalosis. Each can be divided into metabolic acidosis and alkalosis and respiratory acidosis and alkalosis.
- Besides physical assessment findings, acid–base imbalances are primarily identified by analyzing three components of ABG results. These three include pH, $PaCO_2$ (dissolved carbon dioxide), and HCO_3 (bicarbonate).
- When caring for clients with acid–base imbalances, or their potential, the nurse collects appropriate data including the results of ABGs, provides interventions to manage actual or potential complications associated with particular imbalances, implements medical orders to eliminate the cause or provide treatment for the imbalance, and monitors the client's response.

CRITICAL THINKING EXERCISES

1. Describe the relationship of water to imbalances in electrolytes, acids, and bases.
2. When assessing a client, discuss data that suggest a fluid volume imbalance.
3. Choose any electrolyte imbalance and discuss its cause, manifestation, laboratory test results, treatment, and nursing responsibilities.
4. Explain the pathophysiology that contributes to acid–base imbalances and how the body attempts to regulate and restore equilibrium.

Suggested Readings

Bullock, B. L. (1996). *Pathophysiology: Adaptations and alterations in function* (4th ed.). Philadelphia: Lippincott-Raven.

Clayton, K. (1997). Cancer-related hypercalcemia: How to spot it, how to manage it. *American Journal of Nursing, 97*(5), 42–48.

Kirton, C. A. (1996). Assessing edema. *Nursing, 26*(7) 54.

Metheny, N. *Fluid and electrolyte balance: Nursing considerations* (3rd ed.). Philadelphia: Lippincott-Raven.

Monahan, F. D., Drake, T., Neighbors, M. (1994). *Nursing care of adults*. Philadelphia: Saunders.

Sherwood, L. (1995). *Fundamentals of physiology: A human perspective* (2nd ed.). St. Paul: West Publishing.

White, V. M. Hyperkalemia. (1997). *American Journal of Nursing, 97*(6), 35.

Additional Resources

International Food Information Council
http://ificinfo.health.org/

Chapter 22

Caring for Clients in Shock

KEY TERMS

Anaphylactic shock
Antidiuretic hormone
Cardiac output
Cardiogenic shock
Catecholamines
Colloid solutions
Corticosteroid hormones
Crystalloid solutions
Distributive shock
Hypercarbia
Hypovolemic shock
Hypoxemia
Hypoxia
Ischemia
Neurogenic shock
Obstructive shock
Oliguria
Positive inotropic agents
Renin–angiotensin–aldosterone system
Septic shock
Shock
Vasopressors

LEARNING OBJECTIVES

On completion of this chapter, the reader will:

- Define shock and list at least four main types.
- List at least five pathophysiologic consequences associated with shock.
- Identify three physiologic mechanisms that attempt to compensate for shock.
- Discuss at least eight signs and symptoms manifested by clients in shock.
- Name three diagnostic measurements used when monitoring clients in shock.
- Give three medical approaches for treating shock.
- List at least six complications of shock.
- Name two nursing diagnoses for clients with shock.
- Discuss the nursing management of clients with shock.

Shock is a life-threatening condition that occurs when arterial blood flow and oxygen delivery to cells and tissues are inadequate. In some cases, the body is able to implement compensatory mechanisms to counteract the effects of shock. In others, shock progresses until therapeutic measures are implemented. If physiologic and therapeutic measures are inadequate, irreversible shock occurs and death follows.

Types of Shock

The four main categories of shock are hypovolemic, distributive, obstructive, or cardiogenic depending on the mechanism that causes it to develop (Table 22–1). More than one type of shock can develop simultaneously.

Hypovolemic Shock

In **hypovolemic shock,** the volume of extracellular fluid is significantly diminished primarily because of a loss or reduction in blood or plasma (water component). Because the intravascular, interstitial, and intracellular fluid volumes are interdependent on each other, a loss from one location results in a similar depletion in others. A deficit of intravascular volume reduces the net circulating volume. Hypovolemic shock can develop when the overall fluid volume is depleted from significant bleeding. This may occur during surgery, after trauma, or after delivery of an infant. Or it may occur from significant fluid loss, as may occur with burns, large draining wounds, reduced fluid intake, suctioning, or disorders in which fluid losses exceed fluid intake, such as diabetes insipidus (see Chap. 56).

TABLE 22-1 **Types of Shock**

Type	Cause	Examples
Hypovolemic shock	Decreased blood volume	• Hemorrhage (frank and internal) • Extreme diuresis • Severe diarrhea or vomiting • Dehydration • Third-spacing
Distributive shock	Redistribution of intravascular fluid from arterial circulation to venous or capillary areas	• Severe allergic reaction • Toxic reaction to gram-negative bacterial infection • Spinal cord injury
Obstructive shock	Impaired filling of the heart with blood	• Cardiac tamponade (see Chap. 31) • Dissecting aneurysm • Tension pneumothorax (see Chap. 28)
Cardiogenic shock	Decreased force of ventricular contraction	• Heart attack • Cardiac arrhythmia (see Chaps. 33 and 34)

Distributive Shock

Distributive shock is sometimes called *normovolemic shock* because the amount of fluid in the circulatory system is not reduced, yet the fluid does not circulate in a way that permits effective perfusion of the tissues. Vasodilation, a prominent characteristic, results in an increase in the space within the vascular bed. Central blood flow is reduced because peripheral vascular areas have exceeded their usual capacity. Three types of distributive shock are neurogenic, septic, and anaphylactic shock.

NEUROGENIC SHOCK

Neurogenic shock results from an insult to the vasomotor center in the medulla of the brain or its connections through nerve fibers that extend from the spinal cord to peripheral blood vessels. The result is a decrease in arterial vascular resistance, vasodilation, and hypotension. Central nervous system conditions, such as spinal cord or head injuries, overdoses of opioids or opiates, tranquilizers, and general anesthetics can cause neurogenic shock.

SEPTIC SHOCK

Septic shock, also called *toxic shock,* is associated with overwhelming bacterial infections. This type of shock is more common in those with gram-negative *bacteremia* (bacteria in the blood), caused by microorganisms such as *Escherichia coli*, species of *Pseudomonas,* and drug-resistant *Staphylococcus aureus*. *Endotoxins,* harmful chemicals released from within the bacterial cell, are probably the major cause of the shock reaction.

ANAPHYLACTIC SHOCK

Anaphylactic shock (see Chap. 42) is a severe allergic reaction that occurs after exposure to a substance to which a person is extremely sensitive. Common allergens include bee venom, foods such as fish and nuts, and drugs such as penicillin.

Obstructive Shock

Obstructive shock occurs when the heart or great vessels are compressed. The compression reduces the space available for blood within the heart. This compromises the volume of blood that enters and leaves the heart en route to the lungs and tissues. Any condition that fills the thoracic cavity with tissue, fluid, or air can lead to obstructive shock. Examples include an increase in fluid or blood within the pericardial sac (cardiac tamponade), air that accumulates between the layers of pleura (tension pneumothorax), or abdominal fluid or air that crowds the diaphragm, thus reducing the size of the thorax.

Cardiogenic Shock

In **cardiogenic shock,** there is ineffective contraction of the heart, which reduces **cardiac output,** the volume of blood ejected from the left ventricle per minute. A myocardial infarction (heart attack) with subsequent heart failure (see Chaps. 33 and 36) is one of the leading causes of cardiogenic shock.

PATHOPHYSIOLOGY

Regardless of its type, many complex events occur when shock develops. There is reduction in cardiac output, decreased arterial blood pressure, increased concentration of intravascular fluid, reabsorption of water by the kidneys (which lowers urine output), decreased exchange of oxygen and carbon dioxide in the lungs, **hypercarbia** (increased carbon dioxide in the blood, also called hypercapnia), **hypoxemia** (decreased oxygen in the blood), and **hypoxia** (decreased amount of oxygen reaching all cells), which compromises vital organs such as the heart, brain, and kidneys.

PHYSIOLOGIC COMPENSATION

Several physiologic mechanisms attempt to stabilize the spiraling consequences of shock. They include the release of catecholamines, activation of the renin–angiotensin–aldosterone system, and production of antidiuretic and corticosteroid hormones.

Catecholamines

To compensate, the body releases endogenous **catecholamines,** *epinephrine* and *norepinephrine,* into the circulation. Epinephrine is secreted by the adrenal medulla and norepinephrine is secreted mainly at nerve endings of sympathetic nerve fibers. Box 22-1 lists the major effects of epinephrine and norepinephrine. The release of epinephrine and norepinephrine results in an increase in heart rate and contractile ability of the myocardium. This is followed by increased venous return to the right atrium and an increase in the amount of blood sent to the lungs. Bronchial dilatation increases the amount of oxygenated air entering the lungs, followed by a more efficient exchange of oxygen and carbon dioxide.

Renin–Angiotensin–Aldosterone System

The **renin–angiotensin–aldosterone system** is a mechanism that restores blood pressure. In response to low renal (kidney) blood perfusion, renin, an enzyme-like substance in the nephrons of the kidneys, is released. It causes a series of chemical reactions that eventually produce angiotensin II, a potent vasoconstrictor, that raises blood pressure. Angiotensin II also stimulates the hypothalamus to signal the adrenal cortex to release aldosterone, a mineralocorticoid that promotes reabsorption of sodium and water by the kidney, which serves to increase blood volume.

Antidiuretic Hormone and Corticosteroid Hormones

Low blood volume also stimulates the pituitary to secrete **antidiuretic hormone** (ADH), also known as *vasopressin,* and *adrenocorticotropic hormone* (ACTH). ADH promotes reabsorption of water that would ordinarily be excreted by the kidney. ACTH stimulates the adrenal glands to secrete **corticosteroid hormones** such as *glucocorticoids* and *mineralocorticoids.* Glucocorticoids help the body respond to stress. Mineralocorticoids, such as aldosterone, conserve sodium and promote potassium excretion and thus have an active role in controlling sodium and water balance.

The faster shock can be reversed, the greater the chance of uncomplicated recovery. Regardless of the cause, prolonged shock is incompatible with life. In few instances is the careful attention to nursing practices and principles more important to recovery than it is in the management of a client in impending or actual shock.

BOX 22-1 Effects of Endogenous Catecholamines

Effect	Outcome
Constriction of arterioles of skin, mucous membranes, subcutaneous tissues	Sends blood to larger blood vessels supplying vitral organs
Dilatation of arterioles of skeletal muscles	Increases blood supply to skeletal muscles
Dilatation of coronary arteries	Increases oxygen to myocardium
Increased contractile ability of myocardium	Increases amount of blood leaving the left ventricle each time ventricle contracts (cardiac output)
Increased heart rate	Increases blood supply to body, especially vital organs
Bronchial dilatation	Increases the amount of air entering the lungs on inspiration
Release of glycogen stored in the liver	Provides energy

Assessment Findings

Signs and Symptoms

The nurse monitors for evidence that blood volume or circulation are becoming compromised. Although shock can develop quickly, there is a period during which early signs and symptoms become evident. Critical assessments include measurements of vital signs, characteristics of peripheral pulses, and changes in mentation, the skin, and urine output.

ARTERIAL BLOOD PRESSURE

In shock, the systolic and diastolic *arterial blood pressure* falls. The fall may be rapid and sudden or slow and insidious.

Hypotension occurs because cardiac output decreases or the vascular bed size increases. For the normotensive (normal blood pressure) adult, the average systolic blood pressure is less than 140 mm Hg. Therefore, a systolic blood pressure of 90 to 100 mm Hg indicates impending shock, whereas 80 mm Hg or below indicates shock.

To determine if shock is present, the client's previous blood pressure must, if possible, be known. Regardless of the numeric figure, a progressive fall in blood pressure is a serious sign. For example, a blood pressure of 120/82 is generally considered normal; but, if an individual with an original blood pressure of 190/112 develops a blood pressure of 120/82, shock may be developing. The physician is made aware of any fall in systolic blood pressure below 100 mm Hg, any fall of 20 mm Hg or more below the client's usual systolic blood pressure, or any trend in progressively decreasing blood pressure.

Direct blood pressure monitoring (intra-arterial) is more accurate than indirect—the usual, auscultatory method using a blood pressure cuff (see Chap. 30)—but it is primarily implemented in critical care areas.

PULSE PRESSURE

Pulse pressure is the numeric difference between the systolic and diastolic blood pressures. If a client has a blood pressure of 120/80, the pulse pressure is 40 mm Hg. A pulse pressure between 30 and 50 is considered normal, with 40 being a healthy average. In shock, the pulse pressure tends to narrow (decrease) as the falling systolic pressure nears the diastolic pressure.

PULSE RATE, VOLUME, AND RHYTHM

As cardiac output decreases, compensatory tachycardia develops to increase cardiac output. In hypovolemic shock, the *pulse rate* and other assessment data are used to identify the severity of shock and estimate the approximate reduction in blood volume (Table 22–2). *Pulse volume* becomes weak and thready as circulating volume diminishes. In later stages, the pulse may be imperceptible. *Pulse rhythm* may change from regular to irregular. Hypoxia, especially when it affects heart tissue, is one of the leading causes of dangerous cardiac arrhythmias such as ventricular fibrillation.

RESPIRATIONS

In shock, tissues receive less oxygen. In response, the body tries to obtain more oxygen by breathing faster. Rapid respirations help move blood in the large veins toward the heart. Respirations are shallow, and grunting may be heard. In early stages, the client is hungry for air, but in profound shock as death nears, the respiratory rate decreases.

TEMPERATURE

Heat-regulating mechanisms are depressed in shock, and heat loss is increased by added diaphore-

TABLE 22-2 **Shock Classification and Estimated Blood Loss**

Assessment Data	Class I	Class II	Class III	Class IV
Pulse rate	<100	>100	>120	>140
Pulse pressure	Normal or increased	Decreased	Decreased	Decreased
Blood pressure	Normal	Normal	Decreased	Decreased
Respirations	14–20	20–30	30–40	>35
Urine output/h	≥30 mL	20–30 mL	5–15 mL	Negligible
Mental status	Slightly anxious	Mildly anxious	Anxious and confused	Confused and lethargic
Blood loss	≤750 mL	750–1,000 mL	1,500–2,000 mL	≥2,000 mL
Percent of total blood volume lost*	≤15%	15–30%	30–40%	≥40%

Adapted from American College of Surgeons. (1993). Advanced trauma life support for physicians.
*Estimates are based on an adult male weighing 70 kg

sis. With the possible exception of septic shock, subnormal temperature is characteristic.

MENTATION

Alteration in cerebral function often is the first sign of inadequate oxygen delivery to the tissues. Mild anxiety, increasing restlessness, agitation, or confusion accompany shock. As the condition deteriorates, the client becomes listless and stuporous and ultimately loses consciousness.

SKIN

In shock, the skin becomes pale, cold, and clammy as peripheral blood vessels constrict to direct blood from the skin to more vital organs, such as the heart, kidneys, and brain. Slow capillary filling (eg < 3 seconds) and cyanosis, especially of the nail beds, lips, and ear lobes, indicates a deficiency of oxygen. In highly pigmented clients, such as African-Americans, cyanosis is more accurately detected by inspecting the color of the conjunctiva and oral mucous membranes. Lack of cyanosis, however, does not prove the absence of hypoxia, because it is one of the last signs to appear.

URINE OUTPUT

Decreased urine output occurs because reduced cardiac output decreases renal blood flow. Vasoconstriction, the body's physiologic response to shock, also contributes to a marked reduction in renal blood flow. In many instances, the rate of urine formation is an important indicator of the status of a client in shock (see Table 22–2). When shock is quickly reversed, urine output usually returns to normal. Continued **oliguria** (decrease in urine formation) indicates renal damage, caused by reduced blood flow to the kidney.

Diagnostic Findings

A diagnosis of shock is supported by arterial blood gas, central venous pressure, and pulmonary artery pressure measurements, which are also used to monitor the client's response to treatment.

ARTERIAL BLOOD GAS MEASUREMENTS

In shock, the PaO_2, partial pressure of oxygen in arterial blood, normally 80 to 100 mm Hg, falls below 60 mm Hg. The $PaCO_2$, the partial pressure of carbon dioxide in arterial blood, may be normal or decreased. Arterial blood gas (ABG) specimens are drawn from a direct arterial puncture or from an indwelling arterial catheter (see Chap. 30). Sometimes used to continuously monitor the oxygenation of clients, a pulse oximeter measures the amount of oxygen that is bound to hemoglobin, or the saturated oxygen (SpO_2). Normally the SpO_2 is 95% to 100%. If the SpO_2 is above 90%, it can be assumed the PaO_2 is 60 mm Hg or above.

CENTRAL VENOUS PRESSURE

Central venous pressure (CVP) is the pressure of the blood in the right atrium or venae cavae. It distinguishes relationships among hemodynamic variables in shock: the venous return, quality of right ventricular function, and vascular tone. CVP measurements, especially trends in readings, are useful in the management of a client in shock (see Chaps. 21 and 30). Normal CVP is 4 to 10 cm H_2O. In hypovolemic shock, the CVP is lower than normal; in cardiogenic shock, it is generally above normal. The trend in CVP measurements is more helpful than an isolated reading.

PULMONARY ARTERY PRESSURE

Although the status of right ventricular function can be evaluated by CVP measurements, left ventricular function cannot. Because left ventricular function is more pertinent to circulation than the right, knowing fluid pressures on the left side of the heart are more meaningful. To assess left ventricular function, a two-, three-, or four-lumen catheter is inserted into the vena cava and advanced through the right atrium and right ventricle into the pulmonary artery (Fig. 22–1). The catheter is connected to a monitor from which the pulmonary artery pressure (PAP) or pulmonary capillary wedge pressure (PCWP) is measured (see Chap. 30). Normal PAP ranges from 20 to 30 mm Hg systolic and from 8 to 12 mm Hg diastolic. Normal PCWP ranges from 4 to

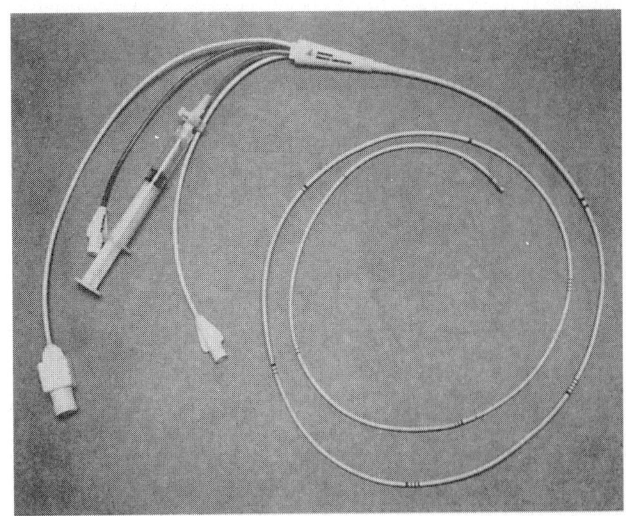

FIGURE 22-1. A four-lumen pulmonary artery catheter.

12 mm Hg. (References may vary slightly on these figures.) In shock, PAP measurements are usually low because they reflect the low volume of blood in the arterial system.

Medical Management

Shock may sometimes be prevented by aggressively treating conditions that predispose to shock. Once it develops, treatment depends on the type and level of shock that exists. Generally, treatment includes one or more of the following: intravenous fluid therapy, drug therapy, and mechanical devices that restore circulation of blood to cells.

Intravenous Fluid Therapy

Intravenous fluids are prescribed to restore intravascular volume. The total volume, type of solution(s), and rate of administration vary according to the etiology. Generally a ratio of 3:1 is followed; that is, 3 liters of fluid administered for every 1 liter of fluid loss. This stabilizes the client, replaces the deficit, and provides a reserve to prevent shock from recurring. Initially, as much as 250 to 500 mL may be infused in 1 hour. Solutions may include **crystalloids,** those containing dissolved substances such as sodium or glucose in water (see Chap. 23); **colloids,** those containing proteins such as albumin, to increase osmotic pressure; and blood and blood products if there has been major blood loss.

Drug Therapy

Medical management of shock is extremely complex; drugs are carefully titrated and used singularly or in combination to improve the client's cardiovascular status. Adrenergic drugs are the main medications used in the treatment of shock. Drugs that have alpha-adrenergic activity increase peripheral vascular resistance and raise blood pressure and are called **vasopressors.** Examples of vasopressors include dopamine (Intropin), norepinephrine (Levophed), and metaraminol (Aramine). Drugs with beta-adrenergic activity increase the heart rate and improve the force of heart contraction are **positive inotropic agents** (inotropic means to affect the force of muscular contraction). Digoxin (Lanoxin), isoproterenol (Isuprel), and dobutamine (Dobutrex) are examples of inotropic drugs. Many drugs have combined alpha- and beta-adrenergic effects. Epinephrine has combined effects and is the drug of choice in anaphylactic shock.

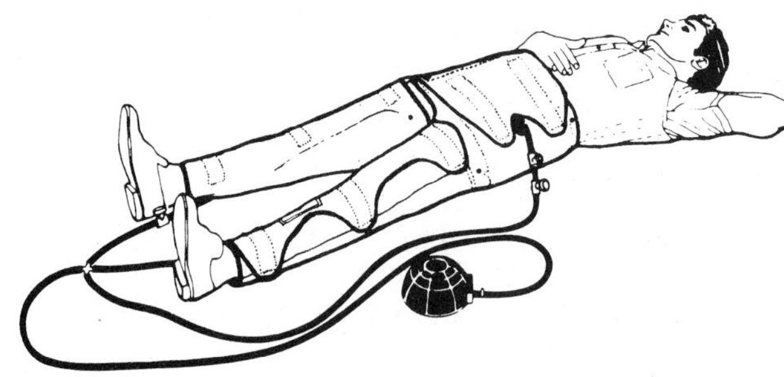

FIGURE 22-2. A pneumatic antishock garment.

Mechanical Devices

Mechanical devices help improve circulation of blood. Those used in the treatment of shock include the intra-aortic balloon pump (IABP) and ventricular assist device (VAD) (see Chap. 36) and the pneumatic antishock garment (PASG), also called military antishock trousers (MAST) (Fig. 22–2). The PASG is used to raise blood pressure mechanically by first responders (paramedics). It also helps to control bleeding. Its use is considered somewhat controversial because applying or removing it incorrectly is life threatening, and air transport facilitates the quick transferral of unstable clients to specialized trauma centers.

Prognosis and Complications

When shock is treated adequately and promptly, the client usually recovers. However the recovery period may be tenuous as a consequence of secondary complications. The complications are almost always a direct result of tissue hypoxia and organ **ischemia,** reduced oxygenation. Life-threatening complications include kidney failure, neurologic deficits, bleeding disorders such as disseminated intravascular coagulation (see Chap. 39), adult respiratory distress syndrome (see Chap. 28), stress ulcers, and sepsis that can lead to multiple organ dysfunction.

NURSING PROCESS
The Client in Shock

Assessment
Assess skin color and temperature, level of consciousness, vital signs every 5 minutes, quality of pulse, capillary perfusion, peripheral pulses, and urine output. The nurse gathers data and identifies early signs and

symptoms of shock. Symptoms of shock are reported immediately. The nurse implements medical therapy and monitors the client's response.

Diagnosis and Planning

The plan for caring for clients predisposed to or in actual shock includes, but is not limited to, the following:

Nursing Diagnoses and Collaborative Problems	Nursing Interventions
Decreased Cardiac Output related to (specify) blood loss, impaired distribution of fluid, impaired circulation, inadequate heart contraction	Establish two intravenous (IV) sites. Administer IV fluids or blood products at rate prescribed and ensure IV catheter(s) are patent. Warm blood product before rapid infusion.
Goal: Client's heart rate will be between 60 and 120 beats/min	
Impaired Tissue Perfusion related to reduced cardiac output *Goal:* The systolic blood pressure will be at least 90 mm Hg, and hourly urine output will be 50 mL or greater.	Assess skin color and temperature. Maintain client in supine position with legs elevated unless there is head injury, heart failure, increased intracranial pressure, possible spinal cord injury, or dyspnea.
	Administer oxygen by the prescribed method and percentage.
	Insert an indwelling urinary catheter.
	Observe for response to treatment or deteriorating condition by continuously monitoring vital signs, cardiac rhythm, level of consciousness, urine output, and peripheral perfusion.
	Give prescribed medications for improving cardiovascular status.
	Reduce or eliminate unnecessary physical activity.
	If a PASG is used, monitor garment pressures and distal pulses and notify the physician if the garment pressure is greater than 30 mm Hg for more than 2 hours. When the client is stable, deflate the garment starting with the abdominal port or a leg section, never remove the entire garment at once.

Evaluation

- The client's vital signs stabilize.
- There is satisfactory tissue perfusion as evidenced by adequate urine output, palpable peripheral pulses, warm, dry skin, and intact sensorium.

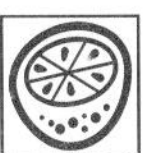

General Nutritional Considerations

Because the metabolism of carbohydrates produces more carbon dioxide that the metabolism of either protein or fat, it is recommended that fat intake increase and carbohydrate intake decrease to reduce the burden on the lungs in clients with respiratory distress syndrome. Protein should provide approximately 20% of total calories with the rest divided evenly between carbohydrates and fat. Avoid overfeeding, which causes overproduction of carbon dioxide.

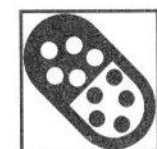

General Pharmacologic Considerations

Ringer's lactate and 0.9% sodium chloride (isotonic solutions) are commonly used to treat hypovolemic shock.

Morphine sulfate may be administered to decrease anxiety and pain.

Dopamine (Intropin) is used in the treatment of shock due to myocardial infarction, trauma, septicemia, renal failure, and cardiac decompensation. This drug must be properly diluted and administered by continuous infusion regulated by an infusion pump.

Administration of vasopressors such as dopamine demands constant nursing supervision. Depending on institutional policy, blood pressure is monitored every 5 minutes with an automatic monitoring device. The rate of infusion is adjusted to maintain a specific blood pressure.

General Gerontologic Considerations

Older adults, particularly those with cardiac disease, are prone to cardiogenic shock.

The older adult has a lower percentage of body water and is more likely to develop hypovolemic shock.

SUMMARY OF KEY CONCEPTS

- Shock is a life-threatening condition that occurs when arterial blood flow and oxygen delivery to cells and tissues are inadequate. Four main types of shock are hypovolemic, distributive, obstructive, and cardiogenic shock.
- When shock occurs, there is a decrease in cardiac output, hypotension, decreased intravascular blood volume, low urine output, inadequate gas exchange in the lungs, and accumulation of carbon dioxide and reduced oxygen at the cellular level.
- To stabilize the client and reverse the consequences of shock, the body releases catecholamines, activates the renin–angiotensin–aldosterone system, and stimulates the release of antidiuretic and corticosteroid hormones.
- Clients in shock generally manifest low blood pressure; narrowed pulse pressure; rapid and shallow respira-

tions; lowered body temperature; confusion and decreased levels of consciousness; cold, clammy and perhaps cyanotic skin; and low output of concentrated urine.

- Arterial blood gas, central venous pressures, and pulmonary artery pressure measurements are used to detect the early stages of shock, determine its severity, and evaluate the response of the client to treatment.
- Medical treatment of shock includes intravenous fluid therapy, drug therapy, and mechanical devices that restore circulation of blood to cells.
- Complications of shock include kidney failure, neurologic deficits, disseminated intravascular coagulation, adult respiratory distress syndrome, stress ulcers, and sepsis.
- Nursing management of clients in shock includes gathering data, identifying and reporting signs and symptoms of shock, implementing medical therapy, planning and providing appropriate nursing care, and monitoring the client's response.
- Nursing interventions include monitoring parenteral fluid therapy, administering prescribed medications, and conserving the client's energy and reducing the work of the heart by eliminating unnecessary activities.

CRITICAL THINKING EXERCISES

1. Correlate the pathophysiologic processes that produce the signs and symptoms of shock.
2. When caring for a client who has the potential for shock discuss the assessment data that are important to report immediately.
3. Explain the therapeutic effects of two different categories of drugs used for treating shock.

Suggested Readings

DeJong, M. J. (1997). Cardiogenic shock. *American Journal of Nursing, 97*(6), 40–41.

Hagland, M. R. (1996). Septic shock: A case study. *Intensive and Critical Care Nursing, 12*(1), 55–59.

Lisanti, P. (1996). Emergency! Anaphylaxis. *American Journal of Nursing, 96*(11), 51.

Sandrock, J. (1997). Managing hypovolemia. *Nursing, 27*(2), 32aa–32bb, 32ee.

Update97 (left ventricular assist device). (1997). *Nursing, 27*(5), 64.

Vonfiolio, L. G., & Noone, J. (1995). Self-test: Recognizing signs of shock. *Nursing, 25*(7), 18, 21.

Additional Resources

American College of Surgeons
55 East Erie Street
Chicago, IL 60611
(312) 664–4050

Chapter 23

Caring for Clients Requiring Intravenous Therapy

KEY TERMS

Blood products
Central venous infusions
Colloid solutions
Crystalloid solutions
Drop factor
Drop size
Electronic infusion device
Emulsion
Hypertonic solution
Hypotonic solution
In-line filter
Infiltration
Infusion pump
Intravenous therapy
Isotonic solution
Macrodrip tubing
Medication lock
Microdrip tubing
Packed cells
Peripheral venous sites
Plasma expanders
Pressure infusion sleeve
Primary tubing
Secondary tubing
Total parenteral nutrition
Unvented tubing
Venipuncture
Vented tubing
Volumetric controller
Whole blood
Y-administration tubing

LEARNING OBJECTIVES

On completion of this chapter, the reader will:

- Explain intravenous (IV) therapy and list three substances commonly infused.
- Differentiate between crystalloid and colloid solutions.
- Describe the difference between isotonic, hypotonic, and hypertonic solutions.
- Discuss the purpose of total parenteral nutrition and name one solution often administered concurrently.
- Explain the difference between whole blood, packed cells, blood products, and plasma expanders.
- List nursing responsibilities implemented before administering IV therapy.
- List three items of equipment essential when administering IV therapy.
- List three types of tubing used to administer IV solutions.
- Name two techniques for infusing IV solutions.
- Explain the difference between an infusion pump and a volumetric controller.
- Give three nursing actions involved in performing a venipuncture.
- Name three venipuncture devices and identify the one most commonly used.
- Name two general sites used for IV therapy.
- Identify three nursing diagnoses common among clients who require IV therapy.
- Discuss the nursing management of clients receiving IV therapy.
- List three complications of IV therapy and three associated with administering blood.
- Discuss the purpose of a medication lock.

Intravenous (IV) therapy, the parenteral administration of fluids and additives into a vein, demands skillful administration techniques, close observation of the client, and a number of special nursing considerations. Solutions (eg, dextrose, plasma expanders, amino acids), whole blood and blood components, and medications are given by the IV route in specific situations.

Purposes of Intravenous Therapy

Intravenous therapy is used to maintain or restore fluid balance when oral replacement is inadequate or impossible, maintain or replace electrolytes, administer water-soluble vitamins, provide a source of calories and nutrients, administer drugs (Box 23–1), and replace blood and blood products.

BOX 23-1 Indications for Administering Drugs intravenously

Drugs are administered IV in the following circumstances:

- When a rapid drug effect is required
- When oral intake is restricted
- When a client cannot swallow or absorb the medication by any other route of administration
- When gastrointestinal absorption is impaired
- When a continuous therapeutic blood level is desired

Types of Solutions

Types of IV solutions that are administered are crystalloid and colloid solutions. **Crystalloid solutions** consist of water and other uniformly dissolved crystals such as salt (sodium chloride) and sugar (glucose, dextrose). **Colloid solutions** consist of water and molecules of suspended substances such as blood cells and blood products (eg, albumin).

Crystalloid Solutions

Crystalloid solutions are divided into isotonic, hypotonic, and hypertonic solutions (Table 23–1), referring to the concentration of dissolved substances in relation to plasma where they are instilled. When administered to clients, the concentration influences the osmotic distribution of body fluid (Fig. 23–1; see Chap. 22).

ISOTONIC SOLUTION

An **isotonic solution** is one that contains the same concentration of dissolved substances as is normally found in plasma. Isotonic solutions are administered to maintain fluid balance when clients cannot eat or drink for a short period of time. Because of its equal concentration, an isotonic solution does not cause any appreciable redistribution of body fluid.

HYPOTONIC SOLUTION

A **hypotonic solution** contains fewer dissolved substances in comparison to plasma. Hypotonic solutions are effective in rehydrating clients experiencing fluid deficits; therefore, they are administered to clients experiencing fluid losses in excess of their fluid intake, such as those who have diarrhea or vomiting. Because hypotonic solutions are dilute, the water in the solution passes through the semipermeable membrane of blood cells, causing them to swell. This can temporarily increase blood pressure because it expands the circulating volume. The water may also pass through capillary walls and become distributed within other body cells and the interstitial spaces.

TABLE 23-1 **Types of Intravenous Solutions**

Solution	Components	Special Comments
Isotonic Solutions		
0.9% saline, also called normal saline	0.9 g sodium chloride/100 mL water	Contains amounts of sodium and chloride in physiologically equal amounts to that found in plasma
5% dextrose and water, also called D_5W	5 g dextrose (glucose/sugar)/100 mL water	Isotonic when infused but the glucose is metabolized quickly, leaving a solution of dilute water
Ringer's solution or lactated Ringer's	Water and a mixture of sodium, chloride, calcium, potassium, bicarbonate, and in some cases, lactate	Replaces electrolytes in amounts similarly found in plasma. The lactate, when present, helps maintain acid–base balance
Hypotonic Solutions		
0.45% sodium chloride, or also called half-strength saline	0.45 g sodium chloride/100 mL water	A smaller ratio of sodium and chloride than found in plasma causing it to be less concentrated in comparison
5% dextrose in 0.45% saline	5 g dextrose and 0.45 sodium chloride/100 mL water	The sugar provides a quick source of energy, leaving a hypotonic salt solution
Hypertonic Solutions		
10% dextrose in water, also called $D_{10}W$	10 g dextrose/100 mL water	Twice the concentration of glucose than present in plasma
3% saline	3 g sodium chloride/100 mL water	The high concentration of salt in the plasma will dehydrate cells and tissue
20% dextrose in water	20 g dextrose/100 mL water	Rapidly increases the concentration of sugar in the blood, causing a fluid shift to the intravascular compartment

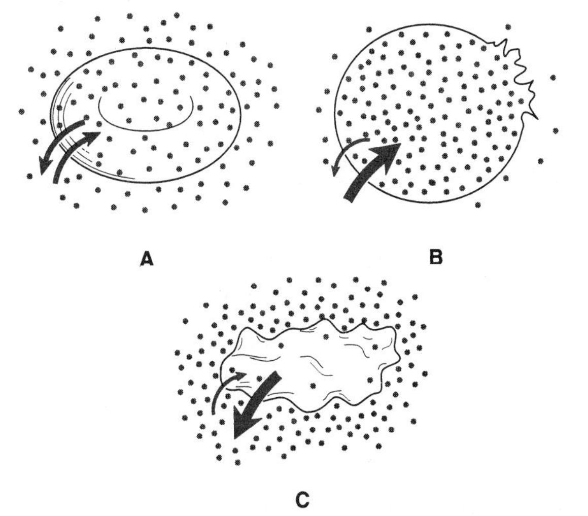

FIGURE 23-1. Osmotic distribution of fluid. (A) Isotonic fluid, (B) Hypotonic fluid, (C) Hypertonic fluid.

HYPERTONIC SOLUTION

A **hypertonic solution** is more concentrated than body fluid. Consequently, it draws fluid into the intravascular compartment from the more dilute areas within the interstitial spaces. Hypertonic solutions are not used very frequently except when it is necessary to reduce cerebral (brain) edema, expand circulatory volume rapidly, or administer nutrition parenterally.

TOTAL PARENTERAL NUTRITION

Total parenteral nutrition (TPN) is a hypertonic solution consisting of nutrients designed to meet nearly all the caloric and nutritional needs of clients who are severely malnourished or who cannot consume food or liquids for a long period of time (Box 23–2). Extremely concentrated, TPN solutions are instilled into the central circulation (see central veins discussed later in this chapter) where they are diluted in a fairly large volume of blood. Because of their immediate dilution, they do not dehydrate cells.

A lipid emulsion is sometimes administered intermittently with TPN. An **emulsion** is a mixture of two liquids, one of which is insoluble in the other, but when combined is distributed throughout as small droplets. A lipid emulsion is a mixture of water and fats in the form of soybean or safflower oil, egg yolk phospholipds, and glycerin, which looks milky white. It provides additional calories and promotes adequate blood levels of fatty acids.

BOX 23-2 Candidates for Total Parenteral Nutrition

Candidates for total parenteral nutrition (TPN) include clients:

- Who have not eaten for 5 days and are not likely to eat during the next week
- Who have had a 10% or more loss of body weight
- Exhibiting self-imposed starvation (anorexia nervosa)
- With cancer of the esophagus or stomach
- With postoperative gastrointestinal complications
- With inflammatory bowel disease in an acute stage
- With major trauma or burns
- With liver and renal failure

COLLOID SOLUTIONS

Colloid solutions are used to replace circulating blood volume because the suspended molecules pull fluid from other compartments. Examples of colloid solutions include blood, blood products, and solutions known as plasma expanders.

Blood

Whole blood and packed cells are probably the most common types of colloid solutions administered. One unit of **whole blood** contains approximately 475 mL of blood cells and plasma with 60 to 70 mL of preservative and anticoagulant added, whereas **packed cells** have most of the plasma removed. Packed cells are preferred for clients who need cellular replacements, but do not need—and may be harmed by the administration of additional fluid. Whole blood and packed cells are typed and crossmatched by the laboratory before administration to ensure that the donor's and recipient's blood types are compatible (Table 23–2).

Blood Products

Several types of solutions contain **blood products,** components extracted from blood (Table 23–3). Blood products are administered to clients who need specific substances, yet do not need all the fluid or cellular components in whole blood.

Plasma Expanders

Plasma expanders are nonblood solutions, such as dextran 40 (Rheomacrodex) and hetastarch (Hespan), that pull fluid into the vascular space. They are used as an economic and virus-free substitute for blood and blood products when treating hypovolemic shock.

Administering Intravenous Therapy

Administering IV therapy includes: (1) selecting and preparing the appropriate equipment, (2) preparing

TABLE 23-2 **Types of Blood Products**

Blood Product	Description	Purpose for Administration
Platelets	Disk-shaped cellular fragments that promote coagulation of blood	Restores or improves the ability to control bleeding
Granulocytes	Types of white blood cells	Improves the ability to overcome an infection
Plasma	Serum minus blood cells	Replaces clotting factors or increases intravascular fluid volume by increasing colloidal osmotic pressure
Albumin	Plasma protein	Pulls third-spaced fluid by increasing colloidal osmotic pressure
Cryoprecipitate	Mixture of clotting factors	Treats blood clotting disorders like hemophilia

the client, (3) selecting the venipuncture site, and (4) performing the venipuncture.

Intravenous Therapy Equipment

Equipment commonly used when administering IV therapy includes the solution, IV tubing, and an IV pole or infusion device. A fluid warmer may be used to raise the temperature of parenteral solutions when it is beneficial to ensure stable body temperature.

The nurse selects and prepares the fluid that will be administered, chooses appropriate tubing, and decides on an infusion technique.

Preparing Intravenous Solutions

Crystalloid solutions are stored in plastic bags containing volumes of 1,000, 500, 250, 100, and 50 mL. Only a few solutions are in glass containers. The physician specifies the type of solution, additional additives, and the volume to be infused in a period of time. To reduce the potential for infection, it is standard practice to replace IV solutions every 24 hours even if the total volume has not been instilled. Before preparing the solution, the nurse inspects the container and determines that the type of solution is the one prescribed, the solution is clear and transparent, the expiration date has not elapsed, no leaks are apparent, and a separate label is attached identifying the type and amount of drugs added to the original solution.

TABLE 23-3 **Blood Groups and Compatible Types**

Blood Groups	Percentage of Population	Compatible Blood Types
A	41%	A and O
B	9%	B and O
O	47%	O
AB	3%	AB, A, B, and O
Rh+	85% whites 95% African Americans	Rh+ and Rh–
Rh–	15% whites 5% African Americans	Rh– only

Intravenous Tubing

The IV tubing consists of a spike for accessing the solution, a drip chamber for holding a small amount of fluid, a length of plastic tubing with one or more ports for instilling IV medications or additional solutions, and a roller or slide clamp for regulating the rate of the infusion (Fig. 23–2).

Despite the common components, the nurse selects from various options in the tubing design. The choice depends on four considerations: (1) whether to use primary, secondary, or Y-administration tubing, (2) whether to use vented or unvented tubing, (3) the drop size indicated, and (4) whether a filter is needed.

PRIMARY, SECONDARY, AND Y-ADMINISTRATION TUBING

Primary tubing is used to administer a large volume of IV solution over a long period of time or a small volume through a medication lock. Primary tubing is generally quite long to span the distance from the solution that hangs several feet above the infusion site. **Secondary tubing,** which is shorter, is used to administer smaller volumes of solution through a port in the primary tubing. **Y-administration tubing** is used to administer whole blood or packed cells (Fig. 23-3). It contains two branches, one for blood and one for isotonic (normal) saline. The two branches extend above a filter that removes blood clots and cellular debris. The normal saline infuses before and after the

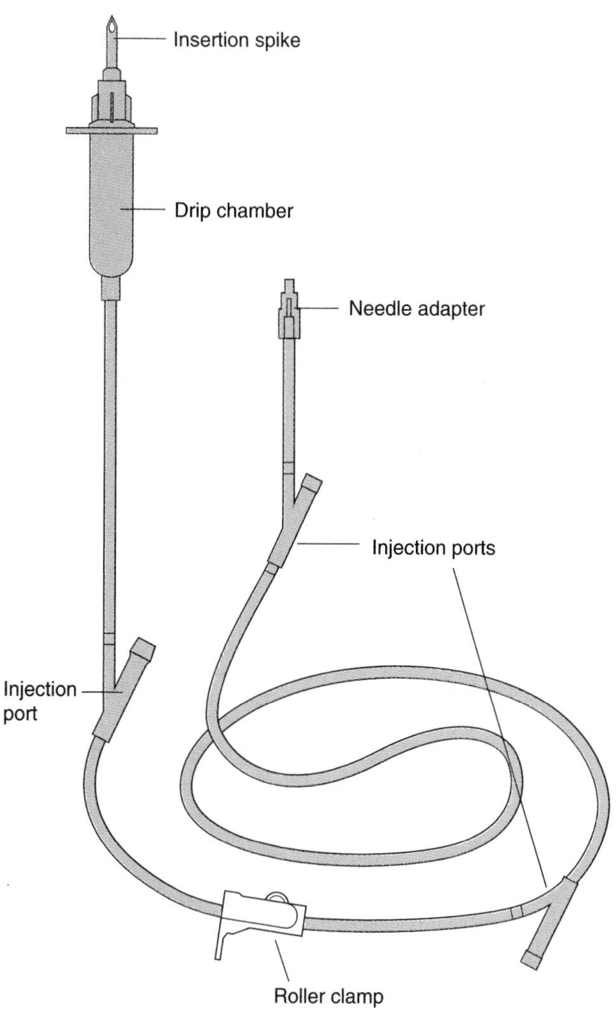

FIGURE 23-2. Basic components of intravenous tubing.

blood is infused, or during the infusion, if a transfusion reaction occurs.

VENTED VS. UNVENTED TUBING

The IV tubing may be vented or unvented. **Vented tubing** draws air into the container of solution, whereas **unvented tubing** does not (Fig. 23–4). Vented tubing is used for administering solutions packaged in glass containers to facilitate its flow; unvented tubing is used for solutions packaged in plastic bags.

DROP SIZE

The opening through which fluid passes from the solution container into the drip chamber determines the **drop size.** The opening is designed by tubing manufacturers to deliver large-sized drops (**macrodrip tubing**) or small-sized drops (**microdrip tubing**). The nurse determines which to use. When a solution infuses at a fast rate, it is usually easier to count larger drops than smaller ones. When the rate must be infused very precisely or at a slow rate, smaller drops are preferred.

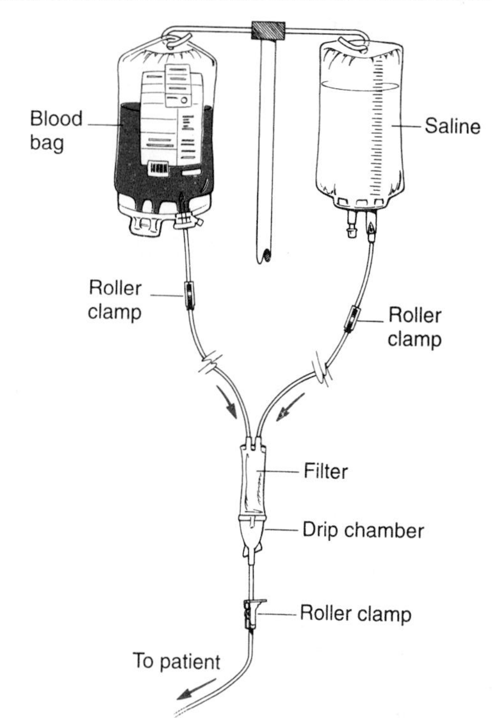

FIGURE 23-3. Blood administration set.

Microdrip tubing, regardless of the manufacturer, delivers a standard volume of 60 drops/mL. However, macrodrip tubing varies in the drop size. Common **drop factors,** the ratio of drops to mL, are 10, 15,

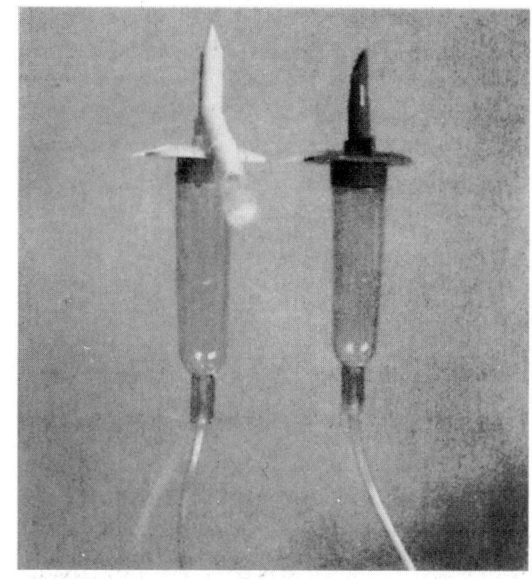

FIGURE 23-4. Vented tubing (left) and unvented tubing.

and 20 drops (gtt)/mL. The nurse determines the drop factor by reading the package label. The drop factor is important in calculating the infusion rate.

FILTERS

An **in-line filter** (Fig. 23–5) is a device that removes air bubbles as well as undissolved drugs, bacteria, and large molecules. Filtered tubing is used when administering TPN, blood and packed cells, and solutions to immunosuppressed or pediatric clients.

Another factor that may affect the type of tubing selected is the technique that will be used to administer the IV solution.

Infusion Techniques

Intravenous solutions are instilled by gravity or with an **electronic infusion device,** a machine that regulates and monitors the administration of IV solutions. In some cases, the use of an electronic infusion device affects the type of tubing used.

The method for calculating the rate of infusion varies depending on the infusion technique (Box 23–3). If the solution is infused by gravity, the rate is calculated in gtt/min. When an electronic infusion device is used, the rate is calculated in mL/h.

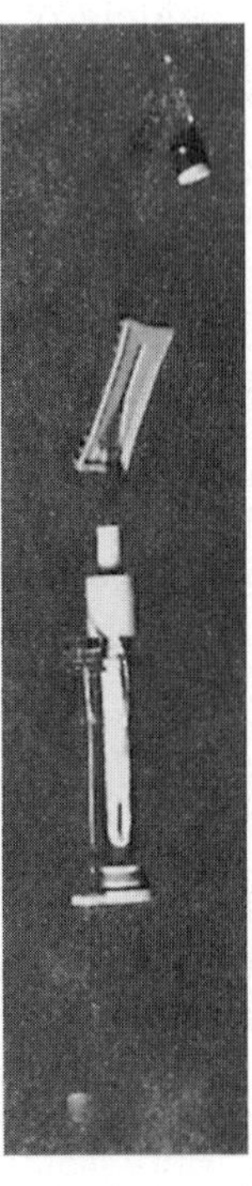

FIGURE 23-5. An in-line filter.

GRAVITY INFUSION

Intravenous solutions can be infused by gravity. The height of the IV solution in relation to the infusion site influences the rate of flow. To overcome the pressure in the client's vein, which is higher than atmospheric pressure, the solution is elevated at least 18 to 24 inches (45–60 cm) above the site of the infusion. The higher the solution, the faster it infuses, and vice versa. The roller clamp is used to adjust the rate of flow. In some cases a **pressure infusion sleeve,** which exerts a squeezing action to facilitate rapid infusion, may be applied around the solution bag.

ELECTRONIC INFUSION DEVICES

The two general types of electronic infusion devices are infusion pumps and volumetric controllers. Both are programmed to deliver a preset volume per hour and sound audible and visual alarms if the infusion is not progressing at the pre-programmed rate. They also produce an audible sound when the infusion container is nearly empty, contains air within the tubing, or senses an obstruction or resistance to delivering the fluid.

Infusion Pump

An **infusion pump** (Fig. 23–6) is a device that exerts positive pressure to infuse solutions. Infusion pumps usually require special tubing that contains a cassette for creating sufficient pressure to push fluid into the vein. The machine adjusts the pressure according to the resistance it meets. This features explains one of its major disadvantages: if the catheter or needle within the vein becomes displaced, the pump may continue to infuse fluid into the tissue.

Volumetric Controller

A **volumetric controller** (Fig. 23–7) is a device that infuses IV solutions by gravity by compressing the tubing at a certain frequency to infuse the solution at a precise preset rate. Volumetric controllers may or may not require special tubing. Some models allow the nurse to program the infusion of more than one solution. In some cases, when one container of fluid finishes infusing, the controller automatically shifts to infuse another.

Refer to Clinical Procedure 23–1 for preparing an IV solution and tubing for gravity infusion.

Venipuncture

A **venipuncture** is the method for gaining access to the venous system by piercing a vein with one of a variety of devices. Clients are given an explanation of the purpose of the procedure at their level of understanding. This is best done *before* the equipment is

BOX 23-3 Formulas for Calculating Infusion Rates

When using an infusion device:	**Example:**
$\frac{\text{Total volume in mL}}{\text{Total hours}} = \text{mL/h}$	$\frac{1{,}000 \text{ mL}}{8 \text{ h}} = 125 \text{ mL/h}$
When infusing by gravity:	
$\frac{\text{Total volume in mL}}{\text{Total time in minutes}} \times \text{drop factor*} = \text{gtt/min}$	$\frac{1{,}000 \text{ mL}}{480 \text{ min}} \times 20 = 42 \text{ gtt/min}$

*The macrodrip drop factor varies among manufacturers.

brought to the client's room. Every effort is made to make the explanation clear, concise, and informative without causing the client undue anxiety. Time is allowed to answer the client's questions. The following points may be included in the explanation: why IV therapy is needed, about how long the procedure will take, the site to be used, the amount of discomfort that normally accompanies insertion of the needle or catheter, and instructions regarding limitation of activities.

Performing a Venipuncture

Venipunctures are performed by nurses who are trained to do so. When performing a venipuncture, the nurse assembles needed equipment, inspects and selects a vein, and inserts the venipuncture device. The following items are necessary when performing a venipuncture: venipuncture device, gloves, tourniquet, antiseptic swabs to clean the skin, antiseptic ointment, a dressing, tape for securing the needle or catheter, dressing, tubing, and solution. An armboard or splint may be needed to prevent dislodging the venipuncture device.

VENIPUNCTURE DEVICES

Several devices are used for accessing a vein: a butterfly needle, an over-the-needle catheter (most

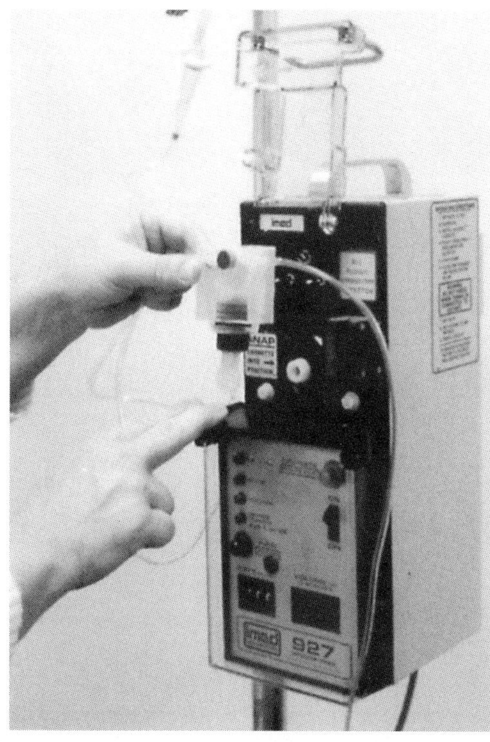

FIGURE 23-6. Infusion pump with specialized tubing and cassette.

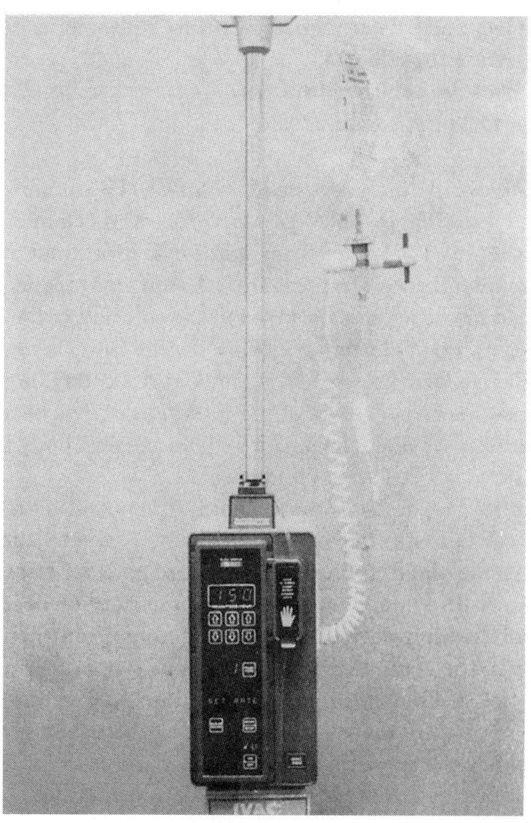

FIGURE 23-7. Electronic infusion controller.

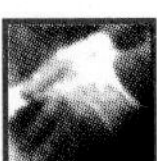

Clinical Procedure 23-1
Preparing Equipment for a Gravity Infusion

PURPOSE

- To maintain or replace body fluid
- To provide a medium for administering intravenous medication

EQUIPMENT

- Solution container
- Tubing
- IV pole or electronic infusion device
- Time strip
- Bedside intake and output record

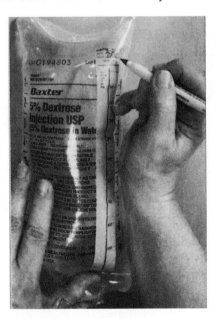

Nursing Action	Rationale
ASSESSMENT	
Check the medical orders for the type, volume, and projected length of IV fluid therapy.	Guides the selection of equipment
Review the client's medical record for information on the risk for infection.	Determines if there is a need for filtered tubing
Read and compare the print on the bag of solution with the medical order or the medication administration record at least three times.	Prevents errors
Check client's identification.	Prevents errors
PLANNING	
Obtain the necessary equipment.	Prevents unnecessary delays in the plan of care
Calculate the rate of flow.	Coordinates administration according to medical orders
Attach a time strip to the container identifying the client's name, room number, date and time, and mark the volume that should infuse in hourly increments.	Facilitates future monitoring
IMPLEMENTATION	
Wash your hands.	Reduces the transmission of microorganisms
Select the appropriate tubing and stretch it once it has been removed from the package.	Straightens the tubing by removing bends and kinks

continued

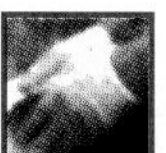

Clinical Procedure 23-1
Continued

Nursing Action	Rationale
IMPLEMENTATION	
Tighten the roller clamp.	Aids in filling the drip chamber

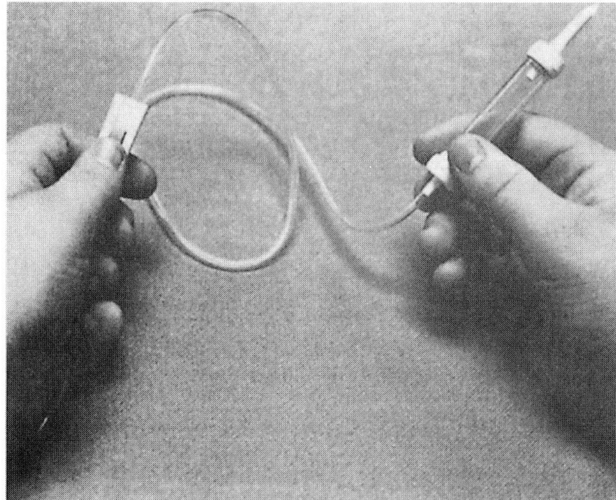

Nursing Action	Rationale
Remove the cover from the access port.	Exposes the spike
Insert the spike by puncturing the seal on the container.	Provides an exit route for fluid

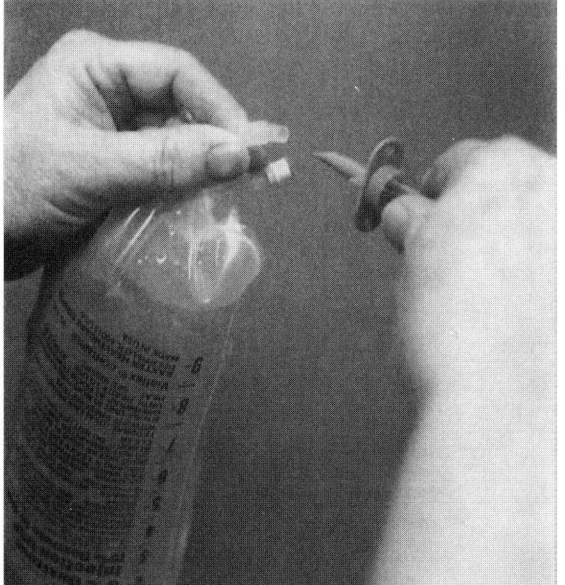

Nursing Action	Rationale
Hang the solution container from an IV pole or suspended hook.	Inverts the container and facilitates proceeding

continued

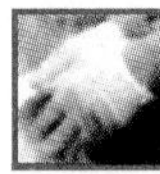

Clinical Procedure 23-1
Continued

Nursing Action	Rationale
IMPLEMENTATION	
Squeeze the drip chamber, filling it no more than half full. 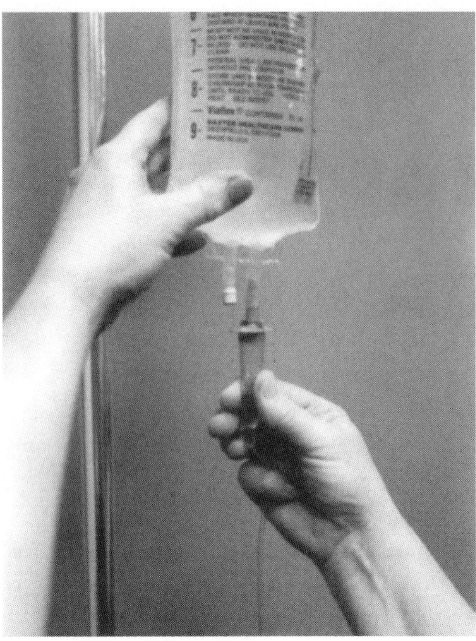	Leaves space to count the drops when regulating the rate of infusion
Release the roller clamp.	Flushes air from the tubing
Invert the ports within the tubing as the solution approaches. 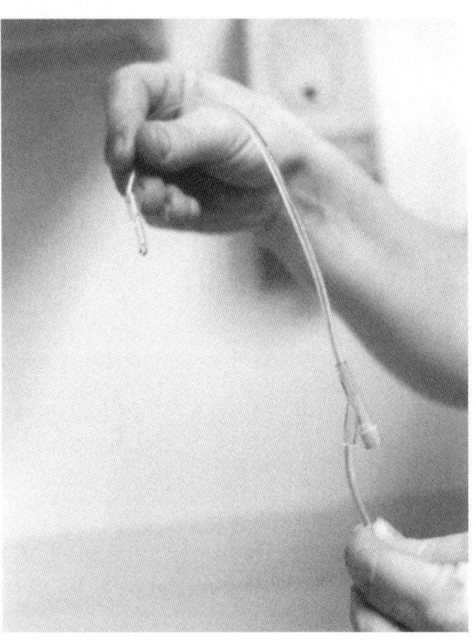	Displaces air trapped in the junction
Tighten the roller clamp when all the air has been removed.	Prevents loss of fluid
Attach a piece of tape or label on the tubing identifying the date, time, and your initials.	Provides a quick reference for determining when the tubing needs to be changed.
Take the solution and tubing to the client's room.	Facilitates administration

commonly used), or a through-the-needle catheter (Fig. 23–8). Regardless of the design, venipuncture devices come in various diameters or gauges; the larger the gauge number, the smaller the diameter. *The diameter of the venipuncture device should always be smaller than the vein into which it will be inserted.* This reduces the potential for occluding blood flow. The 18-, 20-, or 22-gauge needles are the sizes most used for adults.

VENIPUNCTURE SITES

Intravenous therapy is administered through peripheral venous sites or central veins. Selection of a vein depends on several factors, such as the client's age, condition of the veins, duration of IV therapy, IV solution ordered, needle or catheter size, and client cooperation.

Peripheral Veins and Central Veins

Peripheral venous sites include the superficial veins of the arm and hand (antecubital fossa, or inner elbow; dorsum, or back, of the hand; and forearm veins; Fig. 23–9). Scalp veins are used in infants. Veins in the foot are avoided because infusions in the lower extremities restrict mobility and increase the risk for forming blood clots.

Central venous infusions are those that deliver solutions into large central veins, such as the vena cava (Fig. 23–10). A central venous catheter is inserted by a physician, when the jugular or subclavian veins are directly accessed, or by nurses specially trained to insert a peripherally inserted central catheter (PICC). Central venous catheters are inserted when providing TPN, monitoring central venous pressure, or administering IV solutions when peripheral veins have collapsed or when long-term IV therapy or thrombophlebitis (inflammation of a vein) and **infiltration** has reduced their availability. After insertion of the catheter, a chest radiograph is taken to confirm catheter placement.

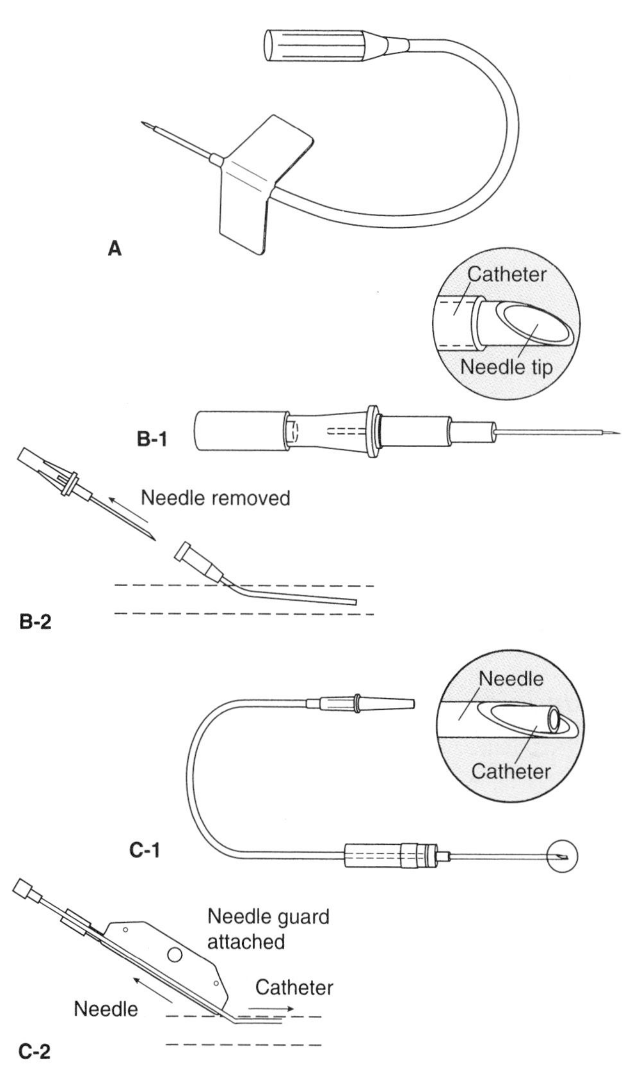

FIGURE 23-8. Venipuncture devices. (A) Butterfly needle. (B-1) Over-the-needle catheter. (B-2) Needle removed. (C-1) Through-the-needle catheter. (C-2) A needle guard covers the tip of the needle, which remains outside the skin.

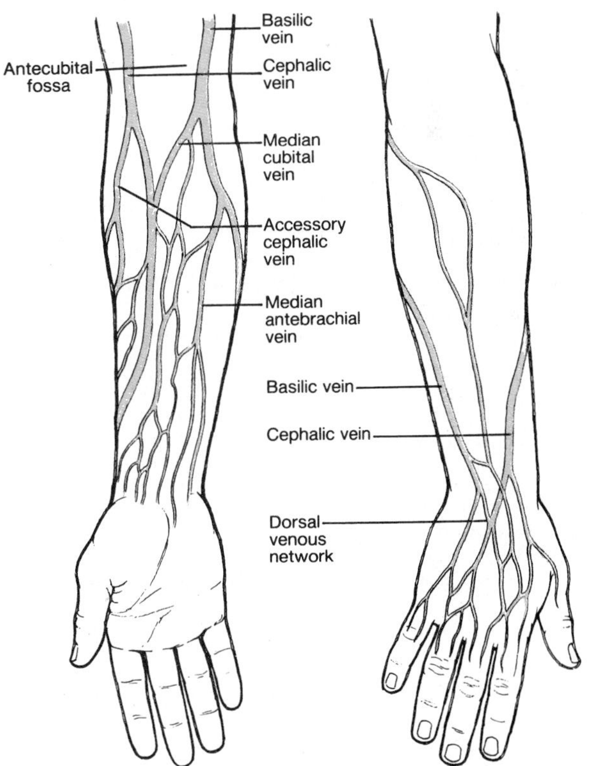

FIGURE 23-9. Venipuncture sites.

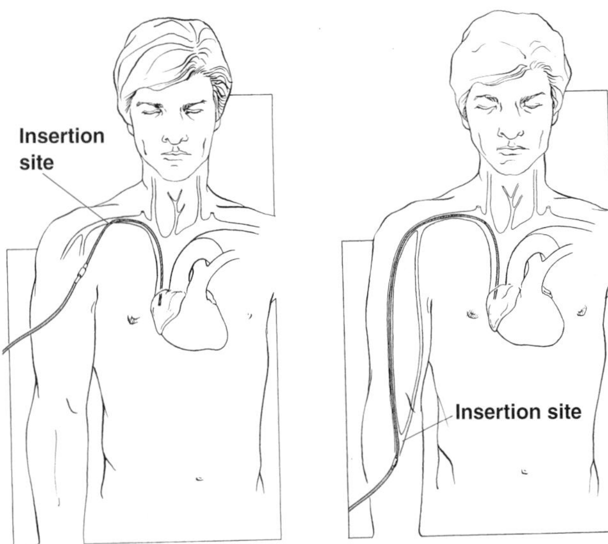

FIGURE 23-10. Examples of central venous catheters. (A) Subclavian insertion, (B) Peripheral insertion.

NURSING PROCESS
The Client Receiving Intravenous Therapy

Assessment

Determine nondominant hand and assess for veins in the forearm that are distant from the wrist and elbow joint. Assess IV site for swelling, warmth, pain, induration. Assess flow rate frequently; assess infusion devices to ensure that they are correctly programmed and functioning properly. Monitor intake and output to determine trends in fluid balance.

Diagnosis and Planning

Nursing care of a client receiving IV therapy includes, but is not limited to the following:

Nursing Diagnoses and Collaborative Problems	Nursing Interventions
Self-Care Deficit (specify type) related to compromised mobility of extremity used for infusion **Goal:** The client will accomplish self-care unhampered by and without disturbing the IV line.	Use a vein in the nondominant hand or arm, if possible and choose a location unaffected by joint movement. Secure IV tubing away from the body. Provide a disposable glove to cover site when washing. Assist client with activities of daily living as needed. Assure client that normal activity will not dislodge the tubing. Place signal device within easy reach of client.
Risk for Infection related to disruption in skin integrity **Goal:** The client will remain free of infection at IV site.	Rotate intravenous sites as per facility policy to prevent infection. Change dressing at intervals outlined in facility policy and more often as indicated. Use aseptic technique when changing dressing, tubing, and bags. Assess site for signs and symptoms of infection. Discontinue infusion and remove cannula if signs and symptoms of infection exist and apply warm soaks to site. Restart infusion in a fresh site.
Risk for Fluid Volume Excess or Deficit related to too rapid or too slow infusion of fluids **Goal:** Fluid balance will be maintained or restored.	Calculate rate of infusion accurately. Monitor time strip hourly. Respond whenever an electronic infusion device sounds an alarm. Record intake and output throughout IV therapy; report marked changes. Assess daily weight and vital signs and other signs of fluid imbalance (see Chap. 21).

Evaluation

- The client is able to use the extremity with minimal inconvenience from the IV infusion.
- The IV site is clean without signs or symptoms of infection.
- The solution infuses at the prescribed rate.

Refer to Nursing Guidelines 23–1 for Administering Total Parenteral Nutrition.

Complications of Intravenous Therapy

There are several complications associated with the infusion of IV solutions. Table 23–4 lists those common when infusing crystalloid solutions and Table 23–5 identifies complications that can occur when administering blood and blood products. Nursing actions are specified in each table.

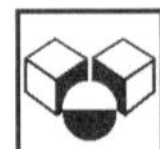

Nursing Guidelines 23-1

Administering Total Parenteral Nutrition

- Weigh client daily.
- Use tubing that contains a filter; however, bypass the filter when administering lipid emulsions to prevent obstructing the filter with large fat molecules.
- Change TPN tubings daily.
- Tape all connections in the tubing to prevent accidental separation and the potential for an air embolism.
- Clamp the central catheter whenever separating the tubing from its catheter connection.
- Use an electronic infusion device to administer TPN.
- Infuse initial TPN solutions gradually (eg, 25–50 mL/h); increase rate according to the agency's standard of care or the physician's medical orders.
- Monitor blood glucose levels regularly to assess the client's ability to metabolize the concentrated glucose.
- Wean client from TPN gradually to avoid a sudden drop in blood sugar.

TABLE 23-4 **Complications of Intravenous Therapy**

Complication	Signs and Symptoms	Cause(s)	Action
Infection	Swelling Discomfort Redness at site Drainage from site	Growth of microorganisms	Change site. Apply antiseptic and dressing to previous site. Report findings.
Circulatory overload	Elevated blood pressure Shortness of breath Bounding pulse Anxiety	Rapid infusion Reduced kidney function Impaired heart contraction	Slow the IV rate. Contact the physician. Elevate the client's head. Give oxygen.
Infiltration (extravasation)	Swelling at the site Discomfort Decrease in infusion rate Cool skin temperature at the site	Displacement of the venipuncture device	Restart the IV. Elevate the arm.
Phlebitis	Redness, warmth, and discomfort along the vein	Administration of irritating fluid Prolonged use of the same vein	Restart the IV. Report the findings. Apply warm compresses.
Thrombus formation	Swelling Discomfort Slowed infusion	Stasis of blood at the catheter, needle tip, or vein	Restart the IV. Report the findings. Apply warm compresses.
Pulmonary embolus	Sudden chest pain Shortness of breath Anxiety Rapid heart rate Drop in blood pressure	Movement of previously stationary blood clot	Stay with the client. Call for help. Administer oxygen.
Air embolism	Same as pulmonary embolus	Failure to purge air from the tubing	Same as for pulmonary embolus, but also place the client's head lower than the feet. Position the patient on left side.

Site Care

Because the venipuncture is a type of wound, it is important to inspect the site at routine intervals observing for signs of infection, infiltration, phlebitis, and thrombus formation (see Table 23–4). Notation of site appearance is documented daily in the client's medical record. A common practice is to change the dressing over the venipuncture site every 24 to 72 hours according to the agency's infection control policy or immediately if complications develop.

Equipment Replacement

Solutions are replaced when they finish infusing or every 24 hours, which ever comes first. Most IV tubing is changed every 72 hours depending on agency policy. Some exceptions include tubing used to administer TPN and tubing used to administer intermittent secondary infusions. Y-tubing used to administer blood can be reused one time for a second unit that immediately follows the first. Medication locks and venipuncture devices are replaced immediately if there is evidence of complications or every 3 days. Central catheters remain in the same site indefinitely.

Discontinuing Intravenous Therapy

Intravenous infusions are discontinued when the solution has infused and no more is scheduled to follow. Refer to Nursing Guidelines 23–2 for Discontinuing an Intravenous Infusion. Alternatively, the venipuncture device may be temporarily capped, and kept patent with the use of a medication lock.

MEDICATION LOCK

A **medication lock** is a sealed chamber that allows intermittent access to a vein. The lock is inserted into the venipuncture device. The vein is kept patent by flushing the lock with saline or heparinized saline. Medication locks are used when the client no longer need continuous infusions, needs intermittent IV medication administration, or may need emergency IV fluids or medications.

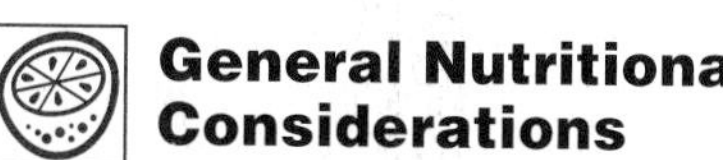

General Nutritional Considerations

When administered parenterally, dextrose provides 3.4 cal/g, not 4 cal/g like carbohydrates consumed orally. Therefore, 1 liter of D_5W, which contains 50 g dextrose, provides a total of 170 calories. Three liters of D_5W infused over 24 hours only provides 510 calories.

TABLE 23-5 **Complications of Blood Transfusion**

Complication	Signs and Symptoms	Cause(s)	Action
Incompatibility reaction	Hypotension, rapid pulse rate, difficulty breathing, back pain, flushing	Mismatch between donor and recipient blood groups	Stop the infusion of blood. Infuse the saline at a rapid rate. Call for assistance. Administer oxygen. Raise the feet higher than the head. Be prepared to administer emergency drugs. Send first urine specimen to laboratory. Save the blood and tubing.
Febrile reaction	Fever, shaking chills, headache, rapid pulse, muscle aches	Allergy to foreign proteins in the donated blood	Stop the blood infusion. Start the saline. Check vital signs. Report findings.
Septic reaction	Fever, chills, hypotension	Infusion of blood that contains microorganisms	Stop the infusion of blood. Start the saline. Report findings. Save the blood and tubing.
Allergic reaction	Rash, itching, flushing, stable vital signs	Minor sensitivity to substances in the donor blood	Slow the rate of infusion. Assess the client. Report findings. Be prepared to give an antihistamine.
Moderate chilling	No fever or other symptoms	Infusion of cold blood	Continue the infusion. Cover and make the client comfortable.
Circulatory overload	Hypertension, difficulty breathing, moist breath sounds, bounding pulse	Large volume or rapid rate of infusion; inadequate cardiac or kidney function	Reduce the rate. Elevate the head. Give oxygen. Report findings. Be prepared to give a diuretic.
Hypocalcemia (low calcium)	Tingling of fingers, hypotension, muscle cramps, convulsions	Multiple blood transfusions containing anticalcium agents	Stop the blood infusion. Start saline. Report findings. Be prepared to give antidote, calcium chloride.
HIV and HbV transmission	Opportunistic infections; elevated antibody titers, abnormal blood cell counts or liver enzyme levels	Blood collected from infected donors that passed screening examinations	Encourage autologous (self) blood collection if possible.

Because simple IV solutions (ie, dextrose in water) are nutritionally and calorically inadequate, clients should not be maintained on them longer than 1 to 2 days.

The composition of TPN formulas are individualized according to the individual client's nutritional requirements and medical condition. Because there are standard concentrations of protein, carbohydrate, and fat in standard volumes, individualization is somewhat limited.

Although IV lipid emulsions offer several advantages (they are isotonic, high in calories and prevent fatty acid deficiency), they are contraindicated for clients with egg allergy, hyperlipidemia, severe liver disease, and acute pancreatitis.

Cyclical TPN, infused over a 10- to 16-hour period with an 8- to 14-hour "rest," is most often used for clients on home TPN or to supplement clients consuming an inadequate oral diet. Cyclical TPN offers the client more mobility, especially if infused during the night, and has the advantage of allowing enzyme and hormone levels to drop to normal levels during the "off" periods. To give the body time to adjust to the decreasing glucose load (eg, prevent rebound hypoglycemia), the infusion should be tapered near the end of each cycle.

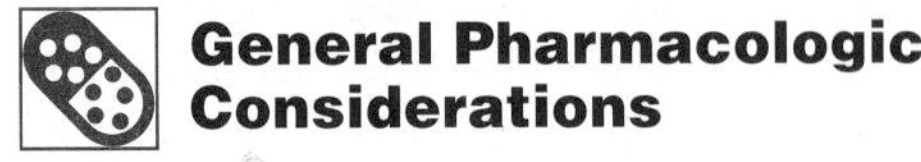

General Pharmacologic Considerations

Read labels carefully on vials containing flush solutions for medication locks. Deaths have occurred when potas-

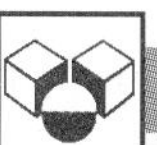

Nursing Guidelines 23-2

Discontinuing an Intravenous Infusion

- Wash your hands.
- Clamp the tubing and remove the tape holding the dressing and venipuncture device in place.
- Don clean gloves.
- Gently press a dry, sterile gauze square over the site (use of an alcohol swab interferes with blood clotting).
- Remove the catheter or needle by pulling it out without hesitation following the course of the vein.
- Continue to apply pressure to the site for 30 to 45 seconds while elevating the forearm to control bleeding.
- Cover the site with a dressing or bandaid.
- Remove gloves and wash your hands.
- Record the time the IV was discontinued, the amount of fluid infused, and the appearance of the venipuncture site.

sium chloride has been used incorrectly to flush a lock or central venous catheter.

Medications are never added to whole blood or to the saline solution used to start the transfusion.

Additive sets and secondary (piggy-back) solution bags are used for intermittent IV drug administration and generally administered in 30 minutes to 2 hours.

Drugs given by the IV route have a more rapid drug effect than when they are given by other routes.

Before adding a drug to an IV solution, the label on the container must be carefully read. Only drugs labeled "for IV use" are given by this route.

Literature must be carefully checked before adding drugs that will be administered by the IV route. Some medications require special dilution or the use of specific diluents or have warnings regarding the maximum dose allowed.

When medications are added to an IV solution, the container is labeled with the name and dose of the medication, the date and time, and the nurse's name who added the medication.

Some IV medications such as dopamine (Intropin) can cause severe tissue damage if they infiltrate. Phentolamine (Regitine) is kept available should dopamine infiltrate. Infiltration is reported to the physician as soon as possible.

Insulin may be added to TPN solutions to facilitate the metabolism of glucose.

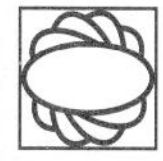

General Gerontologic Considerations

IV solutions usually are given at a slower rate because many older adults have cardiac or renal disorders.

The older adult's skin may be traumatized by the application of a tourniquet. Placing a hand towel or washcloth or the sleeve of the gown over the area may reduce skin trauma.

Because veins of older adults tend to be rigid, difficulty may be encountered during a venipuncture. Poor skin turgor may make it difficult to keep the skin taut over the vein when stabilizing the vein during venipuncture.

Confused or disoriented clients are observed at frequent intervals because excessive movement or pulling on the IV line may dislodge the needle or catheter.

Older adults are more prone to fluid overload and are closely observed for signs and symptoms of this complication.

SUMMARY OF KEY CONCEPTS

- IV therapy is the parenteral administration of fluids and additives into a vein. Substances that are commonly infused include solutions of water and various nutrients, blood and blood products, and medications.
- Crystalloid solutions are composed of water and uniformly dissolved crystals such as salt (sodium chloride) and sugar (glucose, dextrose). Colloid solutions are mixtures of water and molecules of suspended substances like blood cells and plasma proteins like albumin.
- An isotonic solution contains the same concentration of dissolved substances as is normally found in plasma; hypotonic solutions contain fewer dissolved substances, and hypertonic solutions contain more dissolved substances.
- Total parenteral nutrition (TPN) involves IV administration of a nutrient solution designed to meet nearly all the caloric and nutritional needs of clients. A lipid emulsion, which is often administered concurrently, provides additional calories and promotes adequate blood levels of fatty acids.
- Whole blood contains plasma, blood cells, some preservative, and an anticoagulant. Packed cells contain the same except some of the plasma has been removed. Blood products contain solutions with components extracted from blood. Plasma expanders are nonblood solutions that can be used in an emergency to increase the intravascular volume.
- Before initiating IV therapy, the nurse selects and prepares the equipment, prepares the client, selects a venipuncture site, and performs the venipuncture.
- Three items essential when preparing IV solutions include the container of solution, the tubing, and an IV pole or electronic infusion device.
- Three types of IV tubing are primary, secondary, and Y-administration tubing. Components that may be varied include tubing with or without a vent, options in drop size, and the use or elimination of an in-line filter.
- IV therapy can be administered by gravity or an electronic infusion device. Two types of electronic infusion devices are: an infusion pump that exerts positive pressure to infuse solutions and a volumetric controller that infuses IV solutions by gravity by compressing the tubing at a precise preset rate.
- Nurses who have been trained to perform venipunctures do the following: explain the purpose of the procedure at the client's level, assemble needed equipment, inspect and select a vein, and insert the venipuncture device.

- When performing a venipuncture, the nurse can use a butterfly needle, an over-the-needle catheter, or a through-the-needle catheter.
- To prevent occluding blood flow around the venipuncture device, one that is smaller than the diameter of the vein is selected.
- IV therapy is administered through peripheral venous sites or central veins.
- When caring for clients receiving IV therapy, nursing diagnoses common in the plan of care include: *Self-Care Deficit* and *Risk for Fluid Volume Excess or Deficit.* Nursing care also includes assessing for IV therapy complications, caring for the venipuncture site, replacing equipment as needed, and discontinuing the infusion when IV therapy is no longer needed.
- Complications associated with IV therapy include infection, circulatory overload, infiltration, phlebitis, thrombus formation, pulmonary embolus, and air embolus. Complications that can occur when administering blood include incompatibility reactions, febrile reaction, sepsis, mild allergic reactions, hypocalcemia, and bloodborne viral disease transmission.
- Clients who no longer need continuous IV therapy, but may need intermittent IV fluid or medication administration, benefit from having a medication lock.

CRITICAL THINKING EXERCISES

1. Determine the rate of infusion for 1,000 mL of solution ordered to infuse by gravity over 8 hours. You have tubing with a drop factor of 15 gtt/mL. Explain how you determine if the solution is infusing according to the calculated rate.
2. Discuss the nursing care of a client receiving IV therapy.
3. Describe one complication of IV therapy and blood administration, identify its cause, signs and symptoms, and appropriate nursing actions.

Suggested Readings

Clark, A. (1997). The nursing management of intravenous drug therapy. *British Journal of Nursing,* **6**(4), 201–206.

Dougherty, L. (1997). Reducing the risk of complications intravenous therapy. *Nursing Standards, 12*(5), 40–42.

Fitzpatrick, L., & Fitzpatrick, T. (1997). Blood transfusion, keeping your patient safe. *Nursing, 27*(8), 34–41.

Gorski, L. A. (1997). Discharge planning for the patient requiring home intravenous antimicrobial therapy. *Orthopedic Nursing, 16*(3), 43–48.

Intravenous therapy handbook. (1996). *Nursing, 26*(10), 48–51.

Konick-McMahan, J. (1997). Discharged with dobutamine. *RN, 60*(4), 24–28.

Masoorli, S. (1997). Managing complications of central venous access devices. *Nursing, 27*(8), 59–63.

Whitson, M. (1996). Intravenous therapy in the older adult: Special needs and considerations. *Journal of Intravenous Nursing, 19*(5), 251–255.

Wood, D. (1997). A comparative study of 2 securement techniques for short peripheral intravenous catheters. *Journal of Intravenous Nursing, 20*(6), 280–285.

Chapter 24

Caring for Perioperative Clients

KEY TERMS

Anesthesia
Anesthesiologist
Anesthetist
Conscious sedation
Dehiscence
Embolus
Evisceration
Intraoperative
Malignant hyperthermia
Paralytic ileus
Perioperative
Phlebothrombosis
Postoperative
Preoperative
Thrombophlebitis

LEARNING OBJECTIVES

On completion of this chapter, the reader will:

- Identify reasons why surgical procedures may be performed.
- Differentiate the phases of perioperative care.
- Outline the preoperative assessments needed to identify surgical risk factors.
- Develop a preoperative teaching plan.
- Describe members of the surgical team and their function.
- Differentiate the types of anesthesia.
- Describe the criteria for clients admitted for ambulatory surgery.
- Define conscious sedation.
- Identify assessments needed to prevent postoperative complications.
- Describe standards of care, nursing diagnoses, and common interventions for the general surgical client in the later postoperative period.

Surgery, no matter how minor, produces stress and puts the client at risk for possible complications. Many variables, such as procedure performed, age of the client, and coexisting medical conditions determine the care needed by clients before, during, and after surgery. However, undergoing anesthesia and disrupting physiologic processes (creation of the surgical wound and the operation itself) subject clients to a common set of problems that require standardized and individualized assessments and interventions. All clients require thorough preoperative education. The goal of the nurse caring for surgical clients is to minimize their anxiety, prepare them for surgery, and assist in their speedy, uncomplicated recovery.

Surgical procedures are performed on an emergency basis or nonurgent or elective basis. Box 24–1 identifies reasons for surgery. Box 24–2 categorizes surgery in terms of the urgency.

Perioperative Care

Perioperative is a term used to describe the entire span of surgery, including what occurs before, during, and after the actual operation. Three phases of perioperative care are:

- **Preoperative:** begins with the decision to perform surgery and continues until the client has reached the operating area.
- **Intraoperative:** includes the entire duration of the surgical procedure, until the client is transferred to the recovery area.
- **Postoperative**: begins with admission to the recovery area and continues until the client receives a follow-up evaluation at home or is discharged to a rehabilitation unit.

Each of these phases requires specific assessments and nursing interventions.

Preoperative Care

Preoperative care requires that the client have a complete assessment. Even in emergent situations, every effort is made to gather as much data as possible. Client needs must be identified to determine if the

BOX 24-1 Reasons for Surgery

Type of Surgery	Purpose	Example
Diagnostic	Removal and study of tissue to make a diagnosis	Breast biopsy Biopsy of skin lesion
Exploratory	More extensive means to diagnose a problem; generally involves the exploration of a body cavity or the use of scopes inserted through small incisions	Exploration of the abdomen for unexplained pain Exploratory laparoscopy
Curative	Removal of diseased tissue or the replacement of defective tissue to restore function	Cholecystectomy Total hip replacement
Palliative	Relieves symptoms or enhances function without cure	Resection of a tumor to relieve pressure and pain
Cosmetic	Correct defects, improve appearance, or change a physical feature	Rhinoplasty Cleft lip repair Mammoplasty

client is at risk for complications during or following the surgical procedure. General risk factors are related to age; nutritional status; weight; use of alcohol, tobacco, and other substances; physical condition; medical problems; and liver and kidney function. Table 24–1 lists risk factors and related complications.

Assessment

Client assessment varies depending on the urgency of the surgery or whether the client is admitted the same day of surgery or at an earlier time. When the client is admitted, the nurse reviews preoperative instructions, such as diet restrictions and skin preparations, to ensure they have been followed. If the client has not carried out a specific portion of the instructions, such as withholding foods and fluids, the surgeon is immediately notified. Time for preoperative assessment, nursing diagnoses, and evaluation of the nursing management may be limited when a client is admitted for ambulatory surgery or admitted shortly before surgery. Recognition of the client's immediate preoperative needs is important, however, and preparation for surgery still includes the use of the nursing process.

When surgery is not of an emergent nature, a thorough history and physical examination are performed. The client is assessed for knowledge of the surgical procedure, postoperative expectations, and ability to participate in the recovery process. Cultural needs also must be considered, specifically in relation to a client's beliefs about surgery, personal privacy, and presence of family members during the preoperative and postoperative phases. There also may be strong cultural feelings

BOX 24-2 Categories of Surgery Based on Urgency

Classification	Examples
Emergency—without delay Client's condition is life-threatening, requires immediate surgery.	Gunshot wound Severe bleeding Small bowel obstruction
Urgent—within 24 to 30 hours Client requires prompt attention.	Kidney stones Acute gallbladder infection Fractured hip
Required—planned for a few weeks or months following decision Client needs to have surgery at some point.	Benign prostatic hypertrophy Cataracts Hernia without strangulation
Elective—Client will not be harmed if surgery is not performed but will benefit if it is performed.	Revision of scars Vaginal repairs
Optional—personal preference	Cosmetic surgery

Adapted from Smeltzer, S. C., & Bare, B. G. (1996). *Brunner and Suddarth's textbook of medical-surgical nursing* (8th ed., p. 360). Philadelphia: Lippincott-Raven.

TABLE 24-1 **Surgical Risk Factors and Potential Complications**

Variable	Potential Complication
Age	
Very young	
Immaturity of organ systems and regulatory mechanisms	Respiratory obstruction, fluid overload, dehydration, hypothermia, and infection.
Elderly	
Multiple organ degeneration and slowed regulatory mechanisms	Decreased metabolism and excretion of anesthetics and pain medications, fluid overload, renal failure, formation of blood clots, delayed wound healing, infection, confusion, and respiratory complications
Nutritional Status	
Malnourished	
Low weight and nutrient deficiencies	Fluid and electrolyte imbalances, cardiac arrhythmias, delayed wound healing, and wound infections
Obese	
Stressed cardiovascular system, decreased circulation, decreased pulmonary function	Atelectasis, pneumonia, formation of blood clots, delayed wound healing, wound infection, delayed metabolism and excretion of anesthetics and pain medication
Substance Abuse	
Altered respiratory function, nutritional status, or liver function	Atelectasis, pneumonia, altered effectiveness of anesthetics and pain medications, drug interactions, drug withdrawal
Medical Problems	
Respiratory	Atelectasis, bronchopneumonia, respiratory failure
Acute and chronic respiratory problems and history of tobacco use	
Cardiovascular	
Hypertension, coronary artery disease, peripheral vascular disease	Hypo- or hypertension, fluid overload, congestive heart failure, shock, arrhythmias, myocardial infarction, stroke, blood clot formation
Hepatic	
Liver dysfunction	Delayed drug metabolism leading to drug toxicity, disrupted clotting mechanisms leading to excessive bleeding or hemorrhage, confusion, increased risk of infection
Renal	
Kidney disease, chronic renal insufficiency, renal failure	Fluid and electrolyte imbalances, congestive heart failure, arrhythmias, delayed excretion of drugs leading to drug toxicity
Endocrine	
Diabetes	Hypoglycemia, hyperglycemia, hypokalemia, infection, delayed wound healing

regarding disposal of body parts and blood transfusions. Table 24–2 lists information important when assessing the preoperative client. If the surgical procedure is an emergency, some tasks may have to be omitted because of the client's condition or need for rapid preparation for surgery. There may not be time to perform a thorough assessment or write nursing diagnoses.

Surgical Consent

Before surgery, the client must sign a surgical consent form or operative permit. This form, when signed, indicates that the client consents to the procedure and understands the risks and benefits as explained by the surgeon. If the client has not understood the explanations, the surgeon is notified before the client signs the permit. This consent must be obtained for any invasive procedure that requires anesthesia and has risks of complications.

If an adult client is confused, unconscious, or not mentally competent, a family member or guardian must sign the consent. If the client is under age 18, a parent or legal guardian needs to sign the consent. A person under age 18 who is living away from home and is self-supporting is regarded as an emancipated minor and is allowed to sign the consent. In an emergency, the surgeon may have to operate without consent. However, every effort is made to obtain consent via telephone, telegram, or fax. The nurse needs to be familiar with agency policies and state laws regarding surgical consent forms.

TABLE 24-2 **Preoperative Assessment**

Review preoperative laboratory and diagnostic studies:

- Complete blood count
- Blood type and crossmatch
- Serum electrolytes
- Urinalysis
- Chest x-ray
- Electrocardiogram
- Other tests related to procedure or client's medical condition such as prothrombin time, partial thromboplastin time, blood urea nitrogen, creatinine, and other radiographic studies

Review the client's health history and preparation for surgery:

- History of present illness and reason for surgery
- Past medical history
  - Medical conditions—acute and chronic
  - Previous hospitalizations and surgeries
  - History of any past problems with anesthesia
  - Allergies
  - Present medications
  - Substance use:
    - Alcohol
    - Tobacco
    - Street drugs
- Review of systems

Assess physical needs:

- Ability to communicate
- Vital signs
- Level of consciousness
  - Confusion
  - Drowsiness
  - Unresponsiveness
- Weight and height
- Skin integrity
- Ability to move/ambulate
- Level of exercise
- Prostheses
- Circulatory status

Assess psychological needs:

- Emotional state
- Level of understanding of surgical procedure and preoperative and postoperative instructions
- Coping strategies
- Support system
- Roles and responsibilities

Assess cultural needs:

- Language—need for an interpreter
- Particular customs related to surgery, privacy, disposal of body parts, and blood transfusions

The consent form must be signed before the client has received any preoperative sedatives. When the client or designated person has signed the permit, an adult witness signs the permit to indicate that the client or designee signed the permit voluntarily. This person is usually a member of the health care team or employee in the admissions department. The nurse is responsible for ensuring that the consent form has been signed and is in the client's chart before the client goes to the operating room (OR).

Preoperative Teaching

Teaching clients about their surgical procedure and expectations before and after surgery is best done during the preoperative period. Clients are more alert and free of pain during this time. Clients and family members are better able to participate in the recovery if they know what to expect. Instructions and explanations are adapted to the client's ability to understand. The teaching plan addresses the client's cognitive abilities. When clients understand what they can do to help themselves recover, they are more likely to follow the preoperative instructions and work with the health care team members.

The information included in a preoperative teaching plan varies with the type of surgery and the amount of time the client is hospitalized. The following are examples of information to include in preoperative teaching: preoperative medications (when it is given and the effects), postoperative pain control, explanation and description of the postanesthesia recovery room or postsurgical area, and information regarding frequency of vital signs and monitoring equipment. The nurse also explains and demonstrates deep breathing and coughing exercises, use of incentive spirometry, how to splint the incision for breathing exercises and moving, position changes, and feet and leg exercises. The client also needs to be informed about intravenous (IV) fluids and other lines and tubes. Sometimes IV fluids are initiated prior to surgery, along with indwelling catheters or nasogastric tubes.

When clients have received demonstrations, it is important they return the demonstrations to practice these skills and provide an opportunity for the nurse to assess if the client understood the instructions. The preoperative teaching time also gives the client the chance to express any anxieties and fears and for the nurse to provide explanations that will help alleviate those fears.

For clients admitted for emergency surgery, there is no time for detailed explanations of preoperative preparations and the postoperative period. However, if the client is alert, brief explanations should be provided. During the postoperative period, the explanations will need to be more complete. Family members require as many preoperative explanations as possible.

With adequate preoperative teaching/learning, it is expected that the client will have an uncomplicated and shorter recovery period. The client is more likely to deep breathe and cough, move as directed, and require less pain medication. The client and family members demonstrate sufficient knowledge of the surgical procedure, preoperative preparations, and postoperative procedures and are able to participate fully in the client's care.

Preoperative Preparation

Preparing a client for surgery is an essential element of preoperative care and includes both physical and psychosocial preparation.

PHYSICAL PREPARATION

Depending on the time of admission to the hospital or surgical facility, some of the physical preparation may be done. The physical preparation includes:

SKIN PREPARATION. Skin preparation depends on the surgical procedure and the policies of the surgeon or institution. To prevent contamination of the surgical area from microorganisms present on hair and to prevent hair from entering the wound where it acts as a foreign body and interferes with healing, shaving, clipping of hair, or depilatory cream may be used for hair removal. Some institutions do not permit shaving of surgical areas because of the risk of injury to the skin, which provides an entry for microorganisms. To cleanse the skin and decrease the number of microorganisms on the skin, plain soap and water or topical antiseptics such as povidone-iodine are used. Most hospitals have guidelines or charts showing the areas of skin to be prepared (Fig. 24–1). Before any skin preparation, the nurse explains the proce-

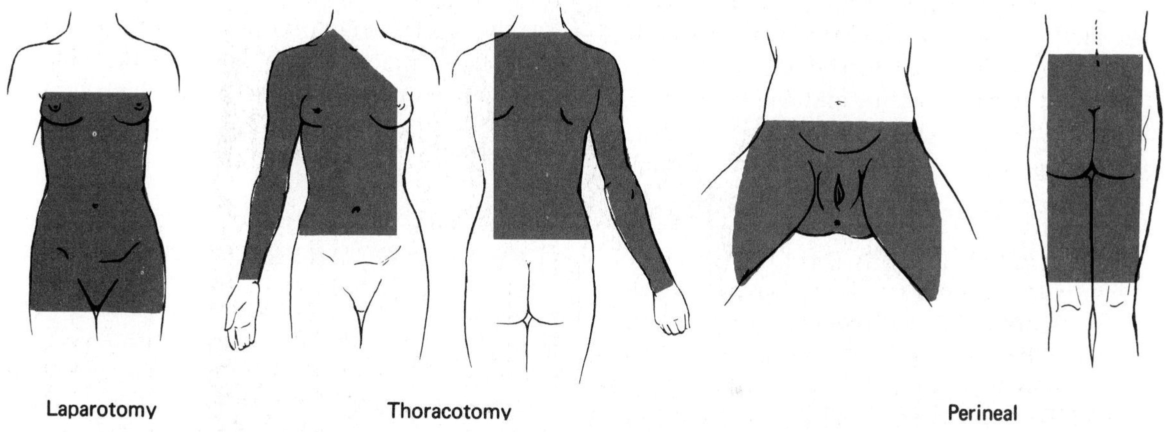

FIGURE 24-1. Areas of skin prepared before laparotomy, thoracotomy, and surgery in the perineal area. Skin preparation is extensive in each of these examples. The procedure of each hospital varies in the designation of the areas to be prepared.

dure. If skin preparation is to be done at home, instructions are given to the client or family.

ELIMINATION. An indwelling urinary catheter may be inserted preoperatively for some surgeries, particularly lower abdominal surgery. A distended bladder creates greater risks of bladder trauma and difficulty in performing the procedure. The catheter keeps the bladder empty during the surgery. If a catheter is not inserted, the client is instructed to void immediately before receiving the preoperative medication.

Enemas may be ordered to clean out the lower bowel, especially if the client is having bowel surgery. Enemas are administered to prevent postoperative impaction and distention or pain associated with straining, remove fecal material before gastrointestinal surgery, prevent involuntary bowel movements during surgery or immediately after, and prevent accidental trauma to the bowel during surgery. A cleansing enema or laxative is prescribed the evening before surgery and may be repeated the morning of surgery. If bowel surgery is scheduled, antibiotics may also be prescribed to reduce intestinal flora.

FOOD AND FLUIDS. The physician gives specific instructions about how long food and fluids are to be withheld before surgery; at least 8 to 10 hours is customary. After midnight the night before surgery, the client is usually not allowed to have anything by mouth (NPO). However, many ambulatory surgical centers allow clear fluids up to 3 or 4 hours before surgery. Before these times, the nurse encourages the client to maintain good nutrition, to help meet the body's increased need for nutrients during the healing process. Protein and ascorbic acid (vitamin C) are especially important in wound healing.

CARE OF VALUABLES. The client is encouraged to give valuables to a family member to take home. However, if this is not possible, they are itemized, placed in an envelope, and locked in a designated area. The client signs a receipt and the nurse notes their disposition on the client's chart. If the client is reluctant to remove a wedding band, gauze is slipped under the ring, then looped around the finger and wrist or adhesive tape is applied over a plain wedding band.

The client also removes eyeglasses and contact lenses. They are placed in a safe location or given to a family member.

ATTIRE AND GROOMING. In general, the client wears a hospital gown and a surgical cap in the OR. Hair ornaments and all makeup and nail polish are removed. Removal of cosmetics assists the surgical team to observe the client's lips, face, and nail beds for signs of cyanosis, pallor, or other signs of decreased oxygenation. If a client has acrylic nails, one is generally removed to attach a pulse oximeter, which measures oxygen saturation (see Chap. 26).

If the client is having minor surgery performed under local anesthesia in a room separate from the general surgical suites, the nurse instructs the client on what clothing and cosmetics to remove and provides appropriate hospital attire. The physician may order thigh-high or knee-high antiembolism stockings or order the client's legs to be wrapped in elastic bandages prior to surgery to help prevent venous stasis during and after the surgery.

PROSTHESES. Depending on agency policy and physician preference, the client removes full or partial dentures. This prevents the dentures from becoming dislodged or causing airway obstruction during administration of a general anesthetic. Some anesthesiologists prefer that well fitting dentures be left in place to preserve facial contours. If dentures are removed, they are usually placed in a denture container and left at the client's bedside or placed with the client's belongings. Other prostheses, such as artificial limbs, also are removed, unless otherwise ordered.

PREOPERATIVE MEDICATIONS

The anesthesiologist frequently orders preoperative medications. Types of medications ordered are shown in Table 24-3.

Before preoperative medications are administered, the nurse checks the client's identification bracelet, asks about drug allergies, obtains the client's blood pressure and pulse and respiratory rates, asks the client to void, and makes sure the surgical consent form has been signed. The nurse also reviews with the client what to expect after receiving the medications. Immediately after receiving the medications, the client is instructed to remain in bed; side rails are placed in the up position, and the call button is placed within easy reach.

PSYCHOSOCIAL PREPARATION

Preparing the client emotionally and spiritually is as important as the physical preparation. Psychosocial preparation should begin as soon as the client is aware that surgery is necessary. Anxiety and fear, if extreme, can affect a client's condition during and after surgery. Anxious clients have a poor response to

TABLE 24-3 **Preoperative Medications**

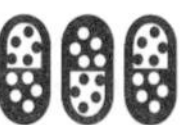

Drug Category/Example	Side Effects	Nursing Considerations/Client Education
Anticholinergics		
Atropine, scopolamine, glycopyrrolate, (Robinul) Used to decrease respiratory tract secretions, dry mucous membranes, and interrupt vaginal stimulation.	Dry mouth Tachycardia Excessive central nervous system stimulation (tremor, restlessness, confusion) followed by excessive central nervous system depression (coma, respiratory depression) Constipation or paralytic ileus Urinary retention Ocular effects: mydriasis, blurred vision, photophobia	Inform the client that a dry mouth may occur, but to refrain from taking oral fluids. Immediately after taking the medications, the client is instructed to remain in bed, side rails are placed in the up position, and the call button is placed in easy reach.
Antiemetics		
Droperidol (Inapsine), promethazine (Phenergan) Used to reduce nausea, prevent emesis and enhance preoperative sedation.	Dry mouth, urinary retention Hypotension, including orthostatic hypotension Extrapyramidal reactions—dyskinesia, dystonia, akathisia, parkinsonism	Inform the client that drowsiness may occur about 20 minutes after administration.
Tranquilizers (hypnotics)		
Diazepam (Valium), flurazam (Dalmane), lorazepam (Ativan) Used to reduce preoperative anxiety and promote induction of anesthesia	Depression of breathing	Inform the client that drowsiness will occur about 20 minutes after administration. Immediately after taking the medications, the client is instructed to remain in bed, side rails are placed in the up position, and the call button is placed in easy reach.
Sedatives		
Midazolam (Vesad), barbiturates: phenobarbital (Nembutal), secobarbital (Seconal), midazolam (Vered) Used to promote sleep, decrease anxiety, and promote the use of anesthesia	Depression of breathing May produce coughing, sneezing, and laryngospasm	Inform the client that drowsiness will occur about 20 minutes after administration. Immediately after taking the medications, the client is instructed to remain in bed, side rails are placed in the up position, and the call button is placed in easy reach. Requires injection, therefore not useful for children because of their small veins.
Opioids (narcotics)		
Morphine, meperidine (Demerol) Used to reduce anxiety and pain, promote sleep, and decrease the amount of anesthesia needed	May slow rate of respiration Hypotension Dizziness, nausea, and vomiting Constipation	Inform the client that drowsiness will occur about 20 minutes after administration. Immediately after taking the medications, the client is instructed to remain in bed, side rails are placed in the up position, and the call button is placed in easy reach.

surgery and are prone to complications. Many clients are fearful because they know little or nothing about what will happen before, during, and after surgery. Fear and anxiety may be resolved by careful preoperative teaching. Careful listening and explanations by the nurse as to what will happen and what to expect can help allay some of these fears and anxieties. The nurse also needs to assess methods used for coping. Religious faith is a source of strength for many clients; therefore, it is important for clients to have contact with their clergy or the hospital chaplain if requested.

PREOPERATIVE CHECKLIST

Most clients are transported to the OR on a stretcher. To provide privacy, safety, and warmth, the nurse covers the client with a blanket and fastens the restraint straps around the client.

Most hospitals or surgical facilities use a preoperative checklist to ensure that all assessments and procedures for the client are complete before surgery. A checklist generally includes:

- *Assessment*: including identification and allergy bracelet on; identification of allergies; listing of current medications; last time the client ate or drank; disposition of valuables, dentures, or prostheses; makeup and nail polish removed; and hospital attire on
- *Preoperative medications*: including route and time administered
- *IV*: including location, type of solution, rate
- *Preoperative preparations*: including, as appropriate, skin preparation, indwelling urinary catheter or nasogastric tube insertion, time and results of enemas or douches, application of antiembolism stockings or wraps, and time and amount of last voiding
- *Chart*: including signed surgical consent, history and physical completed by physician, old records with chart, test results (eg, electrocardiogram, complete blood count, urinalysis, type and screen or type and crossmatch for blood transfusions)
- *Other information*: as required by agency policy
- *Signature(s)*: of nurse and other personnel involved with preparing the client for surgery and transporting the client to the OR

When the preoperative checklist is complete, the client is ready to go to the operating suite. Personnel from the OR assist in the transfer of the client to the stretcher, then to the OR or surgical holding area.

Intraoperative Care

The intraoperative period begins when the client is transferred to the operating table. The surgical team is responsible for the care of the client during this time.

Surgical Team

The surgical team consists of an anesthesiologist or anesthetist, the surgeon and assistants, and the intraoperative nurses.

The **anesthesiologist** is a physician who has completed 2 years of residency in anesthesia. This person is responsible for administering anesthesia to the client and for monitoring the client during and after the surgical procedure. The anesthesiologist assesses the client preoperatively, writes preoperative medication orders, informs the client of the options for anesthesia, and explains the risks involved.

The **anesthetist** may be a medical doctor who administers anesthesia but has not completed a residency in anesthesia, a dentist who administers limited types of anesthesia, or a registered nurse who has completed an accredited nurse anesthesia program and passed the certification examination (Certified Registered Nurse Anesthetist [CRNA]). An anesthetist is supervised by an anesthesiologist and is able to assess the client preoperatively, discuss options for anesthesia, write preoperative medication orders, administer anesthesia, and monitor the client during and after surgery. The anesthesiologist and anesthetist are not sterile members of the surgical team, meaning that they wear OR attire but they do not wear sterile gowns or work within the sterile field.

The *surgeon* heads the surgical team and is a physician, oral surgeon, or podiatrist with specific training and qualifications. The surgeon is responsible for determining the surgical procedure required, obtaining the client's consent, performing the procedure, and following the client postoperatively.

Surgical assistants are classified as either first, second or third assistants. The first assistant assists in the surgical procedure and may be involved with the preoperative and postoperative care of the client. This person may be another physician, a surgical resident, or a registered nurse who has received appropriate approval and endorsement from the American Operating Room Nurses and the American College of Surgeons. Second or third assistants are registered nurses, licensed practical nurses, or surgical technologists who assist the surgeon and first assistant. All assistants are sterile members of the surgical team—they wear sterile gloves and gowns over OR attire and work within the sterile field.

Intraoperative nurses include the *scrub nurse* and *circulating nurse.* The scrub nurse wears a sterile gown and gloves and assists the surgical team by handing instruments to the surgeon and assistants, preparing sutures, receiving specimens for laboratory examination, and counting sponges and needles. The circulating nurse wears OR attire but not a sterile gown. Responsibilities include obtaining and opening wrapped sterile equipment and supplies before and during surgery, keeping records, adjusting lights, receiving specimens for laboratory examination, and coordinating activities of other personnel, such as the pathologist and radiology technician.

Anesthesia

Anesthesia is the partial or complete loss of the sensation of pain with or without the loss of consciousness. Surgical procedures are performed with general, regional, or local anesthesia.

GENERAL ANESTHESIA

General anesthesia produces loss of sensation, reflexes, and consciousness by acting on the central nervous system. Vital functions such as breathing, circulation, and temperature control are not regulated physiologically when general anesthetics are used. General anesthetics are administered as IV, intramuscular, inhaled, or rectal medications. General anesthesia has four distinct but overlapping stages:

- *Induction or beginning stage*: This short period of time is crucial for producing unconsciousness. The client experiences dizziness, detachment, a temporary heightened sense of awareness to noises and movements, and a sensation of "heavy" extremities and not being able to move them. This phase is produced by IV or inhaled anesthetics. When unconsciousness occurs, the client's airway is secured with an endotracheal tube.
- *Maintenance of surgical anesthesia*: During this stage the client is maintained in an unconscious state, ranging from light to deep, depending on the depth of anesthesia required for the surgery. Generally this stage is maintained with a combination of IV and inhaled anesthetics. The client's vital functions are closely monitored.
- *Emergence from surgical anesthesia*: This stage is critical for the client as the anesthetics are carefully withdrawn. Generally the client wakes enough to follow commands and demonstrate the ability to breathe independently. The endotracheal tube is frequently removed while the client is in the OR, but in some cases, may be left in place for much of the recovery period.
- *Recovery period*: This period can be brief or long. Many of the effects of general anesthesia take some time to be eliminated completely. Clients often do not remember much about the initial recovery period.

Throughout the duration of and recovery from anesthesia the client is closely monitored for effective breathing and oxygenation, effective circulatory status including blood pressure and pulse within normal ranges, effective regulation of temperature, and adequate fluid balance.

REGIONAL ANESTHESIA

Regional anesthesia uses local anesthetics to block the conduction of nerve impulses in a specific region. The client experiences loss of sensation and decreased mobility to the specific area that is anesthetized. The client does not lose consciousness. Depending on the surgery, the client may be given a sedative before the local anesthetic, to promote relaxation and comfort during the procedure. Types of regional anesthesia include local anesthetics, spinal anesthesia, and conduction blocks. Table 24–4 describes regional anesthesia.

TABLE 24-4 **Regional Anesthesia**

Type of Regional Anesthesia	Anesthetic Uses and Effects	Examples
Local anesthesia	Provides local loss of sensation; used primarily for dental procedures, eye surgeries, and minor surgical procedures. Administered topically, or via local infiltration when medicine is injected into and under the epidural surface around the area to be treated.	procaine (Novocaine) lidocaine (Xylocaine) bupivacaine (Marcaine) dibucaine (Nupercaine)
Spinal anesthesia	Local anesthetic is injected into the subarachnoid space of the lumbar area (usually L4 or L5). This space contains cerebrospinal fluid. This process anesthetizes spinal nerves as they exit the spinal cord. This type of anesthesia is used for surgical procedures involving the abdomen, perineum, and lower extremities.	procaine (Novocaine) lidocaine (Xylocaine) tetracaine (Pontocaine)
Epidural block	Local anesthetic is injected into the extradural space near the spinal cord. Several spinal nerves are anesthetized at the same time. Although similar to spinal anesthesia, the headache that frequently follows spinal anesthesia does not occur. However, greater technical competence is required.	Anesthetics used for epidural blocks are the same as above. Opioids such as morphine or fentanyl may be added to enhance the anesthetic effect and to provide analgesia when the block has worn off.
Peripheral nerve block	Local anesthetic is injected in a specific body region and directed at a particular nerve or group of nerves. Peripheral nerve blocks are named according to the region in which the anesthetic is injected. Examples are brachial plexus block, ulnar nerve block, and sciatic nerve block. Injection of peripheral nerve blocks requires a high level of technical competence.	lidocaine (Xylocaine) mepivacaine (Carbocaine) bupivacaine (Marcaine)

Advantages of regional anesthesia include less risk for respiratory, cardiac, or gastrointestinal complications. The client needs to be monitored for signs of allergic reactions, changes in vital signs, and toxic reactions. In addition, the anesthetized area must be protected from injury while sensation is absent. The client is at risk for injuries and burns.

The Operating Room Environment

The OR or surgical suite environment is physically isolated from other areas of the hospital or surgical clinic. This restricts access to the area, so that only authorized OR personnel and surgical clients are in the area. Within the surgical suite air is filtered and positive pressure maintained to reduce the number of possible microbes that can cause infection. There are also separate clean and contaminated areas. Surgical suites are designed to be efficient, in that the needed equipment and supplies are immediately available for use. Generally the furniture is made of stainless steel for easy cleaning and disinfecting. The temperature in the OR is kept below 70°F to provide a cooler environment that does not promote bacterial growth, to offer more comfort for OR personnel working in bright lights and wearing OR attire, and to maintain a temperature that enhances client comfort and safety.

Operating room personnel wear specific attire that decreases the opportunity for microbial growth. There is strict adherence as to where clothes are changed, what is worn in the OR, and what protective attire personnel must wear. Table 24–5 identifies typical OR attire. In addition, OR personnel must report any symptoms of infection they are experiencing, because colds, sore throats, and skin infections are potential sources of infection to the client.

TABLE 24-5 **Operating Room Attire**

Attire	Scrubs—tops, pants with cuffs, jackets with cuffs. Changing rooms are located near the operating room; personnel change into OR Attire before entering the OR and take OR attire off when they leave.
Mask	Masks are worn at all times when in the OR; they are changed between surgical procedures or if they become wet.
Headgear	Headgear is worn so that the hair and hairline is covered. Beards must also be covered.
Shoes	OR personnel wear shoes that are comfortable. Agencies vary in specific requirements. Shoe covers are also worn over the shoes. The conductive covers provide an electrical ground.

Nursing Management

Nursing management during the intraoperative period depends on routine tasks performed by nursing personnel in surgery as well as on variables such as type of surgery performed, type of anesthesia used, client's age and condition, and occurrence of complications.

Asepsis in the OR is the responsibility of all OR personnel. The risk of infection is high because of the break in skin integrity from the surgical incision. The client's own pathogens, plus those of the OR, create an unsafe environment if aseptic technique is not strictly adhered to. Protocols for asepsis are strictly followed to protect the client as much as possible.

The safety and protection of the client during surgery is essential. Assessment of the client in the OR is largely based on the type or extent of surgery, the client's age, and any preexisting conditions. Depending on circumstances, assessment before the administration of the anesthetic may include blood pressure, pulse, respiratory rate, and level of consciousness; evaluation of the client's general physical condition; examination for the presence of catheters and tubes; and review of the client's chart, including a signed operative permit; administration of preoperative medications (time, dose, client response); voiding; skin preparation; carrying out other preoperative orders; and laboratory and diagnostic tests.

POSSIBLE INTRAOPERATIVE COMPLICATIONS

Operating room nurses assess the client continuously and protect the client from potential complications, including:

- *Infection*: Strict aseptic technique is followed before and during surgery. If a break in technique is noted, it is immediately brought to the attention of the surgeon and OR personnel. Clients are also at risk for the retention of foreign objects in the wound. The scrub nurse and circulating nurse count surgical instruments, gauze sponges, and sharps to prevent this problem. The circulating nurse records the counts on the intraoperative record.
- *Fluid volume excess or deficit*: The anesthesiologist usually adds fluids to the IV lines, but the circulating nurse may also perform this function. The circulating nurse is responsible for recording and keeping a running total of IV fluids administered. If the client has an indwelling catheter, urine output is measured during surgery.
- *Injury related to positioning*: The client is positioned on the OR table according to the type of surgery. Careful positioning and monitoring help to prevent

interruption of blood supply and nerve injury secondary to prolonged pressure, nerve injury related to prolonged pressure, postoperative hypotension, dependent edema, and joint injury related to poor body alignment.

- *Hypothermia*: During the procedure, the client is at risk for hypothermia related to the low temperature in the OR, administration of cold IV fluids, inhalation of cool gases, exposure of body surfaces for the surgical procedure, opened incisions/wounds, and prolonged inactivity. For some surgeries, the body temperature is deliberately lowered to make the procedure safer (Smeltzer & Bare, 1996).
- **Malignant hyperthermia:** This disorder is manifested by a rapid and progressive rise in body temperature. There is an uncontrolled increase in muscle metabolism and heat production in response to stress and some anesthetic agents. Symptoms include tachycardia, tachypnea, cyanosis, fever, muscle rigidity, diaphoresis, mottled skin, hypotension, irregular heart rate, decreased urine output, and cardiac arrest. Prevention of malignant hyperthermia is essential because the mortality rate is high. Clients at risk include "those with bulky, strong muscles, a history of muscle cramps or muscle weakness and unexpected temperature elevation and an unexplained death of a family member during surgery that was accompanied by a febrile response" (Smeltzer & Bare, 1996, p. 388). The circulating nurse closely monitors the client for signs of hyperthermia. If the client's temperature begins to rise rapidly, anesthesia is discontinued and the OR team implements measures to correct physiologic problems, such as fever or arrhythmias.

Nursing interventions to prevent or reverse hypothermia include warming intravenous fluids to body temperature; replacing wet drapes and gowns with dry ones; warming the client gradually; monitoring the client's temperature and other vital signs constantly; maintaining the client's oxygenation; and assessing the client's fluid balance.

Postoperative Care

The postoperative period designates the time the client spends recovering from the effects of anesthesia. Factors such as the client's age and nutritional status, preexisting diseases, type of surgery performed, and length of anesthesia may affect the duration of this period and the type and extent of nursing management. Immediately after completion of the surgical procedure, the client is transported to the postanesthesia care unit (PACU) also known as the recovery room located near the OR (Fig. 24–2). The nursing staff is specifically knowledgeable in the care of clients recovering from anesthesia. Specialized equipment is available to monitor and treat the client. Surgical and anesthesia personnel are immediately available for any emergencies.

Nursing Management During the Immediate Postoperative Period

The circulating nurse or anesthesiologist reports pertinent information regarding the surgery including any complications that occurred to the nurses in the PACU. The most important aspect of nursing management is close observation and monitoring of the client during emergence from anesthesia.

IMMEDIATE POSTOPERATIVE CARE

Initial assessment of the client postoperatively includes airway patency; effectiveness of respirations; presence of artificial airways, mechanical ventilation, or supplemental oxygen; circulatory status; vital signs; wound condition including dressings and drains; fluid balance including IV fluids, output from catheters and drains, and ability to void; level of consciousness; and pain. The nurse's major responsibilities during the client's PACU stay are to ensure a

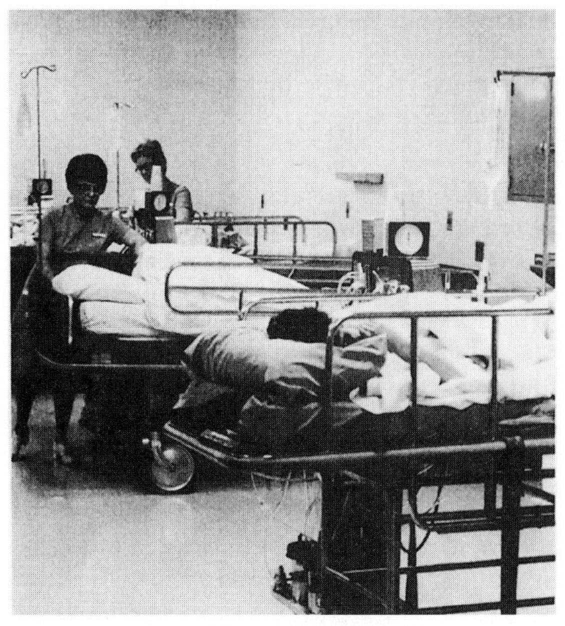

FIGURE 24-2. The client in the PACU is under the continuous surveillance of highly skilled personnel. (Photograph by D. Atkinson)

patent airway; help maintain adequate circulation; prevent or assist with the treatment of shock; maintain proper position and function of drains, tubes, and IV infusions; and monitor for potential complications.

POSTOPERATIVE COMPLICATIONS

During the first 24 hours after surgery, the nurse closely observes the client for signs of hemorrhage, shock, hypoxia, vomiting, and aspiration.

Hemorrhage

Hemorrhage can be internal or external. If the client loses a large amount of blood, the client will exhibit signs and symptoms of shock (see Chap. 22). The nurse inspects dressings frequently for signs of bleeding and checks the bedding under the client because blood may pool under the body and be more evident on the bedding than on the dressing. If the bleeding is internal, it may be necessary to return the client to surgery for ligation of the bleeding vessels. Blood transfusions may be necessary to replace the blood lost. When bleeding occurs, the nurse notes the amount and color of the blood on the chart. Bright red blood signifies fresh bleeding; dark, brownish blood indicates older blood. Reinforce dressings if they are soiled or saturated. A written order is needed to change dressings. The nurse also must be aware of any wound drains and the type and amount of drainage expected. If expected, explain to the client that the drainage is normal and does not indicate a complication. Incontinence pads are placed under the client if drainage occurs.

Shock

Fluid and electrolyte loss, trauma (both physical and psychological), anesthetics, and preoperative medications may all play a part in causing shock. Signs and symptoms include pallor, fall in blood pressure, weak and rapid pulse rate, restlessness, and cool, moist skin. Shock must be detected early and treated promptly because it can result in irreversible damage to vital organs such as the brain, kidneys, and heart.

Narcotics are not administered to a client in shock until a physician evaluates the client. The client in shock should remain flat. Some physicians advocate elevation of the legs to enhance the flow of venous blood to the heart. The treatment of shock varies and depends on the cause, if known. Blood, plasma expanders, parenteral fluids, oxygen, and medications such as adrenergics may be used.

Hypoxia

Factors such as residual drug effects or overdose, pain, poor positioning, pooling of secretions in the lungs, or obstructed airway predispose the client to hypoxia (decreased oxygen). Oxygen and suction equipment must be available for immediate use. The nurse observes the client closely for signs of cyanosis and dyspnea. Breathing may be obstructed if the tongue falls back and obstructs the nasopharynx. If this occurs, insert an oropharyngeal airway (Fig. 24–3). Position the client on his or her side to relieve nasopharyngeal obstruction. Restlessness, crowing or grunting respirations, diaphoresis, bounding pulse, and rising blood pressure may indicate respiratory obstruction. If a client cannot effectively breathe, mechanical ventilation is used.

Vomiting

Postoperative vomiting can be caused by the anesthetics used; by drugs administered before, during, or immediately after surgery; or by the surgery itself. Some clients experience nausea and vomiting when taking fluids for the first time after surgery. Others vomit in the immediate postanesthesia period, before they have even attempted to take oral fluids.

During the early postoperative period, the client needs to have an emesis basin within easy reach. The nurse monitors the amount and nature of the emesis and observes the client for signs and symptoms of dehydration and electrolyte imbalance (see Chap. 21). If vomiting is severe or prolonged, the nurse notifies

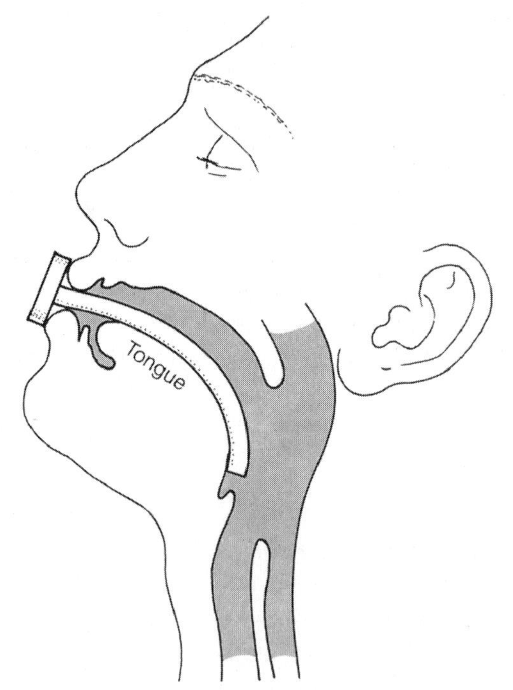

FIGURE 24-3. Oropharyngeal airway in place. The airway prevents the tongue of the unconscious client from blocking the air passages. As long as the airway is unobstructed and in place, air has a free route between the pharynx and the outside.

the physician. Once the client is examined by a physician, oral feedings may be temporarily discontinued, IV fluids administered, and, in some instances, a nasogastric tube inserted and connected to suction. An antiemetic agent may be given if nausea and vomiting persist.

Aspiration

A danger of aspiration from saliva, mucus, vomitus, or blood exists until the client is fully awake and able to swallow. Suction equipment must be kept at the client's bedside until the danger of aspiration no longer exists. The nurse closely observes the client for difficulty swallowing or handling of oral secretions. Unless contraindicated, the client is placed in a side-lying position until oral secretions can be swallowed.

Nursing Management During the Later Postoperative Period

The later postoperative period begins when the client arrives in the hospital room or postsurgical care unit. Because many postoperative problems can be anticipated and prevented or minimized, it is important that nurses approach the care of the client in a systematic, standardized manner. See Nursing Standards for Care of the Postsurgical Client for standards of care, commonly used nursing diagnoses, collaborative problems, and nursing interventions.

Assessment of the client postoperatively includes assessment of respiratory function; evaluation of the client's general condition; measurement and recording of vital signs; assessment of cardiovascular function and fluid status; assessment of pain level; assessment of bowel and urinary elimination; and inspection of dressings, tubes, drains, and IV lines.

RESPIRATION

The nurse focuses on promoting gas exchange and preventing atelectasis. Hypoventilation related to anesthesia, postoperative positioning, and pain is a common problem. Pre- and postoperative instructions include teaching the client to deep breathe and cough and how to splint the incision to minimize pain. Clients who have abdominal or thoracic surgery have greater difficulty taking deep breaths and coughing. Some clients require supplemental oxygen. Nursing management to prevent postoperative respiratory problems includes early mobility, frequent changes in position, deep breathing and coughing exercises, and use of incentive spirometer.

Hiccups (*singultus*) may also interfere with breathing. They result from intermittent spasms of the diaphragm and may occur after surgery, especially abdominal surgery. They may be mild and last for only a few minutes. Prolonged periods of hiccups not only are unpleasant but may cause pain or discomfort and may result in wound dehiscence or evisceration, inability to eat, nausea and vomiting, exhaustion, and fluid, electrolyte, and acid–base imbalances. If hiccups persist, the nurse needs to notify the physician.

CIRCULATION

The nurse must assess the client's blood pressure and circulatory status frequently. Although problems with postoperative bleeding decrease as the recovery time advances, the client may still be at risk for bleeding. Some clients experience syncope when moving to an upright position. To prevent this (and the danger of falling), the nurse has the client slowly move to an upright or standing position.

The client is also at risk for impaired venous circulation related to immobility. When clients lie still for long periods without moving their legs, blood may flow sluggishly through the veins (venous stasis) predisposing the client to venous inflammation and clot formation within the veins (**thrombophlebitis**), or clot formation with minimal or absent inflammation (**phlebothrombosis**). These two conditions most frequently occur in the lower extremities. If the clot travels in the bloodstream (an **embolus**) it has the potential to obstruct circulation to a vital organ such as the lungs and cause severe symptoms and possibly death.

To prevent venous stasis and other circulatory complications, the nurse encourages the client to move legs frequently and do leg exercises, does not use pillows under the knees or calves unless ordered, avoids pressure to the client's lower extremities, applies elastic bandages or antiembolism stockings as ordered, ambulates the client as ordered, and administers low-dose subcutaneous heparin every 12 hours as ordered (frequently ordered for clients who have had abdominal, pelvic, or thoracic surgery and are over 40 years of age).

PAIN MANAGEMENT

Most clients experience pain after an operation and a range of analgesics are usually ordered postoperatively. The most severe pain occurs during the first 48 hours after surgery. Pain creates varying degrees of anxiety and emotional responses. If accompanied by great fear, the degree of pain can increase. It is important that clients receive pain and discomfort relief. When patient-controlled analgesia (PCA) is used, clients administer their own analgesic (see Chap. 20).

The nurse must assess the client for adverse effects of analgesics, timing of the medication in relation to other activities, effect of other comfort measures, contraindications, and source of the pain. The need for pain medications depends on the type and extent of the surgery and the client. Pain unrelieved by medication may signal a developing complication, which underscores the need for a thorough assessment of the cause and type of pain (see Chap. 20).

FLUIDS AND NUTRITION

Intravenous fluids usually are administered after surgery. Length of administration depends on the type of surgery performed and the client's ability to take oral fluids. The nurse monitors the IV fluid flow rate and adjusts the rate as needed. The nurse also assesses the client for signs of fluid excess or deficit (see Chap. 21) and notifies the physician if these signs occur.

Many clients complain of thirst in the early postoperative recovery period. Because anesthesia slows peristalsis, ingesting liquids before bowel activity resumes can lead to nausea and vomiting. Pain medications also may cause nausea and vomiting. See Nursing Guidelines 24–1 for factors to consider before resuming oral fluids.

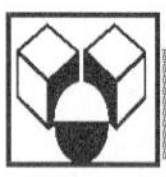

Nursing Guidelines 24-1:

Resuming Oral Fluids After Surgery

Most clients can begin to take fluids within 4 to 24 hours after surgery, unless the surgery has involved the gastrointestinal tract. The nurse must check to make sure that the physician's orders allow fluids to be given.

- If not allowed oral fluids, the client may use mouth rinses and a cool, wet cloth or ice chips against the lips to relieve dryness.
- Before giving fluids, the nurse assesses that the client has recovered sufficiently from anesthesia to be able to swallow. The nurse asks the client to try swallowing without drinking anything. If this can be done, the nurse may offer the client a small sip of water or a few ice chips.
- The nurse gives only a few sips of water or ice chips at a time. Fluids are introduced slowly and given in small amounts to prevent vomiting from occurring. Fluids can be given through a straw so the client does not have to sit up. However, once the client is able to sit up, straws are discouraged because clients tend to swallow air as well, which can lead to abdominal distention and gastric discomfort.
- If vomiting occurs, the nurse reassures the client that this should cease in a short time. The nurse offers mouthwash to remove the taste of anesthetics and vomitus. Antimetics are given as indicated.

Once peristalsis has returned and clear liquids are tolerated, dietary intake is increased. The dietary progression (eg, from clear liquids to a full, solid diet) often depends on the type of surgery performed, the client's progress, and physician preference. IV fluids usually are discontinued when the client is able to take oral fluids and food and nutritional needs are met.

SKIN INTEGRITY/WOUND HEALING

A surgical incision is a wound or injury to skin integrity. There are three modes of wound healing:

- *Primary intention*: The wound layers are sutured together so that wound edges are well approximated. This type of incision generally heals within 8 to 10 days, with minimal scarring.
- *Secondary intention*: Granulating tissue fills in the wound for the healing process. The skin edges are not approximated. This method is used for ulcers and infected wounds. This type of wound healing is slow, although new products have assisted in faster healing.
- *Tertiary intention*: The approximation of wound edges is delayed secondary to infection. When the wound is drained and clean of infection, the wound edges are sutured together. The resulting scar is wider than that with primary intention.

The key to healing is adequate blood flow. Healing is delayed when the blood supply to the wound site is poor. Excessive tension or pulling on wound edges also can delay healing. The nurse must be alert for signs and symptoms of impaired circulation, such as swelling, coldness, absence of pulse, pallor, or mottling, and report them immediately. The nurse must be careful when changing dressings to avoid damaging new tissue as well as causing the client unnecessary discomfort. Packings and dressings that adhere to the wound bed may be soaked with normal saline to assist in easier removal. The client must be closely monitored for signs and symptoms of wound infection such as increased incisional pain; redness, swelling, and heat around the incision; purulent drainage; fever and chills; headache; and anorexia. Treatment of wound infections includes antibiotics, wound treatment, and measures to promote healing such as adequate nutrition and rest.

Other complications of wound healing are dehiscence and evisceration. Wound **dehiscence** is the separation of wound edges without the protrusion of organs. **Evisceration** occurs when there is complete separation of the wound and protrusion of organs. These complications are most likely to occur within 7 to 10 days following surgery. Predisposing factors for wound disruption include: malnutrition, particularly insufficient protein and vitamin C; defective suturing; unusual strain on the incision such as from severe coughing or sneezing, prolonged vomiting, dry heaves, and hiccuping; obesity; enlarged abdomen; and abdominal wall weakened by other surgeries. The client may complain of something "giving away." Pinkish drainage may appear suddenly on the dressing. If wound disruption is suspected, the nurse places the client in a position that puts the least strain on the operative area. If evisceration occurs, the nurse should place sterile dressings moistened with normal saline over the protruding organs and tissues. For any wound disruption, the physician needs to be notified immediately.

ACTIVITY

When possible, ambulatory activities are started shortly after surgery. Factors such as pain tolerance, response to analgesics, general physical condition, and the desire to participate affect the client's ability to be active. Some clients need encouragement, and the importance of increasing activities is stressed. The nurse assists the client to a sitting position at the side of the bed. If dizziness occurs and is more than momentary, the client is returned to a supine position. When the client is able to stand, the nurse assists and supports the client. Assistance with ambulation is continued until it is determined that the client can walk independently. Some clients experience moderate to severe fatigue after surgery. For these clients, the nurse plans care so that activities such as ambulation and personal care are spaced throughout the day.

If the client has received regional anesthesia, activity may initially be restricted. Unless ordered otherwise, the client who has received spinal anesthesia remains flat for 6 to 12 hours. The nurse turns the client from side to side at least every 2 hours. As the anesthesia wears off, the client begins to have a pins-and-needles sensation in the anesthetized parts and pain is felt in the operative area. Clients who develop a headache after spinal anesthesia may have to remain lying flat for a longer period. At first, the client experiences numbness and a feeling of heaviness in the anesthetized area. It may be necessary to reassure the client that the numbness is typical and will subside in a short time.

ELIMINATION: BOWEL

Constipation may occur after the client begins to take solid food and is caused by inactivity, diet, or narcotic analgesics. Some clients experience diarrhea, which may be caused by diet, medications such as antibiotics, or the surgical procedure. The nurse maintains a record of bowel movements and notifies the physician if either of these problems occurs.

Abdominal distention results from the accumulation of gas (flatus) in the intestines because of failure of the intestines to propel gas through the intestinal tract by peristalsis. Contributing factors include manipulation of the intestines during abdominal surgery, inactivity after surgery, interruption of normal food and fluid intake, swallowing of large qualities of air, and anesthetics and medications given during or after surgery. If the symptoms are mild, they can be treated with nursing measures. Clients who are permitted out of bed are encouraged and assisted to ambulate. Sometimes walking, plus privacy in the bathroom, enables the client to expel the gas. The nurse encourages clients to change position frequently and to eat as normally as possible within the allowed dietary limits. If discomfort is severe or is not relieved promptly by nursing measures, the physician needs to be contacted.

Sometimes a serious condition called **paralytic ileus** occurs in which the intestines are paralyzed and, thus, peristalsis is absent. Fluids, solids, and gas do not move through the intestinal tract. Bowel sounds are absent, the abdomen is distended, and abdominal pain often is severe. Vomiting also may occur. If the client complains of severe abdominal pain, assessment includes inspecting the abdomen for distention, palpating for rigidity, and auscultating for bowel sounds. If bowel sounds are absent or sound abnormal or the abdomen is distended or rigid, the nurse notifies the physician immediately. A nasogastric tube usually is inserted and food and fluids withheld until bowel sounds return.

Acute gastric dilatation, a condition in which the stomach becomes distended with fluids, is a complication similar to paralytic ileus. The client may regurgitate small amounts of liquid, the abdomen appears distended, and, as the condition progresses, symptoms of shock may develop. Treatment includes inserting a nasogastric tube, applying suction, and removing the gas and fluid. Some surgeons routinely use suction of the gastrointestinal tract to prevent paralytic ileus and acute gastric dilatation.

ELIMINATION: URINARY

Some clients experience difficulty voiding after surgery, particularly lower abdominal and pelvic surgery. Operative trauma in the region near the bladder may temporarily decrease the sensation of the need to void. Fear of pain also causes tenseness and difficulty voiding. If the client has an indwelling catheter, the nurse monitors urine output frequently. If the client does not have a catheter, the nurse assesses the client's ability to void and measures urine output. If the client is unable to void within 8 hours following surgery, the physician is notified unless there are catheterization orders. Signs and symptoms of bladder distention include restlessness, lower abdominal pain, discomfort or distention, and fluid intake without urinary output.

PSYCHOSOCIAL CARE

Many clients experience anxiety and fear following surgery, as well as an inability to cope with changes in body image, lifestyle, and other factors. The nurse needs to assess what the client is experiencing and how the client is dealing with those issues. Offer referrals for counseling, support groups, and social services. The nurse needs to be an effective listener, identify areas of concern, and work with other health care professionals to assist the client and family to work through the problems.

CLIENT AND FAMILY TEACHING

Before discharge, the client needs to receive instructions on how to carry out treatments at home. It is important that the client and family understand the prescribed treatment regimen. Each client is evaluated to determine the ability to carry out his or her own care and to determine specific needs, such as supervised home care (visiting nurse, other health care agencies and personnel), supplies (eg, dressings, tape, ostomy supplies, crutches), special dietary needs, or adjustments to the living environment (eg, special bed, portable commode, wheelchair access).

The nurse develops a teaching plan to meet the client's individual needs. It may include the following:

- Follow the physician's instructions regarding cleaning the incision, applying the dressing, bathing, diet, and physical activity.
- Notify the physician if any of the following occur:
  - Chills or fever, drainage from the incision (some drainage may be expected in certain cases)
  - Foul odor or pus coming from the incision
  - Redness, streaking, pain, or tenderness around the incision
  - Other symptoms not present when discharged from the hospital (eg, vomiting, diarrhea, cough, chest or leg pain)
- Take medications as prescribed. Do not omit or change the dose unless advised to do so by the physician.
- Do not take nonprescription medications unless approved by the physician.
- Keep all postoperative appointments.
- Tell the physician about any problems that occur during the recovery period.

Nursing Standards for Care of the Postsurgical Client*

Nursing Diagnoses, Collaborative Problems, and Goals
Nursing Interventions

Standard I: Respiratory function is maintained.

Risk for Altered Respiratory Function and Potential Complication: Atelectasis/Pneumonia related to immobility, effects of anesthesia and analgesics, and pain

Goal: Lungs are clear and respirations are full and unlabored.

Monitor respiratory rate and characteristics. Auscultate lung sounds once a shift or more often if indicated. Help client turn and deep breathe every 1 to 2 hours. Reinforce use of incentive spirometer. Show client how to splint incision before coughing. Assess client's ability to mobilize secretions; suction if necessary. Administer oxygen as ordered. Refrain from administering narcotic analgesics if respiratory rate is less than 12. Encourage early ambulation.

Standard II: Circulatory function is maintained.

Potential Complication: Fluid/Electrolyte Imbalance

Goal: The nurse will manage imbalances in fluid and electrolytes.

Assess intake and output during the post-operative period. Ensure that IV fluids are infusing at the prescribed rate and that the IV site is patent. Assess vital signs frequently. Monitor lab values. Monitor postoperative intake and output for at least 48 hours or until all drains and tubes have been removed, client is tolerating oral intake and urine output is normal. Report discrepancies in intake and output, hypotension, dizziness, palpitations, or abnormal lab values. (see Chap. 21 for additional information on management of fluid and electrolyte imbalance.)

Potential Complication: Hemorrhage and Hypovolemic Shock

Goal: The nurse will manage and minimize hemorrhage and/or shock.

Monitor for signs or symptoms of shock: tachycardia, hypotension, decreased urine output, cold clammy skin, restlessness. Keep head of bed flat unless contraindicated. Maintain patent IV line. Assess the surgical site for excessive external bleeding. Reinforce dressing or apply pressure if bleeding is frank. Monitor for internal bleeding: peri-incisional hematoma and swelling, abdominal distention if abdominal surgery was performed, excessive bloody output in wound drainage collection devices, falling hemoglobin and hematocrit, orthostatic hypotension, and signs of impending shock. (See Chap. 22 for additional information on management of shock.) Report findings immediately.

Standard III: Pain and discomfort are recognized and effectively treated.

Pain related to surgical incision and manipulation of body structures

Goal: The client will experience relief of pain.

Assess pain level using an established scale (visual or numerical). Determine source of pain (incision, body position, flatus, IV lines or drainage tubes, distended bladder, etc.).

Provide pain medication and evaluate effectiveness in one-half hour after administration.

Reposition client to improve comfort and teach client about nonpharmacologic methods of pain relief such as breathing exercises, relaxation techniques, and distraction. (See Chap. 20 for additional information on pain management.)

Altered Comfort (nausea and vomiting) related to effects of anesthesia or side effect of narcotics

Goal: The client will report increased comfort and relief of nausea and vomiting.

Encourage client to breathe deeply to help eliminate inhaled anesthetics.

Help the client sit up and turn head to one side while vomiting to avoid aspiration.
Record intake and output. Offer small sips of flat ginger ale or cola, or ice chips if permitted.
Administer antiemetics as ordered.
Provide mouth care, fresh linens after vomiting.
Monitor intake and output and assess for signs or symptoms of dehydration or electrolyte imbalance (see Chap. 21).
Risk for Sleep Pattern Disturbance related to difficulty in assuming comfortable position secondary to surgery, unusual environment, noise, and interruptions
Goal: The client will report enhanced sleep pattern.
Identify factors contributing to poor sleep (noise, room temperature, position, daytime sleeping, hospital routines). Reduce environmental distractions—use night lights, close door. Schedule nursing activities to coincide with client's schedule.
Teach client progressive relaxation techniques and deep breathing exercises to facilitate sleep. Provide back rub. Assist with hygiene and provide clean gown and linens. Limit daytime sleeping and encourage increased daytime activity.
Collaborate with physician about sleeping medication if other methods fail.

Standard IV: Client safety is maintained.

Risk for injury related to decreased alertness secondary to effects of anesthesia and pain medication.
Goal: The client will remain free of injury.
Place bed in low position and elevate side rails. Place call bell in reach.
Ensure that tubings are long enough or properly secured to allow for movement. Inspect drainage tubes for kinks.
Ensure that all equipment is functioning properly.
Provide emesis basin, tissues, ice chips (if allowed), bedpan and urinal within easy reach. Instruct clients to call for assistance with any activity.

Standard V: Wound healing is promoted and wound management is provided.

Risk for Infection related to break in skin integrity (surgical incision, wound drainage devices)
Goal: Evidence of uncomplicated wound healing is present (intact edges, granulation tissue, lack of induration or swelling at site).
Inspect surgical site and periincisional drain sites for signs or symptoms of infection (redness, warmth, tenderness, separation of wound edges, purulent drainage).
Wash hands before and after dressing changes; follow aseptic or sterile technique. Change wet dressings frequently (first dressing change is usually done by surgeon). Use skin barrier to protect skin and wound from irritating drainage. Avoid using excessive tape.
Keep drainage tube exit sites clean.
Prevent excess tension on drainage tubes by securing tubes to dressing.
Empty collection devices frequently to promote drainage; note characteristics of drainage.
Teach client to splint wound when coughing or changing position.

Standard VI: Complication potential is continuously assessed and complications are immediately and effectively treated if they occur.

Potential Complication: Deep Vein Thrombosis
Goal: The nurse will manage and minimize risk of phlebitis/thrombosis.
Reinforce need to perform leg exercises every hour while awake. Instruct client not to cross legs or prop pillow under knees.
Apply compression and antiembolic stockings as ordered.
Monitor for signs and symptoms of thrombophlebitis: calf pain, tenderness, warmth, or redness; swelling of the extremity, low-grade fever. Notify physician if such signs or symptoms occur and maintain bed rest until client can be further evaluated.
Ambulate or encourage client to ambulate for a few minutes each hour while awake. Avoid prolonged sitting, and poorly fitting, constrictive antiembolic hose.
Do not massage calves or thighs.
Administer anticoagulant medication as ordered and monitor lab values for therapeutic levels.
Potential Complication: Acute Urinary Retention
Goal: The nurse will manage and minimize risk of urinary retention.
Assess for bladder distention, discomfort, and urge to void. Encourage client to try to void within the first 4 hours after surgery. Assess volume of first voided urine to determine adequacy of output (voiding frequent, small amounts indicates retention of urine with elimination of overflow only).
If client has difficulty voiding in the bedpan or using the urinal in bed, stand male clients (if allowed) and ambulate female clients to bathroom (if allowed).
If client is unable to void within 8 hours of surgery, consult with physician regarding instituting intermittent catheterization until voluntary voiding returns.
Potential Complication: Paralytic Ileus
Goal: The nurse will manage and minimize risk for developing postoperative paralytic ileus.
Assess bowel sounds every shift or more often if indicated. Assess returning bowel function as evidenced by passage of flatus or stool.
Maintain NPO status until bowel sounds return.
Report large amounts of emesis (more than 300 mL).
Provide client with moistened gauze to wet lips and tongue until oral intake is allowed.
Assist with passage of nasogastric tube, if ordered.

Standard VII: Gastrointestinal function is maintained.

Risk for Colonic Constipation related to effects of anesthesia, surgery (manipulation of abdominal organs), side effects of narcotics, decreased intake of fluids and fiber
Goal: The client will have regular bowel movements.
Once bowel sounds have returned and the client resumes oral intake, encourage intake of sufficient fluids and fiber. Encourage ambulation to promote peristalsis.
Encourage use of bathroom if possible. Provide privacy if client must use bedside commode or bedpan.
Administer bulk forming laxatives or stool softeners prophylactically if ordered.
Notify physician if there is no bowel movement within 2 to 3 days after surgery.

Standard VIII: Self-care and mobility are encouraged as appropriate.

Activity Intolerance related to decreased mobility and weakness secondary to anesthesia and surgery
Goal: The client will regain strength and activity tolerance.
Encourage progressive activity. Help client to dangle legs over bedside the evening of surgery or the next morning, if allowed, followed by sitting out of bed for 15 minutes (or more if tolerated). Progress to ambulation in room and hallway. Collaborate with client in establishing goals for increasing ambulation.

Help client with hygiene activities the evening of surgery and encourage increased self-care as appropriate.
Schedule regular rest periods.

Standard IX: Psychosocial needs are recognized and effectively managed.

Anxiety related to unfamiliar environment, loss of privacy, threat to biologic integrity and fear secondary to illness and surgery
Goal: The client will share anxieties and report increased psychological comfort.
Assess level of anxiety by asking client to rate level on a scale of 0 to 10. Explore reasons for anxiety (concerns about health, financial status, family coping, impact on independence) and provide information and reassurance. Provide referrals if appropriate.
Encourage client to use anxiety reduction techniques (see Chap. 13).
Determine how environment can be modified to improve relaxation (keeping curtains closed or open, reducing noise, moving client closer to nurses station, etc.).
Assess anxiety level after interventions.

Standard X: Discharge instructions including follow-up care and home health services are provided.

Risk for Ineffective Management of Therapeutic Regimen related to incomplete knowledge of wound care, activity and diet restrictions, medications, reportable signs and symptoms, and follow-up care
Goal: The client or family will demonstrate ability to provide wound care, restate specific instructions regarding diet and activity, identify signs and symptoms of complications, and identify needed follow-up care.
Explain, demonstrate, and provide written instructions about care of surgical wound. Observe client or family perform care. Discuss signs and symptoms of wound infection and instruct client and family to contact health care provider if they develop.
Describe and provide written instructions about activity restrictions and time when normal activity can resume.
Include information on walking, bending, lifting, climbing stairs, bathing, showering, driving a car, and engaging in sexual activity.
Explain need for adequate nutrition and fluids and how to manage constipation, which can result from decreased intake, decreased activity, and narcotic pain relievers.
Review all medications to be taken including dose, route of administration, intended effect, side effects, and duration of prescription.
Review signs and symptoms of complications such as shortness of breath, fever, productive cough, weakness, new or unusual pain, pain unrelieved by medication, calf tenderness and swelling, and wound drainage.
Evaluate the client's and family's understanding of discharge instructions.

*These standards apply to all postsurgery clients; however, other standards may also apply. The suggested nursing diagnoses and the interventions described do not represent all possible diagnoses or interventions and are intended to represent a minimum standard of care for the general surgical client. Clients undergoing specialized surgeries such as neurosurgery, open heart surgery, extensive abdominal surgery, organ transplantation, orthopedic surgery, etc. may require additional or different diagnoses and interventions. Refer to specific chapters for additional care.

Resources

Carpenito, L. J. (1997). *Nursing diagnosis: Application to clinical practice* (7th ed.). Philadelphia: Lippincott-Raven.
Nettina, S. (1996). *The Lippincott manual of nursing practice.* Philadelphia: Lippincott-Raven.

Ambulatory Care

Many surgeries and procedures are frequently performed in outpatient settings and ambulatory surgical centers. There is a greater need for nurses to be familiar with ambulatory surgery and conscious sedation.

Ambulatory Surgery

Ambulatory surgery is sometimes referred to as same day surgery or outpatient surgery. It is defined as surgery that requires less than 24 hours of hospitalization. These short-term admissions may be as brief as 1 or 2 hours, or they may extend to an overnight stay. Ambulatory surgical units are either located within a hospital or in a separate building owned by the hospital. Others may be freestanding, privately owned facilities that are not affiliated with a hospital.

There has been a significant increase in the number of surgical procedures performed as ambulatory surgery in the past decade. This is related to advances in surgical techniques, methods of anesthesia, prospective reimbursement, managed care, and changes in provisions in Medicare and Medicaid (Smeltzer & Bare, 1996).

A client who is admitted for ambulatory surgery meets the following criteria:

- The client is not critically ill.
- The surgical procedure is not extensively long and does not require many hours of general anesthesia.
- The client has few, if any, coexisting and disabling illnesses.
- The client is expected to recover quickly and requires minimal specialized care immediately following surgery.
- The client and/or family is able to provide adequate postoperative care.

Generally, clients are discharged from an ambulatory surgical unit by mid-afternoon or early evening. If a complication develops, the client is transferred to an inpatient hospital unit.

Conscious Sedation

Many diagnostic and short therapeutic procedures formerly performed on an inpatient basis are now performed on an outpatient basis. Clients are sedated but not unconscious during the procedure. *Sedation* refers to a pharmacologically induced state of relaxation and emotional comfort. *Analgesia* is the absence or relief of pain. **Conscious sedation** describes a state in which clients are free of pain, fear, and anxiety and able to tolerate unpleasant procedures while maintaining independent cardiorespiratory function and the ability to respond to verbal commands and tactile stimulation (American Society of Anesthesiologists, 1996). Diagnostic and therapeutic procedures that require sedation and analgesia, such as bone marrow biopsy, endoscopy, cardiac catheterizations, or magnetic resonance imaging and computed tomography scanning, take place in a variety of settings. Clients are often discharged shortly after the procedure. The responsibility for ensuring client safety and comfort during the sedation process rests with the nurse who is directly involved with the client's care. Although numerous types of patient monitoring equipment are available, no piece of equipment replaces the careful observations of the nurse.

Presedation Evaluation

The *presedation evaluation* determines which clients are appropriate for administration of sedative medications and is similar to the preoperative evaluation. Past adverse reactions to sedative medication are considered. Age and weight help determine the amount of medication needed.

Sedative Medications

Nurses who care for clients receiving sedation must be aware of the effects, side effects, and desired doses of sedative medications. Benzodiazepines, opioids, sedative-hypnotics, and barbiturates are the classes of drugs used in conscious sedation (Table 24–6). These medications can cause nausea, dizziness, euphoria or depression, flushed skin, coughing, jerking movements, and unusual eye and tongue movements. Although harmless, these side effects can be frightening for the client. Because virtually all sedative medications carry a risk of respiratory depression, the nurse must also be prepared for respiratory or cardiopulmonary arrest.

A class of drugs called *antagonists* reverse the effects of narcotics or benzodiazepines and are readily available whenever these medications are used. If reversal drugs are required, it is imperative that the client be observed for an extended period because the

TABLE 24-6 **Drugs Used to Sedate Clients for Diagnostic and Therapeutic Procedures**

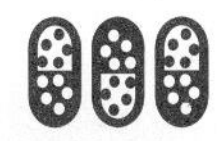

Drug Category/ Examples	Side Effects	Nursing Considerations
Opioids meperidine hydrochloride (Demerol) morphine sulfate fentanyl (Sublimaze)	Respiratory depression, central nervous system (CNS) depression, hypotension, nausea, vomiting, constipation, histamine release, headache, restlessness, tachycardia, seizures, increased intracranial pressure, decreased urination, rash, hives, pain at injection site, bronchospasm, laryngospasm	Use with caution in clients with asthma, hepatic or renal disorders, seizure disorders. Useful for sedation for painful procedures. May cause hypotension in clients with acute myocardial infarction.
Benzodiazepines midazolam hydrochloride (Versed) diazepam (Valium) lorazepam (Ativan)	Respiratory depression, cardiac arrest, hypotension, bradycardia, tachycardia, nausea, vomiting, bronchospasm, laryngospasm, blurred vision, diplopia, pain and local reaction at injection site, hiccups, amnesia, paradoxical excitement	Use with caution in clients with hypersensitivity reactions to other opioid agonists. Respiratory depression may persist beyond period of analgesia. Should not be used in clients with increased intracranial pressure. Theophylline may antagonize the sedative effects of midazolam. Increased adverse effects when administered with narcotics. Causes profound retrograde amnesia. No analgesic effect.
Sedative-hypnotics chloral hydrate	Respiratory depression, nausea, vomiting, diarrhea, hallucinations, rash, urticaria, paradoxical excitement, fever, headache, confusion	Use with caution in clients with congestive heart failure, renal impairment, pulmonary disease, hepatic failure. Should not be used in clients with narrow-angle glaucoma, hepatic or renal impairment, gastritis, peptic ulcer disease or severe cardiac disease.
Barbiturates pentobarbital (Nembutal)	Respiratory depression, laryngospasm, cardiac arrhythmias, bradycardia, hypotension, CNS excitement or depression, pain at injection site, thrombophlebitis at IV site, hallucinations	Use with caution in patients with porphyria. Can cause false-positive urine glucose using Clinitest method. Should not be given to clients with marked liver impairment or porphyria. Use with caution in patients with hypovolemic shock, congestive heart failure, hepatic impairment, respiratory dysfunction, renal dysfunction.

reversal effects are nearly always shorter than the effects of the drugs being reversed. This results in resedation. Flumazenil (Romazicon) reverses benzodiazepines and naloxone (Narcan) reverses narcotics.

Phases of the Sedation Process

The three phases of the sedation process include (1) the *titration* of sedative medications, which is the administration of multiple small doses of medication until the desired drug effect is achieved; (2) the performance of the diagnostic or therapeutic procedure; and (3) the recovery phase. Monitoring for complications is required during each phase.

Levels of sedation range from slight drowsiness to anesthesia, and unpredictable absorption, metabolism, and excretion of medications make the client vulnerable to complications of undersedation or oversedation. Increased vigilance is needed during titration of medications and recovery because the client has the greatest potential to become more deeply sedated during these phases because there is no painful stimulus. Even when the client does not seem to be sedated at the end of the procedure, late sedation may develop from continued drug uptake, delayed excretion, pharmacodynamics, or the lack of stimulation. In addition to monitoring for adverse effects of medications, the nurse monitors for complications of the procedure itself.

NURSING PROCESS
The Client Undergoing Conscious Sedation

Assessment

Before the sedation process, the nurse gathers important client data, records baseline vital signs and oximeter readings, and provides education to clients and their families. Education covers instructions specific to the procedure being performed, preparations for the procedure, sensations likely to be experienced (pain, discomfort, cramping, gagging, nausea), and common side effects of the medications.

During the sedation process, assess the client continually. Monitor heart rate, respiratory rate and pattern, blood pressure, oxygen saturation level, and level of consciousness at all times. Cardiac rhythm should be monitored in clients who are at risk for arrhythmia or cardiovascular compromise. If the client's vital signs deviate significantly during sedation, the nurse collects additional information to help determine if those deviations are secondary to an adverse reaction to the sedation or to the procedure itself. When the client shows signs of distress (ie, deviation in vital signs, respiratory compromise), the nurse immediately reports these signs to the physician and provides interventions such as suctioning, gentle tactile stimulation, or administration of oxygen and continues to monitor the client's response. Monitoring these parameters must be carried out until the client's level of consciousness and vital signs are at baseline. These observations are documented at intervals specified by the institution.

Diagnosis and Planning

Additional nursing care includes but is not limited to the following:

Nursing Diagnoses and Collaborative Problems	Nursing Interventions
Risk for Ineffective Breathing Patterns secondary to effect of sedative medications	Position the head to allow for maximum ventilation and to prevent airway compromise.
Goal: The client will have a normal respiratory pattern	Observe for signs and symptoms of distress related to inappropriate head position (stridor, increased respiratory effort), and reposition airway as indicated.
Risk for injury related to sedation	Provide for client safety by ensuring that bed rails are in the up position, assisting with ambulation, and carefully observing all activities.
Goal: The client will remain safe and uninjured	Monitor for return to presedation level of consciousness, and discharge client in the care of an individual who has received thorough instructions regarding client safety.

After the procedure, the nurse continues to monitor the client's recovery and begins assessing his or her readiness for discharge.

Evaluation and Expected Outcomes

- Stable cardiovascular function and a patent airway
- Easily aroused
- Intact protective reflexes
- Able to talk
- Able to sit up unaided
- Adequate hydration

CLIENT AND FAMILY EDUCATION

After it has been determined that the client meets the appropriate discharge criteria, the nurse provides discharge instructions. Because sedative medications affect memory for events surrounding their administration, review discharge instructions with an adult who will be responsible for the client after discharge. Provide education verbally and in writing. Instruct the client not to drink alcoholic beverages for a specified period after the procedure and to resume prescription and nonprescriptions medications when appropriate. Pain medications may have an additive effect with the sedative medications that were administered so tell the client when it is appropriate to begin taking such medications. Provide dietary instructions and encourage the client to drink plenty of fluids. Give specific activity guidelines; the client should temporarily refrain from activities that depend on physical coordination, such as driving or operating machinery. Tell the client to telephone the physician with any concerns about untoward effects of the medications or complications of the procedure.

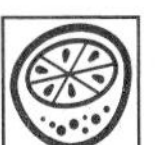

General Nutritional Considerations

Progress the diet as soon as possible after surgery to promote an adequate oral intake. Encourage clients who are anorectic or nauseated to consume small, frequent feedings; high-protein, low-fat liquids may be better tolerated than traditional meals.

If possible, schedule pain medications enough in advance to allow the client a pain-free mealtime.

Normal weight loss during the early postoperative period is about half a pound daily. Weight gain during this period signifies fluid accumulation.

Protein, calories, vitamins A and C, and zinc are important for wound healing and immune system functioning; actual requirements depend on the client's nutritional status, the extent of surgery, and the development of complications.

Unlike the stomach, which does not regain motility for 24 to 48 hours after surgery, the small intestine resumes peristalsis and the ability to absorb nutrients within several hours postoperatively. If the client is malnourished, hypermetabolic, or not expected to resume an oral intake within a few days, a needle-catheter jejunostomy tube may be inserted during surgery so enteral feedings can be given.

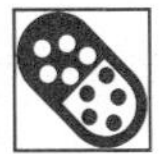

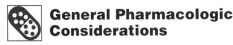

General Pharmacologic Considerations

The preoperative medication is given precisely at the time prescribed by the anesthesiologist. If the preoperative medication is given too early, the optimum potency will be reached before it is needed; if the drug is given too late, the drug action will not begin before the anesthesia is initiated.

Postoperative pain reaches its peak between 12 and 36 hours after surgery and diminishes significantly after 48 hours.

Antiemetics such as promethazine (Phenergan) or prochlorperazine (Compazine) can potentiate the hypotensive effects of the opioids.

During the postoperative period, the client is closely monitored for adverse reactions to the narcotic analgesics such as respiratory depression, decreased blood pressure, nausea, excessive drowsiness, agitation, or hallucinations. Naloxone (Narcan) can be given to counteract narcotic induced respiratory depression.

Some clients experience acute anxiety before surgery. The physician may prescribe a tranquilizer or sedative. The nurse must notify the physician if the medication does not appear to be effective.

The evening before surgery a hypnotic drug may be ordered to ensure rest. The effects of the medication are documented on the client's chart.

The use of PCA does not eliminate the need for frequent observation of the client for effectiveness of the analgesic. Blood pressure, pulse, and respiratory rates are monitored at frequent intervals. A decrease in the blood pressure or respiratory rate is brought to the physician's attention immediately.

Antibiotics may be ordered before as well as after surgery. The antibiotic must be given at specified intervals to maintain consistent therapeutic blood levels.

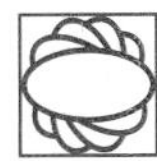

General Gerontologic Considerations

A major adverse reaction to anesthesia in the older adult is decreased mental functioning, which can be manifested as delirium.

Medications such as the opioids and the barbiturates may cause confusion and disorientation in the older adult even when given in standard doses.

The respiratory depressive effects of the opioids may be increased in the older adult.

Sometimes the risk of surgery is greater in older adults because they may have disorders (eg, cardiac or renal disease) that interfere with recovery.

A detailed history of medications is important because some medications persist in the body for a period of time and may interfere with administration of anesthetic agents or medications given before, during, or after surgery.

A diminished ability to hear, see, and understand may interfere with preoperative and postoperative teaching. Explanations and demonstrations may need to be repeated.

Older adults usually receive smaller doses of preoperative, intraoperative, and postoperative medications, especially those that affect the central nervous, cardiovascular, and renal systems.

Older adults are prone to postoperative complications such as shock, atelectasis, pneumonia, paralytic ileus, gastric dilatation, and venous stasis.

Postoperative ambulatory activities are essential but planned according to the client's tolerance, which usually is less than that of a younger person.

The convalescent period usually is longer for the older adult. The client may require positive reinforcement throughout the postoperative period as well as extensive discharge planning.

If the older adult lives alone or with a spouse who also is older or who is ill or infirm, additional consideration is given to discharge planning. It may be necessary to use the services of relatives or friends, a public health nurse, a visiting nurse, or home health care personnel during the convalescent period. In some instances, it is necessary to admit the client to a skilled nursing facility for convalescent care.

A loss of subcutaneous tissue and thinning of the skin accompany the aging process. This, in turn, may lead to stress-producing situations, such as poor wound healing, tissue breakdown caused by excessive pressure on a part, or inadequate development of granulation tissue in healing wounds.

SUMMARY OF KEY CONCEPTS

- A surgical procedure may be performed to obtain a biopsy specimen or establish a diagnosis, for exploratory evaluation, to remove a diseased organ or structure, to relieve pain or pressure, or for cosmetic reasons.
- Perioperative care includes what occurs before, during, and after surgery. There are three phases: preoperative, intraoperative, and postoperative.
- Clients at risk for surgery include the very young and the elderly, malnourished or obese clients, those who are substance abusers, and clients who have other medical problems.
- A preoperative teaching plan includes information about the procedure and what is expected of the client before and after the procedure.
- Immediate preoperative preparations include signing the surgical consent, preparing the skin, having the client void, giving the client nothing by mouth, providing surgical attire, caring for the client's valuables, asking the client to remove makeup and jewelry, and administering preoperative medications.
- Nursing responsibilities during the intraoperative period include maintaining aseptic technique, adding fluids to IV lines, monitoring intake and output, assessing the client, and transferring the client to PACU.
- Members of the surgical team include the anesthesiologist or anesthetist, the surgeon, the surgical assistants, and the scrub nurse and circulating nurse.
- Anesthesia provides a partial or complete loss of sensation of pain with or without loss of consciousness. Anesthesia can be general, regional, or local.
- Ambulatory surgery is common and is performed on clients who are not critically ill, do not require a long period of anesthesia, are relatively healthy, and will be able to manage the postoperative care.
- Conscious sedation allows clients to undergo painful diagnostic or therapeutic procedures while remaining awake enough to follow commands. Clients require careful assessment throughout the sedation process.
- Nursing responsibilities in the immediate postoperative period include maintaining a patent airway and adequate circulation, preventing shock, making accurate assessments, and maintaining IV lines, tubes, and drains.
- Nursing management in the later postoperative period focuses on standard care to prevent and assess complications and assist the client to meet physical and psychosocial needs. This includes promoting optimum respiratory function, adequate circulation and tissue perfusion; assessing bladder and bowel function; performing wound care; assisting the client to reduce fear, and providing effective client and family teaching.
- Major complications that may occur in the immediate postoperative period are hemorrhage, shock, hypoxia, and aspiration. Later complications include pneumonia, wound infection, deep vein thrombosis and paralytic ileus.

CRITICAL THINKING EXERCISES

1. The nurse has checked to make the sure the client's surgical consent is signed and on the chart the evening before surgery. When the nurse assesses this client, he reports that he is uncertain about having the surgery and that he really does not understand what is expected or what it means for the long term. What steps should the nurse take? What needs to be documented?
2. The client reports to the nurse that her family has lost several family members unexpectedly during surgery and that she is very scared about her upcoming surgery. What actions should the nurse take in relation to this information? What should the nurse document?
3. A client is 5 days postop. He complains of incisional pain, feeling warm, and nauseated. What assessments should the nurse make? What needs to be documented?

Suggested Readings

American Society of Anesthesiologists Task Force on Sedation and Analgesia by Non-anesthesiologists. (1996). The American Society of Anesthesiologists: Practice guidelines for sedation and analgesia by non-anesthesiologists. *Anesthesiology, 84*(2), 459–471.

Bostrom, B. M., Ramberg, T., Davis, B. D., & Fridlund, B. (1997). Survey of postoperative patients' pain management. *Journal of Nursing Management, 5*(6), 341–349.

Carpenito, L. J. (1997). *Nursing diagnosis: Application to clinical practice* (7th ed.) Philadelphia: Lippincott-Raven.

Clement, S. B. (1997). Postoperative considerations: Geriatric surgical patients and cardiovascular function. *Today's Surgical Nurse, 19*(5), 19–22.

Dennison, R. D. (1997). Nurse's guide to common postoperative complications. *Nursing,* 27(11), 56–59.

Drury, B. L. (1997). Alternative therapies for postoperative pain. *Nursing Spectrum, 7*(17), 20.

Kleinpell, R. M. (1997). Improving telephone follow-up after ambulatory surgery. *Journal of Perianesthesia Nursing, 12*(5), 336–340.

Nettina, S. (1996). *The Lippincott manual of nursing practice.* Philadelphia: Lippincott-Raven.

Reed, J. A, Lesiuk, N., & MacQuarrie, V. (1997). Managing postoperative gas pain. *Canadian Nurse, 93*(8), 43–45.

Ries, D. T. (1997). From surgery to home. *Nurse Education, 22*(2), 11, 14.

Smeltzer, S. C., & Bare, B. G. (1996). *Brunner and Suddarth's textbook of medical-surgical nursing* (8th ed.). Philadelphia. Lippincott-Raven.

Walsh, J. (1993). Postop effects of OR positioning. *RN 56*(2), 50.

Additional Resources

Consumer Health
http://www.ahcpr.gov:80/consumer/surgery.html

Surginet
http://www.surginet.org

Chapter 25

Caring for Dying Clients

KEY TERMS

Acceptance
Anger
Anticipatory grieving
Bargaining
Denial
Depression
Grieving
Hospice
Near death experience
Nearing death awareness
Palliative treatment
Respite care
Waiting for permission phenomenon

LEARNING OBJECTIVES

On completion of this chapter, the reader will:

- Describe attitudes of society and health care workers toward death.
- Discuss outcomes of informing a client about a terminal illness.
- Discuss how hopefulness can be maintained during a terminal illness.
- Describe emotional reactions the dying client experiences.
- Identify how the dying client can ensure his or her wishes for terminal care are carried out.
- Describe physical phenomena that occur during the dying process.
- Summarize psychological events dying clients have reported.
- Discuss the nursing management of the dying client and the family.

"Of all human experiences, none is more overwhelming in its implications than death. Yet, for most of us, death remains a shadowy figure whose presence is only vaguely acknowledged" (DeSpelder & Strickland, 1992, p. 5). Earlier in this century, many people died in their homes, surrounded by family and loved ones. Later, it became more common to die in a hospital or nursing home. Then, in the 1970s, the hospice movement promoted care of dying clients in their homes or in hospice settings, providing a more dignified and supportive climate. Also, education about death has helped health care professionals be better informed about dying and death and to incorporate this knowledge into the care given to clients.

Increased technology and aggressive treatment have, in some ways, distorted the reality of dying and death for health care providers. For some, death signifies their failure to save lives and to be healers. However, death is a natural and universal experience, a part of life, and a component of health care. It is essential that health care providers acknowledge death as the final stage of growth and development (Kübler-Ross, 1975) and that they explore their own mortality and feelings about dying and death. This is the only way that they can then provide care and comfort to dying clients and their families.

Nurses who care for dying clients share emotional pain with clients and families (Fig. 25–1). Denying death creates a barrier to becoming involved with the client and family and interferes with personal growth. Death can occur in all health care settings; therefore, facing the death of clients is necessary for nurses. It is not partial to a particular age group or population, can be slow and tortuous, or very sudden and unexpected. Preparation for an expected death and care for grieving family members following an unexpected death is often very different. It is important to recognize that nursing care always requires sensitivity and compassion for the client, family, and significant others.

The Dying Client

Although most individuals recognize that death is inevitable, they do not spend time getting ready until actually faced with the prospect. Factors the nurse needs to be involved with when caring for the dying client include informing the client, sustaining hope,

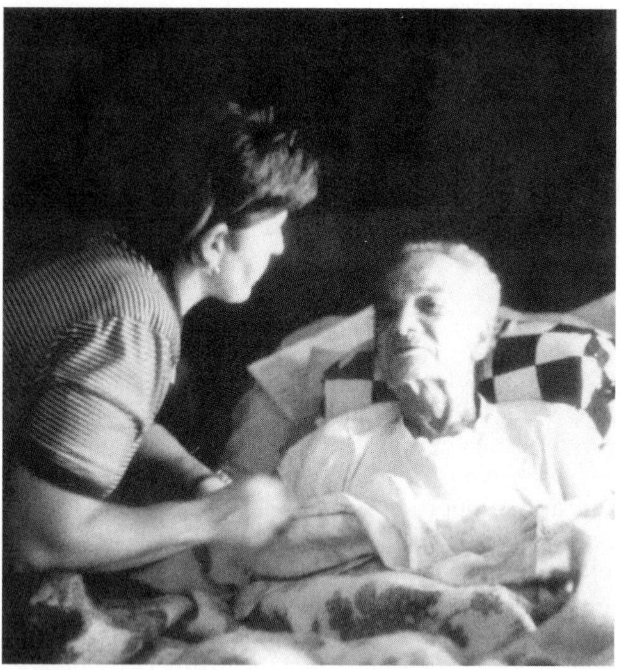

FIGURE 25-1. A hospice nurse gets physically and emotionally close to a dying client. (Courtesy of Visiting Nurse Association of Southwest Michigan)

assisting the client and family with emotional reactions, and recognizing the client's right to make final decisions.

Informing the Dying Client

Nurses honor the dying client's right to know the seriousness of the condition. The physician usually has the responsibility for informing clients of the nature and gravity of their illness. Even though some informed clients may react negatively at first, outcomes of being frank include:

- Maintaining a client–nurse relationship based on honesty rather than on the false pretense that recovery will occur
- Upholding the client's autonomy and the right to determine how to spend the remainder of her or his life
- Providing the client with the opportunity to complete unfinished business—to prepare for and arrange legal and personal affairs and complete any remaining tasks or goals
- Facilitating the use of the client's inner resources and determination to survive and prolong life, often referred to as the "will to live"
- Promoting meaningful communication between the client and family

It is important for all members of the health care team to be aware of what the client has been told regarding the prognosis of her or his illness. Lack of this knowledge greatly interferes with the nurse's relationship with the client. For example, the nurse may avoid all but the most superficial topics of conversation, out of uncertainty about how to respond if asked, "Am I going to die?" Some feel that regardless of how others might try to conceal the truth, most clients gradually recognize clues that their illness is terminal. Avoidance alone tends to confirm their suspicions that they are dying. When uninformed clients are given the opportunity, they may give hints of their awareness of approaching death. Some may even indicate they are ready to discuss dying. If the nurse refutes the comments with a reply such as, "Don't talk like that," it conveys a message that the subject of dying is uncomfortable for the nurse. Often, the client will then avoid the subject in all future interactions.

Sustaining Hopefulness

It is important that a spirit of hopefulness be communicated. Hopefulness implies the right of dying clients to believe the health care team will make their remaining life meaningful, to use whatever treatment and comfort measures are appropriate, and to dignify the approaching death. Hope should not be confused with unrealistic optimism. When clients are informed that their condition is terminal, they must also understand that the health care team is still dedicated to providing **palliative treatment,** treatment that reduces physical discomfort but does not alter the progress of the disease.

Assisting With Emotional Reactions

Although dying clients respond to terminal illnesses in unique ways, studies show that a common emotional pattern develops. Elisabeth Kübler-Ross, a physician who has studied death and dying extensively, described a series of five reactions—denial, anger, bargaining, depression, and acceptance—that dying clients often demonstrate. Clients do not always follow these stages in order. Some regress then move forward again, whereas others may be in several stages at once (eg, a client who is angry as well as depressed).

The first stage, **denial**, is a psychological defense mechanism in which a person refuses to believe that certain information is true. Dying clients usually first deny that the diagnosis is accurate. A common response is "No, not me; there must be some mistake."

They may imagine that the test results are erroneous or reports have been confused. Denial of the diagnosis may be followed by a refusal to accept that the condition is actually terminal.

During the second stage, **anger**, clients ask, "Why me?" The client may say, "I'm still young. My children still need me. Why did *I* get this disease?" Their anger may be displaced onto others such as the physician, nurses, family, or even God or it may be expressed in less obvious ways, such as complaining about their care or blaming anyone and everyone for the slightest aggravation.

The third stage, **bargaining,** is an attempt to postpone death. Usually a bargain is secretly made with God or some higher power. Clients attempt to negotiate a delay in dying until a particularly significant event has occurred. They may say, "If I can just live until my daughter graduates from high school, I will accept death when it eventually comes."

The fourth stage is marked by **depression.** As clients realize the reality of their situation, they may mourn their potential losses such as separation from their loved ones, the inability to fulfill their future goals, or loss of control.

In the fifth stage, **acceptance,** dying clients accept their fate and make peace spiritually and with those with whom they feel close. Clients may begin to detach themselves from activities and acquaintances and seek to be with only a small circle of relatives or friends.

Supporting Final Decisions

The nurse provides options of where and how terminal care may be provided, respects the client's and family's choices, and facilitates their preferences. As long as the dying client remains competent (retains the ability to understand the consequences of his or her choices), the client has the right to request or refuse a variety of options. Problems arise when clients become incompetent before indicating their wishes about terminal care. Consequently, dying clients may be victims of decisions they would ordinarily oppose. Therefore, some individuals write down their wishes, called *advance directives*, in a living will or legally designate someone to have durable power of attorney.

During this emotional turmoil, the dying client often has to make some tough decisions. Under a federal law called The Patient Self-Determination Act, passed in 1990, all health care facilities in the United States funded by Medicare must inform clients on admission of their right to refuse medical treatment and their right to prepare an advance directive. Most agencies supply the necessary forms.

LIVING WILLS

A *living will* is a written or printed statement describing the wishes of a person concerning her or his own medical care when death is near (Fig. 25–2). Generally, a living will describes a desire to avoid being kept alive by artificial means or use of heroic measures. It is not a legal document, and as such, is not binding under the law. Rather, it serves as an informal directive, which others may or may not feel compelled to follow. However, many physicians try to abide by their clients' wishes if they are known or stated in writing.

DURABLE POWER OF ATTORNEY

Some states are now encouraging individuals to appoint someone to have *durable power of attorney* for their health care. This procedure makes it possible for another person, selected by the client, to make medical decisions on the client's behalf when the client is no longer able to do so. It allows competent individuals to identify exactly what life-sustaining measures they want implemented, avoided, or withdrawn, and offers reassurance that their wishes will be carried out. The appointee cannot exercise this authority at any other time or in any other matters. For obvious ethical reasons, the client's physician or other health care workers may not be designated as durable power of attorney. When a durable power of attorney document exists, it is brought to the institution at each admission and a photocopy attached to the chart.

Care of the Dying Client

Some clients who are terminally ill spend their last days in an acute care setting, using the best technology and resources available. Others prefer to be at home, with or without assistance from hospice home care. Others choose a hospice or extended care facility. Regardless of the setting, clients need to know that their symptoms, particularly pain, will be controlled and that they will be kept a part of the planning process for their care.

Home Care

In the early stages of a terminal illness, the client generally remains at home. Nurses often coordinate community services and secure needed home equipment. Many clients report experiencing greater emotional and physical comfort in their own home. They have greater security and personal integrity within a familiar environment. Guilt feelings also may be lessened when family members are involved in caring for the client. In

ADVANCE DIRECTIVE
Living Will and Health Care Proxy

Death is a part of life. It is a reality like birth, growth and aging. I am using this advance directive to convey my wishes about medical care to my doctors and other people looking after me at the end of my life. It is called an advance directive because it gives instructions in advance about what I want to happen to me in the future. It expresses my wishes about medical treatment that might keep me alive. I want this to be legally binding.

If I cannot make or communicate decisions about my medical care, those around me should rely on this document for instructions about measures that could keep me alive.

I do not want medical treatment (including feeding and water by tube) that will keep me alive if:
- I am unconscious and there is no reasonable prospect that I will ever be conscious again (even if I am not going to die soon in my medical condition), or
- I am near death from an illness or injury with no reasonable prospect of recovery.

I do want medicine and other care to make me more comfortable and to take care of pain and suffering. I want this even if the pain medicine makes me die sooner.

I want to give some extra instructions: *[Here list any special instructions, e.g., some people fear being kept alive after a debilitating stroke. If you have wishes about this, or any other conditions, please write them here.]*

The legal language in the box that follows is a health care proxy. It gives another person the power to make medical decisions for me.

I name ______________________________, who lives at ______________________________

______________________________, phone number ______________________________,

to make medical decisions for me if I cannot make them myself. This person is called a health care "surrogate," "agent," "proxy," or "attorney in fact." This power of attorney shall become effective when I become incapable of making or communicating decisions about my medical care. This means that this document stays legal when and if I lose the power to speak for myself, for instance, if I am in a coma or have Alzheimer's disease.

My health care proxy has power to tell others what my advance directive means. This person also has power to make decisions for me, based either on what I would have wanted, or, if this is not known, on what he or she thinks is best for me.

If my first choice health care proxy cannot or decides not to act for me, I name ______________________________

______________________________, address ______________________________,

phone number ______________________________, as my second choice.

FIGURE 25-2. Advance directive. (Reprinted with permission of Choice in Dying [formerly Concern for Dying/Society for the Right to Die], New York)

addition, children can interact more frequently and may be helped to understand death with less fear.

A negative factor of home care is the burden placed on the primary caregiver. If prolonged, the role of primary caregiver can be very isolating and physically exhausting because the responsibility for providing care continues 24 hours a day, day after day. Home care nurses need to periodically assess the toll on the physical and emotional health of the caregiver. **Respite care,** or care for the caregiver, may be arranged to provide periodic relief.

Hospice Care

In 1967, Dr. Cicely Saunders founded St. Christopher's Hospice in Sydenham, England. This hospice has served as a model for hospice care in the United States. A **hospice** is a facility for the care of the terminally ill where dying clients live out their final days with comfort, dignity, and meaningfulness in a caring environment. Hospice care emphasizes helping clients *live* however they wish until they die. Clients receive services that relieve their physical symptoms and emotional distress and promote spiritual support. Pain is liberally controlled. In the United States, the hospice philosophy has been implemented in various ways. In general, the majority of hospice clients, who usually have 6 months or less to live, are cared for in their own homes. A multidisciplinary team of hospice professionals and volunteers provides support to the dying client and caregivers. Services include personal care, homemaking services, companionship, and support programs for family members and significant others including individual counseling during and after the death of the client (grief counseling).

Institutionally Based Palliative Care

Some institutions provide palliative care to terminally ill clients who cannot maintain independent living. This care, too, is often referred to as hospice care. These units may be located in hospitals, long-term care facilities, or other separate facilities. Nurses and other health care personnel give 24-hour care. Factors that influence the decision to use institutionally based palliative care include increased weakness or immobility of the client who then requires more assistance than can be provided at home, inability of the client to manage elimination needs, uncontrolled or inadequately controlled pain or nausea, the inability of the family to provide an adequate level of care, too complex and demanding care, or the caregiver is too exhausted to provide care. Many of the rules that govern traditional hospital and long-term care are relaxed for palliative care units. Visiting hours and ages of visitors are not restrictive. In addition, the family is encouraged to bring in personal items for the client to enjoy and value.

Acute Care

Hospitals offer acute care with a 24-hour staff of nurses and other medical personnel, readily available resuscitative equipment, and access to a greater variety of medications than those in long-term care. However, it is probably the most expensive form of terminal care and often the time and attention afforded to the supportive care of dying clients may be limited.

Signs of Approaching Death

Physical Events

Death generally occurs gradually over a period of hours or days. Cells deteriorate from an underlying lack of sufficient oxygen, which leads to multisystem failure. Signs of impending death that alert the nurse that the client will die shortly include:

- *Cardiac dysfunction.* Failing cardiac function is one of the first signs that a client's condition is worsening. At first, heart rate increases in a futile attempt to deliver oxygen to cells. The apical pulse rate may reach 100 or more beats per minute. Cardiac output, the amount of blood pumped by the heart per minute, may decrease because a fast heart rate impairs the ability of the heart to fill with blood. This may diminish the heart's own oxygen supply, which causes the heart rate to decrease and blood pressure to fall.
- *Peripheral circulation changes.* Reduced cardiac output compromises peripheral circulation and impaired celluar metabolism produces less heat. The skin becomes pale or mottled, nail beds and lips may appear blue, and the client may feel cold.
- *Pulmonary function impairment.* Failure of the heart's pumping function causes fluid to collect within the pulmonary circulation. Breath sounds become moist. Oxygen does not diffuse very well and carbon dioxide is not adequately exhaled, compounding the state of generalized hypoxia (low oxygenation).
- *Central nervous system alterations.* With hypoxia, the brain is less sensitive to accumulating levels of carbon dioxide; therefore, periods of apnea (no breathing) may occur. Pain perception may be diminished; the client may stare blankly through partially open eyes; and the senses may become impaired, although hearing tends to remain intact the longest. Eventually, the client becomes insensitive to all but extreme pressure.
- *Renal impairment.* Low cardiac output causes urine volume to diminish and toxic waste products to accumulate.
- *Gastrointestinal disturbances.* Peristalsis slows, causing gas and intestinal contents to accumulate. This buildup may stimulate the vomiting center, resulting in nausea and vomiting.
- *Musculoskeletal changes.* Reflexes become hypoactive. Urinary and rectal sphincter muscle control are lost, causing incontinence of urine and stool. The jaw and facial muscles also relax. As the tongue falls to the back of the throat, noisy respirations occur. The accumulation of secretions in the respiratory tract, coupled with noisy respirations, is referred to as the *death rattle.* A brief period of restlessness may occur just before death.

Psychological Events

If the stage of acceptance has been reached, some terminally ill clients may look forward to dying because it will end their suffering. However, it has been observed that some may forestall dying when they feel that their loved ones are not yet prepared to deal with their death. This has been described as the **waiting for permission phenomenon** because death often occurs shortly after a significant family member communicates that he or she is strong enough and ready to "let go." Nurses need to support family members at this time because they may feel as though they have given up and let their loved one down.

Near death experiences, in which the client almost dies but is resuscitated, have been reported for some time. People who have experienced near death report similar events, such as floating above their body, moving rapidly toward a bright light, seeing familiar individuals who have already died, feeling warm and peaceful, being told that it is not time yet for them to die, and regretting having to return to their resuscitated body.

Another phenomenon, **nearing death awareness** (Mallison, 1993), is characterized by the dying clients' premonition of the approximate time or date of their death. In addition, just before death, clients may reach out, point, or open their arms as if to embrace someone or call them by name.

Nursing Management

The initial assessment is centered on the client's basic physical needs, such as pain, breathing, nutrition, hydration, and elimination, then goes on to include the psychosocial needs of the client and family. It is important that unnecessary assessments not be repeated, to allow the client to rest. Frequent checks can be made without being physically intrusive. This frequency provides security, so that the client does not feel abandoned.

Nursing care of the dying client is focused on providing palliative care to the client and support to family members and significant others. Client comfort is the primary goal, with the major long-term goal being that the client will die with dignity. Other client goals include control of pain, maintenance of basic physiologic functions, relief of fears and anxieties, completion of unfinished business, and acceptance of death. Having the client's family remain cohesive and supportive is another goal, as is providing a safe and secure environment.

Pain Control

The primary objective of pain control for the dying client is to block pain without suppressing the client's level of consciousness or breathing. The nurse generally gives pain medications on a routine schedule to avoid causing the client to experience intense discomfort followed by a period of heavy sedation. Regular dosing sustains a plateau of continuous pain relief and prevents exhausting the client, who must use additional energy to cope with severe pain (see Chap. 20). Often other medications such as mild tranquilizers or antidepressants are prescribed to reduce fear and anxiety, which intensify pain. Other techniques such as imagery, humor, and progressive relaxation (see Chap. 11) are useful in potentiating the effects of pain medication.

Breathing

The dying client may have difficulty breathing; therefore, it is helpful to place the client in a Fowler's position to ease breathing. If the client is unable to cough and raise secretions, the nurse gently suctions the client. Suctioning will *not* clear the lungs or make breathing easier if the client has pulmonary edema (fluid in the lungs from heart failure). In this case, the physician may prescribe a sedative to relieve the anxiety created by the feeling of suffocation. Oxygen may eventually be used.

Food and Fluids

If the client is able to take oral fluids and food, nourishment should be offered frequently in small amounts and served at the appropriate temperature. The nurse needs to encourage the family to bring in foods that the client likes or that have been a tradition within the family's diet.

Impaired Swallowing

Difficulty in swallowing, gastric and intestinal distention, and vomiting create a potential for aspiration of fluids, as well as a decrease in food intake. Medications for controlling nausea and vomiting should be administered an hour or so before meals. The nurse and family should not insist that the client eat or drink if these symptoms cannot be controlled. Weight loss and inadequate intake need to be reported so alternative nutritional and fluid administration routes may be considered. If drooling occurs, the nurse may elevate and turn the client's head to the side or suction the oral cavity.

Temperature Regulation

Skin temperature drops as death nears and the client may describe feeling cold. Cotton socks, light blankets, and other light clothing may be given if the client feels chilled. Gentle massaging of the arms and legs transfers body heat from the hands to the skin surface and improves circulation. Touch also provides emotional support and communicates personal concern.

Skin and Tissue Integrity

A drop in blood pressure and rapid heart failure leads to poor tissue and organ perfusion. The skin needs to be protected from breakdown by changing the client's position at least every 2 hours. The nurse needs to consult with the physician about administering intramuscular injections to clients with poor tissue perfusion because this may cause inadequate drug absorption and decreased effectiveness.

Self-Care and Activity

Physical activity is not always well tolerated by the dying client. The nurse may need to assist with personal hygiene. The client needs to be clean, well groomed, and free of unpleasant odors to promote dignity and self-esteem. Oral care and ice chips are given because mouth breathing makes the oral mucous membranes and lips dry. Petroleum jelly helps keep the lips lubricated. Glycerin applications should be avoided because they tend to pull fluid from the tissue and eventually accentuate the drying problem.

Sleep

A disturbance in the sleep pattern may occur because of anxiety, fear, pain, or other environmental stimuli, such as bright lights and disturbing noise. Cluster necessary client care activities to avoid awakening the client and to protect the client from a steady stream of health care workers or visitors. When possible, turn off or dim the lights at night and keep noise to a minimum. The radio, television, or recordings of the client's favorite music may mask the continuous hum of equipment and monitors.

Elimination

Normal elimination is promoted by offering a bed pan or assisting the client to the bathroom or bedside commode. Incontinence of the bowel or bladder may occur because of the client's disease process or because the client is near death. Absorbent pads are used when control is lost and the client cleaned thoroughly. Obtain an order for an indwelling or external catheter, particularly if skin breakdown is a problem.

Fear, Social Isolation, Hopelessness, and Powerlessness

Because the dying client tends to become isolated from others (Fig. 25–3), the nurse needs to spend time exclusive of when it is necessary to provide physical care. It is important for the nurse to be flexible and to interrupt physical care if and when the client indicates a need for companionship, support, and communication. During unplanned, spontaneous moments, clients often bring up fears or concerns that should not be ignored or rushed. Interest and a willingness to listen may be communicated by sitting down, leaning forward in the direction of the client, and making direct eye contact. Nodding, responsive comments such as "Yes" or brief periods of silence encourage the client to continue verbalizing.

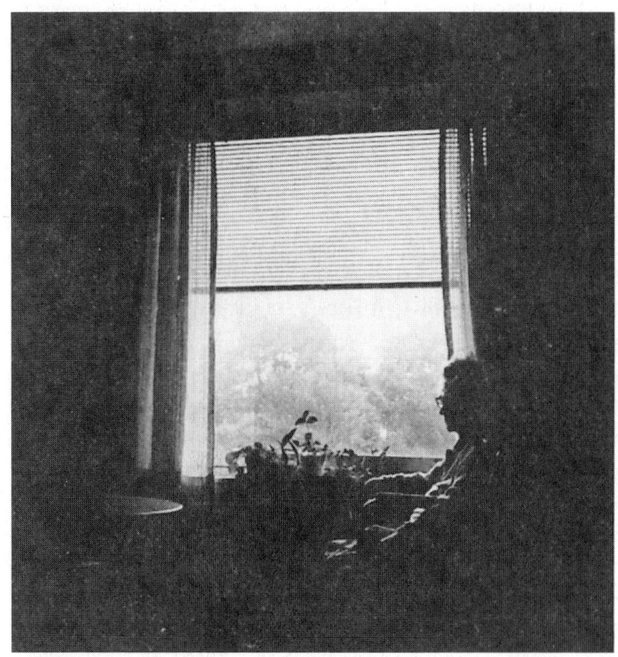

FIGURE 25-3. The dying client tends to become isolated from others. (Photograph by D. Atkinson)

Grieving

Grieving is a painful yet normal reaction that helps individuals cope with loss and leads to emotional healing. **Anticipatory grieving** occurs *before* death, when the dying client and family begin to consider the impact of their potential loss. People express grief in a variety of ways: some become depressed and cry; some are angry and hostile; and some develop physical symptoms, such as anorexia and insomnia. Family members may withdraw emotionally from the dying client because they find the experience too painful, whereas others draw closer, realizing they have only a short time to be with their loved one. It is the nurse's responsibility to facilitate the grieving process and help the client and family deal with their emotions. To do this, nurses may empathically share perceptions of what the client and family are experiencing by saying something like, "It must be a very helpless feeling." Once the client and family sense they can speak freely, the nurse needs to listen in a nonjudgmental manner and avoid criticism or giving advice.

Spiritual Distress

Religious beliefs and cultural customs influence attitudes about death. Clients may find great comfort and support from their religious faith and may want to be visited by someone associated with their religion. If clients indicate a desire for this, clergy need to be notified. If asked, the nurse may pray with clients or assist as indicated. When clients are too ill to express their wishes, the family needs to be asked about spiritual care.

Family Coping

People often find it difficult to communicate frankly with a dying person. Failure to verbalize feelings, express emotions, and show tenderness for the dying family member is often a source of regret for grieving relatives. Therefore, families need to feel that they can express their feelings with nurses who are compassionate listeners. If family members are encouraged and listened to in their frank communication, they may feel more prepared to carry on a similarly honest dialogue with the dying client. Once feelings are mutually expressed and communication barriers are broken, both relatives and the client often experience comfort in the meaningful relationship between them.

If possible, it is important for the family to have a room where they can talk with other relatives, cry, and rest. Sitting with the family for a short time, expressing concern for their welfare, and listening to their concerns provides strong emotional support. The nurse explains measures taken to provide comfort and pain relief for the dying client. It is helpful for the nurse to explain that as death draws near, the dying client may appear to become detached and unaware of those nearby, and may slip into unconsciousness before death. The nurse is likely to be with the dying client and family at the moment of death. Some families may want to remain for a time with the body of the deceased. Therefore, the nurse allows a period of privacy before giving postmortem care. If family members or relatives seem unusually distraught, the nurse remains with them until a clergy member or other family member or friend arrives to be with them.

NURSING PROCESS
The Dying Client

Assessment

Assess the client's and family's feelings about losses, isolation, grief, hopelessness, and distress. Observe family and client communication and coping patterns, strengths, and supports. Assess spiritual and cultural beliefs and practices. Determine family's ability to provide care at home.

Diagnosis and Planning

The following plan of care is intended as a guide and should not be limited to this information.

Nursing Diagnoses and Collaborative Problems	Nursing Interventions
Risk for Spiritual Distress related to fear of death, grief, loss of faith, denial, bargaining, or anger **Goal:** The client will discuss spiritual beliefs in relation to his or her illness and impending death.	Acknowledge the client's fear and feelings. Listen and communicate therapeutically (see Chap. 9) when client brings up subject of impending death. Determine cultural rituals and beliefs about death and facilitate any activities the client desires that are compatible with his or her beliefs. Suggest contacting the client's or hospital's spiritual advisor.
Anticipatory Grieving related to functional losses and impending death **Goal:** The client will verbalize grief and identify support systems.	Assess stage of grieving and coping methods. Provide opportunities for client and family to share their feelings. Reinforce the client's self-esteem. Focus on the present.

	Encourage the client to resolve any conflicts. Identify support systems. Refer client to support groups and other resources.
Fear related to physical pain and concerns that needs will not be met **Goal:** The client will express trust that needs will be met.	Discuss client's fears with client and family. Encourage client to make decisions about care. Plan care with client and family that addresses fears. Discuss pain management program including adjuncts to medication that promote comfort (see Nursing Guidelines 20-1).
Risk for Hopelessness and Powerlessness related to terminal illness and loss of control **Goal:** The client will find comfort and value in the present and take part in decisions involving care.	Emphasize life accomplishments. Encourage reminiscing. Help client identify attainable goals and focus on present. Encourage verbalization of values and spiritual beliefs. Encourage sharing and emotional intimacy with family members and provide privacy to enhance interactions. Convey caring, acceptance, and support. Encourage client to make decisions about care.
Risk for Impaired Home Maintenance Management related to insufficient knowledge **Goal:** The client and family will feel competent in managing terminal care	Evaluate home care needs and discuss with family and client. Provide visual, oral, and written education about use of specialized equipment. Provide education about pain management, especially pain medication, evaluating pain, and avoiding oversedation. Provide information about community resources.
Pain chronic related to disease progression **Goal:** The client will verbalize adequate relief of pain or the ability to tolerate a decreased level of pain.	Implement Nursing Standards for Managing Pain (see Box 20–1).
Breathing Pattern, Ineffective related to hypoxia, decreased lung expansion, and pain **Goal:** The client will not experience severe dyspnea.	Monitor breathing patterns. Position client for maximum respiratory effort. Monitor for changes in level of consciousness, orientation, anxiety, restlessness, and air hunger. Apply supplemental oxygen as ordered. Assess ability to clear secretions. Suction oropharyngeal airway gently as indicated. Assess for pain; medicate client as ordered. Schedule activities in order to provide adequate rest periods. Provide reassurance during acute episodes of dyspnea.
Nutrition, Altered, Less Than Body Requirements related to inability to eat and increased metabolic needs caused by disease process **Goal:** The client will participate in dietary selections and maintain present weight.	Encourage client to select foods that she or he can tolerate. Assist client to select foods that provide calories. Suggest liquid drinks that supplement diet. Refer client to dietician.
Risk for Impaired Skin Integrity for related to poor nutrition, immobility, and incontinence **Goal:** The client's skin will remain intact.	Assess general condition of skin. Assess client's nutritional status. Reposition client at least every 2 hours. Encourage client to ambulate if possible, and to be out of bed. Increase tissue perfusion by massaging around affected areas. Clean, dry, and moisturize skin as indicated.

Evaluation and Expected Outcomes

- The client is able to discuss spiritual beliefs in relation to death.
- The client and family grieve and become reconciled to impending death.
- The client is able to express feelings about losses and impending death.
- The client participates in decisions about care.
- The client expresses that needs are met.
- The client is able to die peacefully and with dignity.
- The client is pain free.
- The client is able to meet nutritional requirements.

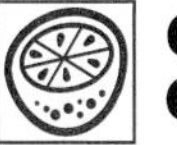

General Nutritional Considerations

Good nutrition becomes a quality of life issue in dying clients. Eating favorite foods with a mealtime companion may stimulate appetite and promote a sense of comfort. However, loss of appetite and weight may be inevitable. "Force feeding" a dying client, either orally or through a tube, may cause nausea and serves no useful purpose. Assure the family that decreased appetite and altered gastrointestinal function are a normal part of the dying process.

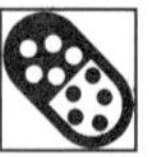

General Pharmacologic Considerations

A priority for the dying client is pain control. Pain relief is best achieved by administering the analgesic on a regular, around-the-clock basis, rather than on an as needed basis.

Pain control often is a great challenge (see Chap. 20) Morphine and meperidine (Demerol) can stimulate the chemoreceptor trigger zone, causing vomiting.

Fears of the client and staff regarding the possibility of the client's developing a tolerance to pain relief medications should be discussed.

Drugs for raising blood pressure, improving tissue and organ perfusion, and correcting cardiac or circulatory problems may be ordered.

General Gerontologic Considerations

Older adults may fear prolonged illness, dependency, and loss of cognitive ability more than death itself.

Older adults are more likely to talk about death and express less fear concerning death than younger adults.

Some older adults who are terminally ill do not want to be alone and fear abandonment by family who cannot cope with the older adult's death.

Older adults may die alone, without the support of family members, relatives, and close friends. The nurse may be the only person to give close emotional support during the final hours of living.

Because of their own unresolved fears concerning death, nurses may administer less emotional support to older dying clients, even though they require as much emotional support as do young and middle-aged clients.

SUMMARY OF KEY CONCEPTS

- Death-denying attitudes among health care workers cause them to neglect the psychosocial needs of dying clients and rob them of an opportunity for personal growth.
- Informing terminally ill clients maintains honest relationships, gives clients the opportunity to plan their remaining time, and provides clients with the chance to complete unfinished business and prepare for death.
- Nurses can communicate hopefulness by demonstrating that the client will not be abandoned, by maintaining quality of care, and by supporting activities the client finds meaningful.
- Dr. Kübler-Ross identified five emotional stages that clients who are dying experience: denial, anger, depression, bargaining, and acceptance.
- A dying client may ensure that desires for terminal care are adhered to by using an advance directive, such as a living will or durable power of attorney for health care.
- Physical signs of impending death include tachycardia followed by bradycardia and hypotension; pale, cool, mottled skin; irregular respiratory rate; moist and gurgling breath sounds; reduced urine production; nausea and vomiting; bladder or bowel incontinence; and diminished level of consciousness.
- The dying process is accompanied by psychological events, such as forestalling death until receiving permission to die from loved ones and family and having near death awareness.
- Nursing management of the dying client and family includes helping with spiritual distress; anticipating grief, fear; hopelessness; home care; pain; breathing; nutrition, and skin care.

CRITICAL THINKING EXERCISES

1. Describe how the nursing care for a younger client dying from acquired immunodeficiency syndrome would be different than the nursing care of an older adult dying from pneumonia.
2. A client with treatable cancer expresses a desire to go to Mexico where they offer coffee enemas and injections with sheep urine as a cure. How would you respond? Would your response be different if the client's cancer were untreatable? Why?
3. If a client wanted to die at home, how would you help the family prepare for terminal home care?

Suggested Readings

Carpenito, L. J. (1995). *Nursing care plans and documentation: Nursing diagnoses and collaborative problems* (2nd ed.). Philadelphia: J. B. Lippincott.

DeSpelder, L. A., & Strickland, A. L. (1992). *The last dance: Encountering death and dying* (3rd ed.). Mountain View, CA: Mayfield.

Durham, E. & Weiss, L. (1997). How patients die. *American Journal of Nursing, 97*(12), 41–46, quiz, 47.

Fanslow-Brunjes, C., Schneider, P. E., & Kimmel, L. H. (1997) Hope: Offering comfort and support for dying patients. *Nursing97, 27*(3), 54–57.

Greenspan, A. J., Lorimar, R. J., Aday, L. A., Winn, R. J., & Baile, W. F. (1997). Terminally ill cancer patients: Their most important concerns. *Cancer Practice, 5*(3), 147–154.

Hankel, C. W. (1993). It's okay to die. *Nursing93, 23,* 96.

Herbst, L. H., Lynn, J., Mermann, A. C., & Rhymec, J. (1995). What do dying patients want and need? *Patient Care, 29*(4), 27–35, 39.

Kübler-Ross, E. (1969). *On death and dying*. New York: Macmillan.

Mallison, M. B. (1993). Decoding the messages of the dying. *American Journal of Nursing, 93,* 7.

Ray, M. C. (1996). Seven ways to empower dying patients. *American Journal of Nursing, 96*(5), (Nurs Pract Extra Ed), 56–57.

Additional Resources

Death, Dying, and Grief
http://www.katsdern.com

Last Acts
http://lastacts.rwjf.org

Compassionate Friends
http://www.compassionatefriends.org

American Association for the Advancement of Palliative Care
http://www.asap.care.com

Association for Death Education and Counseling
http://www.adec.o

6

Caring for Clients With Respiratory Disorders

Chapter 26

Introduction to the Respiratory System

KEY TERMS

Adenoids
Alveolus (pl. alveoli)
Arytenoid cartilages
Bronchioles
Bronchus (pl. bronchi)
Carina
Cricoid cartilage
Diaphragm
Diffusion
Epiglottis
Ethmoid sinuses
Glottis
Hilus
Hypercapnia
Hypocapnia
Hypoxemia
Hypoxia
Larynx
Maxillary sinuses
Mediastinum
Nasal septum
Nasopharynx
Oropharynx
Paranasal sinuses
Parietal pleura
Perfusion
Pharynx
Pleura
Pleural space
Respiration
Sphenoid sinuses
Thyroid cartilage
Tonsils
Trachea
Ventilation
Visceral pleura
Vocal cords

LEARNING OBJECTIVES

On completion of this chapter, the reader will:

- Describe the structures of the upper and lower airway.
- Explain the normal physiology of the respiratory system.
- Differentiate respiration, ventilation, diffusion, and perfusion.
- Define forces that interfere with breathing, including airway resistance and lung compliance.
- Describe the process of oxygen transport.
- Identify the elements of a respiratory assessment.
- List diagnostic tests that may be performed on the respiratory tract.
- Discuss preparation and care for clients having respiratory diagnostic procedures.

Respiratory disorders and diseases are common, ranging from mild to life-threatening. The respiratory system provides oxygen for cellular metabolic needs and removes carbon dioxide, a waste product of cellular metabolism. Disorders that interfere with breathing or the ability to obtain sufficient oxygen greatly affect a client's respiratory status and overall health status.

Respiratory Anatomy

Upper Airway

The upper airway (Fig. 26–1) consists of the nose, paranasal sinuses, pharynx, and larynx.

NOSE

The nose is divided into two passages separated by the **nasal septum.** The nasal mucosa warms and humidifies inspired air. Mucus secreted from the nasal mucosa traps small particles, such as dust and pollen. This helps to prevent irritation and contamination to the lower airway. The mucosa also contains olfactory sensory cells that are responsible for the sense of smell.

PARANASAL SINUSES

The **paranasal sinuses** are extensions of the nasal cavity located in the surrounding facial bones (see Fig. 26–1). They lighten the weight of the skull and give resonance to the voice. The two frontal sinuses lie within the frontal bone that extends above the orbital cavities. The ethmoid bone, located between the eyes, contains a honeycomb of small spaces called the **ethmoid sinuses.** The sphenoidal sinuses lie behind the nasal cavity. The **maxillary sinuses** are found on either side of the nose in the maxillary bones. These

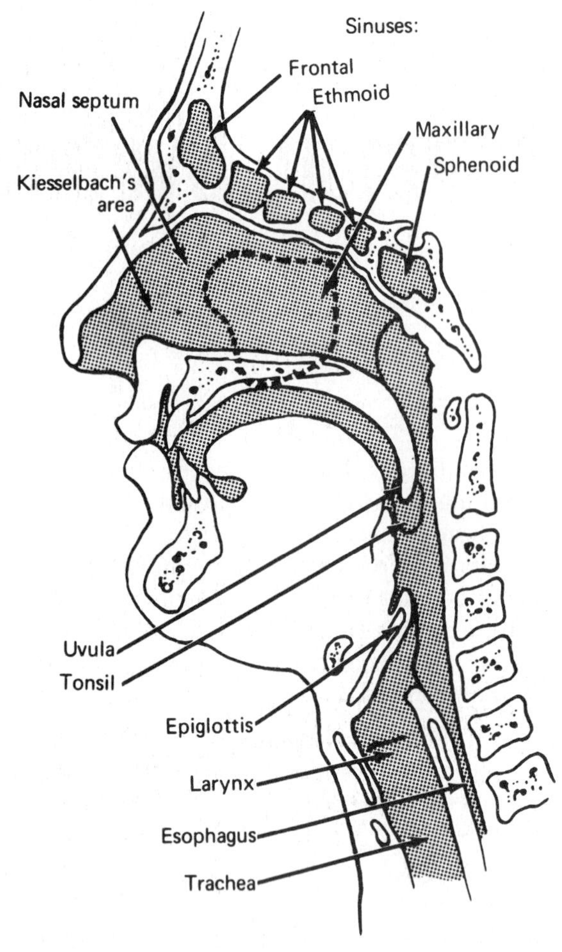

FIGURE 26-1. Major structures of the nose and throat.

are the largest sinuses and the most accessible to treatment. The lining of the sinuses is continuous with the mucous membrane lining of the nasal cavity. The mucus traps particles that the cilia sweep toward the pharynx. IgA antibodies in the mucus protect the lower respiratory tract from infection.

The olfactory area lies at the roof of the nose. The cribriform plate forms part of the roof of the nose and the floor of the anterior cranial fossa. Trauma or surgery in this area carries the risk of injury or infection in the brain.

PHARYNX

The **pharynx,** or throat, carries air from the nose to the larynx, and food from the mouth to the esophagus. The pharynx is divided into three continuous areas: the nasopharynx (near the nose), the oropharynx (near the mouth), and the laryngopharynx (near the larynx). The **nasopharynx** contains the adenoids and the openings of the eustachian tubes. The eustachian tubes connect the pharynx to the middle ear and are the means by which upper respiratory infections spread to the middle ear. The **oropharynx** contains the tongue. The muscular nature of the pharynx allows for closure of the epiglottis during swallowing and relaxation of the epiglottis during respiration.

Tonsils and adenoids, which do not contribute to respiration, are found in the upper airway. **Tonsils** consist of two pairs of elliptically shaped bodies of lymphoid tissue on either side of the upper oropharynx. They protect the body from infection. **Adenoids,** also composed of lymphoid tissue, are found in the nasopharynx. Chronic throat infections often lead to the removal of tonsils and adenoids. In adults, adenoids may shrink and become nonfunctional.

LARYNX

The **larynx,** or voice box, is a cartilaginous framework between the pharynx and the trachea. Its primary function is to produce sound. When air passes through the vocal cords, they vibrate to produce different frequencies. The pharynx, palate, tongue, teeth, and lips mold the sounds made by the vocal cords into speech. The larynx also protects the lower airway from foreign objects because of its ability to facilitate coughing. Other important structures in the larynx include the **epiglottis**, a cartilaginous valve flap that covers the opening to the larynx during swallowing; the **glottis**, an opening between the vocal cords; and the **vocal cords**, folds of tissue within the larynx that vibrate and produce sound as air passes through (Fig. 26–2). Table 26–1 reviews the structures of the larynx.

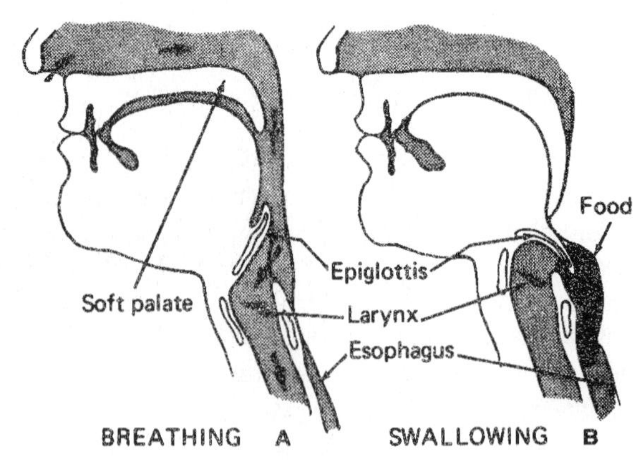

FIGURE 26-2. (*A*) During swallowing, the soft palate elevates to close off air from the nose. Breathing is interrupted momentarily. (*B*) The larynx rises, and its opening is shut off by the epiglottis until the food has passed down into the esophagus.

TABLE 26-1 **Structures of the Larynx**

Structure	Description
Epiglottis	Valve flap of cartilage that covers the opening of the larynx during swallowing
Glottis	Opening between the vocal cords in the larynx
Thyroid cartilage	Largest cartilage in trachea; part of it forms the Adam's apple
Cricoid cartilage	Only complete cartilaginous ring in the larynx, located below the thyroid cartilage
Arytenoid cartilages	Used in vocal cord movement with the thyroid cartilage
Vocal cords	Ligaments that are controlled by muscular movement that produce vocal sounds

(From Smeltzer, S. C., & Bare, B. G. [1996]. *Brunner and Suddarth's textbook of medical-surgical nursing* [8th ed.]. Philadelphia: Lippincott-Raven.)

Lower Airway

The lower respiratory tract consists of the trachea, bronchi, bronchioles, lungs, and alveoli (Fig. 26–3). Accessory structures include the diaphragm, rib cage, sternum, spine, muscles, and blood vessels.

TRACHEA

The **trachea** is a hollow tube composed of smooth muscle and supported by C-shaped cartilage. The trachea transports air from the laryngeal pharynx to the bronchi and lungs. The trachea bifurcates (divides) at the **carina** (lower end of the trachea) to form the left and right bronchi. Stimulation of the carina causes coughing and bronchospasm (spasm of bronchial smooth muscle causing narrowing of the lumen).

BRONCHI

The right mainstem **bronchus** is shorter, more vertical, and larger than the left mainstem bronchus. For these reasons, aspiration of foreign objects is more

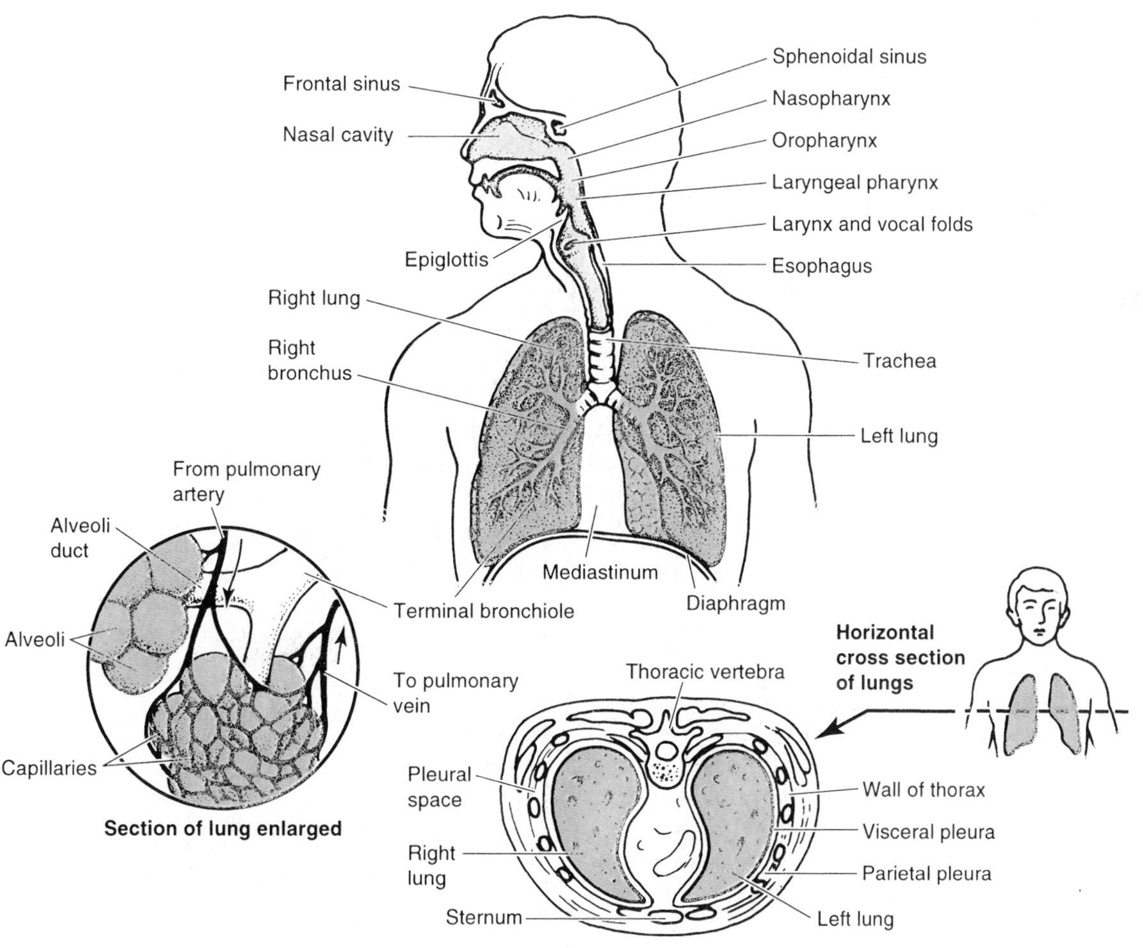

FIGURE 26-3. Respiratory tract.

likely to occur in the right mainstem bronchus and right upper lung. Mucous membrane continues to line this portion of the respiratory tract. Cilia sweep mucus and particles toward the pharynx.

The right and left mainstem bronchi divide into secondary bronchi. There are three secondary right bronchi and two secondary left bronchi, each supplying air to the three right lobes and two left lobes of the lung. The entrance of the bronchi to the lungs is called the **hilus** of the lungs.

LUNGS

The lungs are the site of the exchanges of gases. The bronchi branch, entering each lobe, and continue to branch to form smaller bronchi, and, finally terminal **bronchioles** (smaller subdivisions of the bronchus).

At the end of the bronchioles are the **alveoli,** which are small clustered sacs. Each alveolus consists of a single layer of squamous epithelium cells. Capillaries surround these thin-walled alveoli, which is where the exchange of oxygen and carbon dioxide occurs.

Adult lungs contain approximately 300 million alveoli, which form the mass of the lungs. A huge network of pulmonary capillaries surrounds the alveoli, providing a large area for gas exchange. The epithelium of the alveoli consists of:

- Type I cells—line most of the alveolar surfaces
- Type II cells—produce surfactant, a phospholipid that alters the surface tension of the alveoli, preventing alveolar collapse during expiration and limiting alveolar expansion during inspiration
- Type III cells—destroy foreign material, such as bacteria

The interstitium lies between the alveoli and contains the pulmonary capillaries and elastic connective tissue. This gives the lungs the ability to have elastic recoil (stretch and relax, returning to resting position). Elastic and collagen fibers allow the lungs to have compliance, which refers to the ability of the lung to expand.

A saclike serous membrane called the **pleura** covers the lungs. The **visceral pleura** covers the lung surface and the **parietal pleura** covers the chest wall. Serous fluid separates and lubricates the visceral and parietal pleura—this is called the **pleural space**. The elasticity of the lung tissue allows the lungs to expand and fill the thoracic cavity. This creates a negative or subatmospheric pressure, which keeps the lungs in an inflated state. If air gets into the space between the lungs and the thoracic wall, the lungs will collapse.

The **diaphragm** separates the thoracic cavity from the abdominal cavity. On inspiration, the respiratory muscles contract. The diaphragm also contracts and moves downward, enlarging the thoracic space and creating a partial vacuum. On expiration, the respiratory muscles relax, and the diaphragm returns to its original position. The **mediastinum** is a wall that divides the thoracic cavity into two halves. This wall has two layers of pleura. The remaining thoracic structures are located between the two pleural layers.

Respiratory Physiology

The main function of the respiratory system is to exchange oxygen and carbon dioxide between the atmospheric air and the blood and between the blood and the cells. This process is called **respiration.** Other terms related to respiration are defined in Table 26-2.

Mechanics of Ventilation

Ventilation is the actual movement of air in and out of the respiratory tract. Air must reach the alveoli for gas exchange to occur. This requires a patent airway and intact and functioning respiratory muscles. Ventilation occurs because of pressure gradients between the atmospheric air and the alveoli. Air flows from an area of higher pressure to an area of lower pressure. During inspiration, the diaphragm contracts and flattens, which expands the thoracic cage and increases the thoracic cavity. The pressure within the thorax decreases to a level below that of the atmospheric pressure. As a result, air moves into the lungs. When inspiration is complete, the diaphragm relaxes, and the lungs recoil to their original position. The size of the thoracic cavity decreases, increasing the pressure to levels greater than atmospheric pressure. Air then flows out of the lungs into the atmosphere.

TABLE 26-2 **Terms Related to Respiration**

Ventilation	Movement of air in and out of the lungs sufficient to maintain normal arterial oxygen and carbon dioxide tensions
Inspiration	Movement of oxygen into the lungs
Expiration	Removal of carbon dioxide from the lungs
Diffusion	Transfer of a substance from an area of higher concentration or pressure to an area of lower concentration or pressure; exchange of oxygen and carbon dioxide across the alveolocapillary membrane and at the cellular level
Perfusion	Flow of blood within the pulmonary circulation
Distribution	Delivery of atmospheric air to the separate gas exchange units in the lungs

Neurologic Control of Ventilation

Several mechanisms control ventilation. The respiratory centers in the medulla oblongata and pons control the rate and depth of ventilation. Central chemoreceptors in the medulla are sensitive to changes in carbon dioxide levels and hydrogen ion concentrations (pH) in the cerebrospinal fluid. Signals are sent to the lungs to change the depth and rate of ventilation. Peripheral chemoreceptors in the aortic arch and carotid arteries respond to changes in the amount of oxygen in the blood, the amount of carbon dioxide in the blood, and the pH. Other controls of respiration are described in Table 26–3.

Gas Exchange

Diffusion is the process of oxygen and carbon dioxide exchange through the alveolocapillary membrane. Concentration gradients determine the direction of diffusion. During inspiration, the concentration of oxygen in the capillaries is lower than that of the alveoli. Therefore, oxygen diffuses from the alveoli to the capillaries to the arteries. As it is transported in the arteries, the concentration of oxygen in the cells is lower. Thus, oxygen diffuses into the cells. As carbon dioxide gradients increase in the cells, carbon dioxide diffuses from the cells into the capillaries and then into the venous circulatory system. As it travels to the pulmonary circulation, the concentration of carbon dioxide is higher than that in the alveoli. Therefore, carbon dioxide is diffused into the alveoli.

The respiratory system usually has sufficient reserves to maintain the normal partial pressures or tension of oxygen and carbon dioxide in the blood during times of stress. Respiratory insufficiency develops if there is too much interference with ventilation, diffusion, or **perfusion** (actual flow of blood within the pulmonary circulation). Abnormalities in these processes can lead to **hypoxia, hypoxemia, hypercapnia,** and **hypocapnia**. Table 26–4 describes these terms.

TABLE 26-3 **Neurologic Control of Respiration**

Control	Description
Hering-Breuer reflex	Stretch receptors located in the alveoli are activated during inspiration, so that inspiration is inhibited and lungs are not overdistended.
Proprioceptors	Breathing is stimulated with exercise. Proprioceptors located in the muscles and joints are activated with movement and cause an increase in ventilation.
Baroreceptors	These receptors in the aortic and carotid bodies respond to changes in arterial blood pressure (BP). Elevated arterial BP causes a reflex hypoventilation; lowered BP causes a reflex hyperventilation.

Alveolar respiration determines the amount of carbon dioxide in the body. An *increase* in carbon dioxide, which is present in body fluids primarily as carbonic acid, *decreases* the hydrogen ion concentration (pH) below the normal 7.4. A *decrease* in carbon dioxide *increases* the pH above 7.4. The pH affects the rate of alveolar respiration by a direct action of hydrogen ions on the respiratory center in the medulla oblongata. The kidneys contribute to the maintenance of a normal pH by excreting excess hydrogen ions; this keeps serum bicarbonate within a normal range. The lungs and kidneys combine to maintain the ratio of carbonic acid to bicarbonate at 1:20, fixing the pH at about 7.4.

In a critically ill client, various homeostatic mechanisms operate to compensate for alterations. In an attempt to maintain normal pH, the lungs eliminate carbonic acid by blowing off more carbon dioxide, or the kidneys excrete more bicarbonate. A client's condition remains compensated if the carbonic acid-to-bicarbonate ratio remains 1:20.

Disturbances in pH that involve the lungs are considered *respiratory*. Disturbances in pH involving other mechanisms are termed *metabolic*. At times, respiratory and metabolic disturbances coexist.

Transport of Gases

The transport of gas occurs in two ways:

- A small amount is dissolved in water in the plasma.
- A greater portion combines with hemoglobin in the red blood cells (oxyhemoglobin).

Dissolved oxygen is the only form that can diffuse across cellular membranes. As this oxygen crosses the cell membranes, it is rapidly replaced by oxygen from

TABLE 26-4 **Conditions Related to Abnormalities in Ventilation, Perfusion, Diffusion, and Distribution**

Condition	Description
Hypoxia	Decreased oxygen in inspired air
Hypoxemia	Decreased oxygen in the blood
Hypercapnia	Increased carbon dioxide in the blood
Hypocapnia	Decreased carbon dioxide in the blood

the hemoglobin. Large amounts of oxygen are transported in the blood as oxyhemoglobin.

Carbon dioxide (CO_2) diffuses from the tissue cells to the blood. This is transported to the lungs for excretion. Most of the carbon dioxide enters the red blood cells. Some of it combines with hemoglobin to form carbaminohemoglobin. Most of it combines with the water within the cells and then exits as bicarbonate ions (HCO_3), which are transported in the plasma to the kidneys. A small portion remains in a dissolved form in the plasma and is called carbonic acid. The formation of carbonic acid yields hydrogen ions. The amount of hydrogen ions determines the pH, which also determines the amount of carbon dioxide to be excreted by the lungs. Refer to Chapter 21 for a review of acid-base balance.

Work of Breathing

Several factors influence the work of breathing. Pressures needed to overcome the forces interfering with breathing determine the amount of respiratory effort needed. Forces that interfere with breathing include airway resistance and lung compliance. Airway resistance is related to airway diameter, rate of air flow, or speed of gas flow. More resistance results as the rate of breathing increases. A narrowed airway results from increased or thick mucus, bronchospasm, or edema. Decreased surfactant, fibrosis, edema, and atelectasis (alveolar collapse) affect lung compliance. Greater pressure gradients are needed when lungs are stiff.

Pulmonary Perfusion

There are two blood supplies for the lungs: the bronchial circulation and the pulmonary circulation.

BRONCHIAL CIRCULATION

The bronchial arteries arise in the thoracic aorta and the intercostal arteries. These arteries supply blood to the trachea and the bronchi. They also supply the lungs' supporting tissues, the nerves, and the outer layers of the pulmonary arteries and veins. This circulation returns either to the left atrium via the pulmonary vein or to the superior vena cava via the bronchial and azygos veins.

The bronchial circulation does not supply the bronchioles or alveoli unless there is an interruption to pulmonary circulation. In that event, it will supply those areas, but the bronchioles and alveoli cannot perform their function of gas exchange (Bullock, 1996).

PULMONARY CIRCULATION

The pulmonary artery transports the venous blood from the right ventricle to the lungs. The pulmonary artery divides into the right and left branches to supply the right and left lungs. The blood circulates through the pulmonary capillary bed, where diffusion of oxygen and carbon dioxide occurs. The blood then returns to the left atrium via the pulmonary veins.

Pulmonary circulation is referred to as a low pressure system (Smeltzer & Bare, 1996). This means that pulmonary perfusion is affected by gravity, alveolar pressure, and pulmonary artery pressure. A person in an upright position will have less perfusion to the upper lobes. When a person is on his or her side, there will be greater perfusion to the dependent side. In addition, increased alveolar pressure can cause pulmonary capillaries to narrow or collapse, impacting sufficient gas exchange. Decreased pulmonary artery pressure results in decreased perfusion to the lungs. Clients with lung and cardiovascular disease may have decreased pulmonary perfusion.

Assessment

History

Obtain information about the client's general health history, frequency of respiratory illnesses, respiratory treatments, medications, last pulmonary tests (chest x-ray, tuberculosis test), family history, allergies, occupation, smoking history, history and nature of cough, description of sputum, wheezing, dyspnea (labored or difficult breathing), exercise tolerance, pain, and level of fatigue.

Physical Examination

The next part of the assessment is the physical examination of the client. Begin with a general examination of the client's overall health and condition. Clients with respiratory problems may show signs of shortness of breath when speaking, or they may have a certain posture or position that helps them breathe. Other observations include skin color; level of consciousness; mental status; respiratory rate, depth, effort, rhythm; use of accessory muscles; and the shape of the chest and symmetry of chest movements.

Inspect the nose for signs of injury, inflammation, symmetry, and lesions. Examine the posterior pharynx and tonsils with a tongue blade and light. Note any evidence of swelling, inflammation, and exudate, plus changes in color of the mucous membranes. Note any difficulty swallowing or hoarseness.

The larynx is inspected either directly with a laryngoscope or indirectly with a light and a laryngeal mirror. Both procedures require a local anesthetic to suppress the gag reflex and reduce discomfort and are performed by a physician or nurse practitioner.

Inspect and gently palpate the trachea to assess for placement and deviation from the midline. Note lymph node enlargement. Examine the anterior, posterior, and lateral chest walls for lesions, symmetry, deformities, skin color, and evidence of muscle weakness or weight loss. The contour of the chest walls is important to assess. Normally the anteroposterior diameter of the chest wall is half the transverse diameter. However, some pulmonary conditions, such as emphysema, change the chest dimensions. Table 26–5 describes some common abnormalities.

An experienced examiner palpates the chest wall to detect tenderness, masses, swelling, or other abnormalities of the chest wall. Tactile or vocal fremitus is the capacity to feel sound through the fingers and palm placed on the chest wall. The palpable vibrations occur when the client speaks. The examiner uses the palmar surface of the fingers and hands to palpate, and asks the client to repeat 99 as she or he moves her or his hands. If the client is healthy and thin, the fremitus will be highly palpable. Conditions that affect fremitus are:

- A thick or muscular chest wall (decreases fremitus)
- Lung diseases such as emphysema and pneumonia (increase fremitus)
- Fluid, air, or masses in the pleural space (decrease fremitus)

TABLE 26-5 **Common Abnormalities of the Chest**

Condition	Description
Kyphosis	Exaggerated curvature of the thoracic spine; congenital anomaly or associated with injuries and osteoporosis
Scoliosis	Lateral S-shaped curvature of the thoracic and lumbar spine
Barrel chest	Anteroposterior diameter increases to equal the transverse diameter; chest is rounded; ribs are horizontal; sternum is pulled forward; associated with emphysema and aging.
Funnel chest	Also known as pectus excavatum; the sternum is depressed from the second intercostal space—more pronounced with inspiration; a congenital anomaly.
Pigeon chest	Also known as pectus carinatum; the sternum abnormally protrudes; the ribs are sloped backward; a congenital anomaly.

The experienced examiner performs percussion of the chest wall to assess normal and abnormal sounds produced by this maneuver. With the client in the sitting position, the examiner places her or his middle finger on the chest wall and taps that finger with the middle finger of the opposite hand. The types of sounds heard with percussion are described in Table 26–6.

Auscultate breath sounds from side to side, moving from the upper to the lower chest (Fig. 26-4). Listen anteriorly and posteriorly. Normal breath sounds include:

- Vesicular sounds—Produced by air movement in bronchioles and alveoli, these sounds are heard over the lung fields. They are quiet, low pitched, with long inspiration and short expiration.
- Bronchial sounds—Produced by air movement through the trachea. These sounds are heard over the trachea. They are loud with longer expiration than inspiration.
- Bronchovesicular sounds—Normal breath sounds heard between the trachea and upper lungs. Their pitch is medium with equal length of inspiration and expiration.

Adventitious or abnormal breath sounds are categorized as crackles or wheezes. Crackles are discrete sounds that result from the delayed opening of deflated airways. Sometimes they clear with coughing. They may be present because of inflammation or congestion. Wheezes are continuous musical sounds that can be heard during inspiration and expiration. They are the result of air passing through narrowed or partially obstructed air passages and are heard in clients with increased secretions.

Friction rubs are identified as crackling or grating sounds heard on inspiration and expiration. These sounds occur when there is inflammation of the pleural surfaces. The sounds are not altered if the client coughs.

Diagnostic and Laboratory Procedures

Arterial Blood Gases

Oxygenation of body tissues depends on the amount of oxygen in arterial blood. *Arterial blood gases* (ABGs) determine the pH of the blood, the oxygen-carrying capacity of the blood, and the the amount of oxygen, carbon dioxide, and bicarbonate ion in the blood. Blood gas studies are frequently ordered when a client is acutely ill or has a history of respiratory disorders. If PaO_2 levels are decreased, body tis-

TABLE 26-6 **Sounds Heard with Chest Wall Percussion**

Sound	Description	Implications
Flat	High pitch, little intensity, decreased duration	Heard when a solid area is percussed, such as with a mass or pleural effusion
Dull	Medium pitch, medium intensity, medium duration	Heard when there is no air or fluid in the lung, ie, atelectasis, lobar pneumonia
Tympanic	High pitch, loud intensity, long duration	Normal over stomach and bowel; abnormal over lungs such as in a pneumothorax
Resonant	Low pitch, loud intensity, long duration	Normal lung sound
Hyperresonant	Lower pitch, very loud, longer duration	Abnormal sounds that occur when free air exists in the thoracic cavity, ie, emphysema, pneumothorax

sues do not receive sufficient oxygen. Table 26–7 presents the descriptions and measures of normal blood gas values. Clients with respiratory disorders can neither get oxygen into the blood nor get carbon dioxide out of the blood. Some conditions that affect ABGs are:

1. Hyperventilation during the collection of ABGs causing elevated PaO_2 levels
2. Hypoventilation with neuromuscular disease, chronic obstructive lung disease (COPD), or insufficient oxygen in the atmosphere causing decreased PaO_2 levels
3. Elevated $PaCO_2$ levels in clients with COPD, inadequate ventilation with a mechanical ventilator, or decreased respiratory rates
4. Decreased $PaCO_2$ levels in clients who are nervous or anxious or who have a condition that causes hyperventilation or a rapid respiratory rate

Pulse oximetry is a noninvasive method of measuring the oxygen content of hemoglobin (SaO_2), using a light beam. The monitoring device attaches to the earlobe or fingertip and connects to the oximeter monitor (Fig. 26–5). Wavelengths of light passing through the earlobe or fingertip produce a readout of the arterial oxygen saturation calculated by the monitor. Normal values are 95% or higher. Refer to Clinical Procedure 26–1.

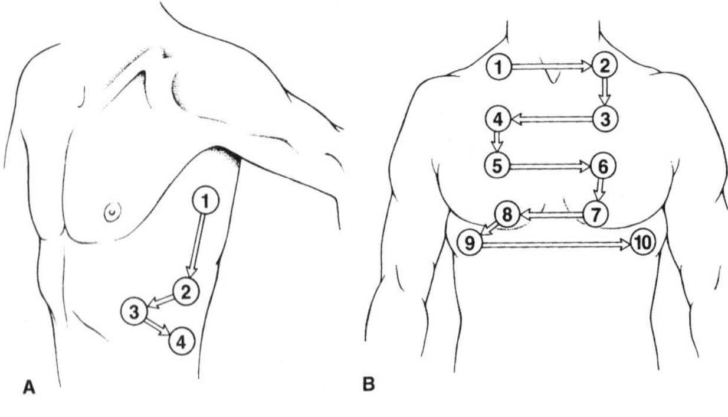

FIGURE 26-4. (*A*) Each side of the chest is auscultated and compared. (*B*) The anterior chest is systematically examined over each lung field.

Tuberculin Skin Test

The *Mantoux test* (*tuberculin skin test*) is commonly done to determine if a client has been infected with *Myobacterium tuberculosis*. It is important to note that this test does not differentiate between active and dormant disease. See Nursing Guidelines 26–1 for administering a Mantoux test.

Pulmonary Function Studies

Pulmonary function studies measure lung ventilation volumes. Measurements are obtained with a spirometer and include:

- *Tidal volume*—volume of air inhaled and exhaled with a normal breath
- *Inspiratory reserve volume*—maximum volume of air inspired at the end of a normal inspiration
- *Expiratory reserve volume*—maximum volume of air exhaled by forced expiration after a normal respiration
- *Residual volume*—volume of air left in the lungs after maximal expiration

TABLE 26-7 **Normal Values for Arterial Blood Gases**

pH	Hydrogen ion concentration; acidity or alkalinity of the blood	7.35–7.45
PaO_2	Partial pressure of oxygen in arterial blood	80–100 mm Hg
$PaCO_2$	Partial pressure of carbon dioxide in arterial blood	35–45 mm Hg
HCO_3	Bicarbonate ion concentration in the blood	22–26 mm Hg
SaO_2	Arterial oxygen saturation or the percent of the oxygen-carrying	95%–100%

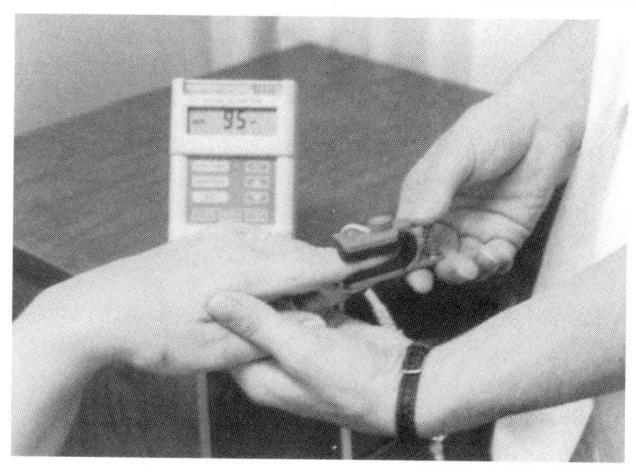

FIGURE 26-5. Spring-tension sensor and microprocessor. (Courtesy of Ken Timby.)

- *Vital capacity*—maximum amount of air expired after maximal inspiration
- *Forced vital capacity*—amount of air exhaled forcefully and rapidly after maximal inspiration
- *Inspiratory capacity*—maximum amount of air inhaled after normal expiration
- *Functional residual capacity*—amount of air left in the lungs after a normal expiration
- *Total lung capacity*—total volume of air in the lungs when maximally inflated

Pulmonary function results vary according to age, sex, weight, and height. The maximum lung capacities and volumes are best achieved when the client is sitting or standing. These studies are done to diagnose pulmonary conditions and to assess a client's respiratory status preoperatively. They are also used to determine the effectiveness of bronchodilators or to screen employees who work in environments that are hazardous to pulmonary health. Refer to the Nursing Guidelines 26–2 for key points related to client care.

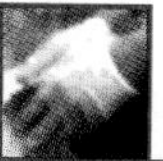

Clinical Procedure 26-1
Pulse Oximetry

PURPOSE	EQUIPMENT
• Monitor client for subtle or sudden changes in SaO_2 • Provide a noninvasive method for monitoring SaO_2	• Pulse oximeter • Sensor probe

Nursing Action	Rationale
ASSESSMENT	
Check the medical orders.	Collaborates nursing activities with medical treatment.
Assess potential sensor sites for quality of circulation, presence of edema, tremor, restlessness, nail polish, or artificial nails.	Determines where best to apply sensor for most accurate results.
Review the medical history for data indicating vascular or other pathology such as anemia or carbon monoxide poisoning.	Pulse oximeter data may be less reliable.
Check prescribed medications for vasoconstrictive effects.	Suggests data from pulse oximeter may be unreliable.
Assess client's understanding of pulse oximetry.	Indicates need for and type of teaching.
PLANNING	
Explain procedure to the client.	Reduces anxiety and promotes cooperation.
Obtain equipment.	Promotes organization and efficiency.
IMPLEMENTATION	
Wash your hands.	Reduces the potential for transmission of organisms.
Position the sensor so that the light emission is directly opposite the detector.	Connects the sensor with the oximeter.
Observe the numeric display, audible sound, or waveform on the oximeter.	Indicates the equipment is functioning.
Set the high and low alarms according to the manufacturer's directions.	Alerts the nurse to assess the client.
Move an adhesive finger sensor every 4 hours and a spring tension sensor every 2 hours.	Prevents skin breakdown.

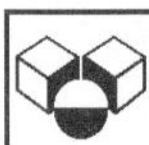

Nursing Guidelines 26-1

Administering and Interpreting a Mantoux Test

- Draw up 0.1 mL intermediate strength purified protein derivative (PPD) in a tuberculin syringe (½-inch 26–27 gauge needle).
- Prepare the injection site on the inner aspect of the forearm, approximately halfway between the elbow and wrist.
- Hold the syringe, bevel up, almost parallel to the forearm.
- Inject the PPD to form a pronounced wheal—this indicates proper intradermal injection.
- Record the site, name of PPD, strength, lot number, and date and time of test.
- Read the test site 48 to 72 hours following the injection by palpating the site for induration. If induration is present, it is measured at its widest width. Erythema (redness) without induration, is not significant. If erythema is present with induration, the induration only is read. The test is interpreted as follows:

  Negative reaction—0 to 4 mm induration. No follow-up needed.
  Questionable reaction—5 to 9 mm induration. If clients are aware of contact with someone with active tuberculosis, this reaction is seen as significant.
  Positive reaction—10 mm or greater of induration

4 mm 10 mm

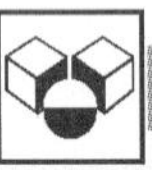

Nursing Guidelines 26-2

Preparing the Client for Pulmonary Function Studies

- Provide explanations of the procedure to decrease anxiety and promote cooperation.
- Assure the client that although the spirometry equipment looks complex, the pulmonary function test is simple.
- Explain to the client that he or she may be tired following the study.
- Remind the client that the tests should not be performed within 2 hours after a meal.
- Tell the client that bronchodilators may be used during the study.
- Inform the client that he or she will use a nose clip during the study so that air cannot escape through the nose.
- Instruct the client to wear loose-fitting clothing.

Sputum Studies

Sputum specimens are examined for the presence of pathogenic microorganisms and cancer cells. Culture and sensitivity tests are done to diagnose infections and prescribe antibiotics. Negative smears of sputum do not always indicate the absence of disease, so collection of sputum for successive days is necessary. Sputum is collected by having the client expectorate a specimen, by suctioning the client, or during a bronchoscopy. Nursing Guidelines 26–3 provides information for the nurse obtaining a sputum specimen.

Radiography

Chest radiographs show the size, shape, and position of the lungs and other structures of the thorax. Physicians use chest x-rays to screen for asymptomatic disease and to diagnose tumors, foreign bodies, and other abnormal conditions. *Fluoroscopy* enables the physician to view the thoracic cavity with all its contents in motion. It more precisely diagnoses the location of a tumor or lesion. A *computed tomographic scan* or *magnetic resonance imaging* is used to produce axial views of the lungs to detect tumors and other lung disorders during early stages of the disease.

Pulmonary Angiography

Pulmonary angiography is a radioisotope study that allows the physician to assess the arterial circulation of the lungs, particularly to detect pulmonary emboli. A catheter is introduced into an arm vein and threaded through the right atrium and ventricle into the pulmonary artery. Contrast medium is rapidly injected

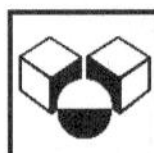

Nursing Guidelines 26-3

Obtaining a Sputum Specimen

- Explain procedure to the client.
- Collect sputum specimen early in the morning or after an aerosol treatment.
- Collect specimen in a sterile specimen container.
- Instruct client to rinse mouth with tap water.
- Instruct client to take several deep breaths, cough forcefully, and expectorate into the container.
- Collect at least 1 to 3 mL (1/2 teaspoon).
- Deliver specimen to laboratory as soon as possible. Container should be transported in sealed plastic bag with requisition.

into the femoral artery and x-rays are taken to see the distribution of the radiopaque material.

Assessment

Assess the client's level of anxiety, and determine what his or her knowledge about the procedure is. Ascertain if the client has any allergies, particularly to iodine, shellfish, or contrast dye.

Diagnosis and Planning

The nursing care of the client undergoing pulmonary angiography includes, but is not limited to, the following:

Nursing Diagnoses and Collaborative Problems	Nursing Interventions
Fear related to lack of knowledge about procedure and expected sensations **Goal:** The client's fear will be reduced or relieved as evidenced by relaxed demeanor and vital signs within normal limits.	Explain the purpose of the study. Explain that site will be cleaned first, which will feel cold. Explain that a feeling of pressure will be experienced as the catheter is inserted into the artery and he or she will experience a warm, flushed feeling and an urge to cough when the contrast medium is injected. Tell the client that strong pressure will be applied to the artery for several minutes after the catheter is removed, followed by the application of a pressure dressing. Explain the need for bed rest for 2 to 6 hours after the study and that his or her extremity will be checked frequently. Give the client an opportunity to ask questions.
PC: Allergic Reaction to contrast medium **Goal:** The client will have minimal problems with allergic reactions.	Ask the client about sensitivity to iodine, shellfish, and contrast dye. Monitor for signs and symptoms of allergic reaction such as itching, hives, or difficulty breathing. Report findings immediately.
PC: Hematoma, Thrombosis, Hemorrhage or Paresthesias **Goal:** The client will experience minimal complications.	Inspect site frequently for swelling, bleeding, or discoloration. Reinforce pressure dressing and notify physician if hematoma develops. Monitor size of hematoma to detect continued bleeding and possible hemorrhage. Palpate distal pulses. Assess capillary refill time frequently. Notify physician if pulses diminish or disappear. Assess skin color and temperature. Monitor vital signs according to policy or more frequently if indicated. Maintain bed rest for 2 to 6 hours without flexing extremity. Monitor extremity for pain, numbness and tingling. Instruct the client to report changes in sensation.

Evaluation and Expected Outcomes

- Fear is decreased.
- Allergic reactions do not occur.
- Minimal swelling or bleeding occurs at the insertion site.
- Circulating status remains intact.
- No complications occur postprocedure.

Lung Scans

There are two types of *lung scans* that may be done for diagnostic purposes—the *perfusion scan* and the *ventilation scan*. Both require the use of radioisotopes and a scanning machine to detect patterns of blood flow through the lungs and patterns of air movement and distribution in the lungs. Perfusion and ventilation scans are particularly useful in diagnosing pulmonary emboli. They are also used to diagnose lung cancer, COPD, and pulmonary edema.

Radioactive contrast media is administered intravenously and by inhalation as a radioactive gas. The radiologist asks the client to change positions as the scanning is done. During inhalation, the client may be asked to hold her or his breath for short periods as scanning images are obtained. It is essential that the client receive adequate explanations before the procedure to reduce anxiety. Assure the client that the amount of radiation from this procedure is less than that of a chest x-ray.

Bronchoscopy

Bronchoscopy allows for direct visualization of the larynx, trachea, and bronchi, using a flexible fiberoptic bronchoscope. The physician introduces the bronchoscope through the nose or mouth, or through a tracheostomy or artificial airway. This procedure is used to diagnose lung disease, treat or evaluate disease, obtain a biopsy of a lesion or tumor, obtain a sputum specimen, perform aggressive pulmonary cleansing, or remove a foreign body. This procedure is very frightening to clients and they require thorough explanations before the procedure. For at least 6 hours before the bronchoscopy, the client abstains from food or drink. This decreases the risk of aspiration, a risk that occurs because the client receives local anesthesia for the procedure. The anesthetic suppresses the swallow, cough, and gag reflexes. The client receives medications before the procedure—usually atropine to dry secretions and a sedative or narcotic. These medications depress the vagus nerve. This is important during a bronchoscopy because if the vagus nerve is stimulated, hypotension, bradycardia, or dysrhythmias may occur. Other potential complications of bronchoscopy include bronchospasm or laryngospasm secondary to edema, hypoxemia, bleeding, perforation, aspiration, cardiac dysrhythmias, and infection.

NURSING PROCESS
The Client Undergoing a Bronchoscopy

Assessment

Assess the anxiety level, knowledge of procedure, baseline vital signs, lung sounds, if the client wears dentures, and when food or fluids were last taken. Determine that the consent form has been signed and witnessed.

Diagnosis and Planning

The nursing care of the client undergoing a bronchoscopy includes, but is not limited to, the following:

Nursing Diagnoses and Collaborative Problems	Nursing Interventions
Fear related to lack of knowledge about what to expect during and after the procedure **Goal:** The client's fear will be reduced or relieved.	Explain that a tube will be inserted through the nose and into the lungs. Inform the client that sedatives will be given to relieve anxiety, reduce secretions, and block the vagus nerve. Explain the purpose to the client. Tell the client that foods and fluids will be restricted after the procedure until the gag reflex returns. Instruct the client to avoid talking, coughing, throat clearing, and smoking after the procedure. Inform client that her or his throat will be irritated for a few days and that blood-tinged mucus is to be expected.
Risk for Aspiration related to diminished gag reflex **Goal:** The client will not aspirate as evidenced by absence of choking, coughing, and clear lung fields.	Assess gag reflex with tongue blade. Keep client NPO until gag reflex returns (usually 2–8 hours). Keep suction equipment available. Maintain client in semi-Fowler's position with head to one side. Encourage client to expectorate secretions frequently. Provide client with a emesis basin. After gag reflex returns, offer sips of water or ice chips initially then progress to soft foods.
PC: Pneumothorax: Dysrhythmia, Bronchospasm **Goal:** The nurse will manage and minimize potential complications.	Monitor respiratory status and compare to baseline assessment. Observe for symmetrical chest movements and auscultate breath sounds. Report hemoptysis, stridor, or difficulty breathing immediately. Monitor heart rate and rhythm and blood pressure.

Evaluation and Expected Outcomes

- Fear is reduced.
- Aspiration is avoided.
- No postprocedure complications develop.

Laryngoscopy

Laryngoscopy provides direct visualization of the larynx. A laryngoscope is used for this procedure. A laryngoscopy is done to diagnose lesions, evaluate laryngeal function, and determine if any inflammation is present. Physicians may also dilate laryngeal strictures and biopsy lesions. Refer to the section on bronchoscopy for nursing management.

Mediastinoscopy

Mediastinoscopy provides visualization of the mediastinum and is done under local or general anesthesia. The physician makes an incision above the sternum and inserts a mediastinoscope. With this procedure the physician can visualize and biopsy lymph nodes. The possible complications include dysrhythmias, myocardial infarction, pneumothorax, and bleeding.

Thoracentesis

A small amount of fluid lies between the visceral and parietal pleurae. When excess fluid or air accumulates, the physician aspirates it from the pleural space by inserting a needle into the chest wall under local anesthesia. This procedure, called *thoracentesis*, also may be used to obtain a sample of pleural fluid or a biopsy specimen from the pleural wall for diagnostic purposes, such as a culture and sensitivity or microscopic examination. Bloody fluid usually suggests trauma. Purulent fluid is diagnostic for infection. Serous fluid is associated with cancer, inflammatory conditions, or heart failure. When a thoracentesis is done for therapeutic reasons, 1 to 2 liters of fluid may be withdrawn to relieve respiratory distress. Medication may be instilled directly into the pleural space to treat infection.

A thoracentesis is done at the bedside or in a treatment or examining room. The client either sits at the side of the bed or examining table, or is in a side-lying position on the unaffected side. If sitting, a pillow is placed on a bedside table and the client rests her or his arms and head on the pillow. The physician determines the site for aspiration by x-ray and percussion. The site is cleansed and anesthetized with local anesthesia. When the procedure is completed, a small pressure dressing is applied. The client remains on bed rest and usually lies on the unaffected side for at least 1 hour to promote expansion of the lung on the affected side. A chest x-ray is done after the procedure to rule out a pneumothorax. Refer to Nursing Guidelines 26–4 for specific nursing management measures. Complications that can occur following a thoracentesis are pneumothorax, subcutaneous emphysema (presence of air in subcutaneous tissue), infection, pulmonary edema, and cardiac distress.

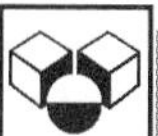

Nursing Guidelines 26-4

Caring for the Client Undergoing Thoracentesis

- Explain procedure to client.
- Assist the client to appropriate position (sitting with arms and head on padded table or in side-lying position on unaffected side) and provide comfort.
- Inform the client about what is happening.
- Maintain asepsis.
- Apply small sterile pressure dressing to the site following the procedure.
- Position client on unaffected side. Instruct the client to remain in this position for at least 1 hour and to remain on bed rest for several hours.
- Check that chest x-ray is done after the procedure.
- Record amount, color, and other characteristics of fluid removed.
- Monitor the client for signs of:

  Increased respiratory rate
  Asymmetry in respiratory movement
  Syncope or vertigo
  Chest tightness
  Uncontrolled cough or cough that is productive of blood-tinged or frothy mucus (or both)
  Tachycardia
  Hypoxemia

Nursing Management

In addition to the specific nursing management associated with individual tests, clients require informative and appropriate explanations of any diagnostic procedures they will experience. It is important to remember that for many of these clients, breathing may in some way be compromised. Their energy levels may be decreased. For that reason, explanations need to be brief yet complete and may need to be repeated. The nurse also facilitates adequate rest periods before and after the procedures.

Following invasive procedures, the nurse must carefully assess clients for signs of respiratory distress, chest pain, blood-streaked sputum, and expectoration of blood. Postprocedure expectations need to be repeated to help reduce the client's anxiety and to ensure the best possible recovery.

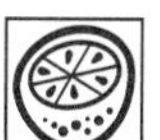

General Nutritional Considerations

The client undergoing a bronchoscopy usually is given nothing by mouth for at least 6 hours before the test to avoid the risk of vomiting and aspiration. Explain the importance of temporary fasting from food and fluids.

Decreased respiratory muscle mass and strength, reduced ventilatory drive, and increased susceptibility to infection are known consequences of malnutrition and severe low body weight; other possible effects include decreased surfactant production and decreased healing after injury. An optimal diet and good nutritional status can help optimize an individual's respiratory status.

Drinking extra fluids may help thin bronchial secretions.

A soft or liquid diet may be ordered for clients who experience pain or difficulty swallowing after a diagnostic procedure such as a laryngoscopy. Cold food and liquids may be better tolerated than hot items.

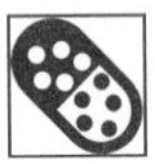

General Pharmacologic Considerations

Clients scheduled for diagnostic tests that involve the use of a contrast medium that contains iodine are questioned about allergies, especially allergies to seafood (which contain iodine) and iodine. If the client appears to have an iodine allergy, the physician is notified before the test. An allergic reaction to iodine can be serious and sometimes fatal.

General Gerontologic Considerations

Although the number of alveoli remains stable with age, the walls of the alveoli become thinner and there are fewer capillaries within the alveoli, resulting in less gas exchange than in a younger adult. The lungs also lose elasticity and become stiffer. These changes place the older adult at increased risk for respiratory disease.

Older clients may have difficulty understanding explanations or directions given by the physician or nurse. It may be necessary to repeat or restate information or directions before or during a diagnostic test.

Older clients may be especially fearful of diagnostic tests because of mental confusion or lack of understanding.

SUMMARY OF KEY CONCEPTS

- The upper airway provides a passageway for air to pass to and from the lungs. The air going in is filtered and humidified.
- The lower airway is responsible for the exchange of oxygen and carbon dioxide at the alveolar-capillary level and for meeting the needs of the body at the cellular level.
- Respiration is the exchange of oxygen and carbon dioxide between the atmospheric air and the blood and between the blood and the cells. Ventilation is the actual movement of air in and out of the respiratory tract. Diffusion is the exchange of oxygen and carbon dioxide across the alveolocapillary membrane and at the cellular level from higher concentrations to lower concentrations. Perfusion is the flow of blood within the pulmonary circulation.
- Airway resistance and lung compliance are forces that interfere with the work of breathing. Airway resistance is related to airway diameter, rate of airflow, or speed of gas flow. Lung compliance is affected by decreased surfactant, fibrosis, edema, and atelectasis.
- Oxygen transport in the blood occurs in two forms: that which is dissolved in the plasma and that in combination with the hemoglobin (oxyhemoglobin). Carbon dioxide combines with red blood cells or is dissolved in plasma for transport in the blood.
- Assessment of the respiratory system includes a thorough health history, particularly the client's smoking history, personal or family history of lung disease, occupational history, history of exposure to allergens, environmental pollutants, and other exposures.
- The physical assessment of the respiratory system focuses on any problems with breathing, presence of a cough, evidence of sputum production or bleeding, signs of wheezing or crackles, and presence of cyanosis.
- Many diagnostic and laboratory studies are done to evaluate a client's respiratory function and breathing ability. Although some are simple and quick, many require invasive techniques and are tiring for the client. Nursing management for these procedures requires careful explanations, provision of comfort, and time for the client to rest.

CRITICAL THINKING EXERCISE

1. Your client had a laryngoscopy and mediastinoscopy today. What are the risks associated with these procedures? What specifically needs to be assessed?

Suggested Readings

Carpenito, L. J. (1995). *Nursing care plans and documentation* (2nd ed.). Philadelphia: J. B. Lippincott.

Faria, S. H., & Taylor, L. J. (1997). Interpretation of arterial blood gases by nurses. *Journal of Vascular Nursing, 15*(4), 128–130.

Fritz, D. J. (1997). Fine tune your physical assessment of the lungs and respiratory system. *Home Care Provider, 2*(6), 299–302; quiz 303–305.

O'Hanlon-Nichols, T. (1998). Basic assessment series: The adult pulmonary system. *American Journal of Nursing, 98*(2), 39–45.

Smeltzer, S. C., & Bare, B. G. (1996). *Brunner and Suddarth's textbook of medical-surgical nursing* (8th ed.). Philadelphia: Lippincott-Raven.

Additional Resources

Lunglinks
http://www.allhealth.edu/lunglinks

Chapter 27

Caring for Clients With Upper Respiratory Disorders

KEY TERMS

Adenoidectomy
Adenoiditis
Aphonia
Coryza
Deviated septum
Epistaxis
Hemoptysis
Hypertrophied turbinates
Laryngitis
Laryngospasm
Nasal polyps
Peritonsillar abscess
Pharyngitis
Rhinitis
Rhinorrhea
Sinusitis
Stridor
Tonsillectomy
Tonsillitis
Tracheostomy
Tracheotomy

LEARNING OBJECTIVES

On completion of this chapter, the reader will:

- Describe the nursing management of clients experiencing infectious or inflammatory upper respiratory disorders.
- Discuss the assessment data required for the nurse to care for a client with a structural disorder of the upper airway.
- Describe the airway problems a client may experience following trauma or obstruction to the upper airway.
- Identify the risk factors that contribute to the development of laryngeal cancer.
- Define the earliest symptom of cancer of the larynx.
- Differentiate the various types of laryngeal cancer.
- Describe measures used to promote alternative methods of communication for a client who has had a laryngectomy.
- Discuss psychosocial issues clients experience following a laryngectomy.
- Identify the possible reasons for a tracheostomy.
- Relate the treatment modalities for clients experiencing short- or long-term problems with airway management.
- Discuss the nursing management of a client with a tracheostomy.

Disorders of the upper airway range from common colds to cancer. The severity depends on the nature of the disorder and the client's physiologic response. Most people experience common colds and sore throats and find them more inconvenient than serious. For others, even the most common disorders of the upper respiratory airway can be of great concern because other physical problems compound the effects of the respiratory disorder.

Infectious and Inflammatory Disorders

The most common upper airway illnesses are infectious and inflammatory disorders. Although it is easy to dismiss these illnesses as unimportant, the average person experiences three to five upper respiratory infections per year.

Rhinitis

Rhinitis is an inflammation of the mucous membranes of the nose. It is often called the common cold, or **coryza.** It may be called acute, chronic, or allergic, depending on its cause. The most common cause of rhinitis is the rhinovirus. More than 100 strains of rhinovirus exist. Colds are rapidly spread by inhalation of droplets and by direct contact, such as hand contact with droplets. Allergic rhinitis is a hypersensitive reaction to allergens, such as pollen, dust, animal dander, or food. For most individuals, rhinitis is not a serious condition. For debilitated, immunosuppressed, or elderly clients, rhinitis may lead to pneumonia and other more serious illnesses.

Symptoms associated with rhinitis include sneezing, nasal congestion, **rhinorrhea** (clear nasal discharge), sore throat, watery eyes, cough, low-grade fever, headache, aching muscles, and malaise. These symptoms continue to some degree for 5 to 14 days. A sustained temperature elevation suggests a bacterial infection or infection in the sinuses or ears. Symptoms associated with allergic rhinitis persist as long as the client is exposed to a specific allergen.

For most clients, treatment for rhinitis is minimal. Antibiotics are not used unless a bacterial infection is identified. Clients are advised to use antipyretics for fever, decongestants for severe nasal congestion, antitussives for a prolonged cough, saline gargles for sore throat, or antihistamines for allergic rhinitis. Desensitization or suppression of the immune response also may be prescribed for allergic rhinitis. Teaching clients about upper respiratory infections helps to prevent infections and minimizes other potential problems. Maintaining a healthy lifestyle is the best prevention. This includes adequate rest and sleep, a proper diet, and moderate exercise. Another important factor is frequent handwashing, which greatly reduces the spread of infection. Box 27–1 presents recommendations for treating rhinitis.

BOX 27-1 Treating Rhinitis

- Rest as much as possible.
- Increase fluid intake to assist in liquefying secretions.
  - Use a vaporizer to help liquefy secretions.
  - Blow nose with mouth open slightly to equalize pressure.
  - Wash hands frequently to avoid spreading infection.
  - Use over-the-counter medications as directed; be aware of possible side effects, especially interactions with food and alcohol.
- Allergic rhinitis:
  - Advise client to be tested for allergen sensitivity.
  - Assess client for exposure to possible allergens.
  - Urge client to avoid specific allergens.
  - Use antihistamines and decongestants as ordered.

Sinusitis

Sinusitis is an inflammation of the sinuses. The maxillary sinus is affected most often. Sinusitis can lead to serious complications, such as infection of the middle ear or brain.

ETIOLOGY AND PATHOPHYSIOLOGY

Sinusitis is caused principally by the spread of an infection from the nasal passages to the sinuses and by the blockage of normal sinus drainage (Fig. 27–1). Interference with the drainage of the sinuses predisposes a client to sinusitis because trapped secretions readily become infected. Allergies frequently cause edema of the nasal mucous membranes, leading to obstruction of sinus drainage and sinusitis. Nasal polyps and deviated septum may also cause impaired sinus drainage.

ASSESSMENT FINDINGS

Signs and Symptoms

Signs and symptoms depend on which sinus is infected and include one or more of the following: headache, fever, pain over the area of the affected sinus, nasal congestion and discharge, pain and pressure around the eyes, and malaise.

Diagnostic Findings

A nasal smear or material obtained from irrigation of the sinus for culture and sensitivity identifies the infectious microorganism and the appropriate antibiotic therapy. Transillumination and radiographs of the sinuses may show a change in the shape or the presence of fluid in the sinus cavity. A thorough history, including an allergy history, usually confirms the diagnosis.

MEDICAL AND SURGICAL MANAGEMENT

Acute sinusitis frequently responds to conservative treatment designed to help overcome the infection. A saline irrigation of the maxillary sinus may be done to remove accumulated exudate and promote drainage. This is accomplished by inserting a catheter through the normal opening under the middle concha, three bones that project from the lateral wall of the chest cavity. Antibiotic therapy is necessary if the infection is severe. Vasoconstrictors, such as phenylephrine nose drops, may be recommended for short-term use to relieve nasal congestion and aid in sinus drainage.

Surgery is often indicated in the treatment of chronic sinusitis. Endoscopic sinus surgery helps in providing an opening in the inferior meatus to promote drainage. More radical procedures, such as the Caldwell-Luc procedure and external sphenoethmoidectomy, are done to

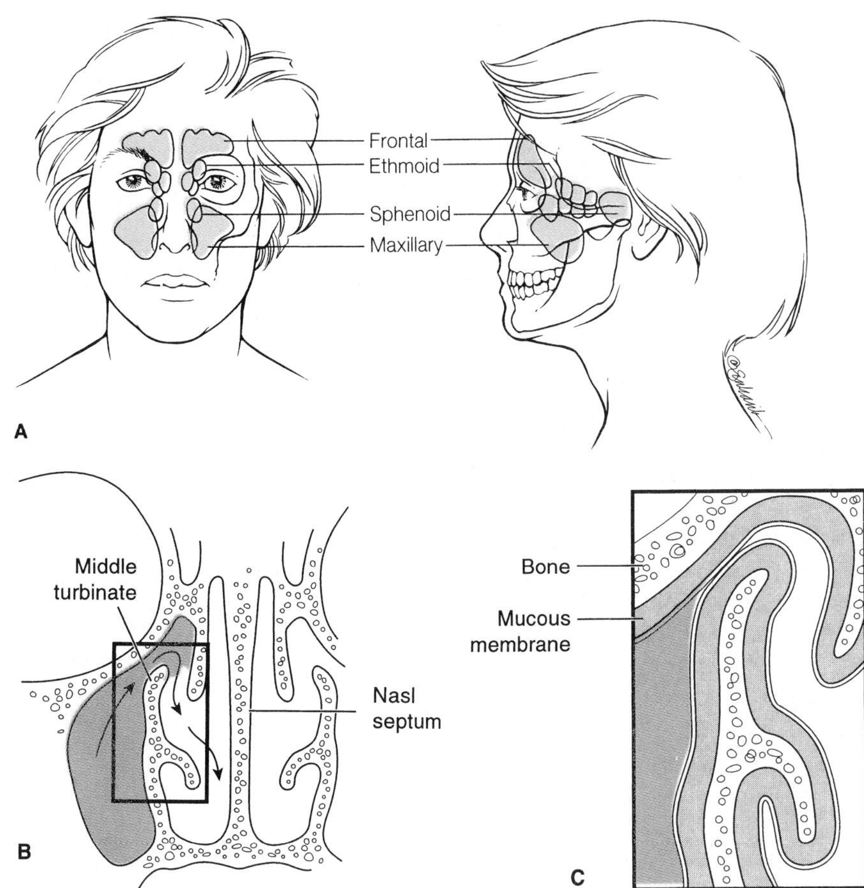

FIGURE 27-1. Edema can cause obstruction of sinus drainage. (*A*) Location of maxillary sinuses. (*B*) The maxillary sinuses normally drain through the openings that lie under the middle turbinates. The opening for the drainage is near the upper portion of the sinus. (*C*) Edema, such as that which commonly accompanies upper respiratory infections, can obstruct the opening and prevent normal sinus drainage.

remove diseased tissue and provide an opening into the inferior meatus of the nose for adequate drainage.

NURSING MANAGEMENT

If the client is receiving medical treatment, inform him or her that humidification, an increase in the fluid intake, and mouthwashes may loosen secretions and increase comfort. Tell the client to take nasal decongestants and antihistamines as ordered.

If the client has undergone sinus surgery, institute the standards for postoperative care (see Chap. 24) and observe the client for repeated swallowing that suggests possible hemorrhage. Because one risk of sinus surgery is damage to the optic nerve, assess the client's visual acuity by asking him or her to identify the number of fingers you are displaying. Monitor temperature at least every 4 hours. Assess client for pain over involved sinuses to determine if postoperative infection or impaired drainage is present. Administer analgesics as indicated and apply ice compresses to involved sinuses to reduce pain and edema.

The client will have nasal packing and a dressing under the nares ("moustache" dressing or "drip pad"). Because the nasal packing forces the client to mouth breathe, encourage oral hygiene and ice chips or small sips of fluids frequently. This will alleviate the dryness caused by mouth breathing. Change the drip pad as needed and report excessive drainage.

Client and Family Teaching

Tell the client not to blow the nose, lift objects more than 5 to 10 lb, or do the Valsalva maneuver for 10 to 14 days postoperatively. Tell the client to remain in a warm environment and to avoid smoky or poorly ventilated areas. Measures that help reduce the incidence or severity of sinusitis include:

- Eat a well balanced diet
- Get plenty of rest
- Engage in moderate exercise
- Avoid allergens
- Seek medical attention promptly if cold symptoms persist longer than 10 days or if nasal discharge is green or dark yellow and foul smelling

Pharyngitis

Pharyngitis is an inflammation of the throat. It is often associated with rhinitis and other upper respiratory infections. Viruses and bacteria cause pharyngitis. The most serious bacteria are the group A beta-hemolytic streptococci that can lead to dangerous cardiac complications, such as endocarditis and rheumatic fever, and harmful renal complications such as glomerulonephritis. Pharyngitis is highly contagious and spreads via inhalation of or direct contamination with droplets.

The incubation period for pharyngitis is 2 to 4 days. The first symptom is a sore throat—sometimes severe. Dysphagia (difficulty swallowing), fever, chills, headache, and malaise accompany the sore throat. Some clients exhibit a white or exudate patch over the tonsillar area and swollen glands. A throat culture reveals the specific bacteria. Rapid identification methods are available to diagnose a beta-hemolytic infection, such as the Biostar or the Strep A optical immunoassay (OIA). These tests are done in clinics and physician offices. Standard 24-hour throat culture and sensitivity tests are done to identify other organisms.

Early antibiotic treatment is the best choice for pharyngitis. This treats the infection and helps to prevent potential complications. Penicillin or penicillin derivatives are generally the antibiotics of choice. Clients sensitive to penicillin receive erythromycin. The client takes antibiotics for 7 to 14 days.

Tonsillitis and Adenoiditis

Tonsillitis is inflammation of the tonsils, and **adenoiditis** is inflammation of the adenoids. Although these disorders are more common in children, they also may be seen in adults.

ETIOLOGY AND PATHOPHYSIOLOGY

The tonsils and adenoids are lymphatic tissues and are common sites of infection. Chronic infection of the tonsils leads to enlargement and partial upper airway obstruction. Primary infection may occur in the tonsils and adenoids, or the infection can be secondary to other upper airway infections. Chronic infection of the adenoids can result in an acute or chronic infection in the middle ear (otitis media). If the causative organism is the group A beta-hemolytic streptococcus, prompt treatment is needed to prevent potential cardiac and renal complications.

ASSESSMENT FINDINGS

Signs and Symptoms

Sore throat, difficulty or pain on swallowing, fever, and malaise are the most common symptoms of tonsillitis. Enlargement of the adenoids may produce nasal obstruction, noisy breathing, snoring, and a nasal quality to the voice.

Diagnostic Findings

Visual examination reveals enlarged and reddened tonsils. White patches may be present on the tonsils if group A beta-hemolytic streptococcus is the cause of the infection. A throat culture and sensitivity test determine the causative microorganism and appropriate antibiotic therapy.

MEDICAL AND SURGICAL MANAGEMENT

Antibiotic therapy, analgesics such as acetaminophen, and saline gargles are used to treat the infection and discomfort associated with tonsillitis. Chronic tonsillitis and adenoiditis may require removal of these structures. **Tonsillectomy** and **adenoidectomy** are the operative procedures. The criteria for performing these procedures are:

- Repeated episodes of tonsillitis
- Hypertrophy of the tonsils
- Enlarged adenoids that are obstructive
- Repeated purulent otitis media
- Hearing loss related to serous otitis media associated with enlarged tonsils and adenoids
- Other conditions, such as asthma or rheumatic fever, exacerbated by tonsillitis (Smeltzer & Bare, 1996)

NURSING MANAGEMENT

Tonsillectomy and adenoidectomy are generally done as outpatient procedures. The preoperative nursing interventions are the same as those presented in Chapter 24.

NURSING PROCESS
The Client Undergoing a Tonsillectomy and/or Adenoidectomy

Assessment

Special attention is placed on the client's hematocrit, platelet count, and clotting time, because postoperative hemorrhage is the greatest risk. Ask the client about bleeding tendencies and the recent use of aspirin, nonsteroidal anti-inflammatory drugs, or other medications that prolong bleeding time. Postoperatively the postoperative standards described in Chapter 24 are implemented.

Diagnosis and Planning

Additional nursing care includes, but is not limited to, the following:

Nursing Diagnoses and Collaborative Problems	Nursing Interventions
Risk for Aspiration related to loss of gag reflex secondary to anesthesia	Following surgery, position client on side with emesis basin to catch drainage until client is alert.

Goals: The client will maintain patent airway with clear breath sounds.	Elevate head of bed 45° when client is fully awake.
The client will expectorate secretions as needed.	Monitor respiratory rate every hour.
	Auscultate breath sounds at least every hour.
	Encourage client to spit secretions into an emesis basin to maintain clear airway.
Risk for Trauma to tissues related to injury to the suture line	Monitor bloody drainage from client's mouth or frequent swallowing.
Goal: The client will demonstrate techniques that decrease the risk of increased bleeding.	Instruct client not to cough, clear the throat, blow nose, or use a straw in the first few postoperative days.
	Encourage client to initially try ice chips, progress to clear cold fluids, and then to popsicles and full liquids as tolerated.
	Instruct client to avoid carbonated fluids and fluids high in citrus content.
	Add soft food, such as gelatin and sherbert, as tolerated after the first 24 hours postoperatively.
Pain related to surgical incision in the throat	Administer analgesics liberally as ordered.
Goals: The client will state that pain is decreased.	Apply ice collar as ordered.
The client will demonstrate improved ability to swallow.	Encourage client to gently gargle with warm saline.

Evaluation and Expected Outcomes

- Aspiration is avoided.
- Breath sounds remain clear.
- Minimal bleeding occurs postoperatively.
- Pain is relieved.
- No complications occur postoperatively.

Client and Family Teaching

Before discharging the client, review the following with the client and family to ensure that the client will be able to manage self-care at home:

- Report any signs of bleeding to the physician—this is particularly important in the first 12 to 24 hours, and then 7 to 10 days following surgery as the throat heals.
- Gently gargle with warm saline or an alkaline mouthwash to assist in removing thick mucus.
- Maintain a liquid and very soft diet for several days postoperatively—avoid spicy foods, and rough textured foods; milk and milk products may increase the amount of mucus produced.

Peritonsillar Abscess

A **peritonsillar abscess** (also called quinsy) is an abscess that develops in the connective tissue between the capsule of the tonsil and the constrictor muscle of the pharynx. It may follow a severe tonsillar infection that is streptococcal or staphylococcal in origin.

The client with a peritonsillar abscess experiences difficulty and pain with swallowing, fever, malaise, ear pain, and difficulty talking. On visual examination, the affected side is red and swollen. The posterior pharynx is also swollen. Drainage from the abscess is cultured to identify the microorganism and sensitivity studies determine the appropriate antibiotic therapy.

Immediate treatment of a peritonsillar abscess is recommended to prevent the spread of the causative microorganisms to the bloodstream or adjacent structures. Penicillin or another antibiotic is given immediately after a culture is obtained and before results of the culture and sensitivity tests are known.

Surgical incision and drainage of the abscess is done if the abscess partially blocks the oropharynx. A local anesthetic is sprayed or painted on the surface of the abscess, and the contents are evacuated. Repeated episodes may necessitate a tonsillectomy.

Nursing management of the client undergoing drainage of an abscess includes placing the client in a semi Fowler's position to prevent aspiration. An ice collar may be ordered to reduce swelling and pain. Fluids are encouraged and the client is observed for signs of respiratory obstruction (eg, dyspnea, restlessness, cyanosis) or excessive bleeding.

Laryngitis

Laryngitis is an inflammation and swelling of the mucous membrane lining the larynx. Edema of the vocal cords frequently accompanies the laryngeal inflammation. Laryngitis may follow an upper respiratory infection and is due to the spread of the infection to the larynx. Excessive or improper use of the voice, allergies, or smoking also cause laryngitis.

Hoarseness, inability to speak above a whisper, or **aphonia** (complete loss of voice) are the usual symptoms of laryngitis. Clients also complain of throat irritation and a dry, nonproductive cough. The diagnosis is made on the basis of the symptoms. If hoarseness persists more than 2 weeks, an examination of the larynx (laryngoscopy) is done. Persistent hoarseness is a sign of laryngeal cancer, and thus merits prompt investigation. Treatment of laryngitis involves voice rest and the treatment or the removal of the cause. Antibiotic therapy may be used if laryngitis is caused by a bacterial infection. If smoking is the cause of the disorder, encourage smoking cessation and refer the client to a smoking cessation program.

Structural Disorders

Epistaxis

Epistaxis, or nosebleed, is a common occurrence. It is not usually serious but can be frightening for the client.

ETIOLOGY AND PATHOPHYSIOLOGY

Nosebleeds are the rupture of tiny capillaries in the mucous membrane of the nose, most commonly in the anterior septum, referred to as Kiesselbach's area. A nosebleed occurs because of trauma or disease, such as rheumatic fever, infection, hypertension, nasal tumors, and blood dyscrasias. Epistaxis that results from hypertension or blood dyscrasias is likely to be severe and difficult to control. Clients who abuse cocaine may have frequent nosebleeds. Foreign bodies in the nose and deviated septum contribute to epistaxis, along with forceful nose blowing and frequent nose picking.

ASSESSMENT FINDINGS

Inspection of the nares using a nasal speculum and light reveals the area of bleeding. A tongue blade is used to examine the back of the throat and a laryngeal mirror is used to examine the area above and behind the uvula.

MEDICAL AND SURGICAL MANAGEMENT

The severity and location of the bleeding determines the treatment. One or a combination of the following therapies is used:

- Direct continuous pressure to the nares for 5 to 10 minutes with head tilted slightly forward
- Ice packs to the nose
- Cauterization with silver nitrate, electrocautery, or application of a topical vasoconstrictor such as 1:1000 epinephrine
- Nasal packing with a cotton tampon
- Pressure with a balloon inflated catheter—inserted posteriorly for a minimum of 48 hours

NURSING MANAGEMENT

The nurse monitors the client's vital signs, and assesses for signs of continued bleeding. The nurse may initiate measures to control bleeding, such as pressure and ice packs. Other treatments must have a physician's order. The client experiencing epistaxis is usually anxious and requires reassurance. If there are underlying conditions causing the epistaxis, the nurse refers the client for medical follow-up. The nurse may also recommend humidification, the use of a nasal lubricant to keep the mucous membranes moist, and the avoidance of vigorous nose blowing and nose picking, or other nasal trauma.

Client and Family Teaching

Before discharge, inform the client and family of the following:

- If epistaxis recurs, apply pressure to nares with two fingers. Breathe through the mouth and sit with head tipped forward slightly to prevent the blood from running down the throat.
- Do not swallow blood; spit out any blood that is oozing from the area. Do not blow the nose.
- If blood has been swallowed, diarrhea and black tarry stools may be seen for a few days.
- Do not attempt to remove nasal packing or to cut the string anchoring the packing.
- Take pain medications as ordered. Do not use aspirin or ibuprofen products until bleeding is controlled.
- Notify the physician if bleeding persists or if any respiratory problems develop.

Nasal Obstruction

The nasal passage may be obstructed, which interferes with the passage of air. Three primary conditions lead to nasal obstruction: deviated septum, nasal polyps, and hypertrophied turbinates.

ETIOLOGY AND PATHOPHYSIOLOGY

Deviated septum is an irregularity in the septum that results in nasal obstruction. The deviation may occur as deflection from the midline in the form of lumps or sharp projections or as a curvature in the shape of an "S." Marked deviation of the nasal septum can result in complete obstruction of one nostril and interference with sinus drainage. A deviated septum may be congenital, but often it is caused by trauma.

Nasal polyps are grapelike swellings that arise from the mucous membranes of the nose. They probably occur as the result of chronic irritation from infection or allergic rhinitis. They obstruct nasal breathing and sinus drainage, which ultimately leads to sinusitis. Most nasal polyps are benign and tend to recur when removed.

Hypertrophied turbinates are enlargements of the nasal concha. This occurs as a result of chronic rhinitis. The hypertrophy interferes with air passage and sinus drainage, and eventually leads to sinusitis.

ASSESSMENT FINDINGS

Signs and Symptoms

Symptoms include a history of sinusitis, difficulty breathing out of one nostril, frequent nosebleeds, and nasal discharge. Clients usually report difficulty breathing through one or both sides of the nose.

Diagnostic Findings

Inspection of the nose with a nasal speculum reveals a left or right deviation of the nasal septum, the number and location of the polyps, or enlarged turbinates.

MEDICAL AND SURGICAL MANAGEMENT

A *submucous surgical resection* or *septoplasty* may be necessary to restore normal breathing and to permit adequate sinus drainage for the client with a deviated septum. This involves an incision through the mucous membrane and the removal of the portions of the septum that cause obstruction. After this procedure, both sides of the nasal cavity are packed with gauze, which remains in place for 24 to 48 hours. A moustache dressing or drip pad is applied to absorb any drainage.

Rhinoplasty, reconstruction of the nose, may also be done at the same time. This procedure enhances the client's appearance cosmetically, but also corrects any structural nasal deformities that interfere with air passage. The surgeon makes an incision inside the nostril and restructures the nasal bone and cartilage. As with septoplasty, the nasal cavity is packed with gauze, and the nose is taped. Application of a nasal splint maintains the shape and structure of the nose and reduces edema. The splint remains in place for at least a week.

Treatment for polyps includes the use of a steroidal nasal spray to reduce the inflammation, or direct injection of steroids into the polyps. If nasal obstruction is severe, the surgeon performs a *polypectomy*, the removal of polyps with a nasal snare or laser under local anesthesia. The polyps are examined microscopically to rule out malignant disease.

Hypertrophied turbinates are often treated with the application of astringents or aerosolized corticosteroids to shrink them close to the nose. Occasionally, one of the turbinates may be surgically removed (*turbinectomy*).

NURSING MANAGEMENT

Surgery for correction of nasal obstruction is usually done on an outpatient basis. The nurse provides thorough explanations throughout the procedures to alleviate anxiety. It is particularly important to emphasize that nasal packing will be in place postoperatively, necessitating mouth breathing, and that ice will be used to reduce pain and swelling.

Place the client in a semi-Fowler's position to promote drainage, reduce edema, and enhance breathing. Inspect the nasal packing and dressings frequently for bleeding. Ask the client to inform you of excessive swallowing, which can indicate bleeding. Monitor vital signs frequently. Provide frequent oral hygiene and saline mouth rinses (when permitted) to help keep mucous membranes moist. Tell the client that it is normal to feel or hear a sucking noise when swallowing; this resolves when nasal packing is removed.

Client and Family Teaching

Prepare the postsurgical client for edema and discoloration around the eyes and nose; it will disappear after a few weeks. Instruct the client in the following measures to prevent bleeding:

- Do not bend over.
- Do not blow nose.
- If sneezing, keep mouth open.
- Avoid contact with nose or surrounding tissue.
- Keep head elevated with an extra pillow when lying down.
- Avoid heavy lifting.
- Do not use aspirin, ibuprofen, alcohol, or tobacco products.

Trauma and Obstruction of the Upper Airway

Fractures of the Nose

A nasal fracture causes swelling and edema of the soft tissues, external and internal bleeding, deformity to the nose, and nasal obstruction. In severe nasal fractures, cerebrospinal fluid, which is colorless and clear, may drain from the nares. This suggests a fracture in the cribriform plate.

The diagnosis of a nasal fracture may be delayed because of the significant swelling and bleeding. As soon as the swelling decreases, the examiner inspects the nose internally to rule out a fracture of the nasal septum or the presence of a septal hematoma. Both of these require treatment to prevent destruction of the septal cartilage. If drainage of a clear fluid is observed, a Dextrostix is used to determine the presence of glucose, which is diagnostic for cerebrospinal fluid. Radiography studies are done to ascertain if there are other facial fractures.

If the fracture is a lateral displacement, pressure applied to the convex portion of the nose reduces the fracture. Cold compresses control the bleeding. If the fracture is more complex, surgery is done after the swelling subsides, usually after several days. The surgeon applies a splint postoperatively to maintain the alignment.

NURSING MANAGEMENT

Nursing management after trauma to the nose is similar to that for nasal obstruction. The nurse instructs the client to keep the head elevated and to apply ice four times a day for 20 minutes, to reduce the swelling and pain. Give analgesics as ordered to alleviate pain. Postoperatively, the nurse assesses the client for:

- Airway obstruction
- Respiratory difficulty—tachypnea, shortness of breath
- Dysphagia
- Signs of infection
- Pupillary responses
- Level of consciousness
- Periorbital edema

In addition, the nurse helps reduce the client's anxiety by answering questions and offering reassurance that the bruising and swelling will subside and the sense of smell will return.

Laryngeal Trauma and Laryngeal Obstruction

ETIOLOGY AND PATHOPHYSIOLOGY

Laryngeal trauma occurs during a motor vehicle accident when the neck strikes the steering wheel or when other blunt trauma occurs in the neck region. Endoscopic and endotracheal intubation may also cause laryngeal trauma. Although not common, a fracture of the thyroid cartilage is also traumatic to the larynx. Laryngeal obstruction is an extremely serious and often life-threatening condition. Some causes of upper airway obstruction include edema due to an allergic reaction, severe head and neck injuries, severe inflammation and edema of the throat, or aspiration of foreign bodies such as food.

ASSESSMENT FINDINGS

Signs and Symptoms

Laryngeal trauma causes neck swelling, bruising, and tenderness. If the tissues surrounding the larynx are greatly swollen, the client will exhibit **stridor,** a high-pitched, harsh sound during respiration, indicative of airway obstruction. The client also has dysphagia, hoarseness, cyanosis, and possible **hemoptysis** (expectoration of bloody sputum). Total obstruction prevents the passage of air from the upper to the lower respiratory airway; choking clients will clutch their throats–the universal distress sign for choking. Partial obstruction results in difficulty breathing. Unless total obstruction is relieved immediately, death occurs from respiratory arrest.

Diagnostic Findings

Laryngoscopy reveals the extent of trauma and internal swelling. Radiographs and oxygenation studies will be performed after a patent airway has been established.

MEDICAL AND SURGICAL MANAGEMENT

Maintenance of a patent airway is crucial. If the client has aspirated a foreign body, the Heimlich maneuver is performed to force the object out of the upper respiratory passages (Box 27–2). Allergic reactions resulting in severe inflammation and edema may be treated with epinephrine or a corticosteroid and possibly intubation. Severe obstruction requires an emergency tracheostomy (surgical opening into the trachea).

NURSING MANAGEMENT

Partial or total obstruction of the upper airway requires immediate recognition and intervention. The Heimlich maneuver is used. If this maneuver fails to dislodge the object, a physician performs an emergency tracheostomy. If edema is the cause of upper airway obstruction, oxygen is given until a physician examines the client. Emergency drugs, a laryngoscope, an endotracheal tube, and a tracheostomy tray are made available for immediate use.

NURSING PROCESS
Care of the Client With Trauma to the Upper Airway

Assessment

Assess airway patency, lung sounds, and respiratory patterns. Monitor the client for signs of increased nasal swelling and bleeding or symptoms of laryngeal edema. Determine if the client's airway is obstructed.

Diagnosis and Planning

The nurse's responsibilities when caring for a client with trauma to the upper airway include, but are not limited to, the following:

Nursing Diagnoses and Collaborative Problems	Nursing Interventions
Ineffective Airway Clearance related to total or partial obstruction of the upper airway	Auscultate lungs and check vital signs.
	Assess cough for effectiveness and productivity.
Goals: The client's airway will be free of obstruction.	Monitor arterial blood gases.
The client will demonstrate improved breath sounds.	Note color changes in nail beds, lips, and buccal mucosa.
	Perform Heimlich maneuver.

Risk for Ineffective Breathing related to nasal obstruction secondary to nasal packing, bleeding, or edema **Goal:** The client will maintain an effective breathing pattern.	Assess respiratory rate and depth. Monitor respiratory pattern. Position client in semi-Fowler's position. Apply ice to nasal area. Assess for dyspnea, use of accessory muscles, retractions, and flaring of nostrils. Immediately report any signs of respiratory difficulty. Have tracheostomy tray available.
Anxiety related to airway obstruction, pain, injury, bleeding, or anticipation of medical or surgical treatments **Goal:** The client will demonstrate decreased anxiety.	Assess level of apprehension. Monitor for increased respiratory rate and irritability. Provide thorough explanations. Comfort client with reassurances, explanations, and presence. Teach relaxation techniques as needed.
Pain related to injury and or surgical incision **Goal:** The client will express pain relief.	Assess level of pain. Implement comfort measures, such as positioning and ice packs. Evaluate effectiveness of pain relief measures.

Evaluation and Expected Outcomes

- Airway is free of obstruction.
- Breathing patterns are improved.
- Anxiety is decreased.
- Pain is relieved.

Malignancies of the Upper Airway

Cancer of the Larynx

With early detection, cancer of the larynx has great potential for cure. Preventive health measures focus on early consultation for persistent hoarseness and other changes in voice quality.

ETIOLOGY AND PATHOPHYSIOLOGY

Cancer of the larynx is most common in people 50 to 70 years of age. Men are affected more frequently than women. The cause of laryngeal cancer is unknown. Carcinogens, such as tobacco, alcohol, and industrial pollutants, are associated with laryngeal cancer. In addition, chronic laryngitis, habitual overuse of the voice, and heredity may predispose a person to laryngeal cancer. Most laryngeal malignancies are squamous cell carcinomas, that is, a malignancy arising from the epithelial cells lining the larynx. The tumor may be located on the glottis (true vocal cords) or above the glottis (supraglottis or false vocal cords) or below the glottis (subglottis).

ASSESSMENT FINDINGS

Signs and Symptoms

Persistent hoarseness is usually the earliest symptom. At first the hoarseness is slight and is often ignored. Later, the client notes a sensation of swelling or a lump in the throat, followed by dysphagia and pain when talking. The client may also complain of burning in the throat when swallowing hot or citrus liquids. If the malignant tissue is not removed promptly, symptoms of advancing carcinoma, such as dyspnea, weakness, weight loss, enlarged cervical lymph nodes, pain, and anemia develop.

Diagnostic Findings

Visual examination of the larynx (laryngoscopy) and biopsy confirm the diagnosis and identify the type of malignancy. In addition, computed tomography scanning and chest radiography are used to detect metastasis and to determine tumor size. The physician also assesses the mobility of the vocal cords. If the mobility is limited, it indicates that the tumor growth is affecting the surrounding tissue, muscle, and airway.

MEDICAL AND SURGICAL MANAGEMENT

Treatment depends on factors such as the size of the lesion, the age of the client, and the presence or absence of metastasis. Medical treatment may include chemotherapy, which appears to have only a minimal effect, and radiation therapy, either alone or in conjunction with surgery.

Surgical treatment includes laser surgery for early lesions or a partial or total laryngectomy. In more advanced cases, total laryngectomy may be the treatment of choice. If the disease has extended beyond the larynx, a radical neck dissection (removal of the lymph nodes, muscles, and adjacent tissues) is performed. Laser surgery may also be used to relieve obstruction in more advanced cases. Table 27–1 provides descriptions of the various types of laryngeal surgery.

A client with a total laryngectomy has a permanent tracheal *stoma* (opening) because the trachea is no longer connected to the nasopharynx. The larynx is severed from the trachea and removed completely. The only respiratory organs in use are the trachea, the bronchi, and lungs. Air enters and leaves through the tracheostomy; the client no longer feels air entering the nose (Fig. 27–2). Because the anterior wall of the

BOX 27-2 The Heimlich Maneuver for Dislodging an Airway Obstruction

- Ask the victim if she is choking.
- Assess the victim's ability to cough and speak.
- If she cannot talk or cough, tell her you can help and place your arms around her waist.
- Make a fist with one hand and place the thumb toward the victim above the umbilicus.
- Hold your fist with the other hand and thrust upward into the abdomen five times.

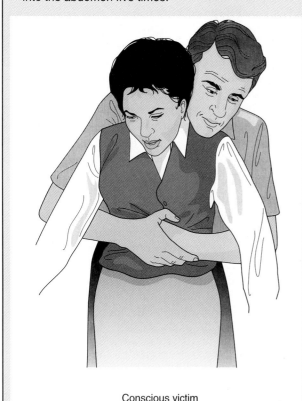
Conscious victim

- If the object is dislodged and the victim can cough effectively, encourage her to cough forcefully to eject the object.
- If the object is not ejected or coughed out and the victim loses consciousness, lower her to the ground.
- Straddle the victim's body and place the heel of one hand on top of the other, position the hands midway between the umbilicus and the xiphoid process.

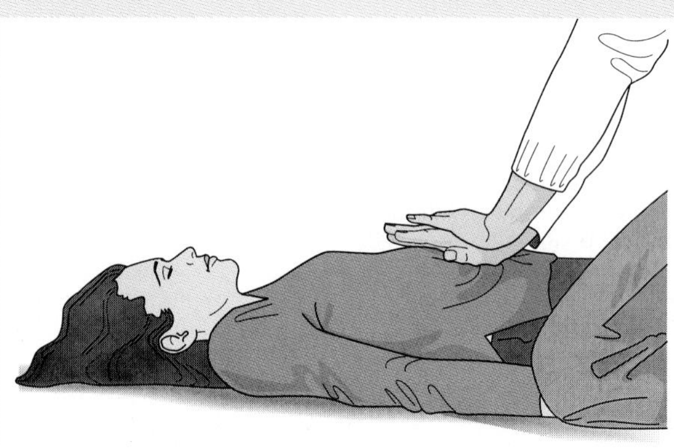
Unconscious victim

- Deliver five forceful thrusts.
- Open the mouth to assess if the object can be swept out with a hooked finger (do not sweep the mouth in children).
- If the airway remains obstructed repeat the procedure.

esophagus connects with the posterior wall of the larynx, it must be reconstructed. Tube feeding facilitates healing by preventing muscle activity and irritation of the esophagus (see Chap. 51 for management of tube feedings).

Loss of the ability to speak normally is a devastating consequence of laryngeal surgery. Communication with others is a basic need. Clients with a malignancy of the larynx require emotional support before and after surgery and help in understanding and choosing an alternative method of speech. Some methods of speech used after a laryngectomy include:

- *Esophageal speech*—a method of speech that requires regurgitation of swallowed air and formation of words with lips
- *Electric larynx*—a throat vibrator held against the neck that projects sound into the mouth; words are formed with the mouth
- *Tracheoesophageal puncture* (*TEP*)—a surgical opening in the posterior wall of the trachea is followed by the insertion of a prosthesis such as a Blom-Singer device. This allows air from the lungs to be diverted through the opening in the posterior tracheal wall to the esophagus and out the mouth.

A speech pathologist works with the client to use an artificial speech device, learn esophageal speech, or speak clearly with a prosthesis. Clients having a partial laryngectomy also may require speech therapy.

TABLE 27-1 **Descriptions of Laryngeal Surgery**

Surgery	Description	Indication	Postoperative Expectations
Partial laryngectomy	The affected vocal cord is removed; other structures left intact.	For early stage laryngeal cancer when only one cord is involved.	Voice will be hoarse; intact trachea; no problems with swallowing; high cure rate.
Supraglottic laryngectomy	Hyoid bone, glottis, and false cords removed; radical neck dissection done on involved side; remaining structures left intact.	For supraglottic tumors.	Voice will be hoarse; tracheostomy postoperatively until glottic airway functions; nutrition administered through nasogastric tube until surgical sites heal; recurrence is possible.
Hemivertical laryngectomy	Thyroid cartilage of trachea is split at midline; one true cord and one false cord are removed along with arytenoid cartilage and half the thyroid cartilage.	When tumor extends beyond the vocal cord but is smaller than 1 cm.	Client will have a tracheostomy and nasogastric tube postoperatively until healed; voice will be hoarse and diminished; client will have an intact airway and the ability to swallow.
Total laryngectomy	Both vocal cords removed along with the hyoid bone, epiglottis, cricoid cartilage, and two or three rings of the trachea; the tongue, pharyngeal walls and trachea remain intact; usually a radical neck dissection is done on the affected side.	When the cancer extends beyond the vocal cords.	Permanent tracheal stoma; prevents aspiration. No voice but ability to swallow remains. Metastasis to cervical lymph nodes is common.
Radical neck dissection	The neck is opened from the jaw to the clavicle from the midline to the interior border of the trapezius muscle. The following are removed: subcutaneous and soft tissue, sternocleidomastoid muscle, jugular vein, and spinal accessory nerve (innervates trapezius muscle—client's shoulder will droop following surgery as the trapezius muscle atrophies). A split thickness skin graft is applied over the carotid artery.	When cancer has metastasized to cervical lymph nodes.	Permanent tracheal stoma. No voice; ability to swallow remains. Client requires physical therapy for neck muscles, along with a prescribed exercise program.

NURSING PROCESS
Care of the Client Undergoing Laryngeal Surgery

Assessment

During the preoperative assessment, determine the client's level of understanding of the diagnosis, the reason for the surgery, and the probable results of the surgery. Begin preoperative teaching and allow the client to express fears about the surgery, the diagnosis, and the potential loss of voice after surgery. Discuss alternative methods of communication and identify which method the client prefers.

After surgery, carefully assess the client for a patent airway and effective airway clearance. Care centers around preventing postoperative complications, managing pain, preventing wound infection, helping the client communicate, and fostering the client's ability to cope with changes in body image. Refer to perioperative standards of care in Chapter 24 for general postoperative care; see Nursing Care Plan 27–1 for care of the client with a tracheostomy.

Determine airway patency, lungs sounds, respiratory rate and rhythm, mental status, and oxygenation. Assess neck incisions and stoma for swelling, bleeding, or subcutaneous emphysema. Monitor vital signs and intake and output. Assess anxiety and pain levels and ability to make needs known.

Diagnosis and Planning

The nursing care of the client undergoing laryngeal surgery includes, but is not limited to, the following:

Nursing Diagnoses and Collaborative Problems	Nursing Interventions
Ineffective Airway Clearance related to inability to cough and raise secretions	Position client on side with head of bed elevated, until fully awake.
Goal: The client's airway remains clear of secretions with effective coughing or suctioning.	Position client in semi-Fowler's or Fowler's position when fully awake.
The client's airway remains patent.	Monitor vital signs, respiratory function, and airway patency at least every 2 hours.

	Auscultate lungs at least every 2 hours. Gently suction laryngectomy or tracheostomy tube as needed. Maintain mist collar to airway at all times.
Impaired Verbal Communication related to removal of the larynx **Goals:** The client will use alternative methods of communication (mouth words, gestures, writing tablet, and computer). The client will effectively communicate needs and other information.	Provide a pad and pen or other means of writing. Identify specific gestures that communicate needs. Respond to client with a normal tone of voice.
Risk for Infection related to impaired skin and tissue integrity and poor physical condition **Goal:** The client will be free of infection as evidenced by temperature within normal limits, intact surgical incision without redness or purulent drainage, and normal white blood cell count.	Maintain aseptic technique when performing wound care and emptying drains. Administer antibiotics as ordered. Monitor vital signs with temperature at least every 4 hours. Report elevated temperatures or changes in surgical wound appearance.
Pain related to tissue trauma following surgery **Goal:** The client will experience tolerable level of pain.	Administer prescribed analgesics liberally. Avoid extreme movements of the head. Support the head when moving or changing position. Place a small pillow or folded towel under the head and shoulders. Avoid the use of full pillows.
Risk for Impaired Oral Mucous Membranes related to nasogastric intubation, oral suctioning, and temporary impaired swallowing **Goal:** The client will maintain intact mucous membranes.	Provide meticulous mouth care at least every 4 hours. Use plain water and oral solutions to rinse mouth. Inspect oral mucous membranes two or three times daily. Gently suction mouth to avoid injury to oral mucous membranes.
Social Isolation related to change in body image, tracheal stoma, and change in or loss of speech **Goal:** The client will socialize with others appropriately.	Demonstrate acceptance of client's changed appearance. Encourage client to maintain or reestablish social relationships. Allow client time to express feelings.

Evaluation and Expected Outcomes

- Client communicates needs effectively.
- Client has no signs or symptoms of infection.
- Airway is patent; PaO_2 is 90% or above.
- Stoma and incisions are clean and intact without bleeding or swelling.
- Pain is relieved.
- Oral mucous membranes are pink, moist, and intact.
- Client willingly engages in social activity.

Client and Family Teaching

Before discharge, instruct the client in the following measures for self-care:

- Place a scarf or gauze dressing loosely over the tube to keep dust and dirt out of the trachea and make the opening less obvious. Avoid fabrics or dressings that fray because small fibers can be drawn into the tube.
- Prevent water from entering the stoma because it will flow down the trachea to the lungs. Swimming is not allowed.
- Take care when bathing. Avoid showers until experienced with care of the stoma. When taking a shower, use hand to keep water away from the stoma. If possible, install a hand-held shower device; when used properly water is less likely to enter the stoma.

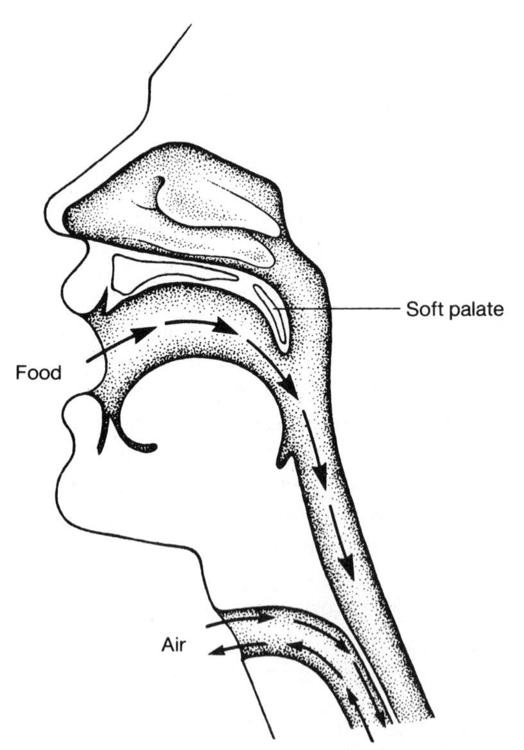

FIGURE 27-2. Air enters and leaves through a permanent tracheal stoma.

- Notify the physician if any of the following occur: fever, progressive weight loss, pain in the operative area, breathing difficulties, difficulty caring for the tracheal stoma, decrease in the size of the stoma, or redness or drainage around the stoma edges.
- Use aseptic and sterile technique when suctioning, cleaning tubes, and caring for stoma.

Treatment Modalities for Airway Obstruction or Airway Maintenance

Clients with serious airway conditions require aggressive treatment to maintain an airway or relieve airway obstruction.

Tracheostomy and Tracheotomy

A **tracheotomy** is the surgical procedure that makes an opening into the trachea. A **tracheostomy** is a surgical opening into the trachea into which a tracheostomy or laryngectomy tube is inserted. A tracheostomy may be temporary or permanent. A permanent opening in the trachea is required for certain disorders, such as a laryngectomy for cancer of the larynx.

Tracheostomy tubes come in several sizes and differ from laryngectomy tubes in their length and diameter. A cuffed tracheostomy tube has a cuff on the lower end that is inflated with air to provide a snug fit (Fig. 27–3).

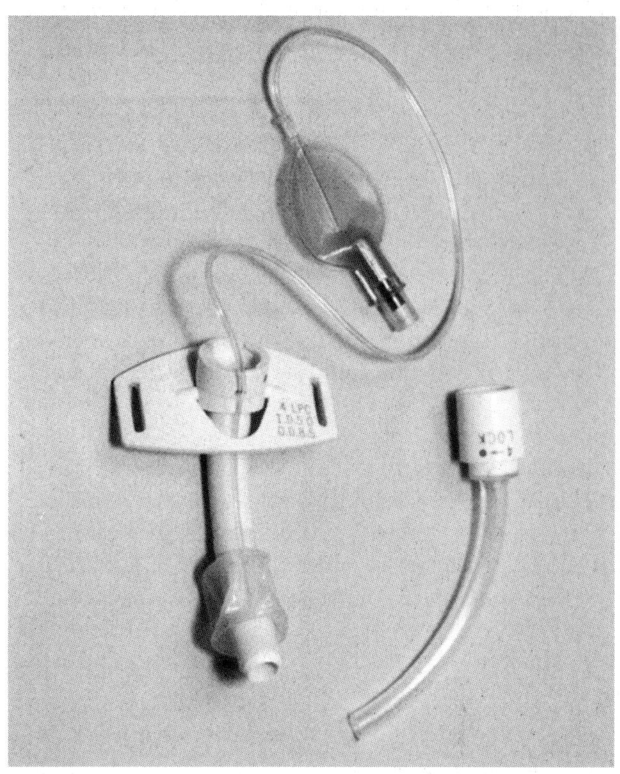

FIGURE 27-3. A cuffed tracheostomy tube. The cuff at the lower end of the tube is inflated with air to provide a snug fit in the trachea.

The cuff prevents aspiration of liquids or the escape of air when a mechanical ventilator is used. The physician specifies the amount of air to be injected into the cuff, usually to achieve a pressure between 20 and 25 mm H_20. The amount of air determines the seating of the cuff in the trachea. Monitor the pressure in the cuff with a pressure gauge at 8-hour intervals. During the immediate postoperative period, the physician may change the tracheostomy tube every 3 to 5 days. Before a tracheostomy tube is inserted into the tracheal opening, the obturator is placed in the tube and then removed as soon as the tube is in place. The outer tube is held snugly in place by tapes inserted in openings on either side of it and tied at the side of the client's neck.

The respiratory passages react to the creation of the new opening with inflammation and excessive secretion of mucus. Copious respiratory secretions are life-threatening and the client cannot be left unattended during the immediate postoperative period because the secretions make frequent suctioning necessary.

Inspired air passes directly into the trachea, bronchi, and lungs without becoming warmed and moistened. This leads to dry secretions that easily form crusts that can break off, obstruct the lower airway, and cause serious respiratory problems. Humidification with a mist collar is usually necessary to prevent drying and incrustation of the mucous membrane in the trachea and the main bronchus.

The long- and short-term complications of tracheostomy include infection, bleeding, airway obstruction due to hardened secretions, aspiration, injury to the laryngeal nerve, erosion of the trachea, fistula formation between the esophagus and trachea, and penetration of the posterior tracheal wall.

NURSING MANAGEMENT

After a tracheostomy is created, monitor vital signs and auscultate breath sounds. Assess skin color, level of consciousness, and mental status. Monitor the client for potential complications. Assess the client frequently for a patent airway because secretions can rapidly obstruct the inner lumen of the tracheostomy tube resulting in severe respiratory difficulty or death by asphyxiation. If the airway is obstructed, the client becomes cyanotic, restless, and frightened.

To facilitate breathing during the immediate postoperative period, position the client as ordered until fully awake. When the client is fully awake and the blood pressure is stable, elevate the head of the bed to about 45°. This position decreases edema and makes breathing easier.

Inspect the tracheostomy carefully and make sure tapes are secure. If not tied securely, the client can cough the tube out, a serious occurrence if the edges of the trachea have not been sutured to the skin, as can be the case in a temporary tracheostomy.

Keep a tracheal dilator at the bedside at all times. If the outer tube accidentally comes out, insert the dilator to hold the edges of the stoma apart until the physician arrives to insert another tube. Never force a tracheal tube back in place. If force is used, the client's trachea may be compressed (by pushing the tube alongside the trachea, thus compressing the trachea, rather than inserting the tube into the stoma). Such action could cause respiratory arrest.

Suction the client to remove secretions that can obstruct the airway (Nursing Guidelines 27–1). Avoid unnecessary suctioning to lessen trauma to the airway. Explain the procedure and tell the client that the catheter will only be inserted for a few seconds.

Keep an extra tracheostomy tube of the same size at the bedside because immediate change may be necessary if the tube becomes blocked with mucus that cannot be removed.

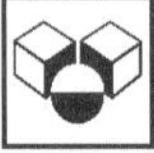

Nursing Guidelines 27-1

Suctioning the Client with a Tracheostomy

- Use sterile equipment (eg, gloves, suction catheter, normal saline) and aseptic technique for tracheal suctioning.
- Place the client in a Fowler's position. Preoxygenate the client for at least 1–2 minutes. Check that suction pressure is at a low setting.
- Open the suction kit, don gloves, lubricate a sterile 10 to 14 French disposable catheter with sterile saline and insert it into the lumen of the tube.
- Do not apply suction while the catheter is inserted down the trachea because this causes irritation to the lining of the trachea.
- Begin intermittent suctioning while slowly withdrawing and rotating the catheter. Do not suction for more than 10 seconds at a time.
- Allow the client to rest and deep breathe before repeating if more suctioning is necessary.
- Discard the suction catheter after use.

Provide routine tracheostomy care as outlined in Clinical Procedure 27–1. Place a gauze dressing under the tube to absorb secretions (Fig. 27–4). Make sure the hospital gown and bed linens never cover the opening of the tracheostomy tube. For additional care, see Nursing Care Plan 27–1.

Endotracheal Intubation and Mechanical Ventilation

An endotracheal tube (Fig. 27–5) is inserted through the client's mouth or nose into the trachea to provide a patent airway for clients who cannot maintain an adequate airway on their own. This includes clients with respiratory difficulty, comatose clients, those undergoing general anesthesia, or clients with extensive edema of upper airway passages.

An endotracheal tube can remain in place for up to 2 weeks. The cuff on the endotracheal tube is inflated to provide a tight seal. The endotracheal tube is attached to a ventilator. Humidification is necessary because air going to the lungs through an endotracheal tube does not pass through the moist mucous membranes of the upper airway.

Accidental removal of an endotracheal tube must be prevented because this can result in laryngeal edema or **laryngospasm** (spasm of the laryngeal muscles, resulting in narrowing of the larynx) and subsequent respiratory arrest. The inflated cuff and placement of tape around the tube attached to the client's cheek secures the endotracheal tube. The proximal end of the tube is marked for determining if downward displacement has occurred.

The tube is removed when the vital capacity is adequate and the client is able to breathe without assistance. Blood gas studies also are used as a guideline for removal. Before removing the tube, the nurse ensures that emergency equipment for respiratory support is available. Depending on hospital policy, the removal of an endotracheal tube is done by the nurse, the respiratory therapist, or the doctor. Suction the pharynx before the cuff is deflated to prevent the aspiration of secretions during extubation. The tube usually is removed with the client in semi-Fowler's position. If laryngospasm occurs, air is administered by positive pressure. Reinsertion of the endotracheal tube by the physician or other trained personnel may be necessary if laryngospasm continues.

Complications that can occur with the use of endotracheal intubation include ulceration and stricture of the trachea or larynx, atelectasis, and pneumonia.

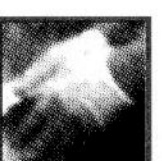

Clinical Procedure 27-1
Tracheostomy Care

PURPOSE	EQUIPMENT
• Maintain a patent airway • Prevent wound infection • Maintain skin integrity around the stoma	• Tracheostomy kit—disposable and sterile gloves, two sterile basins, drape, gauze pads, pipe cleaners, cotton-tipped applicators, stoma dressing, twill ties • Hydrogen peroxide or other solution as indicated by agency policy • Normal saline

Nursing Action	Rationale
ASSESSMENT	
Follow procedure and schedule for providing tracheostomy care.	Provides continuity of care.
Assess the condition of the dressing and the skin around the tracheostomy tube.	Evaluates need for dressing change and skin care.
Assess the client's understanding of the procedure.	Provides an opportunity for health teaching.
PLANNING	
Obtain a tracheostomy kit, hydrogen peroxide, and normal saline.	Promotes organization and efficient time management.
Remove the caps.	Prepares nonprepackaged items—able to maintain sterility.
IMPLEMENTATION	
Wash your hands.	Removes colonizing microorganisms. Prevents transferring microorganisms to the lower airway. Reduces the potential for contaminating sterile supplies.
Position client in a supine or low Fowler's position.	Facilitates access to the tracheostomy tube.
Using a clean glove, remove the soiled stomal dressing and discard it, glove and all, in appropriate receptacle. Wash your hands again.	Follows principles of asepsis. Reduces the transmission of microorganisms.
Open the tracheostomy kit without contaminating the contents. Don sterile gloves—keep the dominant hand sterile. Pour hydrogen peroxide and normal saline into respective containers.	Provides access to supplies and maintains their sterility. Follows principles of asepsis; the hand used to pour solutions is now considered contaminated.
Unlock the inner cannula by turning it counterclockwise and place it in the hydrogen peroxide. Clean the inside and outside of the cannula with pipe cleaners.	Loosens protein secretions and reduces the numbers of colonizing microorganisms. Removes gross debris.
Rinse the cleaned cannula in the normal saline. Tap the rinsed cannula against the edge of the basin and wipe the excess solution with a gauze square.	Removes remnants of hydrogen peroxide. Removes large droplets of fluids.
Replace the inner cannula and turn it clockwise within the outer cannula.	Secures the inner cannula.
Clean around the stoma with an applicator moistened with peroxide. Do not wipe over an area once it is cleaned.	Removes secretions and colonizing microorganisms from the tracheal opening.
Place a sterile stomal dressing around the tracheostomy tube. Change the tracheostomy ties by placing the new ones on first, and removing the soiled ones last. Tie the two new ends snugly, but not tightly, at the side of the neck.	Absorbs secretions and keeps the stomal area clean. Holds the tracheostomy tube in place. Prevents accidental extubation. Prevents skin impairment.
Discard all soiled supplies, remove gloves, wash hands.	Follows principles of asepsis.
Position client for comfort and safety.	Demonstrates concern for client's well-being.

(Adapted from Timby, B. K. [1996]. *Fundamental skills and concepts in patient care* [6th ed.]. Philadelphia: Lippincott-Raven.)

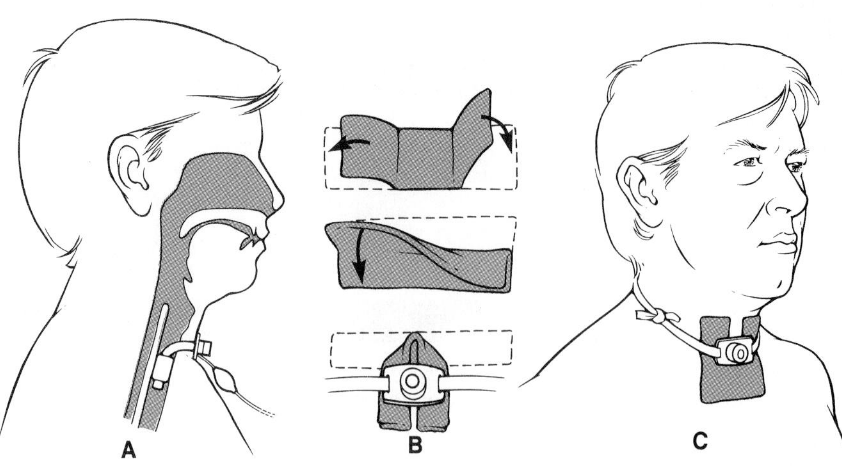

FIGURE 27-4. Tracheostomy tube dressings. (*A*) The cuff of the tracheostomy tube fits smoothly within the tracheal wall. (*B*) This shows how to fold a 4 × 4 gauze square to provide a comfortable neck pad and to collect mucus. (C) Gauze tracheostomy dressings also are available. Tapes hold the outer tube in place and are tied at the side of the client's neck.

NURSING CARE PLAN 27-1
The Client With a Tracheostomy

Potential Problems and Nursing Diagnoses	Nursing Management	Outcome Criteria
PC: Hypoxia, Hemorrhage, Displaced Tracheostomy Tube, Accidental Extubation	Monitor for signs and symptoms of respiratory distress including difficulty breathing, diminished or absent breath sounds, use of accessory muscles, asymmetrical chest wall movements.	Complications are avoided or managed.
	Assess for subcutaneous emphysema (air trapped in the tissues) around the stoma, neck, and chest.	
	Suction as needed. Provide humidification to keep secretions loose.	
	Keep tracheostomy ties secure but not too tight (one finger should slip easily under ties).	
	Monitor pulse oximetry or arterial blood gas results.	
	Administer oxygen as ordered.	
Risk for Ineffective Airway Clearance related to increased secretions, possible occlusion of inner cannula	Elevate head of bed 30°to 45°. Ensure that inspired air is humidified. Encourage client to cough and deep breathe.	The tracheostomy tube and natural airways remain patent.
	Suction as needed.	
	Provide tracheostomy care each shift.	
Risk for Altered Nutrition: Less than Body Requirements related to difficulty swallowing, disease process, and alteration in taste.	Assess the client's ability to swallow. Keep head of bed elevated for meals.	Body weight is maintained.
	Monitor weight weekly or prn.	
	Discuss importance of adequate intake in wound healing.	
	Check stoma and suctioned secretions for food particles that may indicate aspiration.	
	Withhold foods if aspiration is suspected and notify physician.	
	Measure intake and output and notify the physician if the urine output falls below 500 mL in 24 hours.	
	Consult with dietitian to provide adequate intake of nutrients.	

continued

NURSING CARE PLAN 27-1
Continued

Potential Problems and Nursing Diagnoses	Nursing Management	Outcome Criteria
Impaired Verbal Communication related to loss of ability to speak	Assess client's ability to use alternative methods of communication; assess reading level, sensory or cognitive impairment. Discuss preferred method (eg, picture boards or written notes) of communicating preoperatively and have client practice before surgery. Pay close attention when client communicates to avoid repetition and frustration for client. Repeat message to ensure understanding. Provide emotional support and encouragement.	Client can communicate needs.
Risk for Infection related to loss of upper airway protection	Keep stoma clean and inspect for signs of infection or skin breakdown. Maintain sterile technique when suctioning and performing tracheostomy care. Position client so that secretions do not pool around stoma. Teach client to exercise care when bathing to avoid contamination of stoma.	No signs or symptoms of infection.
Anxiety related to change in bodily structure and function and impact on lifestyle	Review the information that was provided preoperatively regarding suctioning and care of stoma. Explain actions before you perform them and include the rationale. Ask client what he or she is most anxious about (inability to care for self, fear of suffocating, change in appearance, impaired ability to communicate, etc) to prioritize issues to work through. Suggest counseling and support groups. Teach anxiety reduction techniques (see Chap. 13)	Decreased anxiety, ability to accept and manage care.
Risk for Ineffective Management of Therapeutic Regimen related to lack of knowledge about tracheostomy care and home support	Teach client how to suction airway, care for tube, and protect stoma. Familiarize client with needed supplies. Teach the client to check for signs and symptoms of infection. Tell client what to do if the tube comes out. Ensure that client has an extra trach tube. Refer client to support groups and home care services.	The client demonstrates ability to care for tracheostomy, suction self, and care for supplies. The client can state how to manage accidental extubation. Home care needs are met before discharge.

NURSING MANAGEMENT

Major goals for the intubated client are to improve ventilations, maintain a patent airway, and communicate needs to others. Monitor vital signs at periodic intervals, depending on the condition of the client and the reason for endotracheal tube insertion. Blood gas studies and pulse oximetry provide an ongoing evaluation of the client's respiratory status. Review the results of these studies and report changes to the physician. Observe the client at frequent intervals for response to respiratory support and complications associated with endotracheal intubation. Evaluate any change in the client's mental status.

Confusion may result from abnormal blood gases or electrolyte imbalances. Sudden restlessness or agitation may indicate obstruction of the endotracheal tube, which can be life-threatening. Auscultate the lungs and observe the symmetrical rise and fall of the chest every 30 to 60 minutes. If breath sounds are not detected bilaterally, notify the physician immediately.

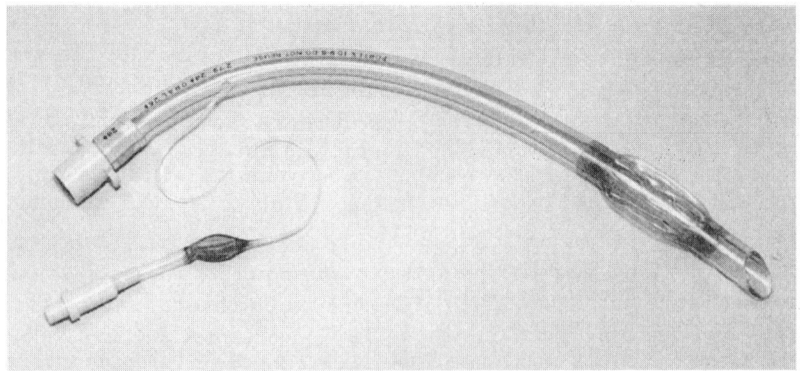

FIGURE 27-5. An endotracheal tube. The cuff on the endotracheal tube is inflated to provide a tight seal.

Keep the inspired air moist through humidification. Clients with endotracheal tubes are unable to cough, secretions are often thick and tenacious, and swallowing reflexes are depressed.

An increase in PCO_2 caused by blockage of the endotracheal tube or malfunctioning of the ventilator may occur secondary to secretions or because the client is biting on the tube. Keep the airway patent at all times using the same suctioning technique as for a tracheostomy. If the client is biting on the tube, a bite block or oral airway may be used to keep the tube patent.

Change the client's position every 2 hours to prevent atelectasis. Give oral care as needed to keep the mouth and lips free of crusts and mucus. Suction the oropharynx and mouth as needed. The teeth may be cleaned with applicators. Inspect the oral cavity at frequent intervals. Report any signs of oral bleeding to the physician.

The client may display anxiety or fear because of the tube, inability to speak, suctioning, and dependence on a machine for breathing. Each time suctioning is needed, reassure the client that the procedure takes only a short time. The client may attempt to remove or pull on the tube if he or she is awake or partially awake. Restraining the client may be necessary. Contact the physician if extreme restlessness is noted. Provide a "Magic Slate" or pencil and paper, and ask questions that can be answered by shaking the head yes or no.

Once the endotracheal tube has been removed, place the client in a high Fowler's or semi-Fowler's position to promote optimal chest and lung expansion. The posterior pharynx may be dry, and the voice may be hoarse. Observe the client at frequent intervals for signs of laryngeal edema and increased respiratory distress. Immediately report any sign of respiratory distress because reinsertion of the endotracheal tube may be necessary.

General Nutritional Considerations

Claims that megadoses of vitamin C cure the common cold generate interest and controversy. Well-controlled studies suggest that large doses of vitamin C neither prevent nor cure colds but may help minimize the severity and duration of symptoms.

A high fluid intake helps thin bronchial secretions.

A nasogastric tube feeding may be ordered for the first 24 to 48 hours after a laryngectomy to avoid irritation to the sutures and reduce the risk of aspiration. When oral intake resumes, small amounts of liquids are offered. The diet is advanced according to the client's tolerance.

Clients who have difficulty swallowing may be able to maintain an oral intake if the texture of the food is altered. A pureed diet, thickened pureed diet, semisolid diet, or soft diet may be needed until a regular diet can be resumed. It may also be necessary to thicken liquids to promote ease of swallowing.

Following a laryngectomy, the client may experience anorexia related to a diminished sense of taste and smell. The appearance of food becomes more important. Attractive food, served in pleasant surroundings and seasoned according to individual taste, may help promote intake. Ensure the client that some sense of taste and smell will return.

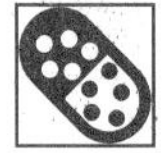

General Pharmacologic Considerations

In some instances, one or more of the drugs contained in multiple-ingredient cold preparations may be contraindicated in certain disorders such as glaucoma, heart disease, hypertension, or prostatic enlargement. Clients with one or more known diseases and who are taking prescription drugs are encouraged to consult the physician before using nonprescription drugs for treatment of a cold.

Aspirin prolongs bleeding time by inhibiting the aggregation (clumping) of platelets. When the bleeding time is prolonged, it takes longer for the blood to clot after a cut, surgery, or injury to the skin or mucous membranes.

Some cold tablets contain antihistamines that thicken nasal secretions. Although this action may temporarily decrease the discomfort of profuse nasal secretions, thickened secretions can block the drainage openings of the sinus cavity, lead to failure of the sinuses to drain adequately, and become a focus for continuing infection.

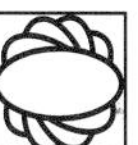

General Gerontologic Considerations

If an older client requires a tracheostomy, the nurse must be alert to possible confusion after the procedure. If the client is confused or does not understand the purpose of the procedure, attempts may be made to pull at the tube or to remove it. Restraining measures may be required.

The common cold may be potentially serious for elderly persons, especially when they have other diseases such as a chronic respiratory disorder or heart disease. Older clients are advised to see a physician if cold symptoms are severe or if breathing is difficult.

After a laryngectomy the older adult may require extra time and instruction to learn esophageal speech, speak with an electric larynx, or use TEP.

SUMMARY OF KEY CONCEPTS

- Infectious and inflammatory disorders of the upper respiratory airway may occur because of allergy, infection, and obstruction. Symptoms include headache, fever, pain, and mild to moderate difficulty breathing.
- Nursing management of clients with upper respiratory disorders caused by infection or allergy and treated medically focuses primarily on relieving symptoms and client and family teaching.
- Many upper respiratory disorders are treated with medications, but surgery may be required if the disorder does not respond to more conservative treatment.
- The nursing assessment of clients with structural disorders of the upper airway includes monitoring vital signs, determining if bleeding is present, assessing airway patency and respiratory patterns, and determining the client's anxiety level.
- Trauma to or obstruction of the respiratory airway may result in mild to severe difficulty in maintaining a patent airway. Complete or partial obstruction of the larynx or oropharynx is an extremely serious and often life-threatening condition.
- Nursing management of those having surgical correction of an upper respiratory obstruction includes maintaining a patent airway and assessing for evidence of increased bleeding.
- Risk factors that contribute to the development of laryngeal cancer include tobacco and alcohol abuse, exposure to industrial pollutants, chronic laryngitis, habitual overuse of the voice, and heredity.
- Persistent hoarseness usually is the earliest symptom of cancer of the larynx. Hoarseness is slight at first and may be ignored. A sensation of swelling or a lump in the throat may be noticed, followed by dysphagia and pain when talking.
- Surgical treatment of cancer of the larynx includes laser surgery and a partial or total laryngectomy. If the disease has extended beyond the larynx, a radical neck dissection is performed.
- After a laryngectomy, communication may be by esophageal speech, throat vibrators, or a surgically implanted prosthesis.
- Clients with a laryngectomy experience a great deal of anxiety as well as difficulty in coping with the diagnosis and surgery. Clients may isolate themselves from others and show signs of anxiety, withdrawal, and depression.
- One of the biggest fears the laryngectomy client has is fear of suffocation. During the immediate postoperative period, nursing tasks must focus on maintaining a patent airway, preventing infection, and meeting the client's physical and emotional needs.
- A tracheostomy may be required for upper airway obstruction, caused by aspiration of food or a foreign object into the trachea, a severe allergic reaction, or infection or edema of the upper respiratory tract.
- Clients with a tracheostomy must be assessed frequently for a patent airway because secretions can rapidly clog the tracheostomy opening, an effect that can result in death by asphyxiation. Clients are not left unattended during the early postoperative period.
- Endotracheal intubation is performed on those who cannot maintain an adequate airway on their own or those having respiratory difficulty, such as clients who are comatose, under general anesthesia, or with extensive edema of upper airway passages, or who are awake but unable to breathe on their own.
- Clients with endotracheal intubation are observed at frequent intervals for response to respiratory support and complications associated with endotracheal intubation.

CRITICAL THINKING EXERCISES

1. A client is seen for a severe pharyngitis. The client is diagnosed with a group A beta-hemolytic streptococcal infection and is placed on penicillin. As the nurse, what discharge instructions are appropriate?
2. A client has an endotracheal tube. Although critically ill, he is somewhat alert and wants to communicate with his family. He has an intravenous line in his right hand and is in a low Fowler's position. What method of communication could you suggest? What suggestions could you give to his family?
3. A neighbor calls you and says that she has had a nosebleed for the past half hour. As you prepare to evaluate her, what steps do you anticipate taking?
4. Your client is scheduled for a partial laryngectomy. What information is appropriate to help him prepare for the postoperative period?

Suggested Readings

Barbarito, C. (1998). Hypertension-induced epistaxis. *American Journal of Nursing, 98*(2), 48.

Boucher, M. A. (1996). When laryngectomy complicates care. *RN, 59*(8), 40–45.

Carpenito, L. J. (1997). *Nursing care plans and documentation: Nursing diagnoses and collaborative problems.* Philadelphia: Lippincott-Raven.

Consult stat. One option when cold symptoms linger on. (1996). *RN, 59(1), 60–61.*

Glass, C. A., & Grap, M. J. (1995). Ten tips for safer suctioning. *American Journal of Nursing, 95*(5), 51–53.

Hatfield, B. O. (1997). Cost effective trach teaching. *RN, 60*(3), 48–49.

Macmillan, C. (1995). Nasopharyngeal suction study reveals knowledge deficit. *Nursing Times, 91*(50), 28–30.

Odom, J. L. (1993). Airway emergencies in the post anesthesia care unit. *Nursing Clinics of North America, 28*(3), 483–491.

Pontieri-Lewis, V. (1997). The role of nutrition in wound healing. *MEDSURG Nursing, 6*(4), 187–192, 221.

Smeltzer, S. C. & Bare, B. G. (1996). *Brunner and Suddarth's textbook of medical-surgical nursing* (8th ed.) Philadelphia: Lippincott-Raven.

Timby, B. K. (1996). *Fundamental skills and concepts in patient care* (6th ed.). Philadelphia. Lippincott-Raven.

Additional Resources

Allergic and Nonallergic Rhinitis
http://www.njc.org

Larynxlink
http://www.larynxlink.com

Dysphagia Resource Center
http://www.dysphagia.com

Tracheostomy
http://housecall.orbisnews.com

Family Village
Tracheostomy On-Line Discussion Groups
http://laran.waisman.wisc.edu

NIH Clinical Center Nursing Department
SOP: Care of the Patient with a Tracheostomy
http://www.cc.nih.gov/nursing/trach.html

Chapter 28

Caring for Clients With Disorders of the Lower Respiratory Airway

KEY TERMS

Acute bronchitis
Asbestosis
Asthma
Atelectasis
Bronchiectasis
Chronic bronchitis
Chronic obstructive pulmonary disease
Emphysema
Empyema
Flail chest
Hemoptysis
Hemothorax
Influenza
Lobectomy
Lung abscess
Orthopnea
Pleural effusion
Pleurisy
Pneumoconiosis
Pneumonectomy
Pneumonia
Pneumothorax
Pulmonary contusion
Pulmonary edema
Pulmonary embolism
Pulmonary hypertension
Segmental resection
Septicemia
Silicosis
Sleep apnea syndrome
Subcutaneous emphysema
Thoracotomy
Tracheitis
Tracheobronchitis
Tuberculosis
Wedge resection

LEARNING OBJECTIVES

On completion of this chapter, the reader will:

- Describe infectious and inflammatory disorders of the lower airway.
- Identify critical assessments needed for a client with an infectious disorder of the lower respiratory airway.
- Define disorders classified as obstructive pulmonary disease.
- Discuss strategies for preventing and managing occupational lung diseases.
- Describe the pathophysiology of pulmonary hypertension.
- List risk factors associated with the development of pulmonary embolism.
- Discuss conditions that may lead to adult respiratory distress syndrome.
- Differentiate acute and chronic respiratory failure.
- Explain why lung cancer is often diagnosed after the disease is advanced.
- Describe the nursing assessments required for a client who experiences trauma to the chest.
- Explain the purpose of chest tubes following thoracic surgery.
- Describe the preoperative and postoperative nursing care for clients undergoing thoracic care.

The exchange of gases and ventilation occur in the lower respiratory tract. The lower airway is subject to a variety of problems and disorders. These disorders compromise the lower respiratory tract's ability to perform its primary functions. If untreated, many of these disorders can lead to respiratory failure. Others become chronic and affect the client's quality of life.

Infectious and Inflammatory Disorders

Acute Bronchitis

Acute bronchitis is characterized by inflammation of the mucous membranes that line the major bronchi and their branches. The inflammatory process may also involve the trachea; it is then referred to as **tracheobronchitis**.

ETIOLOGY AND PATHOPHYSIOLOGY

The most common cause of acute bronchitis is a viral infection, but bacterial infections and chemical irritation from noxious fumes are also implicated. Typically starting as an upper respiratory tract infection, the inflammatory process extends into the tracheobronchial tree and is followed by an increase in the amount of mucus produced by the secretory cells of the mucosa. The disease may be complicated by the development of bronchial asthma.

ASSESSMENT FINDINGS

Signs and Symptoms

Signs and symptoms initially include fever, malaise, and a dry, nonproductive cough that later becomes productive of mucopurulent sputum. Clients experience paroxysmal attacks of coughing and may also report wheezing. Acute bronchitis may be complicated by laryngitis and sinusitis. Moist inspiratory crackles may be heard when the chest is auscultated.

Diagnostic Findings

A sputum sample is collected for culture and sensitivity testing to rule out bacterial infection. A chest film also may be done to detect additional pathology, such as pneumonia.

MEDICAL MANAGEMENT

Acute bronchitis usually is self-limiting, lasting for several days. It is treated with bed rest, antipyretics, expectorants and antitussives, and plenty of liquids. Humidifiers assist in keeping the mucous membranes moist because dry air aggravates the cough. Secondary bacterial invasion occasionally occurs and the previously mild infection becomes a serious condition, accompanied by a persistent cough and the production of thick, purulent sputum. These secondary infections usually subside as the bronchitis subsides, but they may persist for several weeks. A broad-spectrum antibiotic is started immediately; it may be changed to a different antibiotic after the results of the sputum culture become available.

NURSING MANAGEMENT

Auscultate the breath sounds. Monitor vital signs every 4 hours, especially if fever is present. Encourage the client to cough and deep breathe every 2 hours while awake and to expectorate rather than swallow sputum. Humidification of the surrounding air loosens bronchial secretions. Change bedding and clothes if they become damp. Offer fluids frequently. Instruct the client to prevent the spread of infection by:

- Washing hands frequently, particularly when handling secretions and soiled tissues
- Covering the mouth when sneezing and coughing
- Discarding soiled tissues in a plastic bag
- Avoiding sharing articles that the client uses

Refer to nursing management of tuberculosis for applicable nursing diagnoses such as *Ineffective Airway Clearance, Pain, Hyperthermia,* and *Fluid Volume Deficit*, and associated interventions.

Pneumonia

Pneumonia is an inflammatory process affecting the bronchioles and alveoli. Although generally associated with an acute infection, pneumonia can also result from chemical ingestion or inhalation, radiation therapy, and the aspiration of foreign bodies or gastric contents.

ETIOLOGY AND PATHOPHYSIOLOGY

Pneumonia is classified according to the etiology and the presenting symptoms. Viral pneumonias are the most common, with type A virus as the usual causative organism. Bacterial pneumonias are not as common, but are more serious. Causative organisms include:

- *Streptococcus pneumoniae*
- *Staphylococcus aureus*
- *Klebsiella pneumoniae*
- *Pseudomonas aeruginosa*
- *Haemophilus influenzae*

Bacterial pneumonias are referred to as typical pneumonias. Atypical pneumonias are those caused by mycoplasmas, *Legionella pneumophila* (causative agent of Legionnaires' disease), viruses, and fungi. Pneumonia caused by *Mycobacterium tuberculosis* is also classified as atypical.

Radiation pneumonia is a result of damage to normal lung mucosa during radiation therapy for breast or lung cancer. Ingestion of kerosene or inhalation of volatile hydrocarbons (kerosene or gasoline) causes a chemical pneumonia. Aspiration pneumonia results when a foreign body or gastric contents are inhaled during vomiting or regurgitation.

Lobar pneumonia is an inflammation confined to one or more lobes of the lung. Patchy and diffuse infection scattered throughout both lungs is called *bronchopneumonia* (Fig. 28–1). Hypoventilation of lung tissue over a prolonged period can occur when a client is bedridden and breathing with only part of the lungs. This results in accumulation of bronchial secretions and may lead to *hypostatic pneumonia*.

Organisms that cause pneumonia reach the alveoli by inhalation of droplets, aspiration of organisms from the upper airway, or less commonly, seeding from the bloodstream. When the organisms reach the alveoli, an intense inflammatory reaction occurs. This produces an exudate, which impairs gas exchange. Capillaries surrounding the alveoli become engorged and cause the alveoli to collapse (atelectasis), further impairing gas exchange and interfering with ventilation. White blood cells move into the area to destroy the pathogenic organisms, filling the interstitial spaces. If untreated, consolidation occurs as the inflammation and exudate increase. Hypoxemia results from the inability of the lungs to oxygenate blood from the heart. Bronchitis, **tracheitis** (inflammation of the trachea), and spots of *necrosis* (death of tissue) in the lung may follow.

In atypical pneumonias, the exudate infiltrates the interstitial spaces, rather than the alveoli directly. The pneumonia is more scattered, as with bronchopneumonia. As the inflammatory process continues, interference with the exchange of gases between the bloodstream and lungs increases. With an increase in the carbon dioxide content of the blood, the respiratory center in the brain is stimulated, and breathing becomes more rapid and shallow.

Without an interruption of the disease process of any type of pneumonia, the client becomes increasingly ill. If the circulatory system cannot compensate for the burden of decreased gas exchange, heart failure may occur. Death due to pneumonia can occur in elderly people and in those weakened by acute or chronic diseases or disorders such as acquired immunodeficiency syndrome (AIDS), cancer, and lung disease, or by prolonged periods of inactivity.

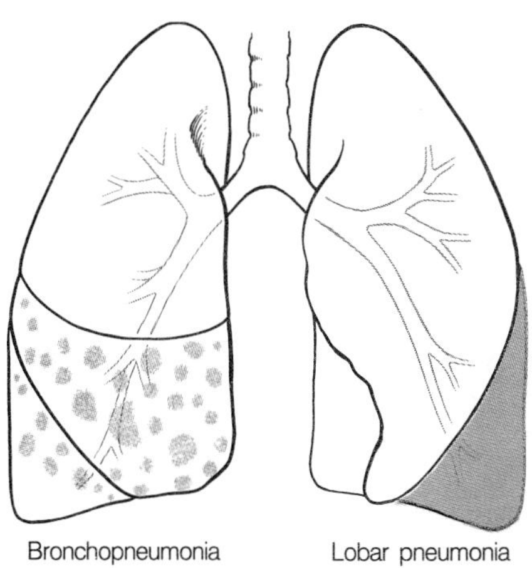

FIGURE 28-1. Distribution of lung involvement in lobar and bronchial pneumonia.

Complications of pneumonia include:

- Congestive heart failure (see Chapter 35)
- **Empyema**—collection of pus in the pleural cavity
- **Pleurisy**—inflammation of the pleura
- **Septicemia**—infective microorganisms in the blood
- Atelectasis
- Hypotension
- Shock

In addition, septicemia may lead to a secondary focus of infection, such as endocarditis (inflammation of the endocardium), pericarditis (inflammation of the pericardium), and purulent arthritis. Recovery, especially from atypical pneumonia, may also be complicated by otitis media (infection of the middle ear), bronchitis, or sinusitis.

ASSESSMENT FINDINGS

Signs and Symptoms

Symptoms vary for the different types of pneumonia. The onset of bacterial pneumonia is sudden. The client experiences fever, chills, a productive cough, and discomfort in the chest wall muscles from coughing. There is also general malaise. The sputum may be rusty colored. Breathing causes pain, and the client tries to breathe as shallowly as possible.

Viral pneumonia differs from bacterial pneumonia in that blood cultures are sterile, sputum may be more copious, chills are less common, and pulse and respiratory rates are characteristically slow. The course of viral pneumonia usually is less severe than that of bacterial pneumonia. In viral pneumonia, the mortality rate is low but rises when bacterial pneumonia occurs as a secondary infection. Many clients with viral pneumonia are weak and ill for a longer period than those with successfully treated bacterial pneumonia.

Diagnostic Findings

Auscultation of the chest reveals wheezing, crackles, and decreased breath sounds. The nail beds, lips, and oral mucosa may be cyanotic. Sputum culture and sensitivity studies identify the infectious microorganism and effective antibiotics for treatment. A chest film shows areas of infiltrates and consolidation. A complete blood count shows an elevated white blood cell count. Blood cultures also may be done to detect microorganisms in the blood.

MEDICAL MANAGEMENT

Medical management involves prompt initiation of antibiotic therapy, hydration to thin secretions, supplemental oxygen to alleviate hypoxemia, bed rest, chest physical therapy, bronchodilators, analgesics, antipyretics, and cough expectorants or suppressants, depending on the nature of the client's cough. If a client is hospitalized with pneumonia, treatment is more vigorous depending on the potential or actual complications. Electrolyte replacement is sometimes necessary secondary to fever, dehydration, and inadequate nutritional intake. If the client experiences severe respiratory difficulty, and thick, copious secretions, intubation may be needed, along with mechanical ventilation.

NURSING MANAGEMENT

Auscultate lung sounds and monitor the client for signs of respiratory difficulty. The client's oxygenation status is best assessed by pulse oximetry, arterial blood gas (ABG) analysis, and quality of breathing. Also assess the client's cough and the nature of the sputum production. Place the client in semi-Fowler's position to aid breathing and increase the amount of air taken with each breath. Encourage increased fluid intake to help loosen secretions and replace fluids lost through fever and an increased respiratory rate. Monitor fluid intake and output, skin turgor, vital signs, and serum electrolytes. Administer antipyretics as indicated and ordered.

Preventing pneumonia is an important role of the nurse. The identification of clients who are at risk for pneumonia provides a means for the nurse to practice preventive care. Nursing Guidelines 28–1 identifies strategies to implement for clients who are at risk for pneumonia. Recommend the pneumococcal vaccine (a vaccine that provides immunity from specific bacterial pneumonias) to clients over 50 years of age or to clients who are at risk because of chronic illness. Because nursing care of clients with infectious lung disorders is similar regardless of the etiology, refer to the nursing management of the client with tuberculosis for nursing diagnoses and additional interventions.

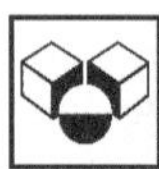

Nursing Guidelines 28-1

Preventing Pneumonia

- Promote coughing and expectoration of secretions if client experiences increased mucus production.
- Change position frequently if client is immobilized for any reason.
- Encourage deep breathing and coughing exercises at least every 2 hours.
- Administer chest physical therapy as indicated.
- Suction client if client is unable to expectorate.
- Prevent aspiration in clients at risk.
- Prevent infections.
- Cleanse respiratory equipment on a routine basis.
- Promote frequent oral hygiene.
- Administer sedatives and opioids carefully to avoid respiratory depression.
- Encourage client to stop smoking and reduce alcohol intake.

Pleurisy

Pleurisy or pleuritis refers to an acute inflammation of the parietal and visceral pleura. During the acute phase of pleurisy, the pleurae are inflamed, thick, and swollen, and an exudate forms from fibrin and lymph. Eventually they become rigid. During inspiration the inflamed pleurae rub together, causing severe, sharp pain.

ASSESSMENT FINDINGS

Respirations become shallow secondary to this excruciating pain. Pleural fluid accumulates as the inflammatory process worsens. The pain decreases as the fluid increases because it separates the pleura. The client develops a dry cough, fatigues easily, and experiences shortness of breath. A friction rub (coarse sounds heard during inspiration and early expiration) is heard during auscultation. Decreased ventilation may result in atelectasis.

Pleurisy generally occurs as a result of a primary condition, such as pneumonia or other pulmonary infections. The inflammatory process spreads from the lungs to the parietal pleura. Pleurisy may also develop with tuberculosis, lung cancer, cardiac and renal disease, systemic infections, and pulmonary embolism. A chest x-ray shows changes in the affected area. Microscopic examination of sputum and a sputum culture may or may not be positive for pathogenic microorganisms. If a **thoracentesis** (removal of fluid from the chest) is performed, a pleural fluid specimen is sent to the laboratory for analysis. Occasionally the physician may perform a pleural biopsy.

MEDICAL MANAGEMENT

The underlying condition dictates the treatment for pleurisy. Analgesic and antipyretic drugs provide relief for pain and fever. A nonsteroidal anti-inflammatory drug such as indomethacin provides analgesia and promotes more effective coughing by the client. Severe cases may require a procaine intercostal nerve block.

NURSING MANAGEMENT

The client has considerable pain with inspiration. Teach the client to splint the chest wall by turning onto the affected side. The client also can splint the chest wall with his or her hands or a pillow when coughing. Provide emotional support to the client to assist in decreasing anxiety.

Pleural Effusion

Pleural effusion is the collection of fluid between the visceral and parietal pleurae and may be a complication of such disorders as pneumonia, lung cancer, tuberculosis, pulmonary embolism, and congestive heart failure (Fig. 28–2). The amount of accumulated fluid may be so great that the lung is partially collapsed on that side, and pressure is placed on the heart and other organs of the mediastinum.

ASSESSMENT FINDINGS

Fever, pain, and dyspnea are the most common symptoms. Chest percussion reveals dullness over the involved area. The examiner may note diminished or absent breath sounds over the involved area when auscultating the lungs. A friction rub may also be heard. A chest x-ray and computed tomographic (CT) scan shows fluid in the involved area. Thoracentesis is sometimes done to remove pleural fluid for analysis and examination for malignant cells.

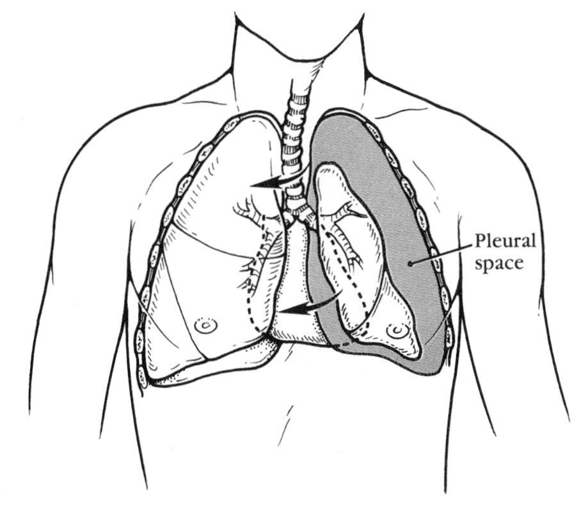

FIGURE 28-2. Pleural Effusion. Fluid has collected in the pleural space and displaced lung tissue. Also note the shift of fluid into the mediastinum and torsion of the bronchus.

MEDICAL MANAGEMENT

The main goal of treatment is to eliminate the cause of pleural effusion. Treatment includes antibiotics, analgesics for pain, cardiotonic drugs to control congestive heart failure (when present), removal of excess pleural fluid by thoracentesis, and surgery for the cancer.

NURSING MANAGEMENT

If a thoracentesis is needed, the nurse prepares the client for this procedure. Nursing Guidelines 26-4 in Chapter 26 outlines the nurse's role during this procedure. The client is usually frightened, and thus it is important for the nurse to provide support throughout the procedure. If the client has a chest tube inserted, refer to Clinical Procedure 28-1.

Lung Abscess

ETIOLOGY AND PATHOPHYSIOLOGY

A **lung abscess** is a localized area of pus formation within the lung parenchyma. As the pus formation increases, necrosis of the tissue occurs. Later, this area collapses and creates a cavity. The infection can extend into the bronchus and pleural cavity. An abscess may occur in the lung parenchyma as a result of aspiration, pneumonia, or a mechanical obstruction of the bronchi, such as a tumor. Other causes of lung abscess include necrosis of lung tissue after an infection and necrotic lesions resulting from inhalation of dust particles. Clients with impaired cough reflex or altered immune function are at risk for lung abscesses.

ASSESSMENT FINDINGS

Signs and symptoms include chills, fever, weight loss, chest pain, and a productive cough. Sputum may be purulent or blood-streaked. The client appears chronically ill. Finger clubbing may occur in chronic cases. Auscultation of the chest reveals dull or absent breath sounds in the area of the abscess. A chest x-ray and CT scan usually locate the abscess. Blood and sputum cultures may be positive for pathogenic microorganisms. Chest percussion detects an area of dullness. In some instances, thoracentesis may be done and the aspirated fluid sent to the laboratory for culture and sensitivity tests.

MEDICAL AND SURGICAL MANAGEMENT

Postural drainage and antibiotics assist in controlling the infection. On occasion a lobectomy may be performed to remove the abscess and surrounding lung tissue.

NURSING MANAGEMENT

Monitor the client for possible adverse effects of antibiotics. Administer chest physical therapy as indicated, and encourage the client to deep breathe and cough frequently. Teach the client to eat a diet high in protein and calories. Provide emotional support, and tell the client that it may take a long time for the lung abscess to resolve.

Empyema

Empyema is a general term used to denote the presence of pus in a body cavity. It usually refers, however, to pus or infected fluid within the pleural cavity (thoracic empyema). Infection may follow chest trauma, such as a stab or gunshot wound, or a preexisting disease, such as pneumonia, tuberculosis, pleurisy, or lung abscess. The pus-filled area may become walled off and enclosed by a thick membrane.

ASSESSMENT FINDINGS

Fever, chest pain, dyspnea, anorexia, and malaise may be present. Auscultation of the chest reveals diminished or absent breath sounds over the affected area. The client appears acutely ill. The affected lung area is distinguished on a chest x-ray.

MEDICAL AND SURGICAL MANAGEMENT

Aspiration of purulent fluid by thoracentesis may be necessary to identify the microorganisms, remove the pus or fluid, and select appropriate antibiotic therapy. Closed drainage may be used to empty the empyemic cavity. **Thoracotomy** (surgical opening of the thorax) is performed, and one or more large chest tubes are inserted. The chest tubes are then connected to an underwater-seal drainage bottle. Open drainage, which necessitates the removal of a section of one or more ribs, may be used when pus is thick and the walls of the empyemic cavity are strong enough to keep the lung from collapsing while the chest is opened. One or more tubes may be placed in the opening to promote drainage. The wound is then covered by a large absorbent dressing, which is changed as necessary. The drainage of pus results in a drop in temperature and general symptomatic improvement.

If empyema is inadequately treated, it may become chronic. A thick coating forms over the lung, preventing its expansion. *Decortication* (removal of the coating) and evacuation of the pleural space allow the lung to re-expand.

NURSING MANAGEMENT

Empyema takes a long time to resolve. Provide emotional support to the client during treatment. Teach the client to do breathing exercises as prescribed. If the client has a chest tube, implement the nursing care as described in Clinical Procedure 28-1.

Influenza

Influenza (flu) is an acute respiratory disease of relatively short duration caused by one of several related and yet distinct viruses. The major strains of the influenza virus are A, B, and C. The virus is able to mutate and produce variants within a given strain. The variants are called subtypes. The viruses that cause influenza are transmitted through the respiratory tract.

Influenza chiefly occurs in epidemics, although sporadic cases appear between epidemics. Because the virus changes, antibodies produced by those who have had influenza are no longer effective against the new subtype, and a different vaccine must be produced. Most clients recover. Fatalities usually are due to secondary bacterial complications, especially among pregnant women, elderly or debilitated clients, and those with chronic conditions, such as cardiac disease and emphysema.

During an epidemic, the death rate from pneumonia and cardiovascular disease rises. Complications include tracheobronchitis, bacterial pneumonia, and cardiovascular disease. Staphylococcal pneumonia is the most serious complication. Table 28–1 lists signs and symptoms of influenza. Diagnosis is based on symptoms. Additional diagnostic studies, such as chest x-ray and sputum analysis, may be performed to rule out other diseases, such as pneumonia.

NURSING MANAGEMENT

Nursing management focuses on prevention of influenza. Annual influenza vaccinations are recommended for people who are at high risk for complications, or those who are exposed daily to many different people, and for health care workers. Each year a new vaccine is developed from three virus strains that are predicted to be present in the coming season.

Clients who are admitted to the hospital with influenza need to be isolated from clients who do not have it. Maintain respiratory precautions when caring for these clients. If a community is experiencing an epidemic, hospitals usually develop policies regarding visitation and admissions.

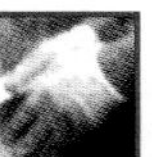

Clinical Procedure 28-1
Maintaining a Water-Seal Drainage System

PURPOSE	EQUIPMENT
• Maintain the integrity of the closed drainage system • Maintain and restore client's optimal respiratory status • Protect client from respiratory injury caused by problem with equipment	• Pair of hemostats • Distilled water • Tape

Nursing Action	Rationale
ASSESSMENT	
Review medical record to determine the client's condition that necessitated inserting a chest tube.	Indicates what to expect in terms of drainage.
Determine if client has one or two chest tubes.	Focuses assessment.
Note the date of chest tube insertion.	Provides a point of reference for evaluation of assessment data.
Check orders for amount of suction ordered, if any.	Provides guidelines for carrying out medical treatment.
PLANNING	
Arrange to assess client as soon as possible after receiving report.	Establishes a baseline and early opportunity for troubleshooting abnormal findings.
Locate tape and container of distilled water.	Facilitates efficient time management for general maintenance of the drainage system.
IMPLEMENTATION	
Introduce yourself. Explain the purpose of the assessment.	Reduces anxiety and promotes cooperation.
Wash your hands.	Maintains asepsis.
Check to see that two hemostats are at the bedside in plain view.	Facilitates checking for air leaks or clamping the chest tube(s) if the drainage system needs to be replaced.
Turn off suction regulator, if one is in use, before assessing the client.	Eliminates noise that can interfere with auscultation of breath sounds.
Assess lung sounds; do not expect to hear breath sounds over deflated lung.	Provides a baseline for future comparisons.
Inspect dressing for signs that it is intact and dry.	Indicates a need for changing dressing.
Palpate skin around chest tube insertion to assess for subcutaneous emphysema.	Indicates subcutaneous air leak.
Inspect all connections to ensure that they are taped and secure.	Indicates that connections are secure.
Reinforce connections if tape is loose.	Prevents accidental separation.
Check that all tubing is unkinked and hangs freely into the drainage system.	Ensures drainage of air and fluid.
Observe fluid level in the water-seal chamber to see if it is at the 2-cm level.	Maintains the water seal.
Add distilled water to the appropriate mark, if low.	Ensures the water seal.
Note if water level rises and falls with each respiration.	Indicates that the tubing is unobstructed and the lung has not completely inflated.
Observe for continuous bubbling in the water-seal chamber.	Indicates an air leak in the tubing or at a connection.
If constant bubbling is noted, clamp hemostats at the chest and a few inches away. Observe if bubbling stops.	Constant bubbling is expected in the suction control center.
Continue releasing and applying the hemostats until the bubbling stops.	Provides a means for determining the location of an air leak within the tubing.

continued

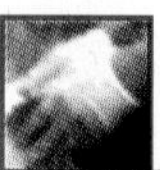

Clinical Procedure 28-1
Continued

Nursing Action	Rationale
Apply tape around the tube above where the last clamp was applied when the bubbling stopped.	Seals the air leak.
Note if the water level in the suction chamber is at 20 cm.	Determines appropriate water level for suction.
Add distilled water to the appropriate mark in the suction control chamber if it has evaporated.	Maintains appropriate amount of suction.
Regulate the suction so that it produces gentle bubbling.	Prevents rapid evaporation and unnecessary noise.
Observe the nature and amount of drainage in the collection chamber.	Provides comparative data. More than 100 mL/hour or bright red drainage is reported.
Keep the drainage system below the chest.	Maintains gravity flow of drainage.
Position the client so as to avoid compressing the tubing.	Facilitates drainage.
Curl and secure excess length of tubing on the bed.	Avoids dependent loops.
Milk tubing to move stationary clots only if absolutely necessary.	Creates extremely high negative intrapleural pressure and is therefore never done routinely.
Encourage deep breathing and coughing at least every 2 hours while awake.	Promotes lung re-expansion.
Instruct client to move in bed, ambulate, and exercise shoulder on side of drainage tube.	Prevents complications associated with immobility.
Never clamp tube for an extended period of time.	Predisposes to pneumothorax; creates extreme air pressure within the lung when there is no avenue for escape.
Insert a separated chest tube within water until it can be reattached and secured to drainage system.	Provides a temporary water seal.
Prevent air from entering the tube insertion site, if the tube should be accidentally pulled out.	Reduces the amount of lung collapse.
Mark the drainage level on the collection chamber at the end of each shift. Never empty the drainage container.	Provides data concerning fluid loss without risk of recollapsing the lung.

TABLE 28-1 **Signs and Symptoms of Influenza**

Incubation Period	1–3 days
Onset	Sudden Abrupt onset of fever and chills Severe headache Muscle aches
Progression	Anorexia Weakness, apathy, malaise Respiratory symptoms: Sneezing Sore throat, laryngitis Dry cough Nasal discharge—rhinitis Conjunctival irritation
Duration	Fever may persist for 3 days, but other symptoms usually continue for 7–10 days Cough may persist longer
Period of contagion	2–3 days beginning with onset of symptoms

Pulmonary Tuberculosis

Pulmonary **tuberculosis** is a bacterial infectious disease caused by *M. tuberculosis*. It primarily affects the lungs, but may also affect the kidneys and other organs. Tuberculosis continues to be a worldwide health issue. Strains resistant to current medications and therapies have occurred secondary to increased immigration, the epidemic of human immunodeficiency virus (HIV), and inadequate public health.

ETIOLOGY AND PATHOPHYSIOLOGY

Tubercle bacilli are gram-positive, rod-shaped, acid-fast aerobic bacilli. Although the bacilli can live in the dark for months in particles of dried sputum, exposure to direct sunlight, heat, and ultraviolet light destroys them in a few hours. The microorganism is difficult to kill with ordinary disinfectants. Tubercle bacilli are killed by pasteurization, a process widely used in preventing the spread of tuberculosis by milk and milk products.

Tuberculosis is most commonly transmitted by direct contact with a person who has the active disease through the inhalation of droplets produced by coughing, sneezing, and spitting. Brief contact does not usually result in infection. In contrast to the number of people who have been infected with the tubercle bacillus, only a small proportion ever become ill. Many factors predispose a client to the development of tuberculosis. Table 28–2 lists factors that place a client at risk for tuberculosis. The incidence of tuberculosis has recently risen, with newer cases of drug resistant microbial forms found to be resistant to drugs.

Tuberculosis is characterized by stages of early infection, latency, and potential for recurrence after the primary disease. The bacilli may remain dormant for many years and reactivate and produce clinical symptoms of tuberculosis.

Early Infection

Bacilli, when inhaled, pass through the bronchial system and implant on the bronchioles or alveoli. Initially, the host does not have any resistance to this infection. Phagocytes (neutrophils and macrophages) engulf the bacilli, but the bacilli continue to multiply. At this time they also spread through the lymphatic channels to the regional lymph nodes to the circulating blood and distant organs. Eventually the cellular immune response limits further multiplication and dissemination of the bacilli.

Immune Activation

When immune activation occurs (usually a full response within 2 weeks), a characteristic tissue reaction results in the formation of a granuloma from epithelial cells merging with the macrophages. The granuloma is referred to as the Ghon tubercle. Lymphocytes surround the granuloma. The central portion of the tubercle undergoes necrosis. The necrosis has a cheesy appearance and is called caseous necrosis. It may liquefy and slough into the connecting bronchus, producing a cavity. It also may enter the tracheobronchial system, promoting airborne transmission of infectious particles.

Healing of the Primary Lesion

The healing of the primary lesion occurs through resolution, fibrosis, and calcification. The granulation tissue of the primary lesion becomes more fibrous and creates a scar around the tubercle. This is referred to as the Ghon complex and is visible with an x-ray.

Latent Period

As the lesion heals, the infection enters a latent period that can persist for many years without producing clinical symptoms. The latent period can last an entire lifetime. However, if the immune response has not been adequate, clinical disease will eventually occur. Clients at particular risk are those with HIV, diabetes, or those on chemotherapy or long-term steroids. Only a small percentage of those infected with tuberculosis will actually have clinical symptoms.

Secondary Tuberculosis

Secondary tuberculosis usually involves reactivation of the initial infection. The person has already had an immune response, and thus the lesions that form tend to remain within the lungs. The course of this phase usually occurs as follows:

- Acute local inflammation with necrosis
- Ulceration of infected lung tissue
- Tubercles cluster together—become surrounded by inflammation
- Exudate fills the surrounding alveoli
- Bronchopneumonia develops
- Tuberculosis tissue becomes caseous—ulcerates into the bronchus
- Cavities form
- Ulcerations heal—scar tissue left around cavity
- Pleura thicken and retract

The course of tuberculosis becomes a cyclical one of inflammation, bronchopneumonia, ulceration, cavitation, and scarring. The tuberculosis gradually

TABLE 28-2 **Risk Factors for Infection With Tuberculosis**

Close contact with an individual with active tuberculosis
Immunocompromised clients:
  Elderly
  Clients with cancer
  Clients on corticosteroid therapy
  HIV-infected clients
Intravenous drug users and alcoholics
Inadequate health care
  Homeless
  Impoverished
  Minorities
Preexisting health conditions, such as:
  Diabetes
  Chronic renal failure
  Malnourishment
Immigrants from countries with high incidence of tuberculosis
Any client within an institution
Individuals living in overcrowded and substandard conditions
Health care workers

(Adapted from Smeltzer, S. C., & Bare, B. G. [1996]. *Brunner & Suddarth's textbook of medical-surgical nursing* [8th ed.]. Philadelphia: Lippincott-Raven.)

spreads throughout the lung fields and into the rest of the respiratory structures, as well as other organs via the lymph system. A client may experience periods of exacerbation, followed by remission. Table 28–3 presents the complications of tuberculosis.

ASSESSMENT FINDINGS

Signs and Symptoms

The onset of tuberculosis is insidious, and early symptoms vary from person to person. An infected person may be asymptomatic for a long time; symptoms may not appear until the disease is advanced. As symptoms develop, they are often vague and can be overlooked. Fatigue, anorexia, weight loss, and a slight, nonproductive cough are the early symptoms of tuberculosis often attributed to overwork, excessive smoking, or poor eating habits. Low-grade fever, particularly in the late afternoon, and night sweats are common as the disease progresses. The cough typically becomes productive of mucopurulent and blood-streaked sputum. Marked weakness, wasting, **hemoptysis** (expectoration of blood from the respiratory tract), and dyspnea are characteristics of later stages of the illness. Chest pain may result from the spread of infection to the pleura.

Diagnostic Findings

Diagnostic tests chiefly consist of tuberculin skin tests, chest x-ray, CT scan, magnetic resonance imaging (MRI), and analysis of sputum and other body fluids. Microscopic examination of sputum and other body fluids identifies the bacilli. A positive tuberculin skin test is evidence that a tuberculous infection has existed at some time somewhere in the body but does not indicate active disease. The chief value of these tests lies in case finding. Refer to tuberculin skin testing in Chapter 26.

Serial microscopic sputum examinations are ordered when tuberculosis is suspected, during and after a course of drug therapy, and after surgical removal of a diseased lobe of the lung. The client is instructed to cough deeply so that the specimen does not consist mainly of saliva. Most clients find that it is easier to raise sputum when they first awaken. It may be necessary to collect specimens on several consecutive days. See Nursing Guidelines 26–3 for strategies in collecting a sputum specimen. Gastric lavage, gastric aspiration, or a bronchoscopy may be used to determine the presence of the tuberculosis bacilli, particularly when a client has had difficulty raising a sputum specimen for examination. Tubercle bacilli may reach the stomach from the lungs when sputum is raised and not expectorated but swallowed. When invasion of other body areas by the tubercle bacillus is suspected, specimens are obtained to confirm the diagnosis.

MEDICAL AND SURGICAL MANAGEMENT

In many cases, drugs have speeded recovery and provided a chance for arresting the disease in clients with advanced lesions, but they do not offer a guaranteed cure. Their usefulness lies in their ability to retard the growth and multiplication of the tubercle bacillus, thus giving the body a chance to overcome the disease. Two factors make drug therapy less than ideal: drug toxicity and the tendency of the tubercle bacillus to develop resistance to the drug. Combined therapy with two or more drugs decreases the likelihood of drug resistance, increases the tuberculostatic action of the drugs, and lessens the risk for toxic drug reactions.

Resistance of the bacilli to drugs is an important factor in the lack of response to medical treatment. Drug therapy usually is carried out while the client is at home. Regular visits to the physician's office or

TABLE 28-3 **Complications of Tuberculosis**

Complication	Pathophysiology
Miliary tuberculosis or hematogenous tuberculosis	If a necrotic Ghon complex erodes through a blood vessel, a large number of organisms invade the blood stream. Clients experience acute illness with fever, dyspnea, and cyanosis, or become chronically ill with systemic symptoms of weight loss, fever, and gastrointestinal disorders. Hepatomegaly, splenomegaly, and generalized lymphadenopathy may be present.
Pleural effusion	If caseous material is released into the pleural space, it triggers an inflammatory reaction. A pleural exudate results.
Tuberculosis pneumonia	Acute pneumonia results when large amounts of bacilli tubercles are discharged from a liquefied necrotic lesion into the lungs or lymph nodes. Symptoms are similar to any bacterial pneumonia, with chills, fever, productive cough, and pleuritic pain.

TABLE 28-4 **Drug Regimen for Tuberculosis**

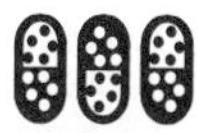

Treatment Period	Drugs Prescribed	Length of Drug Therapy
Initial treatment	isoniazid (INH) rifampin (RIF) pyrazinamide (PZA) (These three medications now in combination tablet)	INH, RIF, PZA for 4 months INH and RIF for additional 2 months
Suspected drug resistance	isoniazid (INH) rifampin (RIF) pyrazinamide (PZA) ethambutol (EMB) or streptomycin (SM)	If sensitive, continue INH and RIF for 6 more months If resistant to INH, use other drugs for 6 months If resistant to RIF, use other drugs for 12–18 months
Prophylactic treatment	isoniazid (INH) May use pyridoxine (vitamin B_6) to minimize side effects	6–12 months

clinic for follow-up care are necessary for assessment of response to therapy. Culture and sensitivity tests may be performed and the adverse effects of the drugs evaluated. Table 28–4 describes the drug regimen used in the management of tuberculosis.

When the disease is located primarily in one section of the lung, that portion may be removed by **segmental resection** (removal of a lobe segment) or by **wedge resection** (removal of a wedge of diseased tissue). If the diseased area is larger, **lobectomy** (removal of a lobe) may be performed. In some cases, the lung is so diseased that **pneumonectomy** (removal of an entire lung) is necessary.

NURSING PROCESS
The Client With Tuberculosis

Antitubercular drugs are given for long periods and without interruption because healing is slow and resistance to drugs is increased by interrupted treatment. The primary focus of nursing management is encouraging the client to adhere to the prescribed medical regimen.

Assessment

Assess the client's breath sounds, breathing patterns, and overall respiratory status. Ask the client if he or she is experiencing any pain with breathing. Inspect sputum for color, viscosity, amount, and for signs of blood. Determine if the client is experiencing other health problems such as fever, dehydration, weight loss, or weakness.

Diagnosis and Planning

The nurse's responsibilities, when caring for a client with tuberculosis include, but are not limited to, the following:

Nursing Diagnoses and Collaborative Problems	Nursing Interventions
Ineffective Airway Clearance related to pain with coughing, inability to cough, and abnormal respirations **Goals:** The client will demonstrate improved breath sounds. The client will demonstrate effective deep breathing and coughing exercises.	Encourage client to deep breathe and cough every 2 hours while awake. Position client in semi-Fowler's position to improve breathing and assist in expectorating mucus. Encourage client to drink 3 to 4 L/day to liquefy and thin secretions. Humidify inspired air. Suction secretions if client is unable to expectorate. Assist client with postural drainage as indicated.
Ineffective Breathing Pattern related to infectious process and pain on inspiration and expiration. **Goals:** The client will regain or maintain an effective breathing pattern. The client's breath sounds will be clear.	Assess respiratory rate and depth. Monitor respiratory pattern. Assess for dyspnea and use of accessory muscles. Position client in semi-Fowler's position. Administer oxygen as indicated.
Pain related to chest expansion secondary to lung infection/inflammation. **Goals:** The client states decreased pain levels and demonstrates ability to use splinting techniques that reduce pain.	Assess pain level. Evaluate effectiveness of pain relief measures. Administer analgesics as indicated. Instruct client in splinting techniques for use during coughing.

Fluid Volume Deficit related to fever, decreased fluid intake, and increased insensible fluid losses. **Goal:** The client will remain hydrated.	Provide 3 to 4 liters of fluid per day. Monitor intake and output. Administer intravenous fluids as indicated.
Altered Nutrition: Less than Body Requirements related to anorexia, fever, pain, or severity of illness **Goal:** The client will attain or maintain preillness weight.	Document client's nutritional status. Assess client's dietary habits. Monitor weight at least twice a week. Encourage small frequent meals high in proteins and carbohydrates.
Hyperthermia related to increased metabolic rate and dehydration secondary to infection **Goal:** The client will demonstrate temperatures within normal range.	Monitor client's vital signs at least every 4 hours. Administer antipyretics as indicated. Provide tepid sponge baths. Change client's bed linens if client is diaphoretic.
Activity Intolerance related to general weakness, respiratory difficulties, fever, and severity of illness. **Goal:** The client will demonstrate increased activity.	Plan and space activities. Provide adequate rest periods. Assist client with activities as required.
Risk for Altered Health Maintenance related to insufficient knowledge of treatments, drug therapies, home care management, and prevention of future infections **Goals:** The client will demonstrate ability to carry out treatment plan, preventive measures, and procedures needed after discharge. The client will identify health risks such as smoking. The client will state value in getting influenza and pneumonococcal vaccines.	Instruct client in self-care activities. Provide information about antismoking strategies and vaccines. Allow client time to return demonstrations of treatments to be done at home.

Evaluation and Expected Outcomes

- The client maintains effective airway clearance and breathing patterns.
- The client reports minimal pain.
- The client is adequately hydrated.
- The client does not experience further weight loss.
- The client demonstrates better activity tolerance and adherence to health maintenance strategies.

Client and Family Teaching

Develop a teaching plan to meet the client's individual needs and include the following guidelines as appropriate:

- Take medications exactly as prescribed. Closely observe the time interval between each dose. Do not skip a dose or take more than the amount prescribed.
- Drugs used to treat tuberculosis must be taken for a long period; complete the entire course of drug therapy to control infection.
- Stress the importance of continuous therapy because lapses in taking the prescribed drugs can result in reactivation of the infection.
- Notify the physician if symptoms worsen or sudden chest pain or dyspnea occurs.
- Drink plenty of fluids.
- Take your temperature once or twice daily or as recommended by the physician. Take the prescribed or recommended drug for reducing fever. If fever continues, contact the physician.
- Discontinue smoking immediately. Avoid exposure to secondhand smoke.
- Eat a balanced but light diet. If more than a few pounds of weight are lost, contact the physician.
- Prevent future infections by following the recommendations for prevention suggested by the physician.
- Explain the importance of routine follow-up care, periodic physical examinations and chest x-rays, and eating a well balanced diet.

Obstructive Pulmonary Disease

Obstructive lung disease describes conditions in which airflow within the lungs is impaired. There is decreased resistance to inspiration and increased resistance to expiration, so that the expiratory phase of respiration is prolonged (Bullock, 1996). **Chronic obstructive pulmonary disease** (COPD) is a broad, nonspecific term that describes a group of pulmonary disorders with symptoms of chronic cough and expectoration, dyspnea, and an impaired expiratory airflow. Bronchiectasis, atelectasis, chronic bronchitis, and emphysema are categorized as COPDs. Asthma is also an obstructive disorder that is more episodic in nature and generally more acute than chronic. **Sleep apnea syndrome** is the cessation of airflow in and out of the lungs during sleep. It can also have obstructive causes.

Bronchiectasis

Bronchiectasis is a chronic disease characterized by irreversible dilatation of the bronchi and bronchioles and chronic infection.

ETIOLOGY AND PATHOPHYSIOLOGY

Causes of bronchiectasis include bronchial obstruction by tumor or foreign body, congenital abnormalities, exposure to toxic gases, and chronic pulmonary infections. When clearance of the airway is impeded, an infection can develop in the walls of the bronchus or bronchiole. This leads to changes in the structure of the wall tissue and results in the formation of saccular dilatations, which collect purulent material. Airway clearance is further impaired, and the purulent material remains, causing more dilatation, structural damage, and more infection (Fig. 28–3).

ASSESSMENT FINDINGS

Signs and Symptoms

Clients with bronchiectasis experience a chronic cough with expectoration of copious amounts of purulent sputum and possible hemoptysis. The coughing becomes worse when the client changes position. The amount of sputum produced during one paroxysm varies with the stage of the disease, but it can be several ounces. When the sputum is collected, it settles into three distinct layers: the top layer is frothy and cloudy, the middle layer is clear saliva, and the bottom layer is heavy, thick, and purulent. Clients also experience fatigue, weight loss, anorexia, and dyspnea.

Diagnostic Findings

Chest x-ray and bronchoscopy demonstrate the increased size of the bronchioles, possible areas of atelectasis, and changes in the pulmonary tissue. Sputum culture and sensitivity identify the causative microorganism and effective antibiotics to control the infection. Pulmonary function studies may also be done.

MEDICAL MANAGEMENT

Treatment of bronchiectasis includes drainage of purulent material from the bronchi, antibiotics, bronchodilators, and mucolytics to improve breathing and help raise secretions; humidification to loosen secretions; and surgical removal if bronchiectasis is confined to a small area.

NURSING MANAGEMENT

Nursing management focuses on instructing the client in postural drainage techniques. Postural drainage helps the client mobilize and expectorate secretions. The position or positions to be assumed depend on the site or lobe to be drained. Figure 28–4

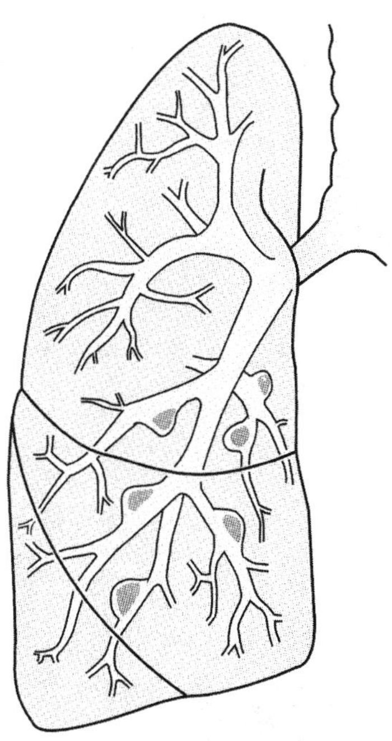

FIGURE 28-3. Bronchiectasis showing abnormal saccular dilatations of the large bronchi that are filled with inflammatory exudate.

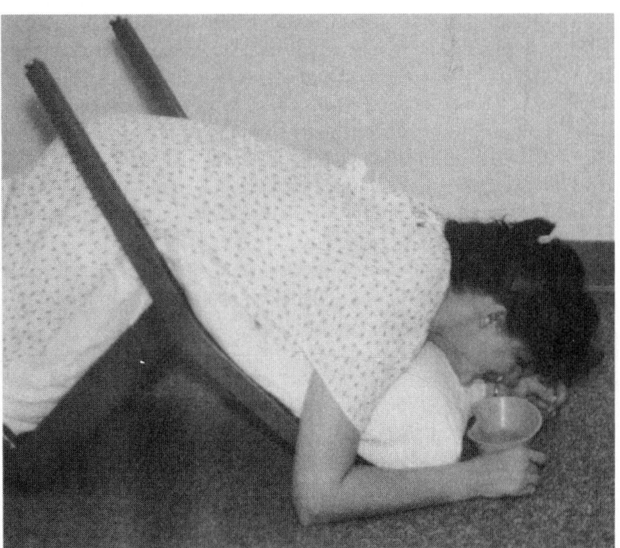

FIGURE 28-4. The exact position assumed by the client during postural drainage depends on the location of the affected areas. The treatment is performed three times a day in each position while the client inhales slowly and blows the breath out through the mouth. It usually take 5 to 15 minutes.

shows the position that will drain the upper segments of both lower lobes. The client remains in this position for 10 to 15 minutes. Chest percussion and vibration may be performed during this time. When complete, the client coughs and expectorates the secretions. This procedure may be repeated. Provide oral hygiene after treatment.

Atelectasis

Atelectasis is the collapse of lung tissue (Fig. 28–5). It may involve a small portion of the lung or an entire lobe. When alveoli collapse, they cannot perform their function of gas exchange. Atelectasis occurs secondary to aspiration of food or vomitus, a mucous plug, fluid or air in the thoracic cavity, or compression on tissue by tumors, an enlarged heart, an aneurysm, or enlarged lymph nodes in the chest. Ill clients may have atelectasis when on prolonged bed rest or from the inability to breathe deeply or cough and raise secretions.

ASSESSMENT FINDINGS

Symptoms of atelectasis are related to the amount of lung tissue involved. Small areas of atelectasis may have few symptoms. With a larger area, cyanosis, fever, pain, dyspnea, increased pulse and respiratory rates, and increased pulmonary secretions may be seen. Although crackling may be auscultated over the affected areas, usually breath sounds are absent. A chest x-ray reveals dense shadows, indicating collapsed lung tissue. Sometimes the x-ray is inconclusive. ABGs and pulse oximetry may be abnormal.

MEDICAL MANAGEMENT

Treatment includes improving ventilation, suctioning, and deep breathing and coughing to raise secretions. Bronchodilators and humidification assist in loosening and removing secretions. Oxygen is administered for dyspnea. Removal of the cause of atelectasis helps to correct the condition.

NURSING MANAGEMENT

Nursing care focuses on the prevention of atelectasis, especially when caused by failure to aerate the lungs properly. Deep breathing and coughing postoperatively can prevent atelectasis. If atelectasis occurs, the nurse encourages the client to take deep breaths and cough at frequent intervals, and instructs the client in the use of an incentive spirometer (Fig. 28–6). Refer to Nursing Guidelines 28–2 for instructing a client in the use of an incentive spirometer.

Chronic Bronchitis

Chronic bronchitis is the persistence of a chronic cough with excessive production of mucus for at least 3 months a year for 2 consecutive years. It is a serious health problem that develops gradually and may go untreated for many years until the disease is well established.

ETIOLOGY AND PATHOPHYSIOLOGY

Chronic bronchitis is characterized by hypersecretion of mucus by the bronchial glands and recurrent or chronic respiratory tract infections. As the infection progresses, there is a significant alteration in the ability of the cilia lining the airway to propel the secre-

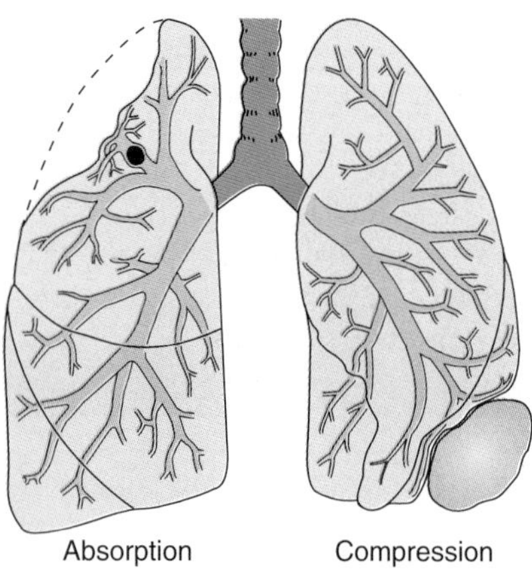

FIGURE 28-5. Atelectasis caused by airway obstruction and absorption of air from the involved lung area on the *left* and by compression of lung tissue on the *right*.

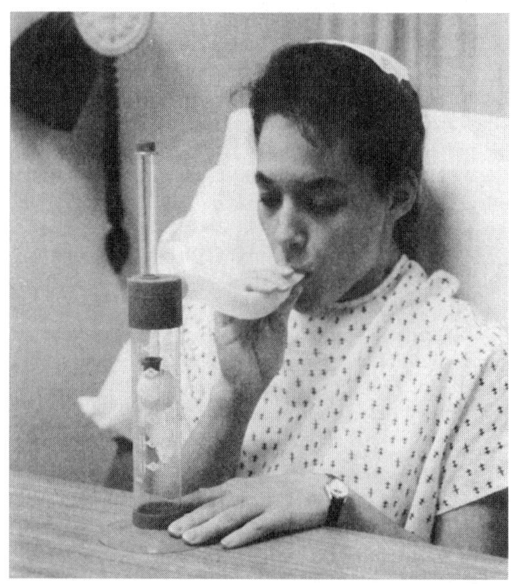

FIGURE 28-6. An incentive spirometer is used to encourage deep breathing.

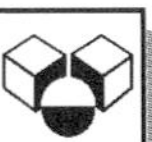

Nursing Guidelines 28-2

Instructions in the Use of an Incentive Spirometer

- Instruct client to sit upright unless contraindicated.
- Mark the goal for inhalation.
- Exhale normally.
- Place mouthpiece in mouth, sealing lips around it.
- Inhale slowly until predetermined volume has been reached.
- Hold breath for 2 to 6 seconds.
- Exhale normally.
- Repeat the exercise 10 to 20 times per hour while awake, or as ordered.
- Do not rush during the procedure. Slow down if dizziness is experienced.

(Adapted from Timby B. K. [1996]. Fundamental skills and concepts in patient care [6th ed.]. Philadelphia: Lippincott-Raven.)

tions upward. Secretions remain in the lungs and form plugs within the smaller bronchi. These plugs become areas for bacterial growth and chronic infection, which increases mucous secretion, and eventually causes areas of focal necrosis and fibrosis. Airway obstruction results from the inflammation of the bronchi.

Multiple factors are associated with chronic bronchitis. Its development may be insidious, or it may follow a long history of bronchial asthma or an acute respiratory tract infection, such as influenza or pneumonia. Air pollution and smoking are significant factors. Smoking causes hypertrophy and hypersecretion of the bronchial glands. The disease may occur at any age, but is most often seen in middle age following years of untreated, low-grade bronchitis. Diagnosis is based on evaluation of the duration of the symptoms, how it began, and the client's occupational history, history of pulmonary disease, and smoking history.

ASSESSMENT FINDINGS

Signs and Symptoms

The earliest symptom is a productive cough of thick white mucus, especially when rising in the morning and in the evening. Bronchospasm may occur during severe bouts of coughing. Acute respiratory infections are frequent during the winter months and may persist for at least several weeks. As the disease progresses, the sputum may become yellow, purulent, copious, and, after paroxysms of coughing, blood-streaked. Cyanosis secondary to hypoxemia may be noted, especially after severe coughing. Dyspnea begins with exertion, but progresses to occurring with minimal activity, and later occurs at rest. Right heart failure results from the hypoxemia, which causes edema in the extremities.

Diagnostic Findings

Diagnostic studies are performed depending on the progression and history of symptoms. Initially the physical examination, chest x-ray, and pulmonary function tests may be normal. As the disease progresses, these findings will become increasingly abnormal. The chest x-ray shows signs of fluid overload and consolidation. Later, the heart is enlarged as right-sided failure develops. Pulmonary function tests demonstrate decreased vital capacity and forced expiratory volume, and increased residual volume and total lung capacity. Diagnostic studies such as bronchoscopy, microscopic examination of the sputum for malignant cells, and lung scan may be performed to rule out cancer, bronchiectasis, tuberculosis, or other diseases in which cough is a predominant feature.

MEDICAL MANAGEMENT

The goals of treatment are to prevent recurrent irritation of the bronchial mucosa by infection or chemical agents, to maintain the function of the bronchioles, and to assist in the removal of secretions. Treatment includes:

- Smoking cessation
- Bronchodilators to dilate bronchi, and reduce airway obstruction and bronchospasm
- Increased fluid intake
- Maintenance of a well balanced diet
- Postural drainage to remove secretions from the bronchi
- Steroid therapy if other treatment is ineffective
- Change in occupation if work involves exposure to dust and chemical irritants
- Filtration of incoming air to reduce sputum production and cough
- Antibiotic therapy

NURSING MANAGEMENT

Nursing management focuses on educating clients in managing their disease. Help clients identify ways to eliminate environmental irritants. This includes smoking cessation, occupational counseling, monitoring air quality and pollution levels, and avoiding cold air and wind exposure that can cause bronchospasm. Preventing infection is another important aspect of care. Instruct clients to avoid others with respiratory tract infections and to receive pneumonia and influenza immunizations. Teach the client to monitor sputum for signs of infection. Instruct clients in the proper use of aerosolized bronchodilators and corticosteroids. Refer to Nursing Guidelines 28–3 for teaching a client how to

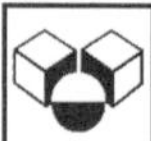

Nursing Guidelines 28-3

Teaching a Client to Use a Metered-Dose Inhaler

Teach the client to:

- Attach the stem of the canister into the hole of the mouthpiece so that the inhaler looks like an "L."
- Shake the canister to distribute the drug within its pressurized chamber.
- Exhale slowly through pursed lips.
- Seal lips around the mouthpiece.
- Compress the canister between thumb and fingers and slowly inhale at the same time.
- Release the pressure on the canister, but continue inhaling as much as possible.
- Withdraw the mouthpiece.
- Hold breath for a few seconds.
- Exhale slowly through pursed lips.
- If second dose is required, wait for a few seconds before repeating procedure.

(Adapted from Timby, B. K. [1996]. Fundamental skills and concepts in patient care [6th ed.]. Philadelphia: Lippincott-Raven.)

use a metered-dose inhaler. Warn against overuse. Instruct the client in postural drainage techniques and measures for improving overall health such as eating a well balanced diet, getting plenty of rest, and engaging in moderate aerobic activity. For clients with lung disease, the amount of aerobic activity should be determined by dyspnea, not heart rate. In other words, clients should exercise at the pace and for the length of time they can tolerate without dyspnea. Refer to nursing management of emphysema for nursing diagnoses and additional interventions.

Pulmonary Emphysema

Emphysema is a chronic disease characterized by abnormal distention of the alveoli. The alveolar walls and alveolar capillary beds also show marked destruction. This process of lung destruction occurs over a long period. By the time the diagnosis is made, the lung damage is usually permanent. Emphysema is a common cause of disability and the most common chronic pulmonary disease.

ETIOLOGY AND PATHOPHYSIOLOGY

The major cause of emphysema is smoking. Contributing factors may also be exposure to secondhand smoke, air pollution, chronic infection, and allergens. A small percentage of clients have a familial tendency for developing emphysema, and exposure to the contributing factors increases their susceptibility to developing emphysema. This predisposition may be due to connective tissue in the lungs failing to be protected from protein digestion by enzymes released from macrophages and leukocytes. The result is damage to the lung tissue.

In emphysema the alveoli of the lungs lose elasticity, trapping air that normally should be expired. On microscopic examination, the walls of the alveoli have broken down, forming one large sac instead of multiple, small air spaces (Fig. 28–7). The capillary bed previously located within the alveolar walls is destroyed and much of the tissue replaced by fibrous scarring. The formation of fibrous tissue and destruction of the alveoli prevent the proper exchange of oxygen and carbon dioxide during respiration.

As the disease progresses, large air sacs (bullae, blebs) may be seen over the lung surface. These sacs can rupture, allowing air to enter the thorax (**pneumothorax**) with each respiration. When this occurs, emergency thoracentesis is performed to remove the air from the thoracic cavity. A chest tube may be inserted to keep additional air from entering. Recurrent episodes of pneumothorax may require surgery to cor-

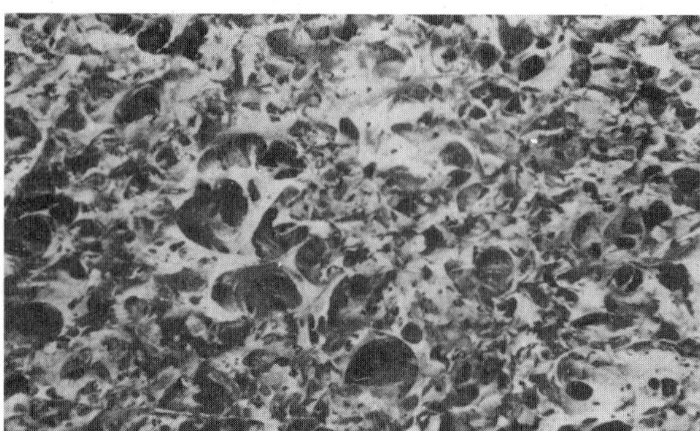

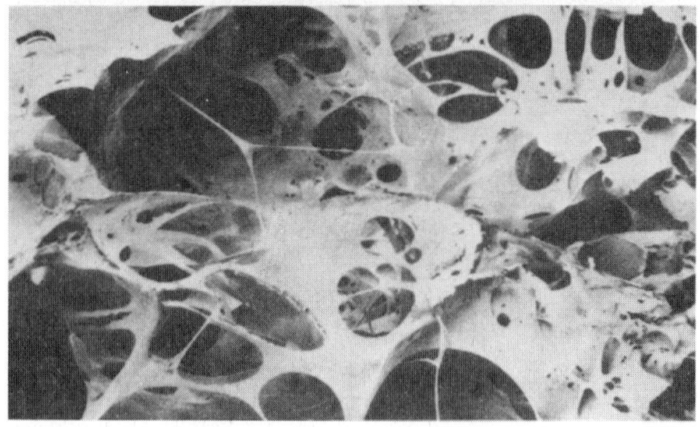

FIGURE 28-7. Scanning electron micrographs of lung tissue. *Top*, normal lung tissue. *Bottom*, emphysematous tissue. (Courtesy of Kenneth Siegesmund, PhD, The Medical College of Wisconsin, Milwaukee)

rect the problem. (See discussions of pneumothorax in the section on penetrating wounds and of chest tubes in postoperative nursing management of the client undergoing thoracic surgery for more information.)

ASSESSMENT FINDINGS

Signs and Symptoms

Shortness of breath that occurs with minimal activity is called *exertional dyspnea*. It is often the first symptom of emphysema. As the disease progresses, the breathlessness occurs even at rest. A chronic cough is invariably present and is productive of mucopurulent sputum. Inspiration is difficult because of the rigid chest cage and the chest is characteristically barrel-shaped (Fig. 28–8). The client uses the accessory muscles of respiration (muscles in the jaw and neck, and intercostal muscles) to maintain normal ventilation. Expiration is prolonged, difficult, and often accompanied by wheezing. In advanced emphysema, respiratory function is markedly impaired. Clients with advanced emphysema characteristically appear drawn, anxious, and pale and speak in short, jerky sentences. When sitting up, they often lean slightly forward and are markedly short of breath. The neck veins may distend during expiration.

In advanced emphysema, memory loss, drowsiness, confusion, and loss of judgment may occur. These symptoms are caused by the markedly reduced amount of oxygen that reaches the brain and the increased amount of carbon dioxide in the blood. If the disorder goes untreated, the carbon dioxide content in the blood may reach toxic levels, resulting in lethargy, stupor, and, eventually, coma. This condition is called *carbon dioxide narcosis*.

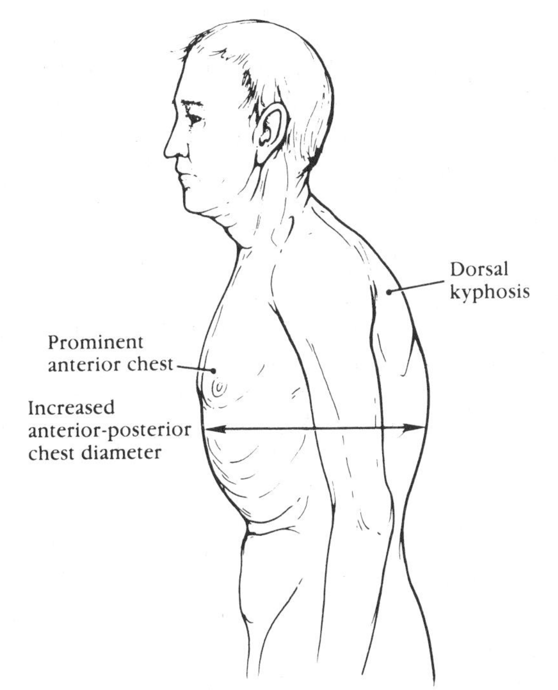

FIGURE 28-8. Barrel chest of emphysema.

Diagnostic Findings

Lung auscultation reveals decreased breath sounds, wheezing, and crackles. Heart sounds are diminished or muffled. Visual inspection shows a barrel-chested person breathing through pursed lips and using the accessory muscles of respiration. Chest x-rays and fluoroscopy demonstrate hyperinflated lung fields. Pulmonary function studies show a marked decrease in overall function, including increased total lung capacity and residual volume, and decreased vital capacity and forced expiratory volume. ABG analysis assesses gas exchange, which almost always reflects hypoxemia and a compensated state of respiratory acidosis.

MEDICAL MANAGEMENT

The goals of medical management include improving the client's quality of life, slowing the disease progression, and treating the obstructed airways. Treatment includes:

- Bronchodilators—to dilate airways by decreasing edema and spasms and improving gas exchange
- Aerosol therapy—nebulized aerosols for inhalation of bronchodilators and mucolytics; inhaled deep within the tracheobronchial tree
- Antibiotics
- Corticosteroids on a limited basis to assist with bronchodilation and removal of secretions
- Physical therapy to increase ventilation—deep breathing, coughing, chest percussion, vibration, and postural drainage

If the client is not helped by the prescribed treatment regimen, progressive loss of sleep, appetite, weight, and physical strength may occur. As the disease progresses, the client may need to curtail physical activities.

NURSING MANAGEMENT

The respiratory center of the brain is sensitive to the level of carbon dioxide in the blood. If the level increases slightly, the respiratory rate and depth increase to eliminate the excess carbon dioxide. If, however, the carbon dioxide level is chronically elevated, the respiratory center becomes insensitive to carbon dioxide changes. Under these circumstances, the level of oxygen in the blood becomes a regulatory factor—the hypoxic drive to respiration. As long as the level of oxygen saturation of the blood is low, a client breathes sufficiently to maintain oxygenation. If oxygen is given at 100% (or any other high concentration) by mask or other means, the hypoxic drive to respiration is lost and the respiratory rate drops, leading to the further retention of carbon dioxide, apnea, and death.

If the client requires oxygen, the safest method of administration is by nasal catheter or cannula, with the oxygen flow rate set at no more than 2 to 3 L/min. If the client's color improves but the level of consciousness decreases, oxygen administration is discontinued and the physician notified; the client may be approaching a state of respiratory arrest.

Therapeutic breathing exercises effectively use the diaphragm, thus relieving the compensatory burden on the muscles of the upper thorax. Clients are taught to let the abdomen rise as they take a deep breath and to contract the abdominal muscles as they exhale. They can feel the correct way to do this by placing one hand on the chest and the other on the abdomen: during abdominal breathing, the chest should remain quiet and the abdomen should rise and fall with each breath. Other exercises include blowing out candles at various distances and blowing a small object, such as a pencil or a piece of chalk, along a tabletop. Clients are encouraged to exhale more completely by taking a deep breath and then bending the body forward at the waist while exhaling as fully as possible. Pursed-lip breathing (ie, breathing with the lips pursed or puckered on expiration) helps to control the respiratory rate and depth and slows expiration. This maneuver may decrease dyspnea and in turn reduce the anxiety that often is associated with breathing difficulties.

NURSING PROCESS
The Client With Obstructive Pulmonary Disorder

Assessment

Assess the client's respiratory status, including respiratory effort, rate, and pattern. Determine if the client is dyspneic at rest and intolerant of activity. Assess the client for signs of infection. Ask the client what she or he does to relieve pulmonary symptoms.

Diagnosis and Planning

Nursing care for a client with chronic pulmonary disaster includes, but is not limited to the following:

Nursing Diagnoses and Collaborative Problems	Nursing Interventions
Ineffective Airway Clearance related to bronchoconstriction, increased mucus production, and ineffective cough **Goal:** The client will maintain a patent airway with clearer breath sounds and an effective cough.	Auscultate breath sounds. Assess respiratory status. Note any dyspnea, restlessness, respiratory distress, or use of accessory muscles. Assist client to rest in position of comfort that also maximizes breathing. Instruct client to use pursed-lip breathing, abdominal breathing, and effective coughing. Assess nature of cough and sputum. Increase fluid intake to 3,000 L/day, if not contraindicated. Administer medications as indicated. Assist in administering inhaled medications. Assist client with postural drainage as indicated. Provide humidification.
Impaired Gas Exchange related to obstructed airways, bronchospasm, or trapped air **Goal:** The client will demonstrate improved ventilation and adequate oxygenation.	Instruct client to use pursed-lip and abdominal breathing. Monitor level of consciousness and mental status. Assess activity level. Monitor ABGs and pulse oximetry. Encourage alternating rest and activity.
Risk for Infection related to increased mucous production and inability to clear secretions. **Goal:** The client will remain free of pneumonia.	Monitor temperature. Review importance of pulmonary exercises including deep breathing, coughing, and changing positions. Instruct client to maintain high fluid intake unless contraindicated. Teach client methods to prevent the spread of infection. Administer antibiotics as indicated.
Activity Intolerance related to fatigue, hypoxemia, and ineffective airway clearance **Goal:** The client demonstrates increased activity tolerance.	Plan rest periods before and after activities. Allow client to perform activities at own rate. Collaborate with occupational and physical therapy to plan and implement an exercise program that promotes endurance.

Evaluation and Expected Outcome

- The client has improved breath sounds.
- Cough is productive and clears mucus.
- ABGs are improved.
- Client practices pulmonary exercises effectively.

- Infections are prevented.
- Client has increased tolerance for activity.

Client and Family Teaching

Education is an important part of therapy aimed at helping clients adjust to their current level of disability and to the potential for increased disability in the future. The primary goal is to prevent or delay progression of the disorder. Explain strategies to slow the disease progression. Emphasize that success depends on strict adherence to the treatment regimen. Motivated clients profit more from available treatments and make the best use of their remaining pulmonary function.

Develop a teaching plan that meets individual needs, and adheres to the following guidelines:

- Take medication exactly as prescribed. Observe the time intervals between medications. Do not skip doses or take more than what is prescribed.
- Maintain close medical supervision.
- Contact the physician if any of the following occur:
  - Adverse drug effects
  - Failure of drugs to relieve symptoms
  - Appearance of new symptoms
  - Increased severity of symptoms
  - Signs or symptoms of respiratory infection
- Drink extra fluids as indicated, unless fluids are restricted.
- Avoid respiratory irritants and people with respiratory infections.
- Eat a well balanced diet.
- Perform breathing exercises as prescribed.
- Take frequent rests during the day. Space activities to prevent fatigue and shortness of breath.
- Avoid dry-heated areas that can aggravate symptoms. Humidify inspired air during the winter months.

Asthma

Asthma is a reversible obstructive disease of the lower airway. Inflammation of the airway and a hyperresponsiveness of the airway to stimuli characterize asthma. The incidence of asthma is increasing, particularly in children and adolescents. Asthma affects almost one-fifth of the population at one time in their lives. Asthma may be fatal, but for most people it accounts for disruptions in school and work attendance and affects choices in careers and activities.

ETIOLOGY AND PATHOPHYSIOLOGY

There are three types of asthma: *allergic asthma* (extrinsic), which occurs in response to allergens, such as pollen, dust, spores, and animal danders; *idiopathic asthma* (intrinsic) associated with factors such as upper respiratory infections, emotional upsets, and exercise; and *mixed asthma*, which has characteristics of allergic and idiopathic asthma. Mixed asthma is the most common form.

Acute asthma occurs as a result of increasing airway obstruction caused by bronchospasm and bronchoconstriction, inflammation and edema of the lining of the bronchi and bronchioles, and production of thick mucus that can plug the airway (Fig. 28–9). Allergic asthma causes the IgE inflammatory response. These antibodies attach to mast cells within the lungs. Reexposure to the antigen causes the antigen to attach to the antibody, releasing mast cell products such as histamine. The manifestations of asthma become evident as this occurs. Other types of asthma are hyperresponsive to the inflammatory changes.

Because the alveoli are unable to expel air, they hyperinflate and trap air within the lungs. The client breathes faster, blowing off excess carbon dioxide. Although the client tries to force the air out, the narrowed airway makes it difficult. Wheezing is usually audible with expiration, resulting from air being forced out of the narrowed airway and from the vibrating mucus.

Other pathophysiologic changes include:

- Interference with gas exchange
- Poor perfusion
- Possible atelectasis
- Respiratory failure if inadequately treated

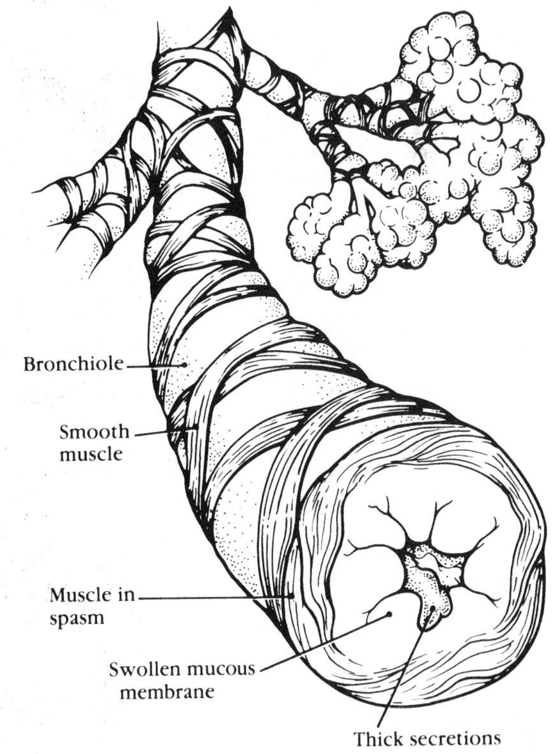

FIGURE 28-9. Bronchial asthma. The bronchiole is obstructed on expiration, particularly by muscle spasms, edema of the mucosa, and thick secretions.

Table 28–5 provides an overview of the pathophysiology of asthma.

Asthma may develop at any age. A significant relationship has been noted between the occurrence of bronchiolitis (inflammation of the bronchioles) in the first year of life and the development of asthma in early childhood. Asthma may be limited to occasional attacks with the client symptom-free between attacks.

ASSESSMENT FINDINGS

Signs and Symptoms

Asthma is typified by paroxysms of shortness of breath, wheezing, and coughing, and the production of thick, tenacious sputum. Duration of the acute episode varies; it may be brief—less than 1 day, or extended, lasting for several weeks.

Most clients are aware of the wheezing and report it as one of their symptoms. Every breath becomes an effort. During an acute episode, the work of breathing is greatly increased, and the client may suffer from a sensation of suffocation. A classic sitting position commonly is assumed, with the body leaning slightly forward and the arms at shoulder height. This position facilitates expansion of the chest and more effective excursions of the diaphragm. Because life depends on the power to breathe, fear accompanies and intensifies the symptoms.

The effort to move trapped air is accompanied by marked prolongation of the expiratory phase of respiration. Coughing commences with the onset of the attack but is ineffective in the early stage. Only as the attack begins to subside is the client able to expectorate large quantities of thick, stringy mucus. The skin usually is pale; if the attack is severe, however, cyanosis of the lips and nail beds may be noted. Perspiration typically is profuse during an acute attack. After spontaneous or drug-induced remission of the episode, examination of the lungs commonly reveals normal findings. Sometimes an acute attack intensifies and progresses to *status asthmaticus* (persistent state of asthma), which can be life-threatening.

TABLE 28-5 **Pathophysiology of Asthma**

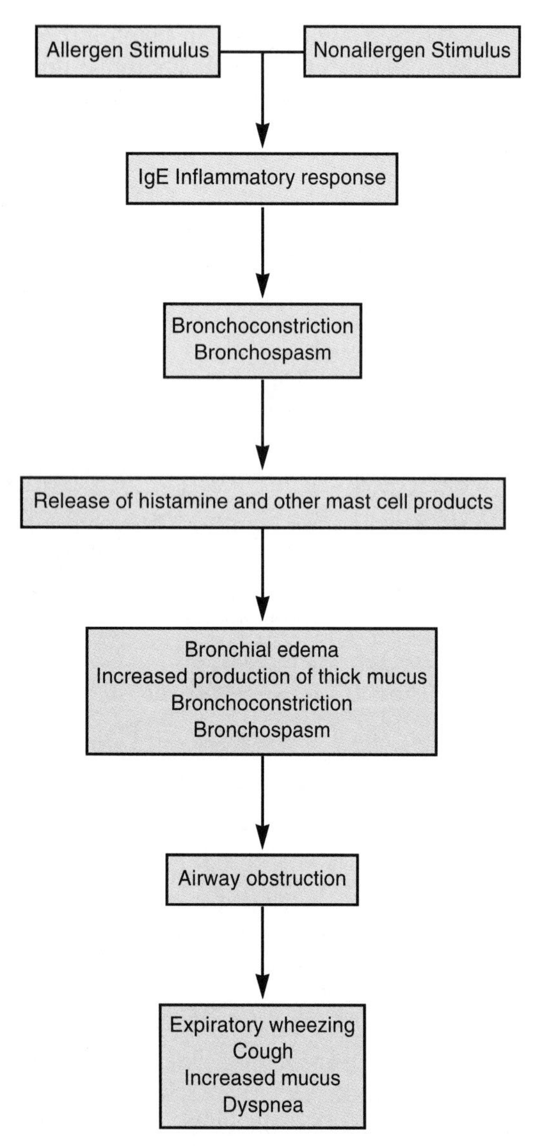

Diagnostic Findings

Auscultation of the chest reveals expiratory and sometimes inspiratory wheezes and diminished breath sounds. Pulmonary function studies, especially the forced expiratory volume, may be abnormal, with the total lung capacity and functional residual volume increased secondary to trapped air. The forced expiratory volume and forced vital capacity are decreased. During acute attacks, blood gases show hypoxemia. The $PaCO_2$ may be elevated if the asthma becomes worse, but generally the $PaCO_2$ is decreased because of the rapid respiratory rate. A normal $PaCO_2$ in the later part of an asthma attack may indicate impending respiratory failure.

MEDICAL MANAGEMENT

Symptomatic treatment is given at the time of the attack. Long-term care involves measures to treat as well as prevent further attacks. An effort must be made to determine the cause of the attacks. If the history and diagnostic tests indicate that allergy is a causative factor, treatment includes avoidance of the allergen, desensitization, or antihistamine therapy. Oxygen usually is not necessary during an acute attack because most clients are actively hyperventilating. Oxygen may be necessary if cyanosis occurs.

Pharmacologic management is classified as rescue therapy and maintenance therapy (Eisenbeis, 1996). Rescue therapy medications treat acute episodes of asthma, whereas maintenance therapy is a daily regimen designed to prevent and control symptoms. Many medications are taken through inhalers (Fig. 28–10). Table 28–6 lists medications used in maintenance therapy.

Humidification of the inspired air is valuable because dehydration of the respiratory mucous membrane may lead to asthmatic attacks. The use of steam or cool vapor humidifiers also has proved effective. Liquefaction of the secretions promotes more effective clearing of the airways and a rapid return to normal. Air conditioners may filter out offending allergens as well as control temperature and humidity.

NURSING MANAGEMENT

Clients are extremely anxious. Reassure the client that someone will remain with him or her during the acute phase of an attack. Administer oxygen as indicated. Put the client in a sitting position. Rest and adequate fluid intake are important. Keep fluids within easy reach, and encourage the client to drink them. Increased fluid intake makes secretions less tenacious and replaces the fluids lost through perspiration. Check the intravenous (IV) site frequently for signs of extravasation. This is especially important during an acute attack because restlessness can result in needle dislodgment. Observe for adverse drug effects, especially when the client is receiving epinephrine or other adrenergic agents such as aminophylline, which may cause palpitations, nervousness, trembling, pallor, and insomnia.

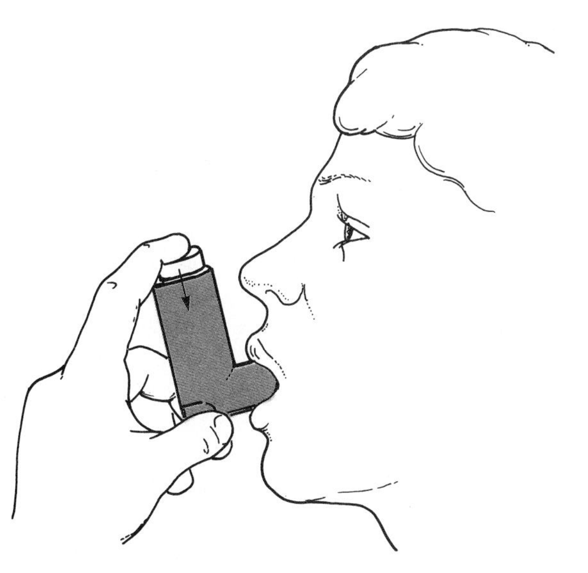

FIGURE 28-10. A respiratory inhalant may be used to deliver a medication directly into the lungs. The client takes a slow, deep breath as the top of the cannister is pressed downward. Each depression of the cannister delivers a metered dose of the drug.

Client and Family Teaching

After the acute asthma attack has subsided, assess the client's level of understanding about the disease process. Ask if the client has a peak flowmeter; if not, obtain one and tell the client to use it to monitor airway obstruction. Explain how to use it:

- Sit upright in bed or chair and inhale as deeply as possible.
- Form a tight seal around mouthpiece with lips.
- Exhale forcefully and quickly.
- Note the reading.

The client can use the peak flowmeter to assess effectiveness of medication or breathing status. Tell the client to seek care if readings fall below baseline. Teach clients correct use of inhalers. Help clients identify triggering events such as dust, smoking, emotional upset, or exposure to irritants such as cleaning fluids or bug sprays. Teach the client relaxation techniques and the therapeutic breathing techniques to ease breathing, as discussed in nursing management of emphysema.

Sleep Apnea Syndrome

Sleep apnea syndrome is characterized by frequent, brief episodes of respiratory standstill during sleep. It is classified according to the presence or absence of respiratory muscle effort:

- Central—air movement absent secondary to cessation of ventilatory efforts
- Obstructive—air movement absent secondary to pharyngeal obstruction; chest and abdominal movement present
- Mixed—combination of central and obstructive sleep apnea within one apneic episode

Sleep apnea is most common in older obese men. They snore loudly during sleep with cessation of breathing for as long as 10 seconds. They awaken suddenly as the PaO_2 level drops, usually with a loud snort. These episodes are frequent, from 10 an hour to several hundred per night (Smeltzer & Bare, 1996). Other symptoms include daytime fatigue, morning headache, sore throat, enuresis, and impotence. Partners may report that the client is different in terms of personality and behavior and that the snoring is pro-

TABLE 28-6 **Maintenance Drug Therapy for Asthma**

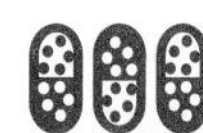

Drug Category/Drug Action	Side Effects	Nursing Considerations
Beta-Agonists		
albuterol (Ventolin) Dilates the smooth muscles of the bronchioles, reduces muscle spasm and therefore increases the size of the airway	Restlessness, apprehension, anxiety, fear, central nervous system stimulation, nausea, arrhythmias, sweating, flushing, paradoxical airway resistance with repeated excessive use	Ensure that client understands technique for administering inhalers. Tell client to not exceed recommended dose, to report chest pain, dizziness, irregular heart rate, difficulty breathing, productive cough, or failure to achieve relief.
Anticholinergics		
ipratropium bromide (Atrovent) Decreases vagal tone to airways resulting in bronchodilation	Nervousness, dizziness, headache, nausea, cough, palpitations, exacerbation of glaucoma and urinary retention	Demonstrate proper use of inhaler. Tell client to report eye pain or visual changes, rash, difficulty voiding.
Corticosteroids		
triamcinolone (Azmacort) Decreases inflammatory response	Inhalants: oral, laryngeal, and pharyngeal irritation and fungal infections*	Tell client not to use during an acute asthma attack and not to use more often than prescribed. If using an aerosolized bronchodilator, administer the bronchodilator first. Tell client to not discontinue medication abruptly.
Mast Cell Inhibitors		
Inhaled cromolyn (Intal) Prevents the release of mast cell products, promoting bronchodilation and decreasing inflammation; ineffective in acute attacks, but very therapeutic if taken regularly.	Dizziness, nausea, throat irritation	Do not use during an acute attack. Follow manufacturer's instructions for administration. Do not discontinue abruptly.

*Corticosteroids administered by other routes and in higher dosages are associated with multiple adverse effects.

gressively worse. The repeated apneic spells have serious effects on the cardiopulmonary system.

Diagnosis is made according to reported symptoms and sleep studies. If the cause is obstructive, surgical procedures are done to relieve the obstruction. If surgery is not an option, clients are advised to lose weight and to avoid alcohol and drugs that depress respirations. Additional treatment includes continuous positive airway pressure (CPAP) with supplemental oxygen at night via a nasal cannula or face mask. Client compliance is often an issue with CPAP. Tracheostomy is a successful treatment; however, this option may be rejected by the client or may be technically difficult if the client is markedly obese. If a tracheostomy is performed, it is plugged during the day.

Occupational Lung Diseases

Exposure to organic and inorganic dusts and noxious gases over a long period can cause chronic lung disorders. **Pneumoconiosis** refers to a fibrous inflammation or chronic induration of the lungs after prolonged exposure to dust or gases. It specifically refers to diseases caused by the inhalation of silica (**silicosis**), coal dust (black lung disease, miners' disease), or asbestos (**asbestosis**). Workers who inhale fiber particles (such as cotton) are also susceptible. Although these conditions are not malignant, they may increase the client's risk for developing malignancies. Table 28–7 describes these specific conditions in more detail.

Dyspnea and cough are the most common symptoms. Those exposed to coal dust may expectorate black-streaked sputum. The diagnosis is based on the history of exposure to dust in the workplace. A chest x-ray may reveal fibrotic changes in the lungs. The results of pulmonary function studies usually are abnormal.

Treatment typically is conservative because the disease is widespread rather than localized. Surgery seldom is of value. Infections, when they occur, are treated with antibiotics. Other treatment modalities include oxygen therapy if severe dyspnea is present, improved nutrition, and adequate rest. Many people with advanced disease are permanently disabled.

The primary focus is on prevention, with frequent examination of those who work in areas where dust is present in high concentration. Laws require that work areas are safe in terms of dust control, ventilation pro-

TABLE 28-7 **Occupational Lung Diseases**

Occupational Lung Disease	Etiology and Pathophysiology	Signs and Symptoms
Silicosis	Inhalation of silica dust. Seen with workers involved with mining, quarrying, stonecutting, and tunnel building. Silica particles inhaled into the lungs cause nodular lesions that enlarge and form dense masses over time. Results in loss of lung volume, restrictive and obstructive lung disease.	Shortness of breath Hypoxemia Obstruction of airflow Right-sided heart failure Edema
Asbestosis	Inhalation of asbestos dust. Laws restrict asbestos use, but old materials still contain asbestos. Asbestos fibers enter the alveoli and cause fibrous tissue to form around them. Pleura also have fibrous changes and plaque formation. Results in restrictive lung disease, decreased lung volume, and decreased gas exchange.	Dyspnea Chest pain Hypoxemia Anorexia and weight loss Respiratory failure
Coal worker's pneumoconiosis	Referred to as "black lung disease." Inhalation of coal dust and other dusts. Initially, lungs clear particles by phagocytosis and transport out of the lungs. When dust inhalation becomes too great, macrophages collect in the bronchioles, leading to clogging of the airways with dusts, macrophages, and fibroblasts. Coal macules eventually form, seen as black dots on x-ray. This results in local emphysema and eventually massive blackened lung lesions.	Chronic cough—sputum production Dyspnea Large amounts of sputum containing black fluid (melanoptysis) Respiratory failure

tective masks, hoods, industrial respirators, and other protection. Workers are encouraged to practice healthy behaviors, such as quitting smoking.

Nursing management of clients with occupational lung disease is basically the same as for clients with emphysema. Many clients require a great deal of emotional support because these diseases may result in permanent disability at a relatively young age.

Pulmonary Circulatory Disorders

Pulmonary Hypertension

ETIOLOGY AND PATHOPHYSIOLOGY

Pulmonary hypertension results from heart disease, lung disease, or both. Resistance to blood flow within the pulmonary circulation causes pulmonary hypertension. The pressure in the pulmonary arteries increases, which in turn increases the workload of the right ventricle. Normal pulmonary arterial pressure is approximately 25/10 mm Hg. In pulmonary hypertension the pressure rises above 40/15 mm Hg and can be higher as the disease progresses. Primary pulmonary hypertension is a rare condition that exists without evidence of other disease. Although there is not an apparent cause, there appears to be a familial tendency. Secondary pulmonary hypertension occurs with other heart and lung conditions, most commonly with COPD.

Complex mechanisms cause pulmonary hypertension. In primary pulmonary hypertension, the inner lining of the pulmonary arteries thickens and hypertrophies, followed by an increase in the pressure in the pulmonary arteries and vascular bed. In secondary pulmonary hypertension, alveolar destruction results in increased resistance and pressure in the pulmonary vascular bed. In both types of pulmonary hypertension, the increased resistance and pressure in the pulmonary vascular bed results in pulmonary artery hypertension. Consequently, strain is placed on the right ventricle, resulting in enlargement and possible failure.

ASSESSMENT FINDINGS

Signs and symptoms

The most common symptoms are dyspnea on exertion and weakness. In clients with secondary pulmonary hypertension, additional symptoms are those of the underlying cardiac or respiratory disease: chest pain, fatigue, weakness, distended neck veins, **orthopnea** (difficulty breathing while lying flat), and peripheral edema.

Diagnostic Findings

An electrocardiogram (ECG) may show right ventricular hypertrophy or failure. ABG analysis results are abnormal. Cardiac catheterization demonstrates elevated pulmonary arterial pressures. The results of pulmonary function studies show an increased residual volume but a decreased forced expiratory volume. Echocardiography may show various abnormalities, such as right ventricular dysfunction and tricuspid valve insufficiency.

MEDICAL MANAGEMENT

Treatment of primary pulmonary hypertension includes the administration of vasodilators and anticoagulants. The primary form of this disorder has a poor prognosis. Therefore, some clients may be considered candidates for heart–lung transplantation. Treatment of secondary pulmonary hypertension includes management of the underlying cardiac or respiratory disease. Oxygen therapy commonly is used to increase pulmonary arterial oxygenation. If right-sided failure is present, other treatments include medications such as digitalis to improve cardiac function, rest, and diuretics.

NURSING MANAGEMENT

Nursing management focuses on recognizing signs and symptoms of respiratory distress. The nurse can reduce the body's need for oxygen by preventing fatigue, assisting with activities of daily living, and administering oxygen, when needed.

Pulmonary Embolism

Pulmonary embolism involves the obstruction of one or more pulmonary vessels. The blockage is the result of a thrombus that forms in the venous system or right side of the heart.

PATHOPHYSIOLOGY AND ETIOLOGY

An embolus is any foreign substance, such as a blood clot, air, or particle of fat that travels in the venous blood flow to the lungs. The clot travels to and occludes one of the pulmonary vessels, causing infarction (necrosis or death) of lung tissue distal to the clot. The infarcted area is later replaced by scar tissue.

The usual source of pulmonary emboli is clots from the deep veins of the lower extremities or pelvis. Emboli also may arise from the endocardium of the right ventricle when that side of the heart is the site of a myocardial infarction or endocarditis. A fat embolus usually occurs following a fracture of a long bone, especially the femur. Other conditions that cause pulmonary emboli include recent surgery, prolonged bed rest, trauma, the postpartum state, and debilitating diseases. Three conditions, referred to as Virchow's triad, predispose a person to clot formation: venostasis, disruption of the vessel lining, and hypercoagulability (Bullock, 1996).

ASSESSMENT FINDINGS

Signs and Symptoms

When a small area of the lung is involved, signs and symptoms usually are less severe and include pain, tachycardia, and dyspnea. Fever, cough, and blood-streaked sputum may also occur. Larger areas of involvement produce more pronounced signs and symptoms, such as severe dyspnea, severe pain, cyanosis, tachycardia, restlessness, and shock. Sudden death may follow a massive pulmonary infarction when a large embolism occludes a main section of the pulmonary artery.

Diagnostic Findings

Serum enzymes typically are markedly elevated. A chest x-ray may show an area of atelectasis. An ECG rules out a cardiac disorder such as myocardial infarction, which produces some of the same symptoms. In addition, a lung scan, CT scan, or pulmonary angiography may be performed to detect the involved lung tissue.

MEDICAL AND SURGICAL MANAGEMENT

Treatment of a pulmonary embolism depends on the size of the area involved and a client's symptoms. IV heparin may be administered to prevent extension of the thrombus and the development of additional thrombi in veins from which the embolus arose. IV injection of a *thrombolytic* drug (one that dissolves a thrombus) may also be used. Anticoagulants commonly are given after thrombolytic therapy. Other measures, such as complete bed rest, oxygen, and analgesics, are used to treat symptoms.

Pulmonary embolectomy, using cardiopulmonary bypass to support circulation while the embolus is removed, may be necessary if the embolus is lodged in a main pulmonary artery. The insertion of an umbrella filter device in the vena cava prevents recurrent episodes of pulmonary embolus. The umbrella filter is inserted by an applicator catheter inserted into the right internal jugular vein and threaded downward to an area below the renal arteries. Another surgical treatment is the insertion of Teflon clips on the inferior vena cava. These clips narrow the channel of the vena cava, allowing blood to pass through on its return to the right side of the heart but keeping back large clots.

NURSING MANAGEMENT

Pulmonary embolism almost always occurs suddenly, and early recognition of this problem is important. Start an IV infusion as soon as possible to establish a patent vein before shock becomes profound. Administer vasopressors such as dopamine or dobutamine as ordered to treat hypotension. Provide oxygen for dyspnea and analgesics for pain and apprehension. Monitor vital signs closely and observe the client at frequent intervals for changes. Institute continuous ECG monitoring because right ventricular failure is a common problem. Monitor fluid intake and output, electrolyte determinations, and ABGs. Assess the client for cyanosis, cough with or without hemoptysis, diaphoresis, and respiratory difficulty. Monitor blood coagulation studies (ie, partial thromboplastin time, prothrombin time, and international normalized ratio) when anticoagulant or thrombolytic therapy is instituted.

Assess the client for evidence of bleeding and relief of the symptoms associated with pulmonary embolism. Because clients with pulmonary emboli will be discharged on oral anticoagulants, instruct them to check for signs of occult bleeding, take medication exactly as prescribed, report missed or extra doses, and keep all appointments for follow-up blood work and office visits.

Pulmonary Edema

Pulmonary edema is an accumulation of fluid in the interstitium and alveoli of the lungs. Pulmonary congestion results when the right side of the heart delivers more blood to the pulmonary circulation than the left side of the heart can handle. The fluid escapes the capillary walls and fills the airways. A client with pulmonary edema experiences dyspnea, breathlessness, and a feeling of suffocation. In addition, the client exhibits cool, moist, and cyanotic extremities. The overall skin color is cyanotic and gray. The client has an incessant productive cough of blood-tinged, frothy fluid. This condition requires emergency treatment. (See Chap. 35 for a discussion of cardiogenic pulmonary edema.)

Adult Respiratory Distress Syndrome

Adult respiratory distress syndrome (ARDS) is a complication that occurs following other clinical conditions. It is not a primary disease. When it occurs, it can lead to respiratory failure and death. It is referred to as noncardiogenic pulmonary edema (pulmonary edema not caused by a cardiac disorder). ARDS is characterized by severe hypoxemia and progressive loss of lung compliance.

ETIOLOGY AND PATHOPHYSIOLOGY

The body responds to injury by reducing blood flow to the lungs. This results in platelet clumping. The platelets release substances such as histamine, bradykinin, and serotonin, which causes localized inflammation of the alveolar membranes, leading to increased permeability of the capillaries surrounding the alveoli. Fluid then enters the alveoli, and pulmonary edema occurs. This decreases gas exchange and metabolic acidosis occurs.

ARDS also causes decreased surfactant production, which contributes to alveolar collapse. The lungs become stiff or noncompliant. Decreased functional residual capacity, severe hypoxia, and hypocapnia result.

Causes of ARDS include chest trauma, shock, drug overdose, drowning, gram negative infections, emboli, and major surgery. Hematologic disorders, pancreatitis, and uremia may also be factors in the development of ARDS. The mortality rate with ARDS is high, particularly if the underlying cause cannot be treated or is inadequately treated.

ASSESSMENT FINDINGS

Signs and Symptoms

Severe respiratory distress develops within 8 to 48 hours after the onset of illness or injury. In the early stages there are few definitive symptoms. As the condition progresses, the following signs are seen:

- Increased respiratory rate
- Shallow, labored respirations
- Cyanosis
- Use of accessory muscles
- Respiratory distress unrelieved with oxygen administration
- Anxiety, restlessness
- Mental confusion, agitation, and drowsiness with cerebral anoxia

Diagnostic Findings

Diagnosis is made according to the following criteria: evidence of acute respiratory failure; bilateral infiltrates on chest x-ray; and hypoxemia evidenced by

PaO_2 less than 50 mm Hg with supplemental oxygen of 50% to 60% (Smeltzer & Bare, 1996). Pulmonary angiography may also be done.

MEDICAL MANAGEMENT

The initial cause of ARDS must be diagnosed and treated. The client receives humidified oxygen. Insertion of an endotracheal tube ensures maintenance of a patent airway. Mechanical ventilation is necessary, using positive end-expiratory pressure (PEEP) to keep the alveoli inflated during expiration and facilitate gas exchange. PEEP may also be used without mechanical ventilation—referred to as continuous positive airway pressure (CPAP), using a tight-fitting oxygen mask. Complications associated with the use of PEEP include pneumothorax and *pneumomediastinum* (air in the mediastinal space).

Hypotension results in systemic hypovolemia. Although the client experiences pulmonary edema, the rest of the circulatory volume is decreased. As the client's fluid status is monitored with a pulmonary artery pressure monitor, IV fluids are carefully administered. Colloids such as albumin may be used to help pull fluids in from the interstitium to the capillaries. Nutritional support is provided with total parenteral nutrition or enteral feedings.

NURSING MANAGEMENT

Nursing management focuses on the promotion of oxygenation and ventilation and prevention of complications. Assessing and monitoring a client's respiratory status are essential. Potential complications include deteriorating respiratory status, infection, renal failure, and cardiac complications. The client is also anxious and requires explanations and support. Additionally, if the client is on a ventilator, verbal communication is impaired. The nurse provides alternative methods for the client to communicate.

Respiratory Failure

Respiratory failure describes the inability to exchange sufficient amounts of oxygen and carbon dioxide for the body's needs. Even when the body is at rest, basic respiratory needs cannot be met. The ABG values that define respiratory failure include a PaO_2 less than 50 mm Hg, a $PaCO_2$ greater than 50 mm Hg, and a pH less than 7.25.

Respiratory failure is classified as acute or chronic. Acute respiratory failure occurs suddenly in a client who previously had normal lung function. In chronic respiratory failure, the loss of lung function is progressive, usually irreversible, and associated with chronic lung disease or other disease. Table 28–8 describes precipitating factors that can result in respiratory failure.

ETIOLOGY AND PATHOPHYSIOLOGY

Acute respiratory failure is a life-threatening condition in which alveolar ventilation cannot maintain the body's need for oxygen supply and carbon dioxide removal. This condition results in a fall in arterial oxygen (hypoxemia) and a rise in arterial carbon dioxide (hypercapnia), which is detected by ABG analysis. Ventilatory failure develops when the alveoli cannot adequately be expanded, when neurologic control of respirations is impaired, or when traumatic injury to the chest wall occurs. Some causes of acute respiratory failure include oversedation, administration of a general anesthetic, head injury, chest trauma, thoracic surgery, upper abdominal surgery, **hemothorax** (blood in the thorax, blood in the pleural space) pneumothorax, and pneumonia. Neurologic diseases such as myasthenia gravis, multiple sclerosis, and amyotrophic lateral sclerosis also may result in acute respiratory failure.

Chronic respiratory failure develops in response to chronic lung disease and other chronic disease. The

TABLE 28-8 **Factors That Precipitate Respiratory Failure**

Precipitating Factor	Example
Pulmonary infection—especially with COPD	Bacterial, viral, or fungal pneumonia
Trauma	Motor vehicle accident Gunshot/knife wound Burns
Infection	Sepsis Wound infection
Cardiovascular event	Myocardial infarction Aortic aneurysm Pulmonary embolism
Allergic reaction	Transfusion reaction Drug allergy Bee sting or other venom
Pulmonary aspiration	Vomitus Near drowning
Surgical procedure	Abdominal or thoracic surgery
Drug reaction	Overdose of barbiturates or narcotics Reaction to anesthesia
Mechanical factor	Pneumothorax Pleural effusion Abdominal distention
Iatrogenic factor	Endotracheal intubation Failure to clear tracheobronchial secretions
Neuromuscular disorders	Guillain-Barré syndrome Multiple sclerosis Muscular dystrophy

underlying disease accounts for the pathology that is seen when the respiratory system fails.

ASSESSMENT FINDINGS

Signs and Symptoms

Apprehension, dyspnea, wheezing, cyanosis, and use of the accessory muscles of respiration are seen in clients with respiratory failure. If the disorder remains untreated, or if treatment fails to relieve respiratory distress, cardiac arrhythmias, hypotension, congestive heart failure, respiratory acidosis, and cardiac arrest occur.

Diagnostic Findings

Diagnosis of respiratory failure is based on symptoms, client history (eg, surgery, known neurologic disorder) and ABG results. Additional tests include chest x-ray and serum electrolyte determinations.

MEDICAL MANAGEMENT

Treatment of respiratory failure focuses on maintaining a patent airway (if upper respiratory airway obstruction is present) by inserting an artificial airway, such as an endotracheal or a tracheostomy tube. Additional treatments include administration of humidified oxygen by nasal cannula, Venturi mask (Fig 28–11), or reservoir mask. Respiratory failure is managed with mechanical ventilation using intermittent positive pressure ventilation. When possible, the underlying cause of respiratory failure is treated.

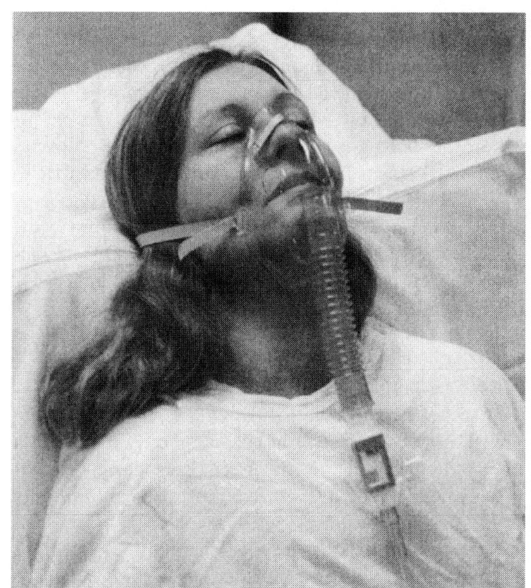

FIGURE 28-11. Venturi mask.

NURSING MANAGEMENT

Because symptoms often occur suddenly, recognition is important. Notify the physician immediately and obtain emergency resuscitative equipment. Respirations and vital signs are quickly assessed and monitored at frequent intervals. Pay particular attention to respiratory rate and depth, the presence or absence of cyanosis, other signs and symptoms of respiratory distress, and the client's response to treatment.

Malignant Disorders

Tumors and growths affecting the respiratory system are usually malignant. The malignancies may be primary in that they arise from the lungs or mediastinum, or they can be secondary metastatic growths from other sites. Treatment of these cancers does not generally stop the progression of the disease. Disability, debilitation, and death are common outcomes from respiratory malignancies.

Lung Cancer

Lung cancer is a very common cancer particularly among cigarette smokers and those exposed to secondhand smoke. The incidence of lung cancer has markedly increased, related to:

- More accurate methods for diagnosis
- The growing population of aging people
- Continued popularity of cigarette smoking
- Increased air pollution
- Increased exposure to industrial pollutants

ETIOLOGY AND PATHOPHYSIOLOGY

There are four major cell types of lung cancer: the large cell or undifferentiated type, the small cell or oat cell type, the epidermoid or squamous cell type, and adenocarcinoma. Many tumors begin in the bronchus and spread to lung tissue, regional lymph nodes, and other sites, such as the brain and bone. Many tumors have more than one type of cancer cells. Table 28–9 differentiates the major cell types of lung cancer.

The exact mechanism for development of lung cancers is unknown; however, the link between respiratory irritants and lung cancer has been established. Prolonged exposure to carcinogens more than likely will produce cancerous cells. Smokers who are able to quit reduce their risk of lung cancer to that of nonsmokers within 10 to 15 years. Lung cancer is more common in men than women. However, the rate of women dying from lung cancer has increased, and in-

TABLE 28-9 **Differentiation of Lung Cancers**

Cell Type	Pathology	Metastasis
Large cell (undifferentiated)	Arise in peripheral bronchi. Do not have well defined growth patterns. First diagnosed as bulky tumor mass.	Metastasize early, usually to the central nervous system.
Small cell (oat cell)	Most malignant form of lung cancer. Arises from bronchi. Hypersecrete antidiuretic hormone by the tumor cells—leads to hyponatremia.	Metastasizes early through the blood stream and lymphatics. Metastasis usually occurs to the mediastinum, liver, bone, bone marrow, central nervous system, adrenal glands, pancreas, and other endocrine organs.
Epidermoid cell (squamous cell)	Arise from bronchi and bronchioles. Slow-growing tumors. Growth spreads into bronchial lumen, causing obstruction.	Epidermoid cells that are well differentiated typically metastasize within the thorax, whereas poorly differentiated epidermoid cells metastasize to the small bowel.
Adenocarcinoma	Most common type of lung cancer. Arises within the peripheral lung tissue. Patchy growth throughout lung fields. Often invade the pleura, leading to malignant pleural effusion.	Early metastasis to the brain, other lung, bone, liver, and adrenal glands.

deed is greater that the rate for women dying from breast cancer. Most clients are older than 40 when the lung cancer is diagnosed.

ASSESSMENT FINDINGS

Signs and Symptoms

The cell type of the lung cancer, the size and location of the tumor, and the degree and location of metastasis determine the presenting signs and symptoms. A cough productive of mucopurulent or blood-streaked sputum is a cardinal sign of lung cancer. The cough may be slight at first and attributed to smoking or other causes. As the disease advances, the client may report fatigue, anorexia, and weight loss. Dyspnea and chest pain occur late in the disease. Hemoptysis is not uncommon. If pleural effusion occurs from tumor spread to the outside portion of the lungs, the client experiences dyspnea and chest pain. Other indications of tumor spread are symptoms related to pressure on nerves and blood vessels. Symptoms include head and neck edema, pericardial effusion, hoarseness, and vocal cord paralysis.

Diagnostic Findings

Early diagnosis of cancer of the lung is difficult because symptoms often do not appear until the disease is well established. The sputum is examined for malignant cells. Chest films may or may not show a tumor. A CT scan or MRI is done if the chest x-ray is inconclusive or to further delineate the tumor area. Bronchoscopy may be done to obtain bronchial washings and a tissue sample for biopsy. A lung scan also may identify the tumor. A bone scan detects metastasis to the bone. The results of a lymph node biopsy may be positive for malignant changes if the lung tumor has metastasized. Mediastinoscopy provides a direct view of the mediastinal area and possible visualization of tumors that extend into the mediastinal space.

MEDICAL AND SURGICAL MANAGEMENT

Treatment depends on several factors. One major consideration is the classification and staging of the tumor. After classification of the tumor, the stage of the disease is determined. Staging refers to the extent of the tumor, the location, and the absence, presence, and extent of metastasis. Other factors that determine treatment are the client's age and physical condition and the presence of other diseases or disorders, such as renal disease and congestive heart failure.

Surgical removal of the tumor may result in a cure in the early stages of the disease. Depending on the tumor's size and location, lobectomy or pneumonectomy is performed.

Radiation therapy may help to slow the spread of the disease and provide symptomatic relief by reducing tumor size, thus easing the pressure exerted by the tumor on adjacent structures. In turn, pain, cough, dyspnea, and hemoptysis may be relieved. In a small percentage of cases, radiation may be curative, but for most, it is a palliative measure. Complications associated with the use of radiation therapy include esophagitis, fibrosis of lung tissue, and pneumonitis.

Chemotherapy may be used alone or with radiation therapy and surgery. The principal effect of chemotherapy is to slow tumor growth and reduce tumor size and the pressure exerted by the tumor on adjacent structures. Chemotherapy is also used to treat metastatic lesions. Most chemotherapeutic regimens use a combination of drugs rather than a single agent and, although not curative, often make the client more comfortable.

The prognosis is poor unless the tumor is discovered in its early stages and treatment begins immediately. Because cancer of the lung produces few early symptoms, the mortality rate is high. Metastasis occurs to the mediastinal and cervical lymph nodes, liver, brain, spinal cord, bone, and opposite lung.

NURSING MANAGEMENT

Management of clients with lung cancer or a tumor of the mediastinum is essentially the same as that for any client with a malignant disease. See Chapter 19 for the nursing management of a client with cancer. See Chapter 24 and nursing management of the client undergoing a thoracotomy for perioperative care.

Mediastinal Tumors

Tumors of the mediastinum in adults often are malignant and metastatic. These tumors include lymphomas, tumors of the thymus, and neurogenic tumors. They are designated as anterior, middle, or posterior, according to their location on the mediastinum. The cause of these tumors has not been identified. Clients may be asymptomatic initially. When symptoms occur, they include chest pain, difficulty swallowing, dyspnea, and orthopnea. Symptoms often are related to pressure of the tumor on other chest structures. Chest x-ray, CT scan, MRI, mediastinoscopy, and biopsy of the lesion identify the tumor. Malignant tumors of the mediastinum are almost always inoperable but may respond to radiation therapy and chemotherapy.

Trauma

All chest injuries are serious or potentially serious. A client with a chest injury must be observed for dyspnea, cyanosis, chest pain, weak and rapid pulse, and hypotension—all signs and symptoms of respiratory distress. Clients with a chest injury need to be examined by a physician as soon as possible.

Fractured Ribs

ETIOLOGY AND PATHOPHYSIOLOGY

Fractured ribs are a common injury and may be caused by a hard fall or a blow to the chest. Automobile and household accidents are frequent causes. Although rib fractures are painful, they usually are not serious unless injury to other structures results; for example, the sharp end of the broken bone may tear the lung or thoracic blood vessels. If the injury involves fractured ribs without complications, the client often is permitted to return home after emergency treatment.

Flail chest occurs when two or more adjacent ribs are fractured in multiple places (more than two), and the fragments are free-floating (Fig. 28–12). The stability of the chest wall is affected and results in a paradoxical chest wall movement. With inspiration the chest expands, but the free-floating segments move inward instead of outward. On expiration the free-floating segments move outward, interfering with exhalation. Intrathoracic pressures are greatly affected, so that movement of air is greatly decreased. Many pathophysiologic phenomena occur as a result.

ASSESSMENT FINDINGS

Signs and Symptoms

Symptoms consist primarily of severe pain on inspiration and expiration and obvious trauma.

Diagnostic Findings

Chest x-rays (usually from several angles) are necessary to confirm the diagnosis.

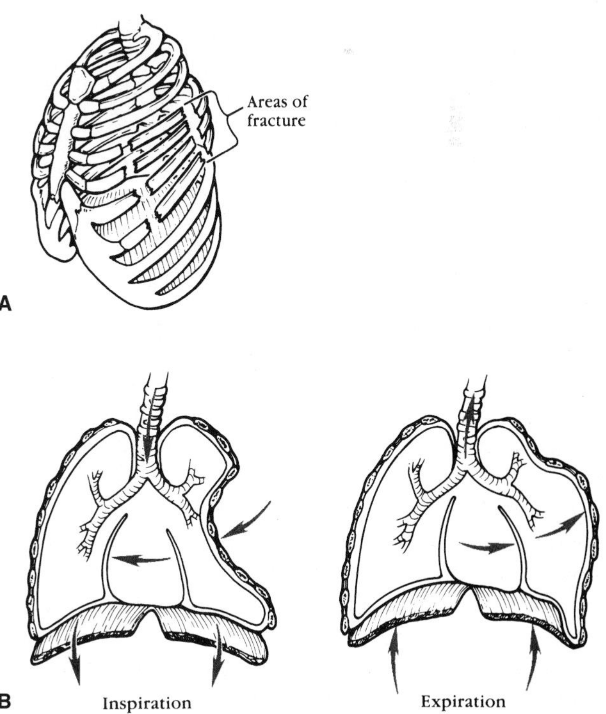

FIGURE 28-12. (A) Chest wall injury that can produce flail chest abnormality. (B) Physiology of flail chest abnormality resulting in paradoxical breathing.

MEDICAL MANAGEMENT

Supporting the chest with an elastic bandage or a rib belt assists in immobilizing the rib fractures. However, this can lead to decreased lung expansion followed by pulmonary complications such as pneumonia and atelectasis. Therefore, the use of these devices usually is limited to multiple rib fractures. Analgesics such as codeine may be prescribed for pain. Sometimes a regional nerve block is used to relieve pain.

Management of flail chest includes supporting ventilation, clearing lung secretions, and managing pain. Other treatment depends on the severity of the flail chest. If a **pulmonary contusion** (crushing bruise of the lung) also exists, fluids are restricted because of the damage to the pulmonary capillary bed. Antibiotics are given to prevent infection, which is common following this type of injury. Endotracheal intubation and mechanical ventilation may be necessary, if a client's respiratory status is greatly compromised.

NURSING MANAGEMENT

With fractured ribs, the nurse may apply the immobilization device after the physician examines the client. Instruct the client about the application and removal of the rib belt or elastic bandage. Stress the importance of taking deep breaths every 1 to 2 hours, even though breathing is painful. Nursing management of clients with more severe injuries is planned and implemented based on client respiratory needs. The nurse assesses and monitors the client for signs of respiratory distress, infection, and increased pain.

Blast Injuries

Compression of the chest by an explosion can seriously damage the lungs by rupturing the alveoli. Death often results from hemorrhage and asphyxiation. Severe respiratory distress with outward evidence of chest trauma is apparent. **Subcutaneous emphysema** (air in subcutaneous tissues) is a common finding because the lungs or air passages have sustained an injury. This condition resembles a superficial swelling. When the area is palpated with the fingers, *crepitation* (a crackling sound) is heard or felt and may be caused by air leaking around the chest tube.

Diagnosis is based on symptoms and physical examination. Additional diagnostic tests, such as chest x-ray and lung scan, may be necessary to identify foreign objects or air in the chest. Treatment includes complete bed rest and the administration of oxygen. Thoracentesis to remove air or fluid may be necessary. Some clients may require surgery and the insertion of chest tubes if severe injury to lung tissue has occurred or if pneumothorax is present. When a client has suffered a blast injury, the most important nursing task is immediate recognition of respiratory distress. Victims of a blast injury are closely observed for early signs of respiratory distress.

Penetrating Wounds

Penetrating wounds of the chest are serious because an opening into the thorax, which on inspiration normally is at negative pressure, creates continuous and direct communication with the outside, which is at positive pressure. An open or penetrating wound permits air to enter the thoracic cavity, causing a pneumothorax (Fig. 28–13). If not recognized and treated promptly, death may occur.

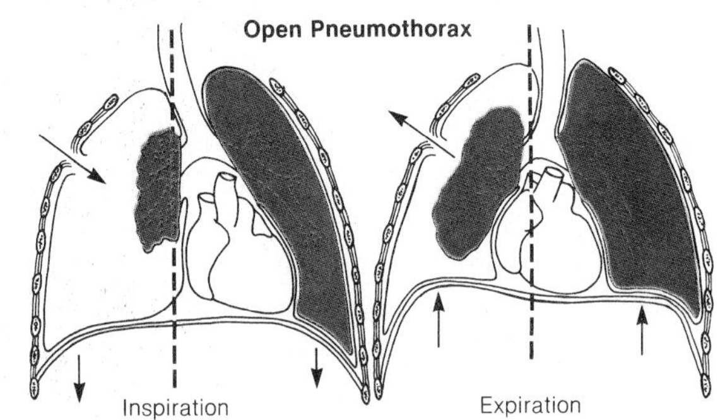

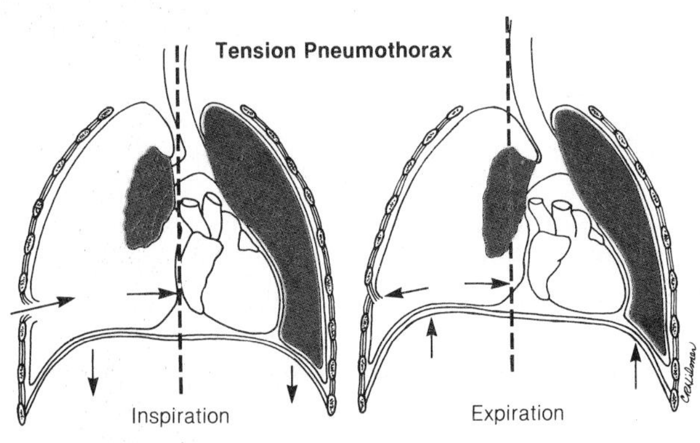

FIGURE 28-13. *Top*, open or communicating pneumothorax. In open pneumothorax, air enters the chest during inspiration and exits during expiration. *Bottom*, tension pneumothorax. In tension pneumothorax, air can enter but not exit chest cavity. As the pressure increases, the heart and great vessels are compressed and the mediastinal structures are shifted toward the opposite side of the chest. The trachea is pushed toward the opposite side of the chest and the unaffected lung is compressed.

If the wound is large, a sucking noise may be heard as air enters and leaves the chest cavity. Depending on the size of the wound, it takes seconds to hours before the lung collapses as the pressure in the thorax reaches atmospheric pressure. Many chest injuries involve both pneumothorax and hemothorax. Subcutaneous emphysema may also be noted.

Diagnosis is based on history of an injury, physical examination, and auscultation of the lungs. Radiographs show the degree of lung collapse and the amount of air or blood in the thoracic cavity.

Air and blood are aspirated from the pleural space by thoracentesis. A chest tube is inserted and attached to an underwater-seal drainage system. A thoracotomy may be required to repair the injury. Foreign bodies, such as a bullet or a knife, that have entered the chest are surgically removed. Their presence in the wound may prevent or slow the entrance of air. Removal before the victim is transported to the hospital may result in continuous sucking of air into the chest, collapse of the lung, compression of the heart and opposite lung, and death.

Emergency treatment of pneumothorax caused by a penetrating wound includes the application of a tight pressure dressing over the injury site to prevent more air from entering the thorax. Immediate evaluation of the client's respiratory status is imperative. Oxygen is given until the physician examines and treats the injury.

Thoracic Surgery

A thoracotomy is a surgical opening in the chest wall. It may be done to:

- Remove fluid, blood, or air from the thorax
- Remove tumors of the lung, bronchus, or chest wall
- Perform a pneumonectomy (removal of a lung), lobectomy (removal of a lobe of the lung), segmental resection (removal of a segment of a lobe), or wedge resection (removal of a small section of the lung)
- Repair or revise structures contained in the thorax, such as open heart surgery or repair of a thoracic aneurysm
- Repair trauma to the chest or chest wall, such as penetrating chest wounds or crushing chest injuries
- Biopsy a lesion
- Remove foreign objects such as a bullet or metal fragments

A thoracentesis may be done as an emergency procedure to remove blood, fluid, or air from the chest. In some instances, it is necessary to perform a thoracotomy to insert chest tubes (tube thoracotomy) to remove air or fluid from the chest during the preoperative period.

PREOPERATIVE NURSING MANAGEMENT

Preparing clients for thoracic surgery includes assessment of vital signs and breath sounds, particularly noting the presence or absence of breath sounds in any area of the chest. The condition of the client dictates the extent of the assessment and obtaining a history. If the surgery is an emergency, physical assessment may be limited to a general statement of the client's condition, a list of emergency measures and treatments done, and vital signs. Refer to perioperative care in Chapter 24.

POSTOPERATIVE NURSING MANAGEMENT

The opening of the thoracic cavity requires special postoperative nursing measures. A significant issue is the interference with normal pressures within the thoracic cavity. When the chest is opened, air from the atmosphere rushes in because of the negative pressure that exists in the thoracic cavity on inspiration. The entrance of air under atmospheric pressure collapses the lungs. The lungs can no longer expand or contract. The anesthesiologist ventilates the client during surgery.

After thoracic surgery, it is usually necessary to drain secretions, air, and blood from the thoracic cavity to allow the lungs to expand. A catheter placed in the pleural space provides a drainage route via a closed or underwater-seal drainage system. Sometimes two chest catheters are placed—one anteriorly and one posteriorly (Fig. 28–14). The anterior catheter (usually the upper one) removes air; the posterior catheter removes fluid.

Chest tubes are securely connected to an underwater-seal system. The tube coming from the client must always be under water. A break in the system, such as from loose or disconnected fittings, allows air to enter the tubing and then the pleural space, further collapsing the lung. All connections are taped carefully to minimize the possibility of air entering the closed system.

When caring for a client with chest tubes, the nurse should be aware of the following:

- Fluctuation of the fluid in the water-seal chamber is initially present with each respiration.
- Fluctuations cease when the lung reexpands. The time for lung re-expansion varies.
- Fluctuations may also cease if:
  - The chest tube is clogged
  - The wall suction unit malfunctions

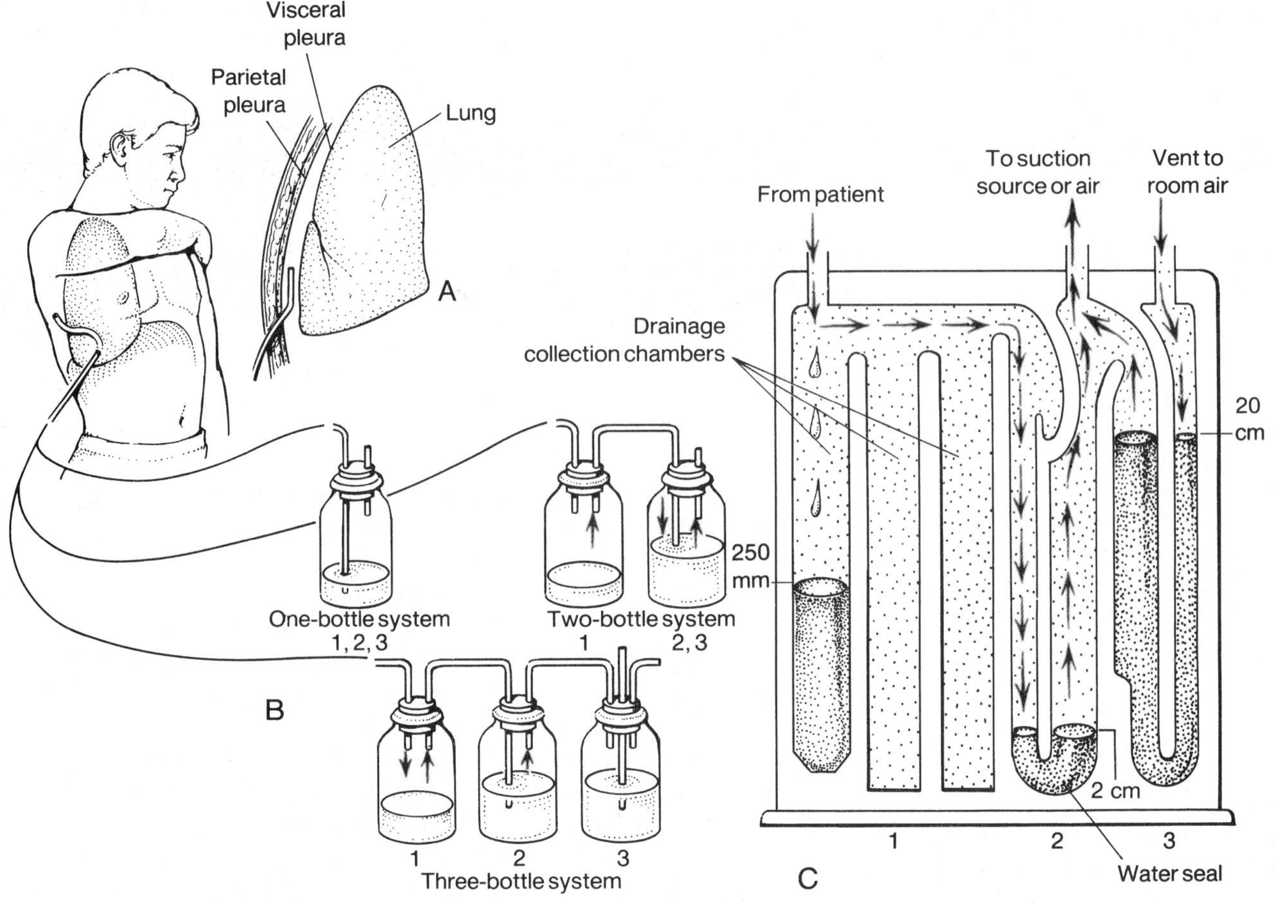

FIGURE 28-14 Chest drainage system. (*A*) Strategic placement of a chest catheter in the pleural space. (*B*) Three types of mechanical drainage systems. (C) A Pleur-Evac operating system: (1) the collection chamber, (2) the water seal chamber, and (3) the suction control chamber. The Pleur-Evac is a single unit with all three bottles identified as chambers.

   - A kink or dependent loop develops in the tubing
- Bubbling in the water-seal chamber occurs in the early postoperative period. If bubbling is excessive, check the system for leaks. If leaks are not apparent, notify the physician.
- Bloody drainage is normal, but it should not be bright red or copious.
- The drainage tube(s) must remain patent to allow the escape of fluids from the pleural space. Clogging of the catheter with clots or kinking, causes drainage to stop. The lung cannot expand, and the heart and great vessels may shift (mediastinal shift) to the opposite side. Malfunctions need to be corrected immediately.
- If a break or major leak occurs in the system, clamp the chest tube immediately with hemostats kept at the bedside. Notify the physician if this occurs.

Refer to Clinical Procedure 28–1 for maintenance of a water-seal drainage system.

NURSING PROCESS
The Client Undergoing Thoracic Surgery

Assessment

Check the underwater-seal drainage system noting amount and color of drainage and if bubbling or fluctuation is present. Assess dressings for drainage and firm adherence to the skin. Inspect the skin around the dressings for signs of subcutaneous emphysema. Assess the client's color, mental status, and heart rate and rhythm, and monitor respiratory rate, depth, and rhythm. Auscultate the chest for normal and abnormal breath sounds. Assess levels of pain and anxiety.

Diagnosis and Planning

Immediate postoperative care includes following the standards outlined in Chapter 24. In addition, the nurse's responsibilities when caring for a client who has had thoracic surgery include, but are not limited to, the following:

Nursing Diagnoses and Collaborative Problems	Nursing Interventions
Ineffective Breathing Pattern related to decreased lung expansion **Goal:** The client will establish an effective respiratory pattern.	Assess respiratory function. Report rapid or shallow respirations, dyspnea, cyanosis, or changes in vital signs. Auscultate breath sounds at least every 4 hours. Note chest excursion. Implement procedure for maintaining chest tube drainage system.
Ineffective Airway Clearance related to inability to cough and raise secretions secondary to lung disease or thoracic trauma **Goal:** The client will effectively clear the airway.	Assist client to deep breathe and cough in an upright position and to use splinting techniques. Assess amount and nature of sputum production. Suction client as indicated.
Pain related to surgical incision and presence of chest tubes **Goal:** The client will report relief of pain.	Assess client's level of pain. Medicate client as indicated. Evaluate effectiveness of pain medications. Provide comfort measures: position changes, back rubs, and support with pillows.
Anxiety related to change in health status and surgery **Goal:** The client will demonstrate reduced anxiety.	Assess client's level of anxiety. Provide time for client to express fears. Provide adequate explanations of procedures and client's questions. Assure client that he or she will be closely monitored postoperatively.
Impaired Physical Mobility related to surgery, pain, and chest tubes **Goal:** The client will move arms and perform arm exercises.	Encourage the client to move arms, slowly increasing movement and exercise as tolerated. Increase exercise level after chest tubes are removed. Perform passive range of motion exercises several times a day. Encourage the client to change position every 2 hours.
Knowledge Deficit regarding surgical procedure, prognosis, other factors **Goal:** The client will verbalize understanding of the surgical procedure and what is expected postoperatively.	Answer client's questions and provide additional information as required. Instruct client regarding postoperative expectations. Provide demonstrations of equipment used postoperatively. Emphasize the importance of deep breathing and coughing.

Evaluation and Expected Outcomes

- Respirations are even and unlabored, chest tubes are functional without air leaks, and oxygen saturation is above 92%.
- Pain is relieved.
- Mobility is maintained.
- Client accurately states what to expect after surgery.

Client and Family Teaching

Develop a teaching plan that includes instructions given by the physician. Include the following guidelines:

- Continue to perform arm exercises to prevent stiffness and pain.
- Eat a well balanced diet, or follow recommended diet.
- Take rest periods throughout the day until fatigue decreases.
- Practice breathing exercises and take frequent deep breaths.
- Contact physician if:
  - Breathing is difficult.
  - Drainage, excessive redness, or pain around incision occurs.
  - Fever develops.
  - Pain occurs elsewhere in the body.
- Avoid infection or irritants.
- Increase activities slowly and avoid fatigue.
- Take drugs as prescribed. Do not omit, increase, or decrease dose.

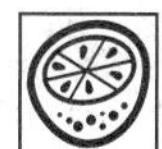

General Nutritional Considerations

Malnutrition among clients with emphysema is multifactorial. Shortness of breath and difficulty in breathing impair the ability to chew and swallow. Inadequate oxygenation of GI cells causes anorexia and gastric ulceration. Slowed peristalsis and digestion contribute to loss of appetite. Labored breathing increases calorie requirements, and eating is not a priority among clients who are anxious about breathing. To correct malnutrition, a high-protein, high-calorie diet is indicated. Because carbohydrates produce more CO_2 when metabolized than either protein or fat (and thus increase the burden on the lungs), carbohydrates are limited and fat is increased.

The diet should consist of approximately 40% carbohydrates, 40% fat, and 20% protein for clients with hypercapnia or those on ventilator support. Small frequent feedings of nutrient and calorie dense foods help maximize intake and lessen fatigue; concentrated liquid supplements are beneficial. Encourage ample fluid intake. Obese clients with emphysema are encouraged to lose weight to improve breathing.

Encourage clients with asthma to consume adequate calories and protein to optimize health and resist infection. Certain vitamins and minerals are important for immune function, especially vitamins A, C, B6, and zinc, and should be liberally consumed. Food allergens that may trigger allergic asthma include milk, eggs, seafood, and fish.

Specially designed enteral formulas are available for clients with respiratory failure; they are high in calories and consist of 40–55% of calories from fat to reduce carbon dioxide production. They should be administered continuously and advanced gradually as tolerated.

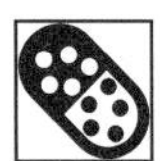

General Pharmacologic Considerations

Antibiotics may be ordered for the client with a respiratory tract infection; a culture and sensitivity test may be performed to identify the causative microorganisms. Once the microorganisms are identified and their sensitivity to various antibiotics is determined, the appropriate antibiotic is prescribed.

The indiscriminate use of nonprescription cough medicines may cause more harm than good. Coughing is the mechanism used by the body to clear the respiratory passages of mucus; depressing the cough reflex may cause a pooling of secretions and lead to further problems. Clients with respiratory disease are advised to check with their physicians before using nonprescription antitussive preparations (drugs used to prevent coughing).

Bronchodilators are used to manage acute breathing disorders, such as acute asthma attacks or reversible bronchospasm.

Examples of bronchodilators include adrenergic drugs, such as epinephrine, isoproterenol (Isuprel), and terbutaline (Bricanyl), and the xanthine derivatives, such as aminophylline and theophylline.

When theophylline or aminophylline are used to manage attacks of acute bronchial asthma and bronchospasm associated with chronic bronchitis and emphysema, serum theophylline levels should be maintained in the therapeutic range between 10–20 mcg/mL. Levels over 20 mcg/mL are associated with toxicity.

Isoniazid (INH) is used in combination with other antitubercular drugs and alone as a prophylactic to prevent the spread of tuberculosis. For example, INH may be give to household members and close associates of those re cently diagnosed with tuberculosis.

Zafirlukast (Accolate) is one of a new classification of ant asthma drugs, the leukotriene receptor antagonists. Th drug is administered to manage asthma symptoms on a ongoing basis. Asthma symptoms should improve withi 1 week of beginning therapy. Zafirlukast is NOT use during an acute asthma attack.

When a narcotic is administered to a client who has ha thoracic surgery, the respiratory rate is counted befor and 20 to 30 minutes after the client receives the med ication. If the respiratory rate falls below 10 breaths pe minute at either time, the physician must be notified im mediately.

Single-dose analgesics are best given before pain reache its maximum intensity. The client is evaluated for drug e fectiveness 30 to 45 minutes after administration. If single-dose analgesic or patient-controlled analgesi fails to provide pain relief, the physician is notified. larger dose or a different drug may be needed or a com plication of surgery may have occurred.

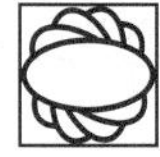

General Gerontologic Considerations

Older adults are more prone to pneumonia and may b more acutely ill with this infection because of concom tant health problems, such as heart disease and dia betes.

Before the flu season begins, the physician may recom mend that a vaccine be administered. Older and debil tated clients are more likely to contract the disease an develop complications.

Older adults, who are more subject to falls, may fractur one or more ribs and be more susceptible to pneumoni after a rib fracture.

During the postoperative period, the older client may b confused and attempt to pull out the chest tubes. Th physician is notified if confusion is apparent. An order fo restraints may be needed.

If confusion occurs, the older client requires more frequer observation and assessment of needs.

The older client may require more detailed explanation o home care management. Adequate time and repeate demonstrations may be necessary.

When possible, a family member is taught postoperativ exercises to ensure proper return of function to the mus cles on the operative side.

For clients over the age of 50, nursing home residents, an debilitated clients, vaccination against pneumococ pneumonia is recommended.

SUMMARY OF KEY CONCEPTS

- Acute bronchitis is characterized by inflammation of th mucous membranes that line the major bronchi an their branches. The inflammatory process frequently ir

volves the trachea and then is referred to as tracheobronchitis.
- Pneumonia is an acute illness caused by infection of the lungs. There is inflammation and edema of the alveoli, resulting in engorgement of the capillaries surrounding the alveoli.
- Pleurisy is an inflammation of the visceral and parietal pleurae. It is usually seen with pneumonia, in which the inflammatory process spreads from the lung to the parietal pleura.
- Pleural effusion is the collection of fluid between the visceral and parietal pleurae.
- A lung abscess, a localized area of pus formation, may occur in the lung parenchyma as a result of the aspiration of a foreign body, vomitus, or infectious material. The localized infection forms a cavity.
- Empyema is a general term used to denote the presence of pus in a body cavity. It most frequently refers to pus within the pleural cavity.
- Influenza (flu) is an acute respiratory disease of relatively short duration caused by one of several related yet distinct viruses.
- The presence of *M. tuberculosis*, the tubercle bacillus, is necessary to cause pulmonary tuberculosis. Tubercle bacilli are aerobic, gram-positive, and acid-fast. They are rod-shaped and can be identified by microscopic examination of sputum and other body fluids.
- Assessment of the client with an infectious or inflammatory disorder of the lower respiratory airway includes: vital signs, weight, lung auscultation, type of cough, amount, color, and consistency of cough, quality, rate, and depth of respirations, location and type of pain, inspection of the skin for cyanosis, flushing, or diaphoresis, and evaluation of mental status.
- Obstructive lung disease describes a group of pulmonary disorders characterized by chronic coughing and expectoration, dyspnea, and reduced expiratory airflow.
- Bronchiectasis is a chronic obstructive disease in which structural changes in the bronchial walls result in saccular changes, which collect purulent material and interfere with expiration.
- Atelectasis is the collapse of lung tissue. It may be limited to a small area of the lung or affect an entire lobe.
- Chronic bronchitis is characterized by hypersecretion of mucus by the bronchial glands as well as chronic infection and obstruction of airflow.
- Pulmonary emphysema is a chronic disorder of the lungs characterized by the following morphologic changes in lung tissue: alveolar sac distention, rupture of alveolar walls, and destruction of the alveolar capillary bed.
- The triad of symptoms of acute asthma includes spasm of the smooth muscle of the bronchi and larger bronchioles, swelling of the mucosal lining, and thick secretions.
- Pneumoconiosis is an inclusive term that describes a lung disease caused by inhalation of particles. The specific diseases are caused by inhalation of silica (silicosis), coal dust (black lung disease, miners' disease), and asbestos (asbestosis).
- Management of occupational lung diseases is focused on prevention. Strategies include dust control, ventilation, protective masks, hoods, industrial respirators, and other protection.
- In primary pulmonary hypertension, the inner lining of the pulmonary arteries thickens. Pressures in the pulmonary arteries and vascular bed are increased. In secondary pulmonary hypertension alveolar destruction results in increased resistance and pressure in the pulmonary vascular bed.
- In pulmonary embolism, a clot occludes one of the pulmonary vessels, causing infarction (necrosis or death). Most pulmonary emboli arise from venous clots in the legs or pelvis, but they may also come from the right ventricle if it is the site of a myocardial infarction. Other conditions that cause pulmonary embolus include recent surgery, prolonged bed rest, leg fracture or trauma, the postpartum state, and debilitating diseases.
- ARDS can lead to respiratory failure and death. It is referred to as noncardiogenic pulmonary edema. Causes include chest trauma, shock, drug overdose, drowning, emboli, and major surgery.
- Acute respiratory failure occurs suddenly in a person who previously had normal lung function. Causes include oversedation, anesthesia administration, head injury, chest trauma, thoracic or abdominal surgery, hemothorax, pneumothorax, and pneumonia. Neurologic diseases such as multiple sclerosis may also cause acute respiratory failure.
- Acute respiratory failure is life-threatening. Alveolar ventilation is not sufficient to maintain necessary oxygen and carbon dioxide exchange, leading to hypoxemia and hypercapnia.
- Chronic respiratory failure occurs in clients with chronic respiratory disorders such as emphysema. Loss of lung function is progressive and usually irreversible.
- Early diagnosis of lung cancer is difficult because symptoms do not appear until the disease is well established.
- Chest injuries are potentially very serious. The client needs to be observed for dyspnea, cyanosis, chest pain, weak and rapid pulse, and hypotension—signs of respiratory distress.
- Thoracic surgery involves opening the thorax and affecting the normal intrathoracic pressures.
- After thoracic surgery, chest tubes are generally placed in the chest and connected to a closed drainage system for the purpose of removing excess air and fluid.
- Postoperative care includes monitoring chest drainage, condition of dressings, respiratory status, and pain level. The nurse encourages the client to deep breathe and cough, splint incision when coughing and moving, and move arms, increasing exercise.

CRITICAL THINKING EXERCISES

1. A client who underwent cholecystectomy (removal of the gallbladder) 2 days ago presses his call button. As you enter his room, he tells you that he is having trouble breathing and has pain. What brief questions would you ask the client before you call the physician?
2. A client has a history of asthma and was admitted to the hospital with uncontrolled diabetes mellitus. What nurs-

ing assessments would you make if the client experiences respiratory distress?

3. An AIDS client has developed pleurisy. His physician instructs him to perform deep breathing and coughing exercises hourly. What can you do to ease the pain and discomfort when he is performing these exercises?

Suggested Readings

Angelucci, P. (1996). A new weapon against ARDS. *RN, 96(11), 22–24.*

Bullock, B. (1996). *Pathophysiology: Adaptations and alterations in function* (4th ed.). Philadelphia. Lippincott-Raven.

Calianno, C. (1996). Action stat: Aspiration pneumonia. *Nursing, 26*(10), 47.

Calianno, C. (1996). Nosocomial pneumonia: Repelling a deadly invader. *Nursing, 26*(5), 34–39.

Carpenito, L. J. (1995). *Nursing care plans and documentation* (2nd ed.) Philadelphia. J. B. Lippincott.

Eisenbeis, C. (1996). Full partner in care: Teaching your patient how to manage her asthma. *Nursing, 26*(1), 48–51.

Eisenhauer, B. (1996). Action stat: Dislodged tracheostomy tube. *Nursing, 26*(6), 25.

Forth, R. (1998). Common questions about obstructive sleep apnea. *American Journal of Nursing, 98*(2), 60–64.

Gaedeke, M. K., & Cross, J. (1996). Action stat: Blunt chest trauma. *Nursing, 26*(2), 33.

Kenny, M. F. (1997). Acute pulmonary edema. *Nursing 27*(11), 33.

Majoros, K. A., & Moccia, J. M. (1996). Pulmonary embolism: Targeting an elusive enemy. *Nursing, 26*(4), 26–31.

Parini, S. M. (1997). Treating tuberculosis. *Nursing 27*(11), 32; hn 20–21.

Smeltzer, S. C., & Bare, B. G. (1996). *Brunner and Suddarth's textbook of medical-surgical nursing* (8th ed.). Philadelphia: Lippincott-Raven.

Timby, B. K. (1996). *Fundamental skills and concepts in patient care* (6th ed.). Philadelphia: Lippincott-Raven.

Additional Resources

Lung Cancer
http://www.erinet.com

The Lung Cancer and Cigarette Smoking Web Page
http://ourworld.compuserve.com/homepages/lungcancer

Oncolink-Lung Cancer
http://oncolink.upenn.edu

Emphysema Patient Resources
http://johns.largnet.uwo.ca/largh/patients/emphysema.html

Pulmonary Disabilities Page
http://people.delphi.com

American Academy of Allergy, Asthma, and Immunology (AAAAI)
http://www.aaaai.org

Teach Your Patients about Asthma: A Clinician's Guide
http://www.meddean.luc.edu

National Asthma Education Program
Office of Prevention, Education, and Control
National Heart, Lung, and Blood Institute
National Institute of Health
Bethesda, MD 2089

7

Caring for Clients With Cardiovascular Disorders

Chapter 29

Introduction to the Cardiovascular System

KEY TERMS

Angiocardiography
Aortography
Arrhythmias
Arteriography
Automaticity
Cardiac index
Cardiac output
Central venous pressure
Conductivity
Contractility
Depolarization
Echocardiography
Electrocardiography
Excitability
Hemodynamic monitoring
Isoenzyme
Left ventricular end-diastolic pressure
Nomogram
Phonocardiography
Polarization
Pulmonary capillary wedge pressure
Refractory period
Repolarization
Rhythmicity
Starling's law
Stroke volume
Telemetry
Vectorcardiography

LEARNING OBJECTIVES

On completion of this chapter, the reader will:

- Describe normal anatomy and physiology of the cardiovascular system.
- Identify and describe focus assessment criteria when caring for a client with cardiovascular problems.
- List common diagnostic tests used to evaluate the client with suspected heart disease.
- Discuss the nursing management of a client undergoing cardiovascular diagnostic tests.

Heart disease is the leading cause of death for adults in the United States. Heart disease interferes with the ability to supply body cells and tissues with oxygen-rich blood and rid the cells of carbon dioxide and wastes. Although human heart transplantation and the temporary use of an artificial heart are available, preserving the natural heart by preventing heart disease is a primary focus.

Anatomy and Physiology

The cardiovascular system consists of the heart, major blood vessels that empty into or exit directly from the heart, and a vast network of smaller peripheral blood vessels. The heart's ability to pump blood is the result of five qualities unique to cardiac tissue:

- **Automaticity**—the ability to initiate its own electrical stimulus
- **Excitability**—the ability to respond to electrical stimulation
- **Conductivity**—the ability to transmit the electrical stimulus from cell to cell within the heart
- **Contractility**—the ability to stretch as a single unit and recoil
- **Rhythmicity**—the ability to repeat the cycle with regularity

Heart Chambers

The heart is a four-chambered muscular pump about the size of a fist (Fig. 29–1). The upper chambers, the right and left *atria* (sing., *atrium*), are receiving chambers for blood. The lower chambers, the right and left *ventricles*, are the pumping chambers of the heart. The

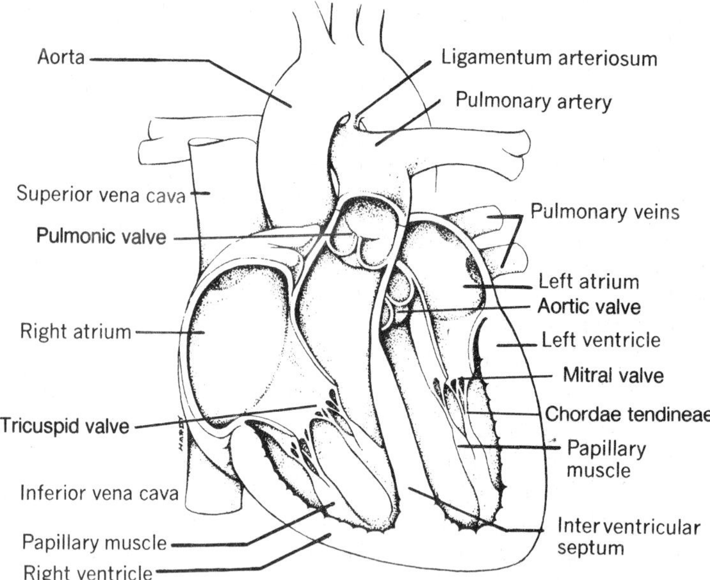

FIGURE 29-1. Structure of the heart.

right side of the heart is separated from the left side, which contains the left atrium and left ventricle, by a thick *septum*, or wall. The right atrium of the heart receives deoxygenated blood from the venous system and the right ventricle pumps that blood to the lungs to be oxygenated. The left atrium of the heart receives oxygenated blood from the lungs and the left ventricle pumps that blood to all the cells and tissues of the body. Therefore, the heart is a double pump, the right side conducts pulmonary circulation, and the left side is responsible for systemic circulation.

The heart lies below and slightly to the left of the midline of the sternum in the mediastinum, a portion of the thoracic cavity that contains the heart, trachea, and blood vessels. The upper portion of the heart is the *base*, and the tip is the *apex*. The right ventricle is directly under the sternum, a location that is significant in cardiopulmonary resuscitation. The lower border of the right ventricle rests on the diaphragm and forms a blunt point that angles to the left side of the body.

Cardiac Tissue Layers

Three distinct layers of tissue make up the heart wall. The outer layer is the *epicardium*. The middle layer, the *myocardium*, consists of muscle tissue, and is the force behind the pumping action of the heart. The inner layer, the *endocardium*, is composed of a thin, smooth layer of endothelial cells. Folds of endocardium form the heart valves. The endocardium is in direct contact with the blood that passes through the heart.

The *pericardium* is a saclike structure that surrounds and supports the heart. Two membranous layers form the pericardium, the outer, tougher, parietal pericardium, and an inner serous layer—the visceral pericardium (also called the epicardium), which adheres to the heart itself. The density of the parietal pericardium safeguards the heart from invasion by infectious microorganisms. Serous fluid fills the pericardial space between the two layers, lubricating the heart and reducing friction with each heart beat.

Heart Valves

The valves of the heart are membranous structures that ensure that blood passes through the heart in a one-way, forward direction. In a normal heart, the valves do not allow blood to backflow, or regurgitate, into the chamber from which it has come.

The two *atrioventricular valves* separate the atria from the ventricles. They prevent blood from returning to the atria when the ventricles contract. These valves are cusped, or leaflike. The valve between the right atrium and right ventricle is the *tricuspid valve*, meaning that it has three cusps. The valve between the left atrium and left ventricle is the *bicuspid*, or two-cusped, valve. The bicuspid valve is also called the *mitral valve*.

Attached to the mitral and tricuspid valves are cordlike structures known as *chordae tendineae*, which in turn attach to two major muscular projections from the ventricles, the *papillary muscles*. When the ventricles contract, the papillary muscles also contract, applying tension on the atrioventricular valves. The contraction of the papillary muscles and the firm support of the chordae tendineae prevent eversion of the valves and regurgitation of blood back into the atria.

The other two valves, called *semilunar valves* because they resemble portions of the moon, prevent blood from flowing back into the ventricles after the heart contracts. The valves are named for the blood vessel into which the blood is deposited. The valve between the right ventricle and pulmonary artery is called the *pulmonary*, or *pulmonic, valve*. The valve between the left ventricle and aorta is the *aortic valve*. As the ventricles contract, blood is forced into the pulmonary artery and aorta. Ventricular contraction is followed by relaxation, and the fall in the pressure in the ventricles cause the pulmonic and aortic valves to close, preventing backflow into the ventricles.

Arteries and Veins

Arteries carry oxygenated blood from the heart, and *veins* return deoxygenated blood to the heart. The smallest arteries are called *arterioles*, and the smallest veins, *venules*. Arteries and arterioles are elastic and dilate or constrict to accommodate changes in blood flow.

Arteries and veins are comprised of three layers. The outer layer, the *tunica adventitia*, consists of connective tissue; the middle layer, the *tunica media*, is composed of smooth muscle; and the inner layer, the *tunica intima*, is composed of endothelial cells. The tunica media is thicker in arteries than in veins, to accommodate the higher blood pressure in the arteries.

Arterioles branch into *capillaries*, which are microscopic vessels that form a connecting network between arterioles and venules. Capillaries are one cell layer thick and are in direct contact with the cells of all tissues. Oxygen and metabolic substances are delivered to the cells through this complex circulatory network. The thin walls, tremendous surface area, and tiny size of the capillaries allow for rapid exchange of gases and metabolic substances between the blood and cells. After this exchange occurs, blood is transported back to the heart via the venules and veins.

Contraction of the heart moves blood from the heart into arteries and arterioles; skeletal muscle contraction compresses veins and propels blood back to the heart. Closure of successive sets of valves within veins keeps the blood from pooling downward under the influence of gravity.

Cardiopulmonary Circulation

The largest veins in the body, the *inferior* and *superior venae cavae* bring venous (deoxygenated) blood from all areas of the body into the right atrium. The coronary sinus in the right atrium is where blood that has been used by the heart itself is deposited. The right atrium fills with blood, and the tricuspid valve opens. Blood then travels into the right ventricle and is pumped into the *pulmonary artery* (the only artery in an adult that carries deoxygenated blood). The pulmonary artery branches to deliver venous blood to the right and left lung. The lungs exchange the oxygen in inspired air for the carbon dioxide in the venous blood. The carbon dioxide is transferred into the alveoli and exhaled. Four *pulmonary veins* then bring the oxygenated blood into the left atrium. Oxygenated blood leaves the left atrium through the bicuspid, or mitral valve. The left ventricle then pumps the blood through the *aorta* to all the body's cells and tissues.

Blood Supply to the Heart

Oxygenated blood is supplied to cardiac muscle by means of the *left coronary artery* and the *right coronary artery*. The openings to the coronary arteries lie just

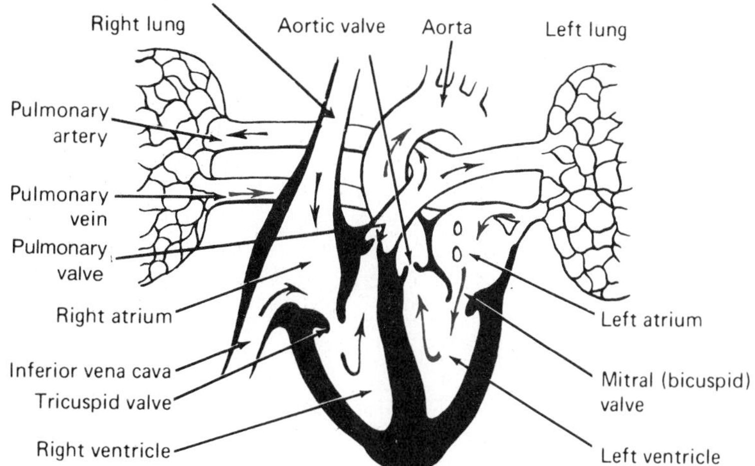

FIGURE 29-2. Blood flow through the heart and lungs. The path can be observed by starting at the venae cavae and following the arrows through the right atrium, right ventricle, pulmonary arteries, pulmonary veins, left atrium, and left ventricle and into the aorta. Red arrows indicate flow of oxygenated blood.

inside the aorta. Thus, the myocardium is the first tissue to be supplied with oxygenated blood with each heartbeat (Fig. 29–3).

The left coronary artery and its branches, the *left anterior descending artery* and *left circumflex artery*, are critical for maintaining the pumping function of the heart because they keep the left atrium and most of the left ventricle perfused with oxygen, enabling the left side of the heart to forcefully pump oxygen-rich blood to the body. The right coronary artery and its branches maintain heart rhythm because they nourish the nerve tissue of the conduction system.

After having distributed oxygenated blood to the myocardial cells, the coronary veins carry away the carbon dioxide produced by cellular metabolism. The coronary veins empty into the coronary sinus in the right atrium. The blood then mixes with blood from the inferior and superior venae cavae and is recirculated to the lungs.

Cardiac Cycle

The term *cardiac cycle* refers to the contraction (*systole*) and relaxation (*diastole*) of both atria and both ventricles (Fig. 29–4). The atria contract simultaneously; then, as they relax, the ventricles contract and relax. The contraction of the left ventricle can be felt as a wavelike impulse (the pulse) in peripheral arteries. The pause between pulsations is ventricular diastole. The contraction of the atria and then the ventricles can be heard with a stethoscope as the "lub-dub" sounds. The sounds are created when the atrioventricular and semilunar valves alternately snap shut.

Both sides of the heart work in unison to accomplish seemingly different goals. Blood enters both atria and as pressure builds from the increasing volume of blood in the atria, the atrioventricular valves open, depositing blood into the ventricles. During atrial systole, the contraction of the upper chambers squeezes the remaining blood into the ventricles. When pressure builds in the ventricles, the atrioventricular valves snap shut.

During ventricular systole, blood is pumped through the semilunar valves into the major vessels exiting the heart. The greater the stretch of the myocardium as the ventricles fill with blood, the stronger the ventricular contraction. This phenomenon is called **Starling's law**. It can be compared to the effect created by stretching a rubber band: the more the rubber band is stretched, the greater the snap when it is released.

Conduction System

The electrical activity of the heart is sustained by the conduction system. The conduction system consists of the sinoatrial (SA) node, the atrioventricular (AV) node, the bundle of His, bundle branches, and Purkinje fibers.

The *SA node* is an area of nerve tissue located in the posterior wall of the right atrium. The SA node is called the pacemaker of the heart because it initiates the electrical impulses that cause the atria and ventricles to contract. Under normal circumstances, it produces impulses between 60 and 100 times per minute; the average is about 72 times per minute. The

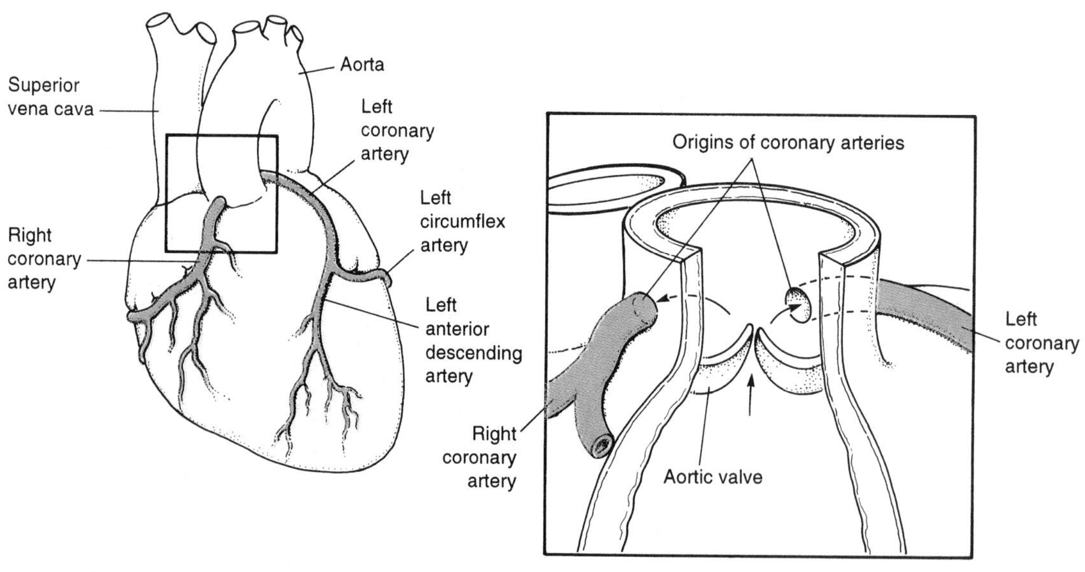

FIGURE 29-3. The coronary arteries, which originate in the aorta, supply the myocardium with oxygenated blood.

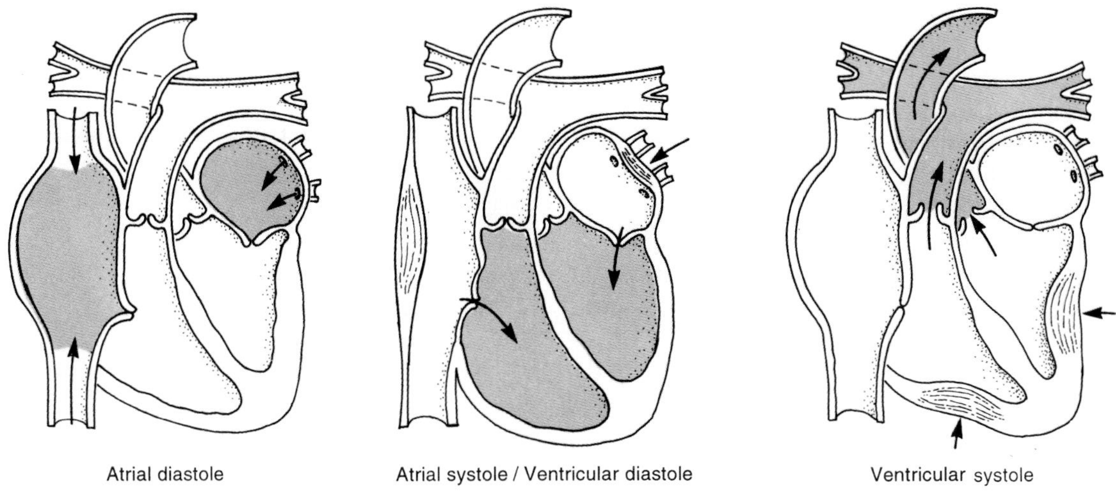

FIGURE 29-4. Pumping cycle of the heart. During atrial diastole, blood from the venae cavae and pulmonary veins fills the atria. During atrial systole, blood is delivered to the ventricles. When the ventricles contract, blood is pumped into the aorta and pulmonary arteries.

SA node initiates impulses faster in response to sympathetic nervous system stimulation and slows in response to parasympathetic stimulation. Other areas in the conduction pathway may initiate an electrical impulse if the SA node malfunctions, but they do so at rates slower than that of the SA node.

In the normal sequence of events, the cardiac impulse starts in the SA node (Fig. 29–5). It spreads throughout the atria over internodal and interatrial pathways. The waves of stimulation through the heart resemble the rings made by a pebble dropped into a pond. Once the cells in the atria are excited, they contract in unison. When the impulse reaches the *AV node*, it is delayed a few hundredths of a second. The impulse then stimulates the ventricles. While the ventricles fill with blood, the impulse travels from the AV node to the *bundle of His*, to the right and left *bundle branches*, and, eventually, to the *Purkinje fibers*. Then both ventricles contract.

During diastole, while the myocardial cells are at rest and before an impulse is generated, the cells are in a *polarized state* (**polarization**). Positive ions predominate outside myocardial cell membranes; negative ions predominate inside. When an electrical impulse is initiated, it spreads from cell membrane to cell membrane, causing a transfer of ions. The positive ions move inside and the negative ions move outside. This process, which corresponds to cardiac muscle contraction, is called **depolarization**. It occurs first in the atria and then in the ventricles. Once depolar-

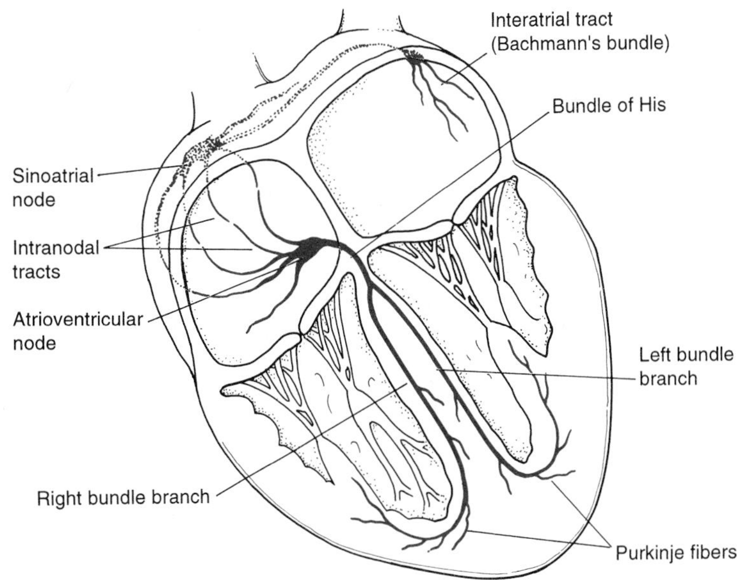

FIGURE 29-5. Electrical conduction system of the heart.

ization has occurred, the ions realign themselves in their original position and wait for another electrical impulse. This process is called **repolarization**. Another normal cardiac impulse cannot be carried out until the ions are again in polarized alignment. The time during which the cells are resistant to electrical stimulation is called the **refractory period**.

Electrolyte balance is important for the proper functioning of all the cells in the body. Normal ranges of potassium and calcium ions are particularly essential for maintaining heart function (see Chap. 21). Excess potassium ions decrease the heart rate and strength of contraction. Cardiac rhythm is disturbed when potassium levels become abnormally low. Excess calcium ions increase and prolong heart contraction. Low serum calcium levels reduce heart function.

Depolarization and repolarization produce electrical changes. Because body tissues conduct current easily, this electrical activity can be detected by electrodes placed on the external surface of the body and recorded by a machine known as the *electrocardiograph (ECG)* (Fig. 29–6).

It is normal for the heart rate and rhythm to fluctuate to accommodate for changes in activity and stimulation from the autonomic nervous system. Box 29–1 highlights factors that alter heart rate and rhythm.

Cardiac Output

Cardiac output is the amount of blood pumped out of the left ventricle each minute. In a healthy adult, cardiac output ranges from 4 to 8.0 L/min (average, about 5 L/min). Volume varies according to body size.

BOX 29-1 Factors That Alter Heart Rate and Rhythm

- Impaired circulation through the coronary arteries
- Hyperthyroidism
- Hypoxia
- Drug effects and side effects
- Stress
- Electrolyte imbalance
- Altered body temperature
- Exercise

The heart adjusts cardiac output to the body's changing needs. During active exercise, athletes may have a cardiac output that is five to seven times the normal amount. Cardiac output can be increased in two ways: by increasing the heart rate and by increasing the **stroke volume**. Stroke volume is the amount of blood pumped per contraction of the heart. The stroke volume averages about 65 to 70 mL. The following formula is used to calculate cardiac output:

cardiac output = heart rate x stroke volume

Assessment of a Client With a Cardiovascular Disorder

History

The initial assessment includes the client's (or family member's) description of the symptoms being experi-

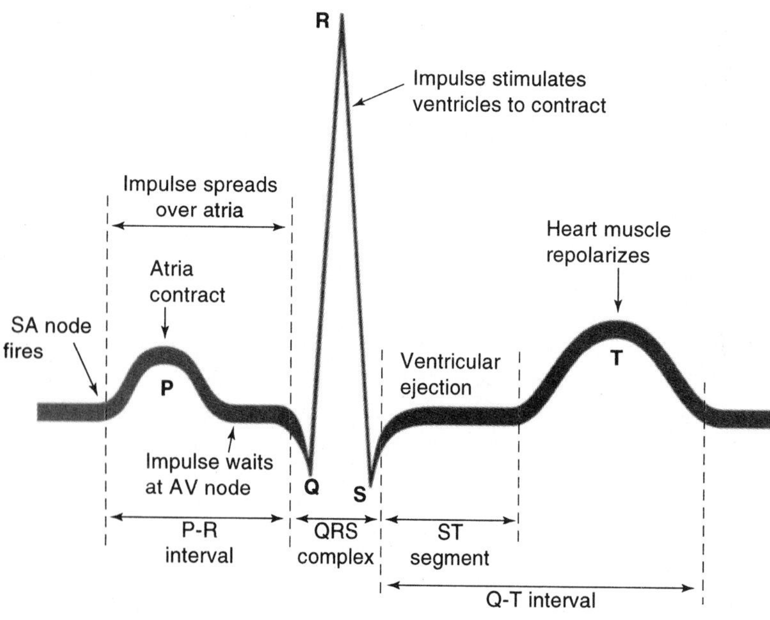

FIGURE 29-6. ECG waves, electrical and mechanical events. An electrical impulse is initiated by the SA node and spreads throughout the conduction system of the heart, causing the P, Q, R, S, and T waves. If the heart responds normally, the atria and then the ventricles contract.

enced before admission and during the admission assessment. A past medical history of angina, myocardial infarction, and any cardiac surgeries is also important to note at this time. The client is asked to identify prescription and nonprescription drugs that are being taken. Adverse effects or drug interactions can contribute to cardiac symptoms. Drug and food allergies are noted because future diagnostic procedures may involve the administration of drugs or substances, such as radiopaque dyes. An allergy to seafood may indicate that the client is also allergic to iodine, which commonly is used in contrast media during various radiographic examinations. If a client is in acute distress, a history may need to be gathered from a family member.

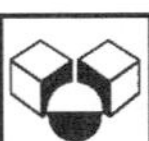

Nursing Guidelines 29-1

Assessing Cardiac Pain

Assessment of pain includes:

- Description of the pain (sharp, dull, squeezing, crushing)
- Location of pain and any radiation
- Duration of the pain. When did it start and end?
- Radiation of the pain to other areas (the pain may or may not radiate)
- Change in the character of the pain (increasing in severity, changing from dull to sharp, etc)
- Intensity of the pain using a scale from 1 to 10, with 1 being characterized as slight pain, and 10 describing the worst pain ever experienced
- Relation of the onset of pain to other factors, such as eating, exercise, or emotions

Physical Assessment

GENERAL APPEARANCE

An appraisal of the client's general appearance may suggest problems that require further exploration. The client's nonverbal behavior and body position may indicate that the client is anxious, depressed, in pain, or uncomfortable.

PAIN

Poor circulation, a common problem in clients with cardiovascular disorders, causes *ischemia* (reduced blood supply) to body organs. A classic sign of ischemia is pain, which is caused by a lack of oxygen in the tissue. Chest pain is a manifestation of ischemia to the heart muscle. Leg pain, especially with activity, can indicate inadequate oxygenation to leg muscles.

When present, pain is evaluated carefully. It is important to obtain as much information as possible. Rapid treatment of pain is extremely important. Nursing Guidelines 29–1 highlights the procedure for assessing pain.

VITAL SIGNS

Temperature, pulse, respiratory rate, and blood pressure are routinely taken on all clients.

Temperature

Fever is characteristic in some types of heart disease. It can accompany the inflammatory response when myocardial cells are damaged after an acute myocardial infarction (heart attack) or infections such as rheumatic fever and subacute bacterial endocarditis. Observe agency policy about taking the temperature rectally on clients with a cardiac disorder. In the past, this method was contraindicated in clients because it was thought to stimulate the vagus nerve and cause bradycardia. Many agencies now have abandoned this restriction.

Pulse Rate

When taking a client's pulse, the nurse notes its rate, rhythm, and quality. Pulse rhythm is the pattern of the pulsations and the pauses between them. A normal pulse is felt regularly with a similar length of pause. The pulse quality refers to its palpated volume. Pulse volume is described as feeling full, weak, or thready, meaning barely palpable. The nurse also determines if a *pulse deficit* is present. Clinical Procedure 29–1 highlights the procedure involved in determining a pulse deficit.

Respiratory Rate

The respiratory rate is counted for 60 seconds. The character of the respirations is observed, noting whether the client's breathing is easy or labored (dyspneic), deep or shallow, noisy or quiet. The use of accessory muscles (neck or abdominal muscles) during respiration is an indication that the client is having difficulty breathing.

Blood Pressure

Cardiac disorders often are associated with changes in blood pressure. If the client is not acutely ill, the blood pressure is taken with the client in the standing, sitting, and lying positions (orthostatic vital signs). These baseline determinations are necessary to monitor the effects of cardiovascular diseases and drugs that can alter the blood pressure during position changes. To ensure an accurate assessment, the nurse selects the cuff width most appropriate for the diameter of the client's arm.

The blood pressure is taken in both arms on admission and at least once daily thereafter. A marked dif-

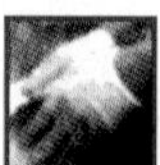

Clinical Procedure 29-1
Assessing Pulse Deficit

A pulse deficit exists when some of the contractions of the heart are not strong enough to create a pulse in the peripheral, radial artery. The assessment of pulse deficit requires two nurses.

Nursing Action	Rationale
Place a watch where the two nurses can readily see it.	Provides accuracy in the measurement of the pulse.
One nurse auscultates the heart over the apex of the client's heart. The proper location is the client's fifth intercostal space, left midclavicular line.	The heart rate is more easily heard over the apex of the heart.
The second nurse palpates the radial pulse, and both nurses begin counting at a predetermined time.	Ensures that both nurses are assessing the pulses simultaneously.
The heartbeat is counted for 1 full minute. The nurses compare the respective heart rates.	A pulse deficit exists if the radial pulse is slower than the apical pulse.

ference in pressure between the left and right arms is reported. When charting, identify the arm used to measure the blood pressure and the client's position at the time it was measured.

Question the client about dizziness or light-headedness when changing positions, such as rising from a sitting or lying position. These symptoms may indicate postural (or orthostatic) hypotension, which may be due to specific drugs or other factors.

CARDIAC RHYTHM

The electrical activity that produces the heart rhythm can be observed continuously with bedside cardiac monitoring. Electrodes are attached to the chest and connected to a machine that displays the cardiac rhythm on an oscilloscope. The components of an ECG are discussed later in the chapter. A paper strip of the cardiac rhythm can be printed and attached to the client's record. Most cardiac monitors sound an alarm and automatically print out abnormal rhythms, called **arrhythmias** or *dysrhythmias*.

A cardiac monitor reveals the heart's electrical activity but not its mechanical activity. A peripheral pulse must be palpated or the apical heart rate auscultated to obtain this information. Comparing the heart rate and rhythm with the information displayed on the monitor is important because the ECG pattern may appear normal in some clients even when mechanical function is abnormal.

Cardiac **telemetry** sends ECG information over radio waves to a monitor that is distant from the client. Telemetry is used by paramedics to communicate information to personnel in the hospital emergency department. It may also be used when a client's condition is stable enough to be transferred from a critical care unit, but continuous monitoring is required. When telemetry is used, the electrodes are attached to a battery pack. The battery is secured inside a pocket on the client's hospital gown (Fig. 29–7).

HEART SOUNDS

Normal Heart Sounds

Auscultation of the heart requires familiarization with normal and abnormal heart sounds. The first

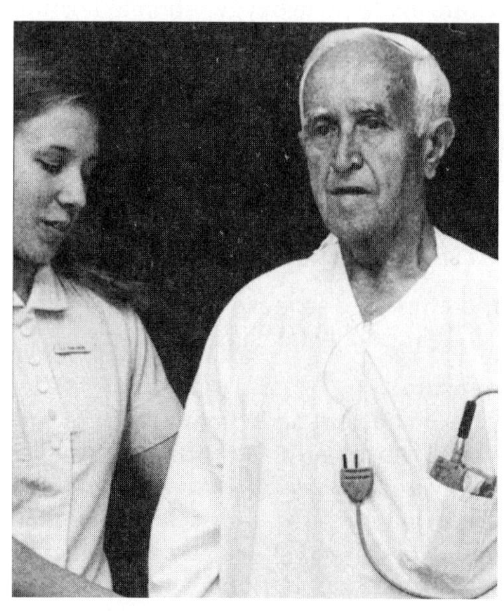

FIGURE 29-7. Cardiac client being monitored by telemetry.

heart sound ("lub"), referred to as S_1, is the closing of the mitral and tricuspid valves. It is heard loudest over the apex of the heart and occurs nearly simultaneously with the palpated pulse. The second heart sound ("dub"), referred to as S_2, is the closing of the aortic and pulmonic valves. It is heard loudest with the stethoscope at the second intercostal space to the right of the sternum.

Abnormal Heart Sounds

All other heart sounds are abnormal and take considerable practice to recognize. A sound that follows S_1 and S_2 is called an S_3 heart sound or a ventricular gallop. When the three sounds are heard together, some say the cadence sounds like "Ken-tuck-y" or "lub-dub-dee." The presence of an S_3, while normal in children, often is an indication of heart failure in an adult. An extra sound just before S_1 is an S_4 heart sound, or atrial gallop. Some say this sound resembles the word "Ten-nes-see" or "lub-lub-dub." An S_4 sound often is associated with hypertensive heart disease.

In addition to heart sounds, auscultation may reveal other abnormal sounds, such as murmurs and clicks caused by turbulent blood flow through diseased heart valves. A rough, grating sound may be caused by a friction rub, which is indicative of pericarditis (inflammation of the pericardium).

PERIPHERAL PULSES

The radial arteries and the major arteries of the leg are palpated bilaterally during the physical assessment (Fig. 29–8).

The presence or absence of these pulses and their strength are recorded.

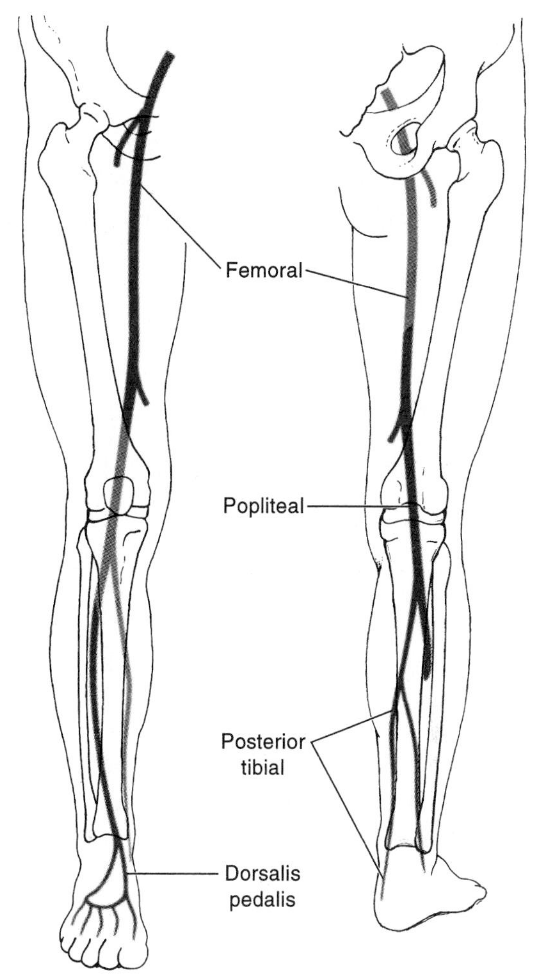

FIGURE 29-8. Major arteries of the leg that can be palpated for pulsation where they come close to the surface.

SKIN

Many clients with cardiac disorders exhibit changes in skin color (ie, cyanosis, pallor). A good light is necessary when assessing skin color. Cyanosis can be detected by carefully noting color changes in the oral mucous membranes as well as on the lips, earlobes, skin, and nail beds. In light-skinned clients, extreme pallor is easy to detect because the skin appears almost bloodless. In dark-skinned clients, a grayish cast to the skin usually indicates pallor.

When assessing the skin, it is important to note whether the skin is warm or cold, dry or clammy. If the client has a problem with peripheral circulation, the arms and legs are inspected for variations in skin color and temperature and compared bilaterally with other areas of the body. Sparse hair growth on the legs and thick toenails can indicate poor circulation. The presence of varicosities (enlargement of veins) is also noted.

PERIPHERAL EDEMA

Edema occurs when blood is not pumped efficiently or when plasma protein levels are inadequate to maintain osmotic pressure. When heart failure occurs, blood accumulates in the great vessels and backs up in peripheral veins. Because it has nowhere else to go, the extra fluid enters the tissues. Dependent parts of the body, such as the feet and ankles, must be examined in particular. Other areas prone to edema are the fingers, hands, and over the sacrum. To assess for edema, the examiner's fingers are gently pressed into the skin and then quickly released. If the marks of the fingers remain, the effect is termed *pitting edema*. Edema is evaluated on a scale of +1 to +4, depending on the depth of the pit and the amount of time it takes the pit to disappear (see Chap. 21). The higher the number, the more pronounced the edema.

WEIGHT

Weight gain can be an indication of edema. A gain in weight often means that edema is increasing. A 2-lb weight gain in a short period of time indicates that the client has an additional liter of fluid in the body. Weight loss often reflects the loss of excess fluid from the tissues and is used to evaluate the effectiveness of drug therapy, especially diuretics. If weight is recorded daily, the client is weighed at the same time, with the same amount of clothing, using the same scale, each day. The weight is recorded as accurately as possible.

JUGULAR VEINS

If the right side of the heart fails to pump efficiently, blood becomes congested in the neck veins (Fig. 29–9). With the client sitting at a 45-degree angle, the head is turned to the left or right to inspect the external jugular vein. Distention of this vein usually indicates increased fluid volume and pressure within the right side of the heart (see Chap. 35).

LUNG SOUNDS

If the left side of the heart fails to pump efficiently, blood backs up into the pulmonary veins and lung tissue. The lungs are auscultated for abnormal and normal breath sounds. With left-sided congestive heart failure, a crackling sound is heard on auscultation. Wheezes and gurgles also may be heard. Wet lung sounds are accompanied by dyspnea and an effort to sit up to breathe. If uncorrected, left-sided heart failure is followed by right-sided heart failure because the circulatory system is a continuous loop.

SPUTUM

Clients with cardiac disease may have a productive or nonproductive cough. Note the type and frequency of the cough and the amount and appearance of the sputum; it can be important in diagnosing heart failure or other pulmonary complications.

MENTAL STATUS

Some clients with cardiac disorders may be alert and oriented; others may be confused and disoriented. Confusion or disorientation can result from a

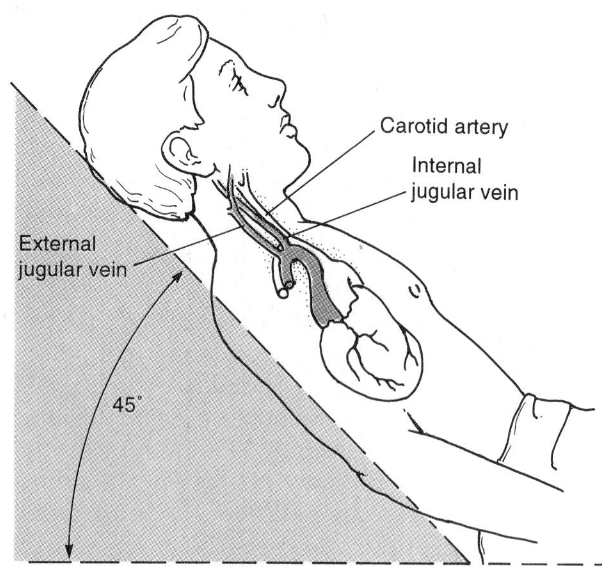

FIGURE 29-9. Jugular vein distention is assessed with th client at a 45-degree angle.

decrease in the oxygen supply to the brain (cerebra ischemia) caused by poor circulation. Chest pain and impaired breathing can create anxiety. Extremes of emotion or an alteration in thought processes is reported to the physician because such an effect could interfere with the client's safety, diagnostic testing, and prescribed therapy.

Diagnostic Studies

LABORATORY TESTS

Various general laboratory tests are used in the diagnosis of heart disease and in monitoring the client's progress. Laboratory tests may be performed daily or every few days. They may be used to monitor the results of therapy.

Blood Chemistry

Laboratory tests that provide a general picture of a client's overall condition and cardiac risks commonly are ordered. Blood chemistries, such as fasting blood glucose and serum electrolyte, cholesterol, and triglyceride levels, may be used as part of the diagnostic analysis.

Serum Enzymes and Isoenzymes

Enzymes are complex proteins produced by living cells that function as catalysts. Catalysts are substances that are capable of producing chemical changes without being changed themselves. An

isoenzyme is one of several forms of the same enzyme that may exist in cells and is capable of being identified separately from others.

When tissues and cells break down, are damaged, or die, great quantities of certain enzymes are released into the bloodstream. The following enzymes are important in cardiac disease.

- Creatine kinase (CK), formerly creatine phosphokinase, and its isoenzymes
- Lactate dehydrogenase (LDH) and its isoenzymes
- Aspartate aminotransferase (AST), formerly serum glutamic- oxaloacetic transaminase.

These enzymes also can be elevated in response to other disorders. Therefore the isoenzymes CK-MB, LDH_1, and LDH_2, are evaluated due to their cardiac specificity.

RADIOGRAPHY AND RADIOISOTOPE STUDIES

Chest radiography and fluoroscopy are used to determine the size and position of the heart and condition of the lungs. These studies are also used to guide the insertion and confirm the placement of cardiac catheters and pacemaker wires. Computed tomography and magnetic resonance imaging are used to determine heart size and detect lung involvement.

Radioisotopes are drugs that are injected into, and travel through, the bloodstream. The radioisotope technetium 99m is used to detect areas of myocardial damage. The radioisotope thallium 201 is used to diagnose ischemic heart disease during a stress test.

ECHOCARDIOGRAPHY

Echocardiography uses ultrasound waves to determine the functioning of the left ventricle and to detect cardiac tumors, congenital defects, and changes in the tissue layers of the heart. High-frequency sound waves, which cannot be heard by the human ear, pass through the chest wall and are displayed on an oscilloscope. The image is recorded and kept as a permanent record.

PHONOCARDIOGRAPHY

Phonocardiography is the graphic representation of normal and abnormal heart sounds. It is used in the diagnosis of valvular and other cardiac disorders. Microphones placed on the chest pick up heart sounds, which are then amplified and converted to electrical impulses. These impulses are relayed to a recorder, which produces a graph of the heart sounds.

ELECTROCARDIOGRAPHY

Electrocardiography is the graphic recording of the electrical currents generated by the heart muscle. This method of studying the heart muscle is especially helpful in identifying cardiac arrhythmias and detecting myocardial damage. Color-coded electrodes matched to corresponding lead wires connect the client to the recording machine. The electrodes are coated with conductive gel and applied to the skin surface (usually on the wrists, ankles, and chest). Computerized ECG machines immediately interpret the tracings, or rhythm strips, which serve as screening devices. The rhythm strips are later interpreted by a physician. The 12-lead ECG is used by the physician to aid in diagnosing heart disease. The nurse can continuously monitor a client's cardiac activity by observing one or more leads.

The ECG pattern consists of waves, intervals, segments, and complexes (see Fig. 29–6). The *P wave* represents the initiation of the electrical impulse that causes depolarization of the atria. The *PR interval* is the period of time it takes from the initiation of the impulse, through the atrial conduction pathways, to the AV node. The *QRS complex*, the collective term for the *Q, R*, and *S waves*, is the measurement of time that it takes for the impulse to spread throughout the ventricles from the AV node to the Purkinje fibers, causing its subsequent depolarization. The *ST segment* represents early repolarization of the ventricular muscle, which ends after the *T wave*. The ST segment is a particularly sensitive indicator of ischemia and myocardial damage. Ischemia causes the ST segment to sag below the baseline (isoelectric line). An elevated ST segment indicates muscle injury. The *QT interval* represents ventricular depolarization and repolarization.

Ambulatory Electrocardiography

Ambulatory ECG, or Holter monitoring, is the recording of an ambulatory client's cardiac rate and rhythm over a 24- to 48-hour period as the client goes about daily activities. The Holter monitor, which is worn on a belt or carried on a shoulder strap, consists of a tape recorder connected to ECG leads attached to the client's chest. During the test period, the client keeps a diary of activities and associated symptoms. At the end of the recording period, the monitor is returned to the hospital or physician and the tape is analyzed. The client's written notes are compared with the recorded information. Ambulatory ECG helps to detect arrhythmias and myocardial ischemia that occur sporadically during activity or rest.

Stress Testing

Stress testing is done to evaluate how the heart functions during exercise. The electrical activity of the heart is assessed with an ECG monitor while the client walks on a treadmill, pedals a stationary bicycle, or climbs up and down stairs.

A resting ECG is taken as a baseline before the test is started. During the test, the speed of the treadmill, the force required to pedal the bicycle, or the pace of stair climbing is gradually increased. The goal is to increase the heart's workload until a predetermined target heart rate is reached. The client's heart rate and rhythm are monitored continuously, and ECG waveforms are recorded periodically. The client's blood pressure and respiratory rate are also assessed. The client is instructed to report the onset of chest pain, dizziness, leg cramps, or weakness. The test is aborted if the client develops chest pain, severe dyspnea, elevated blood pressure, confusion, or arrhythmias. The ECG tracings obtained during the test are interpreted by the physician. Radioisotopes may also be used during a stress test to provide additional information.

CARDIAC CATHETERIZATION

Cardiac catheterization provides a means for measuring fluid pressures within the chambers of the heart and collecting blood samples to analyze the oxygen and carbon dioxide content. A long flexible catheter is inserted from a peripheral blood vessel in the groin, arm, or neck into one of the great vessels and then into the heart. Cardiac catheterization may be carried out on the left side of the heart by way of an artery or on the right side by way of a vein.

Because risks are associated with this procedure, the client or a responsible family member must sign a consent form. If a contrast medium is to be used during the study, the client is asked again about allergies because a reaction could be life-threatening. Food and fluids are restricted for at least 6 hours before the test, and the client is given a sedative. The skin over the catheter insertion site is shaved and cleansed with an antiseptic. The presence and quality of peripheral pulses and skin color and temperature are documented before the start of the procedure.

General anesthesia is not used, although the client is sedated. The client is positioned supine on a padded table in a room equipped with radiography and fluoroscopy. The procedure usually takes 1 or more hours.

The client is alert and often anxious about the procedure. The nurse prepares the client by explaining what will be experienced during the procedure. There is slight discomfort from the vascular incision and insertion of the catheter. As the catheter enters the chambers of the heart and contacts conduction tissue, an irregular heart rhythm may develop accompanied by a fluttering feeling in the chest. In addition, coughing may occur if the catheter is passed into the pulmonary artery. These sensations pass quickly and are no cause for alarm. If the contrast medium is injected, the client is warned that the injection may produce a warm sensation. The room is darkened at intervals during the test to facilitate the use of the fluoroscope. This may not be necessary if a fluoroscopic image amplifier, or image intensifier, is used.

The client is monitored by ECG, and resuscitative equipment is available if a serious arrhythmia develops. When the catheter is withdrawn, a sterile pressure dressing is placed over the insertion site. A sandbag may be applied over the dressing to provide additional pressure to prevent bleeding. Pulmonary edema and air embolism are rare complications. The client's temperature may be elevated for a few hours after the test. Clients who have cardiac catheterization as an outpatient may be discharged as soon as 6 hours after the procedure. Box 29–2 highlights discharge instructions for clients who have had a cardiac catheterization.

ARTERIOGRAPHY

Coronary Arteriography

The most common use of a left-side cardiac catheterization is to determine the degree of blockage of the coronary arteries by performing **arteriography**

BOX 29-2 Discharge Instructions for Clients Having Cardiac Catheterization

- Rest for the next 3 days, and avoid heavy lifting, strenuous activity, or sports during this time.
- Do not drive or climb stairs for the next 24 hours.
- Do not take a tub bath until the puncture site is healed.
- Change the bandage in 24 hours; continue changing the bandage until a crust or scab forms over the puncture site.
- You may experience some soreness at the puncture site; however, if it becomes worse, notify your physician.
- If pain or swelling of the puncture site occurs, notify your physician.
- If the puncture site begins to bleed, hold pressure over the site and call 911 or another emergency services number.

while the catheter is in place. Contrast medium is injected into each coronary artery. Occlusive heart disease is indicated if one or more coronary arteries appear narrow or do not fill. Clients with coronary artery disease who are considered candidates for invasive treatment procedures must undergo cardiac catheterization and coronary arteriography.

After the catheter is removed, the insertion site is inspected for bleeding, tenderness, hematoma formation, and inflammation. The client is kept on bed rest for the rest of the day. Flexion, or bending, of the arm or leg used for catheter insertion is avoided. Vascular assessments distal to the insertion site continue at frequent intervals. Absent distal peripheral pulses, cool toes, and pale or cyanotic arms and legs indicate arterial occlusion, usually from a blood clot. These signs as well as a rapid or irregular pulse rate indicate a medical emergency and must be reported immediately to the physician.

Angiocardiography

In **angiocardiography**, a radiopaque dye is injected into a vein, and its course through the heart is recorded by a series of radiographic pictures taken in rapid succession. The pictures reveal the size and shape of the heart chambers and great vessels and the sequence and time of their filling with dye. Angiocardiography is used particularly to diagnose congenital abnormalities of the heart and great vessels. It usually is performed when simpler diagnostic measures fail to provide the necessary information. The client fasts for at least 3 hours before the test. A sedative and an antihistaminic medication usually are administered before the client is taken to the radiography department.

Aortography

Aortography detects aortic abnormalities such as aneurysms (abnormal dilatation of a blood vessel wall) and arterial occlusions. When aortography is performed, contrast medium is injected and radiographic films are taken of the abdominal aorta and major arteries in the legs. Distribution of the contrast medium may also be observed as it is circulated to other vessels, such as the renal arteries.

Peripheral Arteriography

Peripheral arteriography is used to diagnose occlusive arterial disease in smaller arteries. Contrast medium is injected into an artery, and radiographic films are taken. After the procedure, the chance for bleeding is greater than after a venipuncture; therefore, a pressure dressing is applied and client activity restricted for about 12 hours. The client is observed for bleeding, cardiac arrhythmias, and the adequacy of peripheral circulation by frequent checking of the peripheral pulses.

HEMODYNAMIC MONITORING

Hemodynamic monitoring is used to assess the volume and pressure of blood within the heart and vascular system by means of a surgically inserted catheter. Methods for hemodynamic monitoring include direct blood pressure monitoring, central venous pressure monitoring, and pulmonary artery pressure monitoring. Such monitoring is used to assess cardiac function and circulatory status, detect fluid imbalances, adjust fluid infusion rates, and evaluate the client's response to therapeutic measures, such as drug therapy.

Direct Blood Pressure Monitoring

Direct blood pressure monitoring requires the placement of a catheter within a peripheral artery (Fig. 29–10). The artery most commonly used is the radial artery. The brachial and femoral arteries may also be used. The catheter tip contains a sensor that measures and transmits the fluid pressure to a transducer, which electronically converts the data to a visual waveform. A monitor continuously displays the waveform and indicates the client's systolic, diastolic, and mean arterial pressures. This type of equipment eliminates the need to auscultate the blood pressure. Direct blood pressure monitoring may be used in clients with severe and sustained hypertension or hypotension and intraoperatively and postoperatively in clients who have undergone cardiac surgery. A three-way stopcock can be attached within the tubing to allow the nurse to periodically draw arterial blood samples for blood gas analysis.

Central Venous Pressure Monitoring

Right atrial pressure, or **central venous pressure** (CVP), is the pressure produced by venous blood in the right atrium. Normal CVP is 2 to 7 mm Hg or 4 to 10 cm H_2O. This measurement is used to detect an excess or a deficit in venous blood volume.

To monitor CVP, a catheter is inserted into a large vein, usually the jugular or subclavian vein in the neck and advanced into the superior vena cava or right atrium. The catheter's proximal end is connected to a three-way stopcock, which controls the direction in which intravenous fluid flows. The stopcock may be mounted on a calibrated tube, called a *manometer* (or the catheter may be attached to a transducer that connects to a computer used to analyze hemodynamic data). The manometer is used periodically to measure fluid pressure. The nurse must be familiar with the type of CVP manometer being used.

When measuring CVP, the nurse makes sure that the zero mark on the manometer is at the level of the client's right atrium; otherwise, an incorrect reading is obtained. The client is positioned supine or with the head slightly elevated but in exactly the

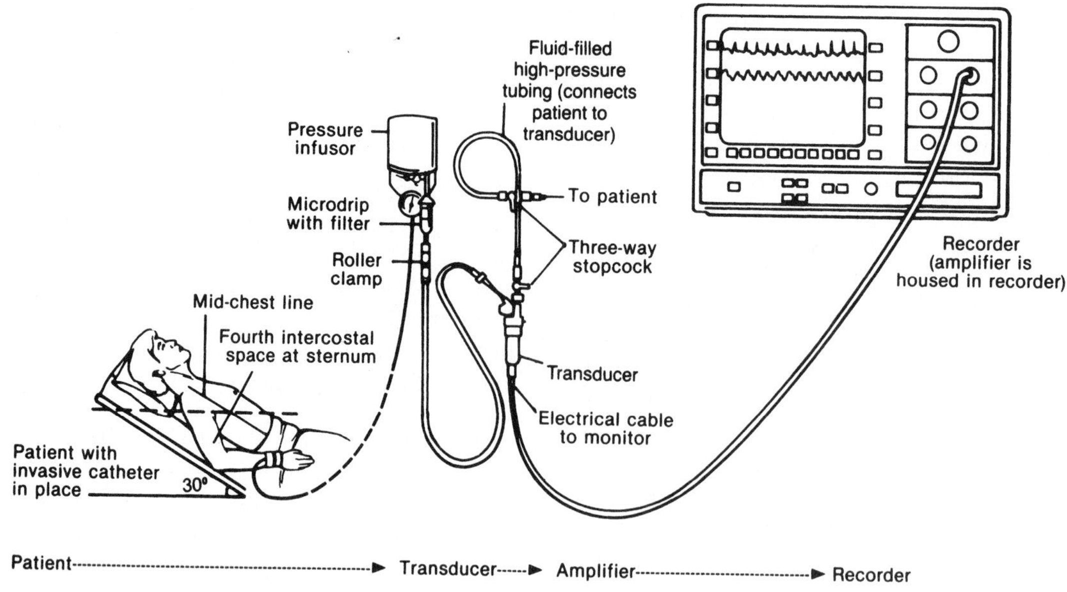

FIGURE 29-10. Blood pressure can be continuously monitored through the radial artery. The indwelling arterial catheter is attached by specialized pressure tubing to a transducer. The transducer is connected to an amplifier/monitor that visually displays a waveform and systolic, diastolic, and mean pressure values. The plumbing system comprises a flush solution under pressure, a continuous flush device, and a series of stopcocks. The stopcocks closest to the insertion site are used to draw blood samples from the artery; the stopcocks located near the transducer are used for zeroing.

same position as during previous measurements. The stopcock is rotated so that the manometer is partially filled with intravenous solution. The fluid in the manometer is then allowed to flow into the client. The fluid stops flowing when the pressure in the manometer equals the pressure in the right atrium. The CVP measurement is obtained by noting the calibrated mark on the manometer that corresponds to the top of the fluid column (Fig. 29–11). The stopcock is then repositioned to resume the infusion of intravenous fluid. Between CVP measurements, the head of the bed can be raised or lowered. The physician orders the frequency of CVP measurements. However, measurements may be obtained any time the nurse suspects a change in the client's fluid status.

Pulmonary Artery Monitoring

By inserting a catheter into the pulmonary artery, pressures and cardiac output can be measured to assess left ventricular function. When in place, the pulmonary artery catheter, a multilumen catheter, can measure both pulmonary artery pressure and right atrial pressure or CVP. Pulmonary artery pressure monitoring aids in the early treatment of fluid imbalance problems, prevents left-sided congestive heart failure or promotes its early correction, and helps monitor the client's response to treatment.

The pulmonary artery catheter is inserted into a large peripheral vein and advanced through the right side of the heart until the distal tip rests in the right or left pulmonary artery. When the small balloon at the tip of the catheter is inflated, the balloon floats forward, eventually wedging in a pulmonary capillary (Fig. 29–12). As the balloon blocks the flow of blood through the capillary, the catheter tip that protrudes from the inflated balloon senses the fluid pressure ahead of it. **Pulmonary capillary wedge pressure** (PCWP) is the retrograde pressure from the fluid on the left side of the heart at the end of left ventricular diastole. Sometimes this is abbreviated LVEDP, for **left ventricular end-diastolic pressure**. The balloon must be deflated immediately after the pressure is measured to avoid pulmonary infarction from prolonged blockage of capillary blood flow.

To measure cardiac output, a syringe with 5 to 10 mL of 5% dextrose in water solution (D5W) is pushed through a port of the catheter. In the past, iced injectate was used, but with the newer computers, injectate at room temperature may be used. A computerized probe measures the temperature change as the fluid exits the catheter within the heart. The com-

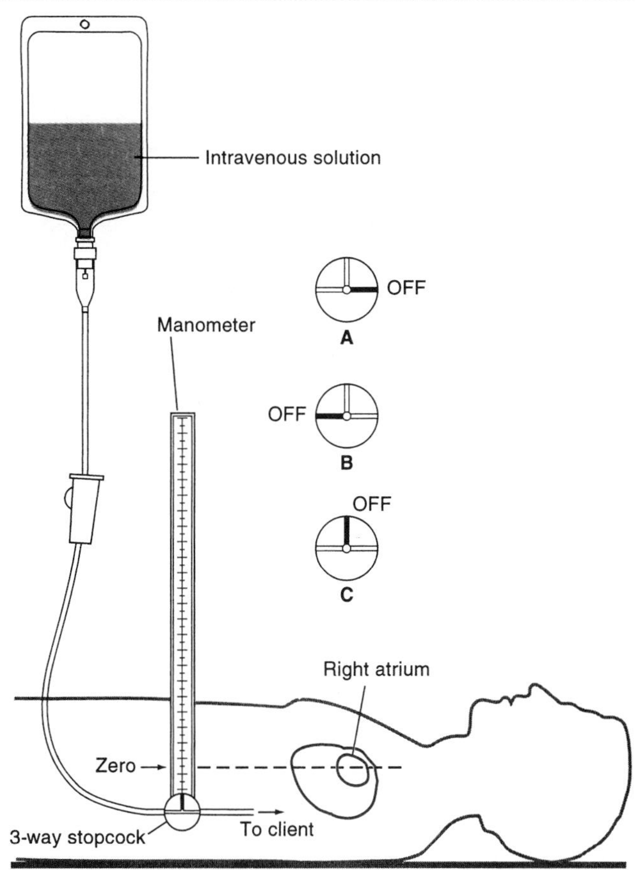

FIGURE 29-11. Central venous pressure measured by a water manometer. The arrow points to the zero mark, which must be at the level of the client's right atrium. (*A*) Stopcock position for filling the manometer. (*B*) Position for measuring the central venous pressure. (*C*) Position for allowing intravenous solution to flow through the tubing to the client, keeping the central venous pressure line patent.

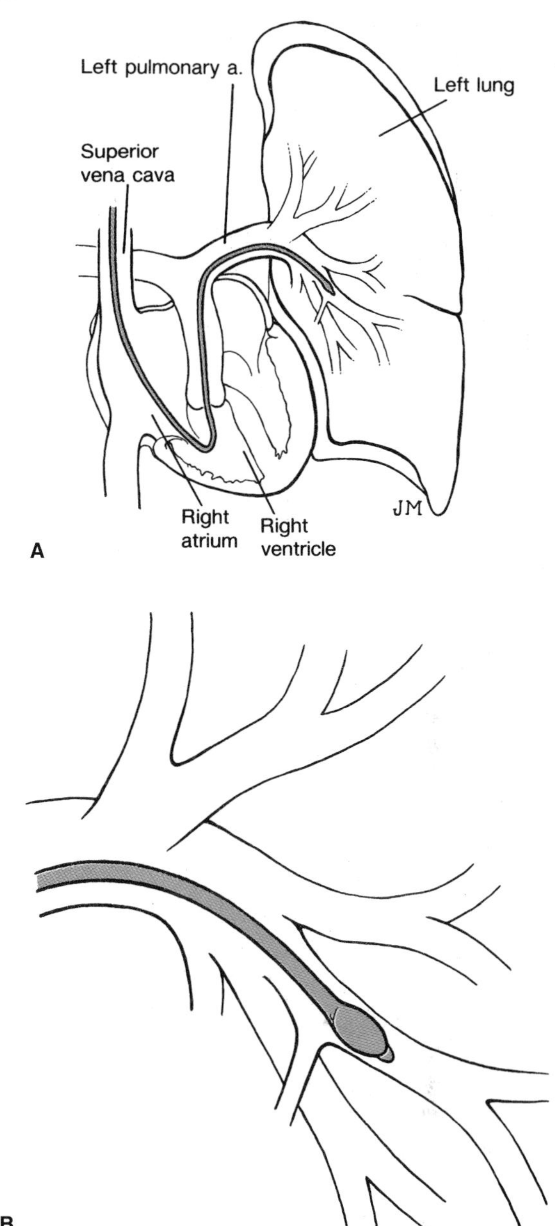

FIGURE 29-12. Fluid status can be monitored with a pulmonary artery catheter. (*A*) Location of the catheter within the heart. The catheter enters the right atrium via the superior vena cava. The balloon is then inflated, allowing the catheter to follow the blood flow through the tricuspid valve, through the right ventricle, through the pulmonic valve, and into the main pulmonary artery. Waveform and pressure readings are noted during insertion to identify the location of the catheter within the heart. The balloon is deflated once the catheter is in the pulmonary artery and properly secured. (*B*) Pulmonary capillary wedge pressure (PCWP). The catheter floats into a distal branch of the pulmonary artery when the balloon is inflated, and becomes "wedged." The wedged catheter occludes blood flow from behind, and the tip of the lumen records pressures in front of the catheter. The balloon is then deflated, allowing the catheter to float back into the main pulmonary artery.

puter then calculates the rate of temperature change with the speed at which the fluid traveled through the heart. A solution that is quite warm after its instillation indicates that the heart's pump function is impaired. If the solution remains close to the instillation temperature, the heart's pump function is working optimally. The computer converts the electronic data into numerical equivalents for cardiac output. The nurse repeats the assessment three to four times in succession and takes the average of the data. Using a formula, the nurse can calculate the **cardiac index**, which reflects the cardiac output in relation to the particular client's body size. The cardiac index is computed by dividing the cardiac output by the client's body surface area. Body surface area is obtained from a **nomogram**, a chart based on height and weight.

NURSING PROCESS
The Client Undergoing Diagnostic Procedures of the Cardiovascular System

Assessment

Some clients undergo diagnostic testing as outpatients; others are tested while they are hospitalized. A thorough initial assessment is necessary to establish accurate baseline data for use before, during, and after a diagnostic procedure. Symptoms often change suddenly. Significant symptoms, such as chest pain or pain in the arms or legs, dyspnea, and changes in heart rate and rhythm or blood pressure, may occur. Any change in the client is reported immediately and recorded before the client undergoes a diagnostic test.

Assess the client's anxiety and knowledge level about the procedure to be performed. Assess baseline vital signs.

Diagnosis and Planning

The nursing care of clients undergoing diagnostic procedures of the cardiovascular system includes but is not limited to:

Nursing Diagnoses and Collaborative Problems	Nursing Interventions
Anxiety related to insecurity **Goal:** The client's anxiety will be reduced.	Greet the client by name and introduce personnel involved in his or her care. Promote a relaxed environment. Allow one person who is supportive to accompany the client as much as possible before, during, or after the test. Orient the client to surroundings. Tell the client when the test will begin and about how long it will take. Keep the client informed of delays in the schedule. Remain in view of the client or establish some other means of contact for assistance.
Knowledge Deficit related to the test's purpose, performance, and after-care **Goal:** The client and family will demonstrate sufficient knowledge on which to provide informed consent and self-care afterwards.	Assess client and family's knowledge concerning test. Provide both verbal and written information concerning the test's purpose, procedure, and after-care. Use language that the client can easily understand. Ask the client and/or family member to paraphrase information. Promote a relaxed environment conducive to asking questions.
Risk for Pain and Activity Intolerance related to ischemia **Goal:** The client's pain will be relieved or controlled within a tolerable level during the diagnostic procedure and activity will be performed without excessive dyspnea or tachycardia.	Assess the client frequently during the diagnostic procedure; notify physician if client develops pain before procedure. Allow for periods of rest. If pain or dyspnea develop stop procedure, assess vital signs, give vasodilator (nitroglycerin) as ordered, and administer oxygen.
Risk for Injury related to untoward reactions during or after diagnostic tests **Goal:** The client's condition will remain stable during and after diagnostic tests.	Assess the client for any of the following: • Dyspnea • Hypo- or hypertension • Cardiac arrhythmias • Mental changes • Pain or discomfort • Cyanosis Collaborate with the physician to restore the client to a stable condition.

Evaluation and Expected Outcomes

- The client is relaxed and feels secure.
- The test is performed uneventfully.
- The client and family have an accurate understanding of the diagnostic testing process and discharge instructions.

General Nutritional Considerations

Food and fluid are withheld before invasive diagnostic procedures and are not resumed until the client is stable and free of nausea and vomiting.

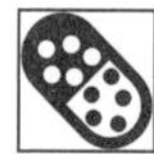

General Pharmacologic Considerations

Medications can affect the blood pressure and the pulse rate and rhythm. When obtaining a medication history, it is important that a list of all prescription and nonprescription medications be obtained from the client or a family member.

When a contrast medium is used during a cardiac catheterization or arteriogram, the patient may feel an intense flushed feeling and the need to void when the dye is injected. Inform the client these feelings will pass within a short period (30 to 60 seconds).

The patient is assessed for iodine or seafood allergy before any diagnostic test requiring an iodinated contrast. Usually a hypoallergenic nonionic contrast may be used if an allergy is suspected.

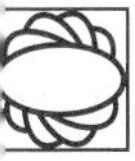

General Gerontologic Considerations

Older clients are more likely to experience confusion and disorientation due to decreased perfusion to the brain that can occur when the cardiopulmonary system is compromised. If so, repeated explanations and reassurances throughout all phases of the nursing process are indicated.

The aging heart is less able to meet the demands placed upon it in times of stress and requires more time to return to base levels after a stressful situation. This inability to handle stress is due to a decrease in cardiac output and contractile strength and a delay in conduction within the heart.

The older adult with renal impairment or who is chronically dehydrated is at increased risk for complications during and after diagnostic studies requiring the use of a dye, because the iodinated contrast is nephrotoxic.

The incidence of cardiac arrhythmias increases with age due to anatomic changes that occur with aging. Arrhythmias are also more serious and difficult to treat in the older adult because organs that are already impaired by aging can be further compromised by the lack of adquate blood supply caused by the arrhythmia.

SUMMARY OF KEY CONCEPTS

- The heart consists of four chambers—two atria and two ventricles. The right and left sides of the heart act as a double pump. The right side pumps blood to the lungs. The left side pumps blood to cells and tissues. The myocardium is the muscular layer of the heart. Heart contraction is called systole; relaxation is called diastole. The right and left coronary arteries supply oxygenated blood to the heart itself. The cells of the heart possess five unique characteristics: automaticity, excitability, conductivity, contractility, and rhythmicity.
- Assessments that are essential when caring for the cardiac client include pain characteristics, vital signs (especially pulse rate and rhythm and blood pressure), presence and quality of peripheral pulses, heart sounds, and presence of edema.
- Some common diagnostic tests performed on clients suspected of having cardiovascular disease include resting ECG, stress test, echocardiography, cardiac catheterization, and coronary arteriography.
- When managing the care of a client undergoing cardiovascular tests, the nurse performs a comprehensive assessment, reports unusual findings, utilizes techniques to relieve anxiety, provides appropriate information and health teaching, and monitors and responds to adverse responses that occur during the tests.

CRITICAL THINKING EXERCISES

1. A client is scheduled to have a pulmonary artery catheter inserted. The client's spouse asks you what the catheter is for, and what will happen once it is placed. How will you respond?
2. You are assisting a client who is undergoing a stress test. The client becomes cyanotic and short of breath. What is your next course of action? What follow-up care will be indicated?

Suggested Readings

Caldwell, M. A., Drew, B. J., & Pelter, M. M. (1996). Chest pain is an unreliable measure of ischemia in men and women during PTCA. *Heart Lung, 25*(6), 423–429

Dvorak-King, C. (1997, November). PA catheter numbers made easy. *RN, 60*, 11.

Ellis, J., Nowlis, E., & Bentz, P. (1996). Modules for basic nursing skills (6th ed.). Philadelphia: Lippincott-Raven.

Hudak, C. M., & Gallo, B. M. (1994). *Critical care nursing: A holistic approach* (6th ed., p. 189). Philadelphia: J. B. Lippincott.

Guyton, A. C. (1996). *Textbook of medical physiology* (9th ed.). Philadelphia: Saunders.

Hochrein, M. A., & Sohl L. (1992, December). Heart smart: A guide to cardiac tests. *American Journal of Nursing, 22*, 22.

Kienast J., & Fitzgerald D. (1997). Identifying and treating femoral artery pseudoaneurysms following invasive cardiac procedures. *MEDSURG Nursing, 6*(2), 95–97, 106.

Kirton, C. (1996, February). Assessing normal heart sounds. *Nursing, 26*,(2), 56–57.

Memmler, R. L., Cohen, B. J., & Wood, D. L. (1996). The human body in health and disease (8th ed.). Philadelphia: Lippincott-Raven.

Montes, P. (1997). Managing outpatient cardiac catheterization. *American Journal of Nursing, 97*(1), 34–37.

Olbrych, D. D. (1993). Interpreting CPK and LDH results. *Nursing, 23*(1), 48–49.

Additional Resources

Nursing Net
http://www.communique.net/-nursgnt/

American Association of Critical Care Nurses
http://www.aacn.org

Heartweb
http://webaxis.com/heartweb/

National Institute of Health Home Page
http://www.nih.gov

Nursing Healthweb
http://www.lib.umich.edu/html/nursing.html

Chapter 30

Caring for Clients With Infectious and Inflammatory Disorders of the Heart and Blood Vessels

KEY TERMS

Cardiac tamponade
Carditis
Doppler ultrasound
Effusion
Emboli
Homan's sign
Hypertrophic cardiomyopathy
Impedance plethysmography
Intermittent claudication
Pericardiectomy
Pericardiocentesis
Pericardiostomy
Petechiae
Plication procedure
Polyarthritis
Precordial pain
Pulsus paradoxus
Splinter hemorrhages
Sympathectomy
Thrombectomy
Vegetations
Venography

LEARNING OBJECTIVES

On completion of this chapter, the reader will:

- List four inflammatory conditions of the heart.
- Identify three organisms that cause infectious conditions of the heart.
- Describe treatment for inflammatory heart disorders.
- Discuss the nursing management of clients with infectious or inflammatory heart disorders.
- Differentiate between thrombophlebitis and thromboangiitis obliterans.
- List three interventions that reduce the risk of thrombophlebitis in the hospitalized client.
- Discuss the nursing management of clients with inflammatory disorders of peripheral blood vessels.

The body uses many defense mechanisms to combat the effects of trauma, disease, and microorganisms. The inflammatory response, the skin and mucous membranes, and the immune system work together to protect the body's cardiovascular system. Despite these protective mechanisms, infections and inflammatory disorders may compromise the cardiovascular system.

Infectious and Inflammatory Disorders of the Heart

Rheumatic Fever and Rheumatic Heart Disease

Rheumatic fever is a systemic inflammatory disease that occurs as a result of group A streptococcal infections of the throat. Rheumatic heart disease refers to the cardiac manifestations of rheumatic fever, in either the acute or later stage.

ETIOLOGY AND PATHOPHYSIOLOGY

Rheumatic fever is often called an autoimmune disorder because it occurs after the body is exposed to a bacterial toxin that is similar to antigens within the body's own tissues. Antibodies mistakenly identify the normal cells in the heart and joints as foreign and, consequently, attack and destroy them (Fig. 30–1).

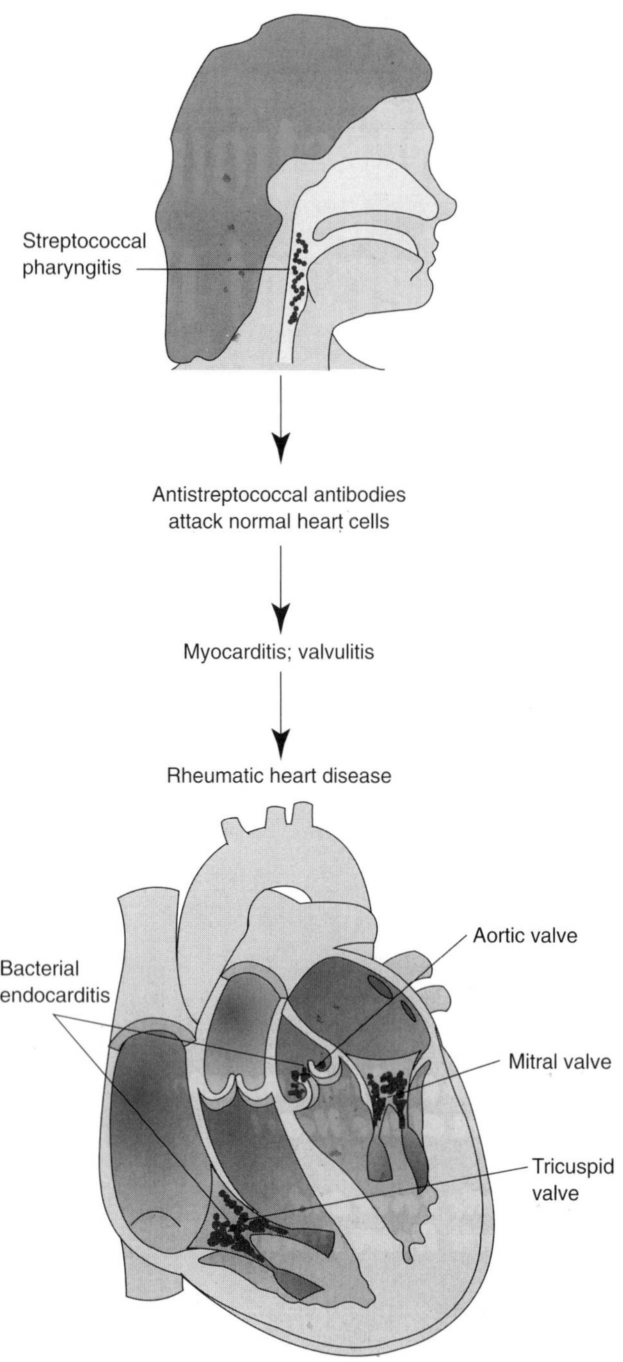

FIGURE 30-1. Rheumatic heart disease and bacterial endocarditis after group A streptococcal pharyngitis.

ASSESSMENT FINDINGS

Signs and Symptoms

Rheumatic fever involves several body systems, including the heart, joints, and nervous system. Some people may experience mild symptoms and fail to seek treatment. Acute rheumatic fever occurs most often among children about 2 to 3 weeks after a streptococcal infection. **Carditis** (inflammation of the layers of the heart), **polyarthritis** (inflammation o more than one joint), rash, subcutaneous nodules and *chorea* (involuntary muscle twitching) are th classic symptoms. Adults do not exhibit the same degree and range of symptoms as young children.

A mild fever, if untreated, continues for severa weeks. The heart rate is rapid because of the fever and abnormal rhythms may occur. A red, spotty rash appears on the trunk but disappears rapidly, leaving irregular circles on the skin in its place. Several joints most commonly the knees, ankles, hips, and shoulders, become swollen, warm, red, and painful. The involvement migrates from joint to joint. Sometimes marble-sized nodules appear around the joints. Motor disturbances cause involuntarily grimacing and an inability to use skeletal muscles in a coordinated manner. Complications may develop. A heart murmur suggests valve damage; a pericardial friction rub is indicative of pericarditis.

Diagnostic Findings

No laboratory test is specific for the diagnosis o rheumatic fever. The results of laboratory tests such as an antistreptolysin O titer, erythrocyte sedimentation rate, and C-reactive protein are elevated, indicating an inflammatory process involving the streptococcal organism. Specific cardiac tests, such as electrocardiography (ECG) and echocardiography, may show structural changes in the valves, the size of the heart, and the heart's ability to contract.

MEDICAL AND SURGICAL MANAGEMENT

Intravenous (IV) antibiotics are given. Penicillin is the drug of choice for group A streptococci, unless contraindicated due to an allergy. Bed rest may be indicated depending on the client's condition. Aspirin is used to control the formation of blood clots that can occur near heart valves. Steroids may be used to suppress the inflammatory response.

The treatment of rheumatic heart disease depends on the extent of damage. If minor, no treatment may be given; if heart failure or life-threatening arrhythmias occur, extensive treatment is necessary. Surgery may be required to treat the complications of carditis, such as constrictive pericarditis and damage to heart valves.

NURSING MANAGEMENT

The nurse administers the prescribed drug therapy and monitors for adverse effects and evidence of the drug's effectiveness. Diversional activities that require minimal activity, such as reading and putting puzzles together, are planned to counteract the boredom of weeks of bed rest. Focused cardiac assessments help to track the progression or improvement of heart involvement. Clients with a history of rheumatic fever are susceptible to infective endocarditis and are told to take prophylactic antibiotics before any invasive procedure, including dental work. Additional nursing management depends on the assessment data.

Infective Endocarditis

Infective endocarditis (formerly called *bacterial endocarditis*) is an inflammation of the inner layer of heart tissue.

ETIOLOGY AND PATHOPHYSIOLOGY

The microorganisms that cause infective endocarditis include bacteria and fungi (Box 30–1). *Streptococcus viridans* and *Staphylococcus aureus* are the bacteria most frequently responsible for this disorder. They are found abundantly on the skin and the mucous membranes of the mouth, nose, throat, and other cavities.

BOX 30-1 Microorganisms That Cause Endocarditis

STREPTOCOCCI	
	Common inhabitant of the mouth and upper respiratory tract. Accounts for up to 80% of cases.
S. viridans	Has a tendency to affect previously damaged heart valves.
STAPHYLOCOCCI	
S. aureus	Virulent strain with high mortality.
S. epidermidis	Associated with dental procedures and valve replacements.
S. faecalis	Causes both acute and subacute infections. Associated with urologic instrumentation in men.
FUNGI	
Candida	Increased incidence in IV drug users. Risk is increased with improper use of antibiotics and steroids.
GRAM-NEGATIVE BACTERIA	
Escherichia coli *Klebsiella* *Pseudomonas*	May travel from gastrointestinal or genitourinary tracts, increased risk in elderly.

Most pathogens find their way into the bloodstream through a cut or break in the skin or mucous membrane. Although anyone can contract endocarditis, clients with a history of rheumatic fever are especially susceptible. Prolonged IV therapy, insertion of cardiac pacemakers, cardiac catheterization, tracheal intubation, cardiac surgery, repeated genitourinary instrumentation (Foley catheters), and IV drug abuse also are portals of entry for the microorganisms that cause endocarditis.

Once the microorganisms infect the heart, they congregate around the heart valves, chordae tendineae, and papillary muscles (see Fig. 30–1). Fibrin, platelets, and blood cells stick to the injured endothelium, forming **vegetations**. The microorganisms bury themselves within the vegetative mass, making them difficult to destroy with antibiotic therapy. The mitral valve is the most common location of vegetations. If the valve leaflets erode and slough, blood leaks between the heart chambers, diminishing the efficiency of the heart as a pump. Heart failure is often a consequence. The vegetations can break off to form **emboli**, mobile masses of tissue that circulate in the bloodstream. Emboli may occlude small blood vessels and interfere with an organ's blood supply.

ASSESSMENT FINDINGS

Signs and Symptoms

Infective endocarditis can have an insidious onset with slight fever, headache, malaise, and fatigue. As the condition advances, purplish, painful nodules may be present on the pads of the fingers and toes. Black longitudinal lines, called **splinter hemorrhages**, can be seen in the nails. The spleen may be enlarged, and tenderness may be apparent on abdominal palpation. A heart murmur caused by malfunctioning valves may be present. **Petechiae**, tiny reddish hemorrhagic spots on the skin and mucous membranes, are signs of embolization. Pronounced weakness, anorexia, and weight loss are common. Symptoms can change suddenly if embolization or heart failure occurs. Emboli to the brain cause cerebrovascular accidents; emboli to the kidneys cause flank pain and renal failure; pulmonary emboli result in sudden chest pain and dyspnea. Clients experiencing heart failure present with dyspnea, hypotension, and peripheral or pulmonary edema.

Diagnostic Findings

Anemia and slight leukocytosis are common findings. Blood cultures identify the microorganism circulating in the blood. Echocardiography reveals the vegetations and impaired pumping quality of the ventricles. Abnormalities in heart rhythm may occur if the vegetations involve a valve that lies close to conduction tissue.

MEDICAL AND SURGICAL MANAGEMENT

High doses of antibiotics are prescribed. The antibiotic is given by continuous or intermittent IV administration over a period of 2 to 6 weeks or longer. If the infection recurs after the drugs have been stopped, antibiotic therapy is resumed. Bed rest is ordered initially. When the client begins to improve, bathroom privileges and increased activity are allowed.

If a heart valve has been severely damaged, and if drug therapy does not adequately support the heart in failure, valve replacement may be necessary. Valve replacement is discussed in Chapter 36.

NURSING MANAGEMENT

Appreciating the danger of the disease without seeing external signs of the damage that is occurring is often difficult for the client. The client needs gentle but firm reminding that activity must be limited. Changes in weight, pulse rate and rhythm, and the appearance of new symptoms is reported.

The prescribed antibiotic is administered around the clock to sustain therapeutic blood levels of the medication at all times. Clients are informed that periodic antibiotic therapy is a lifelong necessity because they will be vulnerable to the disease for the rest of their lives.

Myocarditis

Myocarditis is an inflammation of the myocardium (the muscle layer of the heart).

ETIOLOGY AND PATHOPHYSIOLOGY

A viral, bacterial, fungal, or parasitic infection causes myocarditis. The myocardium also can become inflamed from the toxins of microorganisms, chronic alcohol abuse, radiation therapy, or autoimmune disorders. Most cases of myocarditis in the United States have a viral origin.

Whatever the damaging agent, an inflammatory response occurs causing the muscle tissue to swell. Swelling interferes with the myocardium's ability to stretch and recoil. Cardiac output is reduced and the circulation of blood is impaired. The myocardium becomes ischemic from a reduced supply of oxygenated blood, predisposing the client to tachycardia and arrhythmias. **Hypertrophic cardiomyopathy** (diffuse enlargement and thickening of the heart) is a complication of myocarditis.

ASSESSMENT FINDINGS

Signs and Symptoms

Clients may complain of general chest discomfort relieved by sitting up, low-grade fever, tachycardia, arrhythmias, dyspnea, malaise, fatigue, and anorexia. The skin may be pale or cyanotic. If the pumping activity of the heart becomes impaired, neck vein distention, ascites, and peripheral edema may be noted indicating right-sided heart failure, or crackles heard in the lungs if the left side fails. An S_3 galloping rhythm or a pericardial friction rub may be heard.

Diagnostic Findings

Serum electrolyte levels and thyroid function studies help to rule out other causes for the client's symptoms. The white blood cell count is slightly elevated. C-reactive protein, a nonspecific antigen–antibody test, is elevated in inflammatory conditions. Cardiac isoenzyme levels are elevated and the ECG may be abnormal. Radioisotope imaging displays abnormal ventricular wall motion and reduced ejection of blood from the heart. Chest radiography shows an overall enlargement of the heart and fluid infiltration in the lungs.

MEDICAL AND SURGICAL MANAGEMENT

Management is aimed at treating the underlying cause and preventing complications. Antibiotics are prescribed if the infecting microorganism is bacterial. Bed rest, a sodium-restricted diet, and cardiotonic drugs (digitalis and related drugs) are prescribed to prevent or treat heart failure. In severe cases of cardiomyopathy, a heart transplant is necessary.

NURSING MANAGEMENT

The nurse monitors the client's cardiopulmonary status to assess for possible complications such as congestive heart failure or arrhythmias. This includes obtaining daily weights, recording intake and output, assessing heart and lung sounds, and monitoring dependent edema. The nurse also maintains the client on bed rest to reduce cardiac workload and promote healing.

Pericarditis

Pericarditis, inflammation of the pericardium, can occur as a *primary condition* (one that develops independently of any other condition) or as a *secondary condition* (one that develops because of another condition). The inflammation can occur with or without **effusion**, the accumulation of fluid within two layers of tissue.

ETIOLOGY AND PATHOPHYSIOLOGY

Pericarditis usually occurs secondary to endocarditis, myocarditis, chest trauma, myocardial infarction (heart attack), or after cardiac surgery. Other contributing causes include tuberculosis, malignant tumors, uremia, and connective tissue disorders.

When the pericardial cells become inflamed, their membranes become more permeable and intracellular fluid leaks into the interstitial spaces (Fig. 30–2). The exudate or effusion can be serous, resembling clear serum; fibrinous, like thick, congealed liquid; purulent, containing pus; or sanguineous, containing blood.

Pericardial fluid accumulation results in acute compression of the heart, or **cardiac tamponade**. The fluid takes up space the heart needs for expanding as it fills (Fig. 30–3). This is reflected by a condition called pulsus paradoxus or paradoxical pulse. **Pulsus paradoxus** is an abnormal drop in systolic blood pressure during inspiration in clients with cardiac tamponade. Because the rigid pericardium limits heart expansion, the increase in capacity of the right ventricle that occurs with inspiration causes a reduction in the capacity of the left ventricle. The smaller capacity reduces the stroke volume from the left ventricle. This is reflected in a sudden drop in systolic blood pressure by 10 or more mm Hg (Clinical Procedure 30–1). As cardiac tamponade progresses, stroke volume is diminished, reducing cardiac output, and resulting in death if uncorrected.

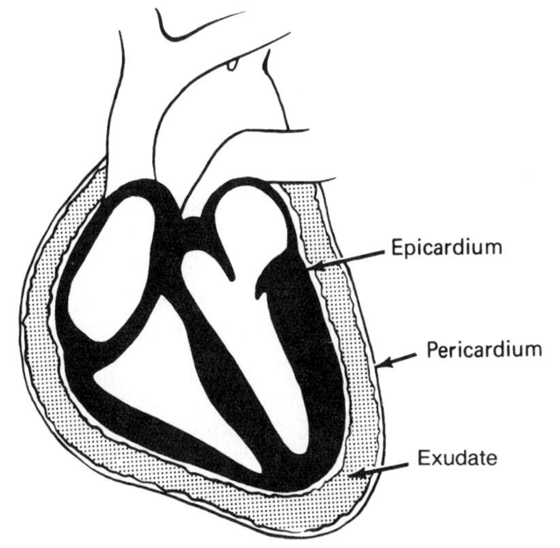

FIGURE 30-2. Pericarditis. Normally, the epicardium and the pericardium slide over each other easily. They are lubricated by a small amount of fluid, which is replaced in pericarditis by thicker material.

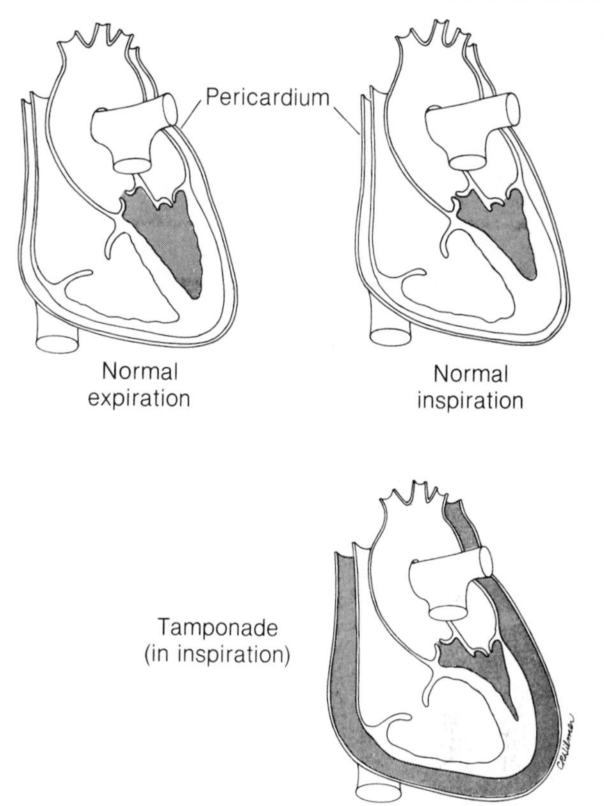

FIGURE 30-3. Effect of respiration and cardiac tamponade on ventricular filling and cardiac output.

ASSESSMENT FINDINGS

Signs and Symptoms

The typical signs and symptoms that accompany an inflammatory response, such as fever and malaise, are present. The client is dyspneic or complains of heaviness in the chest. One chief characteristic is **precordial pain** (pain in the anterior chest overlying the heart). It may be slight or severe and can be mistaken for esophagitis, indigestion, pleurisy, or myocardial infarction. Moving and deep breathing worsen the pain; sitting upright and leaning forward relieve the pain. In contrast, the pain of acute myocardial infarction remains unchanged regardless of position, movement, or breathing. A pericardial friction rub, a scratchy, high-pitched sound, is a diagnostic sign. Heart sounds, muffled by the accumulating fluid, are difficult to hear. Respiratory symptoms occur as the enlarged heart crowds the airway passages and lung

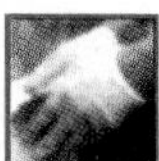

Clinical Procedure 30-1
Assessment of Pulsus Paradoxus

Pulsus paradoxus is an abnormal symptom common in cardiac tamponade or pericarditis. Normally, the systolic arterial pulse falls 4 to 5 mm Hg during inspiration. An inspiratory decrease in the pulse of more than 10 mm Hg is considered abnormal.

Nursing Action	Rationale
Advise client to breathe normally throughout the procedure.	Provides information; decreases chance of error.
Inflate blood pressure (BP) cuff 20 mm Hg above systolic pressure. Begin to slowly deflate cuff, note when the first BP sound (Korotkoff's) is heard.	During deflation, it will become evident that some sound will be audible during expiration but not during inspiration.
Continue to deflate the cuff until BP sounds are heard during both inspiration and expiration.	Disorders that restrict the ability of the heart to contract cause a dramatic fall in the systolic blood pressure during inspiration.
Measure the difference in mm Hg between the first BP sound during expiration and the first BP sound heard during both inspiration and expiration.	

tissue and respirations become rapid and labored. There is severe hypotension, and weak pulse quality.

Diagnostic Findings

The ST segment of the ECG is elevated, but cardiac isoenzyme levels are normal. The heart may appear enlarged on chest radiography. Echocardiography demonstrates a wide gap between the pericardium and the epicardium, indicating that the space is filled with fluid. Hemodynamic monitoring values are abnormal. Pericardial fluid may be cultured, but if the cause of the pericarditis is nonbacterial, the test results often are nondiagnostic.

MEDICAL AND SURGICAL MANAGEMENT

Myocardial infarction must be ruled out. Treatment depends on the underlying cause. Rest, analgesics, antipyretics, nonsteroidal anti-inflammatory drugs, and sometimes corticosteroids are prescribed. **Pericardiocentesis**, needle aspiration of fluid from between the visceral and parietal pericardium, may be necessary when cardiac output is severely reduced. A small drainage catheter can be left in place. Needle aspiration is hazardous because the needle can puncture the myocardium, a branch of a coronary artery, or the pleura.

In cases where pericardiocentesis and catheter drainage are inadequate, an opening or window is made in the pericardium (**pericardiostomy**) to allow the fluid to drain. Constrictive pericarditis is treated surgically by removing the pericardium (**pericardiectomy** or *decortication*) to allow more adequate filling and contraction of the heart chambers.

NURSING PROCESS
The Client With Pericarditis

Assessment

Ask the client about the nature of the pain and what worsens it. Assess for a pericardial friction rub by asking the client to briefly hold his or her breath while auscultating heart sounds; a pericardial friction rub will not disappear when the breath is held. Assess for signs and symptoms of cardiac tamponade (Fig. 30–4) and decreased cardiac output.

Diagnosis and Planning

The care of the client with pericarditis includes, but is not limited to, the following:

Nursing Diagnoses and Collaborative Problems	Nursing Interventions
Pain related to pericardial inflammation **Goal:** Client will be free of pain or pain will be tolerable 30 minutes after analgesic is administered.	Assess pain status frequently. Assist client to a position of comfort. Administer anti-inflammatories and analgesics, as needed. Evaluate pain level after medications are given, notify physician if pain is not relieved. Reassure client that pericardial pain does not indicate a heart attack.
Potential Complication: Decreased Cardiac Output	Monitor frequently for changes in vital signs and hemodynamic parameters. Assess lung

Goal: The nurse will manage and minimize symptoms of decreased cardiac output.

sounds every 8 hours. Assess peripheral pulses, level of consciousness, and anxiety level. Assess for signs of cardiac tamponade such as tachycardia, pulsus paradoxus, restlessness, and distended neck veins. Administer supplemental O_2. Have emergency pericardiocentesis tray available.

Evaluation and Expected Outcomes

- The client states pain is relieved.
- Vital signs are stable and there is no arrhythmia.

If pericardiocentesis is performed, the nurse reinforces the information provided by the physician, witnesses the client's signature on the consent form, prepares the equipment at the bedside, and obtains baseline vital signs for comparison after the procedure. The amount of fluid removed by pericardiocentesis is measured, recorded, and described. Specimens obtained during pericardiocentesis for cancerous cells or culture are properly labeled and sent to the laboratory. The site is covered with a sterile dressing and inspected for bleeding or leakage of fluid. As the dressing becomes moist, it is reinforced or changed. Significant changes in breathing, heart rate and rhythm, and blood pressure are reported because they could indicate complications. Relief of respiratory symptoms, return of the heart rate and blood pressure to more normal levels, strong pulse quality, and increased urine output are signs to monitor because they indicate that pericardiocentesis was therapeutic.

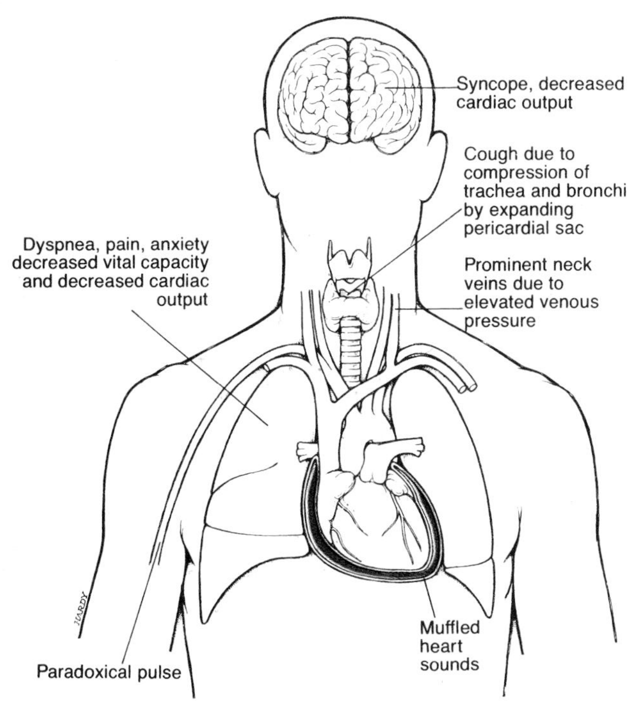

FIGURE 30-4. Assessment for cardiac tamponade due to pericardial effusion.

Client and Family Teaching for Clients With Infectious and Inflammatory Disorders

Explain the procedures required during therapy and the importance of each treatment modality to the client and family. Provide an opportunity for them to ask questions. Inform clients with endocarditis and other infectious or inflammatory disorders of the heart of the necessity for continued follow-up care, as they will always be at risk for endocarditis. Inform those with a history of rheumatic fever, congenital valve disorders, or prosthetic valve replacements to see their physician if fever, malaise, or other symptoms of infection occur. Instruct clients with damaged heart valves concerning the need for antibiotics just before, and for a short time after, an event that might cause bacteremia, such as dental surgery. Make sure clients who are prescribed antibiotics understand that they must take the full dose for the full time. Noncompliance with the drug regimen can hinder the complete destruction of the pathogen.

Explain how medication is to be taken. Identify the potential adverse effects and what signs need to be reported. Provide written instructions or pamphlets explaining the prescribed drugs if they are written in language the lay person can understand. Find discreet ways of quizzing the client, such as asking, "How often must you take this drug?" to evaluate if the instructions have been understood. Document the information that has been provided and evidence of the client's understanding. Frequently prescribed drugs for infectious or inflammatory disorders of the heart can be found in Table 30–1.

Inflammatory Disorders of the Peripheral Blood Vessels

Thrombophlebitis

Thrombophlebitis is an inflammation of a vein accompanied by clot formation.

ETIOLOGY AND PATHOPHYSIOLOGY

Venous stasis (slowed circulation), altered blood coagulation, and trauma to the vein predispose clients to

TABLE 30-1 **Drugs Used in the Treatment of Infectious and Inflammatory Disorders of the Heart**

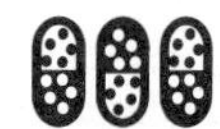

Drug Category/Drug Action	Side Effects	Nursing Considerations
Anticoagulants		
heparin sodium (Hepalean) Inhibits thrombus and clot formation by blocking the conversion of prothrombin to thrombin and fibrinogen to fibrin.	Hemorrhage, bruising, thrombocytopenia, alopecia, chills, fever, increased chance of hemorrhage with oral anticoagulants	Monitor results of partial thromboplastin time (PTT) and clotting times. Apply pressure to all intramuscular injection sites, monitor for epistaxis, other forms of bleeding, have protamine sulfate on unit in case of overdose.
Nonsteroidal Anti-inflammatory Drugs		
aspirin Inhibits the synthesis of prostaglandins causing analgesia and anti-inflammatory action. Antipyretic action is not understood. Inhibits platelet aggregation.	Nausea, epigastric pain, occult blood loss, anaphylaxis, tinnitus, dizziness, increased risk of bleeding especially if given with anticoagulants	Ascertain allergy to aspirin, give drugs with food, do not crush or chew enteric-coated or sustained-release tablets. Aspirin is not drug of choice for children.
Corticosteroids		
cortisone (Cortone Acetate) Exerts anti-inflammatory and immunosuppressive effects.	Headaches, mood swings, ulcers, hypertension, fluid and electrolyte disturbance, amenorrhea, muscle weakness, hyperglycemia in clients with diabetes. Masks signs and symptoms of infection.	Do not discontinue abruptly, taper dosage. Limit exposure to clients with infectious diseases, monitor for salt, water retention, monitor for increased glucose levels.
Antibiotics		
penicillin G potassium (Pfizerpen) Inhibits cell wall synthesis in susceptible organisms, causing cell death.	Anaphylaxis, glossitis, gastritis, sore mouth, nausea, vomiting, diarrhea, rash, fever, superinfection, phlebitis	Ascertain if penicillin allergy exists, monitor for 30 min after first parenteral dose given, assess IV site for pain and signs or symptoms of phlebitis.

thrombophlebitis. Factors that contribute to clot formation include inactivity, reduced cardiac output, compression of the veins in the pelvis or legs, and injury. Some drugs and chemicals that are given IV also irritate the vein. Elderly clients with heart and blood vessel disease are susceptible to thrombophlebitis. The risk for clot formation is increased among women who take oral contraceptives, although the exact triggering mechanism is not known. Women who take oral contraceptives and smoke are at even higher risk.

When the inner lining of the vein is irritated or injured, platelets clump together, forming a clot. The presence of the clot interferes with blood flow, causing congestion of venous blood distal to the blood clot. Sometimes collateral vessels are able to recirculate the blood blocked by the clot. The presence of accumulated waste products in the blocked vessel irritate the vein wall, initiating the inflammatory response. The increased permeability of cells and the convergence of leukocytes and lymphocytes cause the area to swell, redden, and feel warm and tender.

ASSESSMENT FINDINGS

Signs and Symptoms

Clients with thrombophlebitis frequently complain of discomfort in the affected extremity. Calf pain that increases on dorsiflexion of the foot is referred to as a positive **Homan's sign**. Along the length of the affected vein there is heat, redness, and swelling. Capillary refill takes less than 2 seconds because of venous congestion. The client often has a fever, malaise, fatigue, and anorexia.

Diagnostic Findings

Most cases of thrombophlebitis are diagnosed on clinical findings alone. **Venography**, using radiopaque dye instilled into the venous system, indicates a filling defect in the area of the clot. **Doppler ultrasound** may detect an area of venous obstruction. The results of Doppler ultrasound are sometimes difficult to interpret because there are so many collateral vessels, and deep veins are especially difficult to assess. **Impedance plethysmography** (IPG) is the preferred test for diagnosing clots within deep veins. During IPG, a sensor records blood volume in the arm or leg before and after inflating a blood pressure cuff to stop venous blood flow. If a clot is present, the blood volumes are nearly the same because venous return is impaired by the clot.

MEDICAL AND SURGICAL MANAGEMENT

Complete rest of the arm or leg is essential to prevent the thrombus from breaking free and floating in the circulation (embolus). Anticoagulant therapy with heparin or oral anticoagulants is prescribed to decrease the incidence of future clot formation (see Table 30–1). People with repeated episodes may be placed on long-term oral anticoagulant therapy. Continuous warm, wet packs are ordered to improve circulation, ease pain, and decrease inflammation.

Surgical intervention may be necessary when a large vein is occluded by a clot or the danger of a pulmonary embolus arises. **Thrombectomy**, the surgical removal of a clot, is performed if the clot interferes with venous drainage from a large vein such as the femoral vein. With danger of pulmonary emboli, surgery on the inferior vena cava may be necessary to reduce the possibility of a clot traveling from the legs to the lungs. Several surgical procedures may be performed on the vena cava: ligation of the vena cava, insertion of an umbrella-like prosthesis in the vena cava (to catch emboli before they reach the heart and lungs), or vena caval plication. A **plication procedure** changes the lumen of the vena cava from a single channel to several small channels through the use of a suture or a Teflon clip.

NURSING MANAGEMENT

One of the most important roles for the nurse is to prevent venous stasis and thrombophlebitis by promoting activity and exercise for at risk clients. Ankle pumping exercises are imperative for clients on bed rest (Fig. 30–5). For inactive clients, apply knee- or thigh-high elastic stockings or use a pneumatic venous compression device that alternately inflates and deflates to support vein walls and promote venous circulation. Assist the client to change positions frequently. Avoid restricting venous blood flow from prolonged sitting or gatching the bed at the knees. For additional nursing management of a client who develops a thrombophlebitis, refer to the nursing process discussion.

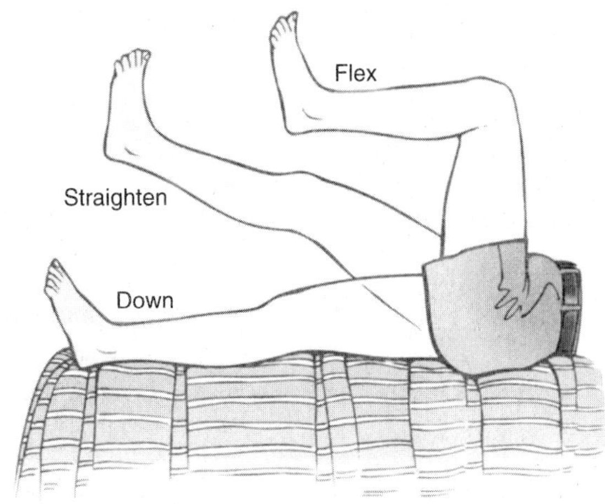

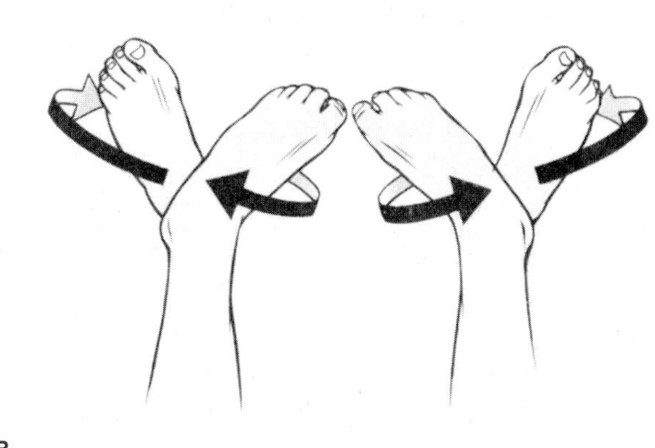

FIGURE 30-5. Leg exercises help prevent thrombophlebitis. (*A*) Have client bend knee, raise the foot, and hold for three seconds. Repeat with each leg 5 times each hour. (*B*) Have client trace circles 5 times with each foot every hour.

NURSING PROCESS
The Client With Thrombophlebitis

Assessment

Determine if Homans' sign is positive. Ask the client whether there is pain or tenderness in the affected extremity. Inspect the color, temperature, and size of the leg (or arm) and compare with the unaffected extremity. Check if a low-grade fever is present and monitor body temperature on a regular basis.

Diagnosis and Planning

The plan of care for a client with thrombophlebitis includes but is not limited to the following:

Nursing Diagnoses and Collaborative Problems	Nursing Interventions
Potential Complication: Embolism (moving clot)	Maintain bedrest; do *not* rub or massage the affected extremity.
Goal: An embolic episode will be managed and minimized.	Administer prescribed anticoagulant therapy. Check and report coagulation test results daily to the physician before administering the next dose. Monitor for signs of bruising or bleeding.
	Elevate the head of the bed, give oxygen, and report chest pain, dyspnea, or tachycardia immediately.
Pain related to imflammation **Goal:** The client's discomfort will be relieved or reduced to a tolerable level.	Administer prescribed analgesia and antiinflammatory agents.
	Support and handle the extremity gently.
Altered Tissue Perfusion related to localized swelling secondary to impaired venous circulation **Goal:** Tissue will have adequate venous and arterial circulation.	Assess peripheral circulation at least once per shift.
	Keep the affected extremity elevated above the level of the heart.
	Apply warm, moist compresses, taking care to protect the skin from being burned.
	Use a thermostatically controlled device, such as a K-pad, to ensure a constant, uniform level of warmth.

Evaluation and Expected Outcomes

- No signs or symptoms of a pulmonary embolus are present.
- Pain is resolved.
- Both extremities are comparable in size, temperature, and color. Homans' sign is negative.

Client and Family Teaching

Teach clients with thrombophlebitis how to prevent recurrences by avoiding prolonged sitting and crossing the legs at the knee, performing active movement, elevating the legs periodically, wearing support hose, and drinking fluids liberally. Inform clients on long-term anticoagulant therapy of the importance of taking the medication exactly as prescribed and having the ordered laboratory tests to determine the effectiveness of therapy. Identify signs that indicate impaired clotting, such as nosebleeds, bleeding gums, rectal bleeding, easy bruising, and prolonged oozing from minor cuts.

Thromboangiitis Obliterans (Buerger's Disease)

Thromboangiitis obliterans is an inflammation of blood vessels that is associated with clot formation and fibrosis of the blood vessel wall. It affects primarily the small arteries and veins of the legs. The arms occasionally are involved.

ETIOLOGY AND PATHOPHYSIOLOGY

The cause of thromboangiitis obliterans has not been established. It is far more common in men than in women, and the onset is usually during young adulthood. Cigarette smoking aggravates the condition.

The affected arteries are prone to spasms that constrict the lumen of the arteries. Inflammatory lesions are found in isolated segments intermixed among healthy areas of the same vessel. The lesions occlude blood flow through the vessel during exercise and at rest. Skin and soft tissue cells experience degrees of hypoxia and anoxia. Some cells die. The necrotic (dead) tissues slough, forming ulcerations. The extent may be so severe that gangrene results. Thrombophlebitis also may be present.

ASSESSMENT FINDINGS

Signs and Symptoms

The client notes that one or both feet are always cold and may report numbness, burning, and tingling in some areas of the feet. **Intermittent claudication** (cramps in the legs after exercise) is a common symptom. Pain occurs at rest when circulation has been seriously impaired. The symptoms usually fluctuate in severity; attacks of acute distress often are followed by remissions.

Cyanosis and redness of the feet and legs may be noted. The skin frequently is a mottled purplish red and appears thin and shiny with sparse hair growth. Shallow, dry leg ulcers in various stages of healing may be seen. Black gangrenous areas may be observed on the toes and heels. The nails are thick. Peripheral pulses may be present during rest but diminish or disappear with activity. Capillary refill is prolonged.

Diagnostic Findings

Doppler ultrasound, IPG, and angiography help to evaluate the location and extent of vessel destruction.

MEDICAL MANAGEMENT

Tobacco in any form is restricted. Buerger-Allen exercises are ordered to stimulate and promote collateral circulation (Nursing Guidelines 30–1). Walking

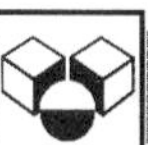

Nursing Guidelines 30-1

Teaching Buerger-Allen Exercises

Tell the client to:

- Lie flat in bed with both legs elevated above the level of the heart for 2 or 3 minutes, then
- Sit on the edge of the bed with the legs dependent for 3 minutes, and
- Exercise the feet and toes by moving them up, down, inward, and outward, then
- Return to the first position and hold it for about 5 minutes.

The exercises are repeated several times during one exercise period and performed periodically throughout the day.

and active foot exercises are allowed as long as they do not cause pain. Analgesics are prescribed to ease pain. If leg ulcers develop, treatment may include the application of moist dressings that are changed when the gauze becomes damp as well as topical antiseptics or antibiotic ointments.

SURGICAL MANAGEMENT

Sympathectomy, the interruption or suppression of some portion of the sympathetic nervous pathway, is performed to relieve vasospasm. If ulcerations occur, wound debridement (removal of necrotic tissue) and skin grafting may be required. If circulation becomes so impaired that gangrene results, amputation may be necessary.

NURSING MANAGEMENT

A thorough history is taken, including a smoking history, the client's symptoms and how long they have been present. A description of the type and degree of pain, and factors that increase or decrease it, are recorded. The affected areas are examined for redness, swelling, and other color changes, such as cyanosis and mottling. The nails and skin are inspected for changes, and the skin temperature above and below the affected area is noted. The presence and quality of peripheral pulses are monitored. Capillary refill time is assessed.

The nurse instructs and supervises the client on performing Buerger-Allen leg exercises (refer to Nursing Guidelines 30–1). When the client is not performing exercises, the legs are kept horizontal or dependent. Elevating the legs increases ischemia and, therefore, contributes to pain. The nurse carries out meticulous wound care if leg or foot ulcers exist.

Client and Family Teaching

Hospitalization for acute problems or complications may occur, but most care is carried out at home. Teach self-care and stress the importance of smoking cessation and performing prescribed exercises consistently. Clients should be instructed to avoid caffeine, tobacco products, and OTC drugs that cause vasoconstriction, such as nasal decongestants. Include instructions for inspecting the fingernails, toenails, and skin on the arms and legs daily; cleaning the arms and legs properly; avoiding trauma to the arms and legs; wearing properly fitting shoes and stockings (or socks); and avoiding prolonged exposure to the cold. When cold weather is unavoidable, advise the client to wear thick socks or insulated boots and gloves to protect the hands and feet from exposure to low temperatures.

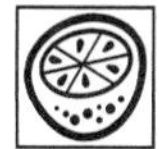

General Nutritional Considerations

A full liquid diet is used in the initial treatment of rheumatic heart disease and progressed as tolerated. Sodium is restricted if the client has edema or is treated with steroids.

Anorexia and weight loss are common side effects of infections; increase calories and protein as needed to replenish losses. Fever increases fluid requirements. Encourage small, frequent feedings to maximize intake.

Encourage weight loss in obese clients with thrombophlebitis.

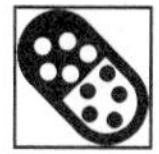

General Pharmacologic Considerations

Most clients with peripheral vascular disease have pain; nonnarcotic analgesics, such as salicylates, may be used to alleviate pain.

Pentoxifylline (Trental) may be used to improve (but not cure) intermittent claudication. This drug decreases blood viscosity and improves blood flow. Common adverse reactions associated with pentoxifylline include nausea, dizziness, headache, and dyspepsia.

Oral anticoagulants (eg, warfarin sodium [Coumadin]) may be prescribed as part of the long-term mangement of venous thrombosis. Frequent monitoring of prothrombin time (PT) is important for clients on warfarin; PT should be 1.5 to 2.5 times the control value (12 to 15 seconds) in order to achieve therapeutic effect of anticoagulant therapy. When PT is reported as an international normalized ratio (INR) factor, the normal range is 2.0 to 4.0.

Vitamin K (phytonadione, Aqua-Mephyton) is given as an antidote for overdose of Coumadin.

Heparin therapy may be instituted for a client with thrombophlebitis. Heparin, an anticoagulant, prevents extension of the thrombus and the development of additional thrombi.

Heparin is measured in units and the dosage is regulated by venous clotting time determinations, such as partial thromboplastin time (PTT) or activated partial thromboplastin time (aPTT). Optimum drug effect is reached when PTT and the aPTT are 1.5 to 2.5 times normal.

Clients receiving an anticoagulant must be observed for signs of bleeding tendency (eg, blood in the urine or stool, easy bruising, bleeding gums, excessive bleeding from minor cuts or scratches).

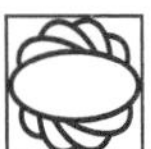

General Gerontologic Considerations

Geriatric clients are at increased risk for the development of infectious or inflammatory disorders of the cardiovascular system. A decreased inflammatory and immune response may prolong recovery.

Discourage older adults from using electric heating devices because of decreased temperature perception due to impaired circulation. Therefore, burns are more likely to occur. Thermal underwear and blankets are alternatives to electric blankets and heating pads for providing warmth.

Older clients who are inactive are encouraged to move about every hour during the day to promote circulation. This is especially important during long automobile or airplane trips.

Rheumatic heart disease may occur in the older adult who had rheumatic fever at an earlier age, or an acute episode may occur later in life. Joint inflammation is more disabling in the older adult who may have some joint deformity or damage from chronic disorders such as osteoarthritis.

A significant number of older adults have peripheral vascular insufficiency that is manifested in weak or absent pedal pulses; cold, clammy feet; thickened toenails; and shiny skin on the lower extremities.

The risk of hemorrhage during heparin therapy is greater in clients 60 years of age or older.

SUMMARY OF KEY CONCEPTS

- Inflammatory conditions of the heart include rheumatic fever, infective endocarditis, myocarditis, and pericarditis.
- Common organisms that cause inflammatory conditions of the heart are streptococci, staphylococci, and viruses.
- The risk of acquiring an infectious or inflammatory heart disorder can be reduced by maintaining intact skin and mucous membranes, obtaining early diagnosis and treatment of bacterial upper respiratory tract infections, and, if there is a history of heart infection, taking prophylactic antibiotics before invasive procedures.
- Clients with rheumatic fever present with a history of an earlier pharyngeal infection followed by carditis, polyarthritis, and chorea. It is treated primarily with antibiotic therapy; penicillin is the drug of choice.
- Infective endocarditis is characterized by fever, vegetations that form on heart valves, and the risk of embolization. Penicillin therapy, aspirin, and corticosteroids are used to treat infective endocarditis.
- The client with myocarditis presents with a fever, chest discomfort, fast and irregular heart rhythm, and dyspnea. An antibiotic is prescribed if the myocarditis is caused by bacteria. Otherwise, treatment consists of bed rest and drugs to maintain cardiac output and prevent rhythm disturbances.
- Assessment findings associated with pericarditis include fever, precordial pain that can mimic myocardial infarction pain, pericardial friction rub, and hypotension. Drugs are prescribed to reduce the inflammation. Pericardiocentesis may be performed; in some cases, pericardiostomy or pericardiectomy is necessary.
- When managing the care of clients with infectious or inflammatory heart disorders, the nurse collects assessment data, administers antibiotic and antiinflammatory drugs and monitors the client's response, keeps the client at rest during actue stages of an illness, assesses for complications and reports them immediately, and provides health teaching to ensure the client's safe self-care.
- Thrombophlebitis is an inflammation of the vein accompanied by a thrombus, or clot. The condition is acute and, after successful treatment, does not result in complications. During the acute inflammation, elevation of the arm or leg promotes comfort.
- Thromboangiitis obliterans is a chronic, progressive inflammatory disorder that is accompanied by clots that form in small arteries and veins. Some clients develop leg ulcers that are slow to heal or become gangrenous. Elevation of the arm or leg produces discomfort.
- The nursing management of clients with inflammatory disorders of peripheral blood vessels includes focused assessments such as checking Homans' sign and physical examination of the skin, nails, and extremities; administering analgesic and anticoagulant therapy; facilitating circulation; preventing tissue injury; and teaching clients how to prevent or manage future episodes.

CRITICAL THINKING EXERCISES

1. A client complains of intermittent claudication, pain when the legs are elevated, and cold, numb feet. The nurse notes several dry ulcerations of the feet.
   Does the client suffer from venous or arterial insufficiency?
   What additional assessment data must be collected?
   What lifestyle habits might predispose the client to this disorder?
2. A client on prolonged antibiotic therapy for endocarditis with valve involvement expresses boredom and despair concerning prolonged antibiotic therapy. The client exhibits a knowledge deficit regarding the need for extensive antibiotic therapy.
   How will you explain the reason for prolonged antibiotic therapy?
   What diversional activities might you suggest to the client?

Suggested Readings

Blake, G. J. (1995). Managing antibiotic prophylaxis for dental and upper respiratory tract procedures. *Nursing, 25*(1), 18, 21.

Blondin, M. M., & Titler. M. G. (1996). Deep vein thrombosis and pulmonary embolism prevention: what role do nurses play? *MEDSURG Nursing, 5*(3), 205–208.

Briant, C., Kutscher, A. H., Jr., & Roye, K. (1997). Pericarditis as a manifestation of Lyme disease. *Journal of Emergency Nursing, 23*(6), 525–529.

Bright, L. D. (1995). Clinical snapshot: Deep vein thrombosis. *American Journal of Nursing, 95*(6), 48–49.

Cantwell-Gab, K. (1996). Identifying chronic peripheral arterial disease. *American Journal of Nursing*, 96(7), 40–46.

Carpenito, L. J. (1997). *Nursing diagnosis: Application to clinical practice* (7th ed.). Philadelphia: Lippincott-Raven.

Dziadulewicz, L., & Shannon-Stone, M. (1995). Postpericardiotomy syndrome: A complication of cardiac surgery. *AACN Clinical Issues, 6*(3), 464–470.

Hatcher, I. (1997). In search of the best anti-embolism devices. *Today's Surgical Nurse, 19*(4), 19–22; quiz 41–42.

Maye, J., & Marshall, N. E. (1996). Penetrating mine injury to the heart with a pericardial tamponade. *CRNA, 7*(1), 25–28.

Nikolic, G. (1995). Myocardial infarction or inflammation? *Heart and Lung, 24*(2), 179–182.

Nunnelee, J. (1997, November). Healing venous leg ulcers. *RN, 60* (11), 38–42.

O'Connor, H. (1996). The treatment of Buerger's disease. *Journal of Wound Care, 5*(10), 462–463.

Page, J. G., & Hubble, M. W. (1996). Recognizing infective endocarditis: Case study of a 28-year-old. *Journal of Emergency Nursing, 22*(1), 24–28.

Prince, S. E., & Cunha, B. A. (1997). Postpericardiotomy syndrome. *Heart and Lung, 26*(2), 165–168.

Additional Resources

American Heart Association
http://americanheart.org

Heart Disease
http://www.merck.com

Cardiac Rehabilitation and Prevention Patient Information
http://www.jhbmc.jhu.edu/cardiology/rehab/patientinfo.html

Chapter 31

Caring for Clients With Valvular Disorders of the Heart

KEY TERMS

Afterload
Annuloplasty
Balloon valvuloplasty
Commissure
Incompetence
Point of maximum impulse
Pulmonary hypertension
Regurgitation
Sequela
Stenosis
Water-hammer pulse

LEARNING OBJECTIVES

On completion of this chapter, the reader will:

- List five disorders that commonly affect heart valves.
- Discuss assessment findings common among clients with valvular disorders.
- Name three diagnostic tests used to confirm valvular disorders.
- Identify consequences of valvular disorders.
- Name five categories of drugs used in the treatment of valvular disorders.
- Give two examples of treatment approaches (other than drug therapy) to correct valvular disorders.
- Discuss the nursing management of clients with valvular disorders.

Each structure of the heart helps to maintain normal cardiac function. The valves promote the forward circulation of blood to sustain an adequate cardiac output (Fig. 31–1).

Disorders of the Aortic Valve

Aortic Stenosis

Stenosis means narrowing. Aortic stenosis is a narrowing of the opening through the aortic valve that occurs when the valve cusps become stiff and rigid (Fig. 31–2).

ETIOLOGY AND PATHOPHYSIOLOGY

In young adults, aortic stenosis is commonly a congenital defect or a consequence of cardiac damage from rheumatic fever and rheumatic heart disease. In older adults, valve changes are caused by progressive deposits of calcium within valve cells that cause the valve to become less elastic.

The stiff valve is unable to open properly and more force is needed to push blood through the narrow opening. The muscular wall of the left ventricle thickens (hypertrophy) in response to the increased work it must perform. The volume of blood passing through the narrowed valve eventually becomes insufficient to nourish the myocardium and other organs.

ASSESSMENT FINDINGS

Signs and Symptoms

A client with aortic stenosis may experience dizziness, fainting, and anginal pain due to insufficient cardiac output. Initially, dyspnea and fatigue are experienced during periods of activity. If the left ventricle is enlarged, the pulsation of the heart felt on the chest wall, called the **point of maximum impulse** (PMI), is displaced laterally or distally. The carotid pulse may feel weak because of a low stroke volume.

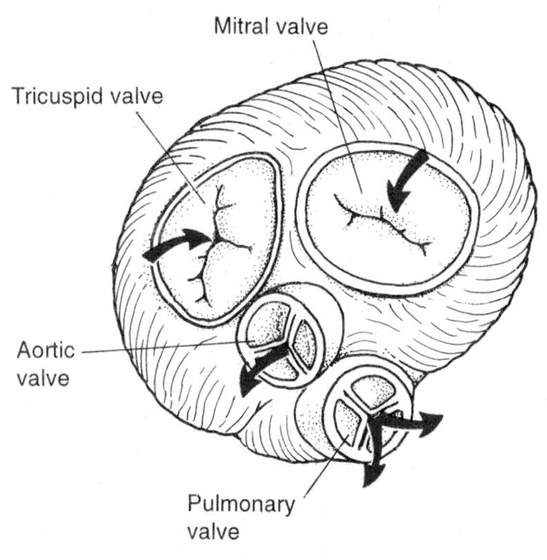

FIGURE 31-1. The tricuspid and mitral valves, located between the atria and ventricles, prevent blood from returning to the atria during ventricular contraction. The aortic and pulmonary valves, referred to as semilunar valves, open as blood is ejected from the ventricles.

The S_2 heart sound is split; that is, there is a definite separation between the sound of the aortic valve and the pulmonic valve closing. The sounds of these two valves closing usually occur in unison or are so closely timed that they seem as one sound. While listening at the second intercostal space to the right and left of the sternum, the S_1 and the split S_2 sound like "lub-t-dub." The sound persists throughout inspiration and expiration and does not disappear when the client sits up during auscultation. This distinguishes the split S_2 from a normal, physiologic splitting. Sometimes other abnormal sounds (eg, a systolic murmur and click) can be identified.

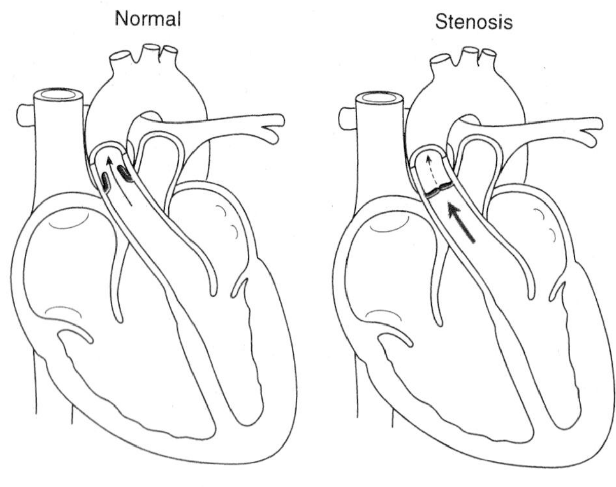

FIGURE 31-2. Aortic stenosis. Blood pools in the left ventricle and cardiac output is reduced because it cannot completely pass through the narrowed valve opening.

Diagnostic Findings

Ventricular enlargement is evident on a chest radiograph. An echocardiogram validates ventricular thickening and calcification of the aortic valve. The height of the R wave on an electrocardiogram (ECG) may be taller than usual, reflecting the large mass and force of contracting muscle. During left-sided cardiac catheterization, the pressure of blood within the left ventricle is higher than usual.

MEDICAL AND SURGICAL MANAGEMENT

Treatment measures focus on maintaining an adequate cardiac output by supporting the heart's pumping actvity. Digitalis, antiarrhythmic drugs, and diuretics are prescribed. Sodium is restricted from the diet. Antibiotics are prescribed to prevent infective endocarditis. Nitroglycerin is beneficial for relieving chest pain.

Balloon valvuloplasty is an invasive, nonsurgical procedure for enlarging a narrowed valve opening. A catheter with a deflated balloon is threaded through a peripheral bood vessel into the heart until the tip is located within the stenotic valve. When in position, the balloon is inflated to stretch the opening. Balloon valvuloplasty is considered a temporary measure for clients too unstable for other surgical treatment, yet whose symptoms cannot be adequately controlled with more conservative measures. The valve opening tends to become narrow again.

Surgery eventually becomes a necessary option. Ideally, aortic valve replacement is performed before the client reaches the late stages of heart failure (see Chap. 35).

NURSING MANAGMENT

The nurse monitors the client's subjective and objective symptoms. Dyspnea, irregular heart rhythms, chest pain, fainting, and confusion are reported immediately because they indicate inadequate cardiac ouput. Bed rest is maintained while these signs and symptoms are present. The pulse rate and rhythm are assessed before administering cardiotonics, such as digitalis, that slow the heart rate and increase the force of the heart's contraction. Such medications are withheld if the heart rate is below 60 beats per minute, because lowering the heart rate may also severely reduce cardiac output. Fluid intake and ouput are measured and the client is weighed to monitor fluid status, because fluid volume excess predisposes the client with impaired circulation to heart failure. Activity is paced to balance with the client's energy and tolerance. For additional nursing interventions, see Nursing Care Plan 31–1: The Client With a Valvular Disorder.

Aortic Insufficiency (Aortic Regurgitation)

Aortic insufficiency occurs when the aortic valve does not close tightly, a condition called valvular **incompetence**.

ETIOLOGY AND PATHOPHYSIOLOGY

An incompetent aortic valve can result from damage to the valve cusps or papillary muscles from rheumatic fever, endocarditis, syphilis, or age-related stretching of the proximal aorta. When blood is pumped through the incompetent aortic valve, some of the blood leaks backward (**regurgitation**) into the left ventricle. This backflow reduces cardiac output and causes fluid overload in the left ventricle. The left ventricle becomes chronically stretched, which hinders its ability to function as an effective pump (see Chap. 35). High fluid pressure in the left ventricle causes the mitral valve to shut early, which interferes with left atrial emptying. The blood in the left atrium backs up into the pulmonary circulation.

Left ventricular enlargement increases the heart's need for oxygen. When the coronary arteries are unable to supply the heart muscle with enough oxygen due to the decreased cardiac output, the myocardium becomes ischemic and anginal pain is experienced. Dizziness and confusion may occur, and left ventricular failure may develop.

ASSESSMENT FINDINGS

Signs and Symptoms

The client remains asymptomatic as long as the left ventricle can sustain adequate circulation. When valve damage affects the left ventricle, the client becomes aware of forceful heart contractions (palpitations). At first, this symptom is apparent only when the client is lying flat or on the left side. In latter stages, dyspnea and chest pain are experienced.

During physical examination, the client's skin may be flushed and moist, especially in the upper regions of the body. The radial pulse of a client with aortic insufficiency is apt to feel quite strong, with quick, sharp beats followed by a sudden collapse of the force, a characteristic called a **water-hammer pulse** or Corrigan's pulse. There is often a wide pulse pressure as the systolic blood pressure tends to be extremely high, whereas the diastolic pressure usually remains low or within normal ranges. The enlargement of the heart displaces the PMI. The chest may heave or rock from the forceful contractions of the enlarged left ventricle. A heart murmur, caused by the turbulence of blood falling back through the dilated aortic valve, also may be heard.

Diagnostic Findings

A cardiac catheterization reveals high left ventricular pressure and the backward movement of blood. A chest radiograph reveals heart enlargement and the aortic valve appears dilated. The ECG presents with tall R waves. Depressed ST segments indicate myocardial ischemia (see Chap. 30). A radionuclide scan comparing blood flow through the heart at rest and during exercise will reveal the severity of disease.

Medical and Surgical Management

Because aortic regurgitation is mild in most people and only slowly progressive, clients may be sustained with drug therepy, using cardiac glycosides or beta blockers and diuretics (Table 31–1). When taken appropriately, prophylactic antibiotics prevent recurrence of infective endocarditis. Clients are advised to modify their lifestyles so as to avoid excessive demands on the heart, such as that which may result from strenuous exercise and emotional stress.

When a client becomes symptomatic, replacement of the diseased aortic valve is considered (see Chap. 36). The less heart damage that occurs before surgery, the better the outcome. If the aorta is diseased, the procedure is more involved because repair involves a vascular graft.

Nursing Management

The nurse prepares clients for diagnostic procedures and monitors them afterward. Changes in heart rate and rhythm, dyspnea, chest pain, and loss of consciousness are reported immediately. Prescribed medications are administered, and the client's response is evaluated. Physical activity is balanced according to the client's tolerance. Before discharge, the nurse explains the need for antibiotic therapy before medical and dental procedures and teaches the client how to maintain a regular assessment of blood pressure as well as methods for controlling hypertension. See Nursing Care Plan 31–1 for nursing diagnoses and collaborative problems common to clients with valvular disorders of the heart.

Disorders of the Mitral Valve

Mitral Stenosis

Mitral stenosis is a narrowing of the valve between the left atrium and the left ventricle (Fig. 31–3).

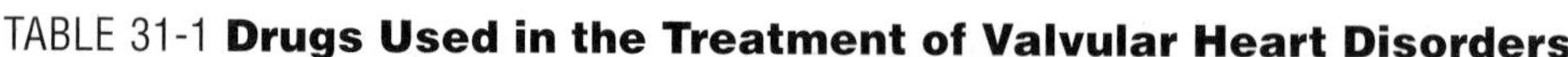

TABLE 31-1 **Drugs Used in the Treatment of Valvular Heart Disorders**

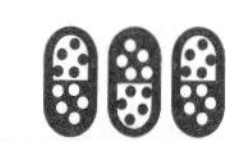

Drug Category/Drug Action	Side Effects	Nursing Considerations
Antibiotics		
penicillin G potassium (Pfizerpen) Inhibits cell wall synthesis in susceptible organisms, causing cell death.	Anaphylaxis, glossitis, gastritis, sore mouth, nausea, vomiting, diarrhea, rash, fever, superinfection, phlebitis	Must ascertain if penicillin allergy exists, monitor for 30 min after first parenteral dose given, assess IV site for pain, and signs and symptoms of phlebitis. Administer oral doses on an empty stomach with a full glass of water.
Anticoagulants		
warfarin sodium (Coumadin) Prevents the formation of thrombi. Prolongs clotting times by interfering with vitamin K-dependent clotting factors.	Increased incidence of bleeding, nausea, leukopenia, alopecia, dermatitis, fever, rash	Monitor complete blood counts and prothrombin time and international normalized ratio (INR) frequently, advise client to wear a Medic Alert tag, instruct client to report any unusual or excessive bleeding.
Cardiac Glycosides		
digoxin (Lanoxin) Increases cardiac output by slowing the heart rate (negative chronotropic action) and increasing the force of contraction (positive chronotropic action).	Fatigue, generalized muscle weakness, agitation, hallucinations (toxic effects on the heart may be life-threatening and require immediate attention) yellow-green halos around images, blurred vision	Assess pulse rate before each dose. Withhold administration if pulse is < 60 or > 120 beats/min. Monitor serum potassium levels; ensure intake of sources of potassium. Administer before meals to promote absorption.
Antiplatelets		
ticlopidine hydrochloride (Ticlid) Decreases clot production by interfering with platelet aggregation.	Dizziness, diarrhea, nausea, abdominal pain, neutropenia, bleeding, rash	Administer drug with meals, monitor white blood cell count and assess for excessive bleeding, relate need for regular, follow-up lab tests. Give drug with food or meals.
Antiarrhythmics		
quinidine (Quinaglute) Alters the action potential of cardiac cells and interferes with electrical excitability of the heart.	Nausea, vomiting, diplopia, new arrhythmias, hemolytic anemia, rash, tinnitus, headache	Monitor for new or worsened arrhythmias. Dosage is reduced in clients with hepatic or renal failure. Monitor blood counts during prolonged therapy.

ETIOLOGY AND PATHOPHYSIOLOGY

Mitral stenosis is a **sequela** (a condition that follows a disease) of heart inflammation caused by rheumatic fever. The condition worsens with each recurrence of endocarditis. The inflammation causes the cusps to stick together and form a thick, rigid scar, called a **commissure** and the chordae tendineae fuse and shorten. The mitral valve is unable to open completely, leading to incomplete emptying of the left atrium. Pooled blood from incomplete emptying contributes to the formation of clots, which puts the client at risk for arterial emboli.

The left atrium enlarges because it has to contract more forcibly to empty itself. Pressure from overfilling is conveyed backward through the blood vessels of the lungs, creating **pulmonary hypertension**. The right ventricle may eventually enlarge from having to pump against the high pressure in the pulmonary system. When the contraction of the right ventricle is no longer able to overcome the resistance in the pulmonary vasculature, venous circulation is impaired as well. The liver becomes congested and edema occurs in the legs.

ASSESSMENT FINDINGS

Signs and Symptoms

It may take many years for a client who has had rheumatic fever to develop mitral stenosis. When symptoms do occur, clients report fatigue and dyspnea after slight exertion. The symptoms become accentuated when unusual demands are placed on the heart (eg, when the client has a fever, during pregnancy). Later, clients experience heart palpitations caused by tachyarrhythmias (rapid arrhythmias). With the onset of pulmonary hypertension, clients

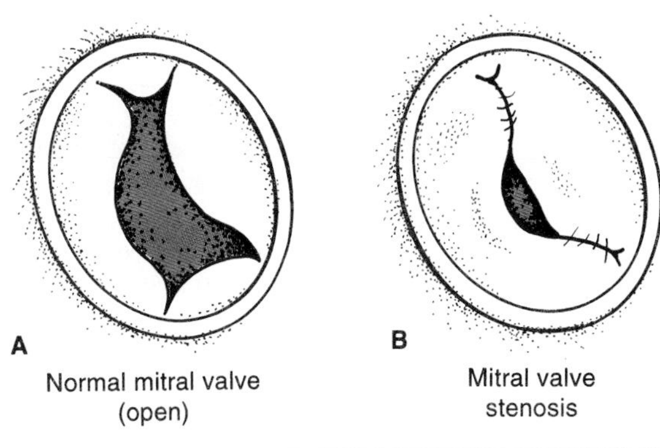

FIGURE 31-3. (*A*) The normal mitral valve opens widely to allow blood to pass from the left atria to the left ventricle. (*B*) Following what is generally an infectious process, the mitral valve leaflets become fused with scar tissue, causing a partially obstructed pathway for the passage of blood.

may become more dyspneic at night and must sleep in a sitting position. A cough productive of pink, frothy sputum may develop.

Changes in heart sounds may be the earliest indication of mitral valve stenosis. S_1 may be extremely loud if the cusps are fused or muffled or absent if the cusps have calcified and are immobile. A murmur described as sounding like a rumbling underground train can be heard at the heart's apex, especially when the client assumes a left lateral position. The systolic blood pressure is low from reduced cardiac output.

If backward pressure through the pulmonary circulation is sufficient to affect the right ventricle, the client's face is flushed; neck vein distention is evident; the liver is enlarged; and there is peripheral edema. Crackles heard in the bases of the lungs are a sign of pulmonary congestion.

Diagnostic Findings

A chest radiograph of a client with mitral stenosis reveals an enlarged left atrium and mitral valve calcification. In advanced stages, the right ventricle is enlarged with signs of fluid congestion in the lungs (pulmonary edema). An echocardiogram demonstrates decreased movement of the mitral valve cusps and changes in the size of the heart chambers. The P wave of the ECG is notched, showing that the left atrium is taking longer to depolarize than the right atrium, due to its increased size.

MEDICAL AND SURGICAL MANAGEMENT

Antibiotic therapy is prescribed to prevent future episodes of infective endocarditis. Preventing or relieving the symptoms of heart failure is an important part of the treatment. A daily aspirin, dipyridamole (Persantine), or an oral anticoagulant may be ordered to avoid clot formation. Arrhythmias, such as atrial fibrillation (quivering of the atrial muscle with insufficient force to pump blood out), are treated with cardiotonic drugs or cardioversion. Cardioversion stops the heart momentarily to allow the sinoatrial node to reestablish itself as the pacemaker.

Not all clients with mitral stenosis are suitable candidates for surgery. Those whose condition is so slight that it does not cause symptoms or so severe or of such long duration that profound changes in the heart and lungs have occurred usually are excluded. The earlier in the disease process that surgery is performed, the greater the likelihood that the symptoms will be relieved. Surgical management of mitral stenosis includes commissurotomy, valvuloplasty, and valve replacement (see Chap. 35).

NURSING MANAGEMENT

The nurse monitors the client's physical condition, prepares the client for diagnostic testing, and provides preoperative and postoperative care, if necessary. Discharge teaching includes information regarding drug therapy, activity modification, signs and symptoms of complications, and when to contact the physician. See Nursing Care Plan 31-1: The Client With a Valvular Disorder for additional nursing management.

Mitral Insufficiency (Mitral Regurgitation)

Mitral insufficiency occurs when the mitral valve does not close completely (Fig. 31–4).

ETIOLOGY AND PATHOPHYSIOLOGY

Mitral insufficiency is associated with rheumatic heart disease and mitral valve prolapse (see Mitral Valve Prolapse). It also is associated with connective tissue disorders, stretching of the valve opening from an enlarged left ventricle, and malfunction of a replaced valve.

When the mitral valve does not close completely, blood flows backward into the left atrium during ventricular systole. The heart can usually compensate for a small amount of blood that backflows into the left atrium, and pulmonary congestion does not occur. If the regurgitation affects the papillary muscles, or the heart is damaged from a myocardial infarction or rupture of a prosthetic valve, the heart is less able to compensate for the increased blood in the left atrium, and pulmonary congestion occurs. The regur-

NURSING CARE PLAN 31-1
The Client With a Valvular Disorder

Nursing Diagnoses and Collaborative Problems	Nursing Interventions	Outcome Criteria
Risk for Decreased Cardiac Output related to tachycardia and hypertension **Potential Complication: Congestive Heart Failure**	Maintain or improve cardiac output by providing rest periods, reducing fever, and relieving anxiety. Support compliance with sodium and fluid restrictions. Monitor the effectiveness of cardiotonic drugs and diuretics.	Cardiac output is adequate as evidenced by absence of chest pain, hypotension, and dizziness.
Activity Intolerance related to decreased cardiac output	Provide complete or partial assistance with ADLs. Allow adequate time for self-care. Intersperse periods of activity with rest.	The client tolerates activity without excessive dyspea or tachycardia.
Risk for Impaired Gas Exchange related to pulmonary hypertension or tachypnea secondary to anxiety	Position in a semi-sitting, sitting, or orthopneic position. Reduce activity. Instruct to inhale deeply and exhale through pursed lips. Administer oxygen if dyspnea is severe.	Arterial saturation remains at ≥95%.
Pain related to ischemia	Provide rest immediately. Administer oxygen temporarily. Give prescribed nitroglycerin or an analgesic. For clients with mitral valve prolapse, assist in assuming positions that relieve pain (see Mitral Valve Prolapse, Nursing Management).	Pain is relieved.
Risk for Infection related to increased susceptibility secondary to previous inflammatory heart disorders	Reassign the care of a susceptible client if the designated caregiver has infectious respiratory symptoms, or have the caregiver wear a face mask and change it frequently. Perform conscientious handwashing. Follow aseptic principles when changing dressings covering impaired skin and vascular insertion sites.	Temperature and white blood cell count remain within normal ranges.
Anxiety related to dyspnea, insecurity, or fear	Keep the call button readily available and answer calls promptly. Remain calm to diffuse apprehension. Limit conversation, but talk in low, soothing tones. Work with the client to reduce respiratory rate. Describe procedures before they are performed. Explain briefly how an intervention will relieve symptoms. Encourage the presence of a supportive family member or friend and give opportunities for discussing fears.	Anxiety is reduced or relieved.
Risk for Impaired Home Maintenance Management related to activity intolerance	Discuss ways to divide major home responsibilities into smaller tasks before discharge. Recommend moving appliances, such as the washer and dryer, and bed to the ground floor to eliminate climbing stairs. Discuss a referral to a community agency that may be able to provide a home health aide.	Home management responsibilities are prioritized with a realistic plan for carrying them out.

continued

NURSING CARE PLAN 31-1

Continued

Nursing Diagnoses and Collaborative Problems	Nursing Interventions	Outcome Criteria
Risk for Ineffective Management of Therapeutic Regimen related to insufficient knowledge of self-care	Give a complete explanation of all treatment modalities such as drug therapy, adequate rest, diet, and fluid restrictions.	Client accurately describes discharge instructions.
	Advise consulting the physician before dental or invasive treatments for prophylactic antibiotic therapy.	
	Caution against lifting heavy objects or straining at stool as these actions precipitate Valsalva's maneuver (forced expiration through a closed glottis), which is accompanied by increased blood pressure and blood volume entering the heart.	
	Teach the client the signs and symptoms of heart failure (see Chap. 35) and to report them immediately.	
	Advise clients to avoid caffeine and OTC medications that contain cardiac stimulants that increase heart rate.	
	Instruct clients to avoid strenuous exercise or competitive sports.	
	Teach stress reduction techniques (refer to Chap. 11) to clients with mitral valve prolapse.	

gitated blood plus the normal amount of blood in the left atrium are pushed into the left ventricle. The left ventricle enlarges because of the excess blood and increased pressure it takes to eject the large volume from the heart. When the left ventricle weakens from functioning under these strenuous conditions, heart failure develops, resulting in decreased stroke volume and cardiac output. At the same time, the function of the left atrium may also be compromised, resulting in pulmonary congestion.

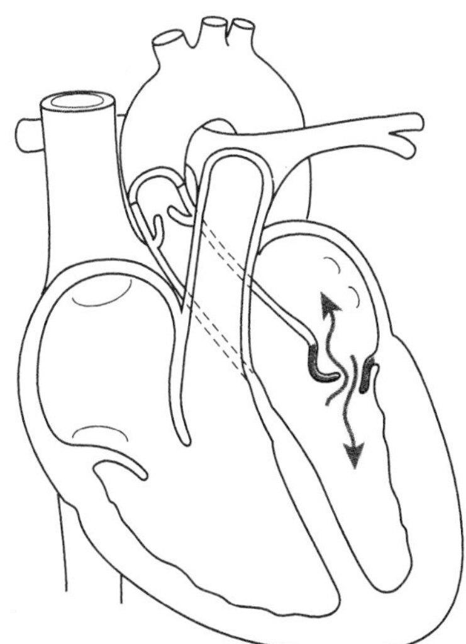

FIGURE 31-4. Mitral insufficiency. The incompetent atrioventricular valve allows blood to return to the left atrium.

ASSESSMENT FINDINGS

Signs and Symptoms

The client typically experiences dyspnea on exertion and fatigue. If pulmonary congestion occurs, the client develops shortness of breath and moist lung sounds typical of left ventricular failure (see Chap. 35).

The client may notice heart palpitations caused by the forceful contraction of the left ventricle as it attempts to empty the excessive volume of blood from its chamber. Tachycardia may also develop as a compensatory mechanism when stroke volume decreases. Hypertension becomes evident if cardiac output is inadequate. A loud, blowing murmur is often heard throughout ventricular systole at the apex of the heart. The S_1 heart sound is diminished because of the incomplete closure of the mitral valve. An S_3 heart sound, if heard, is an early sign of impending heart failure.

Diagnostic Findings

Echocardiography is the best technique for identifying structural changes in the mitral valve. Chest radiography shows enlargement of the chambers on the left side of the heart. Radionuclide angiography provides information on the volume of regurgitated blood. ECG reflects cardiac enlargement, papillary muscle or chordae tendineae dysfunction, and various associated arrhythmias (eg, atrial fibrillation).

MEDICAL AND SURGICAL MANAGEMENT

Medical treatment includes medications such as digitalis and those that prevent thrombus formation. Prophylactic antibiotics are prescribed to avoid future episodes of infective endocarditis. Vasodilators are ordered to reduce arterial vascular resistance, or **afterload** (the pressure against which the left ventricle must pump). This maximizes stroke volume and reduces the work of the left ventricle. An intra-aortic balloon pump, which provides counterpulsation to the contraction of the left ventricle, can be used in an emergency to stabilize a client in left ventricular failure (see Chap. 35).

Surgery to correct mitral insufficiency includes **annuloplasty,** repair of the valve leaflets and their fibrous ring. This procedure may be accompanied by the implantation of a biologic or prosthetic valve to restore unidirectional blood flow (see Chap. 36).

NURSING MANAGEMENT

The nurse closely monitors blood pressure, heart rate and rhythm, heart sounds, and lung sounds. The client is weighed to determine changes in fluid balance. If sodium is restricted, the nurse works with the client and dietitian to find seasonings and foods that are palatable. Medications are administered to treat symptoms. Signs of right- or left-sided heart failure are reported immediately. The nurse emphasizes the need for prophylactic antibiotics and periodic health assessments. Refer to Nursing Care Plan 31-1: The Client With a Valvular Disorder for more specific nursing interventions.

Mitral Valve Prolapse

In mitral valve prolapse, the valve cusps enlarge, become floppy, and bulge backward into the left atrium (Fig. 31–5).

ETIOLOGY AND PATHOPHYSIOLOGY

The cause of mitral valve prolapse is not completely understood, but it has been associated with some connective tissue disorders and coronary artery disease. It is more common in young women than in men and can be inherited.

Changes in the mitral valve tissue layers cause the cusps to distend. The billowing cusps stretch the papillary muscles as they balloon backward into the left atrium. The stretching of the papillary muscles may cause local ischemia and atypical chest pain (see Assessment Findings). As the papillary muscles provide less support to the mitral valve, valvular incompetence occurs. Structural changes predispose the valve to damage during infective endocarditis.

Some clients with mitral valve prolapse may also have increased levels of catecholamines (ie, epinephrine, norepinephrine), abnormal catecholamine regulation, and decreased intravascular volume, which causes symptoms that mimic severe anxi-

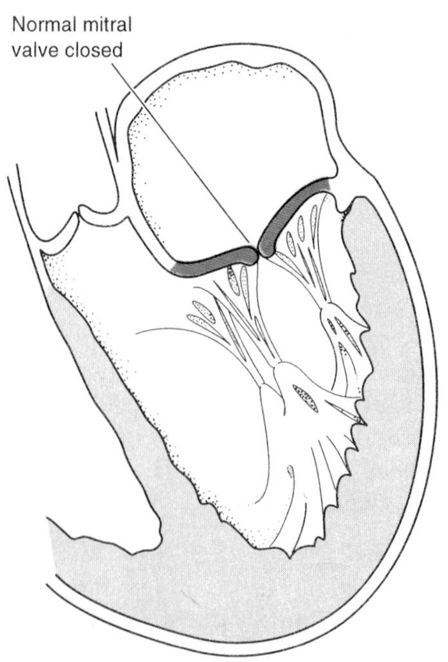

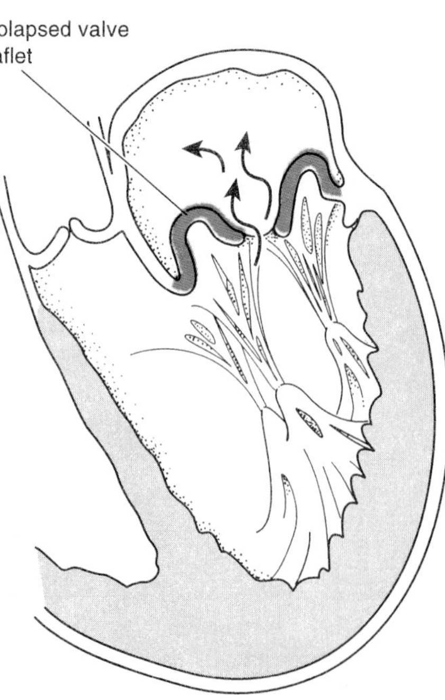

FIGURE 31-5. In mitral valve prolapse, the floppy valve leaflets allow blood to regurgitate, or move in retrograde fashion, from the left ventricle to the left atria.

ety (eg, tachycardia, palpitations, breathlessness, dizziness).

ASSESSMENT FINDINGS

Signs and Symptoms

Many clients with mitral valve prolapse are asymptomatic. When symptoms are present, they include chest pain, palpitations, and fatigue. The chest pain is different from that of angina: its onset does not correlate with physical exertion, its duration is prolonged, and it is not easily relieved. Some clients also experience symptoms that resemble anxiety or panic such as a rapid and irregular heart rate, shortness of breath, light-headedness, difficulty concentrating, and a fear that the symptoms indicate impending death. Auscultation of heart sounds reveals a characteristic click during ventricular systole that may develop into a systolic murmur. Symptoms of mitral insufficiency may also be manifested (see earlier discussion).

Diagnostic Findings

Echocardiography shows abnormal movement of the mitral valve. The ECG is essentially normal, eliminating myocardial infarction as a cause for the chest pain.

MEDICAL AND SURGICAL MANAGEMENT

Many clients with mitral valve prolapse require no treatment except periodic antibiotic therapy before invasive procedures. Tachyarrhythmias are controlled with such drugs as beta blockers, calcium channel blockers, and digitalis. Antianxiety medication may be prescribed to prevent panic attacks. Medications to reduce platelet aggregation (eg, a single daily aspirin or ticlopidine [Ticlid]) are prescribed to prevent thrombus formation. If symptoms become severe, valve replacement may be considered.

NURSING MANAGEMENT

Chest pain is relieved by having the client lie flat with the legs elevated and supported against a wall or couch at a 90-degree angle for 3 to 5 minutes to facilitate volume changes within the heart. Other recommendations include increasing activity when tachycardia occurs to eliminate the initiation of extra, ineffective beats to make up for reduced cardiac ouput and to lower levels of catecholamines. To relax or decrease shortness of breath, the nurse instructs the client to breathe deeply and slowly and then exhale through pursed lips. Clients are advised to avoid caffeinated beverages, to avoid contributing to an already rapid heart rate, and over-the-counter medications that contain stimulating chemicals. If hypertension is not a problem, the client is encouraged to drink an adequate volume of fluid and continue moderate use of salt to maintain intravascular fluid volume. The use of alcohol is discouraged because withdrawal can cause cardiac stimulation. Clients who are prescribed minor tranquilizers are warned not to stop the medication abruptly or they may experience stimulating withdrawal symptoms. Additional nursing management depends on other assessment data. See Nursing Care Plan 31-1: The Client With a Valvular Disorder.

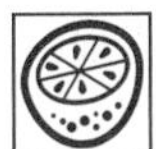

General Nutritional Considerations

Because approximately 75% of the sodium in the typical American diet comes from processed foods, clients who need to limit their sodium intake are encouraged to substitute homemade foods for mixes and prepared items. High-sodium foods to avoid include canned fish, meat, poultry, soup, vegetables, and vegetable juices; smoked and processed meats; sauerkraut; commercial mixes; instant rice and pasta mixes; casserole mixes; instant and quick-cooking cereals; condiments such as catsup, relish, pickles, barbecue sauce, soy sauce, and Worcestershire sauce; and seasoning salts.

Salt substitutes replace sodium with potassium or other minerals and may taste bitter. Low-sodium salt substitutes may contain up to half as much sodium as regular table salt. Neither type should be used without the physician's approval.

Foods that liquefy at room temperature, such as ice cream, ice milk, gelatin, ice pops, and sherbet are counted as liquids when fluid intake is restricted.

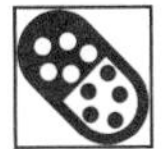

General Pharmacologic Considerations

Clients receiving an oral anticoagulant are closely monitored for episodes of bleeding, melena (blood in the stool), easy bruising, and oozing from superficial injuries, such as cuts from shaving or bleeding from the gums after brushing the teeth.

Oral anticoagulant therapy requires close monitoring of prothrombin time (PT). Therapeutic PT levels are 1.5 to 2.5 times the control value. When the PT is reported as an international normalized ratio (INR), the normal range is 2.0 to 4.0.

Beta blockers can aggravate chronic obstructive pulmonary disease and contribute to hypoglycemia in insulin-dependent adults. Some diuretics can deplete the body's potassium, resulting in hypokalemia.

When administering beta blockers, the apical pulse is taken prior to administering the drug. If the heart rate is less than 50 beats per minute, withhold the drug and notify the primary health care provider.

Patients taking beta blockers must be monitored closely for signs and symptoms of overdosage: bradycardia, severe dizziness, drowsiness, and bluish discoloration of the palms and/or the fingernails. Notify the primary health care provider immediately if these symptoms appear.

When administering quinidine observe the client for symptoms of cinchonism (quinidine toxicity), which include ringing of the ears, headache, nausea, dizziness, and fever.

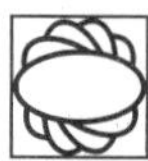

General Gerontologic Considerations

Older adults may require lower doses of cardiac glycosides because of their metabolic changes. The more medications older adults take, the more likely they are to have dangerous interactions. The heart rate and blood pressure of older adults taking beta-blockers must be monitored closely, as the adverse effects of bradycardia and hypotension can cause confusion and falls.

Fluid and electrolyte imbalances resulting from diuretic therapy in older adults can cause fatigue and weakness, which may be confused as a worsening of the symptoms related to valvular disease.

Calcification of heart structures, especially valvular tissue and the proximal aorta, increases with aging, putting older adults at higher risk for dangerous arrhythmias and heart failure with subsequent alterations in cardiac output.

Syncope and falls resulting from decreased cardiac output occur more readily in older adult clients.

SUMMARY OF KEY CONCEPTS

- Aortic stenosis, aortic insufficiency, mitral stenosis, mitral insufficiency, and mitral valve prolapse are common valvular disorders.
- Valvular disorders collectively impair the forward movement of blood, resulting in retrograde congestion in the heart chambers and blood vessels proximal to the diseased valve. They also decrease cardiac output.
- Common assessment findings include abnormal heart sounds, displacement of the PMI, changes in peripheral pulse quality, tachyarrhythmias, syncope, and chest pain. With the onset of complications, dyspnea, moist lung sounds, neck vein distention, peripheral edema, and weight gain become apparent.
- Valvular disorders are best diagnosed using echocardiography, chest radiography, and cardiac catheterization.
- Categories of drugs used to prevent and treat complications of valvular heart disorders include antibiotics, anticoagulants, antiplatelets, cardiac glycosides, antiarrhythmics, and diuretics. Coronary and peripheral vasodilators occasionally are prescribed.
- Balloon valvuloplasty is an invasive, nonsurgical procedure used to temporarily dilate a stenotic heart valve; valve replacement is a more permanent treatment.
- Complications commonly seen in clients with valvular disease include left- and right-sided heart failure, arrhythmias, and embolization.
- The nursing management of clients with valvular disorders includes a comprehensive cardiopulmonary assessment, promoting adequate cardiac output and oxygenation of blood, administering prescribed drugs and monitoring their effectiveness, facilitating activity within the client's level of tolerance, preventing or relieving severe anxiety, and providing health teaching to prevent future complications.

CRITICAL THINKING EXERCISES

1. Compare and contrast stenosis of the aortic and mitral valves or insufficiency of these same valves.
2. You are assisting a newly admitted client with a diagnosis of mitral stenosis into his hospital room. The individual in the bed next to this client has a diagnosis of tracheobronchitis. The roommate has a humidifier at the bedside and receives frequent aerosol therapy treatments.
   What is the potential problem in this situation?
   What measures are appropriate to correct the situation?

Suggested Readings

Chase, S. (1997). Antiarrhythmics. *RN, 60*, 5.

Davis, J. S. (1995). Small BM Advances in the treatment of aortic stenosis across the lifespan. *Nursing Clinics of North America, 30*(2), 317–332.

Hayes, D. D. (1997). Mitral valve prolapse revisited. *Nursing 27*(10), 34–39; quiz 40.

Holloway, S., & Feldman, T. (1997). An alternative to valvular surgery in the treatment of mitral stenosis: Balloon mitral valvotomy. *Critical Care Nurse, 17*(3), 27–36.

Hudak, C. M., & Gallo, B. M. (1994). Critical care nursing: A holistic approach (6th ed.). Philadelphia: J. B. Lippincott.

Karch, A. (1998). *1998 Lippincott's nursing drug guide.* Philadelphia: Lippincott-Raven.

Lazzara, D., & Sellergren, C. (1996). Chest pain: Making the right call when the pressure is on. *Nursing, 26*(11), 42–53.

Memmler, R. L, Cohen, B. J., & Wood, D. L. (1996). *The human body in health and disease* (8th ed.). Philadelphia: Lippincott-Raven.

McGrath, D. (1997). Clinical snapshot: Mitral valve prolapse. *American Journal of Nursing, 97*(5), 40–51.

Scordo, K. A. (1997). Mitral valve prolapse syndrome. Nonpharmacologic management. *Critical Care Nursing Clinics of North America, 9*(4), 555–564.

Strimike, C., & Wojcik, J. (1998). Stopping atrial fibrillation with ibutilide. *American Journal of Nursing, 98*(1), 32–34.

Additional Resources

1997 Heart and Stroke Guide
http://www.amhrt.org/hs97

Heart Homepage
http://www.hearthome.com/

Facts about Mitral Valve Prolapse
http://www.skylinefamilypractice.com/mvp.html

Mitral Valve Regurgitation
http://study.haifa.ac.il~vstern/heartvlv.h

Chapter 32

Caring for Clients With Disorders of Coronary and Peripheral Blood Vessels

KEY TERMS

Aneurysm
Angina pectoris
Arteriosclerosis
Atherectomy
Atheroma
Atherosclerosis
Bruit
Collateral Circulation
Coronary artery bypass graft
Coronary occlusion
Coronary thrombosis
Embolus
Hyperlipidemia
Infarct
Ischemia
Laser angioplasty
Percutaneous transluminal coronary angioplasty
Peripheral vascular disease
Phlebothrombosis
Plaque
Thrombolytic agents
Thrombosis
Thrombus
Transmyocardial revascularization
Varicosities
Vein ligation
Vein stripping
Ventricular assist device

LEARNING OBJECTIVES

On completion of this chapter, the reader will:

- Distinguish between arteriosclerosis and atherosclerosis.
- List the risk factors associated with coronary artery disease and discuss which factors can be modified.
- Discuss the symptoms, diagnosis, and treatment of coronary artery disease.
- Discuss the symptoms, diagnosis, and treatment of myocardial infarction.
- Describe the nursing management of clients with an acute myocardial infarction.
- Discuss the symptoms, diagnosis, and treatment of Raynaud's disease.
- Discuss the symptoms, diagnosis, and treatment of thrombosis, phlebothrombosis, and embolism.
- Describe the nursing management of clients with an occlusive disorder of peripheral blood vessels.
- Discuss the symptoms, diagnosis, and treatment of varicose veins.
- Describe the nursing management of clients undergoing surgery for varicose veins.
- Discuss the symptoms, diagnosis, and treatment of an aortic aneurysm.
- Describe the nursing management of clients with an aortic aneurysm.

Cardiovascular disease is the leading cause of death in the United States. Occlusive disorders of the coronary arteries and resulting complications are largely responsible for this statistic. Occlusive disorders of peripheral blood vessels also affect many Americans. Uninterrupted blood flow is essential to cells and tissues. The most common causes of occlusive vascular diseases include atherosclerosis, arteriosclerosis, clot formation, or vascular spasm.

Arteriosclerosis and Atherosclerosis

Arteriosclerosis refers to the loss of elasticity or hardening of the arteries. **Atherosclerosis** is a condition in which the lumen of the artery fills with fatty deposits (chiefly composed of cholesterol) called **plaque** or **atheroma**. Arteriosclerosis and atherosclerosis affect many parts of the body (heart, brain, kidneys, and extremities) and cause a variety of disorders (myocardial infarction [MI], cerebrovascular accidents, renal failure). The rate at which arterial changes occur in various organs or structures varies.

ETIOLOGY AND PATHOPHYSIOLOGY

Arteriosclerosis and atherosclerosis accompany the aging process. Many factors affect the rate of onset and, overall severity of these conditions. As cells within the arterial tissue layers degenerate due to aging, calcium is deposited within the cytoplasm. The calcium causes the arteries to become less elastic. As the left ventricle contracts sending oxygenated blood from the heart, the rigid arterial vessels fail to stretch. This potentially reduces the volume of oxygenated blood delivered to organs.

Hyperlipidemia or high blood fat levels trigger atherosclerotic changes. Factors such as gender, heredity, diet, and level of activity individually or collectively influence hyperlipidemia. For example, some clients inherit genetic codes that replicate cells with reduced numbers of receptors for binding with cholesterol; therefore, they are more likely to develop high lipid levels. Clients who consume a high-fat diet may saturate all available cholesterol receptors, which also results in hyperlipidemia. A client with elevated lipid levels who also has other risk factors, such as cigarette smoking, stressful lifestyle, diabetes mellitus, or hypertension, is at risk for the accelerated buildup of fatty plaque deposits beneath the intimal layer of the arteries.

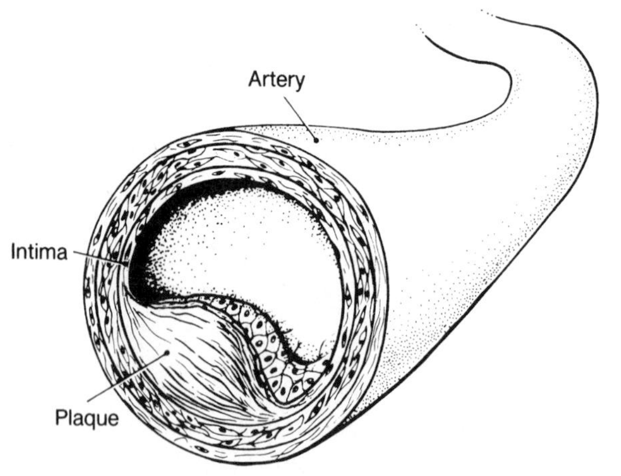

FIGURE 32-1. Schematic of an atheromatous plaque. A central area of necrosis and hemorrhage into the area both impinge on the lumen of the vessels.

Microscopic injury in blood vessel walls may occur because of carbon monoxide from cigarette smoke, catecholamine release from stress, hyperglycemia from diabetes mellitus, or increased pressure from hypertension. The body responds to the injury by activating the inflammatory response. Monocytes migrate to the site of injury and deposit themselves under the endothelial cells of the tunica intima. The monocytes then attract and accumulate lipid (fatty) material. The enlarging lesion elevates the endothelium of the artery wall and narrows the lumen (Fig. 32–1). Atherosclerotic vessels are unable to produce endothelial-derived relaxing factors and the ability of the artery to dilate is impaired. As the subendothelial atheroma enlarges, the intimal layer may split and expose the lesion. As blood flows through the vessel, platelets become trapped in the roughened wall and initiate the clotting mechanism. When this occurs in a coronary artery, the resulting mass is called **coronary thrombosis**.

Occlusive Disorders of Coronary Blood Vessels

Coronary occlusion is the closing of a coronary artery, reducing or totally interrupting blood supply to the area distal to the occlusion. Coronary artery disease precedes coronary occlusion. If the occlusion is not treated, an MI occurs. Symptoms generally do not occur until at least 60% of the arterial lumen is occluded.

Coronary Artery Disease

Coronary artery disease (CAD) refers to the arteriosclerotic and atherosclerotic changes taking place in the coronary arteries that supply the myocardium. The disease may not be diagnosed until individuals are late middle age or older, but the vascular changes most likely began occurring at a much younger age.

ETIOLOGY AND PATHOPHYSIOLOGY

Coronary artery disease is thought to be due to many factors, rather than a single cause. Inherited and behavioral risk factors for the development of coronary artery disease appear in Box 32–1. Men are affected at a younger age than women; however, the

BOX 32-1 Coronary Artery Disease Risk Factors

Inherited	Behavioral
Increased age	Smoking
Male gender	Sedentary lifestyle
Diabetes mellitus	Obesity
Increased lipid levels	Competitive, aggressive personality
Genetic predisposition	
Hypertension	High-fat diet

incidence rises in postmenopausal women and becomes similar to that in men.

A progressively diminishing oxygen supply to cells may actually stimulate **collateral circulation**—arterial channels that form to supply the ischemic area. Branches of the coronary artery below the narrowed segment may even dilate. At rest, ample blood flow may be maintained despite considerable CAD. The condition may go unrecognized, particularly among those with a sedentary lifestyle. However, during situations that increase myocardial oxygen demand (exercise or emotional stress), the compromised coronary arteries are unable to adequately oxygenate the myocardium. When the myocardial tissue becomes **ischemic** (deprived of oxygen), clinical manifestations of CAD, such as chest pain of cardiac origin (**angina pectoris**), occur. *Coronary insufficiency* describes a clinical condition in which cardiac pain is frequently more severe than that of typical angina, but death of the heart muscle does not occur.

ASSESSMENT FINDINGS

Signs and Symptoms

In mild CAD, clients are asymptomatic or complain of feeling fatigued. The most prominent symptom is chest pain or discomfort that occurs during periods of activity or stress. The classic symptom is sudden pain or pressure, which may be most severe over the heart (precordial) or under the sternum (substernal). Pain may radiate to the shoulders and arms, especially on the left side, or to the jaw, neck, or teeth. Some clients describe discomfort other than pain, such as indigestion, or a burning, squeezing, or crushing tightness in the upper chest or throat. Box 32–2 highlights the different types of angina pectoris.

Some clients present with signs suggesting hyperlipidemia. They may be obese and hypertensive. Findings suggest that an obese person with an apple-shaped body (carries most of the weight in the abdomen) is at higher risk for CAD than someone with a pear-shaped body (carries most of their weight below the hips). The pulse may be higher than usual at rest and become irregular with exercise. An opaque white ring about the periphery of the cornea, called *arcus senilis* (Fig. 32–2), is due to a deposit of fat granules but may only be apparent in older adults. *Xanthelasma*, a raised yellow plaque on the skin of the upper and lower eyelids (Fig. 32–3), suggests lipid accumulation. Although research is ongoing, some cardiolo-

BOX 32-2 Types of Angina

	Stable Angina	Unstable Angina	Variant Angina (Prinzmetal's)
CAUSE	75% coronary occlusion accompanying exertion, elevated heart rate or blood pressure, eating a large meal	Progressive worsening of stable angina; more than 90% coronary occlusion	Arterial spasm in normal or diseased coronary arteries
SYMPTOMS	Chest pain lasts ≤ 15 minutes; may radiate; characteristics of pain severity, frequency, and duration are similar with each episode	Increased frequency, severity, and duration of chest pain; poorly relieved by rest or oral nitrates; risk for MI within 18 months of onset	Chest pain at rest; attacks usually occur between midnight and 8 AM; ST elevation rather than depression. Pain tends to come and go over a period of 3 to 6 months, then diminishes over time
TREATMENT	Rest, sublingual nitrates, antihypertensives, lifestyle changes	Sedation, IV nitroglycerin, oxygen, antihypertensives, anticoagulant or antiplatelet therapy, revascularization procedures	Nitrates or calcium channel blockers

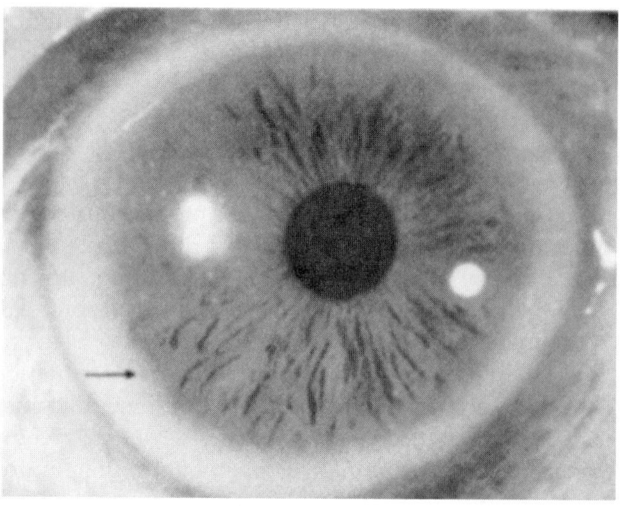

FIGURE 32-2. Arcus senilis, an opaque ring in the periphery of the cornea, is a sign of systemic fat deposits. (Photo courtesy of Kellogg Eye Center, University of Michigan)

gists indicate a relationship between a diagonal crease in the earlobe and the risk for CAD.

Diagnostic Findings

The serum cholesterol and triglyceride levels are elevated. Exercise electrocardiogram (ECG) or stress testing may reveal ST segment depression, arrhythmias, and exercise-induced hypertension. Narrowing of one or more coronary arteries is shown during coronary arteriography.

MEDICAL AND SURGICAL MANAGEMENT

Treatment of CAD includes drugs that produce arterial vasodilation, such as the nitrates (eg, nitroglycerin and isosorbide dinitrate). Beta-adrenergic blocking agents, which decrease myocardial oxygen consumption by reducing heart rate and increasing the diameter of peripheral arteries, are also used in the treatment of CAD. Calcium channel blocking agents are used in the treatment of CAD, although research has shown that they may not be of much benefit. The physician selects the drug that produces the best results for the individual.

Drugs such as angiotensin-converting enzyme (ACE) inhibitors and diuretics, as well as stress management, are used to control hypertension. Nicotinic acid (Niacin) in pharmacologic doses (eg, not the dosage in multivitamins) helps increase high-density lipoprotein (HDL), the beneficial type of cholesterol, and lowers low-density lipoprotein (LDL), undesirable cholesterol. Blood sugar is kept regulated and weight loss is encouraged. Prevention of further plaque formation is attempted by lowering elevated cholesterol and triglyceride levels through diet, exercise, and, in extreme cases, drugs. Factors that contribute to arterial constriction, like nicotine from cigarettes, are eliminated. Some physicians advise taking one aspirin tablet daily to prevent thrombi from occurring. Nonstrenuous but active, regular exercise, prescribed after stress testing, can promote collateral circulation.

Invasive but nonsurgical procedures are done to reopen narrowed coronary arteries. For clients who fit specific criteria, **percutaneous transluminal coronary angioplasty** (PTCA) is performed. In this procedure, a balloon-tipped catheter is inserted through the skin and threaded from a peripheral artery into the diseased coronary artery under local anesthesia (Fig. 32–4). Under fluoroscopy, the catheter is threaded within the area of stenosis and the balloon inflated with controlled pressure. Inflation of the balloon compresses the atherosclerotic plaque, increasing the diameter of the artery. Arterial rupture, MI, and abrupt reclosure are complications of this procedure. Repeating the procedure is often necessary because the plaque tends to renarrow the artery.

Coronary *stents* are also placed into the coronary artery. These small, metal tubes with rectangular openings, are inserted using a guide catheter and balloon. The balloon and stent are expanded near the area of plaque, widening the arterial lumen by squeezing the plaque up against the arterial wall. The stent also keeps the lumen open for a longer period than traditional PTCA.

For clients whose plaques are no longer soft and pliable a **laser angioplasty** is performed. A guide catheter is threaded into the diseased coronary artery to the narrowed area. A laser tip is inserted through the catheter. The laser is activated. It converts electrical energy into ultraviolet light. The light vaporizes the plaque. An **atherectomy**, using a tiny motor-driven, circular blade inserted through a ballooned coronary catheter may also be performed when plaque has

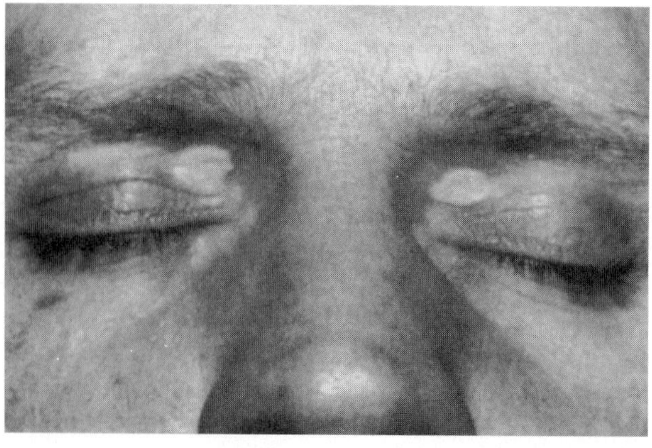

FIGURE 32-3. Xanthelasma, yellowish plaques about the eyelids, is a sign of lipid accumulation. (Photo courtesy of Kellogg Eye Center, University of Michigan)

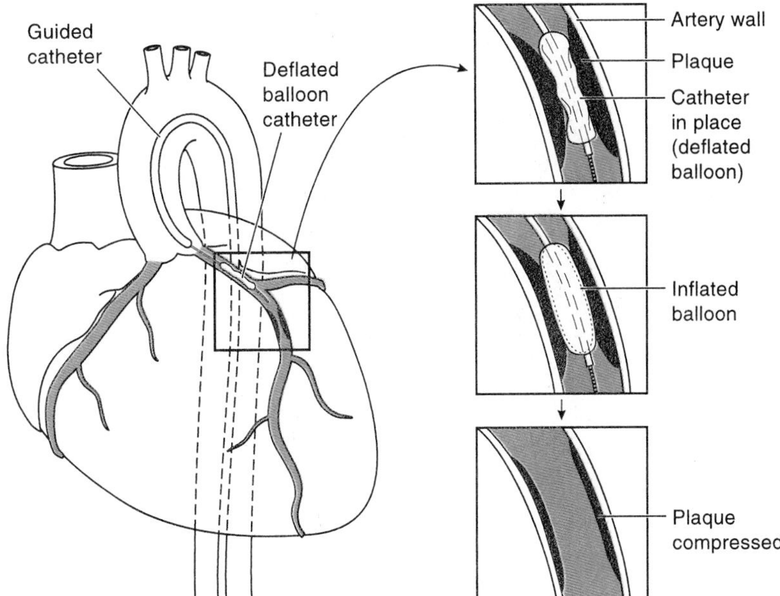

FIGURE 32-4. A coronary artery can be opened by compressing soft plaque with a balloon catheter.

reached a stage of calcification. As the plaque is shaved from the lining of the artery, the shredded tissue is held within the guide catheter to prevent embolization.

Coronary artery bypass graft (CABG) surgery (see Chap. 36) is a technique for revascularizing the myocardium. The results tend to last longer than PTCA, laser angioplasty, or atherectomy.

A newer technique, **transmyocardial revascularization,** may provide clients who are not candidates for CABG surgery a higher quality of life. The procedure involves a laser that creates channels in the myocardium experiencing ischemia (distal to the occluded coronary artery). The channels created by the laser allow the ischemic myocardium to absorb the oxygenated blood that seeps into the area. Therefore, the myocardium receives oxygen, not by a coronary artery, but from the blood that seeps into the space between the cells.

NURSING MANAGEMENT

Assess the characteristics of chest pain and administer prescribed drugs that dilate the coronary arteries. If rest, drugs, and oxygen do not relieve the pain, notify the physician. Help clients learn how to reduce CAD risk factors that are modifiable and instruct them on the administration and side effects of antianginal drugs. Emphasize that severe, unrelieved chest pain indicates a need to be examined by a physician without delay.

The basic preparation of clients who undergo invasive, nonsurgical procedures such PTCA and atherectomy procedures is similar to that for clients who have surgery (see Chap. 24). Cleanse and remove hair from skin insertion sites (one for the coronary artery catheter and the other for an arterial line through which the blood pressure will be directly monitored). Withhold anticoagulant therapy before the procedure, to decrease the chance of hemorrhage.

Monitor all vascular sites for bleeding postprocedure and assess distal pulses. Observe the client's mental status as cerebral emboli can occur. Measure urine output. Administer analgesics for discomfort. Report any of the following data immediately: severe chest pain, abnormal heart rate or rhythm, mental confusion or loss of consciousness, hypotension, urine output less than 30 to 50 mL/h, or a cold, pulseless extremity.

Client and Family Teaching

Educating clients in ways they can modify their risk factors is a critical element in the care of clients with CAD. A low-fat diet and regular aerobic exercise can significantly reduce the risk of CAD. Provide clients with material regarding diet (see General Nutritional Considerations at the end of this chapter) and refer them to a dietitian for assistance in meal planning. Encourage activity and inform clients that regular exercise such as walking and gardening are sufficient to obtain health benefits. Refer clients to smoking cessation programs and discuss medications that can help them quit (see Chap. 16). Explain that these modifications can benefit their overall health and well-being as well as their cardiac health.

Myocardial Infarction

An **infarct** is an area of tissue that dies (necrosis) due to inadequate oxygenation. An MI or heart attack occurs when there is prolonged, 100% occlusion of

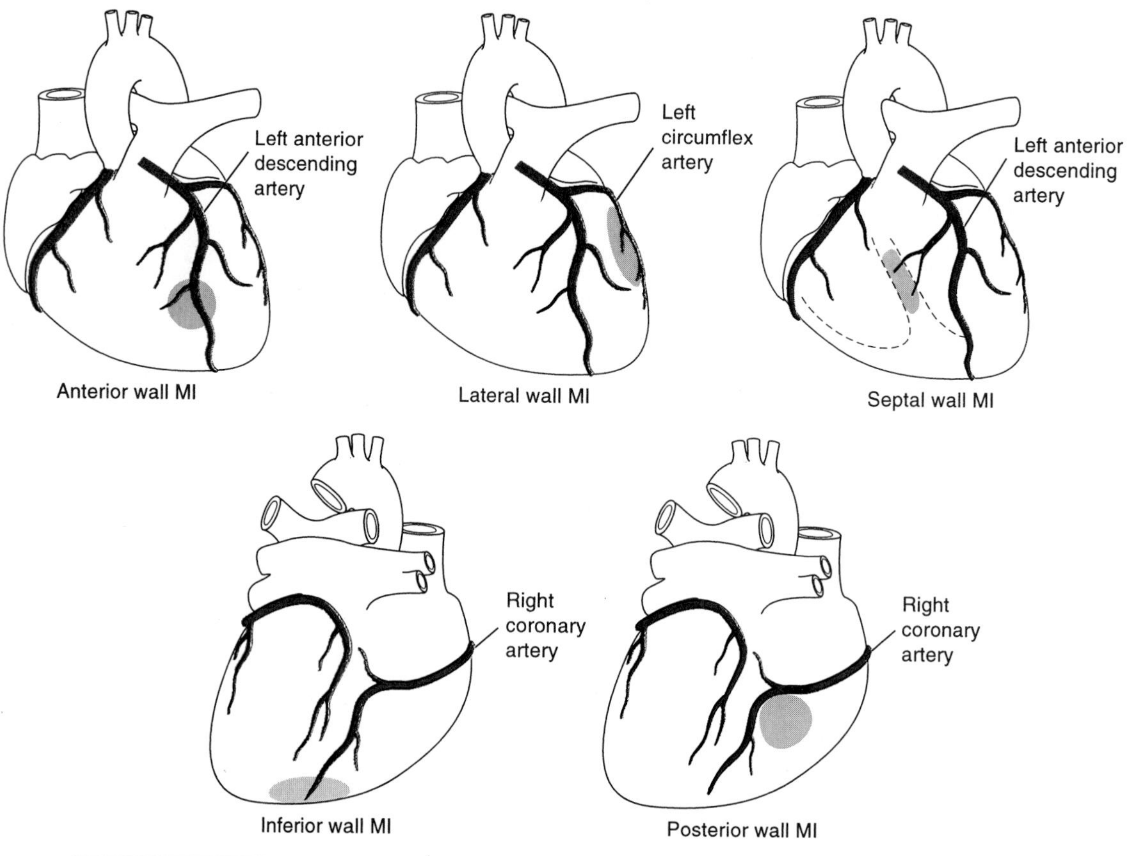

FIGURE 32-5. Zones of myocardial infarction based on the coronary artery that becomes occluded.

coronary arterial blood flow (Fig. 32–5). The larger the necrotic area, the more serious the damage. An infarct that extends through the full thickness of the myocardial wall is called a transmural infarction or Q wave MI. A partial thickness infarct is called a subendocardial infarction, or non-Q wave MI.

Each coronary artery supplies a different area of the myocardium. The zone of necrosis is identified according to the area of myocardium supplied by the respective coronary artery.

ETIOLOGY AND PATHOPHYSIOLOGY

The most common cause of an MI is a coronary thrombosis. Thrombosis is usually secondary to arteriosclerotic and atherosclerotic changes in the coronary arteries. Arterial spasms and calcium emboli (dislodged from a calcified aorta) may also cause an MI.

Once an area of the myocardium has been damaged and destroyed, the cells in that area lose their special functions of automaticity, excitability, conductivity, and contractility, and rhythmicity. Consequently, arrhythmias and heart failure are common consequences of an MI.

Injury to the myocardium triggers the inflammatory response. The permeability of cell membranes is disrupted and the damaged cells release intracellular enzymes and electrolytes into the extracellular fluid. Loss of intracellular potassium and the accumulation of lactic acid from anaerobic cellular metabolism affect depolarization and repolarization of myocardial cells. Dangerous arrhythmias can develop during this time because the affected areas are electrically unstable.

The infarction process can take up to 6 hours to complete. There are three zones of tissue damage. The first zone consists of a central area of necrotic, dead, myocardial cells. A second zone of injured cells surrounds this zone that may live if the blood supply to the area is restored. The third zone is the ischemic area that will probably live if circulation is restored. Thrombolytic drugs (clot busters) are given during this 6-hour window of opportunity to re-establish blood flow and save as many myocardial cells as possible.

Leukocytosis and a mild elevation in body temperature follow in 3 to 7 days. New capillaries begin to grow to establish collateral circulation to the infarcted area, but it takes 2 or 3 weeks before there is significant blood flow to the area. A "cardiac patch" made up of collagen fibers begins to form within the first 2 weeks of the infarct, but it takes as long as 3 months for the scar to grow firm. The scar tissue does not function as the myocardium it replaced; it does not stretch and contract like the original tissue. Lack of resiliency impairs the heart's ability to pump effectively and heart failure is always a lifelong, potential complication.

COMPLICATIONS

Arrhythmias

Any number of arrhythmias (see Chap. 33) may occur during the acute phase. More than half the deaths from MI occur within 72 hours. Some abnormal rhythms can be fatal within a few minutes. Early detection and treatment of dangerous arrhythmias reduces the fatality rate.

Cardiogenic Shock

Cardiogenic shock, which has a high mortality rate, occurs when 40% of the left ventricle has lost the ability to pump effectively. Its onset may be sudden or the condition may develop over hours or days. The sooner shock is detected (monitoring with a pulmonary artery catheter) and treatment instituted, the better the client's chances of survival. This complication has been successfully treated using medications, ventricular assist devices, and an intra-aortic balloon pump (see Chap. 35).

Ventricular Rupture

Ventricular rupture occurs when a soft necrotic area from a transmural or interventricular septal MI ruptures. Dyspnea, rapid right heart failure, and shock result. *Hemopericardium* (blood in the pericardium) and cardiac tamponade follow. The prognosis for ventricular rupture is poor, although survival is possible.

Ventricular Aneurysm

A *ventricular aneurysm* is a bulging of the portion of the heart affected by the MI. This area of poorly contractile tissue predisposes the heart to failure. Blood trapped in the projection tends to form thrombi, which may be released into arterial circulation. The aneurysm may burst, resulting in hemorrhage and death.

Arterial Embolism

Clots can form in the cavity of the ventricular aneurysm (mural thrombi) or tissue debris can break free. If they enter the systemic arterial circulation, they may occlude a peripheral artery. Symptoms depend on the location of the affected artery. Arteriotomy (opening of an artery) and embolectomy (removal of an embolus) may be necessary; a client who has recently suffered an MI, however, is a poor surgical risk.

Venous Thrombosis

Venous thrombosis arises mostly in the veins of the lower extremities and the pelvis. The use of antiembolism stockings and regularly performed foot and leg exercises helps to prevent thrombus formation. Anticoagulants also are given.

Pulmonary Embolism

Most pulmonary emboli arise from venous thrombi in the lower extremities and the pelvis. They also may arise from the right ventricle after an MI. The onset of a pulmonary embolism is usually sudden with chest pain, dyspnea, and cyanosis being the first symptoms. The sputum may be tinged with blood. Treatment depends on the size of the infarcted pulmonary area, the age and condition of the client, and the seriousness (or extent) of the MI.

Pericarditis

Pericarditis may be mild or severe. The mild form may not require treatment (see Chap. 30). If a pericardial effusion develops, the client is observed closely for signs of cardiac tamponade; pericardiocentesis is done to remove excess fluid.

Mitral Insufficiency

If the papillary muscles are involved in an MI and the mitral valve leaflets are compromised, mitral insufficiency may occur. In this condition, blood not only flows forward into the aorta but also backward into the left atrium through an incompetent mitral valve (see Chap. 31).

ASSESSMENT FINDINGS

Signs and Symptoms

Symptoms vary but typically include sudden, severe pain in the chest. Most clients are aware of its seriousness and are apprehensive. The pain is usually substernal and may or may not radiate to the shoulder, arm, teeth, jaw, or throat. The pain is more severe and of longer duration than anginal pain. Some describe the sensation as squeezing or crushing. Unlike anginal pain, rest or sublingual nitrates do not relieve the pain of MI. If untreated, it may last for several hours or as long as 1 or 2 days. Finally, it becomes a soreness or an ache before it disappears entirely. A few experience little or no pain and may never know that they have had an MI until it is detected by an ECG weeks, months, or years later.

Clients appear pale and diaphoretic. Nausea may be followed by vomiting. They may be hypotensive and faint. The pulse is rapid and weak and may be irregular. Signs of left-sided heart failure (eg, dyspnea, cyanosis, and cough) may appear if the pumping of the left ventricle is sufficiently impaired.

Diagnostic Findings

Laboratory tests include a series of serum enzyme and isoenzyme levels, which are elevated (Box 32–3). In addition to standard cardiac enzymes, serial levels of troponin, a protein necessary for the proper contraction of myocardial cells, may be elevated. The white blood cell count and the erythrocyte sedimentation rate increase about the third day due to the inflammatory response triggered by the injury to myocardial cells. The blood sugar may be elevated in clients with diabetes (and those without) because of their response to a major stressor.

Following an MI, characteristic changes appear in the ECG within 2 to 12 hours after the infarction but may take as long as 3 days to develop. These changes include ST segment elevation, T wave inversion, and the appearance of a Q wave (Fig. 32–6).

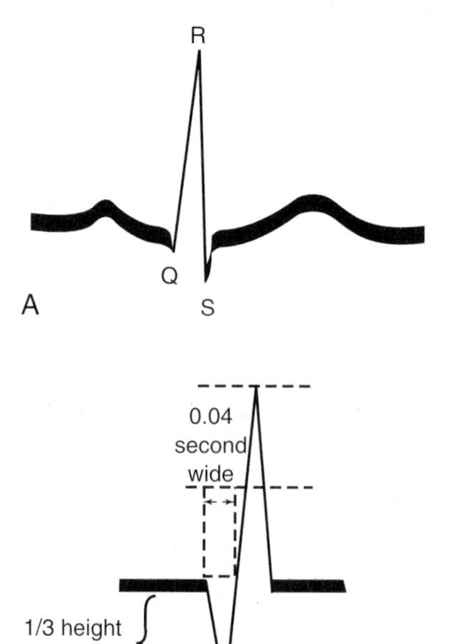

FIGURE 32-6. (*A*) Normal QRS complex. (*B*) The presence of a pathologic Q wave is indicative of a transmural myocardial infarction.

MEDICAL MANAGEMENT

Treatment is directed toward reducing tissue hypoxia, relieving pain, treating shock (if present), and correcting arrhythmias if they occur.

Thrombolytic Therapy

If the client is seen within 6 hours of the onset of the occlusion, re-establishing coronary artery blood flow can reduce the area of infarct. Treatment may include the administration of **thrombolytic agents**. Drugs such as streptokinase, urokinase, and recombinant tissue plasminogen activator (r-TPA), dissolve the thrombus occluding the coronary artery, thus restoring the circulation of oxygenated blood to the myocardium. Depending on how stable the client is, thrombolytic therapy may be followed with PTCA or CABG after the risk for bleeding has been reduced. Box 32–4 highlights guidelines for the administration of thrombolytics.

BOX 32-3 Enzyme Elevation following an Acute Myocardial Infarction

CK-MB (Creatine Kinase)
Rises 4 to 12 hours after infarction, peaks in 24 hours, and returns to normal in 3 to 4 days.

AST (Aspartate Transaminase)
Increases 6 to 12 hours after infarction, peaks in 36 hours, and returns to normal in 3 to 4 days.

LDH_1 and LDH_2 (Lactic Dehydrogenase)
Rises 24 to 48 hours after infarction, peaks in 3 to 6 days, and returns to normal in 7 to 14 days. If **LDH_1** to **LDH_2** ratio is greater than 1.0 it is indicative of myocardial damage.

Symptomatic Treatment

Drug therapy includes analgesics for pain, nitrates or other vasodilating drugs to improve blood flow, diuretics to reduce circulating blood volume, sedatives to promote rest and reduce anxiety, anticoagulants to prevent additional thrombus formation, and drugs to treat arrhythmias (Table 32–1). Oxygen is ordered to treat or prevent hypoxemia. Complete bed rest is initially prescribed but is not recommended for uncomplicated MIs after the first 24 hours. Activity is adjusted according to the extent of the MI, the occurrence of complications, and the client's response to therapy. Smoking is forbidden during the acute phase and permanent cessation is advised. Intake of fat, sodium, and calories are restricted. The intra-aortic balloon pump may be used for clients who develop severe left ventricular failure (see Chap. 35).

BOX 32-4 Contraindications for Thrombolytic Agents

- Chest pain longer than 6 hours' duration
- Coagulation disorders
- Uncontrolled hypertension
- Recent hemorrhagic cerebrovascular accident
- Active internal bleeding
- Recent major surgery
- Pregnancy

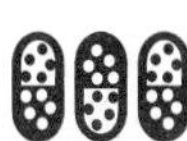

TABLE 32-1 **Drugs Used in the Treatment of Myocardial Infarction**

Drug Category/Drug Action	Side Effects	Nursing Considerations
Vasodilators		
nitroglycerin Relieves chest pain by dilating coronary arteries. Reestablishes blood flow around thrombi.	Headache, dizziness, orthostatic hypotension, tachycardia, flushing, nausea, hypersensitivity	Assess the client for hypotension. Monitor for pain relief. Monitor the client for headache and flushed skin.
Beta-adrenergic Blockers		
propranolol (Inderal) Prevents or inhibits sympathetic stimulation, decreasing myocardial oxygen demand. Used to prevent anginal attacks.	Hypotension, bradycardia, bronchospasm, congestive heart failure, depression, impotence	Administer drugs with meals, do not discontinue medication abruptly. Monitor for fluid retention, rash, difficulty breathing. Monitor blood glucose in clients with diabetes.
Thrombolytics		
alteplase (Activase); recombinant tissue plasminogen activator (r-TPA) Reestablishes blood flow to ischemic areas by dissolving thrombi.	Contraindicated in clients with history of cerebrovascular accident and bleeding tendencies, cardiac arrhythmias, hypotension, bleeding at venous or arterial access sites, nausea and vomiting	Increased risk of hemorrhage if given with heparin. Monitor prothrombin time and partial thromboplastin time; apply pressure to control superficial bleeding.
Anticoagulants		
heparin sodium (Hepalean) Inhibits thrombus and clot formation by blocking the conversion of prothrombin to thrombin and fibrinogen to fibrin.	Hemorrhage, bruising, thrombocytopenia, alopecia, chills, fever	Increase chance of hemorrhage with oral anticoagulants. Given subcutaneously or IV. Apply pressure to all intramuscular injection sites, monitor for epistaxis, other forms of bleeding, have protamine sulfate on unit in case of overdose.
Calcium Channel Blockers		
diltiazem (Cardizem) Relieves angina by improving blood supply to the myocardium by dilating coronary arteries and reducing myocardial oxygen demand. Decreases myocardial contractility, reduces arrhythmias.	Hypotension, dizziness, congestive heart failure, pulmonary edema, nausea	Check blood pressure and heart rate before each dose. Withhold drug in the presence of hypotension, observe for signs and symptoms of congestive heart failure and fluid overload.
Diuretics		
furosemide (Lasix) Decreases work of the heart by promoting the excretion of sodium and water thus reducing circulating blood volume.	Dizziness, dehydration, blurred vision, anorexia, diarrhea, nocturia, polyuria, thrombocytopenia, orthostatic hypotension, hypokalemia	Weigh the client daily. Measure intake and output. Monitor serum potassium, and replace potassium with bananas, orange juice, or prescribed supplement.

SURGICAL MANAGEMENT

A CABG procedure (see Chap. 36) is done to reopen blocked coronary arteries surgically. In clients who are experiencing cardiogenic shock, a **ventricular assist device** may be implanted or cardiomyoplasty, a new procedure for grafting skeletal muscle to replace a dysfunctional area of myocardium, may be used (see Chap. 35).

NURSING PROCESS
The Client With an Acute Myocardial Infarction

Assessment

Most deaths from acute MI occur in the first hours after the onset of pain, so rapid, thorough, and ongoing assessment is essential. A thorough history from the client or family member is necessary to establish baseline data. The history includes a description of the pain with regard to location, type, duration, intensity, and whether it radiates to other areas, such as down the arm or to the jaw. A medical history, including a drug history, also is important because other disorders, such as diabetes mellitus and hypertension, may alter or require additional treatment modalities. Take vital signs frequently. Auscultate heart and lungs, and note the cardiac rate and rhythm. Assess peripheral pulses with particular attention to their amplitude. Note pallor, diaphoresis, nausea, cyanosis, and apprehension. Monitor cardiac output by assessing urine volume and color.

Diagnosis and Planning

The care of the client with an acute MI includes, but is not limited to, the following:

Nursing Diagnosis and Collaborative Problems	Nursing Interventions
Pain related to imbalance of myocardial oxygen supply and demand; ischemia. **Goal:** The client will be free of pain.	Assess pain status frequently. Administer narcotic analgesia and nitrates as ordered. Administer oxygen therapy. Provide for physical and emotional rest—promote a quiet, restful environment.
PC: Hemorrhage **Goal:** The nurse will manage and minimize bleeding.	During and after administration of a thrombolytic drug, observe the client closely for signs and symptoms of bleeding: blood in the urine or stool; bruising; epistaxis; abdominal pain (which may indicate intra-abdominal bleeding); or change in the level of consciousness, mood, or behavior (which may indicate intracranial bleeding). Avoid intramuscular and IV injections and arterial punctures during therapy and until risk for excessive bleeding at the puncture sites has subsided.
PC: Arrhythmias **Goal:** The nurse will manage and minimize arrhythmias.	Place the client on a cardiac monitor and closely observe for arrhythmias. Be prepared to perform cardiopulmonary resuscitation (CPR, see Clinical Procedure 32-1).
Risk for Decreased Cardiac Output related to arrhythmias, decreased contractility related to myocardial damage **Goal:** The client will maintain adequate cardiac output as evidenced by stable vital signs, heart rate within 60 to 100 beats/min, lungs clear, adequate urine output ($\geq$ 30 mL/h).	Assess for signs and symptoms of decreased cardiac output hourly, or as often as indicated by client condition. Monitor heart rhythm. Promote rest. Administer oxygen and nitrates as ordered and indicated. Carry out procedures in a confident manner. Discourage Valsalva's maneuver.
Anxiety and **Fear** related to possible death, concern over actual/potential lifestyle changes, worry concerning family situations **Goal:** Client will have decreased anxiety and fear as evidenced by verbal expressions of decreased anxiety.	Allow client to express fears and anxieties. Carry out procedures in a calm, relaxed manner. Promote uninterrupted blocks of time for client to rest, sleep, or visit with family members. Check on client frequently and answer call lights promptly. Acknowledge feelings of grief over perceived or actual lost lifestyles. Administer sedatives and antianxiety medications as indicated.

Evaluation

- Pain is eliminated.
- There is no evidence of bleeding and arrhythmias are controlled.
- Vital signs are stable and urine output is adequate.
- Anxiety is reduced.

Client and Family Teaching

Assess client and family learning needs. Depending on the physician's prescribed therapy, cover those subjects that are appropriate for each individual client. Family members may be too exhausted

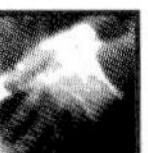

Clinical Procedure 32-1
Performing Cardiopulmonary Resuscitation

PURPOSE	EQUIPMENT
• To establish artificial ventilation of the lungs and circulation of the blood.	• Pocket mask, if available

Nursing Action	Rationale
Attempt to arouse the client; shake him and call his name.	May restore consciousness.
Notify emergency personnel if client does not respond.	Advanced life support may be needed if basic life support is not sufficient.
Open airway with head-tilt, chin-lift.	Moves tongue away from airway.
Remove objects or emesis from mouth.	Objects or vomitus could be forced into airway during rescue breathing.
Ascertain whether client is breathing by looking and listening for air.	Establishes need for rescue breathing.
If no breathing, pinch nose shut and give two rescue breaths through mouth, using a one-way valve pocket mask, if available.	Provides client with oxygen to sustain life.
Feel for a carotid pulse. If none is felt, administer cardiac compressions at a rate of five compressions to one rescue breath (80–100 compressions a minute). (*administer 15 cardiac compressions to two rescue breaths if performing one-rescuer CPR).	Depressing the sternum compresses the heart, forcing blood into the aorta and pulmonary artery, maintaining circulation and blood pressure.
Check effectiveness of CPR after 1 minute (pupils responding to light, pulse at carotid artery, improved skin color).	Establishes adequate blood flow to brain. Client will have a spontaneous pulse when heart begins to beat on its own.
Continue with CPR, enlisting help when needed. Do not interrupt CPR for more than 6 to 7 seconds.	CPR should not be interrupted to sustain circulation.

from spending time at the hospital to assimilate much information. Help family members conserve their own energy by staggering relief vigils in pairs or meeting their own physical needs for sleep and food. Give the family the names of nurses if they have questions after discharge. Verbal Information should be provided as well as written. Include instructions regarding:

- Medication regimen: importance of drug therapy, dose, time taken, adverse drug effects
- Type and amount of activity allowed: prescribed exercise program, resumption of sexual activity (Box 32–5)
- Rehabilitation programs: where located, types, cost
- Diet, how to read food labels, what food labels indicate
- How to monitor pulse rate and blood pressure
- Symptoms that should be reported to a physician as soon as possible
- How to avoid stressful situations
- Importance of continued medical supervision

BOX 32-5 Sexual Guidelines Following Myocardial Infarction

- Check with the physician before resuming sexual activity.
- Avoid sex with anyone other than your usual partner.
- Avoid sexual positions that require supporting your own weight.
- Get adequate rest before sexual intercourse.
- Have sex in the same environment used before the MI.
- Postpone sex for 2 to 3 hours after eating a heavy meal or consuming alcohol.
- Use a short-acting nitrate, if the physician approves, before intercourse.
- Begin with moderate sexual foreplay.
- Use medium water temperatures when bathing or showering before or after sexual activity.

Occlusive Disorders of Peripheral Blood Vessels

Occlusive disorders of the peripheral blood vessels are collectively termed **peripheral vascular diseases**. Common disorders include Raynaud's disease, thrombosis, phlebothrombosis, and embolism.

Raynaud's Disease

Periodic constriction of the arteries that supply the extremities characterizes Raynaud's disease. The condition is much more common in young women than in men.

ETIOLOGY AND PATHOPHYSIOLOGY

The underlying cause of Raynaud's disease is not entirely clear. In some, it seems *idiopathic* (no explainable reason); in others, it is secondary to connective tissue diseases, such as scleroderma, lupus erythematosus, or rheumatoid arthritis (see Chap. 66).

Raynaud's disease is characterized by brief spasms of the arteries and arterioles in the fingers (most common sites), toes, nose, ears, or chin. The spasms last approximately 15 minutes and cause temporary ischemia to the tissues. The vessels then dilate widely, apparently to compensate for the restriction. Patchy areas of necrosis occur if the ischemia is prolonged.

The anatomy of the arteries and arterioles is normal. One theory explaining the vasospasms is impaired prostaglandin release. Several types of prostaglandins (chemicals stored in cellular membranes) can cause vasoconstriction or vasodilation. One type is linked to the typical vasodilation, increased capillary permeability, and pain accompanying an inflammatory response.

ASSESSMENT FINDINGS

Signs and Symptoms

Attacks occur intermittently and with varying frequency but especially after exposure to cold. The hallmark symptoms of arterial insufficiency include ischemia, pain, and paresthesia. The hands become cold, blanched, and wet with perspiration. Numbness and tingling also may occur. Awkwardness and fumbling are noted, especially when fine movements are attempted. After the initial pallor, the hands, especially the fingers, become deeply cyanotic and begin to ache. An attack can be relieved by placing the hands in warm water or by going indoors where it is warm. Eventually the vasospasm is relieved, and blood rushes to the part. The skin in the deprived areas becomes flushed, swollen, and warm, and the person has a sensation of throbbing pain.

In the early stages of the disease, the hands usually appear normal between attacks. The disease does not necessarily progress to cause severe disability. The symptoms are often mild and may even improve spontaneously. When the disease is severe and of long duration, cyanosis of the fingers persists between the attacks and skin changes gradually occur. Painful ulcers and superficial gangrene may develop at the fingertips. The fingers are especially vulnerable to infection. Healing of even minor lesions is often slow and uncertain.

Diagnostic Findings

There are no specific laboratory studies to confirm a diagnosis of Raynaud's disease. Diagnosis is made by a history of the symptoms and an examination of the involved extremities. Laboratory blood tests are ordered to confirm or rule out an accompanying connective tissue disorder.

MEDICAL AND SURGICAL MANAGEMENT

Treatment involves avoiding factors that precipitate attacks. Smoking is contraindicated because it causes vasoconstriction. Drug therapy with peripheral vasodilators, such as isoxsuprine (Vasodilan), may be attempted but results usually are less than desired. Other drugs, such as nifedipine (Procardia), are being used investigationally for this disorder. An intravenous (IV) infusion of prostaglandin E may provide temporary relief.

Sympathectomy may be performed; however, due to the disappointing results, the procedure is performed less frequently than in the past. If gangrene develops, the affected areas are amputated.

NURSING MANAGEMENT

Once an episode of pain occurs, there are several ways that the attack can be aborted. If warming the hands in water is impossible, the client is encouraged to imagine them being warmed in some way such as being held near a roaring fire. The mind can alter the physiology of blood flow. Another technique is to teach clients to imitate the exercise snow skiers use called the McIntyre maneuver. While standing, clients are instructed to swing their arms behind and then in front of their bodies at a rate of about 180 times per minute. The swinging motion distributes blood to the distal areas of the fingers.

Client and Family Teaching

Instruct clients with Raynaud's disease to avoid situations that contribute to the ischemic episodes. Explain that injuries may heal slowly. If clients smoke, it is imperative that they stop because nicotine causes vasoconstriction and increases the frequency of episodes. Advise clients to wear wool socks and mittens during cold weather. Over-the-counter drugs, such as nasal decongestants, cold remedies, and drugs for the symptomatic relief of hay fever, are avoided. Advise clients to wear work gloves while doing household chores like gardening and washing dishes to prevent accidental injury. Inform clients on how to perform nail care to avoid injury; include points like soaking the hands or feet before trimming nails, trimming nails straight across, and using the services of a podiatrist for the treatment of corns or calluses. If a sympathectomy is done, emphasize that the areas from which sympathetic stimuli have been removed no longer perspire. Instruct the client that applying cream to prevent excessive dryness of the skin may be helpful.

Thrombosis, Phlebothrombosis, and Embolism

A **thrombus** is a stationary clot. **Thrombosis** is a state in which a clot has formed within a blood vessel. **Phlebothrombosis** is the development of a clot within a vein without inflammation. Phlebothrombosis and thrombophlebitis have similar symptoms and treatment (see Chap. 30). An **embolus** is a moving mass (clot) of particles either solid or gas within the bloodstream.

ETIOLOGY AND PATHOPHYSIOLOGY

Thrombosis in the venous system most often occurs in the lower extremities and generally is associated with disorders or circumstances that cause venous stasis. For example, inactivity, immobility, or trauma to a blood vessel commonly predispose to clot formation. Orthopedic surgical procedures increase the incidence of deep vein thrombosis of the lower extremities. Atherosclerosis, endocarditis, pooling of blood in a ventricular aneurysm, and arrhythmias like atrial fibrillation can precipitate arterial thrombosis and subsequent embolization.

When a thrombus forms or an embolus reaches a blood vessel that is too small to permit its passage, there is partial or total occlusion of blood flow through the vessel.

ASSESSMENT FINDINGS

Signs and Symptoms

When an arterial clot is present, symptoms arise from ischemia to the tissues that depend on the obstructed vessel for their blood supply. If *total* occlusion exists, the extremity suddenly becomes white, cold, and extremely painful. Arterial pulsations are absent below the area of obstruction. Numbness, tingling, or cramping also may be present, and surrounding blood vessels go into spasm. Loss of sensation and ability to move the part follows these symptoms. Symptoms of shock frequently occur if a large vessel has been obstructed. When a small vessel is occluded, symptoms of ischemia, such as pallor and coldness, occur but are less severe.

Clients with phlebothrombosis may have few, if any, symptoms because inflammation is absent. The signs and symptoms of deep vein thrombosis usually include pain, swelling, and tenderness of the affected extremity, and mild fever. A positive Homans' sign, pain on dorsiflexion of the foot, may be present. A thrombus may become a mobile embolus and lodge in a distal blood vessel, like the pulmonary capillaries, causing symptoms related to the organ to which circulation has become impaired. (Refer to the discussions of pulmonary embolism in Chap. 28 and cerebral embolism in Chap. 45.)

Diagnostic Findings

Arteriography or venography (also called phlebography) using a contrast dye identifies the point of obstruction. Doppler ultrasonography is used to detect abnormalities in peripheral blood flow. Plethysmography measures volume changes within the venous or arterial system.

MEDICAL AND SURGICAL TREATMENT

Treatment depends on whether an artery or a vein is occluded and the degree of occlusion (partial or complete).

Arterial Occlusive Disease

If an artery is completely occluded, treatment *cannot* be delayed. The physician may order an immediate IV injection of heparin to prevent the development of further clots or the extension of those already present. An attempt may be made to improve circulation by administering vasodilating drugs. A sympathetic nerve block (injection of a local anesthetic into the sympathetic ganglia) may relieve vasospasm. Narcotics may relieve pain and ease the client's apprehension. A thrombolytic agent may be prescribed if the client has experienced a pulmonary embolism or the embolus is occluding a large arterial vessel.

If circulation to the extremity cannot be restored, a thrombectomy, embolectomy, endarterectomy (removal of the lining of an artery), or insertion of a bypass graft is necessary. The nursing management of thrombectomy, embolectomy, endarterectomy, and bypass grafting is discussed in Chapter 36.

Venous Occlusive Disease

Venous thrombosis is treated with bed rest, elevation of the extremity, local heat, analgesics for pain, and intermittent subcutaneous injections or continuous IV heparin therapy, followed by oral anticoagulants once the heparin has achieved a therapeutic effect. Deep vein thrombosis may necessitate surgical removal of the clot (thrombectomy).

NURSING MANAGEMENT

Obtain a history of the symptoms and identify the characteristics of the client's pain. Assess for Homans' sign by having the client dorsiflex each foot. Examine the extremities and compare skin color, temperature, capillary refill time, and tissue integrity. Measure each calf. Palpate peripheral pulses; use a Doppler ultrasound device (Fig. 32–7) if pulses cannot be palpated. Mark the location of each peripheral artery with a soft-tipped pen to facilitate its relocation. Immediately report any change in the quality of a peripheral pulse or the sudden absence of a pulse. Any color change (line of demarcation) above or below the area of occlusion can be outlined with a soft-tipped pen to establish a data base for future comparisons. Monitor the client's response to anticoagulation therapy.

Monitor IV infusions of heparin hourly. Monitor partial thromboplastin time if heparin is administered and prothrombin time when oral anticoagulation is prescribed. Therapeutic response and daily dosage are determined by these values. Be alert for signs of bleeding and keep protamine sulfate on hand for reversing heparin, and vitamin K for reversing oral anticoagulants. Additional nursing management is directed toward increasing arterial or venous blood flow, relieving pain, preventing complications, and providing thorough teaching before discharge.

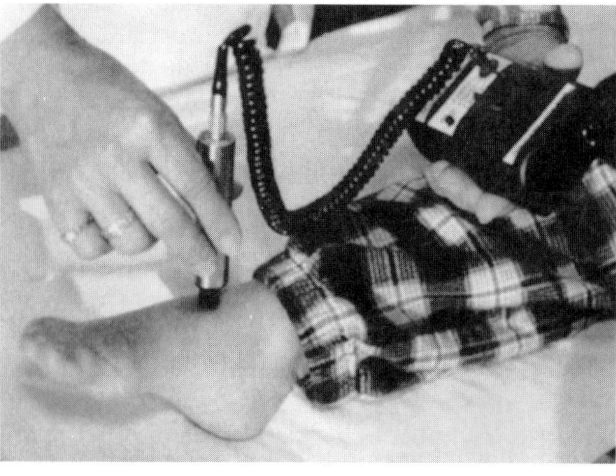

FIGURE 32-7. A hand-held Doppler is used to identify blood flow in an artery with weak or absent pulsations.

Client and Family Teaching

To prevent a recurrence of thrombosis, embolism, and phlebothrombosis, inform clients to avoid prolonged periods of inactivity (especially sitting), elevate the legs periodically, and walk or do isometric leg exercises at frequent intervals if sitting is unavoidable. Recommend wearing antiembolism stockings to prevent venous stasis (especially if the client has venous leg ulcers). Instruct the client to apply these stockings before assuming a dependent position or after elevating the extremities for several minutes. Add that antiembolism stockings need to be removed and reapplied twice a day or as recommended by the physician. Inform those who must take continued anticoagulants to observe for signs of unusual bleeding and to keep appointments for laboratory tests.

Disorders of Blood Vessel Walls

Varicose Veins

Varicose veins are dilated, tortuous veins (**varicosities**). The saphenous veins of the legs are commonly affected because they lack support from surrounding leg muscles. Both sexes suffer equally from this disorder. Varicose veins also may occur in other parts of the body, such as the rectum (hemorrhoids) and the esophagus (esophageal varices).

ETIOLOGY AND PATHOPHYSIOLOGY

There is a familial tendency for varicose veins. The valves of the veins become incompetent in early adulthood, resulting in the development of varicosities. In others, anything that constricts or interferes with venous return contributes to the formation of varicose veins. Prolonged standing compromises venous return as blood pools distally with gravity. Obesity and pressure on blood vessels from an enlarging fetus, liver, or abdominal tumor contribute to venous congestion. Thrombophlebitis sometimes leads to the development of varicose veins because the valves of the veins may be damaged during the inflammatory process.

Normally, the action of leg muscles during movement and exercise aids venous return. When the valves within veins become incompetent (Fig. 32–8), blood accumulates rather than being propelled efficiently to the heart. The congestion stretches the veins. Over time, they are unable to recoil and remain in a chronically distended state. Venous hypertension

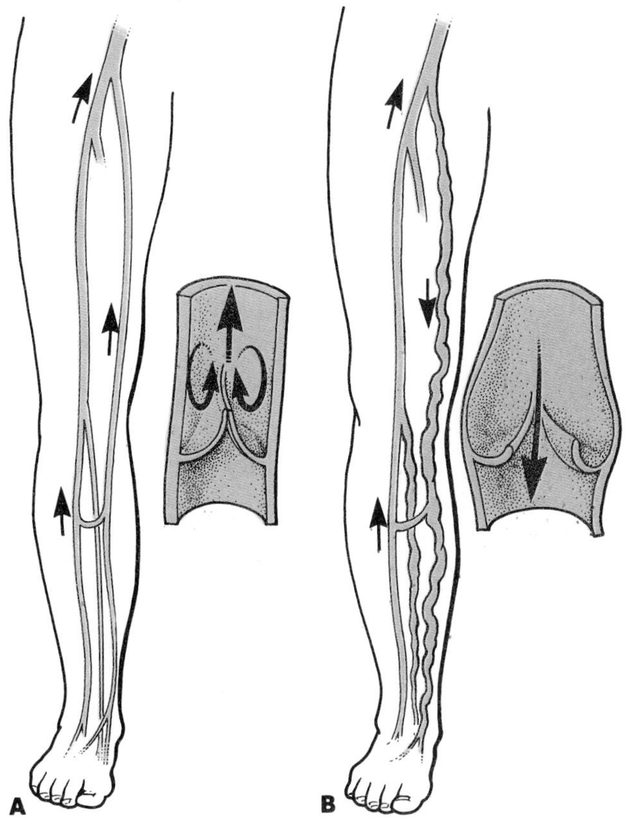

FIGURE 32-8. Varicose veins. (*A*) Normal vein with competent valves. (*B*) Incompetent valve with tortuous, dilated segment.

then forces some fluid to move into the interstitial spaces of surrounding tissue. Venous congestion and local edema may diminish arterial blood flow, resulting in impaired cellular nutrition. Even minor skin or soft tissue injuries easily become infected and ulcerated. The healing of such lesions is slow and uncertain.

ASSESSMENT FINDINGS

Signs and Symptoms

Often the condition first manifests itself when other factors impair venous return. The legs feel heavy and tired, particularly after prolonged standing. The client may say the discomfort is relieved with activity or elevation of the legs.

The veins of the legs look distended and torturous and can be seen under the skin as dark blue or purple swellings. The feet, ankles, and legs may appear swollen. The skin may be slightly darker in the areas of impaired circulation. There may be signs of skin ulcerations in various stages of healing. Capillary refill may be abnormal.

Diagnostic Findings

The *Brodie-Trendelenberg test* is performed for diagnostic purposes. The client lies flat and elevates the affected leg to empty the veins. A tourniquet is then applied to the upper thigh, and the client is asked to stand. If blood flows from the upper part of the leg into the superficial veins when the tourniquet is released, the valves of the superficial veins are considered incompetent. Ultrasonography and venography also are used to detect impaired blood flow.

MEDICAL MANAGEMENT

Treatment of mild varicose veins includes exercise (walking, swimming), weight loss (if needed), the wearing of support stockings, and the avoidance of prolonged periods of sitting. The defective vein may be *sclerosed* or occluded by injecting a chemical that sets up an inflammation within the vein wall. Eventually adhesions form and blood flow must find an alternate route through collateral veins.

SURGICAL MANAGEMENT

Surgical treatment for severe or multiple varicose veins consists of **vein ligation** with or without **vein stripping**. The affected veins are ligated (tied off) above and below the area of incompetent valves. For better results, the ligated veins are severed and removed (stripped). The entire great saphenous vein, which extends from the groin to the ankle, may be removed.

NURSING MANAGEMENT

Assess the skin, distal circulation and peripheral edema. Ask the client to rate the level of discomfort and ability to do active and isometric leg exercises. Refer to Chapter 24 for routine perioperative care.

The client returns from surgery with a gauze dressing covered by elastic roller bandages on the operative leg. If swelling in the operative leg(s) impairs circulation, remove and rewrap the roller bandage. Inspect dressings for signs of active bleeding. Elevate the foot of the bed in the immediate postoperative period to aid venous return. Remind the client to alternately contract and relax the muscles in the lower legs. If the client's active exercise is inadequate, consider using pneumatic venous compression stockings, which cover the leg from the foot to the thigh and periodically inflate and release air, simulating isometric muscle contraction. Ambulate the client as soon as possible to promote venous circulation, reduce edema, and prevent venous thrombosis. When bleeding is no longer a problem, apply antiembolism stockings in place of the elastic roller bandage. Provide an adequate fluid intake to decrease the potential for thrombosis.

Client and Family Teaching

Identify factors that impair venous circulation such as wearing elastic girdles, tight belts, using round garters or rolling and twisting nylon stockings, and standing or sitting for prolonged periods; suggest alternative measures that will promote venous return. Stress that the client should avoid sitting with the knees crossed. Describe appropriate foot and nail care. Recommend active or isometric exercises and elevation of the extremities at frequent periods during the day. Show the client how to apply and remove elastic support stockings. Encourage weight loss if indicated. Explain that any open areas of skin need to be examined and treated by the physician.

Aneurysms

An **aneurysm** is a stretching and bulging of an arterial wall. Aneurysms of the aorta (aortic arch, thoracic, abdominal) are the most common (Fig. 32–9), but aneurysms can be found in other arteries, such as those in the leg and brain.

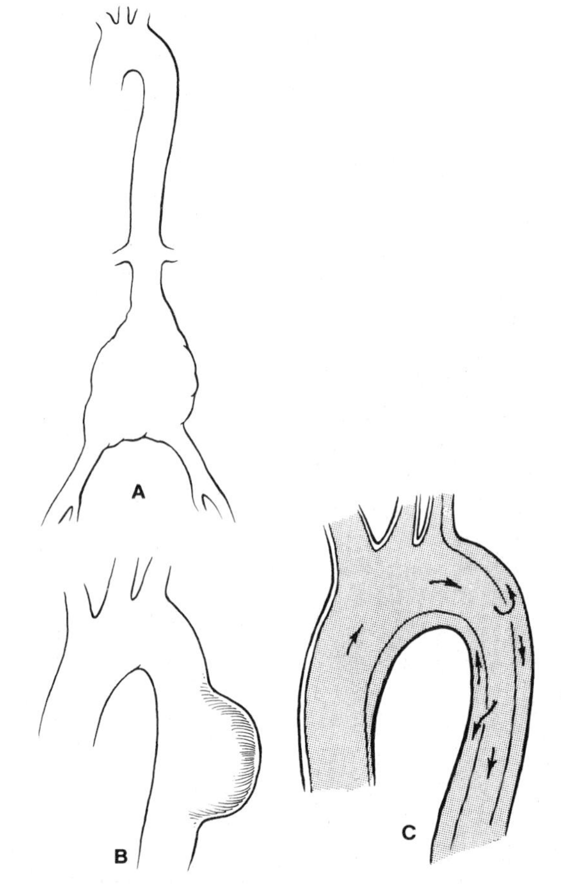

FIGURE 32-9. Aneurysms. (*A*) Fusiform aneurysm of the abdominal aorta characterized by weakening and distention about the entire circumference. (*B*) Sacciform aneurysm in which an isolated area protrudes. (*C*) Dissecting aneurysm identified by one or more tears through which blood accumulates between the layers of the arterial wall.

ETIOLOGY AND PATHOPHYSIOLOGY

Arteriosclerosis, hypertension, trauma, or a congenital weakness can affect the elasticity of the tunica media (middle layer of the artery wall), causing a portion of the vessel to bulge. Once formed, some aneurysms lay down layers of clots, blocking the vessel until blood flow stops. Most aneurysms enlarge until they rupture. Loss of a large volume of arterial blood leads to shock and death if not controlled. Some tear and leak blood into surrounding cavities, like the thorax or abdomen. Blood within a dissecting aneurysm is unavailable to arteries that branch off the aorta. When blood flow decreases or stops, tissue necrosis occurs.

ASSESSMENT FINDINGS

Signs and Symptoms

Many aneurysms go unnoticed by the individual until they are found during a physical examination or the client has a massive hemorrhage. Some cause pain and discomfort and symptoms related to pressure on nearby structures. For example, a thoracic aortic aneurysm can cause bronchial obstruction, dysphagia (difficulty swallowing), and dyspnea. An abdominal aortic aneurysm can produce nausea and vomiting from pressure exerted on the intestines, or it may cause back pain from pressure on the vertebrae or spinal nerves. Most individuals are hypertensive. A pulsating mass may be felt or even seen around the umbilicus or to the left of midline over the abdomen. A **bruit** (purring or blowing sound) can be auscultated over the mass. Circulation to tissue may be impaired.

Symptoms of a dissecting aneurysm vary and depend on whether a branching artery has been occluded or a tear has occurred in the aortic wall. Many clients become suddenly and acutely ill. There may be a marked difference in the blood pressures of the left and right arms, or the blood pressures of the left and right legs may be quite unequal. Severe pain and signs of shock usually are present but symptoms can be less severe in some instances. Because symptoms vary, diagnosis may be difficult.

Diagnostic Findings

Radiographs can demonstrate aneurysms when the arterial wall contains deposits of calcium. Aortography identifies the size and exact location of the aneurysm.

MEDICAL AND SURGICAL MANAGEMENT

Medical treatment includes administering antihypertensive drugs to keep the blood pressure low.

Aneurysms are treated surgically whenever possible; no other cure exists. They are repaired by bypass or replacement grafting. A dissecting aneurysm or rupture of an aneurysm is a surgical emergency.

NURSING MANAGEMENT

The nurse helps to control hypertension by keeping activity low and stressful situations to a minimum. Straining during a bowel movement, coughing, or changing positions is avoided. Blood pressure, pulse, hourly urine output, color, level of consciousness, and characteristics of pain are monitored for signs of hemorrhage or dissection. The nurse prepares the client for diagnostic testing and operative interventions. Afterward, the client is monitored for shock and adequate tissue perfusion. See Chapter 36 for the nursing management of a client undergoing cardiovascular surgery.

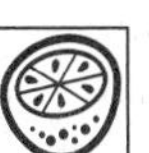

General Nutritional Considerations

Total serum cholesterol is a measure of all cholesterol; its value as a screening tool is limited because it does not distinguish between "bad" and "good" cholesterol. LDL, cholesterol, known as "bad" cholesterol, increases the risk of coronary heart disease. High LDL levels are associated with obesity and excessive intake of calories, saturated fat, total fat, and cholesterol. HDL, the "good" cholesterol, is inversely correlated with coronary heart disease. Smoking cessation, weight loss, exercise, and small amounts of alcohol increase HDL levels.

The National Cholesterol Education Program urges all Americans over the age of 2 to follow a Step One Diet to reduce their risk of heart disease. It is also the initial treatment for hypercholesterolemic clients who have not yet modified their diets. Recommended food choices include:

- 6 oz or less per day of lean meat, fish, and skinless poultry. Red meat is limited to three to four times per week and all visible fat is removed. Dried peas and beans are recommended as a low-fat protein source for meatless meals.
- 3 egg yolks or less per week; egg whites are used freely.
- 1% or skim milk and yogurt; skim milk cheeses.
- 6 teaspoons or less of added fats per day (margarine, oils, salad dressings), including that used in cooking. Hydrogenated fats are avoided; the softer the margarine the better. Olive and canola oils are preferred because they are highest in monosaturated fats.
- More fruits and vegetables
- Whole grain breads and cereals
- Low-fat desserts such as gelatin, sherbet, angel food cake, and fruit

Clients who fail to achieve desired cholesterol levels after 3 months of good compliance with the Step One Diet are progressed to the Step Two Diet, which limits saturated fat and cholesterol more severely.

Weight reduction lowers LDL cholesterol, increases HDL cholesterol, reduces cardiac workload, and has the added benefits of reducing triglycerides, lowering blood pressure, and reducing the risk for diabetes. Eating less fat enhances weight loss.

Antioxidants in the diet, like vitamin E and beta carotene, may help prevent the oxidation of cholesterol within the artery wall and the subsequent series of events that lead to plaque formation. Relatively newly recognized antioxidant phytochemicals (naturally occurring "plant chemicals"), such as flavonoids in citrus fruit and resveratol in red wine, show promise in protecting against heart disease. Because researchers are only beginning to identify and understand how phytochemicals function, the best advice for now is to eat more fruits and vegetables, and the greater variety the better.

Omega-3 fatty acids, abundant in fish oils, lower serum triglycerides and decrease platelet aggregation. Populations who eat fish frequently have a lower incidence of heart disease; however, fish oil supplements have not been demonstrated to be either safe or effective.

Soluble fiber, most abundant in oats, various brans, citrus fruits, carrots, and dried peas and beans, helps lower serum cholesterol by promoting cholesterol excretion. Rich sources of fiber are also low in fat and are good sources of vitamins, minerals, and phytochemicals.

Folic acid is being investigated for its role in heart disease prevention through its effect on homocysteine metabolism. Foods high in folic acid include enriched cereals, brewer's yeast, dried peas and beans, orange juice, and asparagus.

Although moderate alcohol consumption increases HDL cholesterol, it also raises blood pressure, impedes weight loss, and appears to increase the risk of breast cancer in women. Men who drink alcohol should limit their intake to 2 drinks or less per day; women who drink should consume less than 1 drink per day. People who do not drink should not be encouraged to do so.

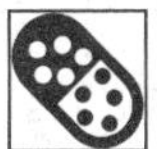

General Pharmacologic Considerations

Aspirin, one tablet (325 mg) daily, may be recommended by the physician for clients with coronary artery disease. It inhibits platelet aggregation, thereby decreasing the ability of the blood to clot. The prothrombin time may be slightly prolonged.

When the client with CAD requires rest and a reduction of anxiety, sedatives or tranquilizers may be prescribed. The physician is notified if the client becomes somnolent and no longer initiates deep breathing, leg exercises, or moving in bed.

All nitroglycerin preparations are stored in their original container and never placed in a container with other drugs.

Each time the tablet, capsule, or ointment is used, the cover or cap must be tightly closed.

The sustained-release form of nitroglycerin is used for prevention (prophylaxis) of anginal attacks, rather than for relief of the pain of an attack. The transdermal systems are pads or disks that are applied to the skin. These systems slowly release nitroglycerin over a period of time. With the topical ointment, a measured amount (in inches) is squeezed from a tube, applied in a uniform layer on the skin, and covered with a plastic wrap.

Nitroglycerin can cause a throbbing headache, flushing, and nausea; usually these effects can be minimized by decreasing the dose. A client not accustomed to taking nitroglycerin should remain seated for a few minutes after taking the medication; some people experience a feeling of faintness.

The vasodilating effects of the oral and topical nitrate preparations are diminished if the drugs are used on a 24-hour continuous basis. Removing the transdermal patch at night and reapplying it in the morning or giving the oral preparation three times a day (rather than around the clock) may prevent a diminished effect.

Before administering thrombolytic agents such as anistreplase or streptokinase, question the client about recent streptococcal infections. Such infections may decrease the effectiveness of anistreplase or streptokinase.

Treatment with a thrombolytic agent must be started within 2 to 6 hours of the onset of symptoms for an MI or within 7 days of other type of thrombi (eg, deep vein thrombosis).

There is an increased risk of bleeding when a thrombolytic agent is administered with heparin. The primary health care provider usually discontinues the heparin with thrombolytic treatment.

An antidote for overdosage of thrombolytic therapy is aminocaproic acid (Amicar).

General Gerontologic Considerations

The incidence of arteriosclerosis and other vascular disorders rises with age. Older clients who take medication should ask their pharmacists to dispense the drug in a container without a childproof cap. This type of cap usually is difficult to remove when the client has arthritis or limited vision.

General physiologic changes of aging predispose clients to occlusive disorders, especially due to atherosclerotic plaque formation. In addition, the pumping ability of the heart decreases with age, increasing the risk of heart failure after an MI.

Coronary artery disease is the most common cause of death in the older adult. However, less than 50% of older adults report chest pain with an acute myocardial infarction, whereas approximately 80% of younger adults report chest pain. Older adults are more likely to have nonspecific symptoms such as dyspnea, confusion, and syncope.

When calcium channel blockers such as nifedipine and verapamil are used to treat angina, a peripheral vasodilating effect may occur. Therefore, they should be given cautiously in older adults who are at greater risk for hypotension.

Older adults are more sensitive to the hypotensive effects of nitrates, probably due to impaired venous valves, diminished baroceptor reflex, and decreased vascular volume.

SUMMARY OF KEY CONCEPTS

- Arteriosclerosis is a hardening of the arteries; atherosclerosis is filling of the artery with fatty plaque. Both interfere with the circulation of oxygenated blood to tissues and organs.
- Some risk factors for developing CAD include a family history, hyperlipidemia, smoking, hypertension, sedentary lifestyle, diabetes mellitus, and being unable to manage stressors. The majority of these can be modified.
- Chest pain, called angina, is the primary symptom of CAD. Diagnosis is made by history, stress ECG, coronary arteriography, and elevated serum lipid levels. Treatment includes reversing cardiac risk factors, eliminating plaque from the arteries, and revascularizing the myocardium.
- Severe, unrelieved chest pain is the hallmark of an MI. The chest pain is accompanied by diaphoresis, pale skin, nausea, and vomiting. Elevated cardiac isoenzymes and later ECG changes confirm the diagnosis. Treatment includes reestablishing coronary artery blood flow, managing the symptoms, and preventing additional complications.
- Nursing management of the client with myocardial infarction includes pain management, monitoring for potential complications such as hemorrhage, maintaining adequate cardiac output, and relieving anxiety and pain.
- One disease caused by arterial vasospasm is Raynaud's disease. It is characterized by skin color variations ranging from pallor due to ischemia; cyanosis due to the buildup of carbon dioxide in tissue; and redness due to rebound dilation of the previously constricted arterioles. Diagnosis is made primarily by the history of the client. The client must avoid factors that cause vasoconstriction such as smoking and chilling. Vasodilating drugs can reduce the symptoms. Imaging techniques can abort attacks.
- Blood vessels also may become occluded by the formation of clots, some of which may break free and travel in the circulation. Occlusion is accompanied by localized symptoms like pain and swelling, and systemic symptoms when circulation to tissues or an organ becomes impaired.
- Nursing management of the client with an occlusive disorder of peripheral blood vessels is directed toward increasing blood flow, relieving pain, preventing complications, and providing thorough teaching.
- Varicose veins form when incompetent valves within the veins cause them to distend with engorged blood. Varicose veins seem to be an inherited trait. Most are diagnosed by appearance alone. Improving venous circulation through elevation of the legs, active exercise, and wearing support stockings is the conservative treatment. In severe cases, one or more veins may be chemically sclerosed or removed surgically.
- Nursing management of the client undergoing surgery for varicose veins is focused on maintaining adequate distal

circulation, controlling pain, preventing injuries, and client teaching.

- An aneurysm is a ballooning of an arterial wall occurring commonly in the aorta. When an aortic aneurysm becomes large, it may produce symptoms like a pulsating abdominal mass or back pain. Aneurysms are often detected when a client is being examined for some other disorder. Controlling hypertension may prevent aneurysms from rupturing; however, only surgical correction will completely relieve the risk for rupture.
- Nursing management of the client with an aortic aneurysm includes controlling hypertension, monitoring for complications, and ensuring adequate tissue perfusion.

CRITICAL THINKING EXERCISES

1. A client presents in the emergency room complaining of substernal chest pain. The client has a history of angina. What assessment criteria will help you differentiate between an anginal attack and an MI? What diagnostic tests will confirm an MI?
2. A client with Raynaud's disease relates to you that she has difficulty reducing attacks during the winter months. What client teaching is indicated in this situation? How can the client reduce the number of ischemic episodes?
3. A client who has had a varicose vein ligation returns to his room following surgery. What assessments are a priority at this time? How can you teach the client to reduce the incidence of further varicose vein formation?

Suggested Readings

Abrams, A. (1998). *Clinical drug therapy: Rationales for nursing practice* (5th ed.). Philadelphia: Lippincott-Raven.

Apple, S. (1996). New trends in thrombolytic therapy. *RN, 59*(1), 30–34.

Ballard, J., Wood, L., & Lansing, A. (1997). Transmyocardial revascularization: Criteria for selecting patients, treatment, and nursing care. *Critical Care Nurse, 17*(1), 42–49, 59.

Carpenito, L. (1997). *Nursing diagnosis: Application to clinical practice* (7th ed.). Philadelphia: Lippincott-Raven.

Fowler, J.P. (1996). How to respond rapidly when chest pain strikes. *Nursing, 26*(4), 42–43.

Hayden, A.M. (1998). Transmyocardial revascularization. *RN, 61* (5), 44–47.

O'Brien, L. (1998). Clinical snapshot. Angina pectoris. *American Journal of Nursing*, 98(1), 48–49.

O'Donnell, L. (1996). Complication of MI: Beyond the acute stage. *American Journal of Nursing, 96*(1), 24–30.

Ondrusek, R. (1996). Spotting an MI before it's an MI. *RN, 59*(1), 26–29.

Ryan, T., Anerson, J., et al. (1996). Guidelines for the management of patients with acute myocardial infarction: A report of the American College of Cardiology/American Heart Association Task Force on Practice Guidelines, Committee on Management of Acute Myocardial Infarction. *Journal of American College of Cardiology 28*, 5.

Sandler, R. (1995). Clinical snapshot: Abdominal aortic aneurysm. *American Journal of Nursing, 95*(1), 38–39.

Strimike, C. (1995). Caring for a patient with an intracoronary stent. *American Journal of Nursing, 95*(1), 40–45.

Wilcox, T. (1997). Angina: Improving the outcome. *RN, 60*(1), 34–40.

Additional Resources

Heart Homepage
http://www.hearthome.com/

Heartweb
http://webaxis.com/heartweb/

Mayo Health Oasis Heart Center
http://www.mayohealth.org

Smart Hearts
http://www.einstein.edu

Heart Disease and Women
http://www.altcard.com

Heart Disease
http://www.merck.com

Cardiac Rehabilitation and Prevention Patient Information
http://www.jhbmc.jhu.ed

Chapter 33

Caring for Clients With Cardiac Arrhythmias

KEY TERMS

Arrhythmia
Asystole
Atrial flutter
Atrial fibrillation
Automatic implantable cardiac defibrillator
Bigeminy
Bradyarrhythmias
Complete heart block
Couplets
Defibrillation
Demand (or synchronous) pacemaker
Elective cardioversion
Fixed-rate (or synchronous) pacemaker
Multifocal PVCs
Pacemaker
Premature ventricular contractions
R on T phenomenon
Sinus bradycardia
Sinus tachycardia
Supraventricular tachycardia
Tachyarrhythmias
Ventricular fibrillation
Ventricular tachycardia

LEARNING OBJECTIVES

On completion of this chapter, the reader will:

- Name and describe six common arrhythmias.
- List three ways arrhythmias are treated.
- Identify four medications to control or eliminate arrhythmias.
- Explain the purpose and two advantages of elective cardioversion.
- Explain when defibrillation is used to treat arrhythmias.
- Name two types of artificial pacemakers and the purpose for their use.
- Describe the nursing management for the client receiving drug therapy, elective cardioversion, defibrillation, or pacemaker insertion.
- Discuss the nursing management of the client with an arrhythmia.

Cardiac rhythm refers to the pattern (or pace) of the heartbeat. This pattern is enabled by the conduction system of the heart and the inherent rhythmicity of cardiac muscle and greatly influences the ability of the heart to pump blood effectively. Cardiac conduction and electrocardiogram (ECG) waveforms are discussed in Chapter 29. The usual cardiac rhythm is called normal sinus rhythm. It is illustrated in Figure 33–1 and its characteristics are listed in Box 33–1. An **arrhythmia** (also called dysrhythmia) is a conduction disorder that results in an abnormally slow or rapid regular heart rate or at an irregular pace. Some arrhythmias do not require treatment, whereas others require immediate intervention because they are potentially fatal. The most common cause of arrhythmias is ischemic heart disease (see Chap. 32). Effects of drug therapy, electrolyte disturbances, metabolic acidosis, and hypothermia can also cause arrhythmias.

Arrhythmias Originating in the Sinoatrial (SA) Node

Sinus Bradycardia

Sinus bradycardia is a regular, but slow, (≤ 60 beats/min) rhythm (Fig. 33–2). It is a pathologic sign in clients with heart disorders, increased intracranial pressure, hypothyroidism, or digitalis toxicity. The danger in bradycardia is that the slow rate may be insufficient to maintain cardiac output. Atropine sulfate is sometimes given intravenously (IV) to increase the heart rate. Healthy athletes and laborers often have heart rates below 60 beats/min; however, this reflects

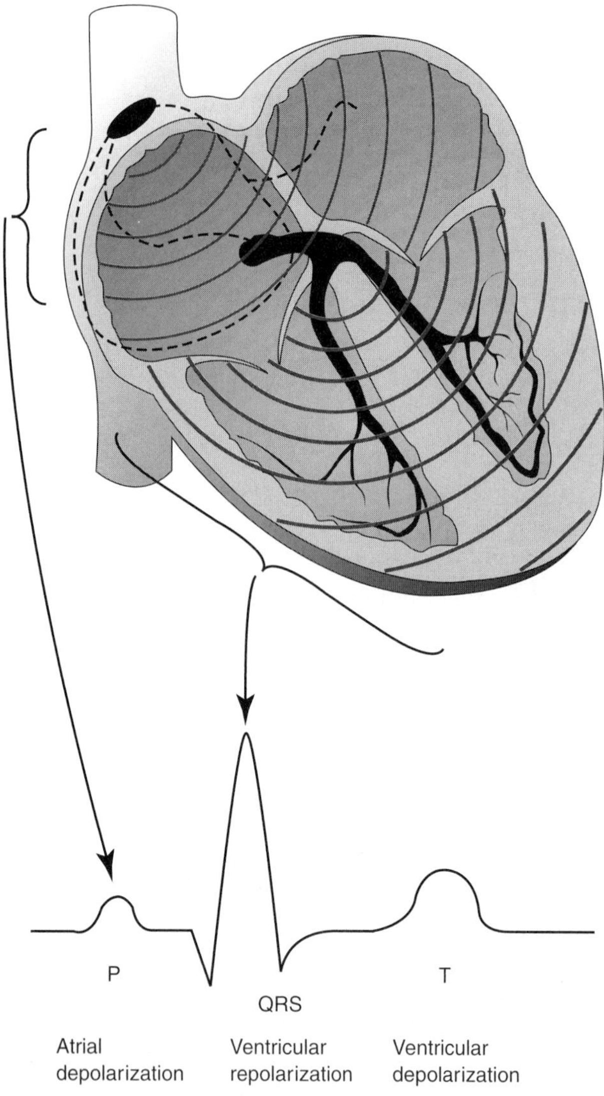

FIGURE 33-1. Normal conduction and ECG waveforms.

a well toned heart conditioned through regular exercise.

Sinus Tachycardia

Sinus tachycardia is a regular but fast (100–150 beats/min) rhythm (see Fig. 33–2). Sinus tachycardia occurs in clients with healthy hearts as a physiologic response to strenuous exercise, anxiety and fear, pain, fever, hyperthyroidism, hemorrhage, shock, or hypoxemia.

Supraventricular Tachycardia

Supraventricular tachycardia (SVT) is an arrhythmia with a dangerously high heart rate (≥ 150 beats/min). At this rate, diastole is shortened and the heart does not have sufficient time to fill. Cardiac output drops dangerously low and heart failure can occur, especially in clients with pre-existing heart disease or damage. Clients with coronary artery disease who have SVT can develop chest pain because coronary blood flow cannot keep up with the increased need of the myocardium imposed by the fast rate. Besides tachycardia and angina, hypotension, syncope, and reduced renal output are signs and symptoms of low cardiac output and impending heart failure. Drugs, such as digitalis, adrenergic blockers, and calcium channel blockers, can be used to slow the heart rate.

BOX 33-1 Characteristics of Normal Sinus Rhythm

- Heart rate between 60 and 100 beats/min.
- Initiated by the sinoatrial (SA) node (upright P wave before each QRS complex).
- Impulse travels to the atrioventricular (AV) node in 0.12 to 0.2 second (the PR interval).
- The ventricles depolarize in 0.12 second or less (the QRS complex).
- Each impulse occurs regularly (evenly spaced).

Atrial Flutter

Atrial flutter (Fig. 33–3) is a disorder in which a single atrial impulse outside the SA node causes the atria to contract at an exceedingly rapid rate (200–400 times/min). The atrioventricular (AV) node conducts only some impulses to the ventricle, resulting in a slower ventricular rate. The atrial waves in atrial flutter have a characteristic sawtooth pattern.

Atrial Fibrillation

In **atrial fibrillation,** several areas in the right atrium initiate impulses resulting in disorganized, rapid atrial activity. The atria quiver rather than contract (Fig. 33–4). The ventricles respond to the atrial stimulus randomly, resulting in an irregular ventricular heart rate. The ventricular response may be too infrequent to maintain an adequate cardiac output. Ibutilide (Corvert) is an antiarrhythmic drug used to convert new-onset atrial fibrillation into sinus rhythm. Atrial fibrillation is also treated with digitalis if the ventricular rate is not too slow or cardioversion is used. Clients who are not candidates for cardioversion and fail to respond to conventional measures experience chronic episodes of atrial fibrillation.

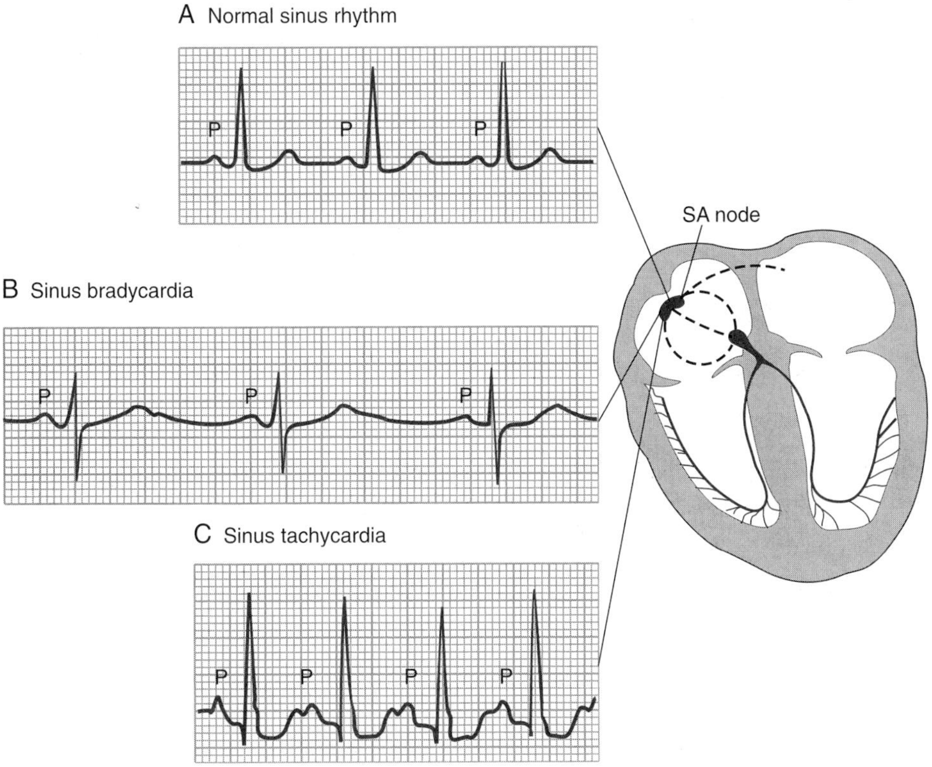

A Normal sinus rhythm

P P P

SA node

B Sinus bradycardia

P P P

C Sinus tachycardia

P P P P

FIGURE 33-2. (*A*) In sinus rhythm, the SA node initiates impulses (P waves) 60 to 100 times/minute. (*B*) In sinus bradycardia, the SA node initiates impulses at 40 to 60 times/minute. (*C*) In sinus tachycardia, the SA node initiates impulses at 100 to 150 times/ minute.

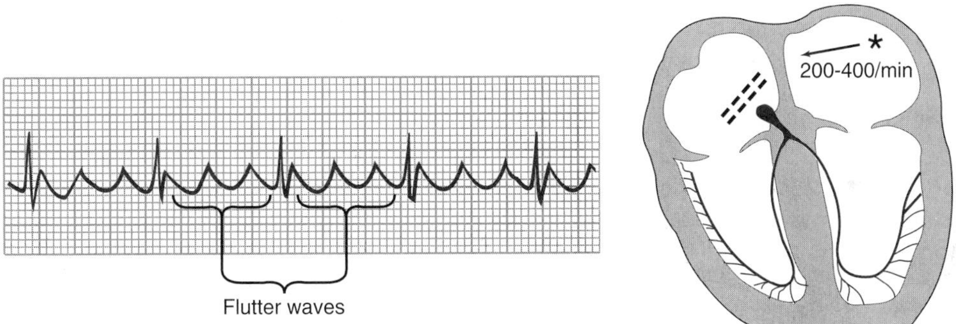

200-400/min

Flutter waves

FIGURE 33-3. Atrial flutter produces sawtooth flutter waves. Most of the atrial impulses are not conducted to the ventricles.

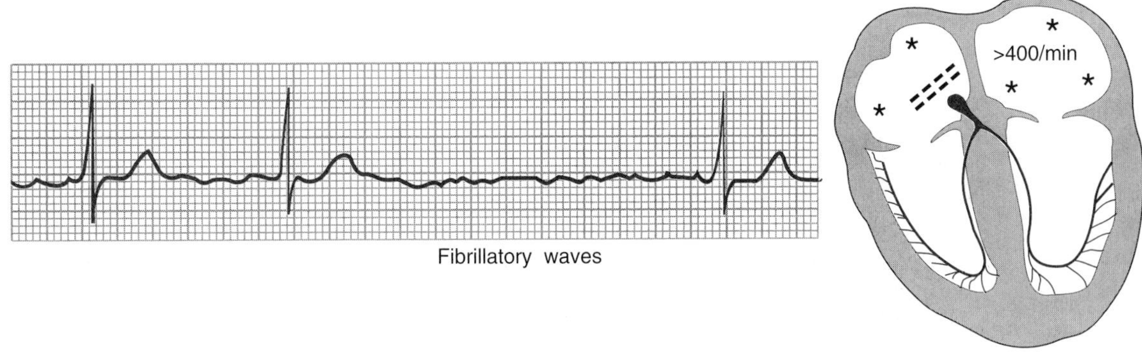

FIGURE 33-4. There are no identifiable P waves in atrial fibrillation. The atrial impulses look like a fine undulating line.

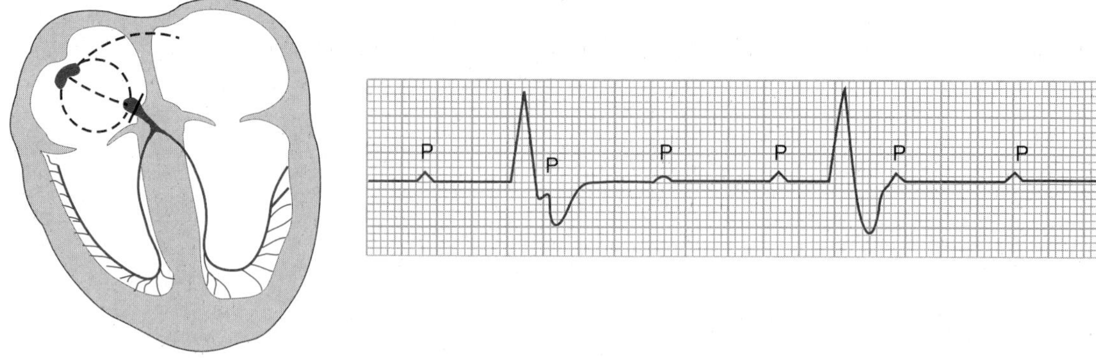

FIGURE 33-5. In heart block, SA initiated impulses are delayed at the AV node or fail to progress altogether. In this example of complete heart block, the ventricles are beating independently of the atria.

Arrhythmias Originating in the Atrioventricular (AV) Node

Heart Block

Heart block refers to disorders in the conduction pathway that interfere with the transmission of impulses from the SA node through the AV node to the ventricles (Fig. 33–5). Heart block may be first degree, second degree, or third degree (also called **complete heart block**). In first- (1°) and second-degree (2°) heart block, the impulse is delayed. In complete heart block, the atrial impulse never gets through and the ventricles develop their own rhythm independent of the atrial rhythm. This rate is usually slow (30–40 beats/min). Pacemaker insertion is the treatment for complete heart block.

Arrhythmias Originating in the Ventricles

Premature Ventricular Contractions

A **premature ventricular contraction** (PVC) is a ventricular contraction that occurs early in the cardiac cycle before the SA node initiates an electrical impulse. No P wave precedes the wide, bizarre looking QRS complex (Fig. 33–6). If the heart rate is very slow, the ventricles can repolarize after a PVC in suf-

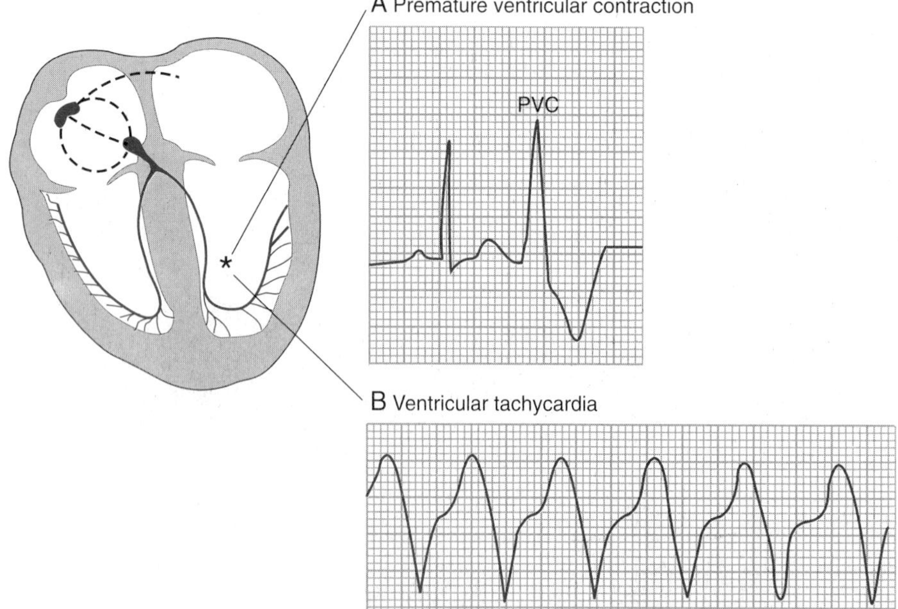

FIGURE 33-6. (*A*) An area outside the normal conduction pathway in the ventricles initiates a premature ventricular contraction. (*B*) Continuous generation of impulses results in ventricular tachycardia.

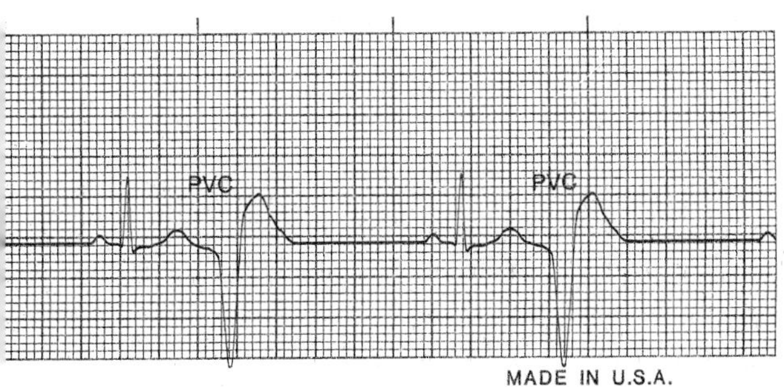

(A) Bigeminy

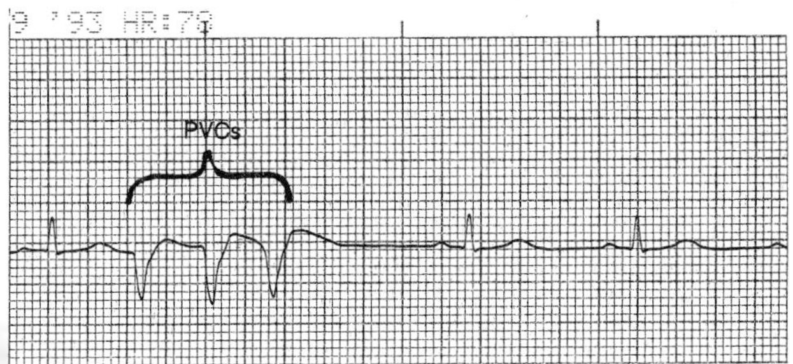

(B) A run of PVCs

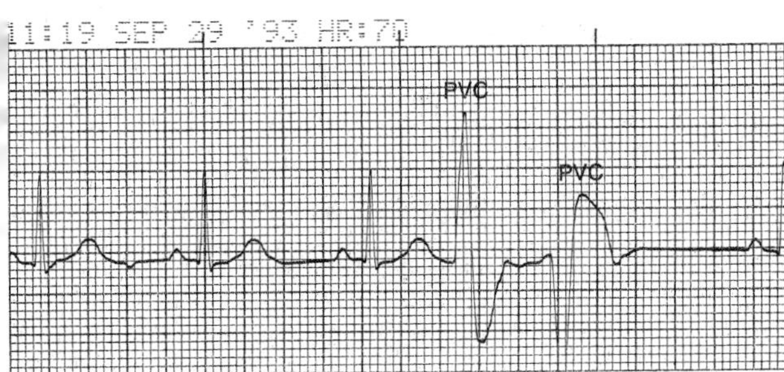

(C) Multifocal PVCs (The PVCs look different)

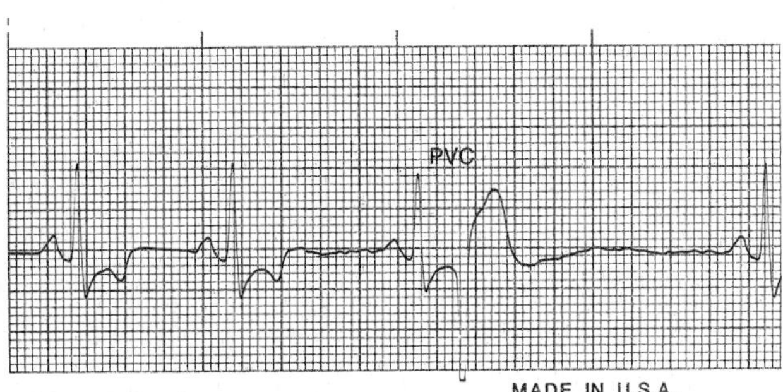

(D) R on T phenomenon

FIGURE 33-7. Some dangerous forms of PVCs include: (*A*) bigeminy, (*B*) short runs of PVCs, (*C*) multifocal PVCs, and (*D*) the R on T phenomenon.

ficient time to receive the atrial stimulus precisely when it is due.

Many people experience PVCs at one time or another. They often cause a flip-flop sensation in the chest, sometimes described as fluttering. The signs and symptoms associated with PVCs include pallor, nervousness, sweating, and faintness. In healthy people, occasional PVCs are *usually* harmless. They may be related to anxiety and stress, fatigue, alcohol withdrawal, or tobacco use. Although PVCs are normally not associated with a specific heart disorder, those whom they frequently trouble should consult a physician. A thorough examination is important in making certain that no heart disease exists.

In the presence of acute heart injury, such as after surgery or in acute myocardial infarction, PVCs that occur in certain patterns suggest myocardial irritability and are precursors of lethal arrhythmias (Fig. 33–7). Box 33–2 outlines types of PVCs considered precursors of life-threatening arrhythmias. When dangerous PVCs occur, the client is given an IV bolus of lidocaine, followed by an IV infusion of the drug.

Ventricular Tachycardia:

Ventricular tachycardia (V-tach) is caused by a single, irritable focus in the ventricle that initiates the heartbeat (see Fig. 33–6). The ventricles beat very fast (150–250 beats/min), and cardiac output is decreased. The client may lose consciousness and become pulseless, depending on the length of time that the arrhythmia is present. V-tach sometimes ends abruptly without intervention, but often requires defibrillation. V-tach may progress to ventricular fibrillation.

Ventricular Fibrillation

Ventricular fibrillation (Fig. 33–8) is the rhythm of a dying heart. PVCs or ventricular tachycardia can precipitate it. The ventricles do not contract effectively and there is no cardiac output. Ventricular fibrillation is an indication for cardiopulmonary resuscitation (CPR) and immediate defibrillation.

BOX 33-2 Premature Ventricular Contractions That Precede Life-Threatening Arrhythmias

PVCs are considered precursors of a life-threatening arrhythmia when the client has:

- Six or more PVCs per minute.
- Runs of **bigeminy** (every other beat is a PVC).
- Two PVCs in a row (**couplets**).
- Runs of PVCs (more than two in a row).
- **Multifocal PVCs** (originating from more than one location).
- A PVC whose R wave falls on the T wave of the preceding complex (**R on T phenomenon**).

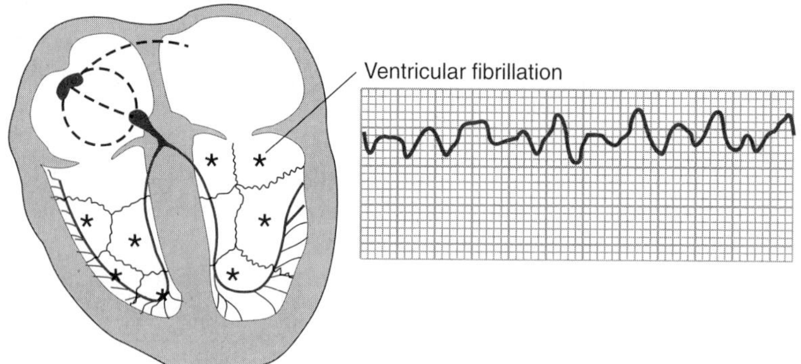

FIGURE 33-8. The ventricles quiver during ventricular fibrillation as shown by a wavy line.

Etiology and Pathophysiology of Cardiac Arrhythmias

Many clinical states predispose to arrhythmias. One of the most common causes of serious arrhythmias is myocardial ischemia, a lack of oxygenated blood to the heart muscle, which can occur secondarily to coronary artery disease, congestive heart failure, inadequate ventilation, and shock. The conduction system is also susceptible to disturbances from anxiety, pain, electrolyte imbalances, valvular heart disease, placement of invasive catheters within the heart, and the effects of drugs. Because of the alteration in rate and rhythm, all arrhythmias affect the pumping action of the heart and cardiac output to some degree.

Assessment Findings

SIGNS AND SYMPTOMS

A client whose arrhythmia causes decreased cardiac output is likely to feel weak and tired, experience anginal pain, or faint. Some with **tachyarrhythmias** (abnormally fast rhythms) describe feeling palpitations or fluttering in their chest. The blood pressure is generally low; the pulse is irregular or difficult to palpate; the rate is unusually fast or slow. The apical and radial pulse rates may differ. The skin may be pale and cool. The client may be disoriented and confused if the brain is not adequately oxygenated, or there may be loss of consciousness and even clinical death.

DIAGNOSTIC FINDINGS

Arrhythmias are identified by a monitor rhythm strip or a 12-lead ECG.

Medical and Surgical Management

Some arrhythmias are not life-threatening and may be untreated. Many are treated with drug therapy and electrical modalities such as elective cardioversion, defibrillation, or temporary or permanent pacing (Table 33–1).

TABLE 33-1 **Characteristics and Treatment of Selected Arrhythmias**

Arrhythmia	Rhythm	Atrial Rate (beats/min)	Ventricular Rate (beats/min)	Treatment
Sinus bradycardia	Regular	< 60	< 60	None unless symptomatic; atropine
Sinus tachycardia	Regular	100–150	100–150	None unless symptomatic; treat underlying disease
Atrial flutter	Usually regular	250–350	75–175	Cardioversion, digitalis, quinidine, propanolol, verapamil
Atrial fibrillation	Grossly irregular	400–600	100–160	Digitalis, quinidine, cardioversion, verapamil
1° AV block	Regular	60–100	30–100	None unless symptomatic
2° AV block	Regular	60–100	30–100	Pacemaker
Complete heart block	Regular	60–100	< 40	Pacemaker
Ventricular tachycardia	Regular	60–100*	150–300	Lidocaine, procainamide, bretylium, cardioversion, defibrillation if pulseless
Ventricular fibrillation	Chaotic	60–100*	400–600	Defibrillation preceded or followed with epinephrine

*Rate may not be distinguishable

Adapted from Kelley, WN, (1996). *Textbook of internal medicine* (3rd ed.). Philadelphia: Lippincott-Raven.

Drug Therapy

Oral and IV antiarrhythmic drugs are used to treat clients who have arrhythmias; however, not all clients with arrhythmias will be on medication. Generally, long-term antiarrhythmic therapy is based on the degree of hemodynamic compromise and the potential for developing a life-threatening arrhythmia. During resuscitation efforts, one or more of the various drugs used in cardiac emergencies are administered (Table 33–2).

Elective Cardioversion

Elective cardioversion is a nonemergency procedure done by the physician to stop rapid, but not necessarily life-threatening, arrhythmias. Cardioversion is

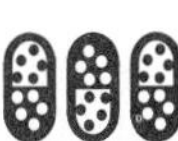

TABLE 33-2 **Emergency Cardiac Drugs**

Drug Category/ Drug Action	Side Effects	Nursing Considerations
epinephrine hydrochloride (Adrenalin) Increases heart rate, force of contraction, and blood pressure. Used in asystole.	Hypertension, arrhythmias, pallor, oliguria	Administer every 5 min during cardiac resuscitation. May cause new arrhythmias. Monitor vital signs and cardiac rhythm.
calcium chloride Increases cardiac contraction in cases of cardiac standstill. Improves weak or ineffective myocardial contractions when epinephrine fails.	Slowed heart rate, tingling, hypotension with rapid IV administration	Give IV. Avoid extravasation; causes tissue necrosis. Monitor cardiac response.
lidocaine hydrochloride (Xylocaine) Suppresses ventricular arrhythmias by decreasing ventricular excitability.	Dizziness, fatigue, drowsiness, nausea and vomiting, vision changes, seizures, hypotension	Monitor cardiac rhythm and vital signs. Keep life support equipment available.
procainamide hydrochloride (Pronestyl) Slows electrical conduction, suppressing ventricular arrhythmias.	Hypotension, rash	Monitor cardiac rhythm and blood pressure frequently.
atropine sulfate Blocks the effects of vagus nerve stimulation. Causes heart rate to increase. Used for bradyarrhythmias.	Palpitations, tachycardia, urinary retention	Monitor for therapeutic and adverse effects. Document heart rate before and after administration.
sodium bicarbonate Neutralizes the acidity of the blood used to counteract the effects of metabolic acidosis in cardiac arrest.	Alkalosis, cellulitis and tissue necrosis if infiltration of IV site occurs.	Obtain arterial blood gas before administration. Flush IV line before and after administration. Monitor therapeutic effects via blood gas analysis.
verapamil hydrochloride (Calan) Given to suppress tachyarrhythmias by inhibiting the movement of calcium ions across cell membranes.	Dizziness, headache, bradycardia, hypotension, heart block	Monitor client's blood pressure, heart rate, rhythm, and output. Keep flat for 1 h after administration. Have equipment for cardioversion and cardiac pacing available.
adenosine (Adenocard) Slows rapid conduction through the AV node, restoring sinus rhythm.	Headache, dizziness, nausea, other arrhythmias, facial flushing, dyspnea, chest pain	Monitor blood pressure and cardiac rhythm continuously and have emergency equipment nearby. Monitor clients frequently, especially those with underlying asthma, chronic obstructive pulmonary disease.
bretylium tosylate (Bretylol) Inhibits the release of norepinephrine. Used for ventricular arrhythmias resistant to other antiarrhythmic agents.	Nausea, vomiting, hypotension, pain at IV injection site	Monitor cardiac rhythm and blood pressure continuously. Keep recumbent.

similar to defibrillation except that the machine that delivers the electrical stimulation waits to discharge until it senses the appearance of an R wave. By doing so, the machine prevents disrupting the heart during the critical period of ventricular repolarization.

The client is sedated for the procedure. Electrodes lubricated with a special gel or moist saline pads are applied to the chest wall. When the discharge button on the paddles (Fig. 33–9) is depressed and the heart is in ventricular depolarization, the electrical energy is released. The electric current completely depolarizes the entire myocardium. As the heart repolarizes, the normal pacemaker regains control and restores continued normal conduction through the heart.

Defibrillation

The only treatment for a life-threatening arrhythmia such as ventricular tachycardia or fibrillation is immediate **defibrillation**. Without it, the client will die. The defibrillator discharges its electrical energy when the discharge button is depressed. It is used during cardiac arrest when there is no identifiable R wave present. The **automatic implantable cardiac defibrillator** (AICD) is used for selected clients with recurrent life-threatening arrhythmias. This unit senses the heart rate (and thus the arrhythmia) and then delivers a spontaneous electrical impulse automatically to correct the arrhythmia (Fig. 33–10).

Pacemaker Insertion

A **pacemaker** is a battery-operated device that provides an electrical stimulus to the muscle of the heart. It is inserted either temporarily or permanently to restore an effective cardiac rhythm. An external (Fig. 33–11) pacemaker, with leads attached to the chest wall (transcutaneous), is a temporary measure until either a transvenous or a permanent pacemaker can be placed. Power for the pacemaker is provided by mercury zinc, lithium, or nuclear-powered (plutonium) batteries. The mercury zinc battery has the shortest life, and the nuclear-powered the longest (8–10 years). Externally charged batteries are also used.

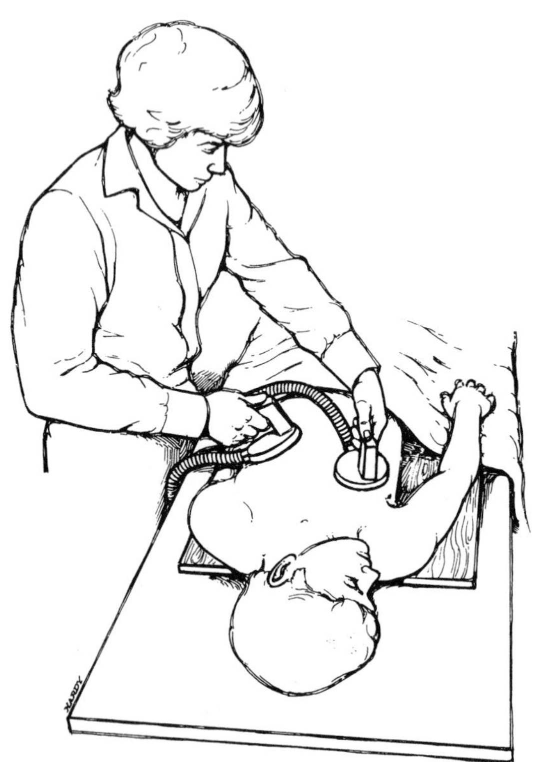

FIGURE 33-9. Paddle placement for cardioversion and defibrillation.

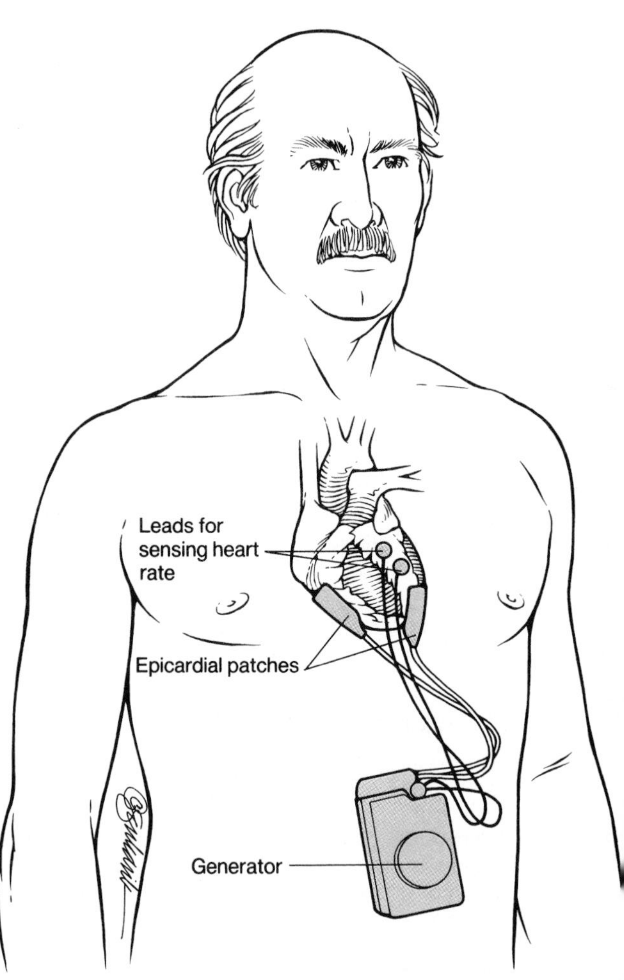

FIGURE 33-10. An automatic implanted cardiac defibrillator (AICD).

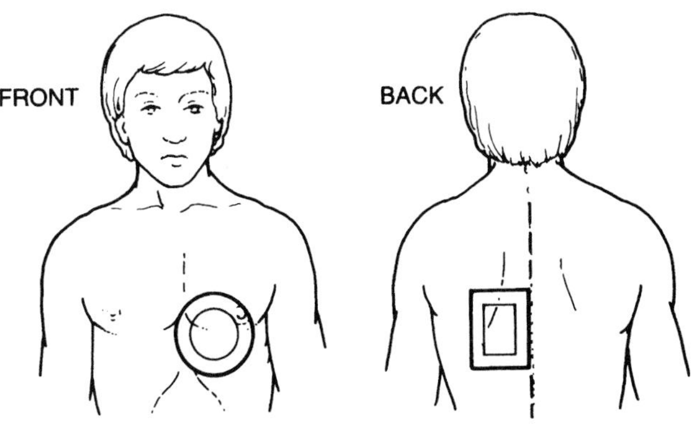

FIGURE 33-11. External pacing pad placement.

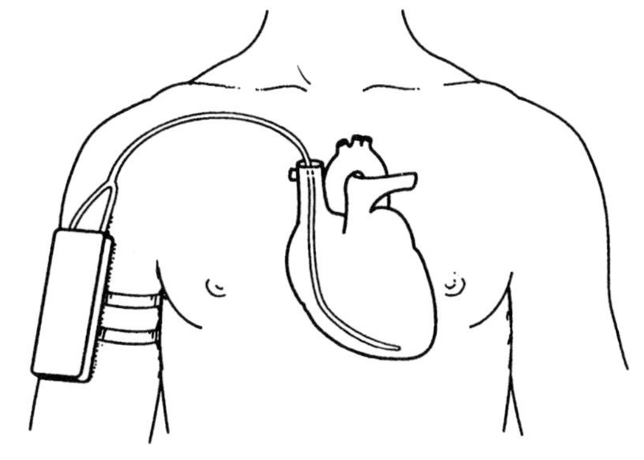

FIGURE 33-12. A transvenous pacemaker.

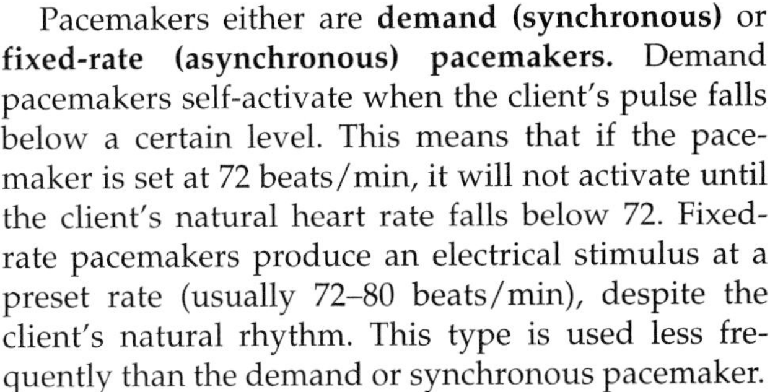

Pacemakers either are **demand (synchronous)** or **fixed-rate (asynchronous) pacemakers.** Demand pacemakers self-activate when the client's pulse falls below a certain level. This means that if the pacemaker is set at 72 beats/min, it will not activate until the client's natural heart rate falls below 72. Fixed-rate pacemakers produce an electrical stimulus at a preset rate (usually 72–80 beats/min), despite the client's natural rhythm. This type is used less frequently than the demand or synchronous pacemaker.

TEMPORARY PACEMAKERS

A temporary pacemaker is indicated in clients with transient **bradyarrhythmias** (slow, abnormal rhythms) such as during an acute myocardial infarction or after coronary artery bypass graft surgery, and with some tachyarrhythmias. Often temporary pacing is done under urgent or emergent circumstances and may even be inserted at the bedside. The electrical lead is introduced through the subclavian, external or internal jugular, or cephalic vein and is threaded first into the right atrium, then into the right ventricle (Fig. 33–12). Fluoroscopy and a cardiac monitor are used to determine the correct placement of the tip of the pacemaker lead.

PERMANENT PACEMAKERS

The most frequent indication for inserting a permanent pacemaker is for complete and some second-degree heart blocks. Occasionally, permanent pacing is used to treat certain tachyarrhythmias that do not respond to treatment or whose treatment results in bradycardia.

The lead is inserted transvenously and the pacing threshold, voltage, and rate are set. One type of pacemaker has leads into both the right atrium and the right ventricle (dual chamber). The implantable pacemaker is then positioned under the skin (Fig. 33–13), usually below the right clavicle, although the left side also can be used. The small incision is closed with sutures. PVCs are more frequent during the early postimplant period, and drug therapy may be ordered to suppress this arrhythmia.

Nursing Management

Clients with symptomatic arrhythmias require careful monitoring and documentation of symptoms, treatment provided, and response to therapy. Many serious arrhythmias are unstable, making frequent rhythm strip observation important. Administering and monitoring the effects of antiarrhythmic drugs is a key nursing responsibility.

Drugs given to restore or control cardiac rhythm are powerful and the therapeutic level is often close to the toxic level. Many have unwanted side effects and are contraindicated in certain conditions. Check

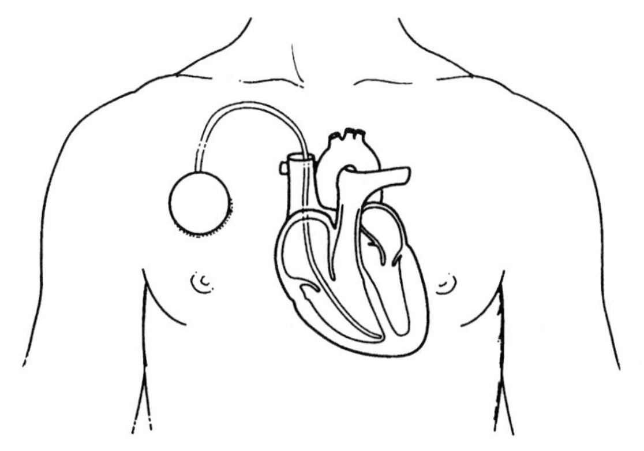

FIGURE 33-13. An internal pacemaker.

drug references, review the client's medical history, including allergies and drug history, and collect data concerning the client's present condition. If there are any questions, communicate with the physician before administering the drug. Determine the desired effect of the drug, the usual dosage and route, side effects, and special administration precautions. Before drug administration, document the blood pressure and the pulse rate and rhythm. Compare the findings with previous data. Clearly label medications added to IV fluid infusions and administer with a controller or infusion pump. Check the site at least hourly or as frequently as the client's response is monitored. Observe the client for adverse drug reactions and response to therapy. If an untoward reaction occurs, notify the physician and continue monitoring the client.

NURSING PROCESS
The Client With an Arrhythmia

Assessment

Review the medical history, including an allergy and drug history. In addition to a general assessment of the cardiovascular system (see Chap. 29), note the trends in heart rate, rhythm, and blood pressure and physiologic changes that occur in response to activity. Record any symptoms expressed by the client, such as dizziness, faintness, or chest pain.

Diagnosis and Planning

Nursing care of the client with an arrhythmia includes, but is not limited to, the following:

Nursing Diagnosis and Collaborative Problems	Nursing Interventions
Decreased Cardiac Output related to arrhythmia or ineffective response to treatment measure **Goal:** The client will maintain adequate cardiac output as evidenced by stable vital signs, no episodes of chest pain, dizziness, syncope, balanced intake and output.	Assess the following as often as client condition warrants: • Vital signs • Intake and output • Pain status • Level of consciousness • Therapeutic response to drug therapy • Tolerance of activity Monitor cardiac rate and rhythm. Maintain physical/emotional rest. Administer oxygen for dyspnea, chest pain, or syncope.
PC: Life-threatening Arrhythmia **Goal:** The nurse will manage and minimize arrhythmias.	Monitor rhythm strip each shift or more often if symptoms develop. Compare the client's rate and rhythm to previously recorded strips to detect changes. Administer antiarrhythmics as prescribed.Prepare the client for defibrillation, cardioversion, or pacemaker insertion. Provide emotional support to the client and family members to lessen fear and anxiety.
Knowledge Deficit related to unfamiliarity with therapeutic regimen **Goal:** The client will state goals of treatment and how to implement care plan.	Assess basic knowledge level of client. Clarify or reexplain the purposes, risks, and benefits of any procedures. Explain the action, side effects, dosage, route, administration, and importance of the medication in controlling the arrhythmia. Teach the client the technique for palpating and counting the radial pulse. Identify the guidelines for withholding the drug and reporting the pulse rate to the physician. Include possible adverse reactions and the importance of continued medical follow-up. Give client and family an opportunity to ask questions. Evaluate effectiveness of client teaching. Give client and family the telephone number of unit to contact if they have questions after discharge.

Evaluation

- Adequate cardiac output is maintained.
- Life-threatening arrhythmias are effectively treated.
- The client and family accurately restate treatment plan.

Elective Cardioversion

Preparation for cardioversion is similar to preparing a client for a surgical procedure. Verify that a consent form has been signed. Restrict food and oral fluids. Ensure that there is a patent intravenous line. Check if scheduled drugs are to be temporarily withheld or if additional drugs to decrease anxiety are to be administered. The physician may order a sedative 30 to 60 minutes before the procedure. Digitalis and diuretics are withheld for 24 to 72 hours before cardioversion because it is believed that their presence in myocardial cells decreases the ability to restore normal conduction and increases the chances of a fatal arrhythmia developing after cardioversion.

Place the cardioverter in the client's room. Check that emergency equipment, such as an oral airway, oxygen, suction, and emergency drugs are on hand.

Just before the procedure, assist the client with bladder or bowel elimination.

Administer a tranquilizer, usually diazepam (Valium) or midazolam (Versed), IV as prescribed. Insert an oral airway once the client is sedated. The desired response to elective cardioversion is a normal sinus rhythm, normal or adequate blood pressure, and strong peripheral pulses in all extremities.

Monitor vital signs every 15 minutes for the first 1 or 2 hours after the procedure and then as ordered. Use continuous cardiac monitoring to evaluate heart rate and rhythm; ECG changes are compared with those present before the procedure.

Defibrillation

Defibrillation is instituted as soon as possible after a dangerous arrhythmia is detected. Until such time, administer CPR to maintain oxygenation and circulation of blood. Defibrillation is performed by a nurse trained in the use of the defibrillator or by a physician.

Remove a nitroglycerin transdermal patch, if present. Protect the skin with saline pads or gel the electrode paddles. Charge the machine. Stand clear of the bed and the client to avoid being shocked when the electric current is administered. Defibrillation may be performed several times in succession. Resume CPR if no pulse is present.

After successful defibrillation, monitor the client's level of consciousness, ECG pattern, blood pressure, and pulse and respiratory rates at frequent intervals. Review laboratory results, such as arterial blood gas analyses and serum electrolytes. Check the paddle application sites for redness and impaired skin integrity. Keep the defibrillator on standby because repeat defibrillation may be necessary.

Even when cardiac activity is restored, the possibility remains that one or more organs have been affected by being deprived of oxygen. Monitor the client's urine output to detect kidney failure and assess for motor weakness or paralysis, memory impairment, and level of consciousness to detect the effects of cerebral anoxia.

Pacemakers

TEMPORARY PACEMAKER

Keep resuscitation equipment in the room because ventricular fibrillation can be mechanically provoked by the tip of the pacemaker lead. Once the pacemaker lead is inserted, attach it to the external pacemaker unit, which is held securely to the client's forearm by means of tape or other anchoring device. Place the unit so that there is no tension on the pacemaker lead. Check the connection several times each day because an improper connection or displacement of the wire from the terminal results in pacemaker malfunction. If the client is confused or restless and movement disturbs the external pacemaker or its lead, notify the physician. Use only grounded electrical equipment in the room. This means that all electrical plugs must have three prongs.

If the client is on a cardiac monitor, an alarm sounds if the client's pulse drops below the lowest level set on the alarm system. The drop in pulse rate may be due to battery failure, internal dislodgment of the pacemaker lead, or a break in the pacemaker lead. The battery of an external pacemaker is easily replaced; keep one or more spare batteries readily available. Dislodgment of the pacemaker lead or a broken wire is reported immediately so that the physician can reposition or reinsert a new one.

PERMANENT PACEMAKER

Place clients on a cardiac monitor and examine the rhythm strip for the pacemaker's characteristic electrical artifact or "spike" identified by a thin, straight stroke (Fig. 33–14). Absence of the spike with a demand pacemaker setting means the impulse is initiated by the natural pacemaker, the SA node. With a fixed-rate pacemaker, there is a spike each time the heart is stimulated. The location of the spike within the series of waveforms is important to note. Report any deviation from the expected pattern. Absence of the spike in a fixed-rate pacemaker may mean faulty monitoring equipment or, more seriously, failure to pace. Other complications include infection, perforation of the ventricular myocardium by the tip of the pacemaker lead, and development of arrhythmias. Box 33–3 highlights necessary dis-

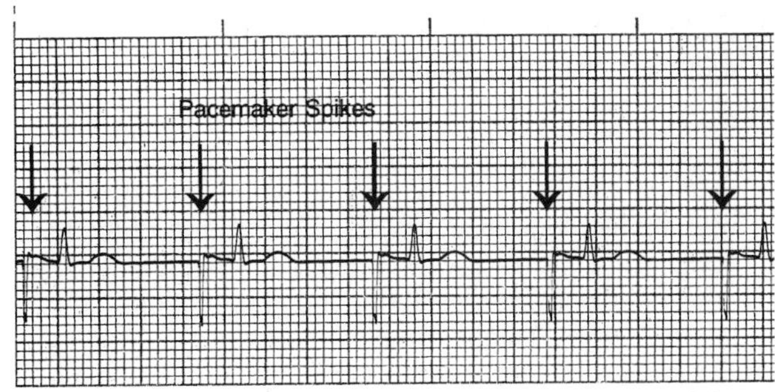

FIGURE 33-14. This rhythm strip shows the characteristic spikes, indicating that the artificial pacemaker is initiating the electrical impulse.

BOX 33-3 Instructions for Clients With a Permanent Pacemaker

Before discharge, instruct the client with a permanent internal pacemaker to:

- Maintain follow-up care.
- Report if the suture line becomes inflamed or sore.
- Avoid injury to the area where the pacemaker is inserted.
- Follow the physician's advice regarding lifting, sports, and exercise.
- Palpate the pulse and count the rate for a full minute daily or when feeling ill.
- Obtain and wear a Medic Alert bracelet or tag identifying that a pacemaker is implanted.
- Be cautious of situations that can cause pacemaker malfunction, such as gravitational force during airplane departures or landings, bumpy automobile rides, high-tension wires, shortwave radio transmissions, telephone transformers, and nuclear magnetic resonance imaging. Move to another location and check the pulse rate if dizziness or palpitations occur.
- Request hand scanning during airport security checks because some pacemakers trigger alarm systems.
- Check with the physician concerning transtelephonic pacemaker checks or when a pacemaker battery change will be necessary in the future.

charge instructions for clients with permanent pacemakers.

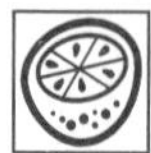

General Nutritional Considerations

During alcohol withdrawal, catecholamines are released and may cause dangerous arrhythmias. Clients who have cardiac risk factors should avoid drinking more than 6 oz of beer or wine a day.

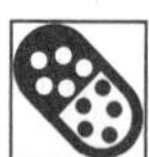

General Pharmacologic Considerations

Administration of lidocaine can result in serious adverse effects, including convulsions and cardiac arrest. An airway should be readily available. If hypotension or additional arrhythmias occur during administration, the IV infusion should be adjusted to the slowest possible rate until the physician can examine the client.

Drug toxicity can occur even when normal doses of digitalis and cardiac glycosides are administered. Signs of toxicity include anorexia; nausea; vomiting; disturbance of vision (eg, halos around dark objects, things or people appear green or yellow); diarrhea; abdominal discomfort; and arrhythmias such as bradycardia, tachycardia, and bigeminal pulse, characterized as one having two beats in close succession followed by a brief pause.

Digitalis toxicity is usually treated by discontinuing the digitalis preparation. Digitalis levels usually return to normal within a short time. However, severe digitalis toxicity resulting in life-threatening overdosage may be treated with immune fab (Digibind) as an antidote for digoxin or digitoxin. Most life-threatening states can be treated with 800 mg digoxin immune fab given IV over 30 minutes.

Take an apical pulse rate before administering oral antiarrhythmic drugs. Withhold the drug and notify the physician if the heart rate is less than 60 beats/min.

The cholinergic-blocking agent atropine may be used to treat the severe bradycardia of complete heart block. A dosage of 0.5 to 1 mg may be given every 1 to 2 hours. A maximum of 2 mg may be given IV. Isoproterenol (Isuprel) also may be used to treat severe bradycardia. When either of these drugs is administered, the pulse rate is closely monitored for drug response.

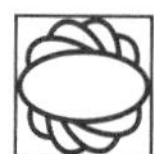

General Gerontologic Considerations

Age increases the risk for arrhythmias from a variety of degenerative changes. The cells in the SA node of older adults continue to decrease and accumulate fat and calcium.

In older adults, stress, exercise, or illness may result in arrhythmias and other cardiac disorders, such as congestive heart failure and myocardial ischemia.

Sinus bradycardia and heart block are common arrhythmias in older clients.

SUMMARY OF KEY CONCEPTS

- Common arrhythmias include sinus bradycardia, characterized by a rate less than 60 beats/min but regular rhythm; sinus tachycardia, characterized by a rate between 100 and 150 beats/min but a regular rhythm; atrial fibrillation and atrial flutter, characterized by a rapid atrial rate and a slower ventricular rate; heart block in which the atria depolarize separately from the ventricles, with each maintaining its own separate rhythm; premature ventricular contractions, ventricular tachycardia and fibrillation, characterized by early ventricular depolarization separate from the influence of the SA node; and cardiac arrest in which there is inadequate cardiac output to sustain cellular function.
- Arrhythmias are treated with drugs, elective cardioversion, defibrillation, and the insertion of a pacemaker. Drugs control or eliminate arrhythmias by depressing the irritability of myocardial tissue and restoring the heart rate to normal range.
- Elective cardioversion is used to restore the normal pacemaker function in nonthreatening arrhythmias. Cardioversion is quicker and avoids potential adverse effects encountered in the use of drug therapy.

- Defibrillation is used at a moment's notice to treat a life-threatening arrhythmia and restore normal sinus rhythm.
- Arrhythmias may be treated with an external or internal pacemaker. A pacemaker is inserted to temporarily or permanently restore a more effective cardiac rhythm.
- Check drug reference and assess the client before drug preparation and administration.
- For cardioversion, the nurse gathers equipment and prepares the client for the procedure. Afterward, the client's heart rate and rhythm are frequently monitored
- When a client requires defibrillation, the nurse places the defibrillator at the bedside, prepares the paddles, and places the paddles in the area of the heart's apex and base. After alerting everyone to stand clear, the current is administered. The process is repeated if there is no response. CPR is resumed whenever necessary. The client is monitored for a return of an arrhythmia and the effects of tissue hypoxia and anoxia.
- When a client receives a pacemaker, its effect on cardiac rhythm is monitored closely and the nurse educates the client in preparation for self-care.
- When caring for a client with an actual or potential arrhythmia, the nurse monitors and documents symptoms, treatment provided, and response to therapy.

CRITICAL THINKING EXERCISES

1. A client for whom an antiarrhythmic has been prescribed returns for a follow-up examination. How would you determine if the client has been compliant with the drug therapy?
2. What information would be essential to document when helping to resuscitate a client who has experienced a cardiac arrest?

Suggested Readings

Abrams, A. (1998). *Clinical drug therapy: Rationales for nursing practice.* Philadelphia: Lippincott-Raven.

Boyer, M. (1997). *Lippincott's need-to-know ECG facts.* Philadelphia: Lippincott-Raven.

Davenport, J., & Morton, P. (1997). Identifying non-ischemic causes of life-threatening arrhythmias. *American Journal of Nursing, 97* (11), 50–55.

Ehrhardt, B., & Glankler, D. (1996). Your role in a code blue. *Nursing96 26*(1), 34–39.

Hademeier, C. (1996). Clinical snapshot: Permanent pacemaker. *American Journal of Nursing, 96*(2), 30–31.

Lazzara, D. (1998). Dealing confidently with deadly arrhythmias. *Nursing, 28*(1), 41–45.

Miracle, V., & Sims, J. (1997). Atrial flutter. *Nursing 27*(5), 41.

Strimike, C., & Wojcik, J. (1998). Stopping atrial fibrillation with ibutilide. *American Journal of Nursing, 98*(1), 32–34.

Yacone-Morton, L. (1995). Cardiovascular drugs: Antiarrhythmics. *RN, 58*(4), 26–31, 33–35.

Additional Resources

Heart Resource Center
http://www.heartinfo.org

Cardiovascular Institute of the South
http://www.cardio.com

Chapter 34

Caring for Clients With Hypertension

KEY TERMS

Accelerated hypertension
Catecholamines
Diastolic blood pressure
Essential hypertension
Hypernatremia
Hypertension
Hypertensive cardiovascular disease
Hypertensive heart disease
Hypertensive vascular disease
Malignant hypertension
Natriuretic factor
Papilledema
Renin-angiotensin-aldosterone mechanism
Secondary hypertension
Systolic blood pressure

LEARNING OBJECTIVES

On completion of this chapter, the reader will:

- Identify two physiologic components that create blood pressure.
- List factors that influence blood pressure.
- Explain systolic and diastolic arterial pressure.
- Define hypertension and identify two groups at risk for developing hypertension.
- List three consequences of chronic hypertension.
- Explain the difference between essential and secondary hypertension.
- Discuss the assessment findings and treatment of hypertension.
- Identify at least four causes of secondary hypertension.
- Discuss the nursing management of clients with hypertension.
- Differentiate between accelerated and malignant hypertension.
- Identify at least four potential complications of uncontrolled malignant hypertension.
- Discuss the medical and nursing management of the client with malignant hypertension.

Blood pressure is the force produced by the volume of blood within the walls of arteries. It is represented by the formula:

BP = CO (cardiac output) × PR (*peripheral resistance*).

The measured pressure reflects the ability of the arteries to stretch and fill with blood, the efficiency of the heart as a pump, and the volume of circulating blood. Blood pressure is affected by age, body size, diet, activity, emotions, pain, position, gender, the time of day, and disease states. Studies of healthy persons show that blood pressure can fluctuate within a wide range and still be normal. It is important to obtain several measurements for comparison.

Arterial Blood Pressure

Arterial pressure is regulated by the autonomic nervous system, the kidneys, and various endocrine glands. When measured, the pressure during systole and diastole is expressed as a fraction. The top number is the systolic pressure and the bottom number is the diastolic pressure. Normal blood pressure for adults ranges from 100/60 to 140/90 mm Hg. Blood pressure tends to increase with age, most likely from arteriosclerotic and atherosclerotic changes in the blood vessels, or other effects of chronic diseases.

Systolic Blood Pressure

Systolic blood pressure is determined by the force and volume of blood ejected from the left ventricle during systole and the ability of the arterial system to distend at the time of ventricular contraction. The walls of the arteries are normally elastic and yield to the force and volume of ventricular contraction. In older clients, systolic blood pressure may be elevated because of loss of arterial elasticity (arteriosclerosis).

Narrowing of the arterioles, either by arteriosclerosis or some other mechanism that causes vasoconstriction, increases peripheral resistance, which in turn increases systolic blood pressure. This resistance can be compared to the slight narrowing of a tube, such as a drinking straw or a garden hose. The narrower the lumen, the greater the pressure needed to move air or liquid through it.

Diastolic Blood Pressure

Diastolic blood pressure reflects arterial pressure during ventricular relaxation and depends on the resistance of the arterioles and the diastolic filling times. If arterioles are resistant (constricted), blood is under greater pressure.

Hypertensive Disease

The term **hypertension** refers to a sustained elevation of systolic arterial pressure of 140 mm Hg or higher, a sustained diastolic arterial pressure of 90 mm Hg or greater, or both. When a cardiac abnormality results from elevated blood pressure, the term **hypertensive heart disease** is used. When vascular damage is present without heart involvement, the term **hypertensive vascular disease** is used. When both heart disease and vascular damage accompany hypertension, the appropriate term is **hypertensive cardiovascular disease.**

Essential and Secondary Hypertension

Hypertension is divided into two main categories: essential (or primary) hypertension and secondary hypertension. **Essential hypertension** is a sustained elevation of blood pressure without any known cause. About 95% of those with hypertension have this type. **Secondary hypertension** is an elevation of blood pressure that results from, or is secondary to some other disorder.

ETIOLOGY AND PATHOPHYSIOLOGY

The exact cause of essential hypertension is unknown. Blood pressure often increases with age and may run in families. African Americans are affected at a higher rate than other ethnic groups. The risk for hypertension is increased by obesity, inactivity, smoking, excessive alcohol intake, and ineffective stress management.

Research into specific factors that contribute to the development of essential hypertension continues. For instance, it is well documented that **hypernatremia** (elevated serum sodium level) increases blood volume, which raises blood pressure. However, a low serum potassium level may actually cause sodium retention because the kidneys try to maintain a balanced number of cations (positively charged electrolytes) in body fluid. Scientists are also investigating the role of calcium in hypertension because serum calcium levels are low in some hypertensive clients.

Essential hypertension may also develop from alterations in other body chemicals. Defects in blood pressure regulation may result from an impairment in the **renin-angiotensin-aldosterone mechanism.** *Renin* is a chemical released by the kidneys to raise blood pressure and increase vascular fluid volume. For those who respond to stress at a heightened degree, hypertension may be correlated with a release of higher than usual **catecholamines,** such ase epinephrine and norepinephrine, which elevate blood pressure. Lastly, some feel that there may be a deficiency of **natriuretic factor,** a hormone produced by the heart, causing arteries and arterioles to remain in a state of sustained vasoconstriction.

Secondary hypertension may accompany any primary condition that affects fluid volume or renal function or causes arterial vasoconstriction. Predisposing conditions include kidney disease, pheochromocytoma (a tumor of the adrenal medulla), hyperaldosteronism, atherosclerosis, the use of cocaine or other cardiac stimulants such as weight control drugs and caffeine, and the use of oral contraceptives.

Regardless of whether a person has essential or secondary hypertension, the organ damage and complications that follow are the same. Hypertension causes the heart to work harder to pump against the increased resistance. Consequently, the size of the heart muscle increases. When the heart can no longer pump adequately to meet the body's metabolic needs, heart failure occurs (see Chap. 35). The extra work and the greater mass increase the heart's need for oxygen. If the myocardium does not receive sufficient oxygenated blood, myocardial ischemia occurs and the client experiences angina.

In addition to the direct effects on the heart, high blood pressure damages the arterial vascular system. It accelerates atherosclerosis. Furthermore, the increased resistance of the arterioles to the flow of blood causes serious complications in other organs of the body, including the eyes, brain, heart, and kidneys. Hemorrhage of tiny arteries in the retina may cause marked visual disturbance or blindness. A cerebrovascular accident may result from hemorrhage or occlusion of a blood vessel in the brain. Myocardial infarction may result from occlusion of a branch of a coronary artery. Impaired circulation to the kidneys results in renal failure among some clients with hypertension.

ASSESSMENT FINDINGS

Signs and Symptoms

Clients may be asymptomatic. The onset of hypertension, considered "the silent killer," is often gradual. Hypertension can be present for years and discovered during a routine physical examination or when the client experiences a major complication. As the blood pressure becomes elevated, clients may identify symptoms such as a throbbing or pounding headache, dizziness, fatigue, insomnia, nervousness, nosebleeds, and blurred vision. Angina or shortness of breath may be the first clue to hypertensive heart disease.

The most obvious finding during a physical assessment is a sustained elevation of one or both blood pressure measurements. The pulse may feel bounding from the force of ventricular contraction. Hypertensive clients may be overweight. Clients often have a flushed face from engorgement of superficial blood vessels. Peripheral edema may be present. An ophthalmic examination may reveal vascular changes in the eyes, retinal hemorrhages, or a bulging optic disk.

Diagnostic Findings

Diagnostic tests are performed to determine the extent of organ damage caused by the hypertension. Electrocardiography, echocardiography, and chest radiography may reveal an enlargement of the left ventricle. Blood tests may show elevated blood urea nitrogen and serum creatinine levels indicating impaired renal function, which may be further validated with excretory urography (intravenous [IV] pyelography). *Fluorescein angiography*, an ophthalmologic test using IV dye, often reveals leaking blood vessels in the retina.

If the cause of the hypertension is secondary to a renal vascular problem, renal arteriography demonstrates narrowing of the renal artery. A 24-hour collected urine specimen detects elevated amounts of catecholamines if the cause of the hypertension is related to dysfunction of the adrenal gland. Blood studies reveal elevated levels of cholesterol and triglycerides, indicating that atherosclerosis is an underlying factor.

MEDICAL MANAGEMENT

The primary objective of therapy with either type of hypertension is to lower the blood pressure and prevent major complications. Table 34–1 presents recommended follow-up based on blood pressure. Initial management depends on the degree of pressure elevation, but generally nonpharmacologic interventions are used first. For mild elevations, weight reduction, decreased sodium intake, moderate exercise, and reduction of other contributing factors, such as smoking

TABLE 34-1 **Recommendations for Blood Pressure Follow-up**

Classification of blood pressure for adults 18 years or older, with recommended follow-up.

Category	Systolic (mm Hg)		Diastolic (mm Hg)	Recommended Follow-up
Optimal*	< 120	and	< 80	Recheck in 2 years
Normal	< 130	and	< 85	Recheck in 2 years
High normal	130–139	or	85–89	Recheck in 1 year
Hypertension *Stage 1* (mild)	140–159	or	90–99	Confirm within 2 months
Stage 2 (moderate)	160–170	or	100–109	Evaluate within 1 month
Stage 3 (severe)	≥ 180	or	≥ 110	Evaluate immediately or within 1 week depending on clinical situation

*Optimal blood pressure with respect to cardiovascular risk is < 120/80 mm Hg. However, unusually low readings should be evaluated for clinical significance.

(From the Sixth Report of the Joint National Committee on Detection, Evaluation, and Treatment of High Blood Pressure, NIH publication, 1997.)

and alcohol use, may return the blood pressure to normal levels. If cholesterol and triglyceride levels are increased, a diet low in saturated fats is recommended.

Depending on the client's response to nonpharmacologic therapy, one of several drugs may be prescribed (Table 34–2). If the blood pressure remains elevated, the dosage may be increased or a second, third, or fourth antihypertensive agent may be added to the regimen (Fig. 34–1). Secondary hypertension often resolves by treating its cause.

TABLE 34-2 **Drugs Used in the Treatment of Hypertension**

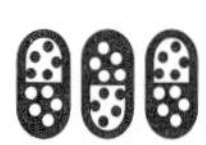

Drug Category/Drug Action	Side Effects	Nursing Considerations
Alpha-Adrenergic Blockers		
prazosin (Minipress) Relaxes vascular smooth muscle by blocking $alpha_1$ receptor sites for epinephrine and norepinephrine.	Hypotension, dizziness, drowsiness, nausea, heart palpitations	Administer first dose just before bedtime to reduce potential for syncope. Monitor for postural hypotension. Caution to change positions slowly.
Beta-Adrenergic Blockers		
propanolol (Inderal) Blocks the effects of catecholamines and decreases renin levels.	Hypotension, bradycardia, bronchospasm, congestive heart failure, depression, impotence	Administer drugs with meals; do not discontinue medication abruptly. Monitor for fluid retention, rash, difficulty breathing. Monitor blood glucose in diabetic clients. Contraindicated in clients with chronic respiratory disorders.
Alpha-Beta Blockers		
labetalol (Normodyne) Blocks alpha, beta, and $beta_2$ adrenergic receptors.	Dizziness, gastrointestinal symptoms, dyspnea, cough, impotence and decreased libido.	Administer with meals. Caution to avoid discontinuing drug therapy abruptly, and to inform anesthesiologist of drug use before surgery to avoid a possible drug–drug interaction.
Diuretics		
furosemide (Lasix) Decreases blood pressure by promoting the excretion of sodium and water thus reducing circulating blood volume.	Dizziness, dehydration, blurred vision, anorexia, diarrhea, nocturia, polyuria, thrombocytopenia, orthostatic hypotension, hypokalemia	Weigh daily. Measure intake and output. Monitor serum potassium. Replace potassium with bananas, orange juice, or prescribed supplement.
Angiotensin-Converting Enzyme (ACE) Inhibitors		
captopril (Capoten) Blocks ACE from converting angiotensin I to angiotensin II (a potent vasoconstrictor). Promotes fluid and sodium loss and decreases peripheral vascular resistance.	Tachycardia, hypotension, gastric irritation, pancytopenia, proteinuria, rash, cough, dry mouth	Reduced excretion in clients with renal failure, first-dose hypotension is common in elderly clients. Administer 1 hour before or 2 hours after meals.
Angiotensin II-Receptor Antagonists		
losartan (Cozaar) Blocks the effects of angiotensin II, relaxes vascular smooth muscle, increases salt and water excretion, and reduces plasma volume.	Orthostatic hypotension; gastrointestinal disturbances; hyperkalemia, respiratory congestion; swelling of face, lips, eyelids, tongue in hypersensitive persons	Assess blood pressure for postural changes. Monitor serum potassium levels. Observe for allergic reactions when beginning drug therapy.
Calcium Channel Blockers		
nifedipine (Procardia XL) Decreases blood pressure by dilating coronary and peripheral arteries.	Hypotension, dizziness, congestive heart failure, edema, atrioventricular block, nausea	Check blood pressure and heart rate before each dose. Withhold drug in the presence of hypotension. Observe for signs and symptoms of congestive heart failure and fluid overload.

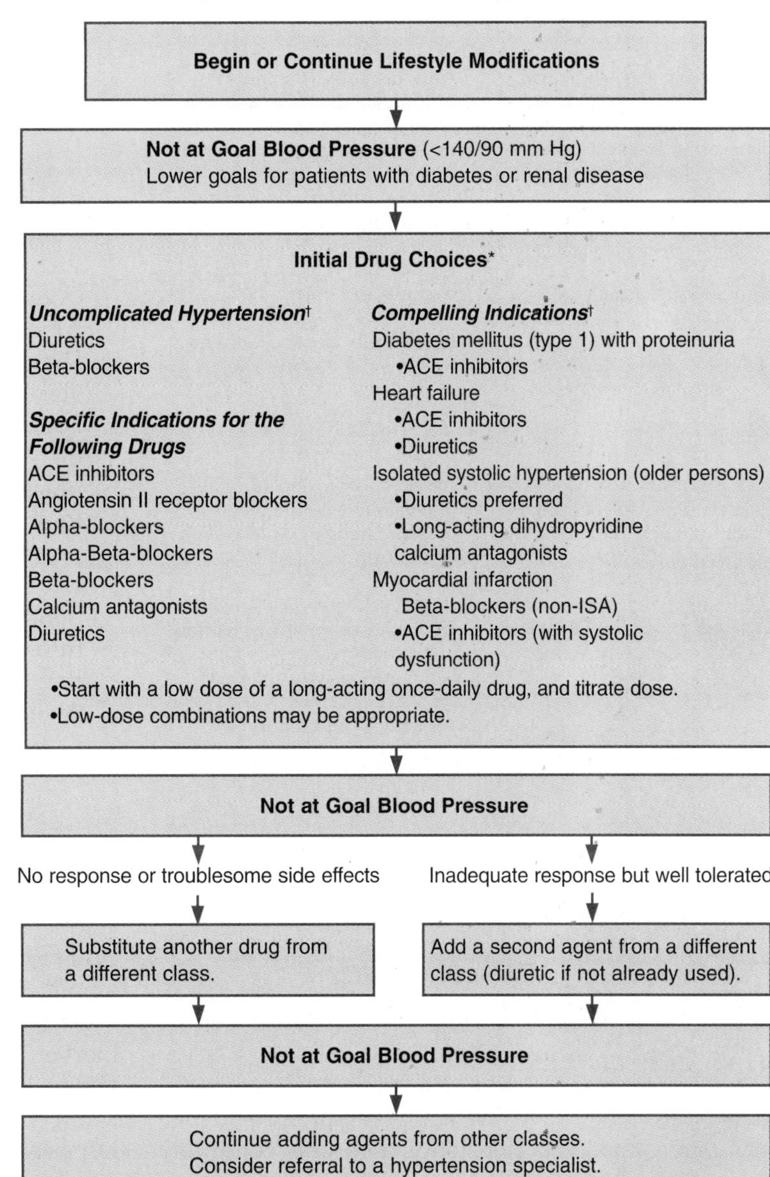

FIGURE 34-1. Individualized step care therapy for hypertension (NIH Publication No. 98-4080, November 1997)

NURSING PROCESS
The Client With Hypertension

Assessment

Clients with hypertension require a complete medical and family history, an assessment of symptoms they have experienced, and careful blood pressure measurement. Using a blood pressure cuff of appropriate size (Table 34–3), take the blood pressure in both arms in a standing, sitting, and then supine position (Clinical Procedure 34–1). Use the same arm and place the client in the same position each time a subsequent reading is taken. The initial assessment of the hospitalized client previously diagnosed and treated for hypertension includes questions about the treatment regimen that is being followed. Additional cardiac assessments are performed (see Chap. 29) depending on the client's medical history and current symptoms.

Diagnosis and Planning

The care of the client with hypertension includes, but is not limited to, the following:

Nursing Diagnosis and Collaborative Problems	Nursing Interventions
Risk for Decreased Cardiac Output, Pain (Angina), and **Activity Intolerance** related to tachycardia and systemic vascular resistance **Goal:** The client will maintain adequate cardiac output as evidenced by heart rate within 60 to 100 beats/min. and adequate urine output. The client will be free of chest pain and able to tolerate moderate activity without discomfort.	Administer oxygen, nitrates, diuretics, antihypertensives as ordered and indicated and document their effects by assessing changes in blood pressure, heart rate and rhythm, urine output, and activity tolerance. Provide rest if tachycardia or dyspnea develops. Restrict nicotine and caffeine.
Risk for Injury related to syncope and dizziness secondary to antihypertensive drugs **Goal:** Client will not experience injury from effects of syncope and dizziness. Client will identify measures to reduce syncopal episodes.	Assess client for postural hypotension by taking blood pressure lying down and then sitting up. Instruct client to rise slowly from a lying or sitting position and to sit on the edge of the bed before rising from bed. Assist with ambulation.

Evaluation and Expected Outcomes

- Adequate cardiac output is maintained.
- No chest pain occurs.
- Able to perform ADLs without fatigue.
- No syncope episodes.

Client and Family Teaching

Many clients fail to adhere to their treatment regimen because they have few, if any, symptoms and feel well. Stress that hypertension is a chronic condition that requires lifelong attention and treatment.

In addition to discussing the dietary measures listed in Box 34–1 and in General Nutritional Considerations, teach clients or family members how to take a blood pressure reading or refer them to a community health service where this is available free or at low cost on a regular basis. Include the following points in the teaching plan:

- Keep a log of the blood pressure measurements for follow-up visits.
- Comply with the treatment regimen involving diet, exercise, and drug therapy.
- Consult cookbooks published or endorsed by the American Heart Association, the American Diabetes Association, or other reliable sources for "heart smart" recipes.
- Follow the directions for medications; never increase, decrease, or omit a prescribed drug unless first conferring with the physician.
- Report adverse effects from medications to the prescribing physician.
- Get medical approval before taking nonprescription drugs.
- Inform all physicians and dentists of medications that are being taken.
- Avoid tobacco and beverages containing caffeine or alcohol, unless permitted by the physician.

Accelerated and Malignant Hypertension

Accelerated and malignant hypertension are more serious forms of elevated blood pressure that develop among individuals with either essential or primary hypertension. **Accelerated hypertension** describes markedly elevated blood pressure, accompanied by hemorrhages and exudates in the eye. If untreated, accelerated hypertension may progress to malignant hypertension. The term **malignant hypertension** describes dangerously elevated blood pressure accompanied by **papilledema** (swelling of the optic nerve at its point of entrance into the eye).

TABLE 34-3 **Recommended Bladder Dimensions for Blood Pressure Cuffs**

Arm Circumference at Midpoint* (cm)	Cuff Name	Bladder Width (cm)	Bladder Length (cm)
24–32	Adult	13	24
32–42	Wide adult	17	32
42–50+	Thigh	20	42

*Midpoint of arm is defined as half the distance from the acromion to the olecranon processes.

(Reprinted with permission. Recommendations for Human Blood Pressure Determination by Sphygmomanometers, ©American Heart Association, 1987.)

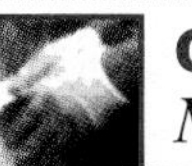

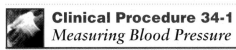

Clinical Procedure 34-1
Measuring Blood Pressure

PURPOSE	EQUIPMENT
• Accurately assess and document blood pressure.	• Blood pressure cuff • Sphygmomanometer • Stethoscope

Nursing Action	Rationale
ASSESSMENT	
Determine in which arm and in what position previous assessments were made.	Ensures consistency.
Review antihypertensive medications.	Helps in analyzing the results of assessment findings.
PLANNING	
Choose a blood pressure cuff that fits the client's arm.	A cuff that is the wrong size will produce a false reading.
Assess the client's blood pressure on the schedule ordered.	Ensures consistency.
IMPLEMENTATION	
Find the client's brachial pulse, position the cuff at least 1 inch above where the pulse is felt.	Pressure applied in the area of the brachial pulse will give most accurate reading.

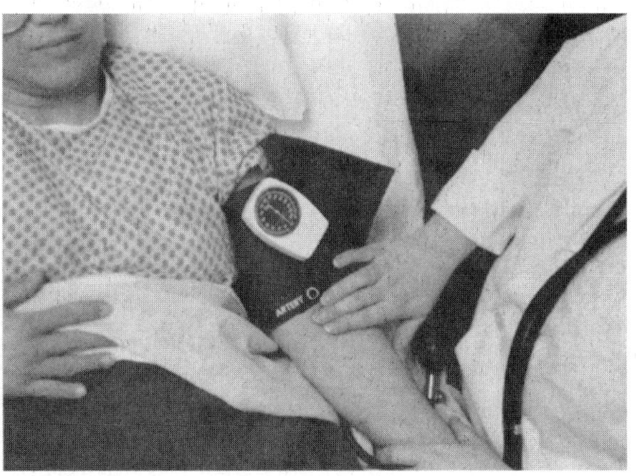

Palpating the brachial artery. (Courtesy of Ken Timby.)

Nursing Action	Rationale
Palpate the radial pulse, inflate the cuff while still feeling the pulse. Note the number on the gauge when the pulse is no longer felt.	To be able to hear the first Korotkoff sound, the cuff must be inflated to a pressure above the point where the radial pulse is no longer felt.
Deflate cuff and wait at least 15 seconds.	A pause allows the blood in the arm to recirculate.
Place stethoscope in ears and on client's brachial artery.	Facilitates hearing Korotkoff's sounds.
Inflate cuff 30 mm Hg above point that radial pulse disappeared.	Increasing pressure above where the pulse was no longer felt ensures a short period of time before the first sounds (corresponding to the systolic pressure) are heard.
Slowly deflate cuff, noting where the first Korotkoff's sounds are heard (systolic) and the point when the last sounds are heard (diastolic).	The systolic blood pressure is the point when the blood first enters the artery. The diastolic blood pressure is recorded as the point where Korotkoff's sounds are greatly muffled or absent.
Quickly release air from the cuff and remove cuff from arm.	Reduces discomfort for the client.
Record the client's blood pressure as a fraction. Use the closest even number. Note the position the client was in and which arm was used.	Measurements are taken consistently for future comparisons.

BOX 34-1 Dietary Guidelines for Healthy Americans

- Total fat should be no more than 30% of total calories.*
- Saturated fatty acid intake should be 8% to 10% of total calories.
- Polyunsaturated fatty acid intake should be up to 10% of total calories.
- Monosaturated fatty acids make up to 15% of total calories.
- Cholesterol intake should be less than 300 mg/day.
- Sodium intake should be less than 2,400 mg/day.
- Carbohydrate intake should make up 55% to 60% or more of calories, with emphasis on increasing sources of complex carbohydrates.
- Total calories should be adjusted to achieve and maintain a healthy body weight.

*Guideline applies to total calories over several days or weeks.
Source: American Heart Association Guidelines.

ETIOLOGY AND PATHOPHYSIOLOGY

Accelerated and malignant hypertension occur in those yet undiagnosed, those who fail to maintain follow-up, or those who are noncompliant with medical therapy. Accelerated and malignant hypertension usually have an abrupt onset and, if untreated, are rapidly followed by severe symptoms and complications. Malignant hypertension is fatal unless the blood pressure is quickly reduced. Even with intensive treatment, the kidneys, brain, and heart may be permanently damaged..

Life-threatening consequences occur when the pressure within the vascular system becomes extremely elevated. Some arterial blood vessels may already have ruptured or will soon. Retinal hemorrhages can lead to blindness. A stroke occurs if vessels in the brain rupture and bleed. If an aneurysm has developed in the aorta from chronic hypertension, it may burst and cause hemorrhage and shock. Cardiac effects include left ventricular failure with pulmonary edema or myocardial infarction. Renal failure also may be forthcoming if the pressure is not reduced.

ASSESSMENT FINDINGS

Signs and Symptoms

Some clients may present with symptoms of confusion, headache, visual disturbances, seizures, and, possibly, coma. The sudden, marked rise in blood pressure may cause chest pain, dyspnea, and moist lung sounds. Renal failure is evidenced by less than 30 mL of urine per hour. The onset of sudden, severe back pain accompanied by hypotension is an indication that an aortic aneurysm is dissecting or has ruptured.

The systolic blood pressure is 160 mm Hg or higher or the diastolic blood pressure is 115 mm Hg or higher. The optic disk (nerve) appears to bulge forward into the posterior chamber due to swelling of the brain. The retinal blood vessels are obscured where they radiate from the bulging disk, making it difficult to identify their continuous pathway. There may be flame-shaped hemorrhages or fluffy white exudates in the retina.

Diagnostic Findings

Diagnostic studies that may prove abnormal include a computed tomographic scan, positron emission tomography scan, or magnetic resonance imaging. Reduction in the blood pressure is a priority at this time and these neurologic tests may be postponed while emergency treatment measures are instituted.

MEDICAL MANAGEMENT

In true hypertensive emergencies, the goal is to lower the blood pressure within 1 or 2 hours by using potent drugs, such as nitroprusside (Nitropress), nitroglycerin, or labetalol (Normodyne) administered IV. If the client's condition is not extremely critical, other alternative antihypertensive drugs, such as nifedipine (Procardia), verapamil (Isoptin), captopril (Capoten), and prazosin (Minipress) are prescribed for oral administration. Oxygen is ordered to reduce hypoxia-induced tachycardia.

NURSING MANAGEMENT

Implement the medical orders promptly to ensure that the blood pressure is lowered as quickly and safely as possible. Mix drugs with IV solution after carefully calculating the dosage. Follow the five rights of medication administration. Administer the medicated solution with an infusion pump or controller. Titrate the rate of infusion according to the client's response and the parameters set by the physician. Check the site and progress of the infusion at least hourly. Apply an automatic blood pressure recording machine to the arm so that the blood pressure is measured every few minutes or assess the blood pressure directly if an arterial catheter is used. Report a systolic pressure of 160 mm Hg or higher or a diastolic pressure of 115 mm Hg or higher immediately. Restrict activity and monitor the client closely for neurologic, cardiac, and renal complications while awaiting medical orders. Keep emergency equipment and drugs in readiness in case additional complications develop. See the Nursing Process: The Client With Hypertension for additional nursing management.

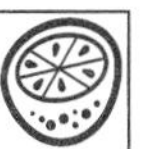

General Nutritional Considerations

For years, standard interventions to control hypertension have been to reduce sodium intake, lose weight if overweight, exercise, and limit alcohol to two or fewer drinks per day. For a significant number of clients with essential hypertension, these measures have the potential to eliminate the need for drug therapy.

Numerous studies show that lowering sodium intake can lower blood pressure. Although some researchers argue that only a small percentage of the population is sensitive to sodium, its restriction is generally accepted as a lifelong component of treatment. All Americans—those with hypertension and those who wish to prevent it—are urged to lower sodium intake to 2,400 mg/day. This is achieved by not adding salt while cooking or at the table and eliminating highly salted processed foods such as smoked, cured, or processed meats; canned vegetables, meats, sauces, and soups; salted snacks such as crackers, potato chips, pretzels, popcorn, and nuts; convenience mixes and instant products, most condiments, and seasoned salts.

Losing weight without reducing sodium intake lowers blood pressure, even if ideal weight is not attained and regardless of the degree of excess weight. Weight reduction is recommended as the initial step in treating overweight clients with mild to moderate hypertension.

In addition to the above recommendations, results of a new study called DASH (Dietary Approaches to Stop Hypertension) shows that eating the right foods can lower blood pressure. Although the study does not identify which dietary components lower blood pressure, it clearly demonstrates that a high intake of fruit, vegetables, and low-fat dairy products, combined with a low intake of total and saturated fat, lowers blood pressure as effectively as drug therapy. In hypertensive clients, the "DASH combination diet" (high in fruits and vegetables combined with fat restriction) lowered systolic blood pressure 11.4 mm Hg and diastolic pressure 5.5 mm Hg. The DASH diet includes:

- 7 to 8 servings of grains
- 4 to 5 servings of vegetables
- 4 to 5 servings of fruit
- 2 to 3 servings of low-fat or nonfat dairy products
- 2 or fewer servings of meat
- 4 to 5 servings of nuts per week
- 2 to 3 servings of added fat per day, and 5 snacks and sweets per week

It is estimated that a population-wide decrease in blood pressure as seen in DASH would reduce the incidence of stroke by 27% and coronary heart disease by 15%.

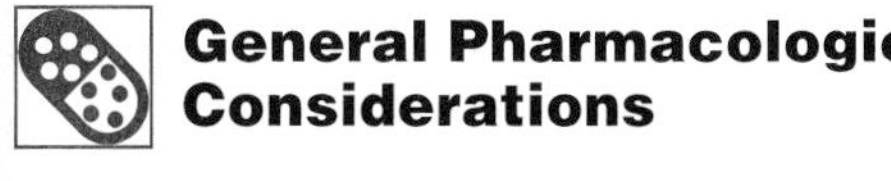

General Pharmacologic Considerations

Drug therapy may include the use of potent antihypertensive agents. The nurse must have a thorough knowledge of possible adverse drug effects. All antihypertensive drugs can cause postural hypotension, which can lead to client falls. Teaching should include tips for managing syncope and dizziness.

Medication controls, but does not cure hypertension. It is important for individuals with hypertension to control body weight, restrict dietary sodium, and learn ways to manage stress appropriately.

ACE inhibitors are used cautiously in patients with renal or hepatic impairment and in older adults.

A sudden drop in blood pressure may occur during the first 1 to 3 hours after the initial dose of an ACE inhibitor. The hypotensive episode may be managed with the administration of normal saline intravenously. This type of hypotensive episode is not an indication to discontinue the drug.

ACE inhibitors may cause a persistent cough that continues until the medication is discontinued.

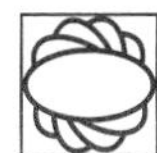

General Gerontologic Considerations

Hypertension caused by arteriosclerosis or atherosclerosis is not uncommon in older adults. This problem may go undiagnosed unless the client sees a physician at regular intervals. Older adults should be encouraged to have their blood pressure checked at least every 6 months. Senior citizen centers and pharmacies frequently offer free blood pressure monitoring.

Because postural hypotension is common in the older adult, correct blood pressure measurement is particularly important. Measurements are obtained while the older person is supine or sitting, and immediately after the patient stands.

Older adults are at increased risk to develop hypokalemia from antihypertensive drugs. Lower doses of hydrochlorothiazide or chlorthalidone can control hypertension and minimize the risk of hypokalemia in the older adult.

SUMMARY OF KEY CONCEPTS

- Blood pressure is the result of the force created by the cardiac output and the peripheral resistance.
- Blood pressure is influenced by age, body size, diet, activity, emotions, pain, position, gender, time of day, and disease states.
- Systolic blood pressure is created by the force and volume of blood ejected from the left ventricle during systole and the ability of the arteries to distend when receiving it. Diastolic pressure is the arterial pressure during ventricular relaxation.
- Hypertension is a sustained systolic pressure of 140 mm Hg or higher, or a diastolic arterial pressure of 90 mm Hg or greater, or both. Two groups that are at risk for developing hypertension are the geriatric population

and those with a family history, especially African Americans.
- Hypertension may develop due to alterations in electrolyte levels, renin secretion, sympathetic nervous system regulation, or insufficient natriuretic factor.
- Chronic hypertension leads to myocardial enlargement, increased myocardial need for oxygenated blood, and acceleration of the atherosclerotic process.
- Essential hypertension is an idiopathic condition (eg, no known cause); secondary hypertension has an underlying cause.
- Many hypertensive individuals are asymptomatic or have mild symptoms such as headache, fatigue, insomnia, and nervousness. However, all have an elevated systolic or diastolic blood pressure, or both. Many demonstrate additional risk factors that contribute to the hypertension, such as obesity and use of tobacco products. Most are diagnosed at the time of a physical examination for other reasons. Treatment begins with lifestyle changes, which may be followed by any number and combinations of drug therapy. Treating the cause of secondary hypertension can reduce the blood pressure.
- The nurse measures the blood pressure accurately and consistently in the same manner. Drugs are administered and the client is monitored for expected and unexpected responses. If diagnostic tests are ordered, the nurse prepares and assesses the client afterward. The nurse provides a great deal of teaching to promote the client's eventual self-care.
- Secondary hypertension may develop from a number of causes, such as an adrenal tumor called pheochromocytoma; primary aldosteronism, as a side effect of oral contraceptives; and from abuse of stimulating substances such as cocaine, amphetamines, Dexedrine, and caffeine.
- Accelerated hypertension is characterized by markedly elevated blood pressure; malignant hypertension is a dangerously elevated blood pressure. Both are accompanied by ophthalmologic changes that indicate extremely high intravascular and rising intracranial pressures.
- If blood pressure is not controlled, stroke, congestive heart failure, myocardial infarction, dissecting or rupture of an aortic aneurysm, and renal failure may ensue.
- In a hypertensive emergency, IV drugs are prescribed by to reduce the blood pressure. The nurse administers them safely and titrates the rate of infusion according to the client's response.

CRITICAL THINKING EXERCISES

1. On admission, you find a client's blood pressure is 210/112 in a supine position. What additional data would be pertinent to collect before reporting the finding to the nurse in charge and the client's physician?
2. To which community resources in your locale would you refer a client with hypertension for support or care following discharge?

Suggested Readings

Abrams, A. (1998). *Clinical drug therapy: Rationales for nursing practice.* Philadelphia: Lippincott-Raven.

Better control of high blood pressure. (1996). *Johns Hopkins Medical Letter, 8*(9), 3.

Calcium channel blockers warrant caution. (1996). *People's Medical Society,15*(6), 4–5.

Carpenito, L. (1997). *Nursing care plans and documentation* (2nd ed.). Philadelphia: Lippincott-Raven.

Chase, S. (1997). Pharmacology in practice: Antihypertensives. *RN, 60*(6), 33–39.

Eaton, L. E., Buck, E. A., & Catanzaro, J. E. (1996). The nurse's role in facilitating compliance in clients with hypertension. *Med-Surg Nursing 5*(5), 339–345, 359.

Ellis, J., Nowlis, E., & Bentz, P. (1996). *Modules for basic nursing skills* (6th ed., vol. 1.). Philadelphia: Lippincott-Raven.

Karch, A. (1998). *1998 Lippincott's nursing drug guide.* Philadelphia: Lippincott-Raven.

Kendler, B. S. (1997). Recent nutritional approaches to the prevention and therapy of cardiovascular disease. *Progress in Cardiovascular Nursing, 12*(3), 3–23.

Kuncl, N., & Nelson, K. (1997, August). Antihypertensives: Balancing risks and benefits. *Nursing, 27*(8), 46–49.

Pettinicchi T. (1996). Action stat! Hypertensive crisis. *Nursing, 26*(8), 25.

Solomon J. (1996). Drug compliance: You can help hypertensive patients. *Office Nurse, 9*(11), 28–31, 34–37.

Ziporyn T. (1996). Nutrition: Shaking up conventional wisdom on salt. *Harvard Health Letter, 22*(2). 6–7.

Additional Resources

American Heart Association
1615 North Stemmons Freeway
Dallas, TX 75201–3480
(214) 748–7212
http://www.amhrt.org

Heart to Heart Volunteers
http://www.csusm.edu/public/guests/bhv/

National Heart, Lung, and Blood Institute
900 Rockville Pike
Bethesda, MD 20892–0002
http://www.nhlbi.nih.gov

Chapter 35

Caring for Clients With Heart Failure

KEY TERMS

Afterload
Aldosterone
Angiotensin
Cardiogenic shock
Congestive heart failure
Cor pulmonale
Digitalization
Exertional dyspnea
Hemopump
Intra-aortic balloon pump
Left-sided heart failure
Orthopnea
Paroxysmal nocturnal dyspnea
Pitting edema
Preload
Pulmonary hypertension
Pulmonary vascular bed
Renin
Right-sided heart failure
Ventricular assist device

LEARNING OBJECTIVES

On completion of this chapter, the reader will:

- Discuss the cause and pathophysiology of heart failure.
- Distinguish between left- and right-sided heart failure.
- List and discuss the symptoms, diagnosis, and treatment of left-sided heart failure.
- List and discuss the symptoms, diagnosis, and treatment of right-sided heart failure.
- Discuss the nursing management of clients with heart failure.
- Discuss the cause and pathophysiology of pulmonary edema.
- List and discuss the symptoms, diagnosis, and treatment of pulmonary edema.
- Discuss the nursing management of clients with pulmonary edema.

The heart is a double pump; the right side pumps deoxygenated blood to the lungs for oxygenation, and the left side pumps oxygen-rich blood into the systemic circulation (Fig. 35–1). This process provides a continuous supply of oxygen and nutrients for cellular metabolism and a mechanism for the elimination of carbon dioxide and metabolic wastes. Disturbances in one part of the heart, if they are severe enough or last long enough, eventually affect the entire circulation.

Heart Failure

Heart failure is the inability of the heart to pump a sufficient amount of blood to meet the body's metabolic needs. The term **congestive heart failure** describes the accumulation of blood and fluid within organs and tissues due to impaired circulation. Because the heart is a double pump, it is possible for either the left or the right ventricle, or both, to become impaired. The terms **left-sided** (*left ventricular*) **heart failure** or **right-sided** (*right ventricular*) **heart failure** describe the location of the pumping dysfunction.

Etiology and Pathophysiology

Acute heart failure is a sudden change in the heart's ability to contract, for example, following a myocardial infarction. More often, heart failure develops gradually as a consequence of some other chronic disorder. Regardless of the etiology, when one of the ventricles fails to pump effectively, the amount of blood entering the atria remains the same but ventricular output is diminished. The net result is that the vascular system becomes overloaded with fluid and cardiac output is reduced.

When cardiac output falls, certain mechanisms occur within the body that are designed to increase stroke volume and raise blood pressure. These compensatory mechanisms often do more harm than good. For example, when cardiac output is low, the sympathetic nervous system raises heart rate and increases the force of myocardial contraction in an effort to eject more blood into the circulation. The in-

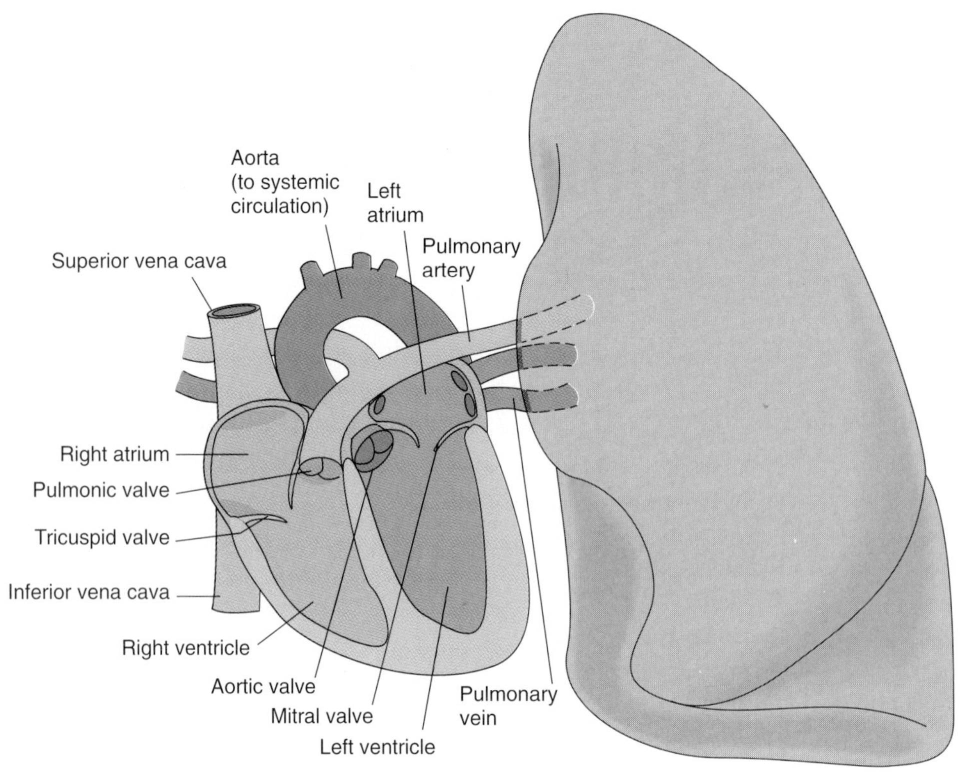

FIGURE 35-1. Right and left cardiac pumps.

creased force and contraction of the heart increases myocardial oxygen demand (the amount of oxygen the heart itself needs to perform its work). Because oxygenated blood is unavailable, the client's condition worsens. Blood vessels constrict in an effort to maintain blood pressure; however, this causes increased resistance against which the failing heart must pump. Another compensatory mechanism is the **renin-angiotensin-aldosterone** mechanism that is initiated in response to decreased blood flow to the kidneys. Renin is released by the kidneys and activates angiotensin. Angiotensin causes vasoconstriction and increased in blood pressure. Angiotensin also stimulates the adrenal gland to secrete aldosterone, which causes sodium and water to be retained, further compromising the client's status by increasing the amount of blood volume the heart must pump.

As cardiac output falls, cells now deprived of oxygen switch from aerobic metabolism to less efficient anaerobic metabolism. Anaerobic metabolism results in an accumulation of lactic acid, which lowers blood pH and can eventually cause metabolic acidosis. In an acidotic state, more oxygen is transferred to the cells, but the amount of oxygenated blood available is quickly exhausted. Figure 35–2 illustrates the compensatory mechanisms that occur in response to low cardiac output.

Left-Sided Heart Failure

Left-sided heart failure produces respiratory distress. If uncontrolled, *pulmonary edema* develops.

ETIOLOGY AND PATHOPHYSIOLOGY

Left-sided heart failure is the result of various conditions that cause the ventricle to overwork and become fatigued. Some conditions predisposing to left-sided failure include:

- High blood pressure secondary to arteriosclerosis and atherosclerosis
- Scar formation following a myocardial infarction
- Prolonged cardiac infections or inflammatory heart conditions
- Hypervolemia accompanying renal failure or rapid infusion of intravenous (IV) fluids
- Tachycardia secondary to hyperthyroidism and hypoxemia

Fluid accumulates in the lungs when the left ventricle fails, creating congestion in the **pulmonary vascular bed** (the capillary network surrounding the alveoli of the lungs). Increased pulmonary vascular bed pressure causes fluid to escape from the pulmonary capillaries into the alveoli. The fluid impairs

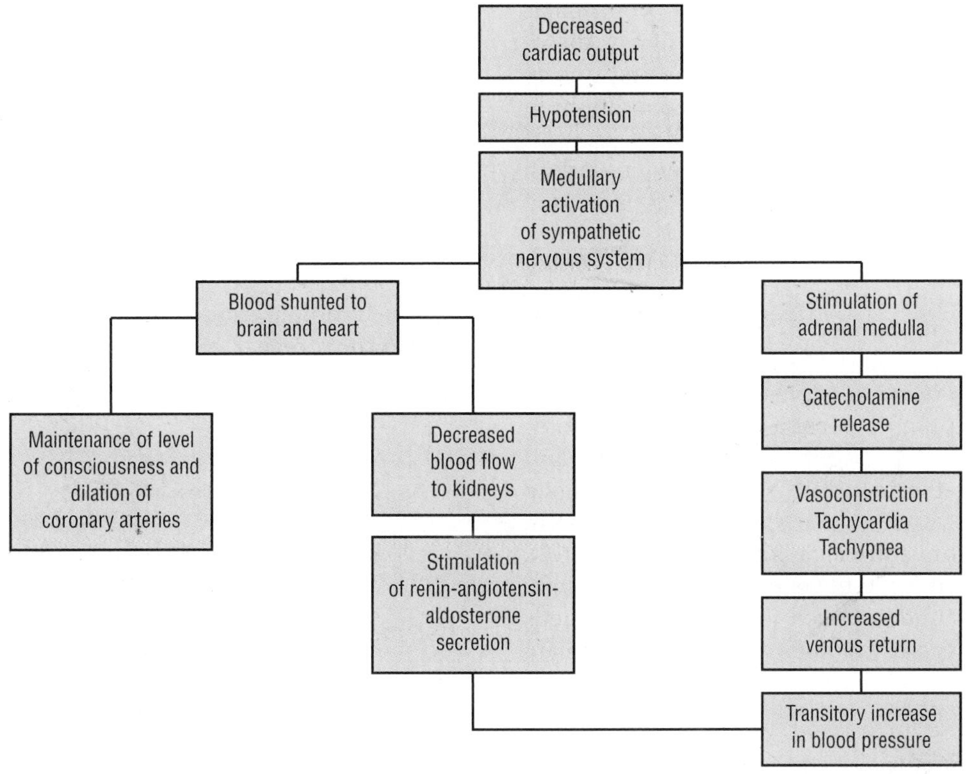

FIGURE 35-2. Compensatory mechanisms of the sympathetic nervous system. Decreased cardiac output triggers a series of compensatory mechanisms within the body in an effort to maintain level of consciousness and blood pressure.

gas exchange, and waste products accumulate in the blood. The client becomes hypoxic (a state of insufficient oxygen within the body).

ASSESSMENT FINDINGS

Signs and Symptoms

Many clients notice unusual fatigue associated with activity. Some find that **exertional dyspnea** (effort at breathing when active) is the first symptom. Inability to breathe unless sitting upright (**orthopnea**) or being awakened by breathlessness (**paroxysmal nocturnal dyspnea**) may prompt the person to use several pillows when in bed or to sleep in a chair or recliner.

The client may have a rapid or irregular pulse. Unless the cardiac output is extremely low, the blood pressure is elevated. A cough, *hemoptysis* (blood-streaked sputum), and moist crackles heard on auscultation are typical respiratory findings. Urine output is diminished. Restlessness and confusion accompany severe hypoxia.

Diagnostic Findings

Chest radiography shows cardiac enlargement and fluid accumulation in the lungs. The increased size of the left ventricle and the ineffective pumping of the heart can be determined by an echocardiogram. At first, arterial blood gas (ABG) analysis may reveal respiratory alkalosis as a result of the client's rapid, shallow breathing. Later, there is a shift to metabolic acidosis as gas exchange becomes more impaired. Serum sodium levels may be elevated. An elevated blood urea nitrogen indicates impaired renal perfusion. If the client is seriously ill, a pulmonary artery catheter may be inserted for hemodynamic monitoring. Cardiac outputs can be measured via the pulmonary artery catheter. Cardiac output is diminished in left-sided heart failure, and pulmonary artery pressure and pulmonary capillary wedge pressure measurements are elevated.

Right-Sided Heart Failure

When the right pump fails, there is congestion of blood within the venous vascular system.

ETIOLOGY AND PATHOPHYSIOLOGY

The major cause of right-sided heart failure is left-sided heart failure. Myocardial infarctions that affect the right ventricle can also cause right ventricular failure. Individuals with chronic respiratory disorders tend to develop right-sided failure first due to cor pulmonale. **Cor pulmonale** is a condition in which the heart (cor) is affected by lung damage (pulmonale). Pulmonary disease impairs oxygen–carbon dioxide exchange in the alveoli, leading to increased carbon dioxide in the blood. By some unknown mechanism, pulmonary arterial vasoconstriction occurs. Prolonged pulmonary arterial vasoconstriction then results in **pulmonary hypertension** (elevated pressure in the pulmonary arterial system). When pulmonary hypertension is present, the right ventricle is forced to pump against a high pressure gradient. Subsequently, the right ventricle enlarges and weakens under the increased workload, leading to failure.

When the right ventricle fails to empty completely, blood is trapped in the venous vascular system. Eventually, the fluid is forced to move into the cells and interstitial spaces of other organs and tissues of the body.

ASSESSMENT FINDINGS

Signs and Symptoms

The client may have a history of gradual unexplained weight gain due to fluid retention. Dependent **pitting edema** (Fig. 35–3) in the feet and the ankles can be observed. This type of edema may seem to disappear overnight but is temporarily redistributed by gravity to other tissues, such as the presacral area. The abdomen may be distended with fluid (ascites) and the liver may be enlarged (hepatomegaly). Jugular veins are often distended due to increased central venous pressure (Nursing Guidelines 35–1). Enlarged abdominal organs often restrict ventilation, creating dyspnea. Clients may observe that rings, shoes, or clothing have become tight. Accumulation of blood in abdominal organs may cause anorexia, nausea, and flatulence. Table 35–1 highlights the differences between left ventricular failure and right ventricular heart failure.

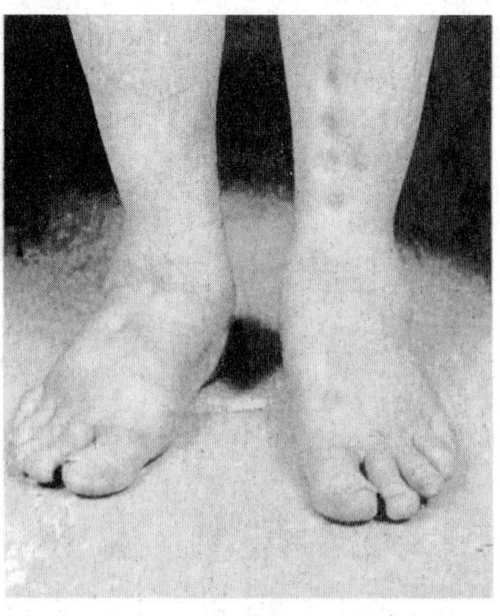

FIGURE 35-3. Pitting edema of feet and lower legs.

Diagnostic Findings

A chest radiograph, electrocardiogram, and echocardiography reveal right ventricular enlargement. Cor pulmonale is confirmed with a lung scan and

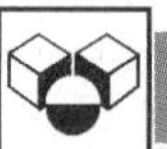

Nursing Guidelines 35-1

Estimating Central Venous Pressure

Central venous pressure is estimated by measuring the height of jugular vein distention.

1. Obtain a centimeter ruler.
2. Help the client to lie flat.
3. Slowly elevate the head of the bed to a 45-degree angle.
4. Locate the sternal angle by placing two fingers at the sternal notch and sliding them down the sternum until they reach a bony prominence.
5. Estimate venous pressure by measuring the vertical distance from the sternal angle (zero cm) to the level of jugular vein distention (cm above zero).

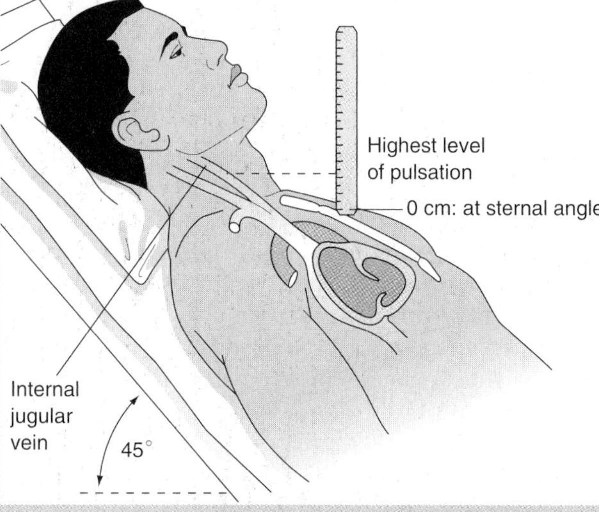

6. Add 5 cm to the ruler measurement to estimate central venous pressure.

Central venous pressure is elevated more than 12 to 15 cm H_2O in clients who have right ventricular heart failure. A more accurate measurement of central venous pressure is obtained by using a central venous catheter.

TABLE 35-1 **Signs and Symptoms of Left and Right Ventricular Failure**

Left Ventricular Failure	Right Ventricular Failure
Fatigue	Weakness
Paroxysmal nocturnal dyspnea	Ascites
Orthopnea	Weight gain
Hypoxia	Nausea, vomiting
Crackles	Arrhythmias
Cyanosis	Elevated central venous pressure
S_3 heart sound	Jugular vein distention
Cough with pink frothy sputum	
Elevated pulmonary capillary wedge pressure	

pulmonary arteriography. Liver enzymes are elevated if the liver is impaired.

Medical Management

The medical management of both left- and right-sided heart failure is directed toward reducing the workload of the heart and improving ventricular output. This is achieved primarily with drug therapy. Activity is limited according to the severity of the client's condition. A low-sodium diet is prescribed and fluids may be restricted. Sedatives or tranquilizers, reduce dyspnea and relieve anxiety. An intra-aortic balloon pump (IABP), left ventricular blood pump (**Hemopump**), or ventricular assist device (VAD) may be used to support left ventricular function until the heart can recover.

DRUG THERAPY

Drug therapy is aimed at improving cardiac output. One or more drugs are prescribed (Table 35–2). Because poorly circulated blood leads to the formation of thrombi and emboli, a daily aspirin, dipyridamole (Persantine), or an oral anticoagulant is prescribed.

INTRA-AORTIC BALLOON PUMP

If acute left ventricular heart failure is accompanied by **cardiogenic shock** (see Chap. 22) an **intra-aortic balloon pump** (IABP) is inserted into the left femoral artery and threaded up to the descending aortic arch (Fig. 35–4). The intra-aortic balloon pump is connected to a machine that is synchronized with the client's ventricular contraction. The balloon inflates during diastole and deflates during systole. Thus, it acts as a secondary pump that supplements the ineffectual contraction of the left ventricle. Inflation of the IABP increases coronary artery, renal artery, and myocardial perfusion. Deflation actually keeps the aorta distended so that cardiac output is improved; the work of the left ventricle is decreased, and peripheral organs are more adequately perfused with oxygenated blood.

LEFT VENTRICULAR BLOOD PUMP

A *left ventricular blood pump* or Hemopump is another treatment that improves cardiac output by supplementing the work of the left ventricle. A motorized device is inserted into the left ventricle. The pump extracts blood that is not ejected from the left ventricle and deposits it into the descending aorta.

LEFT VENTRICULAR ASSIST DEVICE

Some clients who develop cardiogenic shock or are awaiting a heart transplant are treated with a **ventricular assist device** (VAD). A VAD uses an outflow and inflow cannula to reroute blood from the left atrium directly into the aorta (Fig. 35–5). By bypassing the weak, ineffective left ventricle, the heart is given time to rest. This can also be used for right-sided failure or a double assist device can be used for biventricular failure when a client is awaiting heart transplantation. The device allows clients to return home until the time of surgery.

Surgical Management

Adults less than 55 years of age are candidates for a heart transplant when medical treatment is unsuccessful. An artificial heart may be used for a brief period while awaiting a donor organ that is compatible with the tissue and blood type of the recipient. Hopes for long-term use of an artificial mechanical heart have been disappointing. In the few cases where this has been attempted, multiple complications, such as malfunction of an artificial valve, the formation of emboli, and stroke, have occurred. This raised ethical questions concerning the quality of the client's life because the artificial heart allows only short periods during which the client could be separated from the large and noisy air compressor that powers the mechanical pump.

In 1993, the Food and Drug Administration approved a procedure called a *cardiomyoplasty* in which the client's own chest muscle (latissimus dorsi) is grafted to the aorta and wrapped around the heart. An electrical stimulator placed in a subcutaneous pouch triggers skeletal muscle contraction (Fig. 35–6). The contraction acts as a counterpulsation mechanism

TABLE 35-2 **Drugs Used to Treat Heart Failure**

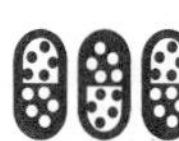

Drug/Drug Action	Side Effects	Nursing Considerations
Cardiac Glycosides		
digoxin (Lanoxin) Increases cardiac output by slowing the heart rate (negative chronotropic action) and increasing the force of contraction (*positive chronotropic action*)	Fatigue, generalized muscle weakness, anorexia, nausea, vomiting, yellow-green halos around images, arrhythmias	Monitor pulse rate before each dose. Withhold administration if pulse is <60 or >110 beats/min. Provide dietary sources of potassium.
Diuretics		
furosemide (Lasix) Promotes the excretion of sodium and water thus reducing circulating blood volume and decreasing workload of the heart	Dizziness, dehydration, blurred vision, anorexia, diarrhea, nocturia, polyuria, thrombocytopenia, orthostatic hypotension, hypokalemia	Weigh the client daily. Measure intake and output. Monitor serum potassium levels. Replace potassium with bananas, orange juice, or prescribed supplement.
Vasodilators		
nitroglycerin Improves stroke volume by reducing **afterload** (systemic vascular resistance); reduces **preload** (filling of the heart with blood) by dilating veins and arteries	Headache, dizziness, orthostatic hypotension, tachycardia, flushing, nausea, hypersensitivity	Assess the client for hypotension. Monitor the client for headache and flushed skin.
Angiotensin-Converting Enzyme (ACE) Inhibitors		
captopril (Capoten) Blocks ACE from converting angiotensin I to angiotensin II (a potent vasoconstrictor); promotes fluid and sodium loss and decreases peripheral vascular resistance	Tachycardia, hypotension, gastric irritation, pancytopenia, proteinuria, rash, cough, dry mouth	Reduced excretion in clients with renal failure, first-dose hypotension is common in elderly clients. Administer 1 hour before meals or 2 hours after meals.
Nonglycoside Inotropic Agents		
dobutamine (Dobutrex) Relieves cardiogenic shock by strengthening the force of myocardial contraction and increasing cardiac output	Headache, hypertension, tachycardia, angina, nausea	Monitor for increased heart rate, elevated blood pressure, and arrhythmias.

similar to the IABP. It augments the ineffective myocardial muscle contraction.

Surgical excision of a portion of the heart muscle in clients who have cardiomegaly is an experimental form of treatment in both North and South America. It is hoped that these techniques will offer other options to individuals who are not candidates for heart transplantation or for whom a donor heart cannot be found.

Nursing Management

Administer drugs carefully because most are quite powerful and an incorrect dose is dangerous. Digitalis is commonly prescribed in frequent and relatively large doses at the beginning of therapy to quickly achieve a therapeutic effect. This is called **digitalization.** Thereafter, a daily, smaller dose is administered to sustain therapeutic blood levels (maintenance dose). Always monitor the heart rate before digitalis administration. Report signs of digitalis toxicity (loss of appetite, nausea, or vomiting; rapid, slow, or irregular heart rate or sudden disturbance in color vision) to the physician.

Monitor serum electrolyte values, especially if the client is receiving diuretics. Some diuretics deplete potassium as well as sodium. Hypokalemia (low serum potassium) is especially dangerous because it

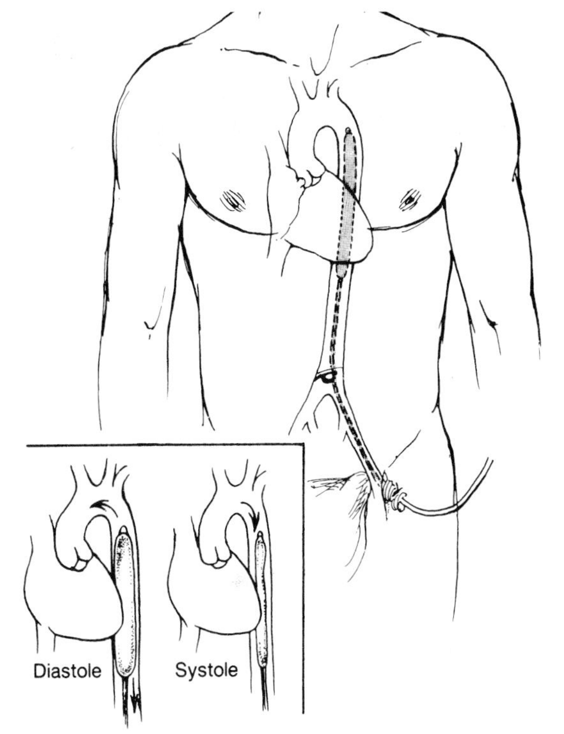

FIGURE 35-4. Intra-aortic balloon pump.

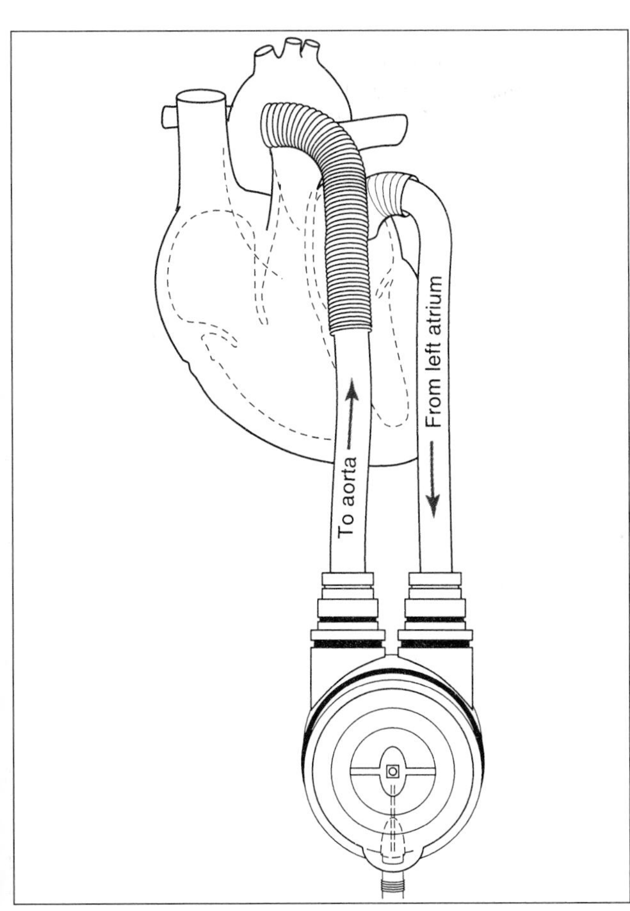

FIGURE 35-5. Ventricular assist device.

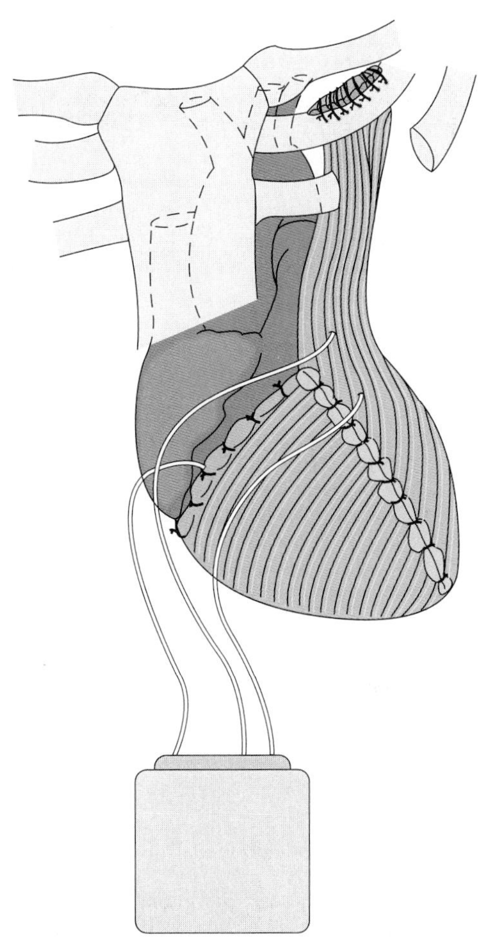

FIGURE 35-6. The latissimus dorsi muscle is dissected and wrapped around the heart itself.

increases the potential for digitalis toxicity. Normal potassium levels can be maintained by increasing the intake of potassium-rich foods (Box 35–1). Monitor serum magnesium levels; hypomagnesemia (low magnesium level) predisposes clients to cardiac arrhythmias.

NURSING PROCESS
The Client With Heart Failure

Assessment

Obtain the client's history of symptoms including activity tolerance and respiratory difficulties during activity and at rest. Assess for dyspnea, moist lung sounds, tachycardia, hypotension, distended neck veins, peripheral edema, reduced urine output, lethargy, and confusion.

Diagnosis and Planning

The nursing care of clients with heart failure includes, but is not limited to, the following:

Nursing Diagnoses and Collaborative Problems	Nursing Interventions
Decreased Cardiac Output related to tachycardia, arterial vasoconstriction, reduced stroke volume, and increased vascular volume **Goal:** The client will have an increase in cardiac output as evidenced by stable vital signs and adequate urine output, and no evidence of arrhythmias, chest pain, dyspnea, confusion, or dizziness.	Assess the following on a regular basis, as often as necessary: Vital signs Heart and lung sounds Intake and output Pulse rhythm and quality Effort of breathing Mental status Presence of edema Administer prescribed medications and observe for desired response—decreased dyspnea, improved lung sounds, diminished peripheral edema, increased urine output. Promote rest; client may be more comfortable with head of bed elevated or sitting in a chair. Reduce environmental stress and assist client in identifying and coping with situations that induce anxiety.
Altered Peripheral Tissue Perfusion related to venous congestion secondary to right-sided heart failure **Goal:** Tissue perfusion will improve as evidenced by decreased edema, decreased pain, improved quality of peripheral pulses.	Assess extremities for edema, cyanosis, peripheral pulses; note degree of edema and location at which it was assessed (pedal, tibial). Elevate extremities and avoid sitting with legs dependent for an extended period. Remove any constrictive clothing including ill-fitting support or antiembolic hose. Inspect edematous extremities for skin breakdown and implement measure to maintain skin integrity.
Impaired Gas Exchange related to pulmonary congestion secondary to decreased cardiac output **Goal:** The client will attain adequate oxygenation status as evidenced by clear lung sounds, decreased work of breathing, pulse oximeter reading above 90%.	Assess the following as often as necessary: • Breath sounds • Color, quantity of sputum • Respiratory rate Maintain in a semi-Fowler's position to maximize lung expansion, but help client change position every 2 hours. Administer oxygen therapy as prescribed. Monitor pulse oximeter readings and report an oxygen saturation of less than 90%. Offer small frequent feedings to avoid gastric distention.
Fluid Volume Excess related to decreased ventricular contractility, decreased renal perfusion, sodium retention **Goal:** The client will achieve fluid balance as evidenced by adequate output, no weight gain, and stable vital signs.	Assess intake and output and weigh the client daily. Administer prescribed diuretics and note response; dosage may be increased if client does not diurese (excrete excess fluid) sufficiently. Observe for symptoms of electrolyte imbalance such as irregular heart rate, confusion, and lethargy. Administer potassium supplements as prescribed and monitor laboratory values. Help client comply with fluid and sodium restriction; space allowed fluids over the course of the day taking into consideration the client's preferences, meal times, and medication administration schedules.
Activity Intolerance related to hypoxia secondary to decreased cardiac output **Goal:** The client will have increased activity tolerance as evidenced by participation in activities of daily living, increased ambulation, and verbal expressions of decreased fatigue.	Assist with activities of daily living; note client's response to activity and provide rest periods. Keep personal items within easy reach. Gradually increase activity and self-care as condition improves. Clients with congestive heart failure often have difficulty sleeping; promote a restful night's sleep by helping client into position of comfort that promotes adequate oxygenation and administering sedatives to reduce restlessness and promote sleep.

Evaluation and Expected Outcomes

- Blood pressure and heart rate return to client's baseline.
- No evidence of edema.
- Respirations are unlabored and lungs are clear.
- Fluid intake approximates output.
- Client is able to participate in activities of daily living within level of tolerance.

CLIENT AND FAMILY TEACHING

Clients with congestive heart failure and their families should be instructed in the disease process, the meaning of the term "failure," the signs and symptoms of impending congestive heart failure such as weight gain, ankle swelling, fatigue, and dyspnea, and the importance of taking all medications regularly. It is also important to teach clients to:

- Measure pulse and blood pressure daily.
- Check weight at the same time each day and using the same scale and to consult a physician if there is more than a 2-lb weight gain.
- Schedule rest periods to reduce or eliminate fatigue and dyspnea.

BOX 35-1 Potassium-Rich Foods

- Potatoes, sweet potatoes, winter squash, tomatoes, tomato juice
- Milk, yogurt
- Dates, bananas, cantaloupes, orange juice, prunes, raisins, prune juice
- Dry beans, peas, lentils
- Peanut butter
- Bran cereals

- Increase activities, such as walking, when able to do so without dyspnea or fatigue.
- Identify and avoid occasions that produce stress.
- Elevate the legs while sitting.
- Follow the diet prescribed by the physician.
- Avoid extreme heat, cold, or humidity.
- Report a heart rate less than 60 or more than 120 beats/min before taking digitalis preparations.
- Contact the physician if symptoms return or there is a sudden increase in swelling in the legs, ankles, or feet.
- Maintain follow-up care.

Pulmonary Edema

Pulmonary edema is fluid accumulation in the lungs that interferes with gas exchange in the alveoli. Pulmonary edema represents an acute emergency. Cardiac arrhythmias and cardiac or respiratory arrest are complications of pulmonary edema.

ETIOLOGY AND PATHOPHYSIOLOGY

Pulmonary edema is a complication of left ventricular failure. Noncardiogenic pulmonary edema, sometimes referred to as adult respiratory distress syndrome (ARDS), also occurs when there is an alteration in the pulmonary capillary membrane from a pulmonary embolism, infections, or blast injuries.

When the etiology is cardiogenic, the left ventricle becomes incapable of maintaining sufficient output of blood with each contraction. The right ventricle, however, continues to pump blood toward the lungs. The pulmonary capillaries and the alveoli become engorged with blood. The lungs can rapidly fill with fluid, and acute respiratory distress develops. As carbon dioxide accumulates, respiratory rate and depth increase. Without treatment, hyperventilation becomes insufficient in preventing respiratory acidosis, which is then followed by metabolic acidosis.

ASSESSMENT

Signs and Symptoms

Clients with acute pulmonary edema exhibit sudden dyspnea, wheezing, orthopnea, restlessness, cough (often productive of pink, frothy sputum), cyanosis, tachycardia, and severe apprehension. Respirations sound moist or gurgling. If a pulmonary artery catheter is in place, the pulmonary artery pressure and pulmonary capillary wedge pressure are elevated, and cardiac output is reduced. While the body responds with arterial vasoconstriction, an adequate blood pressure may be temporarily sustained; however, the client eventually becomes hypotensive and peripheral pulses disappear.

Diagnostic Findings

Chest radiographs show pulmonary infiltration with fluid. ABGs indicate severe hypoxemia (low PaO_2) and hypercapnia (high $PaCO_2$) and a pH less than 7.35.

MEDICAL MANAGEMENT

Every effort is made to relieve lung congestion as quickly as possible because pulmonary edema can be fatal. Relief of symptoms is accomplished by the administration of medications that improve myocardial contractility and decrease preload. Ventilation is supported with supplemental oxygen or mechanical ventilation. If the cause of the heart failure and pulmonary edema is a condition that can be corrected surgically, such as a mitral valve disorder, the client is supported medically while being prepared for surgery.

Drug Therapy

Inotropic agents, such as dobutamine or digitalis, are administered IV to improve the force of ventricular contraction. To reduce myocardial oxygen consumption, drugs that reduce venous return to the heart (diuretics) and those that promote vasodilation, (nitrates or calcium channel blockers) are prescribed.

Intravenous morphine sulfate is often given to lessen anxiety. Morphine seems to help relieve respiratory symptoms by depressing higher cerebral centers, thus relieving anxiety and slowing the respiratory rate. Morphine also promotes muscle relaxation and reduces the work of breathing.

Oxygenation

To facilitate gas exchange, oxygen is administered. A mask rather than nasal cannula is needed to deliver maximum percentages of oxygen. If respiratory failure occurs, the client is intubated and oxygen is administered under continuous positive airway pressure (CPAP) or with mechanical ventilation with positive end-expiratory pressure (PEEP).

Invasive Measures

If the client does not respond to medical measures, invasive procedures, such as the IABP, blood pump, or VAD, are used to sustain the client's life.

NURSING MANAGEMENT

Establish an IV line immediately (if one is not already in place) for administration of drugs. Administer oxygen and apply a pulse oximeter to the client's finger, earlobe, or bridge of the nose to monitor oxygenation. Suction the airway as needed and provide frequent mouth care if mechanical ventilation is used. Assess heart rate and rhythm and frequently monitor blood pressure. Assess pulmonary artery pressures, cardiac output, and central venous pressure. Insert a urinary catheter to evaluate the client's response to diuretics. Provide alternative methods for verbal communication if the client is intubated.

Effective resolution of pulmonary edema requires both medical and nursing management. The nursing diagnosis, interventions, and goals for a client with pulmonary edema are similar to those for the client experiencing congestive heart failure. Refer to the discussion that accompanies heart failure for additional nursing management.

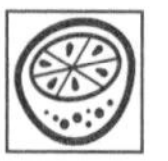

General Nutritional Considerations

Until edema resolves, severe heart failure is treated with a sodium restriction of 500 to 1,000 mg/d. To achieve this level of restriction, daily food choices are limited to 6 oz of meat, 8 oz of milk, specially prepared low-sodium breads, low-sodium cereals and grains, distilled water for drinking and cooking, and low-sodium margarine and salad dressings. Processed and commercially prepared foods are eliminated, as are vegetables with naturally occurring sodium such as beets, celery, carrots, and "greens." Fresh, frozen and canned fruit and fruit juices are not restricted.

Clients with mild heart failure may tolerate as much as 3,000 mg of sodium daily, which is achieved by not adding salt to food and avoiding processed food.

Encourage overweight clients to lose weight to reduce cardiac workload. Be aware that edema can mask clinical signs of malnutrition; weight is not a reliable indicator of nutritional status.

Dyspnea and nausea related to enlarged abdominal organs interfere with appetite and intake. Provide five to six small meals of soft or easy to chew foods and encourage the client to rest after eating. Spicy, gas-forming, and high-fiber foods are avoided to lessen heartburn and flatulence.

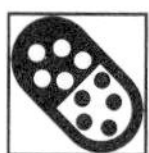

General Pharmacologic Considerations

Many clients with mild heart failure can be managed with the thiazide diuretics such as hydrochlorothiazide or chlorthalidone. Severe heart failure usually requires a loop diuretic such as furosemide.

Certain ACE inhibitors such as captopril, fosinopril, or ramipril may be used to treat heart failure in clients who have not responded to digitalis and diuretics.

Digitalis preparations are potent drugs that are capable of causing various toxic effects. The margin between a therapeutic effect and drug toxicity is narrow. Thus, the client should be observed for signs of digitalis toxicity, not only during the initial period of therapy, but also throughout the entire hospitalization.

For clients taking diuretics, discharge instructions should include a discussion of the signs and symptoms of electrolyte and water loss and the importance of adhering to the medication schedule prescribed by the physician. The client also is instructed to eat foods high in potassium.

Clients receiving emergency drug therapy for acute pulmonary edema are observed for the effectiveness of drug therapy and any adverse effects of the drugs administered. Many of the medications given for this disorder are given IV and occasionally in large doses, hence the importance of client observation. Drugs that are administered are morphine, aminophylline, digoxin (or other digitalis preparations), and vasopressors for hypotension.

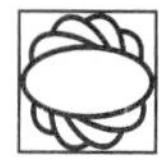

General Gerontologic Considerations

In many older clients dyspnea on exertion is the earliest symptom of heart failure. Older adults may also experience a change in mental status, particularly confusion.

The heart is not exempt from the process of aging. With advancing age, cardiac reserve is lessened, and the heart becomes less able to withstand the effects of injury or disease.

In older adults, vascular changes can lead to heart failure by interfering with the blood supply to the heart muscle and by causing the heart to pump blood through vessels that have become narrowed and inflexible.

A thorough drug history from a new client or the family is essential because many older adults take digitalis preparations for cardiac disorders. Due to changes in the gastrointestinal, renal, and hepatic systems of older adults, nurses must carefully monitor clients for therapeutic effects and adverse reactions. Older adults are at greater risk for toxicity due to decreased ability of the kidney to excrete the drug.

If, for financial reasons, a client is unable to prepare or purchase special foods and needed medications, a social service worker or other community agent is contacted for financial assistance.

SUMMARY OF KEY CONCEPTS

- Heart failure develops when the heart becomes an inefficient pump. This can happen when other conditions weaken or diminish its contractile force and alter the ejected volume of blood.
- When the heart fails, ventricular output falls and circulatory pathways become overloaded with fluid. Left-sided failure produces respiratory effects, whereas right-sided heart failure causes systemic effects.
- Left-sided heart failure is characterized by exertional dyspnea, a cough that may produce blood-streaked sputum, moist lung sounds, and reduced urine output. ABG analysis indicates impaired gas exchange.
- Treatment of left-sided heart failure is directed at reducing the workload of the heart and improving ventricular output. This is achieved primarily with drugs that reduce preload (the volume of venous blood entering the heart); use of cardiotonics to strengthen ventricular contraction; and drugs that reduce afterload (peripheral vascular resistance), such as vasodilators.
- Left ventricular function may be supported with the use of invasive devices such as an IABP, blood pump, or VAD.
- Individuals in right-sided heart failure manifest signs of peripheral fluid retention such as dependent edema, neck vein distention, hepatomegaly, ascites, and dyspnea due to crowding of the diaphragm with abdominal fluid and tissue. Right-sided failure is treated similarly to left-sided heart failure.
- The nursing management of the client with heart failure includes measures to increase cardiac output, improve tissue perfusion, improve gas exchange, achieve fluid balance, and increase activity tolerance.
- The nursing management of the client with pulmonary edema includes administering medications and oxygen, monitoring vital signs, monitoring for complications, and assisting with communication.
- Pulmonary edema is a complication of left-sided heart failure in which the lungs fill rapidly with fluid. Ventilation is extremely impaired because gases cannot diffuse through the fluid medium. The client hyperventilates to compensate, but as carbon dioxide is retained, respiratory acidosis and metabolic acidosis develop. Death is inevitable if the condition is not reversed.
- A person with pulmonary edema experiences sudden dyspnea with moist, gurgling respirations. The client is apprehensive due to the feeling of suffocation. ABG analysis indicates severe hypoxemia and hypercapnia. Potent diuretics and inotropic agents are administered IV. The client may require endotracheal intubation and mechanical ventilation.

CRITICAL THINKING EXERCISES

1. Discuss how the care of a client with right-sided heart failure differs from the care of a client with left-sided heart failure.
2. Describe assessment findings characteristic of right-sided and left-sided heart failure.
3. A client diagnosed with heart failure presents with the following assessment data:

    T 99.1, P 100, R 42, and BP 110/50
    Crackles in both bases of lungs
    Complaints of nausea
    Pulse oximeter reading of 89%
    Enlarged, soft abdomen

Which assessment findings need immediate attention? Why?

Suggested Readings

Bove L. (1995). Now! Surgery for heart failure. *RN, 58*(5), 26–30.

Carpenito, L. J. (1997). *Nursing diagnosis: Application to clinical practice.* Philadelphia: Lippincott-Raven.

Dracup, K., Dunbar, S., & Baker, D. (1995). Rethinking heart failure. *American Journal of Nursing, 95*(7), 22–27.

Ellis, J., Nowlis, E., & Bentz, P. (1996). *Modules for basic nursing skills* (6th ed., vol. 1) Philadelphia: Lippincott-Raven.

Janowski, M. (1996). Managing heart failure. *RN, 59*(2), 34–38.

Karch, A. M. (1998). *Lippincott's nursing drug guide.* Philadelphia: Lippincott-Raven.

Lee, M. (1996). Drugs and the elderly: Do you know the risks?. *American Journal of Nursing, 96*(7), 24–31.

O'Donnell, L. (1996). Complications of MI: Beyond the acute stage. *American Journal of Nursing, 96*(9), 24–30.

Orden Wallace, C. (1998). Emergency: Acute pulmonary edema. *RN, 61*(1), 36–40.

Redeker, N., & Sadowski, A. (1995). Update on cardiovascular drugs and elders. *American Journal of Nursing, 95*(9), 34–40.

Yacone-Morton, L. (1995). First-line therapy for CHF. *RN, 58*(2), 38–43.

Additional Resources

Heartbytes
http://www.geocities.com/Heartland/Hills/2571/heartbytes.htm#chf

Chapter 36

Caring for Clients Undergoing Cardiovascular Surgery

KEY TERMS

Annuloplasty
Cardiopulmonary bypass
Commissurotomy
Coronary artery bypass graft
Embolectomy
Endarterectomy
Extracorporeal circulation
Thrombectomy
Valvuloplasty

LEARNING OBJECTIVES

On completion of this chapter, the reader will:

- Identify the purpose of cardiopulmonary bypass.
- Name five indications for cardiac surgery.
- Identify three techniques to correct valvular disorders.
- Describe how coronary artery blood flow is surgically restored.
- Describe two methods for controlling bleeding from heart trauma.
- List five problems associated with heart transplantation.
- Discuss the preoperative preparation of a client undergoing cardiovascular surgery.
- Discuss the nursing management of clients undergoing cardiac surgery.
- List three types of surgery performed on central or peripheral blood vessels.
- Discuss the nursing management of clients undergoing vascular surgery.

Few attempts at cardiac surgery were made until the 1950s. Initially, hypothermia and crude mechanisms for oxygenating blood outside the body were used. In the 1960s, the technique for mechanically circulating and oxygenating blood outside the body, called **extracorporeal circulation** or **cardiopulmonary bypass** (Fig. 36–1), was developed. Removing blood from the venae cavae, circulating it through an oxygenator, and returning it to the aorta or femoral artery now provides a nearly bloodless area during heart surgery.

Cardiac Surgical Procedures

Valvular Repairs

Heart valves need surgical repair or replacement if they become narrowed (stenosed) or stretched (incompetent) (see Chap. 31). One method of repair is **commissurotomy** (opening adhesions in the valve cusps), which is done without direct visualization of the valve. This procedure is performed by means of a thoracotomy. A purse-string suture is placed in the wall of the heart, an incision is made, and the surgeon's finger or a metal dilator is inserted into the narrowed valve, stretching its opening. The purse-string suture is then pulled tight to prevent the escape of blood. Cardiopulmonary bypass is not required but is usually kept available for immediate use if complications occur or if direct visualization is required to repair the valve. **Valvuloplasty** (valve repair) and **annuloplasty** (repair of the fibrous ring that encircles the valve) tighten an incompetent valve. The diseased valve also can be excised and replaced with a prosthetic ball and cage, pivoting disk, or biologic valve from an animal or a human cadaver (Fig. 36–2).

Myocardial Revascularization

A **coronary artery bypass graft** (CABG) procedure increases the supply of blood to the myocardium by bypassing the occluded portion of the vessel with a

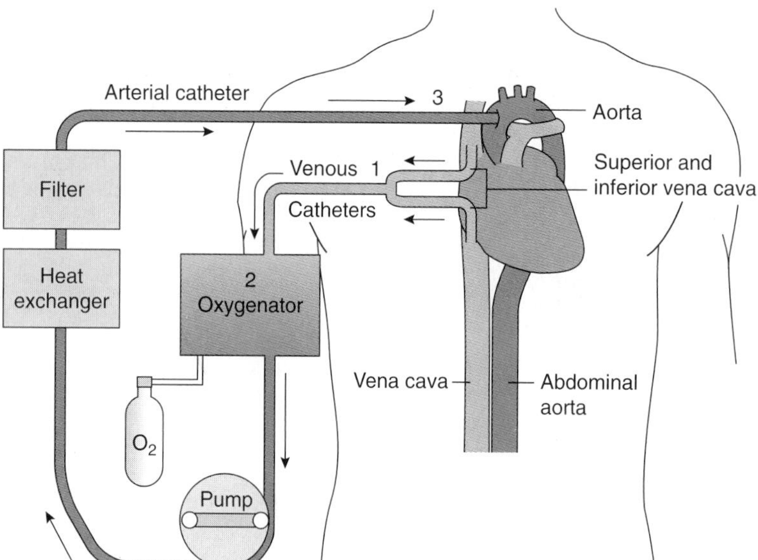

FIGURE 36-1. During cardiopulmonary bypass, venous blood is drained from the vena cavae and oxygenated externally before being pumped into arterial circulation.

donor vessel. The donor vessel is obtained from either the saphenous vein in the leg or from the internal mammary artery. When using a section of saphenous vein, one end is grafted within the aorta and the other is sutured below the blockage in a coronary artery (Fig. 36–3). If the internal mammary artery is used, the proximal end is either left in place or removed from its site of origin. One or more bypasses are done at the same time. There seems to be a longer period during which cardiac symptoms are relieved after CABG surgery as opposed to alternative methods, such as percutaneous transluminal coronary angioplasty (PTCA) for treating coronary artery disease (see Chap. 32).

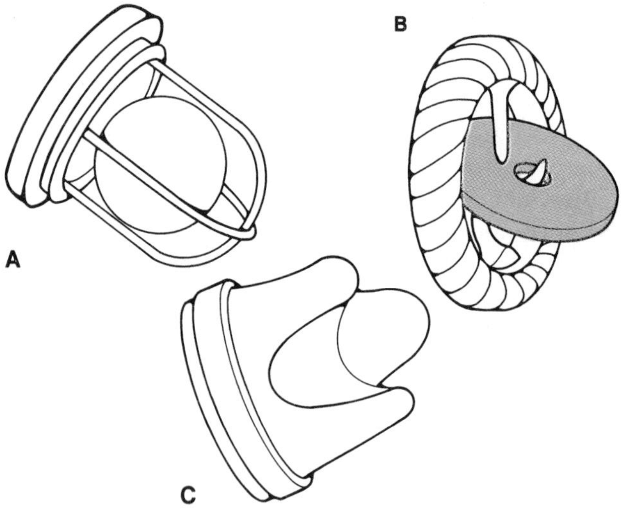

Repair of Ventricular Aneurysm

An aneurysm of the ventricular wall develops when an infarcted area of myocardium balloons outward.

FIGURE 36-2. Common mechanical and biologic valve replacements. (*A*) Caged ball valve (Starr-Edwards/mechanical). (*B*) Tilting-disk valve (Medtronic-Hall/mechanical). (C) Porcine heterograft valve (Carpenter-Edwards/ biologic).

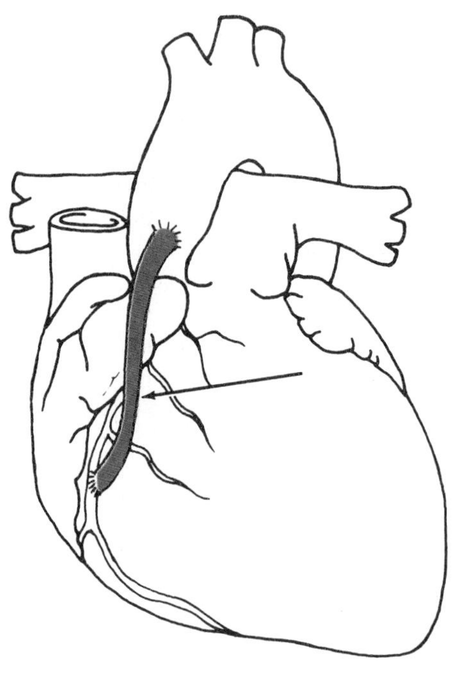

FIGURE 36-3. Section of saphenous vein is used to bypass a narrowed section of a coronary artery.

Thrombi commonly form within the crater of the bulging tissue. A ventricular aneurysm is the most lethal complication among clients who survive the acute stage of a myocardial infarction. Because the motion of the myocardium may rupture the aneurysm, an emergency procedure may be performed to suture the weakened area. If it is possible to wait, the stretched tissue is excised 4 to 8 weeks after the myocardial infarction when scar tissue has formed. If surgery is performed too early, it is difficult to differentiate healthy from necrotic tissue, and sutures placed in necrotic tissue are usually not retained.

Removal of Heart Tumors

Primary tumors of the heart, both benign and malignant, are rare. The clinical course and operative procedure depend on the type of tumor and its location within the heart. Benign tumors typically extend from a pedicle or stem, making their removal uncomplicated. Malignant tumors are more difficult to remove, and the prognosis is extremely poor.

Repair of Heart Trauma

A nonpenetrating injury of the chest, such as being crushed against a steering wheel, may cause bruising and bleeding of the heart. Because the heart is enclosed by the pericardium, blood accumulates in the pericardial space, resulting in cardiac tamponade. Sometimes traumatic cardiac tamponade is treated conservatively with bed rest. The inactivity and increased pressure from blood within the pericardium may stop the bleeding. More often than not, the client will need to have the blood aspirated from the pericardial sac, in which case pericardiocentesis is performed (see Chap. 30). One aspiration is sufficient in most cases, but if bleeding continues, open thoracotomy is indicated to control blood loss.

A penetrating injury, such as a stab wound, also causes leakage of blood into the pericardium. A tear in the pericardium often seals with a clot, whereas a tear in the myocardium continues to bleed. Large tears necessitate surgery. If the wound is severe enough to cause immediate shock from hemorrhage, the prognosis is poor.

Heart Transplantation

Heart transplantation is indicated for cardiomyopathy (severe weakness of cardiac muscle) and end-stage coronary artery disease. It is performed only when other treatment modalities fail. Many factors are considered when selecting transplant recipients. Criteria include the general condition of the client's other vital organs, the client's age and emotional outlook, the presence of other chronic diseases, and the availability of support systems. Once a client is accepted as a candidate for transplantation, his or her name and tissue type are placed on a computerized recipient list. Tissue typing is necessary to match the recipient with a donor. According to the United Network of Organ Sharing (UNOS), a patient who is on mechanical life support in an intensive care unit is given first priority when a donor organ becomes available. Many problems are associated with heart transplantation including the scarcity of donor organs, tissue rejection, postoperative infection, postoperative psychosis, and cost.

When a donor heart becomes available, it must be removed from the donor and transplanted within 6 hours of being harvested. The ventricles and anterior portions of the recipient's right and left atria are removed and their counterparts from the donor heart are sutured in place (Fig. 36–4). Recipients are given immunosuppressive drugs such as cyclosporine (Sandimmune) to prevent organ rejection. The client is closely observed for signs of organ rejection (eg, elevated white blood cell count, electrocardiographic [ECG] changes, fever), and is placed in protective isolation because an infection can be life-threatening.

Care of the Client

PREPARATION FOR SURGERY

The client having cardiac surgery requires an extensive preoperative medical evaluation. Cardiopul-

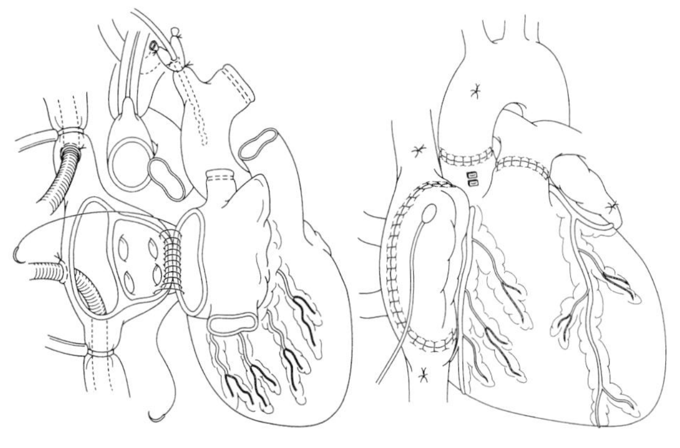

FIGURE 36-4. The donor heart is attached to the posterior walls of the transplant recipient's left and right atria.

monary evaluation includes chest radiography, ECG, exercise ECG (stress test), pulmonary function studies, echocardiography, laboratory blood tests, and coronary arteriography. Most of these studies are performed on an outpatient basis. Cardiac medications may be discontinued 1 or 2 days before surgery. To prevent perioperative complications, an anticoagulant and antibiotic may be prescribed. An anesthesiologist or anesthetist evaluates the client preoperatively and explains the type of anesthesia that will be used. The physician explains the risks and benefits of the procedure and obtains the client's informed consent. The client is sedated the night before and the morning of surgery. Invasive monitoring devices, such as a pulmonary artery catheter and an arterial line, are inserted before surgery.

NURSING MANAGEMENT

Preoperative Care

Obtain the client's medical and surgical history and perform a physical examination (see Chap. 29). The focus of nursing care in the preoperative period is client and family education and includes, but is not limited to, the following:

Nursing Diagnoses and Collaborative Problems	Nursing Interventions
Knowledge Deficit related to unfamiliarity with diagnostic tests, preoperative preparations, and postoperative care	Assess client and family's knowledge concerning procedures.
Goal: The client and family will understand the purpose, preparation, and after-care of tests and surgery.	Provide both verbal and written information concerning the surgical procedure and after-care, using language that the client can understand.
	Ask the client or family member to explain surgery before signing consent form.
	Explain coughing, deep breathing, and leg exercises. Teach the use of an incentive spirometer, splinting the incision to cough.
	Promote a relaxed environment conducive to asking questions.
Anxiety related to fear of surgery	Assess anxiety level using open-ended questions to promote response.
Goal: Client will develop realistic expectations concerning surgery.	Clarify misconceptions concerning surgery.
	Acknowledge emotions and expressions of fear.
	Provide thorough explanations.
	Demonstrate competence when performing skills.

Postoperative Care

Many clients after open-heart surgery are brought directly from the operating room to the intensive care unit by the anesthetist and other members of the operating team. The anesthetist provides the nurse with a comprehensive report and remains until the client is attached to all invasive monitoring devices and stabilized. The nurse thoroughly and systematically assesses the client to provide baseline data. A major nursing responsibility at this time is monitoring the client for signs and symptoms of potential complications, such as hemorrhage and shock, thrombus or embolus formation, cerebral anoxia, cardiac arrhythmias, fluid overload, electrolyte imbalance, respiratory failure, and cardiac tamponade.

Most clients require mechanical ventilation for several hours after cardiac surgery. Compare the ventilator settings with the parameters set by the physician for the percentage of oxygen, rate of machine ventilations, tidal volume, and amount of positive pressure. Inspect the endotracheal tube to make sure it is properly secured and the balloon, which correlates with the internal cuff, is inflated. When the endotracheal tube is properly in place, the client is unable to speak and lung sounds are heard bilaterally. Continue close observation of the client's respiratory status after weaning from the ventilator. Monitor oxygenation by pulse oximetry or arterial blood gas analysis.

Monitor the ECG for disturbances in heart rate and rhythm. Document rhythm each shift or if an arrhythmia occurs. Observe all surgical dressings and drains for bleeding. Inspect chest tubes frequently, making sure that they are not compressed and that the drainage is flowing freely. Hourly observation of the amount of chest tube drainage is required; notify the physician if it exceeds 100 mL/h or is bright red. A Swan-Ganz (pulmonary artery) catheter is used to assess cardiac output, measure pulmonary artery pressure, pulmonary capillary wedge pressure, and central venous pressure. The client's arterial blood pressure is monitored directly and continuously; the arterial line also serves as a direct means for obtaining arterial blood samples for blood gas analyses. Assess the presence and quality of peripheral pulses, skin color, and capillary refill to evaluate circulation. Report laboratory results of partial thromboplastin time, serum electrolytes, complete blood count, hemoglobin, and arterial blood gas analysis as they become available.

Assess the client's fluid status frequently during the immediate postoperative period. Record fluid intake and output hourly. Measure urine specific gravity to determine the client's hydration and how well the kidneys are concentrating urine. Urine output may be initially increased if the client was given osmotic diuretics during cardiopulmonary bypass. This situation corrects itself in a few hours. The client also may have hemoglobinuria (hemoglobin in the urine) because lysis of blood cells can occur during prolonged cardiopulmonary bypass.

Note the client's level of consciousness, neurologic status, and ability to move. Restlessness in an unconscious client can indicate hypoxia or pain. Speak to the client as you perform care, even if he or she still appears sedated. Provide as restful an atmosphere as possible. Support the family and keep them informed of the client's progress.

NURSING PROCESS
The Client Recovering From Cardiac Surgery

Assessment

Assess hemodynamic, respiratory and neurologic criteria as described above as frequently as necessary depending on client's condition and facility policy.

Diagnosis and Planning

Many nursing diagnoses are potentially applicable to the cardiac surgery client (Box 36–1). Common nursing diagnoses and care of the client in the postoperative period include, but are not limited to, the following:

Nursing Diagnoses and Collaborative Problems	Nursing Interventions
Risk for Ineffective Airway Clearance related to ineffective cough and accumulation of secretions within airway **Goal:** Client will have a patent airway as evidenced by noiseless respirations and clear lung sounds	Assess lung sounds every 4 hours or as often as indicated by client condition. Keep airway free of mucus; suction when respirations are noisy. Administer humidified oxygen. Encourage client to cough and expectorate secretions once extubated. Prevent strain on chest incision by teaching client to splint when coughing.
Risk for Impaired Gas Exchange related to retained secretions, hypoventilation secondary to pain, displacement of chest tubes **Goal:** Client maintains adequate gas exchange as evidenced by ABGs within normal limits, no dyspnea or tachycardia.	Assess the following as often as necessary: Lung sounds, heart rate, level of consciousness Pulse oximetry Arterial blood gas results Administer oxygen as prescribed. Elevate head of bed as much as possible. Hyperoxygenate with 100% oxygen prior to suctioning; do not suction for more than 10 to 15 seconds. Promote rest and decrease anxiety. Notify physician if oxygen saturation falls below 90%.
Risk for Decreased Cardiac Output related to impaired ventricular contraction **Goal:** The client will maintain an adequate cardiac output as evidenced by stable vital signs, alert, adequate urine output, and no arrhythmias, chest pain, dyspnea, confusion, or dizziness. Cardiac output readings are within normal limits.	Assess the following on a regular basis, as often as necessary: Vital signs Heart and lung sounds Intake and output Pulse rhythm and quality Effort of breathing Mental status Presence of edema Promote rest, administer prescribed sedatives. Administer medications as prescribed. Assess incisions for redness, warmth, swelling, or purulent drainage.
Risk for Infection related to impaired skin integrity **Goal:** The client will remain free of infection.	Practice conscientious handwashing. Change dressings that are moist or loose. Use aseptic technique when changing dressings, intravenous tubing, bags, or other equipment. Administer prophylactic antibiotic therapy at prescribed time to maintain therapeutic blood levels. Implement infection control precautions for the client who is immunosuppressed.

Evaluation and Expected Outcomes

- The airway is clear, oxygenation is adequate, pulse oximetry is 90% or higher.
- Cardiac output measurements are within normal limits.
- The client shows no signs or symptoms of infection.

Client and Family Teaching

Discharge may be as early as 5 days after surgery. The client and family may have concerns about the medical regimen required after discharge. Depending on such factors as the type of surgery performed, client's degree of recovery, and treatment regimen prescribed by the physician, include information concerning:

- Medication and dietary instructions
- Wound care instructions
- Importance of follow-up care, periodic evaluation of progress, lifelong adherence to certain treatment regimens

BOX 36-1 Possible Nursing Diagnosis for Clients Following Cardiac Surgery

Activity Intolerance
Altered Family Processes
Anxiety
Constipation
Fluid Volume Deficit
Fluid Volume Excess
Hypothermia
Impaired Verbal Communication
Risk for Perioperative Positioning Injury
Risk for Peripheral Neurovascular Dysfunction
Risk for Impaired Skin Integrity
Self-Care Deficit
Sleep Pattern Disturbance

- Purpose of a structured cardiac rehabilitation program (when prescribed and available)
- Monitoring of pulse rate, blood pressure, weight
- Activity progression and exercise
- Stress reduction

Central or Peripheral Vascular Surgical Procedures

Vascular Grafts

Just as grafts are used to bypass a diseased section of a coronary blood vessel, vascular grafts are used to bypass or replace diseased sections of major systemic blood vessels such as the aorta or femoral arteries. The replacement graft may be made of synthetic fiber, such as Dacron or Teflon, or may be human tissue harvested from cadavers. A clamp is placed above and below the affected area and the diseased blood vessel is removed. The replacement graft is then sewn in place, and the clamps are removed (Fig. 36–5). Depending on the area involved, cardiopulmonary bypass may be necessary.

Embolectomy and Thrombectomy

When a major vessel is occluded by thrombi or emboli, a **thrombectomy** (removal of a thrombus) or **embolectomy** (removal of an embolus) is performed. The vessel is opened above the clot, the clot is removed, and the vessel is sutured closed. This type of surgery may be an emergency because complete occlusion results in loss of blood supply to an area.

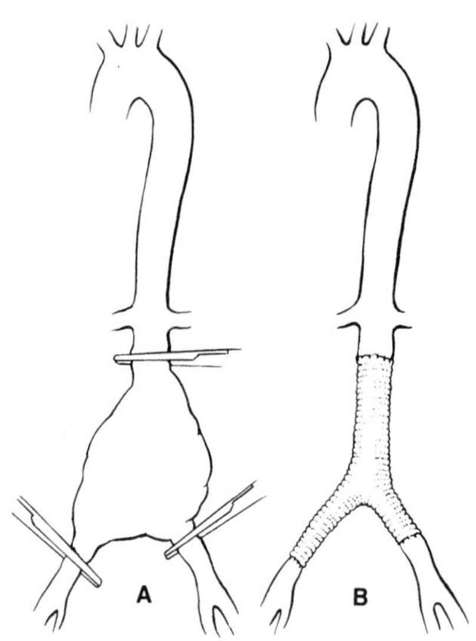

FIGURE 36-5. (*A*) Aneurysm clamped off before removal (*B*) Replacement with a graft.

Endarterectomy

Endarterectomy is the resection and removal of the lining of an artery (see Chap. 45). This type of surgery is performed to remove obstructive atherosclerotic plaques from the carotid, femoral, or popliteal arteries.

Care of the Client

NURSING MANAGEMENT

Preoperative Care

When the client requires emergency surgery, identify the most pertinent data, current signs and symptoms, allergies, and medications. Determine when the client last consumed food or fluids.

If the client is stable and nonemergency surgery is scheduled, obtain a medical and surgical history (see Chap. 29). Evaluate the characteristics of the client's pain or discomfort (ie, location, type, intensity, duration). Palpate the peripheral pulses and mark them with a skin pen. Analyze the level of the client's and family's understanding of the perioperative plan of care. Assess the client's level of anxiety.

Postoperative Care

Monitor the client postoperatively to determine recovery from anesthesia and detect developing complications. The general care of clients in the postoperative period is found in Chapter 24. It is important after vascular surgery to monitor circulation. Palpate the peripheral pulses or use a Doppler device if the pulses are not palpable. Report signs and symptoms of inadequate tissue perfusion, such as a weak pulse, cold or cyanotic extremity, or mottling of the skin, to the physician immediately.

Blood pressure and pulse rate are normally evaluated in both arms after thoracic surgery. A decrease in blood pressure, an increase in the intensity of abdominal or chest pain, narrowing of the pulse pressure, or a rise in pulse rate may indicate internal hemorrhage at the graft site. Decreased urine output may indicate occlusion of the renal artery.

If the client has had a carotid endarterectomy, perform a neurologic assessment every 30 minutes, including evaluation of level of consciousness, size of pupils and their reaction to light, movement in both arms and legs, verbal response, and thought processes. The nursing care of the client in the postoperative period after central or peripheral vascular surgery includes, but is not limited to, the following:

Nursing Diagnoses and Collaborative Problems	Nursing Interventions
PC: Hemorrhage and **decreased cardiac output** related to external loss of blood from surgical procedures and internal deficits related to third-spacing of tissue fluid. **Goal:** Client will maintain adequate blood and tissue volumes as evidenced by adequate urine output, normal vital signs, and hemodynamic pressures within normal limits.	Assess for the following as often as necessary: Drainage from chest tubes Vital signs—initially every 15 minutes until stable Hourly intake and output Chest pain or discomfort Peripheral pulses every 30 minutes for the first 24 hours after surgery, then every 1 to 2 hours Monitor level of consciousness. Monitor dressing and chest drains for signs of fresh or excessive bleeding. Assess skin color and temperature. Monitor hemodynamic parameters every 4 hours or as often as ordered.
Risk for Impaired Tissue Perfusion related to tissue swelling and impaired blood flow **Goal:** Client will maintain peripheral pulses in operative extremity; no dependent edema; capillary refill times less than 3 seconds. Operative extremity is warm, with appropriate color, and Homan's sign is negative.	Assess the following as often as necessary: Pulses Capillary refill times Edema Position extremity above level of heart. Avoid pressure on extremity. Avoid flexing the knee or placing pillows under the knee unless specifically ordered (impairs blood flow and causes thrombosis). Apply antiembolic stockings or automatic venous compression device.
Risk for Paralytic Ileus related to intestinal handling during surgery, effects of narcotics and other medications **Goal:** The client will be free of paralytic ileus as evidenced by active bowel sounds, bowel movements, no abdominal distention.	Assess for the following as often as necessary: Bowel sounds Abdominal distention Patency of nasogastric tube if present Ask client to report passing flatus. Promote activity or reposition the client in bed as often as indicated by the client's condition. Encourage fluid intake if not contraindicated by client's condition. Administer stool softeners or cathartics as prescribed.

Client and Family Teaching

Assess the ability of the client and family to participate in teaching and care during the postoperative period. Develop a teaching plan and include the following:

- Provide instructions about the dosage regimen of anticoagulant therapy and the importance of immediately reporting bleeding episodes to the physician.
- Emphasize the importance of wearing support stockings.
- Inform the client who has had a vascular graft taken from a leg to protect that leg from tissue damage (eg, avoiding injury and prolonged exposure to cold).
- Involve the dietitian if the client must reduce elevated serum cholesterol levels.
- Stress the importance of follow-up care and adherence to the medical treatment prescribed by the physician.

Once teaching has been provided, assess the client's retention and comprehension of discharge instructions.

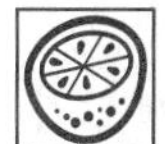

General Nutritional Considerations

Clients with atherosclerosis and elevated serum cholesterol and triglyceride levels should follow a low-fat, low saturated-fat, or low-cholesterol diet (see General Nutritional Considerations in Chap. 31); additional diet modifications may be necessary to control other risk factors, such as hypertension, diabetes, and obesity.

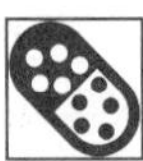

General Pharmacologic Considerations

Narcotic analgesics may be used preoperatively to lessen anxiety and sedate the client. Clients who are relaxed and sedated when anesthesia is given require a smaller dose of anesthetic.

If the client is taking digitalis to improve myocardial contractility, the drug may be discontinued before surgery to decrease the risk of digitalis-induced arrhythmias.

Anticoagulant drugs may be discontinued several days before cardiac surgery to allow the body to re-establish normal clotting patterns.

Many types of drugs may be administered before and after cardiac or blood vessel surgery (eg, antibiotics, anticoagulants, vasopressors, diuretics, electrolytes, cardiotonics). The nurse reviews the dose, route of administration, and adverse effects of each drug given because many of these drugs have narrow margins of safety.

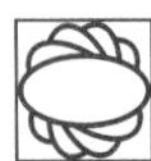

General Gerontologic Considerations

Narcotics must be given with caution in older adults because the respiratory system of the older adult is more sensitive to the depressant effect of narcotic analgesics.

Anticholinergic drugs such as atropine and scopolamine are used cautiously (if at all) in older adults because they are at greater risk for adverse reactions.

The older adult is prone to postoperative confusion. This confusion may manifest as disorientation, paranoia, aggression, or visual hallucinations.

Many older adults are poor surgical risks and have other concurrent medical problems, such as diabetes, heart failure, cardiac arrhythmias, hypertension, and poor renal function. These clients require close observation during the postoperative period.

SUMMARY OF KEY CONCEPTS

- Before nonemergency surgery, the client is evaluated medically with diagnostic tests. Previous cardiac medications are discontinued and replaced with drugs that will reduce potential surgical complications. The surgeon provides the client with information necessary for informed consent. Invasive monitoring devices are inserted. A member of the anesthesia team evaluates the client and directs the client's preparation according to the type of anesthetic that will be used.
- Many surgical procedures are done using cardiopulmonary bypass, which removes venous blood, oxygenates it, and returns it to the aorta so the surgeon can operate in a bloodless area.
- Clients for whom cardiopulmonary bypass is used are at risk for thrombus and embolus formation, fluid and electrolyte imbalance, tissue anoxia, pulmonary complications, and blood-borne infections.
- Cardiac surgery is done to repair damaged valves, improve coronary artery blood flow, repair ventricular aneurysms, remove tumors from the heart, repair penetrating and nonpenetrating chest injuries, and replace the heart with a transplanted organ.
- Valvular disorders are corrected by performing a commissurotomy, reconstructing valves, or replacing damaged valves with a prosthetic or biologic substitute.
- Impaired blood flow to the myocardium can be restored by grafting a vein or artery from an area of adequate blood flow to a location below the stenotic coronary artery.
- A ventricular aneurysm is repaired by excising the thin, bulging area in the wall of the heart.
- The technique used to remove a tumor from the heart depends mostly on the tumor's location and type. Benign tumors are more easily removed and, statistically, have a better prognosis than malignant tumors.
- Thoracotomy may be done to repair heart trauma and control hemorrhage. Sometimes bleeding is controlled by pressure from blood accumulating within the pericardium. If cardiac tamponade develops, a pericardiocentesis may be necessary.
- When heart transplantation is performed, the ventricles and anterior portions of the recipient's right and left atria are removed, and their counterparts from the donor heart are sutured in place.
- Nursing problems of clients undergoing cardiac and vascular surgery include high risk for ineffective airway clearance, potential for impaired gas exchange, alteration in tissue perfusion, and pain and anxiety related to surgical procedures.
- A candidate for heart transplantation faces the odds of not finding or matching a donor organ, organ rejection, infection, postoperative psychosis, and tremendous costs.
- Vascular surgery may be done to replace a diseased vessel with a synthetic device or cadaveric tissue, remove a thrombus or embolus from within a blood vessel, and resect or remove the lining of a vessel.
- Nursing management of the client undergoing vascular surgery includes assessment for hemorrhage, impaired tissue perfusion, and paralytic ileus.

CRITICAL THINKING EXERCISES

1. While caring for a client who is recovering from CABG surgery, the following data are gathered: The client has leg pain, which he rates as 8 on a scale of 1 to 10; his respiratory rate is 30 breaths per minute at rest; there is dried blood on the thoracic dressing; the client's throat is sore after being weaned from mechanical ventilation; and he is concerned because he has not had a bowel movement in 3 days. Which assessment finding should be the major concern for the nurse at this time?

2. The client with a thoracotomy incision has a weak cough, shallow respirations, and diminished breath sounds. What interventions would you perform?

Suggested Readings

Bernat, J. J. (1997). Smoothing the CABG patient's road to recovery. *American Journal of Nursing 97*(2), Continuing Care Extra Education, 22–27.

Bezanson, J. (1997). Respiratory care of older adults after cardiac surgery. *Journal of Cardiovascular Nursing, 12*(1), 71–83.

Bruni, K. R., Hoffman, G. T., & Hoosier-Paty, D. M. (1996). The quality of life of the limb-threatened patient after lower-extremity revascularization. *Journal of Vascular Nursing, 14*(4), 99–103.

Dziadulewicz, L., & Shannon-Stonem M. (1995). Postpericardiotomy syndrome: A complication of cardiac surgery. *AACN Clinical Issues, 6*(3), 464–470.

Edwards, R., Turnbull, N., & Abullarade, C. (1996). Nursing management and follow-up of the postoperative vascular patient in a clinic setting. *Journal of Vascular Nursing, 14*(3), 62–67.

Eillis, M. F. (1997). Low cardiac output following cardiac surgery: Critical thinking steps. *Dimensions of Critical Care Nursing, 16*(1), 48–55.

Henderson, L. J., & Kirkland, J. S. (1995). Angioplasty with stent placement in peripheral arterial occlusive disease. *AORN Journal, 61*(4), 671–677, 679, 682–685.

Lacey, K. O., Gusberg, R. J., Krumholz, H. M., & Meier, G. H. (1995). Outcomes after major vascular surgery: The patients' perspective. *Journal of Vascular Nursing, 13*(1), 8–13.

Lindsay, P., Morin, J., Harkness, C., Doucette, P., Bickerton, L., & Sherrard, H. (1997). Educational and support needs of patients and their families awaiting cardiac surgery. *Heart Lung, 26*(6), 458–465.

Maxwell, L. E. (1996). Acute pain management: Evaluation of the effectiveness of intravenous patient-controlled analgesia with vascular patients. *Canadian Journal of Cardiovascular Nursing, 7*(1), 10–14.

Moore, S. M. (1997). Effects of interventions to promote recovery in coronary artery bypass surgical patients. *Journal of Cardiovascular Nursing, 12*(1), 59–70.

Nelson, S. (1996). Pre-admission education for patients undergoing cardiac surgery. *British Journal of Nursing, 5*(6), 335–340.

Possanza, C. (1996). What you should know about coronary artery bypass graft surgery. *Nursing, 26*(2), 48–50.

Rossi, M. S. (1995). The octogenarian cardiac surgery patient. *Journal of Cardiovascular Nursing, 9*(4), 75–95.

Wikblad, K., & Anderson, B. (1995). A comparison of three wound dressings in patients undergoing heart surgery. *Nursing Research, 44*(5), 312–316.

Additional Resources

NYU Health System
Division of Cardiothoracic Surgery
http://cvsurg.med.nyu.edu

Aneurysm and AVM Support Page
http://www.westga.edu

8

Caring for Clients With Hematopoietic and Lymphatic Disorders

Chapter 37

Introduction to the Hematopoietic and Lymphatic Systems

KEY TERMS

Agranulocytes
Bone marrow
Erythrocytes
Erythropoiesis
Erythropoietin
Granulocytes
Hematopoiesis
Hemoglobin
Leukocytes
Leukocytosis
Leukopenia
Lymph
Lymph nodes
Lymphatics
Lymphocytes
Monocytes
Phagocytosis
Plasma
Platelets
Stem cells

LEARNING OBJECTIVES

On completion of this chapter, the reader will:

- Explain hematopoiesis and name two structures involved in it.
- Name three types of blood cells produced by bone marrow and discuss the function of each.
- List at least five components of plasma.
- Name three plasma proteins and explain the function of each.
- Identify the four blood groups and discuss the importance of transfusing compatible types.
- Explain the function of the lymphatic system and its role in hematopoiesis.
- Discuss the pertinent assessments of the hematopoietic and lymphatic systems when obtaining a health history and conducting a physical examination.
- Name at least five laboratory and diagnostic tests conducted for disorders of the hematopoietic or lymphatic systems.
- Discuss the nursing management of clients with hematopoietic or lymphatic disorders.

Hematopoiesis is the manufacture and development of blood cells. The primary structure of the hematopoietic system is the bone marrow, where most blood cells are produced. However, the lymphatic system, which includes the thymus gland and the spleen, also plays a role in hematopoiesis.

Hematopoietic System

Anatomy and Physiology

Blood consists of cells suspended in a fluid called plasma (Fig. 37–1). Three types of blood cells are produced in the bone marrow; each type of blood cell has specialized functions.

BONE MARROW

Bone marrow is the substance in the interior of the long bones and spongy bones of the skeleton. There are two types of bone marrow: red marrow and yellow marrow. Red marrow is primarily found in the ribs, sternum, skull, clavicle, vertebrae, proximal ends of the long bones, and iliac crest; it manufactures blood cells and hemoglobin. Yellow marrow consists primarily of fat cells and connective tissue and does not participate in the manufacture of blood cells. The fat cells, however, can be replaced by hematopoietic cells under conditions involving intense stimulation.

ERYTHROCYTES

Erythrocytes (red blood cells) are flexible, anuclear (lack a nucleus), biconcave disks covered by a thin

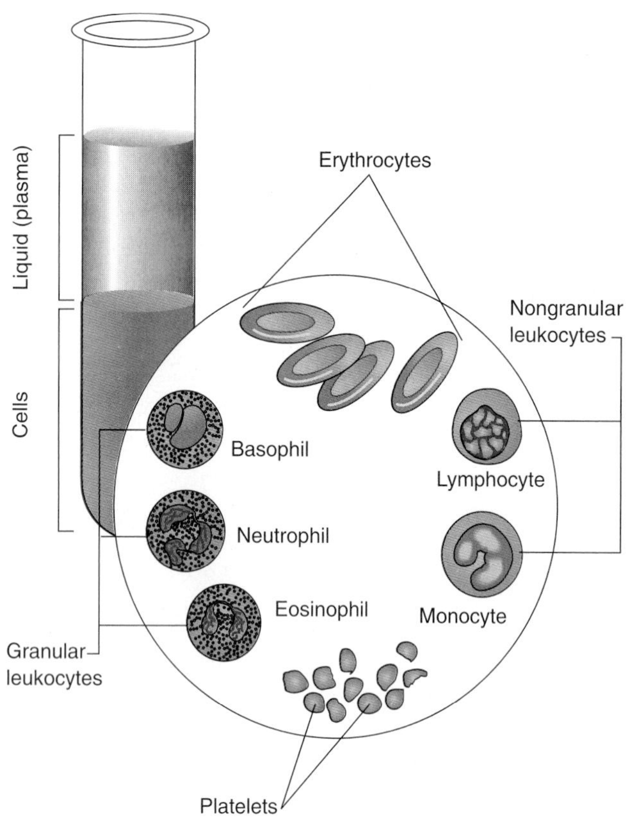

FIGURE 37-1. Liquid and cellular components of blood.

membrane that allows oxygen and carbon dioxide to pass freely through it. The flexibility of erythrocytes allows them to change shape as they travel through capillaries. Their major function is to transport oxygen to and remove carbon dioxide from the tissues.

The production of erythrocytes is called **erythropoiesis** the rate of production is regulated by a hormone released by the kidneys called **erythropoietin.** Erythrocytes arise from **stem cells** (undifferentiated cells) in the red bone marrow and go through several stages of maturation before they are released into the blood. In the early stage they contain a nucleus and are called *erythroblasts*. As the cell matures, it loses its nucleus and is released into the circulation.

The normal number of erythrocytes is between 3.6 and 5.4 million/µL. This number varies with age, sex, and altitude. Infants have more erythrocytes than adults, and women have fewer erythrocytes than men. People who live at high altitudes or engage in strenuous activity have an increased number of erythrocytes.

The red color of blood is caused by **hemoglobin,** an iron-containing pigment, attached to erythrocytes. The *heme* portion of the molecule freely binds with oxygen, forming a substance called oxyhemoglobin. Hemoglobin carries oxygen to the cells of the body. In adults, the normal amount of hemoglobin is 12 to 17.4 g/dl. As erythrocytes pass the lungs, the hemoglobin picks up oxygen and releases carbon dioxide. Oxygenated blood is bright red and is carried by arteries, arterioles, and capillaries to all body tissues. After oxygen has been released from the hemoglobin for use by the tissues, the hemoglobin is called *reduced* (or deoxygenated) *hemoglobin*. The blood becomes dark red and is returned by the veins to the heart and lungs, where carbon dioxide is released and the blood is reoxygenated. Erythrocytes circulate in the blood for about 120 days after which the spleen removes them; the liver removes severely damaged erythrocytes. When erythrocytes are destroyed, the iron component of hemoglobin is returned to the red marrow and reused. The residual pigment is stored in the liver as bilirubin and excreted in bile.

LEUKOCYTES

Leukocytes (white blood cells) are divided into two categories: **granulocytes,** which contain cytoplasmic granules, and **agranulocytes**, which do not contain cytoplasmic granules. Leukocytes protect the body from invading microorganisms and manufacture antibodies. The normal leukocyte count is between 5,000 and 10,000/mm^3. An increase above the normal number of leukocytes is called **leukocytosis;** a decrease is called **leukopenia**. The differential leukocyte count is shown in Table 37–1.

Granulocytes

Granulocytes, also called polymorphonuclear leukocytes, are divided into three subgroups: *neutrophils*, *basophils*, and *eosinophils*. Neutrophils are the number one defense against bacterial infection. They are also called microphages and are active in controlling pyogenic (pus-forming) infections by **phagocytosis** (the ingestion and digestion of bacteria and foreign substances). Immature neutrophils, called band cells, circulate in peripheral blood. Basophils are active in allergic contact dermatitis (immediate hypersensitivity) and some delayed hypersensitivity reactions. Eosinophils phagocytize foreign material. Their numbers increase in allergies, some dermatologic disorders, and parasitic infections.

Agranulocytes

Agranulocytes are divided into two groups: **lymphocytes** and **monocytes.** Lymphocytes are divided

TABLE 37-1 **Differential White Blood Cell Count**

	Percent of Total WBCs	Numeric Range (µL)
Neutrophils	60–70	3,000–7,000
Basophils	1–4	50–400
Eosinophils	0.5–1	25–100
Lymphocytes	20–40	1,000–4,000
Monocytes	2–6	100–600

into *B lymphocytes* (or B cells, immunoglobulins), which provide humoral immunity, and *T lymphocytes* (or T cells), which provide cellular immunity (or cell-mediated response). B lymphocytes produce antibodies against foreign antigens, and T lymphocytes interact with foreign cells and release a substance called *lymphokine*, which enhances the actions of phagocytic cells. Monocytes combat severe infections by phagocytosis and contribute to the immune response. Monocytes are antigen presentation cells. They phagocytize debris and stick to abnormal antigens and carry them to T lymphocytes. T lymphocytes engage B lymphocytes to make the appropriate antibody (see Chap. 40).

PLATELETS

Platelets (*thrombocytes*) are disklike, nonnucleated cells. They are round, flat, or oval. Platelets are manufactured in the red bone marrow and play a role in hemostasis. When a blood vessel is injured, platelets migrate to the injury site. A substance released from the platelets causes them to adhere and form a plug, or clot, that occludes the injured vessel. They have a short life span of about 7.5 days. The normal platelet count is 150,000 to 350,000/mm^3.

PLASMA

Plasma is the liquid, or serum, portion of blood. It consists of 90% water and 10% proteins. Besides blood cells, plasma contains and transports proteins (albumin, globulins, and fibrinogen), prothrombin, pigments, vitamins, carbohydrates, lipids, salts, electrolytes, minerals, enzymes, and hormones.

PLASMA PROTEINS

Albumin, which is formed in the liver, is the most abundant protein in plasma. Under normal conditions, albumin cannot pass through a capillary wall. Consequently, albumin helps maintain the osmotic pressure that retains fluid in the vascular compartment.

Globulins are divided into three groups: alpha, beta, and gamma. The gamma globulins are also called immunoglobulins. Globulins function primarily as immunologic agents; they prevent or modify some types of infectious diseases. Like albumin, they help maintain osmotic pressure in the vascular compartment.

Fibrinogen, the largest plasma protein, plays a key role in forming blood clots. It can be transformed from a liquid to fibrin, a solid that controls bleeding.

BLOOD GROUPS

There are four blood groups or types: A, B, AB, and O. Blood type is determined by heredity. Each blood group has a protein on the red cell membranes. Group A has A antigen, group B has B antigen, group AB has A and B antigen, and group O has no antigen. Antibodies in an individual's plasma react with incompatible antigens: group A has anti-B antibodies; group B has anti-A antibodies; group AB has no antibodies; and, group O has anti-A and anti-B antibodies. People with type O blood are universal donors because they do not have *antigens* on the red cell membrane. People with type AB blood are universal recipients because they do not have *antibodies* in their plasma that will react with types A, B, and O.

The Rh factor is a specific protein on the red cell membrane. If the protein is present, the person is Rh positive. If the protein is absent, the person is Rh negative.

When blood is transfused, donor blood must be compatible with the recipient's blood. The donor's blood is typed and labeled at the time of donation. When a blood transfusion is needed, the recipient's blood is typed and crossmatched (matched for compatibility with the donor blood). Donor and recipient blood are considered compatible if there is an absence of clumping or *hemolysis* (destruction of erythrocytes) when both samples are mixed in the laboratory. The recipient is given blood of the same type and the Rh factor. In an emergency, type O blood can be given to recipients with type A, B, AB, or O (see Chap. 23 and Table 23–3). People with Rh-positive blood can receive Rh-positive or Rh-negative blood because Rh negative indicates the Rh factor is missing; those with Rh-negative blood, however, must never receive Rh-positive blood regardless of whether the blood type is compatible. Various types of transfusion reactions are discussed in Chapter 23.

Lymphatic System

Anatomy and Physiology

The lymphatic system includes the thymus gland, spleen, and a network of lymphatic vessels, lymph nodes, and lymph. This system of **lymphatics** circulates interstitial fluid and carries it to the veins (Fig. 37–2). Along the pathway, the lymphatic system filters and destroys pathogens and removes other potentially harmful substances.

THYMUS GLAND

The thymus gland is lymphatic tissue in the upper chest that contains undifferentiated stem cells released from bone marrow. Once the undifferentiated cells migrate to the thymus gland, they develop into *T lymphocytes* because they are thymus derived (Fig. 37–3).

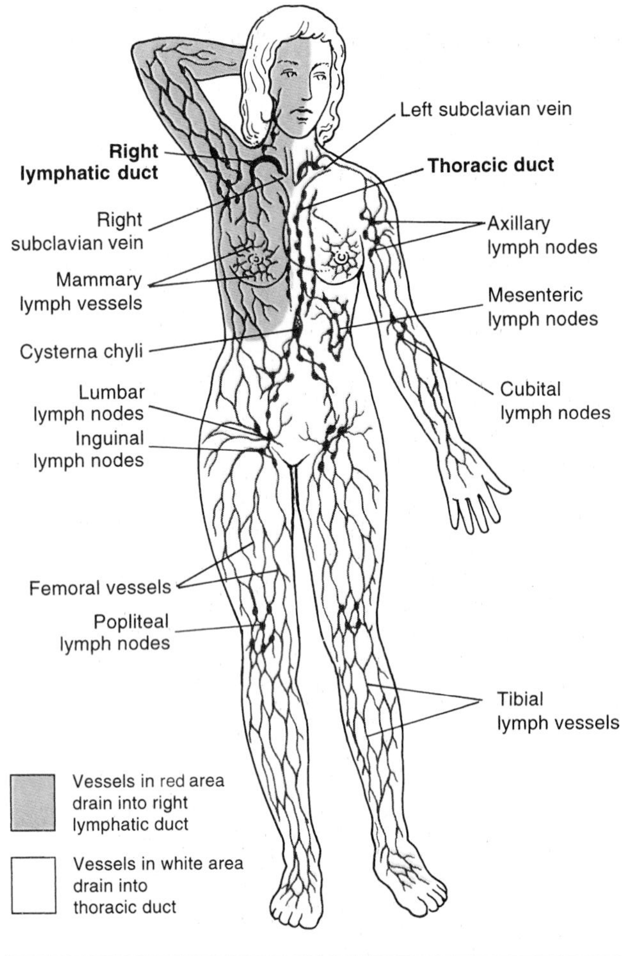

FIGURE 37-2. The lymphatic system.

SPLEEN

The spleen is the largest lymphatic structure. It lies in the abdomen beneath the diaphragm and behind the stomach. The spleen is a reservoir of blood and contains phagocytes that engulf damaged erythrocytes and foreign substances.

LYMPH NODES

Lymph nodes, glandular tissue along the lymphatic network, are clustered in the axilla, groin, and neck and the large vessels of the thorax and abdomen. The nodes are connected by lymphatic ducts through which lymph flows. The lymph nodes contain both T lymphocytes and B lymphocytes (released from the bone marrow but do not reach the thymus gland) within the smaller nodules of each lymph node.

LYMPH

Lymph is fluid that has a composition similar to plasma. It flows through lymphatics by contraction of skeletal muscles. Lymph enters each node by way of the afferent lymph duct, passes through the node, and leaves by the efferent lymph duct (Fig. 37–4). As lymph passes through the node, macrophages attack and engulf foreign substances like bacteria and viruses, abnormal body cells, and other debris.

Assessment

The nurse collects data by taking a health history, examining the client, and monitoring the results of laboratory tests.

Health History

The health history includes the client's description of signs and symptoms. If abnormalities are present, the nurse determines when the signs or symptoms began and their severity and frequency. In relation to the hematopoietic and lymphatic systems, it is especially important to establish if the client:

- Experiences prolonged bleeding from an obvious injury
- Has unexplained blood loss as in rectal bleeding, nosebleeds, bleeding gums, or vomiting blood
- Feels fatigued with normal activities
- Becomes dizzy or faints
- Bruises easily
- Is easily chilled
- Has frequent infections
- Feels discomfort in the axilla, groin, or neck
- Has difficulty swallowing with localized throat tenderness
- Has had surgery with lymph node removal or splenectomy, treatment for cancer, or has renal failure—all of which may affect blood cell volume or lymphatic circulation

The nurse takes a drug history of prescribed and nonprescribed medications. Some antibiotics and cancer drugs contribute to hematopoietic dysfunction. Aspirin and anticoagulants can interfere with clot formation. Because industrial materials, environmental toxins, and household products can also affect blood-forming organs, any exposure to these agents is explored. Foreign travel to countries where malaria or parasitic round worms are common is explored. A dietary history should be obtained because compromised nutrition interferes with the production of blood cells and hemoglobin.

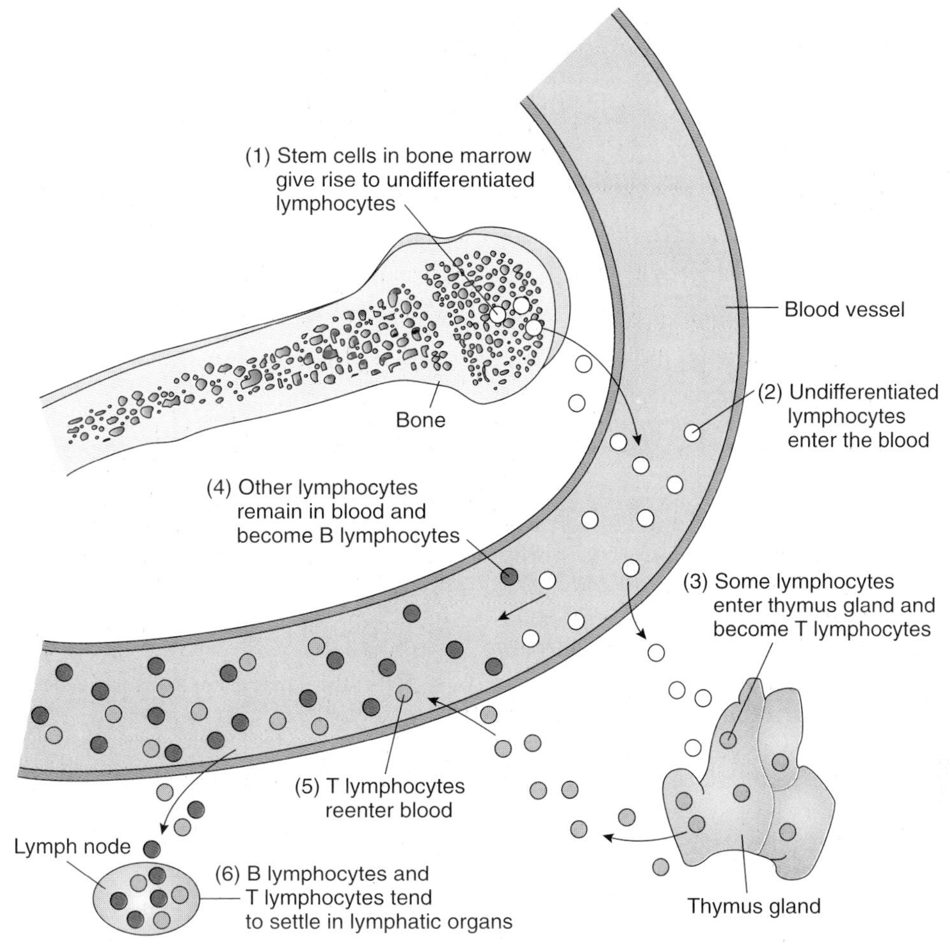
(1) Stem cells in bone marrow give rise to undifferentiated lymphocytes
Blood vessel
Bone
(2) Undifferentiated lymphocytes enter the blood
(4) Other lymphocytes remain in blood and become B lymphocytes
(3) Some lymphocytes enter thymus gland and become T lymphocytes
(5) T lymphocytes reenter blood
Lymph node
(6) B lymphocytes and T lymphocytes tend to settle in lymphatic organs
Thymus gland

FIGURE 37-3. Transformation of T and B lymphocytes.

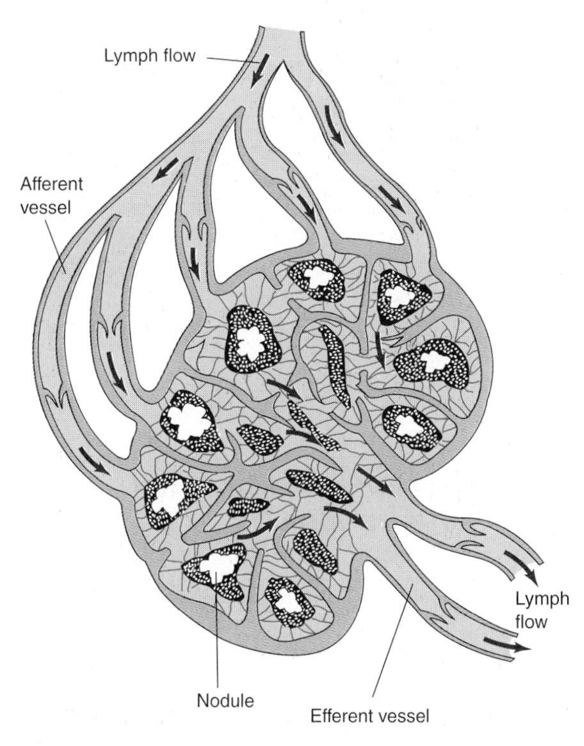
Lymph flow
Afferent vessel
Lymph flow
Nodule
Efferent vessel

FIGURE 37-4. Flow of lymph through a lymph node.

Physical Assessment

Physical assessment includes inspection of the skin with particular attention to color (eg, normal, extreme redness, pallor), temperature, and the presence of ecchymosis or other lesions. A rapid pulse rate can indicate reduced erythrocytes or inadequate hemoglobin levels.

Lymph nodes in the neck are palpated for tenderness or swelling. The size, location, and characteristics of symptomatic lymph nodes are noted. The skin adjacent to the node is examined for redness, streaking, and swelling. The tonsils are inspected for size and appearance. The extremities are examined to determine if they are of similar size; obstruction of lymphatic circulation can cause unilateral enlargement.

LABORATORY AND DIAGNOSTIC TESTS

Blood samples are obtained by puncturing a vein, finger, or earlobe. Laboratory tests include a complete blood count and tests concerning the client's blood clotting status such as prothrombin time, fibrinogen level, activated partial thromboplastin time, D-dimer test for fibrin, fibrin degradation products, and factor assays.

A *bone marrow aspiration*, a procedure in which bone marrow is removed under local anesthesia, is performed to determine the status of blood cell formation. The marrow is examined for the types and percentage of cells and their relation to cells ready to be released into the circulation. The nurse assists the physician, supports the client during a bone marrow aspiration, and monitors his or her status afterward (Nursing Guidelines 37–1).

The *Schilling test* is performed to diagnose pernicious anemia, macrocytic anemia, and malabsorption syndromes. Radioactive vitamin B_{12} is given orally, followed in 1 hour by an injection of nonradioactive B_{12}. All urine is collected for 24 to 48 hours after the client receives the nonradioactive B_{12}. Little or no vitamin B_{12} in the urine indicates absence of the intrinsic factor, or defective malabsorption of vitamin B_{12} from the intestinal tract.

Lymphatic disorders are diagnosed using procedures such as a lymph node biopsy, ultrasound of the spleen or selected lymph nodes, and lymphangiography (radiographic examination using contrast media). Additional diagnostic tests include radiography, computed tomography, bone scan, and magnetic resonance imaging. Although they are not specific for hematologic or lymphatic disorders, they are used to rule out other disorders or note changes in organs that have a direct or indirect relationship to a hematologic or lymphatic disorder.

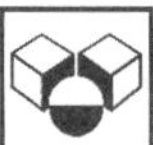

Nursing Guidelines 37-1

Assisting With a Bone Marrow Aspiration

- Inform the client of the plan and approximate time for the bone marrow aspiration and allow time for answering questions.
- Witness the client's signature on a consent form.
- Check the client's medical record for history of allergies, especially to local anesthetics or latex.
- Obtain a sterile bone marrow aspiration tray and add the type and strength of local anesthetic the physician orders.
- Determine the site from which the physician intends to obtain the sample of bone marrow.
- Position the client on his or her back or side to facilitate access to the aspiration site.
- Suggest distraction techniques to avoid focusing on the pressure or discomfort associated with puncturing the bone.
- Label the specimen and ensure its delivery to the laboratory.
- Follow Standard Precautions when there is a potential for contact with blood from the client, equipment, and bedside environment.
- Limit the client's activity for approximately 30 minutes after the procedure.
- Monitor the puncture site at frequent intervals for signs of continued bleeding; change or reinforce the dressing as needed.
- Report prolonged bleeding, unusual pain at the site, and signs of an infection.

Nursing Management

The nurse collects appropriate data to assist the physician in diagnosing hematologic or lymphatic disorders and the client's response to treatment. Before any diagnostic testing, the nurse determines the client's knowledge of the procedure and offers a description of the test routine, what tasks are necessary for participation in the test, and what discomfort is likely to be experienced.

Gloves are worn when collecting specimens. After collection, the specimen is checked for the correct label and immediately taken to the laboratory. When the test involves a puncture, the area is assessed for excessive bleeding. Pressure or a pressure dressing is applied to the site as needed. Vital signs are monitored to assess the client's recovery. The physician is notified regarding adverse responses. Test results are analyzed and reported promptly.

General Nutritional Considerations

In addition to iron, vitamin B_{12}, and folic acid, several other nutrients are involved in erythrocyte production. Vitamin C enhances the absorption of folic acid and iron. Vitamin B_6 serves as a coenzyme in hemoglobin formation, and copper is involved in the transfer of iron from storage to plasma. Hemoglobin is made from protein, as are the enzymes involved in red blood cell production. The exact roles of vitamin A and E are not clear.

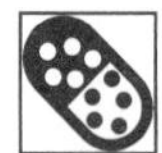

General Pharmacologic Considerations

Many pharmacologic agents affect the hematopoietic system, causing a decrease in various blood components.

Clients taking medications that depress the hematopoietic system, particularly thrombocytes and leukocytes, are monitored closely for signs of leukopenia (fever, sore throat, chills) and thrombocytopenia (unusual or easy bleeding, oozing from injection sites, bleeding gums, dark tarry stools).

The drug epoetin alfa (Epogen) can be used to stimulate the production of red blood cells.

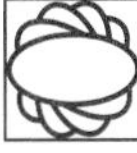

General Gerontologic Considerations

The components of blood change only slightly with age. Red blood cells become slightly less flexible and diminish slightly in number.

With age, lymphocytes decrease in number causing a decrease in resistance to infection.

The Schilling test may pose a problem in the elderly if proper collection of the 24-hour specimen is not possible due to cognitive problems or urinary incontinence.

SUMMARY OF KEY CONCEPTS

- Hematopoiesis is the manufacture and development of blood cells. Two structures involved in hematopoiesis are bone marrow and lymphatic tissue.
- Bone marrow produces erythrocytes, leukocytes, and platelets. Erythrocytes transport oxygen to and remove carbon dioxide from tissues. Leukocytes protect the body from invading microorganisms and manufacture antibodies. Platelets play a role in hemostasis.
- Plasma, the liquid portion of blood, contains plasma proteins, vitamins, glucose, electrolytes, enzymes, hormones, and other chemical substances.
- There are three plasma proteins: (1) albumin helps maintain the osmotic pressure that retains fluid in the vascular compartment; (2) globulin prevents or modifies some types of infectious diseases; (3) fibrinogen is important in forming blood clots.
- The four blood groups are A, B, AB, and O. Clients must receive compatible blood types in transfusions because incompatible blood will result in a life-threatening transfusion reaction.
- The lymphatic system circulates interstitial fluid and carries it to the veins. The lymphatic system filters and destroys pathogens and removes other potentially harmful substances that are present in lymph.
- When obtaining a health history from a client who may have a hematopoietic or lymphatic disorder, the nurse collects data that pertain to the client's present symptoms, especially those that indicate depletion of erythrocytes and hemoglobin, frequent or chronic infections, bleeding disorders, or medical and surgical conditions that cause similar problems. Drug and dietary histories are obtained with particular attention to drugs that can affect blood cell formation or alter the ability to control bleeding. Potential exposure to infectious agents is determined by inquiring about foreign travel.
- While assessing the client physically, the nurse notes the characteristics of the skin, heart rate, tenderness or enlargement of areas around clusters of lymph nodes, and a difference in the size of one extremity compared with the other.
- Common laboratory and diagnostic tests ordered to detect or monitor the treatment of hematopoietic and lymphatic disorders include complete blood count, bone marrow aspiration, lymph node biopsy, ultrasound of the spleen, and lymphangiography.
- Nursing management of clients with hematopoietic and lymphatic disorders includes appropriate data collection, adequate preparation for laboratory and diagnostic tests, proper collection and handling of laboratory specimens, monitoring the client for adverse effects after diagnostic procedures, and prompt reporting of changes in the client's condition and test results.

CRITICAL THINKING EXERCISES

1. Explain the process of blood cell formation.
2. Describe the nurse's responsibilities when assisting with a bone marrow aspiration.
3. After notifying the physician of the following blood count values: 80,000 platelets; 2,400,000 RBCs; and 24,500 WBCs, what precautions are appropriate to institute? What should be added to the nursing plan of care?

Suggested Readings

Borton, D. (1996). WBC count and differential: Reviewing the defensive roster. *Nursing, 26*(9), 26–32.

Campbell, K. (1997). Types of bone marrow and stem-cell transplant. *Nursing Times, 93*(7), 44–46.

Fischbach, F. T. (1996). *A manual of laboratory & diagnostic tests* (5th ed.). Philadelphia: Lippincott-Raven.

Higgins, C. (1996). Leukocytes and the value of the differential count test. *Nursing Times, 92*(20), 34–35.

Memmler, R. L., Cohen, B. J., & Wood, D. L. (1996). *The human body in health and disease* (8th ed.). Philadelphia: Lippincott-Raven.

Roberts, A. (1995). Systems of life. The lymphatic system: 1. *Nursing Times, 91*(2), 29–31.

Roberts, A. (1995). Systems of life. The lymphatic system: 2. *Nursing Times, 91*(6), 37–39.

Roberts, A. (1995). Systems of life. The lymphatic system: 3. *Nursing Times, 91*(10), 35–37.

Additional Resources

American Physiological Society
gopher://gopher.uth.tmc.edu:3300/1

Chapter 38

Caring for Clients With Disorders of the Hematopoietic System

KEY TERMS

Agranulocytosis
Anemia
Aplasia
Blood dyscrasias
Coagulopathy
Erythrocytosis
Leukocytosis
Leukopenia
Pancytopenia
Thrombocytopenia

LEARNING OBJECTIVES

On completion of this chapter, the reader will:

- Explain the meaning of the term blood dyscrasia.
- List at least five types of anemia including two examples of inherited types.
- Identify nutritional deficiencies that can lead to anemia.
- Discuss clinical problems clients experience with any type of anemia.
- Discuss the factors that cause sickling of erythrocytes and its adverse effects.
- List five activities a person with sickle cell disease can do to reduce the potential for a sickle cell crisis.
- Explain the term erythrocytosis, give one example of a characteristic disease, and list three possible complications that can result.
- Explain how forms of leukemia are classified.
- List clinical problems or nursing diagnoses common among clients with leukemia.
- Explain the term pancytopenia and give one example of a disorder that represents this condition.
- Discuss the meaning of coagulopathy and name two coagulopathies.
- Discuss nursing responsibilities when managing the care of clients with coagulopathies.

Blood dyscrasias, abnormalities in the numbers and types of blood cells, and bleeding disorders develop from both treatable and chronic pathologic processes; some etiologies are life-threatening. Despite the pathology, many blood disorders have similar symptoms and require similar diagnostic tests.

Anemia

Anemia is a decrease in the number of erythrocytes and a lower than normal hemoglobin level. A consequence of anemia is a decrease in the amount of oxygen carried to body tissues. Anemia is caused by blood loss, inadequate nutrition, and genetic or acquired disorders.

Hypovolemic Anemia

Loss of blood volume results in a decrease of blood cells. Because erythrocytes are the most abundant type of blood cell, the most critical consequence is *hypovolemic anemia.*

ETIOLOGY AND PATHOPHYSIOLOGY

Hypovolemic anemia is caused by a sudden loss of a large volume of blood or a gradual loss of small amounts of blood over a prolonged period. When the body is unable to increase the production of erythrocytes to compensate for the loss, cellular function is compromised due to an inadequate supply of oxygen and an accumulation of carbon dioxide.

ASSESSMENT FINDINGS

Signs and Symptoms

Acute hypovolemic anemia from severe blood loss is evidenced by signs and symptoms of hypovolemic shock: extreme pallor, tachycardia, hypotension, reduction in urine output, and altered consciousness (see Chap. 22). Symptoms of anemia from chronic blood loss include pallor, fatigue, feeling chilled, postural hypotension, and rapid heart and respiratory rate.

Diagnostic Findings

Laboratory confirmation of acute or chronic anemia includes reduction in the complete blood count, hemoglobin, and hematocrit levels.

MEDICAL MANAGEMENT

Treatment of sudden, severe bleeding involves replacement of blood by transfusions. If blood loss is chronic, as from bleeding uterine tumors and hemorrhoids, the underlying condition is treated. Depending on how much blood is lost, treatment includes blood transfusion or the administration of oral, intravenous (IV), or intramuscular (IM) iron to help the body compensate for the loss of hemoglobin. Oxygen therapy is sometimes necessary if the anemia is severe.

NURSING MANAGEMENT

The nurse gathers pertinent data, manages acute bleeding, limits activity to conserve oxygen stores, administers blood and other IV fluids, gives medications to combat shock, and prepares the client for surgery if indicated. The plan of care for a client with hypovolemic anemia includes, but is not limited to, the following:

Nursing Diagnosis and Collaborative Problems	Nursing Interventions
PC: Hypovolemia and **PC: Hypoxemia** **Goal:** The nurse will monitor and manage low blood volume and reduced oxygenation.	Monitor intake and output accurately each shift or every hour; report urine output less than 30 to 50 mL/hr Assess vital signs every 2 to 4 hours or more often if indicated; report systolic pressure less than 90 mm Hg and heart rate above 100 beats/min Monitor oxygen saturation on a continuous basis; report sustained levels of less than 90% Use Standard Precautions to examine and test body fluids for evidence of blood loss. Apply direct pressure to site of bleeding or apply pressure to a proximal artery as an alternative in the case of hemorrhage. Place client in a modified Trendelenburg position if hypovolemic shock develops. Administer IV fluids and blood as prescribed; be prepared to increase the rate of infusion if hemorrhage and shock occur. Give oxygen to maintain oxygen saturation at or above 90%. Supplement parenteral fluids with oral fluids if possible.
Activity Intolerance related to reduced cellular capacity to carry oxygen **Goal:** The client will tolerate essential activity as evidenced by a heart rate of less than 100 beats/min and a respiratory rate of under 28 breaths per minute.	Limit the client's nonessential physical activities; provide periods of rest. Distribute essential tasks over a long period of time. Administer oxygen during periods of rapid breathing or tachycardia.
Risk for Altered Body Temperature related to decreased energy due to anaerobic metabolism **Goal:** The client's body temperature will remain at 98.6°F ±1°.	Provide additional body warmth by using more blankets or bed clothing; warm blankets before applying. Raise the temperature or humidity; close door or curtains to control drafts.

Iron Deficiency Anemia

Iron deficiency anemia develops when there is an insufficient amount of iron to produce hemoglobin.

ETIOLOGY AND PATHOPHYSIOLOGY

Because iron is necessary for the production of hemoglobin, iron deficiency anemia occurs when (1) heme cannot be recycled due to blood loss, (2) dietary intake of iron is insufficient, (3) absorption of iron from food is inadequate, and (4) the need for iron exceeds the reserves.

Even when a healthy diet is consumed, less than 10% of the iron is absorbed. Individuals whose nutrition is compromised due to unhealthy dieting or who cannot afford to eat a healthy diet, those who lack knowledge about nutrition, or those who have malabsorption disorders are at great risk for iron deficiency anemia. The need for iron increases during periods of rapid growth, pregnancy, and throughout the female reproductive years when intermittent blood loss occurs during menses.

Reduced hemoglobin, for whatever the reason, compromises the oxygen carrying capacity of red blood cells. Without sufficient oxygen, cells must switch to anaerobic metabolism which is less efficient in comparison to aerobic metabolism, to produce energy and sustain functions at the cellular level.

ASSESSMENT FINDINGS

Signs and Symptoms

Most individuals with iron deficiency anemia have reduced energy, feel cold all the time, and experience fatigue and dyspnea with minor physical exertion. The heart rate is generally rapid even at rest.

Diagnostic Findings

The complete blood count, hemoglobin, hematocrit, and serum iron are decreased. A blood smear reveals erythrocytes that are *microcytic* (smaller than normal) and *hypochromic* (lighter in color than normal). Other laboratory and diagnostic tests (eg, stool examination for occult blood) reveal the source of the blood loss.

MEDICAL MANAGEMENT

Treatment is aimed at determining the cause of the anemia and, when possible, eliminating it. Correction of a faulty diet by adding foods high in iron is an important aspect of treatment (see General Nutritional Considerations at the end of the chapter). In some instances an IM injection of iron or an oral iron supplement is prescribed. In severe cases a blood transfusion is necessary.

NURSING MANAGEMENT

The nursing focus is to improve the nutritional intake of iron. The nurse takes a dietary history and collaborates with the dietitian to resolve dietary deficiencies (see Chap. 15 to review the food pyramid and information in the General Nutritional Considerations at the end of the chapter). The nurse implements medical treatment that involves oral or parenteral iron supplementation. Intramuscular administration of iron is given by the Z-track technique (Clinical Procedure 38–1). For a review of blood transfusions, see Chapter

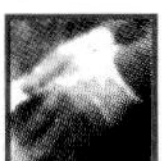

Clinical Procedure 38-1
Intramuscular Injection by Z-Track Technique

PURPOSE

- To seal medication within intramuscular tissue
- To prevent tissue irritation
- To avoid staining skin and subcutaneous tissue

EQUIPMENT

- Parenteral drug (example iron dextran (InFeD)
- 3-mL syringe with a 22-gauge, 1½- or 2-inch needle
- Replacement needle of same gauge and length
- Clean gloves
- Alcohol swab
- Bandaid or gauze square and tape

Nursing Action	Rationale
ASSESSMENT	
Check the medical orders.	Collaborates nursing activities with medical treatment.
Read and compare the label on the drug container with the medical order or medication administration record at least three times.	Prevents errors.
Check the identity of the client using the identification bracelet.	Prevents errors.
Determine how much the client understands about the purpose and technique for the procedure.	Provides an opportunity for health teaching.
Inspect the dorsogluteal site.	Determines if the muscle is of adequate size and there is no evidence of current tissue trauma.
PLANNING	
Obtain the necessary equipment.	Prevents unnecessary delays in the plan of care.
IMPLEMENTATION	
Wash your hands.	Reduces the transmission of microorganisms.
Fill the syringe with the prescribed amount of drug and change the needle.	Prevents tissue contact with the irritating drug.

continued

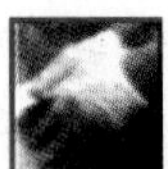

Clinical Procedure 38-1
Continued

Nursing Action	Rationale
Draw up an additional 0.2 mL of air within the syringe.	Ensures that the entire dose of medication will be administered.
Attach a needle that is at least 1½ to 2 inches long.	Helps deposit the drug deep within the muscle.
Don gloves.	Prevents contact with blood.
Position the client on the abdomen or side depending on which injection site is used.	Facilitates identifying injection landmarks.
Using the side of your hand, pull the tissue laterally about 1 inch (2.5 cm) until it is taut.	Creates the potential for sealing the drug with the muscle.

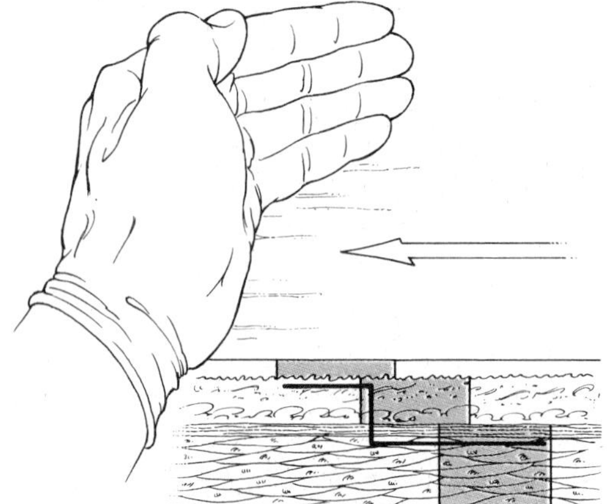

Nursing Action	Rationale
Swab the site with an alcohol pledget.	Removes some transient microorganisms.
Insert the needle at a 90-degree angle while continuing to hold the tissue laterally.	Directs the tip of the needle deeply within the muscle.
Steady the barrel of the syringe with the fingers and use the thumb to manipulate the plunger.	Avoids releasing the tissue being retracted with the nondominant hand.

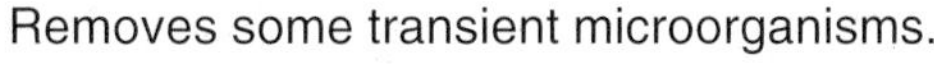

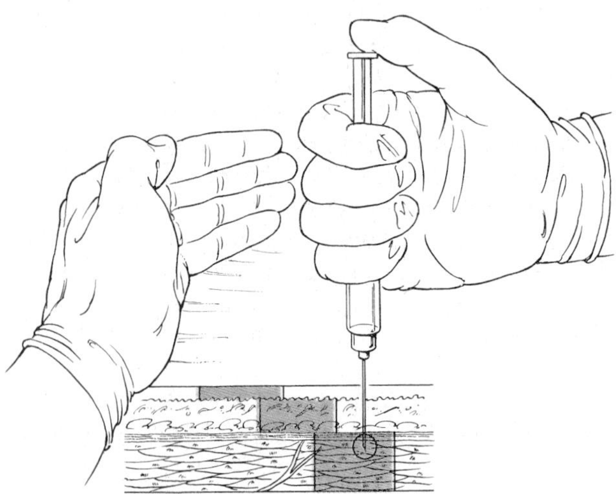

Nursing Action	Rationale
Aspirate for a blood return.	Determines if the needle is within a blood vessel.
Instill the medication by depressing the plunger with the thumb.	Deposits the medication into the muscle.
Wait 10 seconds with the needle in place and the skin still held taut.	Provides time for the medication to be distributed in a large area.

continued

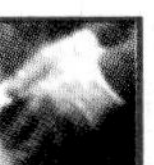

Clinical Procedure 38-1
Continued

Nursing Action	Rationale
Withdraw the needle and immediately release the taut skin.	Creates a diagonal path that prevents leaking into the subcutaneous and dermal layers of tissue.

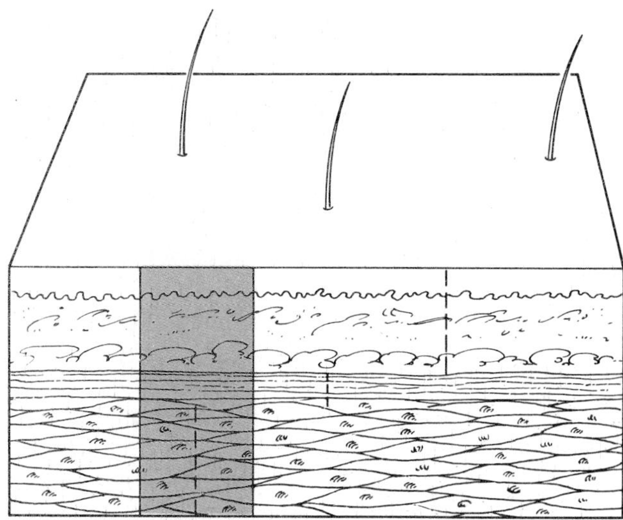

Nursing Action	Rationale
Apply direct pressure to the injection site with a gauze square, but do not rub it.	Controls bleeding, but does not alter the location of the medication.
Cover the injection site with a bandaid or gauze square and tape.	Absorbs blood, should it continue to ooze.
Discard the syringe without recapping the needle.	Reduces the potential for a needle stick injury.
Remove your gloves and wash your hands.	Removes microorganisms.
Document the medication administration.	Maintains a current record of client care.

23. Discharge instructions include pacing activities to minimize fatigue and information concerning oral medications and medical follow-up to determine if the client's hemoglobin level stabilizes within normal limits.

Client and Family Teaching

The nurse instructs the client who takes an oral iron supplement to:

- Dilute liquid preparations of iron with another liquid such as juice and drink with a straw to avoid staining the teeth.
- Take iron with food or immediately after a meal to avoid gastric distress.
- Avoid taking iron simultaneously with an antacid which interferes with iron absorption.
- Check with the physician or pharmacist about combining iron with other prescribed or over-the-counter medications to determine appropriate absorption of each.
- Drink orange juice or take other forms of vitamin C with iron to promote its absorption.
- Expect that iron colors stool dark green or black.
- Consult the prescribing physician if constipation or diarrhea develops.
- Keep medications containing iron out of the reach of small children for whom an accidental poisoning may be fatal.

Sickle Cell Anemia

Sickle cell anemia is so named because erythrocytes become sickle or crescent shaped when there is an inadequate supply of oxygen in the blood (Fig. 38–1).

ETIOLOGY AND PATHOPHYSIOLOGY

Sickle cell anemia is caused by an abnormal form of hemoglobin (hemoglobin S). It is a hereditary dis-

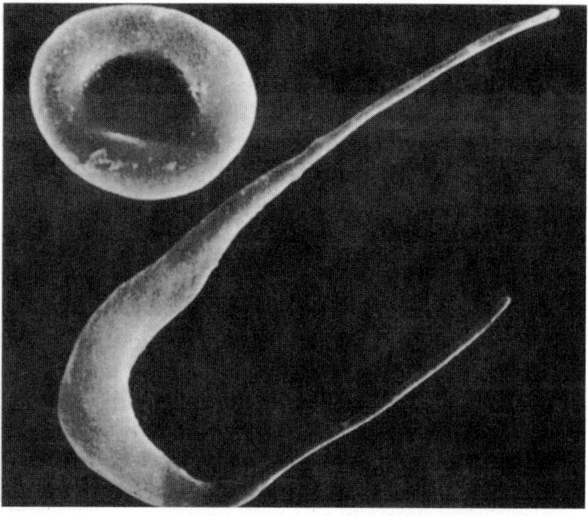

FIGURE 38-1. Normal erythrocyte (upper left) and sickled cell.

ease found primarily in African Americans but also occurs in people from Mediterranean and Middle Eastern countries. To manifest the *sickle cell disease,* a person must inherit two defective genes—one from each parent—in which case, all of the hemoglobin is inherently abnormal. If only one gene is inherited, the individual carries *sickle cell trait.* The hemoglobin of individuals who have sickle cell trait is about 40% affected. Consequently, they are at less risk for developing signs and symptoms than their diseased counterparts. Many more people have sickle cell trait than have sickle cell disease. An abnormality in the hemoglobin shortens the life span of affected erythrocytes and they become hemolyzed (destroyed). The spleen becomes obstructed and infarcted with the excess volume of dead erythrocytes. Once the spleen is damaged, there is increased risk for infection. The bone marrow enlarges to compensate for the continuous need to produce more erythrocytes. The persistent anemia causes tachycardia, dyspnea, cardiomegaly (enlargement of the heart), and arrhythmias. Vascular occlusion induces severe pain in the ischemic tissue. On occasion, the sickle-shaped cells lodge in small blood vessels where they block the flow of blood and oxygen to the affected tissue. Stroke is a common complication, even in young children.

ASSESSMENT FINDINGS

Signs and Symptoms

Evidence of the accelerated rate of erythrocyte destruction is manifested by jaundice caused by hyperbilirubinemia (excess bilirubin pigment in the blood); secondary consequences may be the development of gall stones (see Chapter 56) or a predisposition to infection when the spleen becomes dysfunctional. Anaerobic metabolism compromises growth of those affected. Chronic leg ulcers develop as a result of the blockage of the small blood vessels of the legs. Priapism (prolonged erection) occurs from delayed emptying of thick blood from the penis (see Chap 60). Other signs and symptoms of anemia are also present.

Sickle cell crisis, a rapidly developing syndrome, results from the blockage of small blood vessels with sickled cells. The reduction in blood flow leads to localized ischemia and severe pain and can cause tissue infarction (necrosis) if the oxygen supply is inadequate. Fever, pain, and swelling of one or more joints are common. Other symptoms also occur depending on the blood vessels involved. Sickle cell crisis can lead to cerebrovascular accident, pulmonary infarction, shock, and renal failure.

Diagnostic Findings

A sickle cell screening test determines the presence of abnormal hemoglobin S (HbS). Hemoglobin electrophoresis determines whether the person has sickle cell disease or carries the sickle cell trait. Reticulocytes, immature erythrocytes, are prematurely released into the bloodstream in an effort to replace the hemolyzed mature erythrocytes.

MEDICAL MANAGEMENT

Treatment is supportive rather than curative. Regular blood transfusions decrease the risk for stroke and other infarction complications. However, transfused blood increases blood viscosity (thickness), which potentially does more harm than good. It can result in sensitization to minor antigens in donor blood—especially when the source of the donor blood is from someone of different ethnic origin. Experimental treatment with hydroxyurea (Hydrea), an anticancer agent, shows evidence that it decreases sickling (Porth, 1994). A few people have been cured of sickle cell disease, using bone marrow transplantation. The possibility of curing sickle cell disease with gene replacement therapy is undergoing research, but practical application of the technique is remote at this time. Clients with sickle cell disease are subject to infections that can be life-threatening. Continuous antibiotic therapy is prescribed for some; every infection, no matter how minor, is treated promptly with antibiotics.

During sickle cell crisis, clients are given narcotic analgesia on a scheduled basis or they self-administer using an IV pump. Oxygen is given for hypoxia. The client is kept on complete bed rest, hydrated with IV fluids, and given blood transfusions. An iron-chelating agent, such as deferoxamine (Desferal), is used to remove excess iron associated with multiple blood transfusions and erythrocyte destruction.

NURSING MANAGEMENT

The nurse promotes comfort during a sickle cell crisis and provides measures to reduce the incidence of sickling. Susceptible individuals are encouraged to obtain genetic testing and counseling before conceiving. The nursing plan for care includes, but is not limited to, the following:

Nursing Diagnosis and Collaborative Problems	Nursing Interventions
Pain related to obstructed blood flow	Administer prescribed analgesia as frequently as allowed and assess client's response.
Goal: The client's pain will be reduced or eliminated as evidenced by rating the pain at the lower end of a numerical scale.	Handle affected joints with care.
	Facilitate a position of comfort and change the position every 2 hours.
	Provide at least 3,000 mL of fluid per day orally or in combination with parenteral solutions.
	Keep skin warm with prewarmed blankets or warm compresses to promote vasodilation. Avoid electric heating devices that can cause a thermal burn.

Client and Family Teaching

To avoid a sickle cell crisis, clients are taught to:

- Consume a liberal amount of fluids.
- Dress warmly in cold temperatures.
- Avoid vigorous physical exercise.
- Avoid leg positions or clothing that cause vasoconstriction.
- Stop smoking or other use of nicotine.
- Avoid travel to places at high altitudes.
- Obtain immunizations for pneumococcal pneumonia and influenza caused by *Haemophilus influenzae*.
- See a physician at the first sign of infection.

Hemolytic Anemia

The term *hemolytic anemia* refers to the consequence of a widely diverse group of conditions, some acquired, some hereditary, and some idiopathic, in which there is chronic premature destruction of erthyrocytes.

ETIOLOGY AND PATHOPHYSIOLOGY

Some examples of conditions that can produce hemolytic anemia are the use of cardiopulmonary bypass during surgery, poisoning by arsenic or lead, invasion of the erythrocytes by the malaria parasite, infectious agents or toxins, and exposure to hazardous chemicals. Other causes include the production of antibodies that destroy erythrocytes. Antibodies can be produced against antigens from another person, such as is seen in blood transfusion reactions, as well as against the body's own erythrocytes.

ASSESSMENT FINDINGS

Signs and Symptoms

Symptoms are similar to those associated with anemia. In its more severe forms, the client is jaundiced and the spleen is enlarged. In some cases, hemolysis is so extensive that shock occurs.

Diagnostic Findings

Erythrocyte fragments are apparent on microscopic examination. When an erythrocyte survival study is performed using radioactive chromium, the life span of erythrocytes is 10 days or less. There is a positive reaction on a direct Coombs' test (direct antiglobulin test) when the hemolytic anemia is due to a transfusion reaction, the use of certain drugs, or the production of antibodies against the erythrocytes.

MEDICAL AND SURGICAL MANAGEMENT

Treatment includes removing the cause (when possible) and administering corticosteroids. In some cases the steroid dose can be reduced and then discontinued after several weeks. Blood transfusions are often necessary. Splenectomy is performed if the client fails to respond to medical treatment.

NURSING MANAGEMENT

The nurse obtains a comprehensive health history to help determine the cause of the hemolysis. Until the cause is determined, the nurse provides supportive care to help the client meet basic needs.

Thalassemias

Thalassemias are hereditary hemolytic anemias. They are divided into two major groups: alpha-thalassemias and beta-thalassemias. Alpha-thalassemias are found in people from Southeast Asia and Africa, whereas beta-thalassemias are found in people from the Po valley in Italy and from Mediterranean islands.

ASSESSMENT FINDINGS

Signs and Symptoms

Clients with alpha-thalassemia typically are asymptomatic, as are those with minor forms of beta-thalassemia. Clients with Cooley's anemia, a severe form of beta-thalassemia, exhibit symptoms of severe anemia and a bronzing of the skin caused by hemolysis of erythrocytes.

Diagnostic Findings

Diagnosis is based on symptoms and on the results of hemoglobin electrophoresis.

MEDICAL MANAGEMENT

Treatment of the various forms of thalassemia is symptomatic. Frequent transfusions are often required. Clients with Cooley's anemia require iron chelation therapy because of the iron deposits in the skin.

NURSING MANAGEMENT

When severe anemia is present, the client is placed on bed rest and protected from contact with those who have an infection. When transfusions are necessary, the rate of administration is closely monitored.

Pernicious Anemia

Pernicious anemia develops when there is a lack of the intrinsic factor, normally present in stomach secretions. The intrinsic factor is necessary for absorption of vitamin B_{12}. Vitamin B_{12}, the extrinsic factor in blood, is required for the maturation of erythrocytes.

ETIOLOGY AND PATHOPHYSIOLOGY

Reduction of intrinsic factor occurs with aging and gastric mucosal atrophy. It also occurs secondary to the surgical removal of the stomach or small bowel resection in which the ileum, the site for vitamin B_{12} absorption, is removed. Without adequate vitamin B_{12}, erythrocytes remain in an immature form. If the condition is not recognized and treated promptly, degenerative changes in the nervous system develop. Sometimes permanent damage occurs before treatment is begun.

ASSESSMENT FINDINGS

Signs and Symptoms

In addition to the usual symptoms of anemia, some clients with pernicious anemia develop *stomatitis* (inflammation of the mouth) and *glossitis* (inflammation of the tongue), digestive disturbances, and diarrhea. The anemia may be so severe that dyspnea occurs with minimal exertion. Jaundice, irritability, confusion, and depression are present when the disease is severe. Mental changes usually disappear with treatment. Numbness and tingling in the arms and legs and ataxia are common signs of neurologic involvement. Vibratory and position sense are sometimes lost.

Diagnostic Findings

Diagnosis is established by the client's history and symptoms and by blood and bone marrow studies. The Schilling test is used to confirm the diagnosis. Microscopic examination of a blood smear reveals many large, immature erythrocytes.

MEDICAL MANAGEMENT

Vitamin B_{12} is given IM in a dose adequate to control the disease. Therapy must continue for life. No toxic effects have been noted from the use of vitamin B_{12}. Oral vitamin B_{12} is seldom effective, except for short intervals. Iron therapy is seldom needed because mature erythrocytes are manufactured and the hemoglobin level is normal when the condition is corrected. Clients with permanent neurologic deficits benefit from physical therapy.

NURSING MANAGEMENT

If glossitis and stomatitis are present, a soft, bland diet relieves the discomfort associated with eating. Small frequent meals are better tolerated than three large meals. Meticulous oral care after eating is essential to remove particles of food that increase soreness.

If a permanent neurologic deficit has occurred, the client is encouraged to move about as much as possible to prevent complications associated with immobility, such as contractures and pressure ulcer formation. Assistance with ambulation is necessary because some clients have difficulty walking and are prone to falling. If behavioral changes occur, close supervision is necessary. The importance of lifelong administration of vitamin B_{12} is emphasized. A family member is taught how to administer vitamin B_{12} injections or the client is referred to a home health nursing service.

Folic Acid Deficiency Anemia

Folic acid deficiency can cause anemia that is characterized by immature erythrocytes.

ETIOLOGY AND PATHOPHYSIOLOGY

A folic acid deficiency is commonly related to an insufficient dietary intake of folic acid (vitamin B_9). Elderly people, alcoholics, clients with intestinal disorders that affect food absorption, those with malignant disorders, and clients who are chronically ill often have a folic acid deficiency because of poor nutrition. Certain drugs, such as anticonvulsants and methotrexate, are folic acid antagonists and interfere with folic acid absorption. Because folic acid requirements are increased in pregnant women and in clients with chronic hemolytic anemias, a folic acid deficiency can exist even when a normal diet is eaten. Prolonged IV therapy and total parenteral nutrition can also result in a folic acid deficiency.

ASSESSMENT FINDINGS

Signs and Symptoms

Severe fatigue, sore tongue that is beefy red, dyspnea, nausea, anorexia, headaches, weakness, and light-headedness occur.

Diagnostic Findings

Blood test results reveal low hemoglobin and hematocrit levels. The serum folate level is decreased. A Schilling test differentiates pernicious anemia and anemia caused by a folic acid deficiency.

MEDICAL MANAGEMENT

Oral or parenteral folic acid supplements are given to increase folic acid intake. Parenteral administration is required for clients with an intestinal malabsorption disorder. A well balanced diet that includes foods high in folic acid content is recommended.

NURSING MANAGEMENT

The client is encouraged to eat foods high in folic acid. The ingestion of soft, bland foods and good oral hygiene are encouraged. If fatigue is a prominent symptom, adequate rest periods are planned between activities.

Erythrocytosis

There are some conditions in which one of the primary characteristics is **erythrocytosis,** an increase in circulating erythrocytes. One of these conditions is polycythemia vera.

Polycythemia Vera

Polycythemia vera is characterized by a greater than normal number of erythrocytes, leukocytes, and platelets. For individuals who live at high altitudes, erythrocytosis is a normal phenomenon and usually requires no treatment.

ETIOLOGY AND PATHOPHYSIOLOGY

Polycythemia vera is associated with a rapid proliferation of blood cells produced by the bone marrow. The cause of this accelerated production is unknown. Polycythemia vera usually has an insidious onset and a prolonged course. Despite the abundance of erythrocytes, their life span is shorter. The dead erythrocytes release intracellular potassium, which can cause hyperkalemia, and uric acid, which causes goutlike joint symptoms. The oxygen-combining capacity of the erythrocytes is impaired, which compromises cellular oxygenation. The increased number of erythrocytes makes the blood more viscous than normal and more likely to develop thrombi in small blood vessels. Complications include hypertension, congestive heart failure, stroke, areas of infarction, and hemorrhage.

ASSESSMENT FINDINGS

Signs and Symptoms

The face and lips are reddish purple. Fatigue, weakness, headache, pruritus, exertional dyspnea, and dizziness are common. Excessive bleeding after minor injuries, perhaps because of the engorgement of the capillaries and veins, occurs. Hemorrhoids develop. Splenomegaly (enlargement of the spleen) is common. The joints become swollen and painful because of elevated uric acid levels.

Diagnostic Findings

The blood cell count, especially erythrocytes, is elevated with a similar rise in the hemoglobin and hematocrit levels. The platelet and white blood cell counts are increased. The serum potassium and blood levels of uric acid are above normal.

MEDICAL MANAGEMENT

Treatment involves measures to reduce the volume of circulating blood, lessen its viscosity, and curb the excessive production of erythrocytes. A *phlebotomy* (opening a vein to withdraw blood) is done several times a week; 500 mL of blood is removed at a time. Anticoagulants are prescribed to reduce the potential for forming clots. Radiophosphorus and radiation therapy can be used to decrease the production of erythrocytes in the bone marrow. Antineoplastic drugs such as mechlorethamine (Mustargen) are given to curb excessive bone marrow activity.

Nursing Management

The nurse observes the client for complications and provides information about drug therapy and techniques for promoting circulation and reducing the potential for forming thrombi. The nursing plan for care includes, but is not limited to, the following:

Nursing Diagnosis and Collaborative Problems	Nursing Interventions
Risk for Altered Tissue Perfusion related to venous stasis and increased blood viscosity.	Advise drinking 3 quarts of fluid per day.
Goal: Tissue will remain oxygenated and free of blood clots as evidenced by the absence of ischemic pain and edema and skin that is warm and intact.	Tell the client to avoid crossing the legs at the knee and wearing tight clothing that impairs circulation.
	Encourage the client to move about and change positions frequently, and to elevate lower extremities as much as possible.
	Teach the client to perform isometric exercises, such as contracting and relaxing the quadriceps and gluteal muscles, during long periods of inactivity.
	Encourage the client to wear thromboembolic stockings or support hose during waking hours.
	Tell the client to rest immediately if chest pain develops.

Leukocytosis

Leukocytosis is an increase in the number of leukocytes above normal limits. Contrary to wound healing when an increase in leukocytes serves a protective mechanism, in some disease conditions such as leukemia the proliferation of leukocytes is detrimental.

Leukemia

Leukemia refers to any malignant blood disorder in which there is an unregulated proliferation of leukocytes, usually in an immature form. There is often an accompanying decrease in production of erythrocytes and platelets. There are four general types of leukemia. They are classified according to the stem cell line in bone marrow that is dysfunctional (Table 38–1). Acute and chronic lymphocytic leukemias result from bone marrow dysfunction that affects lymphoid stem cells; the primary marrow dysfunction in acute and chronic myelocytic leukemia is in myeloid stem cells (Fig. 38–2).

ETIOLOGY AND PATHOPHYSIOLOGY

The cause of leukemia is unknown, although factors such as exposure to toxic chemicals and radiation, viruses, and certain drugs are known to precipitate the disorder. In some cases there is a genetic correlation. Although there is a rampant increase in leukocytes, there are many more immature than mature cells. Because of their immaturity they are ineffective in fighting infections. The rapid proliferation of leukocytes results in a decreased production of erythrocytes and platelets. Severe anemia eventually occurs, and the reduction of platelets leads to bleeding. The excessive numbers of leukocytes infiltrate the spleen, liver, lymph nodes, and brain if unchecked.

TABLE 38-1 **Types of Leukemia**

Type	Cellular Characteristics	Age of Onset
Acute lymphocytic (ALL)	Increased immature lymphocytes Normal or low granulocytes Low erythrocytes Low platelets	Younger than 5; uncommon after 15
Chronic lymphocytic (CLL) Most common type in adults	Same as above, but erythrocyte and platelet count may be normal or low	Older than 40
Acute myelogenous (AML)	Decrease in all myeloid formed cells: monocytes, granulocytes, erythrocytes, and platelets	Occurs in all age ranges
Chronic myelogenous (CML) Genetic link in 90% to 95% of cases	Same as above, but greater number of normal cells than acute form	Older than 20, but incidence increases with age

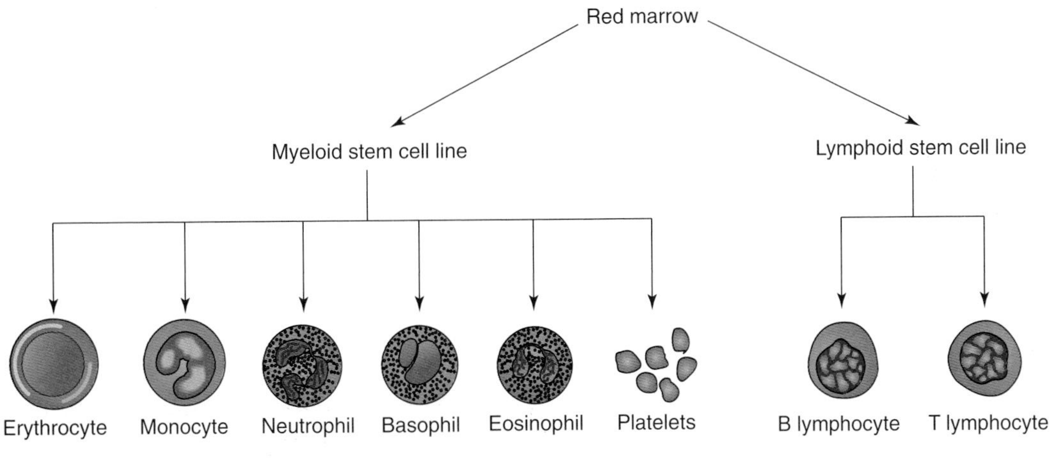

FIGURE 38-2. Maturation of myeloid and lymphoid stem cells.

ASSESSMENT FINDINGS

Signs and Symptoms

Infections, fatigue from anemia, and easy bruising are hallmarks of leukemia. At the onset of leukemia, particularly in acute lymphocytic leukemia, a fever is present, the spleen and lymph nodes enlarge, and internal or external bleeding develops. Common sites from which bleeding occurs include the nose, mouth, and gastrointestinal tract.

Diagnostic Findings

The leukocyte count is low, normal, or high, but the number of normal leukocytes is decreased. There is a consequent decrease in the number of erythrocytes and platelets.

MEDICAL MANAGEMENT

Drug therapy is the primary weapon for arresting leukemia. The type of drug or combination of drugs depends on the form of leukemia. As a result of years of research, successful drug protocols using one or combinations of antineoplastic drugs have been developed.

Erythrocyte and platelet transfusions are necessary to treat the anemia and decrease in platelets. Antibiotics are given when secondary infections develop.

Bone marrow transplantation and stem cell transplantation have increased survival for some clients. Their source is either *autologous* (from oneself) or *allogenic* (from another). Stem cells are harvested by removing them from peripheral blood, obtaining bone marrow, or by collecting cord blood from a newborn. Malignant stem cells are removed from an autologous specimen before transplant. Toxic drugs or radiation are administered prior to the transplant, which renders the client extremely susceptible to infection. The client remains hospitalized for several weeks to observe if normal blood cells are eventually produced, to detect signs of *graft versus host disease* in which the foreign donor cells destroy the recipient's tissues and organs, and to protect the client who is immunosuppressed from acquiring a life-threatening infection.

NURSING MANAGEMENT

The drugs used to treat leukemia are highly toxic and can impair the formation of all blood cells and other healthy cells. Administering antineoplastic agents often results in *alopecia* (loss of hair), nausea, vomiting, diarrhea, excessive bleeding, anorexia, stomatitis, and oral ulcerations. Antiemetics are used to control nausea and vomiting. The nurse offers small, frequent feedings of bland food (which reduces oral irritation) and frequent sips of cool water to maintain fluid and nutrition levels.

NURSING PROCESS: *The Client With Leukemia*

Assessment

Initial assessment includes a history of symptoms experienced as well as current symptoms. Joint pain and other symptoms associated with leukocyte infiltration of the central nervous system (eg, headache, confusion) can occur. Because uric acid levels increase during chemotherapy, the nurse observes the client for signs and symptoms of kidney, ureteral, or bladder stones and encourages a high fluid intake to prevent crystallization of uric acid. The nurse monitors IV fluid therapy for clients who are unable to meet and maintain normal food and fluid intake. Prolonged episodes of inadequate food intake require total parenteral nutrition.

Diagnosis and Planning

The nursing care for a client with leukemia includes, but is not limited to, the following:

Nursing Diagnosis and Collaborative Problems	Nursing Interventions
Risk for Infection related to compromised immunity	Monitor temperature at least once per shift.
Goal: The client will be free of infection as evidenced by a normal temperature, no signs of an infectious disorder.	Assess the client for signs of infection, such as swelling and tenderness, which can appear in any area or organ of the body.
	Institute protective isolation precautions when the client is severely immune suppressed.
	Implement neutropenic precautions (Box 38-1).
	Ensure that any staff person, family member, or visitor who is ill temporarily discontinues direct contact with the client.
PC: Hemorrhage	Monitor the platelet count.
Goal: Bleeding will be managed and minimized	Inspect the skin for signs of bruising and petechiae.
	Report melena, hematuria, or epistaxis (nosebleeds).
	Handle the client gently when assisting with care to avoid bruising.
	Apply prolonged pressure to needle sites or other sources of external bleeding.
	Provide spongy toothettes for oral hygiene and soft foods.
	Advise males to use an electric razor.
	Implement physician's orders for transfusions of blood and platelets.
Activity Intolerance related to hypoxia	(See discussion that accompanies anemia.)
Risk for Body Image Disturbance related to hair loss secondary to chemotherapy	Suggest wearing a cap, scarf or wig until the hair grows back.
Goal: The client will cope with hair loss.	
Anxiety and **Fear** related to unfamiliar experiences and unknown prognosis	Encourage the client to talk about the disorder and the effect it has had on him or her and the family.
Goal: The client's anxiety and fear will be relieved as evidenced by the client's report of emotional comfort.	Explain the plan of care and treatment procedures.
	Give encouragement and emotional support, and foster hope without implying unrealistic expectations.

Evaluation and Expected Outcomes

- The client does not acquire an infection.
- Blood loss is controlled.
- The client tolerates activity.
- The client adapts to changes in body image.
- The client copes with anxiety and fears.

Client and Family Teaching

If medication is to be taken at home, the nurse explains the dosage schedule because compliance is essential to treat the disease successfully. If untoward effects occur, every effort is made to control the symptoms while continuing chemotherapy. The following points are included in a teaching plan:

- Frequent examinations of the blood and sometimes the bone marrow are necessary to monitor the results of therapy. (Emphasis is placed on the importance of these examinations as an aid to staying well rather than on the possible complications from drug therapy.)
- Take precautions to avoid physical injury.
- Avoid exposure to people who have an infection such as a head cold.
- Seek medical care promptly if excessive bleeding or bruising or symptoms of illness or infection occur.

BOX 38-1 Neutropenic Precautions

To help prevent infection in clients with neutropenia:

- Place the client in a private room.
- Wash hands *without fail* before touching the client; encourage client to remind all staff and visitors to wash hands.
- Tell the client to wash his or her hands before and after eating and after using the bathroom.
- Encourage the client to shower daily.
- Place a mask over the client's mouth and nose if leaving the room; minimize amount of time spent in crowded areas.
- Ensure that no raw fruits or vegetables are served.
- Minimize the number of invasive procedures performed (schedule all blood work to be drawn at one time of the day; discontinue invasive lines as soon as possible).
- Tell the client not to handle flowers.

- Obtain sufficient rest and eat an adequate diet to prevent secondary infections.
- When feeling well, continue usual activities unless the physician instructs otherwise.
- If sores in the mouth occur contact the physician as soon as possible. Do not self-treat this problem.
- Contact the physician immediately if any of the following occur: severe nausea with prolonged vomiting, severe diarrhea, fever, chills, excessive bleeding or bruising, cough, chest pain, cloudy, urine, rash, blood in the stool or urine, severe headache, extreme fatigue, increased respiratory rate or difficulty breathing, and rapid pulse rate.
- Follow the physician's recommendations to monitor temperature and weight.
- Keep all clinic or office appointments.

Multiple Myeloma

Multiple myeloma is a malignancy involving plasma cells, lymphocyte-like cells in the bone marrow. The prognosis is poor, with an estimated survival of 1 to 5 years.

ETIOLOGY AND PATHOPHYSIOLOGY

The exact mechanism that triggers the disorder is unknown. The disorder is associated with aging and rarely occurs before the age of 40. The immature plasma cells proliferate in the bone marrow, forming single or multiple *osteolytic* (bone-destroying) tumors. The malignant plasma cells release an abnormal protein called M-type globulin. The excess production of plasma cells reduces the production of erythrocytes, leukocytes, and platelets. Later, the cancerous plasma cells infiltrate the liver, spleen, soft tissues, and kidneys.

ASSESSMENT FINDINGS

Signs and Symptoms

The first symptom is usually vague pain in the pelvis, spine, or ribs. As the disease progresses, the pain becomes more severe and localized. When bone marrow is replaced by tumors, pathologic fractures occur. In addition, resistance to infection is decreased, probably because of a decrease in antibody formation—a function of lymphocytes. Bone marrow destruction causes anemia. Renal calculi and renal failure ultimately occur.

Diagnostic Findings

Skeletal radiographic studies reveal punched-out bone lesions and bone marrow. Serum calcium levels are elevated due to bone destruction. Urine samples are positive for M-type globulin (Bence Jones protein). The uric acid level is elevated due to cellular destruction.

MEDICAL MANAGEMENT

Steroids, melphalan (Alkeran), cyclophosphamide (Cytoxan), and radiation are used to decrease the tumor mass and lessen bone pain. Pain is controlled with analgesics; stronger analgesics are reserved for the terminal stages of the disease. Allopurinol (Zyloprim) is used to prevent uric acid crystallization and subsequent renal calculus formation.

Anemia is treated with blood transfusions, and infections are managed with antibiotics. Back braces are necessary when the spine is involved, and body casts are used when involvement is extensive and pathologic fractures occur.

NURSING MANAGEMENT

The client is frequently assessed for signs of infection, excessive fatigue, and pain in new areas. The nurse assists the client with ambulation because immobility can worsen loss of calcium from the bone. Up to 4,000 mL of fluid are provided to prevent renal damage from hypercalcemia and the precipitation of protein in the renal tubules. Signs suggestive of calculus formation in the kidney, ureters, or bladder are documented and reported (see Chaps. 63 and 64).

Safety is paramount because any injury, no matter how slight, can result in a fracture. When pain is severe, position changes and bathing are delayed until an administered analgesic has reached its peak concentration level and the client is experiencing maximum pain relief.

Agranulocytosis

Agranulocytosis (as opposed to **leukopenia,** a reduction in white blood cells) refers specifically to a decreased production of granulocytes, including neutrophils, basophils, and eosinophils. A decrease in granulocytes places the client at risk for infection.

ETIOLOGY AND PATHOPHYSIOLOGY

The most common cause of agranulocytosis is toxicity from drugs such as sulfonamides, chloramphenicol (Chloromycetin), antineoplastics, and some psychotropic medications.

ASSESSMENT FINDINGS

Signs and Symptoms

Fatigue, fever, chills, headache, and opportunistic infections in the mouth, throat, nose, rectum, or vagina can develop.

MEDICAL MANAGEMENT

Treatment includes removal of the causative factor such as discontinuing the drug that is producing agranulocytosis. The prognosis is related to the cause and severity of the condition. When the cause can be determined and promptly removed, the client usually recovers. Some clients improve after receiving filgrastim (Neupogen), a drug that supplies human granulocyte colony-stimulating factor.

NURSING MANAGEMENT

The nurse determines the names of all drugs (prescription and nonprescription) used within the past 6 to 12 months. Protective isolation is necessary if the leukocyte count is extremely low. Visitors or staff with any type of an infection are restricted from close client contact until the infection has cleared.

Pancytopenia

Pancytopenia refers to conditions such as aplastic anemia in which numbers of all marrow-produced blood cells are reduced.

Aplastic Anemia

Aplastic anemia is more than just a deficiency of erythrocytes—although on rare occasions that is the case. Its name is derived from the word *aplasia,* a word that means "failure to develop." Usually it is manifested by insufficient numbers of erythrocytes, leukocytes, and platelets, collectively described as pancytopenia.

ETIOLOGY AND PATHOPHYSIOLOGY

Aplastic anemia is a consequence of inadequate stem cell production in the bone marrow. In some cases, the cause of the disorder is never determined but it may be autoimmune (self-destroying) in nature (see Chap. 41). In many cases, the bone marrow becomes dysfunctional as a result of exposure to toxic chemicals, radiation, and drug therapy with anticancer drugs and some antibiotics. Clients with aplastic anemia are very ill, and the death rate is high if the bone marrow has been severely damaged.

ASSESSMENT FINDINGS

Signs and Symptoms

Clients with aplastic anemia experience all the typical characteristics of anemia (weakness and fatigue). In addition, they have frequent opportunistic infections plus coagulation abnormalities that are manifested by unusual bleeding, small skin hemorrhages called *petechiae,* and *ecchymoses* (bruises). The spleen becomes enlarged with an accumulation of the client's blood cells destroyed by lymphocytes that failed to recognize them as normal cells or with an accumulation of dead transfused blood cells.

Diagnostic Findings

The blood cell count shows insufficient numbers of blood cells. A bone marrow aspiration confirms that the production of stem cells is suppressed.

MEDICAL MANAGEMENT

In some instances, withdrawal of the causative agent allows the bone marrow to regenerate and assume normal function. Transfusions of whole blood, packed cells, and platelets are given to boost circulating blood cells. Antibiotics are administered to prevent or treat infection. High doses of corticosteroids that suppress the immune system are given in cases of an autoimmune connection. Bone marrow transplantation is considered if a matching donor can be found; otherwise, stem cell transplantation is an alternative.

NURSING MANAGEMENT

The nurse assesses the client for signs of severe anemia, infection, and bleeding tendencies. Every effort is made to prevent infection. If the leukocyte count is extremely low, the nurse implements special isolation procedures, such as restricting visitors and using a laminar airflow room.

Soft foods and oral hygiene techniques are modified to avoid bleeding from the gums. The nurse collaborates with the physician concerning alternative routes for drugs administered parenterally. If that is not possible, the nurse applies additional pressure to any punctures from injections or sites where IV fluids are administered and discontinued. Clients are monitored closely during blood transfusions because the risk for a reaction increases with the repeated introduction of foreign cells from multiple blood donors.

Coagulopathies

The term **coagulopathy** refers to conditions in which a component that is necessary to control bleeding (Fig. 38–3) is missing or inadequate. Two common examples are thrombocytopenia and hemophilia. For information on disseminated intravascular coagulation (DIC), a condition in which hypercoagulation (excessive clot formation) is followed by diffuse bleeding as clotting factors are exhausted, refer to texts on trauma and critical care nursing.

Thrombocytopenia

Thrombocytopenia is a lower than normal number of platelets or thrombocytes.

ETIOLOGY AND PATHOPHYSIOLOGY

Thrombocytopenia occurs when platelet manufacture by the bone marrow is decreased or platelet destruction by the spleen is increased. It accompanies leukemia and other malignant blood diseases and is caused by severe infections and certain drugs. Idiopathic thrombocytopenia purpura is thrombocytopenia without a known cause.

ASSESSMENT FINDINGS

Signs and Symptoms

Thrombocytopenia is evidenced by *purpura*, small hemorrhages in the skin, mucous membranes, or subcutaneous tissues. Bleeding from other parts of the body, such as the nose, oral mucous membrane, and the gastrointestinal tract, also occurs. Internal hemorrhage, which can be severe and even fatal, is possible.

Diagnostic Findings

Diagnosis is based on symptoms, a low platelet count, and abnormal bleeding and clotting times. In some instances bone marrow aspiration is performed. A health history sometimes reveals agents that are associated with drug-induced thrombocytopenia.

MEDICAL AND SURGICAL MANAGEMENT

When possible, the cause is eliminated. Corticosteroids provide symptomatic relief until the platelet count returns to normal. Transfusions of platelets or whole blood are given in a hemorrhagic emergency. If spontaneous recovery does not occur, splenectomy is necessary to stop destruction of platelets in the spleen. Removal of the spleen results in a rise in the platelet count and relief of symptoms.

Clients with idiopathic thrombocytopenia often recover spontaneously. If the cause can be removed or

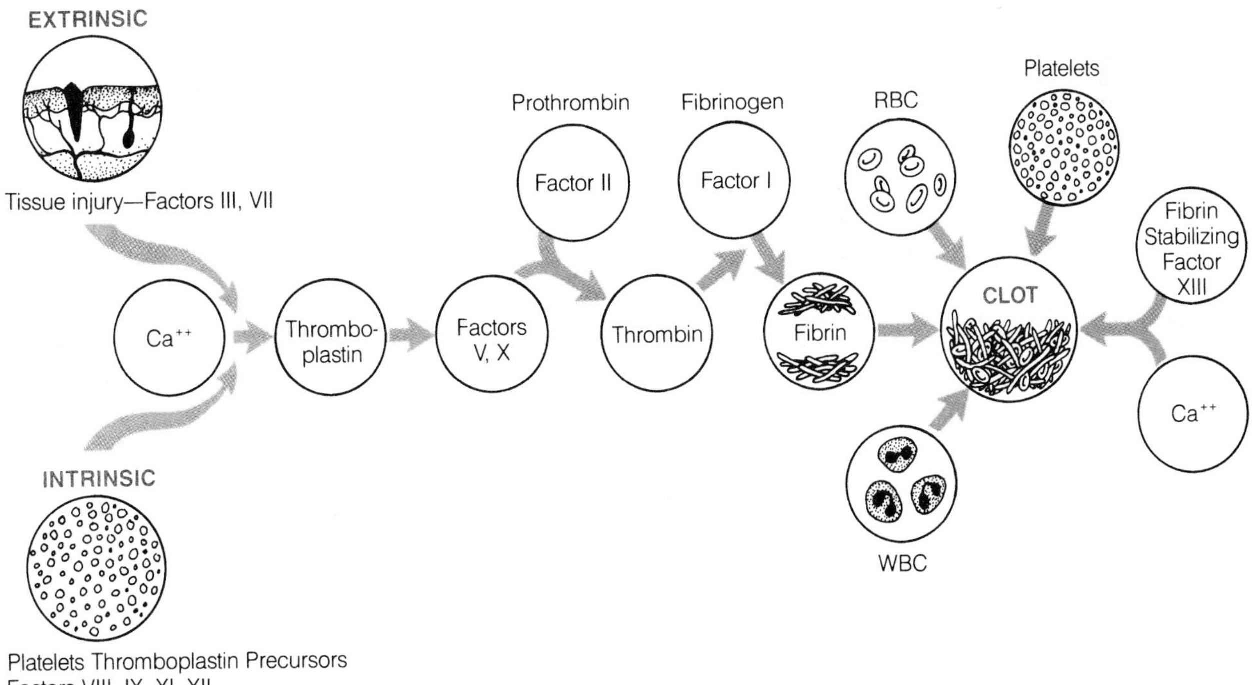

FIGURE 38-3. The process of clot formation. Clotting factors are identified by name and Roman numeral or by Roman numeral alone.

treated, the prognosis is good. Thrombocytopenia in conjunction with illnesses such as leukemia has a poor prognosis.

NURSING MANAGEMENT

Refer to nursing interventions for managing and minimizing bleeding and hemorrhage discussed in the nursing management of leukemia. If corticosteroid therapy is instituted, the client is observed for adverse drug effects. The dose and frequency of steroid medication is gradually tapered before being discontinued to avoid adrenal insufficiency or crisis (see Chap. 56).

Hemophilia

Hemophilia is a disorder involving clotting factors. There are three types of hemophilia: hemophilia A, B, and C. Hemophilia A, the most common type, results from a deficiency of factor VIII (refer to Fig. 38–3). There also is a less serious form of hemophilia A, von Willebrand's disease, in which the amount and quality of factor VIII is diminished. Hemophilia B, or Christmas disease, is a deficiency of factor IX. Hemophilia C, also known as Rosenthal's disease, is a milder form of factor IX deficiency.

ETIOLOGY AND PATHOPHYSIOLOGY

Hemophilia is inherited from mother to son as a sex-linked recessive characteristic. Daughters can inherit the trait, but seldom develop the disease. Women with the trait, however, can transmit it to male offspring.

The severity of the condition depends on the type of hemophilia inherited. Bleeding typically is noted in infancy and childhood. Milder forms can go unrecognized for years. Life expectancy is considerably shortened by the disease; many hemophiliacs do not reach adulthood. Clients with mild hemophilia may lead full and productive lives despite the illness. The human immunodeficiency virus and hepatitis virus have been transmitted to hemophiliacs through transfusion of blood and blood products. The testing of donated blood has markedly reduced the risk for acquiring bloodborne pathogens.

ASSESSMENT FINDINGS

Signs and Symptoms

The disease is manifested by persistent oozing and sometimes severe bleeding that occurs spontaneously or after an injury. Bleeding in joints eventually damages the joint and leads to deformity and limitation of motion.

Diagnostic Findings

Diagnosis is based on the history of symptoms and laboratory tests such as coagulant factor assay, which show a deficiency of factor VIII or IX.

MEDICAL MANAGEMENT

Treatment includes transfusions of fresh blood, frozen plasma, factor VIII concentrate and anti-inhibitor coagulant complex for hemophilia A, factor IX concentrate for hemophilia B, and the application of thrombin to the bleeding area. Other measures used to help control bleeding are direct pressure over the bleeding site and cold compresses or ice packs.

Relatively minor surgical procedures, such as tooth extraction, carry considerable risk and are best performed in a hospital. Transfusions usually are necessary even when minor surgery is performed.

NURSING MANAGEMENT

The nurse obtains a comprehensive health history that includes current symptoms and treatment for the bleeding disorder. The client is questioned regarding when the last episode occurred, its location (eg, mouth, rectum, skin), duration, and what treatments, if any, were necessary.

The joints and mobility are assessed. The skin is inspected for purpura or hemorrhagic areas. Before the blood pressure is taken, the client is asked if the use of a blood pressure cuff ever produced bleeding under the skin or in the arm joints. The temperature is taken tympanically to avoid oral or rectal injuries. The urine and stools are checked for signs of bleeding.

Overall care includes preventing trauma, managing and minimizing bleeding episodes, reducing pain or discomfort, conserving energy, and helping the client learn ways to prevent further bleeding episodes. When transfusion of products such as whole blood, plasma, or antihemophilic factor are required for bleeding episodes, the client is closely observed for signs that bleeding has been controlled. The physician is kept informed of the client's progress because additional treatment modalities are often necessary.

Client and Family Teaching

It is appropriate to educate the client and family in the following ways:

- Explain the treatment regimen to the client and family.
- Eliminate aspirin because this drug can increase bleeding tendencies.
- Avoid activities that can result in injury.

- Wear a Medic Alert bracelet and inform the dentist and others, when appropriate, of the condition.
- Bleeding in internal organs or structures initially produces only vague symptoms. Notify the physician promptly if pain, discomfort, or obvious bleeding from the nose, rectum, in vomitus, or elsewhere occurs.
- Use a soft toothbrush and rinse the mouth with warm water between and after meals.
- Support painful joints on pillows.

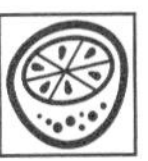

General Nutritional Considerations

Meat, egg yolk, oysters, shellfish, and the dark meat of chicken and poultry are sources of heme iron; its absorption is influenced by body need only. Nonheme iron found in plants represents the largest type of iron in the diet. Good sources include enriched and whole grain breads, iron-fortified cereals, legumes, nuts, greens, and brewer's yeast. The absorption of nonheme iron is enhanced by vitamin C (citrus fruits and juices, strawberries, green peppers, tomatoes), heme iron, certain animal proteins, and gastric acidity. Tea and coffee and various binding agents like bran in whole grains and phosphates in legumes inhibit the absorption of nonheme iron. To maximize nonheme iron absorption, a rich source of vitamin C should be consumed at every meal and coffee and tea should be avoided around and during mealtime.

Anemia and the gastrointestinal symptoms of B_{12} deficiency can be reversed by folic acid; however, neurologic symptoms continue and, if untreated, can be irreversible. It is imperative that the correct cause of megaloblastic anemia be ascertained before treatment begins.

Foods rich in folic acid include enriched breads, fortified cereals, organ meats, broccoli, green leafy vegetables, asparagus, milk, eggs, orange juice, and dried peas and beans. Vitamin C helps convert folic acid to its active form.

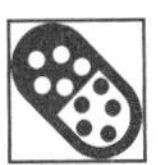

General Pharmacologic Considerations

Because some drugs (eg, antacids, tetracyclines, vitamin C) interact with oral iron, the client should consult the physician before taking other drugs.

The absorption of oral iron is decreased when the drug is taken with coffee, tea, eggs, or milk.

The use of meperidine (Demerol) is avoided when treating pain in clients with sickle cell crisis. The liver converts meperidine to normeperidine which is toxic. Grand mal seizures can occur.

Antineoplastic agents produce many serious adverse effects. The nurse must be thoroughly familiar with the dose, administration, and adverse effects to accurately administer these drugs and competently assess the client for untoward reactions.

For folic acid anemia, therapy is usually 1 mg oral folic acid daily. An injectable form is available if absorption is a problem.

To correct iron deficiency anemia, 200 mg ferrous sulfate is given three times per day, 1 hour before meals. Therapeutic response is monitored through periodic hemoglobin and hematocrit counts.

Liquid iron preparations are available if the client is unable to swallow tablets.

The most expensive and potentially dangerous method for replacing iron is by transfusion.

Pernicious anemia is treated with 100 g vitamin B_{12} IM daily for 2 weeks, then 100 g IM monthly.

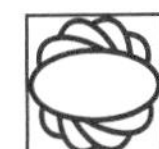

General Gerontologic Considerations

Iron deficiency anemia is not normal in older adults because the body does not eliminate excessive iron causing total body iron stores to increase with age. If the older adult is anemic, blood loss from the gastrointestinal or genitourinary tract is suspected.

Although the most successful treatment is seen in the young, acute leukemia is primarily a disease of the older adult. Acute lymphocytic anemia occurs at a rate four times higher in older adults than in children.

Pernicious anemia (vitamin B_{12} deficiency) accounts for approximately 9% of all anemias in the older adult. Because neurologic damage and dementia may occur before any hematologic changes are found, early detection is critical. The older adult with neurologic decline or dementia must be assessed for pernicious anemia.

Older adults are particularly susceptible to drug-induced hemolytic anemia because they often take more drugs than young people. Discontinuing the offending drug usually corrects the anemia.

Because older adults could forget to take the medicine or could take more than the prescribed amount, instruction or supervision in drug taking is important. These drugs are toxic, and adherence to the prescribed regimen is essential.

Anemia caused by a dietary iron deficiency occurs in older adults for many reasons: living on a fixed income, inability to shop for food, and lack of energy or motivation to prepare complete meals. These clients require a thorough evaluation of their dietary habits and education in the methods of preventing iron deficiency anemia.

SUMMARY OF KEY CONCEPTS

- Blood dyscrasia refers to conditions in which there are abnormalities in the numbers and types of blood cells and bleeding disorders.
- Anemia, a condition in which the number of erythrocytes and the hemoglobin level are lower than normal, results in reduction in the amount of oxygen carried to body cells.

- Different types of anemia include: hypovolemic, iron deficiency, pernicious, and folic acid anemias, which are acquired, and sickle cell anemia and thalassemia, which are inherited.
- Nutritional anemias develop from inadequate intake or absorption of iron, vitamin B_{12}, and folic acid.
- Regardless of the type of anemia, symptoms include fatigue, chills, and tachycardia. Other accompanying signs and symptoms are specific to the type of anemia the client has.
- Sickling is induced by an inadequate supply of oxygen in the blood and when the pH of blood is lowered. The sickle-shaped cells lodge in small blood vessels where they block the flow of blood and oxygen delivery to the affected tissue.
- To reduce the potential for sickling and sluggish circulation, clients should keep well hydrated, avoid vigorous physical exercise, dress warmly, eliminate sources of nicotine, and avoid high altitudes.
- Erythrocytosis refers to an increase in circulating erythrocytes. Erythrocytosis is potentially dangerous because the excessive cells make blood viscous and increase the risk for developing thrombi in small blood vessels.
- Clients with leukemia are at risk of several problems: infections, fatigue from anemia, and bleeding.
- Multiple myeloma is a malignancy involving plasma cells, lymphocyte-like cells, in the bone marrow. The defective plasma cells form bone-destructive tumors and suppress the formation of normal blood cells. Eventually the malignant plasma cells infiltrate the liver, spleen, soft tissues, and kidneys.
- Pancytopenia refers to conditions in which all of the marrow-produced blood cells are reduced. Aplastic anemia, a type of pancytopenia, is manifested by insufficient numbers of erythrocytes, leukocytes, and platelets.
- The term coagulopathy refers to conditions in which a component that is necessary to control bleeding is missing or inadequate. Two examples are thrombocytopenia and hemophilia.
- When caring for clients with coagulopathies, the nurse is responsible for preventing trauma, managing and minimizing bleeding episodes, reducing pain or discomfort, conserving energy, and helping the client learn ways to prevent further bleeding episodes.

CRITICAL THINKING EXERCISES

1. List hematopoeitic disorders that are associated with anemia and an etiology of each.
2. Discuss the problems that clients with anemia, leukemia, or thrombocytopenia have in common. What nursing interventions can be used regardless of the particular disorder?

Suggested Readings

Baylock, B. (1996). Focus on wound care. Sickle cell leg ulcers. *Med-Surg Nursing, 5*(1), 41–43.

Bullock, B. L. (1996). *Pathophysiology: Adaptations and alterations in function* (4th ed.). Philadelphia: Lippincott-Raven.

Campbell, K. (1997). Leukaemia: Advances in treatment. *Nursing Times, 93*(9), Professional Development, 9–14.

Campbell, K. (1996). The principles of bone marrow and stem cell transplantation. *Nursing Times, 92*(48), 34–36.

Ignatavicius, D. D., Workman, M. L., & Mishler, M. A. (1995). *Medical-surgical nursing: A nursing process approach* (2nd ed.). Philadelphia: Saunders.

Marchiondo, K., & Thompson, A. (1996). Pain management in sickle cell disease. *MEDSURG Nursing, 5(1), 29–33.*

Porth, C. M. (1994). *Pathophysiology: Concepts of altered health states* (4th ed.). Philadelphia: J. B. Lippincott.

Simko, L. C., & Lockhart, J. S. (1996). Action stat! Heparin-induced thrombocytopenia and thrombosis...white clot syndrome. *Nursing, 26*(3), 33.

Additional Resources

Joint Center for Sickle Cell and Thalassemic Disorders
Brigham & Women's Hospital
Massachusetts General Hospital
120 Longwood Avenue
Suite 327 LI
Boston, MA 02115
(616) 432–8490
http://cancer.mgh.harvard.edu/medOnc/sickle.htm

National Hemophilia Foundation
The SoHo Building
110 Green Street
Room 406
New York, NY 10012
http://home.earthlink.net/~hemo/

Oncolink
http://www.oncolink.upenn.edu

Oncology Nursing Society
http://www.nauticom.net/www/onsmain/

International Cancer Alliance (ICA)
http://www2.ari.net/icare

Chapter 39

Caring for Clients With Disorders of the Lymphatic System

KEY TERMS

Epstein-Barr virus
Hodgkin's disease
Infectious mononucleosis
Lymphadenitis
Lymphangitis
Lymphatics
Lymphedema
Lymphoma
Non-Hodgkin's lymphoma
Reed-Sternberg cell

LEARNING OBJECTIVES

On completion of this chapter, the reader will:

- Explain the cause and characteristics of lymphedema.
- Discuss the role of the nurse when managing the care of clients with lymphedema.
- Describe nursing interventions for promoting the resolution of lymphangitis and lymphadenitis.
- Explain the nature of infectious mononucleosis and how it is transmitted.
- List suggestions the nurse can offer to those who acquire infectious mononucleosis.
- Define the term lymphoma and name two types.
- Name the type of malignant cell diagnostic of Hodgkin's disease.
- List three forms of treatment used to cure or promote remission of lymphomas.
- Name at least four nursing problems that are addressed when caring for clients with Hodgkin's disease and non-Hodgkin's lymphoma.

Lymph is similar in composition to tissue fluid and plasma. A system of vessels called **lymphatics** carries fluid from body tissues to the veins. Disorders of the lymphatics are infectious, inflammatory, occlusive, or malignant.

Occlusive, Inflammatory, and Infectious Disorders

Lymphedema

Lymphedema results from an obstruction of lymph circulation.

ETIOLOGY AND PATHOPHYSIOLOGY

Lymphedema can be congenitally acquired although it is not manifested until adolescence or early adulthood. Women are affected more often than men. The condition can be secondary to others, such as mastectomy (see Chap. 59), burns and radiation, or cancer. Lymphedema can follow repeated bouts of phlebitis and streptococcal infection. With each attack, scar tissue accumulates, occlusion occurs, and fluid becomes trapped in small, "fibrous" lakes. An infestation of filarial worms causes *elephantiasis*, a form of lymphedema that occurs in the tropics.

The obstruction of lymphatic vessels causes fluid to accumulate in the tissue of the affected part. The edema, when massive, results in deformity and poor nutrition to tissues. Lymphedema usually occurs in the legs, arms, and genitalia.

ASSESSMENT FINDINGS

Signs and Symptoms

The skin in the affected area swells, especially in a dependent position. Pitting is evident, but the tissue remains soft in the early stages. The skin eventually becomes firm, tight, and shiny. Elevation does not diminish the swelling. The skin also appears thickened, rough, and discolored. Because tissue nutrition is impaired, ulcers and infection can occur.

Diagnostic Findings

Lymphangiography reveals the degree and extent of blockage.

MEDICAL AND SURGICAL MANAGEMENT

Treatment is generally symptomatic. The affected part is elevated to promote lymphatic drainage. An elastic stocking or sleeve is worn when the leg or arm is in a dependent position. Massage starting at the toes or the fingers and moving toward the body and active exercises are helpful. A mechanical pulsating air-pressure device can be applied to the arm or leg at prescribed intervals. The alternating filling and emptying "milk" the lymph upward.

Sometimes the obstruction of lymphatics can be relieved with surgery. Congenital lymphedema responds poorly to surgical intervention. In some cases, the lymphedema persists despite treatment.

NURSING MANAGEMENT

The nurse inspects and measures the affected area to assess the extent of enlargement and condition of the skin. The client is encouraged to move and exercise the affected arm or leg to enhance the flow of lymph from the affected area. The nurse instructs clients to elevate legs when sitting and how to apply and use elastic garments and mechanical devices.

Extensive emotional support is necessary when the edema is severe. The client's self-esteem is often decreased, which can lead to social withdrawal. The nurse supports the client's self-image by suggesting certain styles of clothing that conceal abnormal enlargement of an arm or leg. For information on client teaching, see the discussion that follows nursing management for clients after a mastectomy in Chapter 59.

Lymphangitis and Lymphadenitis

Lymphangitis is inflammation of lymph channels. When the lymph nodes near the lymph channels are also affected, the condition is called **lymphadenitis.**

ETIOLOGY AND PATHOPHYSIOLOGY

An infectious agent, commonly streptococcal microorganisms, usually causes both conditions. The lymphatic structures manifest typical signs of inflammation: redness, swelling, discomfort, and compromised function.

ASSESSMENT FINDINGS

Signs and Symptoms

Red streaks follow the course of the lymph channels and extend up the arm or leg. Fever also may be present. When lymphadenitis is present, the lymph nodes along the lymphatic channels are enlarged and tender on palpation. Diagnosis is made by visual inspection and palpation.

MEDICAL MANAGEMENT

A broad-spectrum antibiotic commonly is ordered.

NURSING MANAGEMENT

The area is inspected two to three times daily and the response to antibiotic therapy noted. Assistance is given if the discomfort interferes with activities of daily living. Elevation reduces the swelling. Warmth promotes comfort and enhances circulation. The physician is notified if the affected area appears to enlarge, additional lymph nodes become involved, or the temperature remains elevated. In severe cases with persistent swelling, the nurse teaches the client how to apply an elastic sleeve or stocking.

Infectious Mononucleosis

Infectious mononucleosis is a disease that affects lymphoid tissues such as the tonsils and spleen. Other organs such as the brain and meninges can be involved as well.

ETIOLOGY AND PATHOPHYSIOLOGY

The **Epstein-Barr virus** causes infectious mononucleosis. This contagious disorder spreads by direct contact with saliva and pharyngeal secretions from an infected person. It is transmitted at the time of kissing; through oral spray during coughing, talking, or sneezing; or through sharing food or cigarettes and other items containing oral secretions. It most commonly affects young adults, especially those in close living quarters, such as in the armed services and college dormitories.

At the time of infection, the virus is engulfed by B lymphocytes, resulting in a display of the antigen on the lymphocyte cell surface. This is followed by an active production of T lymphocytes so as to create antibodies. The T lymphocytes infiltrate tissue, particularly the spleen, causing it to enlarge. Force to the abdomen can cause the spleen to rupture when it is enlarged.

ASSESSMENT FINDINGS

Signs and Symptoms

Fatigue, fever, sore throat, headache, and cervical lymph node enlargement typically occur. The tonsils ooze white or greenish gray exudate. Pharyngeal swelling can compromise swallowing and breathing. Some develop a faint red rash on their hands or abdomen. The liver and spleen become enlarged. The symptoms persist for several weeks.

Diagnostic Findings

The leukocyte and differential cell counts demonstrate lymphocytosis. A positive slide agglutination test (Monospot, Mono-test, Monostican) is presumptive evidence that the symptoms are due to the Epstein-Barr virus. A rise in the Epstein-Barr virus antibody titer and a heterophil agglutination test result of 1:224 or greater is conclusive for infectious mononucleosis.

MEDICAL MANAGEMENT

The infection is usually self-limiting. Bed rest, analgesic and antipyretic therapy, and increased fluid intake are recommended. Corticosteroid therapy is prescribed if complications such as hepatic involvement occur.

NURSING MANAGEMENT

The throat is inspected for the extent of inflammation or edema. Lymph nodes are gently palpated to detect swollen lymph nodes. Fluids are encouraged. The client is advised to rest as much as possible. If the client expresses concern over prolonged time off from work or school, the nurse takes time to listen and helps the client cope with the anxiety and concerns.

Lymphomas

The term **lymphoma** applies to a group of cancers that affect the lymphatic system. The types of lymphoma are classified by the microscopic appearance of the malignant cells and how quickly the malignancy spreads. Two of the most common forms of lymphoma are Hodgkin's disease and non-Hodgkin's lymphoma. Acquired immunodeficiency virus (AIDS)-related lymphoma occurs in those who have been infected with the human immunodeficiency virus.

Hodgkin's Disease

Hodgkin's disease is a malignancy that affects the lymph nodes.

ETIOLOGY AND PATHOPHYSIOLOGY

Although the exact cause of Hodgkin's disease is unknown, it appears that a virus alters the production and normal characteristics of lymphocytes. One virus that has been closely implicated in Hodgkin's disease is the Epstein-Barr virus. Initially there is a normal inflammatory and immune response to the virus after which the lymphocytes acquire malignant properties.

The malignant cell typical of Hodgkin's disease is the **Reed-Sternberg cell.** The disease is more common in men than in women and most frequently occurs during late adolescence and young adulthood. Some clients survive 10 or more years; others die in 4 to 5 years. A cure is possible when the disease is localized to one section of the body. Clients who receive treatment usually have remissions that last for months or even years. Death results from respiratory obstruction, cachexia, or secondary infections.

ASSESSMENT FINDINGS

Signs and Symptoms

Early symptoms of Hodgkin's disease include painless enlargement of one or more lymph nodes. The cervical lymph nodes are the first to be affected. As the nodes enlarge, they press on adjacent structures, such as the esophagus or bronchi. As retroperitoneal nodes enlarge, there is a sense of fullness in the stomach and epigastric pain. Marked weight loss, anorexia, fatigue, and weakness occur. Low-grade fever, pruritus, and night sweats are common. Sometimes marked anemia and thrombocytopenia develop, causing a tendency to bleed. Resistance to infection is poor, and staphylococcal skin infections and respiratory tract infections often complicate the illness.

Diagnostic Findings

Performing a biopsy of an affected lymph node or nodes identifies the presence of Reed-Sternberg cells. Lymphangiography, chest radiography, computed tomography, or magnetic resonance imaging demonstrate the size of lymph nodes and the spread of the disease within the thorax, abdomen, or pelvis. A bone marrow aspiration and biopsy indicate abnormalities of other blood cells. After diagnosis, the disease is staged from stage I to stage IV, based on the number of positive lymph nodes and the involvement of other organs (Table 39–1). Staging helps determine treatment.

MEDICAL MANAGEMENT

Treatment of Hodgkin's disease includes localized radiation to affected lymph nodes and

TABLE 39-1 **Stages of Hodgkin's Disease**

Stage	Involvement
I	Single lymph node region
II	Two or more lymph node regions on one side of the diaphragm
III	Lymph node regions on both sides of the diaphragm but extension is limited to the spleen
IV	Bilateral lymph nodes affected and extension includes spleen plus one or more of the following: bones, bone marrow, lungs, liver, skin, gastrointestinal structures, or other sites

chemotherapy therapy with combinations of antineoplastic drugs (Table 39–2). Antibiotics are given to fight secondary infections. Transfusions are prescribed to control anemia. If resistance to treatment develops, autologous bone marrow or peripheral stem cells are harvested followed by high doses of chemotherapy that destroy the bone marrow (see Chaps. 19 and 38). A transplant is performed after separating the normal stem cells from the malignant cells in the harvested specimen.

NURSING MANAGEMENT

The nurse implements interventions to ensure a patent airway, maintain or restore skin integrity, improve nutrition, facilitate activities of daily living, prevent opportunistic infection, reduce anxiety, support coping mechanisms, and explain treatment modalities and home care.

TABLE 39-2 **Chemotherapy Regimens for Hodgkin's Disease**

Regimen	Drugs
ABVD	Adriamycin (doxorubicin), bleomycin (Blenoxane), vinblastine (Velban), dacarbazine (DTIC)
MOPP	mechlorethamine (Mustargen), Oncovin (vincristine), prednisone (Meticorten), procarbazine (Matulane)
MOPP/ABV	Alternation of drugs from both regimens
For partial remission or relapse within 1 year	
CBV	cyclophosphamide (Cytoxan), BCNU (carmustine), Veposid (etoposide)
BEAM	BCNU (carmustine), etoposide (Veposid), cytosine arabinoside-e, melphalan (Alkeran)

NURSING PROCESS: *Care of the Client With Hodgkin's Disease*

Assessment

A general physical examination is performed to detect problems such as marked weight loss, impaired ventilation, bleeding tendencies, and skin infections.

Diagnosies and Planning

The care of a client with Hodgkin's disease includes, but is not limited to, the following:

Nursing Diagnoses and Collaborative Problems	Nursing Interventions
Risk for Ineffective Airway Clearance and **Risk for Impaired Gas Exchange** related to compression of trachea secondary to enlarged cervical lymph nodes **Goal:** The client's breathing will remain adequate to maintain blood saturation of 90% or greater.	Assess respiratory status each shift and prn. Keep the neck in midline and place the client in high Fowler's position if respiratory distress develops. Administer oxygen if blood saturation is consistently less than 90%. Place an endotracheal tube, laryngoscope, and bag-valve mask at the bedside for emergency intubation.
Risk for Infection related to immunosuppression secondary to impaired lymphocytes and drug or radiation therapy **Goal:** The client will be free of infection as evidenced by absence of fever and symptoms of secondary infection.	Restrict visitors or personnel with infections from client contact. Practice conscientious handwashing and follow other principles of medical and surgical asepsis. Institute infectious disease precautions if normal white blood cells are suppressed to dangerous limits.
Risk for Impaired Skin Integrity related to pruritus, inadequate nutrition, and inactivity **Goal:** The client's skin will remain intact throughout care.	Encourage or assist with changing positions at least every 2 hours. Use mild soap for bathing, rinse well, and pat dry. Apply ice to the skin for brief periods, cool sponge baths, or cotton gloves if itching is intolerable. An oral or topical antipruritic medication is often necessary. Trim nails short to avoid scratching when itching occurs. Change bedding as soon as possible if night sweats occur.

	Lift rather than pull client across sheets when changing positions.
	Support and protect bony prominences.
	Collaborate with physician to avoid drugs administered by the parenteral route.
Activity Intolerance and **Self-Care Deficit** related to anemia and generalized weakness from disease	Divide care into manageable sessions.
	Provide rest periods between activities.
Goal: The client will tolerate essential activities as evidenced by heart and respiratory rates within normal limits.	Perform priority activities first.
	Assist client with whatever activities of daily living are unmanageable independently.

Evaluation and Expected Outcomes

- Breathing pattern is normal.
- The client shows no signs or symptoms of infection.
- Skin remains intact.
- The client is able to perform essential activities.

Client and Family Teaching

Teach clients with Hodgkin's disease to:

- Keep appointments for medical follow-up.
- Take prescribed medications as directed and report side effects to the physician.
- Avoid crowds or people who have infectious diseases.
- Wash hands frequently and avoid oral contact with germ-laden objects.
- Contact the physician if breathing becomes labored.
- Eat small amounts frequently or include a liquid nutritional supplement between meals and at bedtime.
- Reduce work schedule to avoid exhaustion. If that is not possible, take frequent rest periods.
- Consult with an employer about sick-leave considerations or a representative from the Social Security Administration about unemployment benefits and disability payments.
- Obtain a disability sticker to facilitate easy access to public buildings and stores to lessen fatigue.

Non-Hodgkin's Lymphomas

Non-Hodgkin's lymphomas are a group of 10 or more malignant diseases that originate in lymph glands and other lymphoid tissue. Examples include lymphosarcoma, Burkitt's lymphoma, and reticulum cell sarcoma. The incidence of non-Hodgkin's lymphomas is six to seven times that of Hodgkin's disease and the number of cases continues to rise.

ETIOLOGY AND PATHOPHYSIOLOGY

No single definitive cause for non-Hodgkin's lymphomas has been found although a genetic link is strongly implicated in some types. An environmental "trigger," such as a viral agent, chemical herbicides, and hair dye, could induce the disease. The administration of immunosuppressive drugs for the prevention of transplant rejection also has been correlated with cases of non-Hodgkin's lymphoma.

In non-Hodgkin's lymphoma chromosomal changes occur in the affected lymphocytes, and lymphoid tissue enlarges to accommodate the proliferative production of malignant cells. The specific subtype of non-Hodgkin's lymphoma is categorized as low, intermediate, or high grade depending on the aggressive pattern of the disease.

ASSESSMENT FINDINGS

Signs and Symptoms

Symptoms of non-Hodgkin's lymphoma depend on the site of lymph node involvement. Lymph node enlargement, which is usually diffuse rather than localized, occurs in cervical, axillary, and inguinal regions.

Diagnostic Findings

The diagnosis and differentiation of the subtypes of non-Hodgkin's lymphoma from Hodgkin's disease depends on microscopic examination of biopsied lymphoid tissue. Additional tests are performed to determine the stage of the lymphoma.

MEDICAL MANAGEMENT

Non-Hodgkin's lymphoma is treated with chemotherapy alone or chemotherapy with radiation therapy. Research continues on using biologic therapy (immunotherapy) to eliminate the malignant cells and bring about remission. To do this, tumor-killing antibodies are attached to radioactive isotopes that seek out atypical cells. Bone marrow and stem cell transplants are considered a potential treatment modality when others are ineffective.

NURSING MANAGEMENT

Nursing care is similar for all clients with lymphoma whether they have non-Hodgkin's or

Hodgkin's disease. Because chemotherapy and radiation kill large numbers of cells, the nurse encourages clients to drink extra fluids (≥ 2,500 mL/d) to excrete the cells destroyed by therapy.

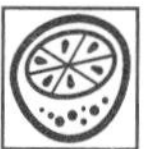

General Nutritional Considerations

The client with ulcerations of the oral mucosa can better tolerate soft, bland food and cold liquids.

Nausea and vomiting often accompany radiation therapy. Food and fluid intake must be maintained. Clear liquids such as carbonated beverages and water, ice pops, and flavored gelatin are offered until nausea subsides. Thereafter, small, frequent meals low in fat help prevent nausea.

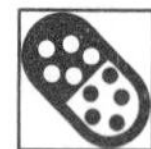

General Pharmacologic Considerations

The incidence of Hodgkin's and non-Hodgkin's lymphoma is increased in those taking the hydantoin drugs, such as phenytoin (Dilantin).

Supportive measures are necessary for clients experiencing toxic effects of chemotherapeutic agents. Bone marrow depression, gastrointestinal disturbances, and alopecia (hair loss) are common toxic effects.

Recognizing and treating adverse drug reactions can help promote an optimal response to therapy.

Clients with Hodgkin's disease are extremely susceptible to toxic effects of medication and to secondary infection due to the combination of treatments (ie, radiation and chemotherapy) plus a weakened immune system from the disease.

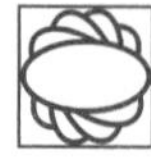

General Gerontologic Considerations

There is an increased risk of malignancies such as lymphoma in older adults primarily from the immunologic changes of aging and from prolonged exposure to carcinogens.

Doxorubicin and methotrexate are not well tolerated among older adults because of toxic effects on the kidney.

Older adults do not respond as well to chemotherapy as younger persons because they are unable to tolerate maximum doses.

The benefits of chemotherapy must be weighed against the adverse reactions that occur in older adults. However, treatment modalities are not based on age alone.

SUMMARY OF KEY CONCEPTS

- Lymphedema results from an obstruction of lymph circulation and can be congenitally acquired or secondary to disorders in which the flow of lymph is impaired.
- Nursing care of clients with lymphedema includes measures to prevent its occurrence when possible. Once the condition develops, the nurse promotes muscle contraction via exercise, elevation, and massage to reduce swelling.
- Conditions such as lymphangitis and lymphadenitis are associated with typical signs of an inflammatory response: redness along the lymphatic channel, localized swelling, tenderness, and compromised use of the affected body part. The nurse administers prescribed antibiotics, uses elevation and warmth to relieve swelling and promote comfort, and instructs the client on the technique for applying an elastic sleeve or stocking if prescribed.
- Infectious mononucleosis is a viral disease that affects lymphoid tissues such as the tonsils and spleen. Direct contact with saliva and pharyngeal secretions spreads the virus from an infected person. The nurse encourages a liberal intake of fluids and advises rest and limitation of activity.
- The term lymphoma applies to a group of cancers that affect the lymphatic system. Two of the most common forms of lymphoma are Hodgkin's disease and non-Hodgkin's lymphoma.
- The malignant cell type of Hodgkin's disease is called a Reed-Sternberg cell.
- The primary modalities currently used for curing lymphomas or promoting remission include:
  - Chemotherapy with antineoplastic drugs
  - Radiation therapy
  - Transplantation of bone marrow or stem cells
- Some common problems among clients with lymphomas include risk for ineffective airway clearance, risk for impaired gas exchange, risk for infection, risk for impaired skin integrity, activity intolerance, and self-care deficit.

CRITICAL THINKING EXERCISES

1. List the differences between lymphedema and lymphoma.
2. Discuss remedial measures the nurse offers the client who has lymphedema.
3. What teaching is indicated for a person who has been diagnosed with Hodgkin's disease?

Suggested Readings

Badger, C. (1996). Treating lymphoedema. *Nursing Times, 92*(11), *Journal of Wound Care Nursing*, 84, 86, 88.

Campbell, K. (1996). Lymphomas: Aetiology, classification, and treatment. *Nursing Times, 92*(9),44–45.

Campbell, K. (1995). Understanding acute and chronic myeloid leukaemia. *Nursing Times, 91*(47), 36–38.

Carter, B. J. (1997). Women's experiences of lymphedema. *Oncology Nursing Forum, 24*(5), 875–882.

Cozad, J. (1996). Infectious mononucleosis. *Nurse Practitioner, 21*(3), 14–16, 23, 27–28.

Farfan, D. (1997). There's always hope. *RN, 60*(6), 31–32.

Harbit, M., & Srinivas, P. B. (1995). Kaposi's sarcoma with elephantiasis associated with AIDS. *Journal of Wound Ostomy Continence Nursing, 22*(5), 223–226.

Hopkins, E. (1996). Sequential compression to treat lymphoedema. *Professional Nurse, 11*(6), 397–398.

Newman, M. L., Passik, S., & Brennan, M. (1996). Lymphedema complicated by pain and psychological distress: A case with complex treatment needs. *Journal of Pain and Symptom Management, 12*(6). 376–379.

Nickalls, S. (1996). Fluid forces...massage, lymphoedema, manual lymph drainage. *Nursing Times, 92*(13), 52–53.

Rivera, L. M. (1997). Blood cell transplantation: Its impact on one family. *Seminars in Oncology Nursing, 13*(3), 194–199.

Servodidio, C. A., & Abramson, D. H. (1997). Lymphoma. *Insight* 22(1), 22–24.

Shaffer, S. (1996). Benign lymphoproliferative disorders. *Seminars in Oncology Nursing, 12*(1), 28–37.

Warmkessel, J. H. (1997). Caring for the patient with non-Hodgkin's lymphoma. *Nursing, 27*(6), 48–49.

Additional References

Lymphoma Research Foundation of America
8800 Venice Boulevard
Suite 207
Los Angeles, CA 90034
(301) 204–7040
http://www.lymphoma.org

Cure for Lymphoma Foundation
http://www.cfl.org/

National Cancer Institute
Office of Cancer Communications
31 Center Drive
MSC 2580
Bethesda, MD 20892–2580

9

Caring for Clients With Immune Disorders

Chapter 40

Introduction to the Immune System

KEY TERMS

Anergy
Antibodies
Antigens
Artificially acquired active immunity
Cell-mediated response
Cytotoxic T cells
Effector T cells
Helper T cells
Humoral response
Immune response
Immunoglobulins
Lymphokines
Macrophages
Memory cells
Microphages
Monocytes
Naturally acquired active immunity
Neutrophils
Passive immunity
Phagocytosis
Plasma cells
Regulator T cells
Stem cells
Suppressor T cells

LEARNING OBJECTIVES

On completion of this chapter, the reader will:

- Explain the meaning of an immune response.
- List two general components of the immune system.
- Discuss the role of T- and B-cell lymphocytes.
- Differentiate between an antigen and antibody.
- Name examples of lymphoid tissue.
- Name three types of immunity and describe how each develops.
- Discuss techniques for detecting immune disorders.
- Describe the role of the nurse when caring for a client with an immune disorder.

The immune system is responsible for protecting the body from invasion by infectious, foreign, or cancerous cells. It does this by activating the immune response. The **immune response** is the protective mechanism that occurs in the presence of atypical or foreign proteins. This response is carried out primarily by lymphocytes, specialized cells located in the blood and lymphoid tissue. These cells search for and destroy unnatural or potentially harmful cells. Hyperactivity of the immune system, as in allergic or autoimmune disorders (see Chap. 41), or a decrease in its function, as in AIDS (see Chap. 42), can be life-threatening.

Structures of the Immune System

The immune system consists of specialized white blood cells and lymphoid tissues.

White Blood Cells

White blood cells (leukocytes) are produced in the bone marrow. Initially they are nonspecific **stem cells** that later differentiate into various types of blood cells including lymphocytes, neutrophils, and monocytes. The function of the various leukocytes is summarized in Table 40–1.

LYMPHOCYTES

Lymphocytes, which are either T-cell or B-cell lymphocytes, comprise 20% to 30% of all leukocytes (Copstead, 1995). T- and B-cell lymphocytes are the primary participants in the immune response. They distinguish harmful substances and ignore those natural and unique to the individual. Figure 40–1 shows the development and role of T- and B-cell lymphocytes.

T-Cell Lymphocytes

The T-cell lymphocytes are manufactured in bone marrow and travel to the thymus gland where they mature to become either regulator T cells or effector T cells. **Regulator T cells** are made up of helper and suppressor cells; **effector T cells** are killer (cytotoxic) cells. **Helper T cells** are especially important in fighting infection. They recognize **antigens,** protein markers on cells, and form additional T-cell clones that stimulate B-cell lymphocytes to produce antibodies against foreign antigens. **Antibodies** are chemical

TABLE 40-1 **Type and Functions of Lymphocytes**

Type	Function
T Cells	
Regulator T cells	
Helper T cells	Recognize antigens; stimulate B cells to produce antibodies
Suppressor T cells	Turn off the immune response
Effector cells	
Cytotoxic cells	Bind to and destroy invader cells; stimulate the release of lymphokines
B Cells	
Plasma cells	Produce antibodies
Memory cells	Convert to plasma cells that will produce antibodies when reexposed to an antigen

substances that destroy foreign agents such as microorganisms. Helper T cells also are called T4 cells or CD4 cells. **Cytotoxic T cells** bind to invading cells, destroy the targeted invader by altering their cellular membrane and intracellular environment, and release chemicals called lymphokines. **Lymphokines** attract neutrophils and monocytes to remove the debris. **Suppressor T cells** limit or turn off the immune response in the absence of continued antigenic stimulation. Because the surface molecules of suppressor and killer T cells are different from those of helper T cells, they sometimes are referred to as T8 or CD8 cells.

The immune response performed by T-cell lymphocytes is called a cell-mediated response. A **cell-mediated response** occurs when T cells survey proteins in the body, actively analyze the surface features, and respond to those that are different from the host by directly attacking the invading antigen. An example of a cell-mediated responses is one that occurs when an organ is transplanted.

B-Cell Lymphocytes

The B-cell lymphocytes mature in the bone marrow and migrate to the spleen and other lymphoid tissues such as the lymph nodes. When stimulated by T cells, the B cells become either plasma or memory cells. **Plasma cells** produce antibodies. **Memory cells** convert to plasma cells on re-exposure to a specific antigen. When activated, B cells accumulate in lymphoid tissues, which explains the phenomena of swollen and tender lymph nodes that accompany infectious disorders and an enlarged spleen in various immune disorders.

Formation of antibodies is called a **humoral response** because it involves substances, namely antibodies, contained in body fluid. Antibodies are more correctly referred to as **immunoglobulins** (Ig) because they are components of gamma globulins, serum (plasma) proteins. There are five classes of immunoglobulins: IgA, IgD, IgE, IgG, and IgM. Each

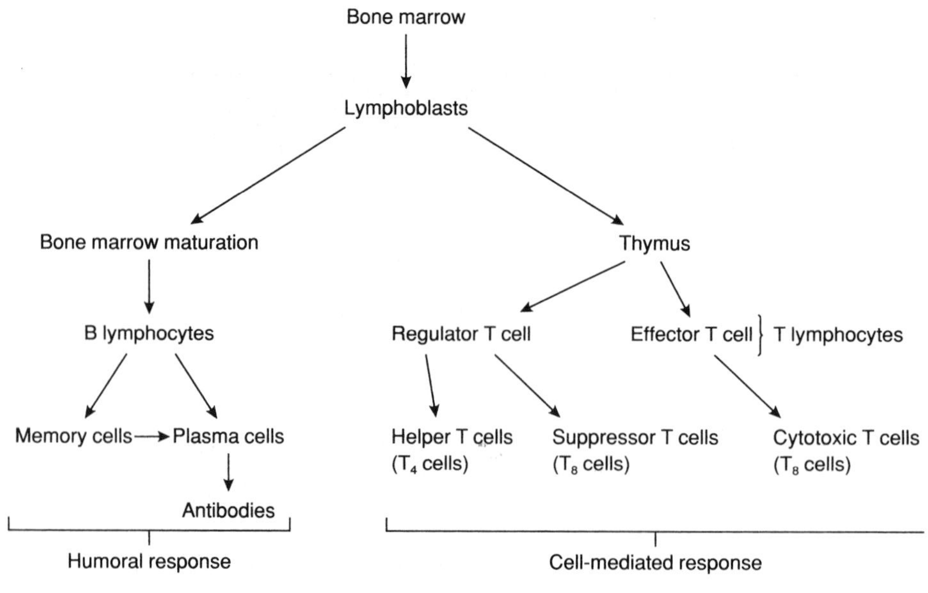

FIGURE 40-1. The development and role of B lymphocytes and T lymphocytes.

immunoglobulin has a separate role in ensuring the maintenance of a healthy state (Table 40–2).

NEUTROPHILS AND MONOCYTES

Neutrophils and **monocytes** are phagocytes, cells that perform phagocytosis. **Phagocytosis** is the process of engulfing and digesting bacteria and foreign material. Phagocytes are stationary (fixed) or mobile. Neutrophils, also called **microphages** because they are small, are present in blood and migrate to tissue as necessary. Monocytes, also called **macrophages** because they are large, are present in tissues such as the lungs, liver, lymph nodes, spleen, and peritoneum (Fig. 40–2). They also migrate following a cell-mediated response. The mononuclear phagocyte system was formerly known as the reticuloendothelial system.

Lymphoid Tissues

Lymphoid tissues (Fig. 40–3), such as the thymus gland, tonsils and adenoids, spleen, and lymph nodes play a role in the immune response and preventing infection (see Chap. 37). Lymphoid tissue is also present on the surface of mucous membranes of the intestine, on alveolar membranes in the lungs, and in the lining of the sinusoids of the liver. Bone marrow is sometimes included as a component of the immune system because it produces undifferentiated stem cells.

THYMUS GLAND

The thymus gland is located in the neck below the thyroid gland. It extends into the thorax behind the top of the sternum. The thymus gland produces lymphocytes during fetal development. It may be the embryonic origin of other lymphoid structures such as the spleen and lymph nodes. After birth, the thymus gland programs T lymphocytes to become regulator T cells or effector T cells. The thymus gland becomes smaller at the time of adolescence but retains some activity throughout the life cycle.

TONSILS AND ADENOIDS

The tonsils are located on either side of the soft palate of the oropharynx. The adenoids are located behind the nose on the posterior wall of the nasopharynx. These tissues filter bacteria from tissue fluid. Because they are exposed to pathogens in the oral and nasal passages, they can become infected and locally inflamed.

SPLEEN

The spleen has both hematopoietic and immune functions. It acts as an emergency reservoir of blood and filters the blood as well. Macrophages present in the spleen remove bacteria and old, dead, or damaged blood cells from circulation.

LYMPH NODES

The lymphatic system consists of vessels similar to capillaries that drain tissue fluid, called lymph. At various areas in the body, the lymphatics converge and drain into larger structures called lymph nodes. The lymph nodes contain B lymphocytes and T lymphocytes and remove bacteria and other foreign par-

TABLE 40-2 **Types of Immunoglobulins**

Type	Percent of Total	Location	Function
IgG	75%	Intravascular and intercellular fluid	Neutralizes bacterial toxins; accelerates phagocytosis
IgA	15%	Body secretions such as saliva, sweat, tears, mucus, bile, colostrum	Interferes with entry of pathogens through exposed structures or pathways
IgM	10%	Intravascular serum	Agglutinates (clusters) antigens and lyses (dissolves) cell walls
IgD	0.2%	Surface of lymphocytes	Binds to antigens; promotes secretion of other immunoglobulins
IgE	0.004%	Surface of basophils and mast (connective tissue) cells	Promotes release of vasoactive chemicals such as histamine and bradykinin in allergic, hypersensitivity, and anti-inflammatory reactions

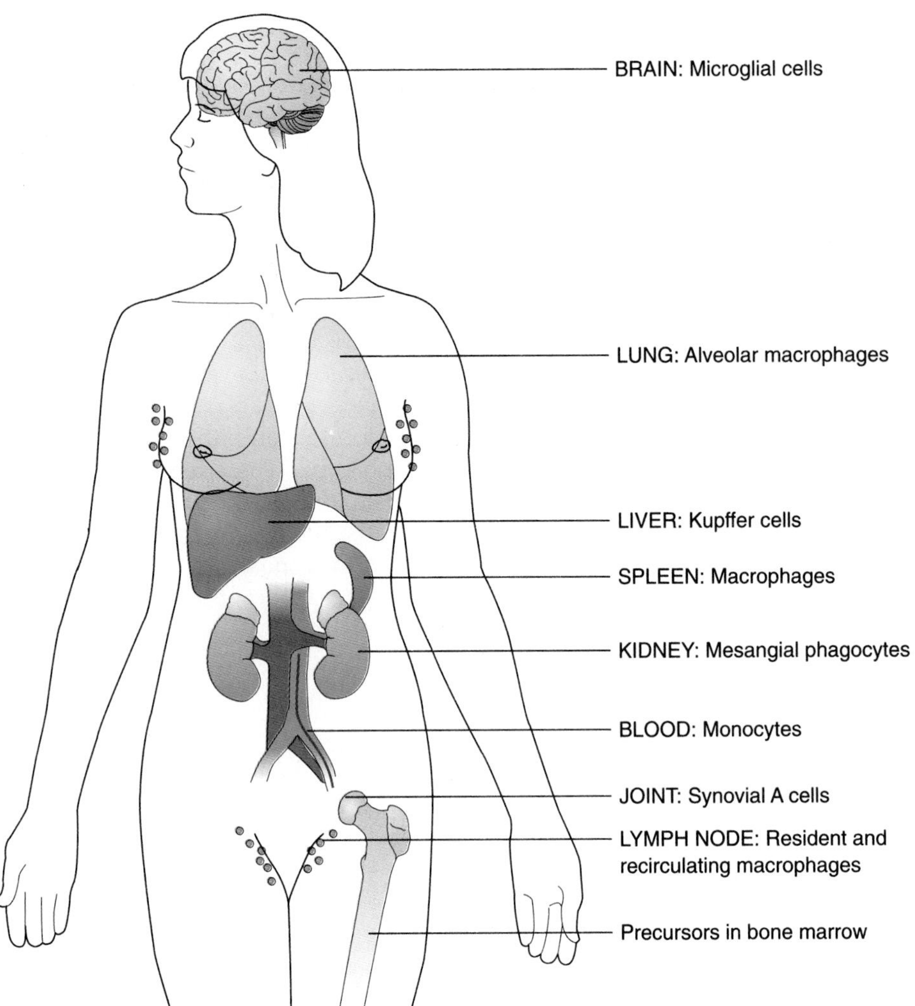

FIGURE 40-2. Locations of phagocytes.

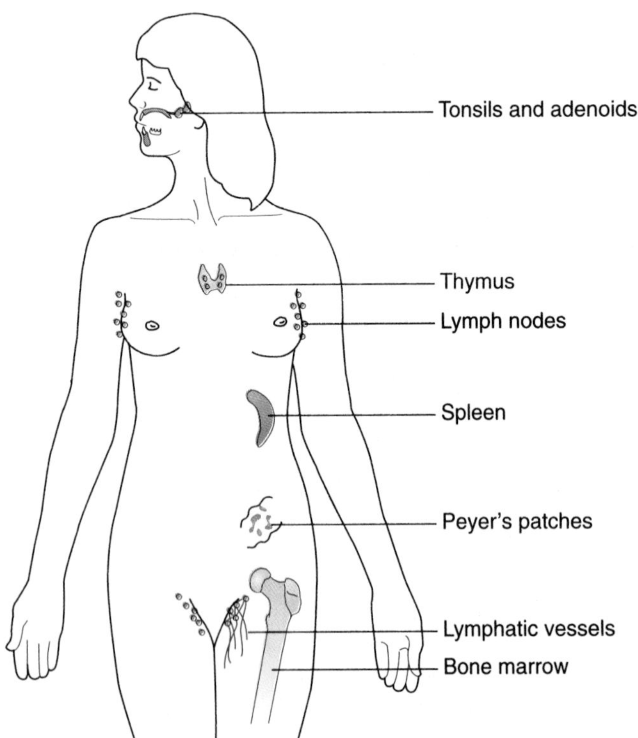

FIGURE 40-3. Lymphoid tissue.

icles from the lymph. Superficial lymph nodes in the axilla, groin, and neck are palpable when enlarged.

Types of Immunity

The three types of immunity are naturally acquired active immunity, artificially acquired active immunity, and passive immunity (Fig. 40–4). Both forms of active immunity require the individual's own production of plasma and memory cells. Passive immunity occurs when ready-made antibodies are provided.

Naturally Acquired Active Immunity

Naturally acquired active immunity occurs as a direct result of infection by a specific microorganism. An example is the immunity to measles that develops after the initial infection. Not all invading microorganisms produce a response that gives lifelong immunity.

Artificially Acquired Active Immunity

Artificially acquired active immunity results from the administration of a killed or weakened microorganism or toxoid (attenuated toxin). The memory cells manufactured by the B lymphocytes "remember" the killed or weakened antigen and recognize it if a future invasion occurs. Refer to Chapter 18 for a recommended schedule for childhood immunizations. Immunizations that are not administered or completed during childhood are recommended for adults. Some immunizations, such as those for tetanus and influenza, require readministration to retain adequate immunity.

Passive Immunity

Passive immunity develops when ready-made antibodies are given to a susceptible individual. The antibodies provide immediate but short-lived protection from the invading antigen. No memory cells are

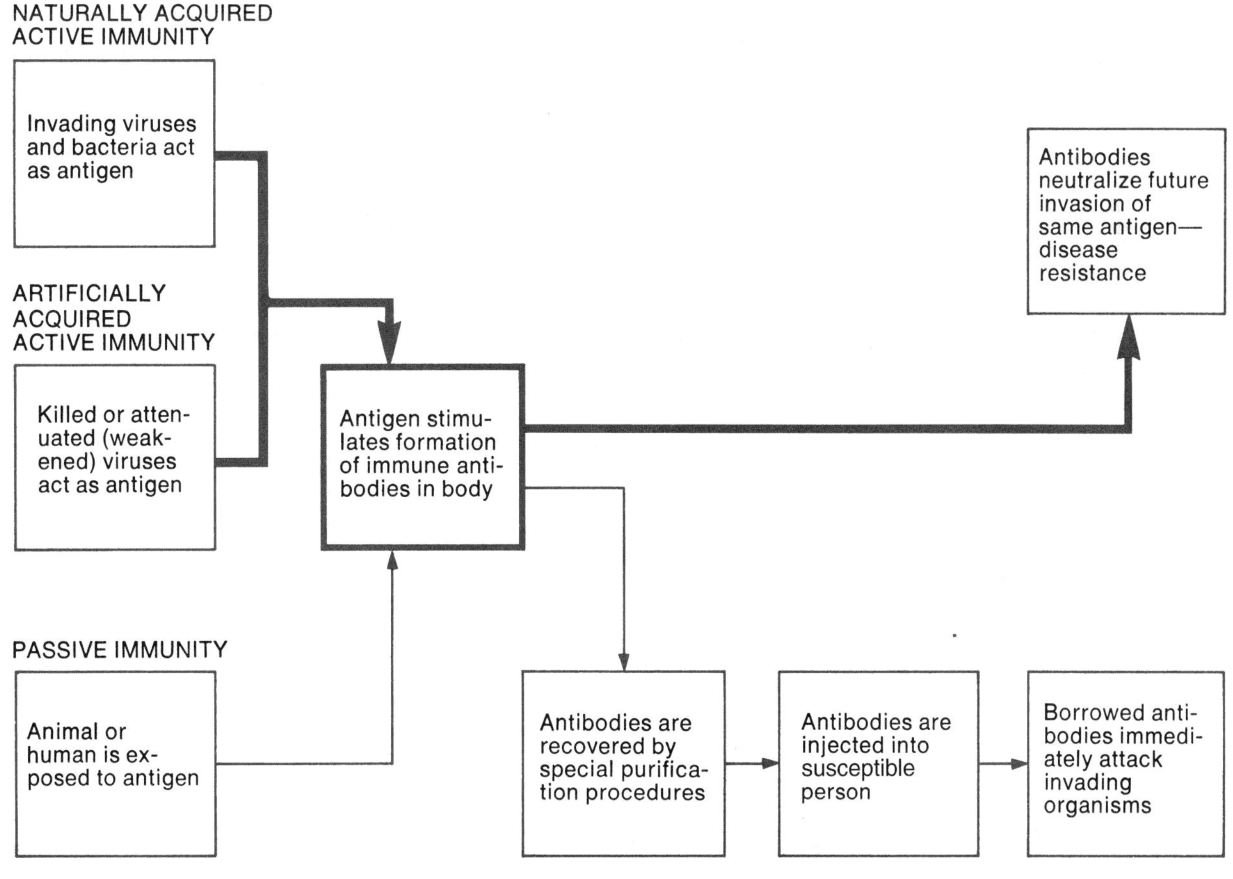

FIGURE 40-4. Active and passive immunity.

produced, and the level of the injected antibodies diminishes over a period of several weeks to a few months.

Ready-made antibodies are obtained from the serum of another organism, either animal or human. Immune serum globulin, also called gamma globulin or immunoglobulins, is recovered from pooled human plasma. Because the pool comprises plasma from more than one donor, the serum is likely to contain a variety of specific antibodies. Human immune serum is used for passive immunization against measles (rubella), pertussis (whooping cough), hepatitis B, chickenpox (varicella), and tetanus.

Newborns receive passive immunity to some diseases for which their mothers have manufactured antibodies. The circulating maternal antibodies cross the placental barrier. As with other forms of passive immunity, infants are protected for only a few months after birth.

Assessment

Obtain a history of immunizations, recent and past infectious diseases, and recent exposure to infectious diseases. Review the client's drug history because certain drugs (eg, corticosteroids) suppress the inflammatory and immune responses. Investigate the client's allergy history. Question the client regarding practices that put him or her at risk for acquired immunodeficiency syndrome (AIDS) (see Chap. 43).

Begin the physical examination with a general appraisal of the client's health. Note whether the client appears healthy, acutely or mildly ill, malnourished, extremely tired, or listless. Record vital signs and weight. Examine the skin for rashes or lesions. Assess the abdomen for an enlarged liver or spleen. Inspect the pharynx for large, red tonsils and purulent drainage. Palpate the lymph nodes in the neck, axilla, and groin for enlargement and tenderness.

Diagnostic Tests

Laboratory tests are used to identify immune system disorders. This generally includes a complete blood count with differential. Protein electrophoresis screens for diseases associated with a deficiency or excess of immunoglobulins. T- and B-cell assays (or counts) and the enzyme-linked immunosorbent assay (ELISA) (see Chap. 42) may be performed. Additional tests are performed when an autoimmune or genetic immune disorder is suspected (see Chap. 41).

Skin tests may be administered. Disease-specific antigens, such as purified protein derivative of the tuberculin toxin, are injected intradermally on the inner aspect of the forearm. The injection area becomes swollen if the client has developed antibodies against the antigen in the past (see Chap. 18). The client is not necessarily actively infectious if the test is positive (see Chap. 28). Skin tests using various common disease antigens like mumps are administered if anergy is suspected. **Anergy** is the inability to mount an immune response. It is a common finding among clients who have AIDS or who are immunosuppressed for other reasons.

Nursing Management

Clearly identify any substances to which the client is allergic. Consult drug references to verify that prescribed medications do not contain substances to which the client is hypersensitive. Explain all diagnostic skin testing procedures. Inform the client when to return to have the results of a skin test interpreted. Ensure that a written consent is obtained before testing for human immunodeficiency virus (HIV); keep the results of HIV testing confidential. Use Standard Precautions whenever there is the potential for contact with blood or body fluids. Follow agency guidelines for controlling infectious diseases or protecting the client who is immunosuppressed. Educate clients regarding immunizations. Provide instructions regarding drug therapy prescribed for disorders involving the immune system.

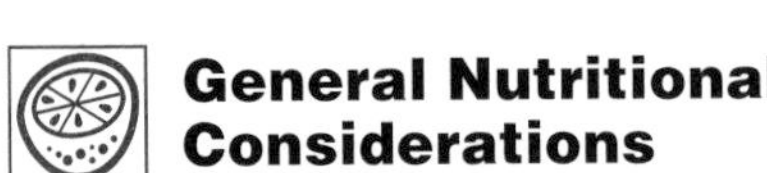

General Nutritional Considerations

Nutrients important in immune system functioning include amino acids; certain fatty acids; the B vitamins; vitamins A, C, and E; and the minerals zinc, iron, copper, magnesium, and selenium. Singly or combined, nutrient deficiencies have the potential to affect almost all aspects of immune system functioning. However, the exact amounts and proportions of nutrients needed for optimal immune system function in healthy people are not yet known. Newer studies clearly indicate that the availability of one nutrient may impair or enhance the action of another nutrient in immune system functioning; nutrient supplements may enhance or suppress immune function through the effects of that supplement on other nutrients. Until more is known about nutrient interactions, the best dietary advice to maximize immune function in healthy people is to eat a moderate diet that is balanced and varied.

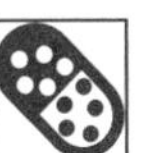

General Pharmacologic Considerations

Some drugs are capable of suppressing immune system function. Examples of these drugs are certain antibiotics, corticosteroids, some of the nonsteroidal anti-inflammatory drugs, and many drugs used in the treatment of cancer.

Intentional suppression of the immune system is used after organ transplantation. Azathioprine (Imuran), cyclosporine (Sandimmune), and muromonab-CD3 (Orthoclone OKT3) are immunosuppressive drugs.

When taking drugs to suppress the immune system, the client has no defense against disease and is at increased risk to develop infection, especially a respiratory or urinary infection. The client is observed for signs and symptoms of infection such as fever, sore throat, productive cough, dysuria, etc.

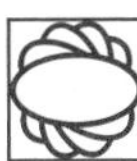

General Gerontologic Considerations

The older client is more likely to have a problem related to the immune system because the activity of the immune system declines during the natural aging process.

Older adults with chronic diseases such as respiratory disorders or cardiac disease should have an annual influenza vaccine and a one-time pneumococcal vaccine.

Although vaccination against viral disorders is recommended for older adults, vaccines are less effective in an older adult than in a younger adult, probably due to the decreased immune response seen with age.

SUMMARY OF KEY CONCEPTS

- The immune response is a protective mechanism that occurs in the presence of atypical or foreign proteins.
- The immune system consists of specialized white blood cells and lymphoid tissues.
- T- and B-cell lymphocytes are the primary participants in the immune response. Neutrophils and monocytes have a supportive role in eliminating inactivated antigens and cellular debris from the body.
- T-cell lymphocytes facilitate a cell-mediated immune response with helper, killer, and suppressor cells. B-cell lymphocytes carry out a humoral immune response by manufacturing antibodies (immunoglobulins) or cells with the potential to do so later.
- An antigen is a protein marker. An antibody is a chemical substance that destroys antigens perceived as harmful.
- Lymphoid tissue includes the thymus gland, tonsils and adenoids, spleen, and lymph nodes. Immune functions are also enhanced by specialized cells on the surface of mucous membranes of the intestine, on alveolar membranes in the lungs, and in the lining of the sinusoids of the liver.
- The immune system can be stimulated to produce three types of immunity: naturally acquired active immunity, artificially acquired active immunity, and passive immunity.
- Active immunity develops when the individual produces self-made antibodies in response to an actual infection or as a consequence of instilling a dead or weakened form of a pathogenic organism. Passive immunity develops when premade antibodies are given to a susceptible individual.
- The presence of immune disorders is determined by obtaining a comprehensive medical history, especially concerning current signs and symptoms, previous infectious disorders or allergic reactions, an immunization history, and exposure to infectious agents, and monitoring the results of diagnostic tests.
- The role of the nurse in caring for clients with immune disorders involves identifying susceptible individuals, performing skin tests, safeguarding the client's health by avoiding substances to which there is a known allergy, administering medications to suppress hyperactive immune responses, and protecting susceptible or immunosuppressed clients from acquiring infectious diseases.

CRITICAL THINKING EXERCISES

1. How would you respond to a friend who tells you that her sister has an immune disorder and asks what this means?
2. Discuss the benefit of obtaining immunizations for common childhood diseases.
3. Explain the type of immunity that develops from receiving a vaccine for hepatitis B, from having chickenpox, and from receiving an injection of gamma globulin.

Suggested Readings

Bottum, C. L., Bacall, D., & Balsam, A. (1995). Prevention update. Better than chicken soup: Encouraging older patients to receive influenza immunization. *Caring, 14*(11), 70–73.

Bullock, B. (1996). *Pathophysiology: Adaptations and alterations in function.* Philadelphia: Lippincott-Raven.

Copstead, L. C. (1995). *Perspectives on pathophysiology.* Philadelphia: Saunders.

Deasy, J. (1997). How the immune system responds to infection. *Journal of the American Academy of Physician Assistants, 10*(5), 73–74, 76, 79–80.

Dudek, S. G. (1997). *Nutrition handbook for nursing practice* (3rd ed.). Philadelphia: Lippincott-Raven.

Fischbach, F. T. (1996). *A manual of laboratory diagnostic tests* (5th ed.). Philadelphia: Lippincott-Raven.

Kaiser, F. E., & Marley, J. E. (1994). Idiopathic CD4+ T lymphopenia in older persons. *Journal of the American Geriatrics Society, 42*(12), 1291–1294.

Memmler, R. L., Cohen, B. J., & Wood, D. L. (1996). *The human body in health and disease* (8th ed.). Philadelphia: Lippincott-Raven.

National Institutes of Health. (1994). *The immune system–how it works.* (Publication No. 94–3229). Bethesda, MD: Author.

Nowak, T. J., & Handford, A. G. (1994). *Essentials of pathophysiology.* Dubuque, IA: Wm. C. Brown.

Post-White, J. (1996). The immune system. *Seminars in Oncology Nursing, 12*(2), 89–96.

Price, S. A., & Wilson, L. M. (1996). *Pathophysiology: Clinical concepts of disease processes* (5th ed.). St. Louis: Mosby.

Smeltzer, S. C., & Bare, B. G. (1996). *Brunner and Suddarth's textbook of medical-surgical nursing.* Philadelphia: Lippincott-Raven.

Westwood, O. M. R. (1997). Nutrition and immune function...part 1. *Nursing Times, 93*(15), 1–6.

Chapter 41

Caring for Clients With Allergic and Autoimmune Disorders

KEY TERMS

Allergen
Allergic disorder
Autoantibodies
Autoimmune disorder
Desensitization
Histocompatible cells
Mast cells

LEARNING OBJECTIVES

On completion of this chapter, the reader will:

- Describe an allergic disorder.
- List five examples of allergic signs and symptoms.
- Name four categories of allergens and give an example of each.
- Give four examples of allergic reactions including two that are potentially life-threatening.
- Describe diagnostic skin testing.
- Name three methods for treating allergies.
- Discuss the nursing management of a client with an allergic disorder.
- Explain the meaning of autoimmune disorder and give at least three examples of related diseases.
- Discuss at least one theory that explains the development of an autoimmune disorder.
- Name three categories of drugs used in the treatment of autoimmune disorders.
- Discuss the nursing management of a client with an autoimmune disorder.

The immune system sometimes responds excessively to substances that are not potentially harmful. When this occurs, individuals manifest allergic and autoimmune disorders.

Allergic Disorders

An **allergic disorder** is characterized by a hyperimmune response to weak antigens that are usually harmless (Table 41–1). The antigens that can cause an allergic response are called **allergens.** Allergies can occur at any age, and the pattern of allergic response can vary in the same person over the years. People may suddenly develop an allergic reaction to a substance with which they have had contact for years. On the other hand, allergic responses to one agent may gradually disappear, to be replaced by sensitivity to another substance. The reason for these changes is not clear.

Types of Allergies

An allergic disorder is manifested in a variety of ways depending on the manner in which the allergen gains entry to the body and the intensity of the response. Organs and structures that are primarily involved in an allergic reaction include the skin, respiratory passageways, and gastrointestinal tract (Table 41–2). Some types of allergic manifestations (eg, allergic rhinitis) cause temporary, localized discomfort, whereas others, such as anaphylaxis and angioedema, are life-threatening.

TABLE 41-1 **Common Allergens**

Type of Allergen	Examples	Common Reaction
Ingestants	Food, drugs (especially penicillin)	Gastroenteropathy, dermatitis, asthma, anaphylaxis, urticaria, angioedema, serum sickness
Inhalants	House dust and mites, insect excrement, animal products (dander, saliva, urine), pollens, and spores	Allergic asthma, dermatitis, rhinitis, hypersensitivity pneumonitis
Contactants	Plant oils, topical medications, occupational chemicals, cosmetics, metals in jewelry and clothing fasteners, hair dyes, latex	Contact dermatitis, rare urticaria or anaphylaxis
Injectant	Drugs, bee venom	Anaphylaxis, angioedema, acute urticaria

Etiology and Pathophysiology

Approximately 10% to 15% of the population develop allergies. The tendency can be inherited. Although members in the same family may have allergies, they may not be sensitive to the same allergens. Allergy-prone individuals may react to more than one type of antigen. For example, some may be sensitive to ragweed pollen and a food product such as eggs.

The first exposure to an allergen does not produce symptoms. However, T-cell lymphocytes process the antigen and present it to B-cell lymphocytes. The B-cell lymphocytes promptly produce IgE antibodies that become attached to basophils or mast cells. **Mast cells** are constituents of connective tissue that contain small amounts of heparin, serotonin, bradykinin, and histamine. With subsequent exposures to the allergen, mast cells and basophils release their vasoactive chemicals, increasing cell permeability (Fig. 41–1). Initially this produces localized reactions such as watery eyes, increased nasal and bronchial secretions, sneezing, vomiting, and diarrhea. Later, additional symptoms such as swelling, itching, and localized redness occur. Histamine causes vasodilation that, if massive, causes hypotension and bronchoconstriction.

Assessment Findings

SIGNS AND SYMPTOMS

Clients often identify a cause and effect relationship between particular substances and their allergic symptoms. Respiratory symptoms can include nasal stuffiness, runny nose, sneezing, coughing, dyspnea,

TABLE 41-2 **Types of Allergies**

Allergy Type	Signs and Symptoms	Medical Management
Allergic rhinitis	Sneezing, itching, nasal congestion, watery nasal discharge, itching and redness of the eyes	Antihistamines, nasal decongestants, corticosteroid nasal spray, immunotherapy, allergen avoidance, eye drops
Contact dermatitis	Itching, burning, redness, rash on contact with substance	Allergen avoidance, wearing gloves, topical or oral antihistamines and corticosteroids
Dermatitis medicamentosa	Sudden generalized bright red rash, itching, fever, malaise, headache, or arthralgias	Discontinuation of drug, antihistamines and topical corticosteroids
Food allergy	Nausea, vomiting, diarrhea, abdominal cramping, malaise, itching, wheezing, rash, cough	Identification and avoidance of allergenic food
Urticaria	Itching, swelling, redness, wheals of superficial skin layers	Topical or oral antihistamines and corticosteroids
Angioedema	Itching, swelling, redness of deeper tissues and mucous membranes	Intubation, subcutaneous epinephrine, aminophylline

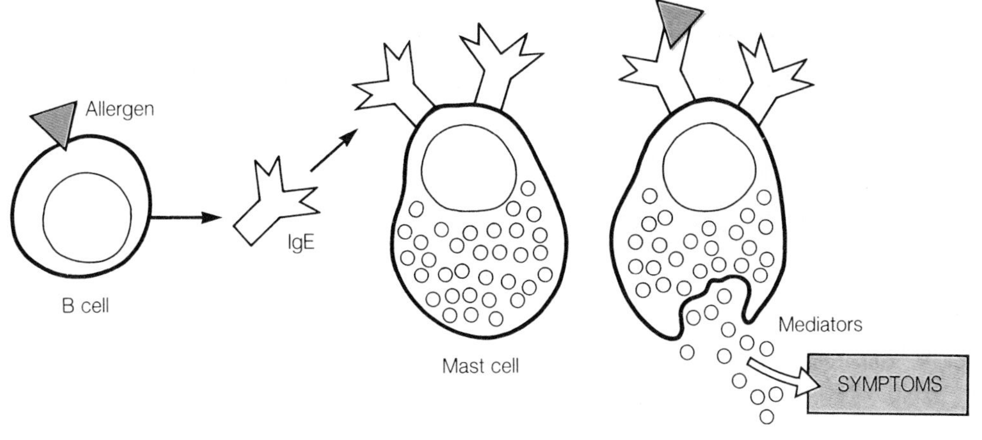

FIGURE 41-1. Process that leads to allergic manifestations.

and wheezing. Skin reactions include hives, rash, and localized itching. Cramping, vomiting, and diarrhea are associated with food allergies. Systemic and potentially fatal effects include shock and airway obstruction caused by swelling. Clients exhibit the same reaction with each exposure to the allergen.

DIAGNOSTIC FINDINGS

Diagnosis of an allergy may be simple and clear-cut or may require multiple tests and an extensive history. The fact that the client may be allergic to more than one substance, and the tendency for symptoms to vary with fatigue, emotional stress, or the seasons, complicates diagnosis.

Various abnormalities in blood tests suggest an allergic disorder. For example, the eosinophil count may be elevated. The radioallergosorbent test (RAST) measures IgE. On a scale of 0 to 5, 2 or greater is a significant measurement.

Specific allergens can be identified by skin testing with extracts of various substances (antigens), such as pollens, animal danders, food, and dust. The three methods of skin testing are the intradermal injection, the scratch or prick test, and the patch test. In the intradermal test, a dilute solution of an antigen is injected intradermally. A positive reaction is based on the size of a raised wheal and localized erythema (redness) that forms where the antigen was injected (Fig. 41–2). The scratch or prick test involves making a scratch on the skin and applying a small amount of the liquid test antigen to the scratch (Fig. 41–3). If a raised wheal or localized erythema appears, a positive reaction to the antigen has occurred. The patch test is used for identifying the offending allergen in allergic contact dermatitis. A concentrated form of the substance is applied to the skin and covered with an occlusive dressing. After 48 hours, the dressing is removed and the area examined for erythema, edema, and vesicles. Food allergens are identified by eliminating all food for several days and then monitoring for symptoms as a new food is added to the diet (Nursing Guidelines 41–1).

Medical Management

The treatment used to relieve the symptoms of an allergy depends on the type of allergy. Besides avoiding

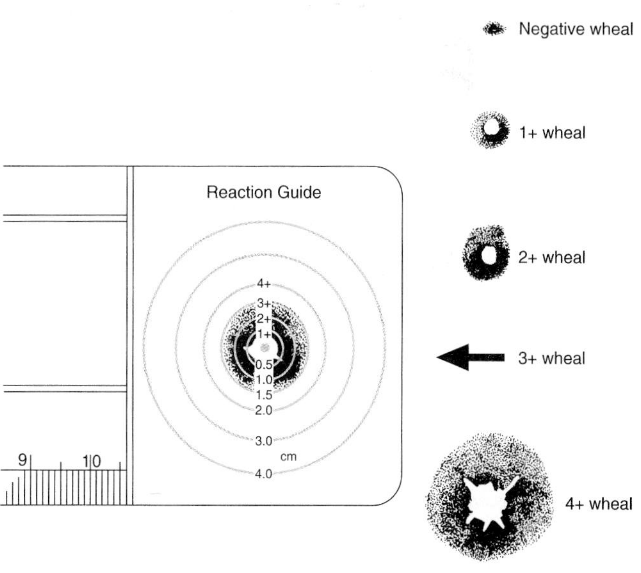

FIGURE 41-2. The wheal that forms after an intradermal skin test is measured to interpret the allergic response. The following scale is used: Negative = soft wheal and minimal redness; 1+ = 5–8 mm wheal and redness; 2+ = 7–20 mm wheal and redness; 3+ = 9–15 mm asymmetrical wheal and redness; 4+ = >12 mm asymmetrical wheal and diffuse redness.

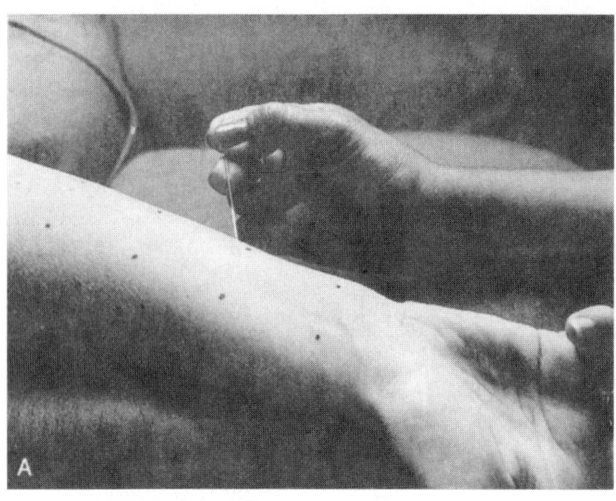

FIGURE 41-3. The prick method of skin testing.

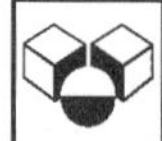

Nursing Guidelines 41-1

Identifying Food Allergens

- Client fasts for 1 to 2 days drinking only distilled water.
- Hypoallergenic foods (such as rice and tapioca) are introduced one at a time.
- Allergenic foods (such as wheat and peanuts) are introduced one at a time in small quantities.
- Client is observed for allergic symptoms after each new food is introduced.

TABLE 41-3 **Drug Therapy for Allergic Disorders**

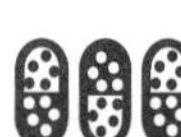

Drug Category/Drug Action	Side Effects	Nursing Considerations
Antihistamines		
diphenhydramine (Benadryl) hydroxyzine (Atarax) terfenadine (Seldane) astemizole (Hismanal) loratidine (Claritin) Block histamine receptors	Common: sedation, dryness of mucous membranes Rare: heart arrhythmias	Caution client not to drive or operate machinery until sedative effects of medication are known; do not combine terfenadine or astemizole with macrolide antibiotics or ketoconazole (life-threatening dysrhythmia may occur).
Nasal Decongestant Agents		
beclomethasone dipropionate (Beconase Nasal Spray) flunisolide (Nasalide) oxymetazoline hydrochloride (Afrin) Vasoconstrict nasal membranes	Headache, transient nasal burning, nasal congestion, sneezing, epistaxis, rebound nasal congestion	Advise client to pump spray 3–4 times before first use and 1–2 times before each daily use to prime. Caution clients using Afrin to avoid using for longer than 3–5 days in a row or rebound nasal congestion may occur.
Oral Decongestant Agents		
(sympathomimetics) pseudoephedrine hydrochloride (Sudafed) Vasoconstrict nasal membranes	Anxiety, nervousness, palpitations Initial sensation of warmth, hypotension or shock, bronchospasm, gastrointestinal (GI) and uterine contractions, urticaria, angioedema Variable; drug-induced lupus, drug fever, pulmonary reactions, lymphadenopathy, hepatic syndromes	Use cautiously in clients with severe hypertension, diabetes, glaucoma, hyperthyroidism, prostatic hyperplasia, coronary artery disease, those taking monoamine oxidase inhibitors, and breast-feeding clients. Avoid taking within 2 hours of bedtime.
Corticosteroids		
dexamethasone (Decadron) hydrocortisone (Cortef) methylprednisolone (Medrol) Regulate immune response; control anti-inflammatory response	Euphoria, insomnia, GI irritation, increased appetite, weight gain, hyperglycemia	Must be tapered down; abrupt discontinuation may lead to acute adrenal insufficiency; give daily doses in the morning with food.

(continued)

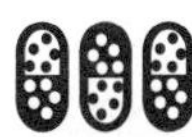

TABLE 41-3 *(Continued)*

Drug Category/Drug Action	Side Effects	Nursing Considerations
Sympathomimetic Agents		
epinephrine (Primatene Mist, Adrenalin Chloride) albuterol (Proventil) theophylline (Theo-Dur) metaproterenol (Alupent) Act on alpha- or beta receptors	Nervousness, tremor, euphoria, palpitations, hypertension, dysrhythmias, headache	Monitor blood pressure and heart rate during use; use caution in those with hypertension, heart disease, diabetes, cirrhosis, or those using digitalis glycosides; May be given orally, subcutaneously, intramuscularly, or by inhalation.

the allergen, many experience symptomatic relief with drug therapy (Table 41–3).

Desensitization is an option also. **Desensitization** is a form of immunotherapy in which the individual is given regular injections of dilute allergen. Repeated exposure to the weak antigen promotes the production of an antibody that blocks IgE. Weekly injections are given until the maximum dose is achieved. Maintenance injections are then administered at longer intervals, usually every 2 to 4 weeks. It may take several years before a treated person experiences significant relief. Following an injection, the client is observed for 30 minutes to assess for allergic symptoms. Epinephrine (Adrenalin) is administered if a severe reaction occurs.

Clients with severe bee sting allergies are advised to carry an emergency kit that contains a premeasured dose of injectable epinephrine. The syringe autoinjects the medication when pressed to the skin. The lateral thigh is the site that is most commonly used (Fig. 41–4).

Nursing Management

Obtain a thorough history from the client with an actual or suspected allergic disorder. Gather data about the client's diet history with particular attention to foods that cause a problem. Determine if others in the family have allergies. Record the client's description of allergic symptoms in detail and the factors that appear to increase or decrease symptoms (ie, exposures, time of year). Identify all prescription and nonprescription drugs taken and those the client reacted to in the past. Be especially alert to allergic manifestations caused by contact with latex (Box 41–1). Examine the skin and describe any rash or eruption that is present.

Closely observe a client with allergies each time a new drug is added to the therapeutic regimen. This includes drugs given by the nurse and drugs used for diagnostic studies, such as radiopaque dyes. Continue to monitor the client when subsequent doses of the new drug are given because reactions may occur with subsequent doses. If an allergic reaction is suspected, do not give the next dose of the drug until a physician sees the client. If an anaphylactic reaction occurs while a drug is being given by a parenteral route, stop administration of the drug and provide life support while the code team is summoned.

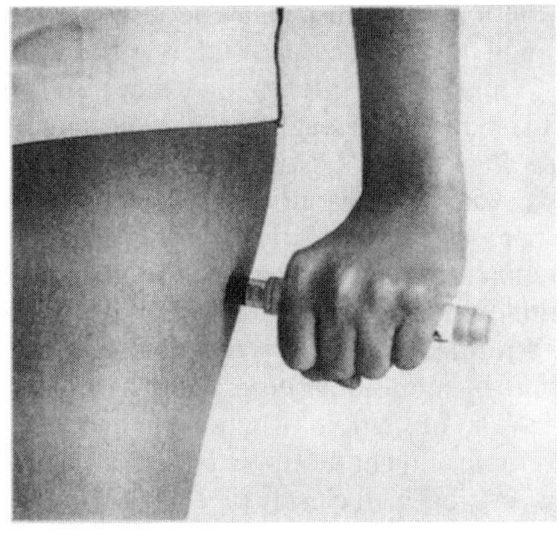

FIGURE 41-4. To avoid an anaphylactic reaction, a premeasured dose of epinephrine is autoinjected into subcutaneous tissue.

BOX 41-1 Products That Contain Latex

Household	Medical
Carpet backing	Gloves
Feeding nipples	Face masks
Pacifiers	Mattresses
Elastic in clothing	Patient-controlled analgesia syringes
Sports equipment	Ambu bags
Balloons	Stethoscope
Erasers	Blood pressure cuff tubing
Toys	Dental devices
Shoe soles	Urinary catheters
Condoms/diaphragms	Tourniquets
Computer mouse pads	Electrode pads
Buttons on electronic equipment	Bulb syringes
Food handled with powdered latex gloves	Syringe stoppers and medication vial stoppers
Handles on racquets, tools, and similar items	Adhesive tape
	Bandages
	Injection ports
	Wound drains

The plan of care for a client with an allergic disorder includes, but is not limited to, the following:

Nursing Diagnoses and Collaborative Problems	Nursing Interventions
PC: Anaphylaxis and Angioedema **Goal:** The nurse will manage and minimize anaphylaxis and angioedema.	Closely monitor the blood pressure, pulse rate, and urine output. Insert an IV line immediately. Administer IV fluids and medications as ordered. Inspect the oral cavity for changes in the appearance of the mucous membranes. Notify the physician immediately if angioedema occurs. Place the client in mid-Fowler's position to allow for full lung expansion and administer high flow rates of humidified oxygen via face mask until a definitive treatment plan is established. If anaphylaxis or angioedema occurs, have another member of the health care team summon help and bring emergency equipment to the bedside. If cardiac or respiratory arrest occurs, administer cardiopulmonary resuscitation.
Altered Comfort: Itching related to histamine release **Goal:** The client will have reduced itching, intact skin.	Administer topical, oral, or IV drugs to control itching. Encourage client to keep nails short to prevent tearing of skin when scratching. Apply skin moisturizers to keep skin soft and prevent cracking. Notify physician if signs of infection or a spread of skin lesions occur.
Impaired Home Maintenance related to inability to work in an environment that produces moderate to severe symptoms **Goal:** The client will maintain the home with reduced allergy symptoms.	Encourage the client to explore alternatives regarding avoiding the offending allergen. Propose the use of air conditioning during summer months, using special furnace filters or electrostatic cleaners to remove the offending allergens from the environment, using hypoallergenic products, and wearing gloves (rubber or plastic) when coming into contact with an offending allergen or irritating substance.

CLIENT AND FAMILY TEACHING

Develop a teaching plan based on the following guidelines:

- Treatment for chronic allergic disorders, such as allergic rhinitis and food allergies, may extend over several years.

- Follow the medical regimen as instructed by the physician.
- If itching is a prominent symptom, keep the nails clean and short; if necessary, wear cotton gloves at night to prevent scratching while sleeping.
- Do not overuse nose drops or sprays for nasal congestion. Use only prescribed or recommended drugs and only in the dosage suggested by the physician.
- Keep a record of the symptoms or lack of symptoms. Bring the record to the physician's office or clinic. This will help the physician determine therapy.
- Keep a record of symptoms or absence of symptoms each time a new food is added to the diet. Add new foods to the diet slowly and one at a time.
- Avoid environmental substances that cause allergic reactions.
- Seek immediate medical attention if symptoms worsen or new symptoms occur.
- Carry identification, such as a Medic Alert card or bracelet, to inform medical personnel of allergies especially if there is a history of anaphylactic reactions.
- Do not miss an immunotherapy appointment because it may require restarting the series of injections.
- Check the prefilled syringes containing epinephrine for an expiration date. The prescription must be refilled and the old prescription discarded on or immediately before this date. Keep the directions for use with the product.

Autoimmune Disorders

Autoimmune disorders are disorders in which natural cells are attacked or destroyed by killer T cells and autoantibodies. **Autoantibodies** are immunoglobulins that target **histocompatible cells,** cells whose antigens match the individual's own genetic code. Diseases are considered autoimmune disorders when they are characterized by unrelenting, progressive tissue damage without any verifiable etiology.

Etiology and Pathophysiology

Several theories have been proposed to explain the cause of autoimmune disorders (Table 41–4). None appears to explain autoimmunity completely, which suggests that more than one mechanism is responsible.

When the immune system fails to recognize histocompatible cells, T and B cells mount a cell-mediated or humoral response. The attack may be localized to one organ or type of tissue or it may be systemic (Box 41–2). Cells, tissues, and organs under attack are damaged or destroyed.

Assessment Findings

SIGNS AND SYMPTOMS

Autoimmune disorders produce a variety of signs and symptoms depending on the tissues and organs affected. The symptoms are characteristically those of an acute inflammatory response. They develop as an-

TABLE 41-4 **Autoimmunity Theories**

Theory	Hypothesis
Cross-antigen theory	Self-antigens that resemble foreign antigens cause T cells to misidentify natural cells and mount an immune attack.
Tissue injury theory	Natural cells are altered by infection, trauma, drugs, and radiation. Consequently they no longer resemble self-antigens.
Viral mutation theory	Viruses alter T-cell receptors that are used to differentiate self from nonself.
Sequestered antigen theory	Some cells, like the lens of the eye, the thyroid, and the brain, are separated from lymphocytes during fetal development. When these cells enter circulation later due to trauma or infection, T cells do not recognize them as "self."
Diminished T-suppressor theory	Immunoregulation is altered as a consequence of reduced numbers of suppressor cells or a shortened life span due to aging and atrophy of the thymus gland.
Genetic instruction theory	Genetic coding for antibody production is altered, which explains the familial pattern to some autoimmune disorders.

BOX 41-2 Examples of Autoimmune Disorders

Organ Specific	Systemic
BLOOD Hemolytic anemia Thrombocytopenia purpura	Lupus erythematosus Scleroderma Rheumatoid arthritis
CENTRAL NERVOUS SYSTEM Multiple sclerosis Guillain-Barré syndrome	
HEART Endocarditis	
MUSCLES Myasthenia gravis	
ENDOCRINE Hashimoto's thyroiditis Juvenile diabetes mellitus	
EYE Uveitis	
JOINT Ankylosing spondylitis	
GASTROINTESTINAL Ulcerative colitis	
RENAL Glomerulonephritis	

tibodies attack normal tissue mistakenly identified as nonself. In some cases, the inflammatory symptoms are episodic. Periods of acute flare-ups alternate with asymptomatic periods. During acute episodes, clients often experience a low-grade fever, malaise, or fatigue. Weight loss may also occur.

DIAGNOSTIC FINDINGS

Diagnostic testing varies depending on the nature of the autoimmune disorder. Overall, an elevation of circulating antibodies is the hallmark for these types of disorders.

Medical Management

Drug therapy using immunosuppressive agents is the mainstay for alleviating the symptoms (Table 41–5). Controlling or limiting side effects of the drugs is a major concern.

Nursing Management

Promote a healthy lifestyle and stress reduction because stress and illness worsen many autoimmune diseases. Encourage good nutrition. Provide information about the illness and medication regimens. Administer prescribed medications and monitor for side effects.

The plan of care for clients with autoimmune disorders includes, but is not limited to, the following:

Nursing Diagnoses and Collaborative Problems	Nursing Interventions
Activity Intolerance related to joint pain and inflammation, malaise, or fatigue **Goal:** The client will perform activities of daily living without extreme fatigue or discomfort.	Encourage rest during periods of severe exacerbations of pain and regular exercise during periods of comfort or disease remission. Provide nonpharmacologic and pharmacologic pain management as ordered by the physician.

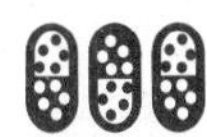

TABLE 41-5 **Immunosuppressive Drug Therapy**

Drug Category/Drug Action	Side Effects	Nursing Considerations
Corticosteroids		
prednisone, methylprednisolone Initiates many immunosuppressive and anti-inflammatory cellular responses.	Euphoria, insomnia, GI irritation, increased appetite, weight gain	Must be tapered; abrupt withdrawal may cause acute adrenal insufficiency.
Cytotoxic Drugs		
azathioprine (Immuran) Suppresses cell-mediated hypersensitivity and alters antibody production.	Oral ulceration, nausea, vomiting, pancreatitis, leukopenia, bone marrow suppression, hepatotoxicity, immunosuppression, thrombocytopenia, rash, hair thinning	Follow hospital policy on administration of cytotoxic drugs. Instruct patients not to take aspirin. Warn patient to report signs of infection, use effective birth control during treatment and 4 months after.
cyclophosphamide (Cytoxan) Interferes with replication of lymphocytes.	Cardiotoxicity, anorexia, nausea, vomiting, oral ulceration, hemorrhagic cystitis, leukopenia, thrombocytopenia, anemia, pulmonary fibrosis, reversible alopecia	Advise clients to void every 1–2 hours while awake and to drink at least 3 liters of fluid per day to reduce risk of cystitis. Do not give drug at bedtime.
methotrexate (Folex-PFS, Mexate-AQ, Rheumatrex) Inhibits cellular replication.	Stomatitis, diarrhea, nausea, vomiting, tubular necrosis, anemia, leukopenia, thrombocytopenia, hepatotoxicity, pulmonary fibrosis, urticaria, photosensitivity, alopecia	Follow hospital policy on administration of cytotoxic drugs. Advise birth control while on medication and to report signs of infection immediately.
Immunosuppressives		
cyclosporine (Sandimmune) Inhibits lymphocytes; exact mechanism of action unknown.	Tremor, gum hyperplasia, nausea, vomiting, diarrhea, nephrotoxicity, leukopenia, thrombocytopenia, hepatotoxicity	Warn to report signs of infection, to take drug at same time every day, to take with meals if it causes nausea, avoid pregnancy, and not to stop medication without physician approval. High risk for anaphylaxis with injection form.
tacrolimus (FK506) Inhibits T-cell activation; exact mechanism of action unknown.	Headache, tremor, insomnia, hypertension, diarrhea, nausea, abnormal renal function, anemia, leukocytosis, thrombocytopenia, hyperkalemia, hyperglycemia, hypomagnesemia, pleural effusion, pain, fever, asthenia	Advise clients to report signs of infection immediately.

Risk for Infection related to immunosuppression and general poor physical condition **Goal:** The client will be free of infection.	Instruct client on signs and symptoms of infection and the increased risk for infection. Instruct client to report signs and symptoms of infection immediately to the physician (cough, shortness of breath, diarrhea, fever). Instruct client on avoidance of high-risk activities, such as being in crowded areas, during periods of immunosuppression.
Disturbance in Self-Concept related to physical changes associated with autoimmune diseases **Goal:** The client will maintain a positive self-concept.	Listen to and validate client's concerns regarding physical changes associated with autoimmune disorders. Provide emotional support as needed. Refer client to community organizations and support groups.

CLIENT AND FAMILY TEACHING

- Notify a health care practitioner of any signs of infection such as a cough, fever, severe diarrhea, mouth lesions, or a sore throat.
- Notify a health care practitioner of any new side effects to prescribed medications.
- Do not stop taking any medications abruptly.

- Avoid crowds or people with infections if taking an immunosuppressant drug.
- Limit stress and use stress reduction techniques such as progressive relaxation or breathing exercises.
- Maintain close follow-up with a physician.

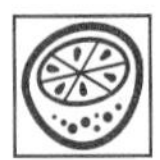

General Nutritional Considerations

The majority of food allergies are caused by milk, eggs, peanuts, soy, and wheat in children, and fish, shellfish, nuts, and peanuts in adults. Glycoproteins are the offending substance.

Once a food allergy has been diagnosed, the only proven therapy is strict elimination of the offending food from the diet. To achieve this, clients need extensive teaching on how to read food labels to identify all sources of the allergen and how to maintain a nutritionally adequate diet.

Food allergies may resolve after several years of excluding the allergen from the diet; however, allergies to peanuts, nuts, fish and seafood tend to be long-lasting and are more likely to cause anaphylactic reactions than other foods.

Clients who are allergic to many foods or to substances pervasive in the food supply (ie, artificial flavors and colors, preservatives) need thorough counseling on how to maintain a nutritionally adequate diet while avoiding the allergen.

Clients who are immunosuppressed secondary to treatment for an autoimmune disorder need teaching about avoiding raw, undercooked, and unwashed foods to avoid infection from microorganisms that reside in food products.

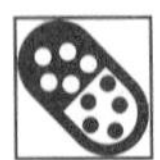

General Pharmacologic Considerations

Most antihistamines cause drowsiness. The client is advised not to drive a car, operate machinery, or perform tasks that require alertness. Some newer antihistamines are not as likely to cause drowsiness.

Clients taking antihistamines are advised not to take them with alcohol or other central nervous system depressants, because additive sedative effects can occur.

Antihistamines are not administered to clients with disorders of the lower respiratory tract. If, for example, these drugs are administered for asthma, a drying effect may occur, making secretions thicker and more difficult to expectorate.

The use of nonprescription eye preparations to reduce redness should be avoided. Itching and redness of the eyes should be evaluated and treated by an ophthalmologist because the symptoms may or may not be caused by an allergy.

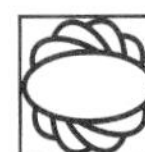

General Gerontologic Considerations

Antihistamines are used cautiously in older clients with prostatic hypertrophy. Older men with prostatic hypertrophy may experience difficulty voiding while taking an antihistamine.

Adverse reactions to the antihistamines, such as dizziness, sedation, and confusion are more common in the older adult. Careful monitoring of the older adult by the nurse or, if an outpatient, by a family member may be necessary.

SUMMARY OF KEY CONCEPTS

- An allergic disorder involves a hyperimmune response to weak antigens that are generally harmless substances.
- Some signs and symptoms of allergic disorders include nasal stuffiness, runny nose, sneezing, coughing, dyspnea, wheezing, hives, rash, localized itching of the skin, cramping, vomiting, diarrhea, shock, and airway obstruction.
- There are generally four categories of allergens: inhalants, ingestants, contactants, and injectants.
- Although there are many types of allergic manifestations, four examples include allergic rhinitis, contact dermatitis, and two that are potentially life-threatening, anaphylaxis (shock) and angioedema.
- There are three methods of skin testing to identify specific allergens to which a person is sensitive: the intradermal injection, the scratch or prick test, and the patch test. All of these techniques involve instilling or applying common allergens to the skin and observing for redness and swelling at the site.
- Three methods for treating a client with an allergic disorder are avoidance of the allergen, drug therapy, and desensitization.
- When caring for a client with an allergic disorder, the nurse gathers a comprehensive history and obtains a detailed description of allergic manifestations and related information that helps to identify the cause. Assistance is provided during and following diagnostic procedures that can result in serious allergic manifestations such as anaphylaxis and angioedema. The nurse responds to emergency situations, promotes relief of allergic manifestations, and provides health teaching to reduce allergens in the home and work environment.
- Autoimmune disorders are similar to allergies except that the immune response is misdirected toward natural cells. Some examples include rheumatoid arthritis, lupus erythematosus, and thrombocytopenia purpura.
- There are many theoretical explanations for why individuals develop autoimmune disorders. One is that when natural cells are damaged in some way by trauma, infection, or other means, the T cells no longer identify them as normal and set about to destroy what they perceive as a threat to self.

- Various types of immunosuppressive drugs are used to reduce the destruction of natural cells. Some drug categories include corticosteroids, cytotoxic drugs, and immunosuppressants.
- When caring for clients with an autoimmune disorder, the nurse implements medical therapy to relieve symptoms and maintain functional tissue, promotes a healthy lifestyle, reduces the potential for opportunistic infections, and uses techniques to help clients cope with living with a chronic, debilitating disease that causes physical changes.

CRITICAL THINKING EXERCISES

1. Discuss ways of avoiding inhaled and ingested allergens.
2. A client complains about being delayed from going home for a half-hour after receiving a desensitizing injection to control his allergies. How would you respond?
3. Discuss three theories that attempt to explain how autoimmune disorders develop.

Suggested Readings

Booth, B. (1995). No time for kid gloves. *Nursing Times, 91*(46), 43–44, 46.

Calianno, C., & Pino, T. (1995). Getting a reaction to anergy panel testing. *Nursing, 25*(1), 58–61.

Chase, S. L. (1997). A new OTC option for allergy sufferers. *RN, 60*(6), 67.

Harwood, S. (1997). Action stat. Anaphylaxis. *Nursing, 27*(2), 33.

Huss, K., Vessey, J. A., & Mason, P. (1996). Primary care approaches. Controlling allergies by assessing risks in the home. *Pediatric Nursing, 22*(5), 432–435.

Kuster, P. A. (1996). Reducing risk of house dust mite and cockroach allergen exposure in inner-city children with asthma. *Pediatric Nursing, 22*(4), 297–305.

Lisanti, P. (1996). Emergency—Anaphylaxis. *American Journal of Nursing, 96*(11), 51.

Mabry, C. S., & Mabry, R. L. (1996). Making the diagnosis of allergy. *Head Neck Nursing, 14*(1), 13–14.

Mudd, K. E. (1995). Indoor environmental allergy: A guide to environmental controls. *Pediatric Nursing, 21*(6), 534–536.

O'Gilvie, W. (1996). Guidance on latex sensitization for the health service. *Nursing Times, 92*(15), 36.

Thompson, G. (1996). Managing latex allergy in hospital patients and health-care workers. *Journal of Wound Care, 5*(10 Suppl.), 1–7.

Titler, M. G., & Steelman, V. M. (1996). Research for practice. Preventing allergic reactions to latex. *MEDSURG Nursing, 5*(2), 111–114, 134.

Additional Resources

American Academy of Allergy, Asthma, and Immunology
611 East Wells Street
Milwaukee, WI 53202
(800) 822-2762
http://www.aaaai.org

Asthma and Allergy Foundation of America
1125 15th Street, NW
Suite 502
Washington, DC 20005
(800) 727-8462
http://www.aafa.org

Chapter 42

Caring for Clients With AIDS

KEY TERMS

Acquired immunodeficiency syndrome
Acute retroviral syndrome
Autologous blood
Directed donor blood
Enzyme-linked immunosorbent assay (ELISA)
Human immunodeficiency virus
Integrase
Kaposi's sarcoma
p24 antigen test
Pneumocystic pneumonia
Polymerase chain reaction (PCR) test
Protease
Protease inhibitor
Retrovirus
Reverse transcriptase
Reverse transcriptase (RT) inhibitor
Reverse transcription
Western blot

LEARNING OBJECTIVES

On completion of this chapter, the reader will:

- Explain the term acquired immunodeficiency syndrome.
- Identify the virus that causes acquired immunodeficiency syndrome.
- Discuss the characteristics of a retrovirus.
- Explain the manner in which HIV is transmitted.
- Name at least four methods for preventing HIV transmission.
- List three criteria for diagnosing AIDS.
- Discuss the pathophysiologic process of AIDS.
- List at least five manifestations of acute retroviral syndrome.
- Name two laboratory tests used to screen for HIV antibodies and one that confirms a diagnosis of AIDS.
- Name two laboratory tests used to measure viral load, and give two purposes for their use.
- Identify two categories of drugs used to treat individuals infected with HIV and give an example of a specific drug in each category.
- Give the criterion for successful drug therapy.
- Discuss the nursing management of a client with AIDS.
- Give examples of information to provide HIV-infected clients.
- Describe techniques for preventing HIV infection among health care workers who care for infected clients.
- Discuss two ethical issues that relate to HIV infection.

The **human immunodeficiency virus** (HIV) profoundly weakens the immune system (Fig. 42–1). **Acquired immunodeficiency syndrome** (AIDS) is a consequence of HIV infection (Fig. 42–2), and the Centers for Disease Control and Prevention estimated that 30.6 million people were infected with HIV worldwide as of June 1997. In the United States, AIDS is currently the leading cause of death among people 25 to 44 years old. If current trends continue, as many as 40 million humans will be HIV positive by the end of the year 2000 (AIDS Action Committee of Massachusetts).

Human Immunodeficiency Virus

The HIV belongs to a family of RNA (ribonucleic acid) viruses that contain an enzyme called reverse transcriptase. HIV is called a **retrovirus** because it copies the viral RNA into deoxyribonucleic acid (DNA), which is the reverse of the usual process.

HIV Replication

Like other viruses, HIV is unable to replicate (duplicate) itself independently. To produce more copies of itself, the HIV becomes a parasite of helper T4 lymphocytes (see Chap. 40). The virus first seeks out and attaches itself to the CD4 surface membrane receptor of the T4 cell. The virus contains two molecules of RNA and three enzymes that govern this process: re-

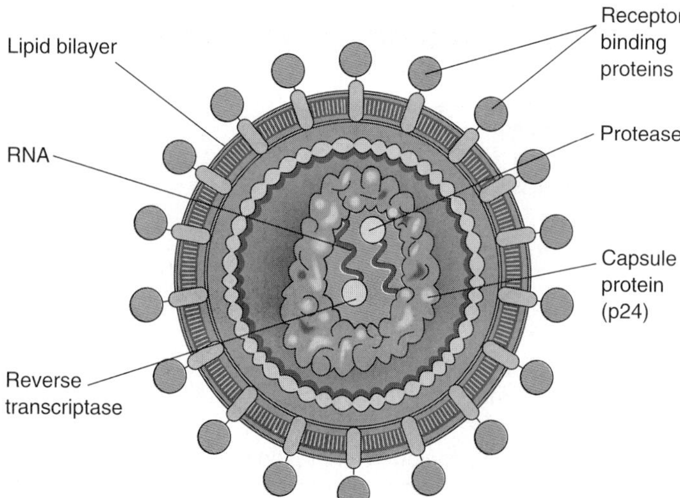

FIGURE 42-1. Structure of a retrovirus.

verse transcriptase, integrase, and protease,. After binding with the cell membrane, the virus enters the host cell (Fig. 42–3).

REPROGRAMMING THE HOST CELL

To survive and multiply, the HIV must alter the cell's genetic code to make more viral particles. To do this, the enzyme **reverse transcriptase** copies the RNA into DNA, a process called **reverse transcription.** DNA tells the cell how to assemble amino acids to form protein substances like the virus. Another viral enzyme, **integrase,** incorporates the reprogrammed DNA—with its new viral code—into the chromosomes within the nucleus of the lymphocyte. The altered DNA now provides the blueprint or cookbook for making clones of HIV and the enzymes it needs to continue reinfecting additional cells. The cell follows the DNA's directions and forms long chains of viral proteins enclosed within a membrane. **Protease,** a third viral enzyme, cuts the long chains, freeing the replicas into the cytoplasm of the cell. Some migrate to the cell wall and form buds. When the buds rupture, they release many copies of the virus that reinfect other cells. More than 10 billion viral particles are released daily. Because mutations occur with some frequency, many different strains of HIV exist and the production of a vaccine is nearly impossible.

HIV Transmission

Casual contact does not transmit the HIV. HIV infection occurs through the transmission of body fluids. Only four body fluids are known to transmit the HIV: blood, semen, vaginal secretions, and breast milk. HIV may be present in saliva and conjunctival secretions,

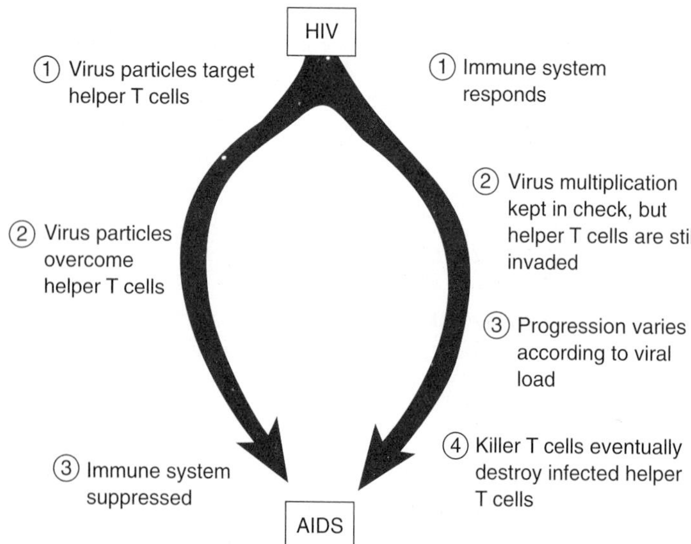

FIGURE 42-2. Cycle of HIV infection and development of AIDS.

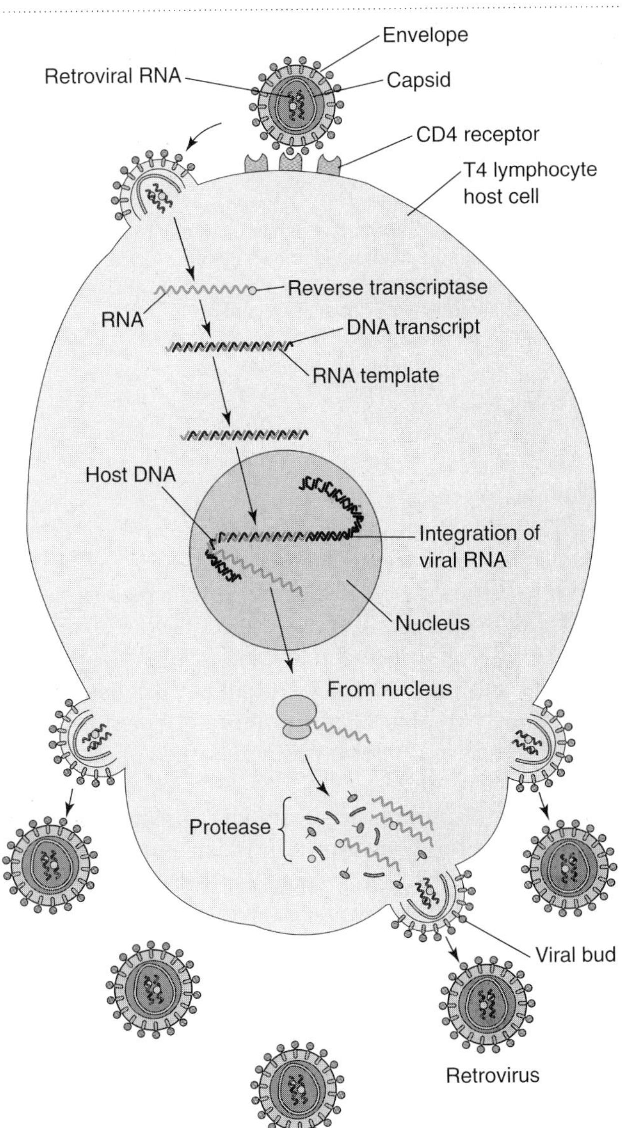

FIGURE 42-3. HIV replication.

but these fluids have not been implicated in HIV transmission. Certain behaviors increase the risk for HIV infection (Box 42–1). The virus can be present for 10 years or more without causing symptoms. During this time the infected person can infect others. An estimated 13,000 infections occur on a daily basis (Stine, 1997).

In 1984, a screening test for donated blood became available. Although screening donated blood for HIV antibodies reduces the risk of HIV infection, antibody screening cannot identify infected blood from donors who have yet to produce a significant amount of antibody. The window of time between the infection (entrance of HIV into the body) and the production of antibodies varies from 1 to 6 weeks. This means that a recently infected person with HIV could donate blood containing the virus, and the screening test would be negative.

BOX 42-1 High-Risk Factors for HIV Infection

- Unprotected vaginal, anal, or oral sex
- Contact with blood and infectious body fluids during medical, surgical, dental, or nursing procedures
- Sharing intravenous needles or syringes
- Receiving nonautologous transfusions of blood or blood products
- Receiving plasma or clotting factors that have not been heat treated
- Contact with infected blood on ear-piercing, tattoo, and dental equipment
- Transmission from infected mothers to infants during pregnancy, birth, or breast-feeding

Prevention of HIV Infection

The transmission of HIV is reduced or eliminated by adhering to the following guidelines:

- Abstain from sexual intercourse.
- Have mutually monogamous sex with an uninfected partner.
- Avoid casual sex with multiple partners.
- During sexual intercourse, use a condom and spermicide that contain nonoxynol 9.
- Abstain from using intravenous (IV) drugs.
- Use a new needle and syringe each time IV drugs are injected.
- Refrain from donating blood if engaged in high-risk behaviors.
- Bank **autologous blood** (self-donated) or **directed donor blood** (specified blood donors among relatives and friends) when preparing for nonemergency surgical procedures (Table 42–1). Some authorities believe that directed blood is no safer than blood collected from public donors because directed donors may not reveal their high-risk behaviors.

Acquired Immunodeficiency Syndrome (AIDS)

AIDS is the end-stage of HIV infection. A person has AIDS when:

- Opportunistic infections develop (Box 42–2), the T4 cell count is or was less than 200 cells/mm^3, and there is a positive HIV test, or

TABLE 42-1 **Guidelines for Autologous and Directed Blood Donation**

Autologous Donation	Directed Donation
Donor must weigh 95 lb.	Donor must weigh 110 lb.
Donor must be at least 14 years old.	Donor must be at least 17 years old.
Exceptions made in medical history	Must meet volunteer donor medical history criteria
Used only for transfusion to donor	Patient's physician must be informed of directed donation.
Blood type does not need to be known at time of donation.	May be transfused to others if not needed by patient
Units that test positive for a disease (other than HIV) will be issued.	Donors should know blood type of patient
Donation frequency may be greater than 1 unit every 56 days	Units that test positive for HIV or hepatitis will not be used
Additional fee to hospital or recipient may be charged for holding blood on reserve.	Additional fees may be charged to the recipient

- Documented weight loss, diarrhea, dementia, and a positive HIV test are confirmed.

Opportunistic infections also occur in people who are not HIV positive; it is the appearance of these infections in those with a markedly decreased T4 cell count that is a criterion for AIDS.

Etiology and Pathophysiology

AIDS is acquired from direct contact with HIV-infected individuals or from indirect contact with infected blood or body fluids. The origin and development of HIV is not clear. One theory is that HIV originated in Africa where it was known as the "wasting disease." It has been proposed that a virus in African monkeys underwent a genetic change or mutation and the virus jumped species from primates to humans.

When HIV infection occurs, it gradually impairs the ability of infected T4 cells to recognize foreign antigens and stimulate B-cell lymphocytes. While massive numbers of viral particles are being released, infected T4 cells are destroyed by the virus itself and by T8 cell lymphocytes that no longer recognize the altered T4 cell membrane as being "self." Although new T4 cells are produced, the process is never as fast as the virus replicates. Eventually, T4 cells become significantly depleted, and immunodeficiency develops. The infected person ultimately dies of an opportunistic infection.

The rate of progression from HIV infection to AIDS is related to the concentration of virus in the blood. For some, the process may take 10 to 12 years. Although most people infected with HIV die of their disease, a few are long-term survivors. Some explanations for long-term survival include infection by a weak strain of HIV and suppression of the virus by stronger than normal killer T8 cells or effective drug treatment.

BOX 42-2 Prevalent Opportunistic Infections

- Pneumocystic pneumonia (PCP)
- Herpes simplex
- Toxoplasmosis
- Tuberculosis
- Salmonellosis
- Histoplasmosis
- Cytomegalovirus infection
- Cryptococcosis
- Coccidioidomycosis
- Cryptosporidiosis
- Candidiasis

Assessment Findings

SIGNS AND SYMPTOMS

When HIV-infected individuals first become symptomatic, the signs and symptoms of **acute retroviral syndrome** (viremia) are often mistaken as "flu" or some other common illness. Some manifestations include fever; swollen and tender lymph nodes; pharyngitis; rash about the face, trunk, palms, and soles of the feet; muscle and joint pain; headache; and nausea, vomiting, and diarrhea. In addition, there may be enlargement of the liver and spleen, weight loss, thrush (candidiasis), and neurologic symptoms such as visual changes and cognitive or motor impairment. Admission of HIV risk behaviors, however, narrows the differential diagnosis.

The client may also present with an opportunistic infection. In women, gynecologic problems may be the chief complaint. Abnormal Papanicolaou smears, genital warts, pelvic inflammatory disease, and persistent vaginitis (see Chaps. 58 and 61) correlate with an HIV infection. **Kaposi's sarcoma,** a rare type of connective tissue cancer common among those with AIDS, may be noted (see Color Plates 1 and 2).

DIAGNOSTIC FINDINGS

The **enzyme-linked immunosorbent assay** (ELISA) is the initial screening test. It is positive when there are sufficient HIV antibodies. Because it is also positive when there are antibodies from other infectious diseases, the test is repeated following an initial positive finding. If a second ELISA is positive, the **Western blot** is performed. A positive Western blot confirms the diagnosis; however, false-positive and false-negative results on both tests are possible.

A total T-cell count, T4 and T8 count, and T4/T8 ratio determine the status of T lymphocytes. A T-cell count of $200/mm^3$ or less is an indicator of AIDS. The **p24 antigen test** and **polymerase chain reaction (PCR) test** measure viral loads. They are used to guide drug therapy and follow the progression of the disease.

Other general laboratory and diagnostic tests are prescribed when opportunistic infections are involved.

Medical Management

Treatment is supportive. Clients with a T4 cell count below 500 $cells/mm^3$ are started on a combination of two antiretroviral drugs: a **reverse transcriptase (RT) inhibitor** and a **protease inhibitor** (Table 42–2). The goal of antiretroviral therapy is to get the viral load below 20,000 and the ideal outcome is "undetectable" levels or 500 copies or less. The RT inhibitor suppresses viral replication within the cell by blocking the development of the DNA copy and the protease inhibitor decreases the release of viral particles into circulation. Combination therapy, known as a drug cocktail, has several benefits:

- Reduced viral load, which slows the rate of disease progression and lengthens survival time
- Diminished rate of viral mutations, which prolongs drug effectiveness
- Reduced resistance to one drug

The physician decides which drugs to prescribe based on the side effect profiles, cost, and interactions of each drug. Antiretroviral medications are very expensive—as much as $10,000 to $15,000 annually. Some social and pharmaceutical companies have compassionate need programs through which antiretroviral drugs are supplied to individuals who cannot afford them.

Besides drugs specific for AIDS, clients require drug treatment or preventive medications for opportunistic infections. To prevent **pneumocystic pneumonia** (PCP), trimethoprim-sulfamethoxazol (Bactrim, Septra) is prescribed. Monthly aerosolized pentamidine isethionate (NebuPent) is also effective. Foscarnet (Foscavir), cidofovir (Vistide), and ganciclovir (Cytovene) are prescribed for cytomegalovirus retinitis. It is usually recommended that HIV infected clients receive pneumococcal vaccine, hepatitis B vaccine, and yearly influenza vaccines. Additional medical management includes treating anorexia, diarrhea, weight loss, and vaginal or oral candidiasis.

Nursing Management

The ongoing health care needs of the client with AIDS focus on preventing infection, maintaining

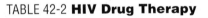

TABLE 42-2 **HIV Drug Therapy**

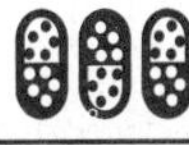

Drug Category/Drug Action	Side Effects	Nursing Considerations
Reverse Transcriptase Inhibitors zidovudine (AZT, Retrovir) Reduces HIV replication by inhibiting the production of the enzyme "reverse transcriptase."	Anemia, nausea, gastrointestinal (GI) pain, diarrhea, myositis, headaches, fever, rash	Monitor blood counts. Administer drug on an around-the-clock schedule, 30 minutes before or 2 hours after meals. Tell client to report extreme fatigue, extreme nausea, vomiting, or rash.
Protease Inhibitors saquinavir mesylate (Invirase) Leads to the production and release of immature, noninfectious viral particles by inhibiting the enzyme "protease," which is necessary to virus maturation.	Headache, nausea, GI pain, diarrhea, elevated creatine phosphokinase	Administer within 2 hours of a full meal. Tell client to report extreme fatigue, lethargy, darkening of urine, changes in stool color, rash, or difficulty breathing.

optimal nutritional status, maintaining a healthy lifestyle, and coping with having an infectious terminal illness.

NURSING PROCESS
The Client With AIDS

Assessment

Obtain a thorough history including risk factors for HIV infection. List all symptoms and explore each thoroughly. Determine the drugs the client currently takes or has taken during previous treatment. Question the client regarding weight loss and weight before becoming symptomatic. Explore the client's past and current dietary intake. Ask about factors that interfere with eating, such as difficulty swallowing or oral discomfort. Ask about elimination patterns and if diarrhea is a problem. Assess the client's mental status and perform a general neurologic assessment (see Chap. 43). Evaluate emotional status. Look for signs of depression and anxiety.

Obtain vital signs and weight. Inspect the oral mucous membranes and all skin surfaces for rashes, skin breakdown, and opportunistic infections such as herpes lesions (see Color Plate 5). Look for Kaposi's sarcoma, which appears as dark purple lesions that may or may not be painful. Assess the client for the presence of peripheral neuropathies (sensation changes in extremities) that can be side effects of antiretroviral medications. Ask if visual changes such as the presence of floaters, spots, and loss of peripheral vision have occurred. Observe for signs of dehydration. Examine the skin and mucous membranes for dryness. Evaluate skin turgor. Note additional signs such as decreased urine output, hypotension, and slow filling of the hand veins. Look for signs and symptoms that indicate a deficit of one or more electrolytes such as excessive thirst, muscle weakness, cramping, nausea, vomiting, cardiac arrhythmias, shallow respirations, and headache. Examine the arms and legs for edema. Auscultate the lungs for normal and abnormal breath sounds. Question the client regarding coughing, sputum production, dyspnea, and orthopnea. Palpate the lymph nodes and abdomen for organ enlargement.

Gather additional data based on the client's complaints or symptoms. Review recent laboratory and diagnostic tests to complete the assessment process. Observe Standard Precautions (see Chap. 18) whenever there is a risk of exposure to blood and body fluids.

Diagnosis and Planning

When caring for a client with AIDS, the plan of care includes, but is not limited to, the following:

Nursing Diagnoses and Collaborative Problems	Nursing Interventions
Risk for Infection (opportunistic) related to immunodeficiency **Goal:** The client will be free of secondary infections.	Follow principles of medical and surgical asepsis. Place in protective isolation if T4 cell count is critically low. Promote hygiene especially before meals and after elimination. Facilitate adequate sleep and nutrition. Prohibit visitors and staff who are ill from contact with the client.
PC: Pneumocystic Pneumonia **Goal:** The nurse will manage and minimize pneumonia.	Auscultate the lungs at least every 4 hours; monitor oxygen saturation. Assist with measures to clear respiratory secretions such as forced coughing, pharyngeal suctioning, aerosol treatments, and chest percussion. Give oxygen as medically prescribed if SpO_2 is 90% or less. Provide mechanical ventilation for acute respiratory failure ($PaO_2 \leq 50$ mm Hg or $PaCO_2 \geq 50$ mm Hg). Administer prescribed antimicrobials.
Risk for Fluid Volume Deficit related to diarrhea secondary to viremia, opportunistic infection, side effects of medication **Goal:** The client will have a balance of fluid intake and output.	Keep a record of intake and output. Measure liquid feces. Offer oral fluids frequently. Withhold foods that are irritating until bowel function improves. Administer prescribed antidiarrheals. Report evidence of dehydration and electrolyte imbalance.
Altered Nutrition: Less than Body Requirements related to anorexia, nausea, diarrhea, or side effects of antiretroviral drugs **Goal:** The client will have an adequate fluid and nutritional intake as evidenced by maintaining admission weight.	Obtain a dietary consult if anorexia is severe. Provide small meals four to six times daily. Give supplementary nourishment between meals. Add hidden calories to beverages and food, such as adding powdered milk to milkshakes or pudding. Suggest significant others bring food from home. Administer prescribed antiemetics, multivitamins and minerals. Consult with the physician concerning tube feedings or total parenteral nutrition if caloric intake is less than adequate.

Risk for Activity Intolerance, Impaired Physical Mobility, and **Self-Care Deficit** related to fatigue, weakness, neurologic involvement **Goal:** The client will tolerate activities of daily living, maintain mobility, and participate in self-care.	Prevent fatigue by spacing activities between periods of rest. Assist with activities of daily living as needed. Accompany the client when ambulating to avoid falls and injuries. Place a commode at the bedside. Provide a walker for ambulatory assistance.
Risk for Impaired Skin Integrity related to impaired capillary blood flow secondary to immobility, skin infections, rash secondary to side effects of drugs **Goal:** The client's skin will remain intact.	Change position every 2 hours. Keep the skin clean and dry. Apply skin moisturizer and gently massage bony prominences with intact skin. Use pressure relieving devices. Clean and dry the perineal area after elimination. Use wipes or a soft washcloth for cleansing.
Altered Oral Mucous Membranes related to inflammation secondary to opportunistic infections **Goal:** The mucous membranes will remain intact.	Provide meticulous oral care after and between meals. Avoid using mouthwashes containing alcohol because they increase irritation. Use mouth rinses with warm (not hot) plain water, normal saline solution, or water and hydrogen peroxide to loosen food particles. Use a soft toothbrush or foam swabs for oral care.
Powerlessness and **Hopelessness** related to poor prognosis of disease **Goal:** The client will control his or her time and make other personal choices; the client will develop a realistic perception of the immediate future.	Give the client opportunities to make choices where choices are possible. Help the client formulate and accomplish short-term goals so that small successes occur more frequently. Discourage clients from seeking unapproved methods of treatment.
Anticipatory Grieving related to potential early death, **Social Isolation** related to rejection by others or death of infected friends, **Altered Family Processes** related to abandonment, **Ineffective Individual Coping** related to stress of coping with an incurable disease **Goal:** The client will work through grief, maintain social contacts with family or friends, and cope effectively with crises.	Be a role model of acceptance for family and friends. Make an effort to touch the client to demonstrate that transmission of the disease through casual contact is exaggerated. Avoid wearing gloves and other barrier garments unnecessarily. Refer the client to an AIDS support group.
Altered Sexuality Patterns related to potential for transmitting HIV **Goal:** The client will practice safer sex.	Remind the client that he or she must inform all sex partners of his or her HIV status. Explain safer sex techniques such as using condoms and maintaining a monogamous relationship.
Altered Thought Processes and **Risk for Injury** related to disorientation and confusion secondary to neurologic involvement **Goal:** The client will become oriented and no injuries will occur.	Orient the client frequently. Use simple language and brief sentences when communicating. Ensure safety by moving the client close to the nursing station. Apply a bed alarm that sounds if the client gets out of bed unassisted.

Evaluation and Expected Outcomes

- Opportunistic infections are treated promptly.
- Infection prevention practices are maintained.
- Optimal nutritional status and fluid balance are maintained.
- Self-care is managed independently when possible.
- Skin and mucous membranes remain intact.
- Effective coping and decision-making are demonstrated.
- Client networks with supportive social system.
- Transmission prevention through safer sex is discussed and practiced.
- Cognition is intact; no trauma is sustained.

CLIENT TEACHING

Develop a teaching plan based on the following guidelines:

- Follow the medication schedule; do not omit or increase the dose without physician approval.
- Comply with the timing of antiviral medications around meals.
- Eat small, frequent, well balanced meals; try to maintain or gain weight. Drink plenty of water.
- Check weight weekly. Report progressive weight loss or loss of appetite to the physician.
- Avoid exposure to people with an infection, including colds, sore throats, upper respiratory tract infections, and childhood diseases (eg, mumps, chickenpox), and those who have recently been vaccinated. Avoid crowds.
- Notify the physician if signs of infection, such as fever, sore throat, diarrhea, respiratory distress, and cough, occur or if signs of a skin, rectal, vaginal, or oral infection appear.
- To prevent bacterial and fungal growths, clean and disinfect areas such as the bathroom, tub, shower, and kitchen surfaces daily.

- Wear gloves and a mask when disposing of animal excreta, such as kitty litter, bird cage liners, and hamster shavings and wash hands thoroughly afterward.
- If necessary, try to rid living area of disease-carrying insects (cockroaches, flies) and rodents (mice, rats).
- Wash all food before cooking; do not eat raw meat, fish, or vegetables or food that has not been completely cooked.
- Frequently dust and vacuum the home, apartment, or room.
- Wash bedding and clothes in hot water and separate from the laundry of others, especially if the bedding and clothes are soiled with body secretions.
- Avoid smoking or exposure to secondhand smoke.
- Personal cleanliness is a must. Bathe or shower daily, wash the hands before and after preparing food, clean the anal and perineal areas after each bowel movement, and wash the hands after voiding or defecating.
- When possible, avoid dry and dusty areas, excessive humidity, and extreme heat or cold. Wear clothing that is appropriate to the weather and temperature.
- Take frequent rest periods, and space activities to prevent fatigue.
- Do not share IV needles, and do not donate blood.
- Inform health care personnel of HIV-positive status.

REDUCING OCCUPATIONAL RISKS

Observe Standard Precautions (see Chap. 18) whenever there is a risk of exposure to blood and body fluids. Follow nursing guidelines for safe handling of needles and sharp instruments (Nursing Guidelines 42–1). The Occupational Safety and Health Administration (OSHA) also recommends the following when caring for all clients regardless of their infectious status:

- Transport specimens of body fluids in leakproof containers.
- Clean and disinfect utility gloves used for cleaning.
- Remove barrier garments (eg, face shields, glasses) as soon as possible after leaving a client's room.

If exposed to the blood of any client, immediately report the incident to the person in charge of employee health. You will be tested for HIV at regular intervals and treated with antiretrovirals depending on the results of tests or the potential for infection. While awaiting the results of diagnostic tests, follow the same sexual precautions as someone who has been diagnosed with AIDS.

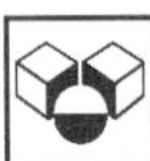

Nursing Guidelines 42-1

Safe Handling of Needles and Sharp Instruments

- Do not become distracted when handling needles and sharp instruments. Concentrate on the task being performed.
- Use a clean tray to pass used or contaminated needles and sharp instruments to another person.
- Keep the container for disposal of needles and sharp instruments close by. When necessary, carry the container to the bedside.
- If a client is uncooperative, ask for assistance when obtaining blood specimens, handling body fluids and secretions, giving injections, or starting IV therapy
- Do not leave uncapped or used needles unattended. Properly dispose of contaminated sharp instruments and needles as soon as they are used.

ETHICAL ISSUES

Ethical issues concerning the care of clients with HIV include confidentiality and the right to work. Never discuss the client's diagnosis or medical management anywhere with anyone. Because of improved drug management that prolongs a productive and essentially healthy life for HIV-infected individuals, many continue to work. It is illegal to prohibit HIV-positive individuals from working or to dismiss them on this basis. Health care workers can continue to practice. Some restrictions may be imposed, however, on performing procedures where blood may be exchanged between a health care worker and client.

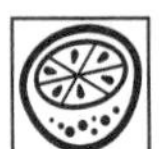

General Nutritional Considerations

HIV has a devastating impact on nutritional status. Progressive weight loss of 30% to 50% of pre-illness weight is not uncommon. Even among clients who do not appear malnourished, loss of muscle mass is common, as are subclinical deficiencies of vitamins and minerals. It is estimated that 80% of people with HIV or AIDS become malnourished; malnutrition may hasten the progression of AIDS through its negative impact on immune system functioning. However, neither weight loss nor malnutrition is an inevitable consequence of HIV. Although nutrition intervention cannot stop the progression of AIDS, it may slow its advance, preserve quality of life, and improve the effectiveness of drug therapy.

Nutrition intervention should begin before the client exhibits weight loss, even if intake appears adequate. Although exact nutritional requirements for HIV and AIDS have not yet been established, calorie and protein needs are increased and multivitamin and mineral supplements are prescribed at amounts greater than normal. Because some nutrients can impair immune system function when taken in large doses, clients are advised against self-prescribing nutrients.

Diet modifications are made to alleviate symptoms that interfere with intake or nutrient utilization. Clients with anorexia are encouraged to eat small, frequent meals of easily digested food and liquids even when they are not hungry. Clients with nausea and vomiting are advised to eat small, low-fat, high-carbohydrate food and liquids. Diarrhea and fat malabsorption improve when residue, lactose, and caffeine are avoided; gluten and sucrose restriction are sometimes necessary. MCT oil minimizes malabsorption and provides readily absorbable calories. Additional fluids are needed to replace fluid and electrolyte losses. Gravies, sauces, and broth added to soft, nonirritating foods promote ease of swallowing in clients with oral or esophageal ulcerations; hot food and liquids are avoided. Some clients require a blenderized or liquid diet.

Numerous enteral products are specifically designed for immunocompromised clients. These formulas are high in protein and low in fat and are enriched with selected ingredients that have been shown to improve immune function, such as omega-3 fatty acids and branched-chain amino acids.

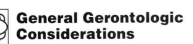

General Pharmacologic Considerations

The most common adverse effects associated with the administration of zidovudine are anemia and granulocytopenia.

Foscarnet is used to treat cytomegalovirus retinitis and is given by controlled IV infusion. Alterations in renal function, fever, nausea, anemia, and diarrhea are the more common adverse effects of this drug.

Administration of didanosine may result in pancreatitis and peripheral neuropathy.

The major adverse effect associated with zalcitabine administration is peripheral neuropathy. Pancreatitis may also occur.

Clients receiving antiviral drugs are informed that these drugs do not cure AIDS but may slow progression of the disease.

General Gerontologic Considerations

According to the Centers for Disease Control approximately 10% of the AIDS cases reported involve those over the age of 50.

Stereotyping older adults as asexual may cause the nurse to neglect to question the older adult about sexual matters, resulting in an inaccurate sexual history.

The dementia caused by AIDS may be mistaken for other dementias commonly associated with older adults.

Older adults with AIDS may lack an adequate support system and feel lonely, anxious, and isolated.

SUMMARY OF KEY CONCEPTS

- Acquired immunodeficiency syndrome (AIDS) is a consequence of an infection with the human immunodeficiency virus (HIV) that may not develop for 10 or more years.
- HIV is a retrovirus that is unable to replicate (duplicate) itself independently. It, therefore, becomes a parasite of helper T4 lymphocytes to make more copies of itself.
- HIV infection occurs through the transmission of four body fluids: blood, semen, vaginal secretions, and breast milk.
- HIV transmission can be avoided by abstaining from sexual intercourse, using barrier methods such as a condom and spermicide during sex, having a mutually monogamous sexual relationship with an uninfected partner, and refraining from IV drug use.
- A person has AIDS when opportunistic infections develop, the T4 cell count is or was 200 cells/mm ^{3} or less, and the HIV test is positive.
- HIV impairs the ability of infected T4 cells to recognize foreign antigens. When sufficient T4 cells are depleted, immunodeficiency develops; the infected person ultimately dies of an opportunistic infection.
- The first symptoms that develop are often mistaken as "flu," but in reality they are manifestations of acute retroviral syndrome (viremia). Some manifestations include fever; swollen and tender lymph nodes; pharyngitis; rash about the face, trunk, palms, and soles of the feet; muscle and joint pain; headache; and nausea, vomiting, and diarrhea.
- The ELISA and Western blot tests determine that a person is infected with HIV based on detecting antibodies in serum. A T cell count of 200/mm^3 or less confirms that the HIV-infected person has developed AIDS.
- The p24 antigen and polymerase chain reaction (PCR) tests measure viral loads. They are used to guide drug therapy and follow the progression of the disease.
- HIV-infected individuals are treated with a combination of two antiretroviral drugs: a reverse transcriptase (RT) inhibitor such as zidovudine (AZT), and a protease inhibitor such as nelfinavir (Viracept). The optimal outcome of drug therapy is "undectectable" viral loads or 500 copies or less. Maintaining a low viral load prolongs life expectancy.
- The nursing management of a client with AIDS includes obtaining a a comprehensive medical history, performing a thorough physical assessment, identifying findings that deviate from normal, developing a plan of care based on actual and potential problems such as the risk for opportunistic infections and the debilitating consequences of the primary infection, and providing health teaching that promotes a healthier lifestyle and prevents infection among others.
- Health teaching may include information about drug therapy, methods for reducing the risk for acquiring opportunistic infections, safer sexual practices, and refraining from IV drug use.
- Health care workers such as nurses can protect themselves from acquiring HIV from clients with known or unknown infectious status by following Standard Precautions, disposing of used needles and sharp instruments appropriately, and transporting specimens of body fluids in leakproof containers.

- Ethically health care workers ensure the confidentiality of any client's diagnosis. If a health care worker is exposed to blood or body fluid, he or she has the right to be tested for HIV antibodies, treated prophylactically with antiretroviral drugs, and remain employed if infected with HIV.

CRITICAL THINKING EXERCISES

1. The family members of a young man with AIDS are fearful of becoming infected if they let him live in their home. What health teaching can you provide?
2. What advice would you give adolescents to reduce their risk for becoming infected with HIV?
3. A nurse on a medical unit sustains a needle stick injury. What actions should the nurse take? What are the responsibilities of the employing agency?

Suggested Readings

Agency for Health Care Policy and Research. (1994, January). *Evaluation and management of early HIV infection. Clinical practice guideline* (Number 7). Rockville, MD: U.S. Department of Health and Human Services.

Cerrato, P. L. (1996). HIV report: Always a death sentence? *RN, 59*(8), 22, 24–28.

Chavez, C. (1996). Passive hyperimmune therapy: Buying time at what cost? *Caring, 15*(8), 48–50.

Consult stat. Choosing a doctor: A life or death decision with AIDS. *RN, 59*(11), 54.

Cuthbert-Allman, C. (1996). Crossing cultural barriers to care for people with AIDS. *Caring, 15*(8), 14–18.

Greif, J. & Golden, B. A. (1995). Home administration of nutritional and medical therapies for persons with AIDS. *Caring, 14*(2), 34–36, 38–39, 41–42.

Hansen, K. N. (1995). HIV testing. *Emergency Medicine Clinics of North America, 13*(1), 43–59.

Highsmith, C. (1997). Painful stimulus: Absorbing and assimilating grief and loss in HIV nursing practice. *Nursing Health Care Perspectives, 18*(5), 232–233.

HIV, hepatitis B, hepatitis C, blood borne diseases nurses' risks, rights, and responsibilities. (1996). *South Carolina Nurse, 3*(2), 35.

Kenny, P. (1996). Managing HIV infection: How to bolster your patient's fragile health. *Nursing, 26*(8), 26–35.

Molaghan, J. B. (1997). Adherence issues in HIV therapeutics. Introduction: The situation. *Journal of the Association of Nurses in AIDS Care, 8*(Suppl), 7–9.

Rabkin, R., & Rabkin, J. (1995). Management of depression in patients with HIV infection. *Caring, 14*(7), 28–30, 32, 34.

Sachs, K. M. (1996). Nutrition for in-home AIDS patients. *Caring, 15*(8), 36–38.

Sherman, D. W. (1996). Taking the fear out of AIDS nursing: Voices from the field. *Journal of the New York State Nurses Association, 27*(1), 4–8.

Stine, G. (1997). *AIDS update 1997.* Upper Saddle River, NJ: Prentice Hall.

Walsek, C., Zafonte, M., & Bowers, J.M. (1997). Nutritional issues and HIV/AIDS: Assessment and treatment strategies. *Journal of the Association of Nurses in AIDS Care, 8*(6), 71–80.

Wormser, G. P. (1996). *A clinical guide to AIDS and HIV.* Philadelphia: Lippincott-Raven.

Additional Resources

National AIDS Clearinghouse
P.O. Box 6003
Rockville, MD 20850
(800) 458–5231

Project Inform
1965 Market Street
Suite 220
San Francisco, CA 94103
(800) 822–7422
http://www.projinf.org/offlinc.html

AIDS Action Committee of Massachusetts
131 Clarendon Street
Boston, MA 02116
(800) 235–2331
http://www.aac.org/

AIDS Treatment Data Network
http://www.aidsnyc.org/network/index.html

AIDS Drug Assistance Programs (ADAP)
2062 Lombard Street
Philadelphia, PA 19146
(215) 545–2212
http://www.critipath.org/docs/adap.htm

National Minority AIDS Council Treatment and Research Advocacy Program
1931 13th Street, NW
Washington, DC 20009–4432
(800) 444–6472
http://www.omhrc.gov/mhr2/progs/94CO212.htm

10

Caring for Clients With Neurologic Disorders

Chapter 43

Introduction to the Nervous System

KEY TERMS

Acetylcholine
Acetylcholinesterase
Arachnoid
Axon
Brain stem
Cauda equina
Central nervous system
Cerebellum
Cerebrum
Decerebrate posturing
Decorticate posturing
Dendrites
Dopamine
Dura mater
Epinephrine
Extrapyramidal
Flaccidity
Medulla oblongata
Meninges
Midbrain
Myelin
Neurilemma
Neuron
Neurotransmitter
Norepinephrine
Parasympathetic nervous system
Peripheral nervous system
Pia mater
Pons
Pyramidal
Subarachnoid space
Sympathetic nervous system
Synapses
Ventricle

LEARNING OBJECTIVES

On completion of this chapter, the reader will:

- Name the two anatomic divisions of the nervous system.
- List the four lobes of the cerebrum.
- Name the three parts of the brain.
- Give two functions of the spinal cord.
- Name two parts of the autonomic nervous system and describe the function of each.
- Describe methods used to assess motor and sensory function.
- List six diagnostic procedures performed to detect neurologic disorders.
- Discuss the nursing management of the client undergoing neurologic diagnostic testing.

The nervous system consists of the brain, spinal cord, and peripheral nerves. It is responsible for coordinating body functions and responding to changes in or stimuli from the internal and external environment. Changes in the functioning of the nervous system have a profound effect on the body.

Anatomy and Physiology

The nervous system is divided into two anatomic divisions: the **central nervous system** (CNS) and the **peripheral nervous system** (PNS). The basic structure of the nervous system is the nerve cell or **neuron** (Fig. 43–1). Neurons are either sensory or motor. Sensory neurons transmit impulses to the CNS, and motor neurons transmit impulses from the CNS.

A neuron is composed of a cell body, a nucleus, and threadlike projections or fibers called **dendrites.** Dendrites conduct impulses to the cell body and are called afferent (to or toward) nerve fibers. A nerve fiber that projects from the cell body, which is usually larger than the dendrites, is called an **axon.** The axon conducts impulses away from the neuron, and therefore, is called an efferent (away from) nerve fiber.

Neurons are separate units and are not directly connected to each other. Impulses travel along neurons, moving from one neuron to the next by means of **synapses,** junctions between the axon of one neuron to the dendrite of another neuron. Transmission of an impulse from one neuron to the next is accomplished by substances called **neurotransmitters** (or neurohormones) (see Chap. 11).

Some axons in the CNS and PNS are covered with a fatty substance called **myelin,** and are called myelinated, or white, nerve fibers. The myelin is covered by a sheath called the **neurilemma.** Myelin serves as an insulating substance for the axon. Axons without myelin are called unmyelinated, or gray, nerve fibers.

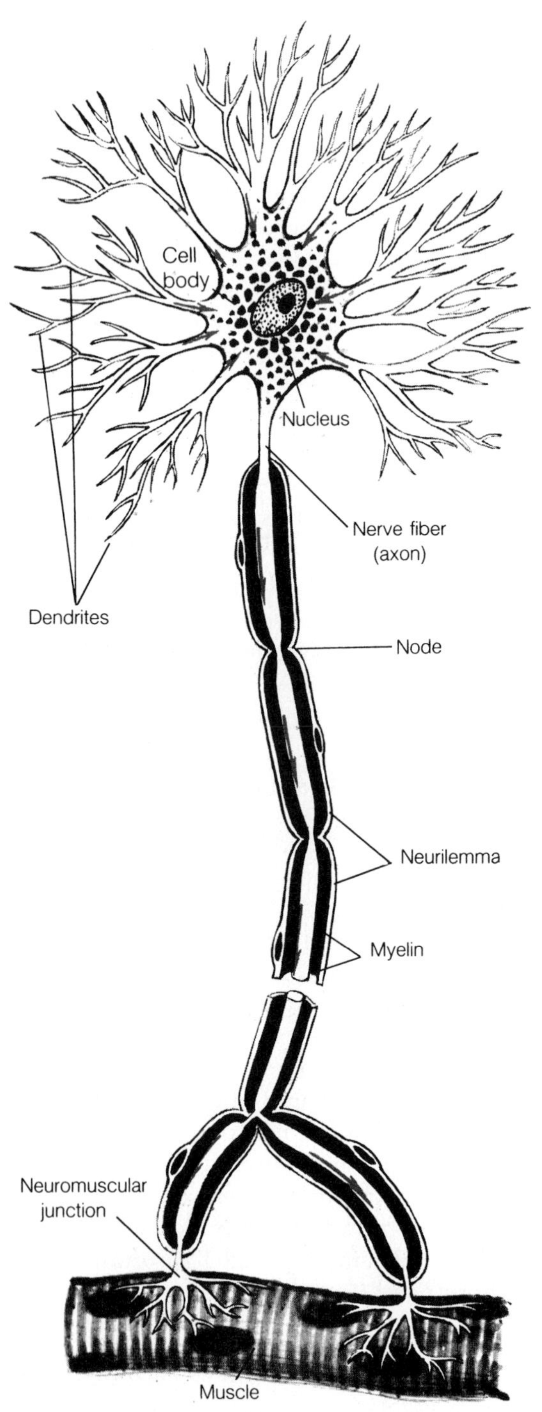

FIGURE 43-1. Diagram of a motor neuron. The arrows show the direction of the nerve impulse.

The Central Nervous System

The CNS consists of the brain and spinal cord.

THE BRAIN

The brain is divided into three parts: the cerebrum, the cerebellum, and the brain stem. The **cerebrum** consists of two hemispheres connected by the corpus callosum, a band of white fibers that acts as a bridge for transmitting impulses between the left and the right hemispheres. Each hemisphere has four lobes: frontal, parietal, temporal, and occipital. The location and primary functions of each lobe are shown in Figure 43–2. The cerebral cortex is the surface of the cerebrum. It contains motor neurons that are responsible for movement and sensory neurons that receive impulses from peripheral sensory neurons located throughout the body.

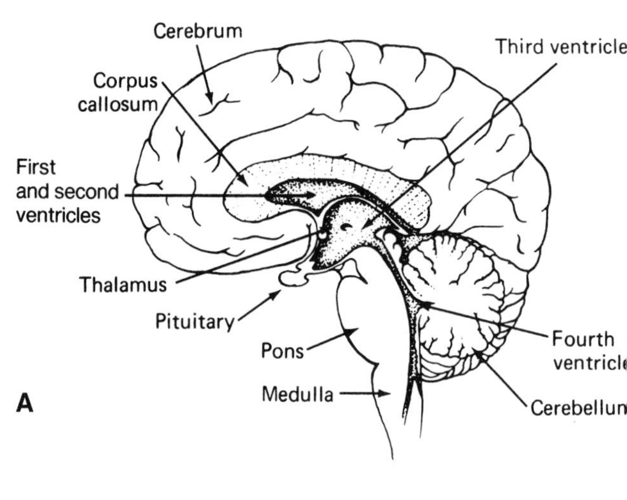

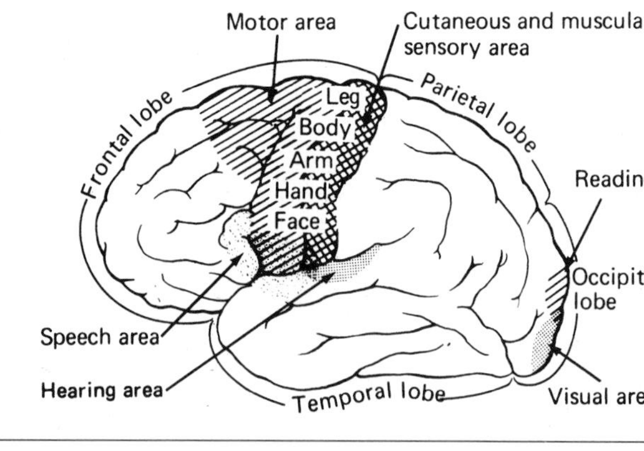

FIGURE 43-2. (*A*) Major structures of the brain. (*B*) Diagrammatic representation of approximate areas of the brain that control various functions.

Motor tracts are **pyramidal** or **extrapyramidal.** Pyramidal motor pathways originate in the motor cortex of the cerebrum, cross over at the level of the medulla, and end in the brain stem and spinal cord. Extrapyramidal fibers originate in the motor cortex and project to the cerebellum and basal ganglia. They do not cross over as they connect to motor neurons in the spinal cord.

The **cerebellum,** which is located behind and below the cerebrum, controls and coordinates muscle movement. The **brain stem** consists of the midbrain, pons, and medulla oblongata. The **midbrain** forms the forward part of the brain stem and connects the pons and cerebellum with the two cerebral hemispheres. The **pons** is located between the midbrain and medulla, and connects the two hemispheres of the cerebellum with the brain stem, spinal cord, and cerebrum. The **medulla oblongata** lies below the pons and transmits motor impulses from the brain to the spinal cord and sensory impulses from peripheral sensory neurons to the brain. The medulla contains vital centers concerned with respiration, heartbeat, and vasomotor activity controlling smooth muscle activity in blood vessel walls.

The brain is protected by the rigid bones of the skull and covered by three membranes or **meninges:** (1) the **dura mater,** the tough, outermost covering; (2) the **arachnoid**, or middle membrane lying directly below the dura; and (3) the **pia mater,** a delicate layer that adheres to the brain and spinal cord. The **subarachnoid space** is between the pia mater and the arachnoid membrane.

Within the brain are four hollow structures called **ventricles** (see Fig. 43–2). The ventricles manufacture and absorb cerebrospinal fluid (CSF), which constantly circulates in the subarachnoid space of the brain and spinal cord. CSF produced in the ventricles passes down into the subarachnoid space of the spinal cord, then up through the basilar cisterns, and over the cerebral hemispheres to the region of the dural venous sinuses where most of the absorption occurs. Acting as a cushion, it protects these structures and helps to maintain relatively constant intracranial pressure.

THE SPINAL CORD

The spinal cord, which is covered by the meninges, is a direct continuation of the medulla and is surrounded and protected by the *vertebrae* (or vertebral column). The spinal cord ends between the first and second lumbar vertebrae, where it divides into smaller sections called the **cauda equina.**

The spinal cord functions as a passageway for ascending sensory and descending motor neurons. The two main functions of the spinal cord are to provide centers for reflex action (Fig. 43–3) and to provide a pathway for impulses to and from the brain. The sensory fibers enter the posterior (dorsal) portion of the cord; the nerve fibers that transmit motor impulses run outward to the peripheral nerves from the anterior (ventral) portion of the cord.

The Peripheral Nervous System

The PNS consists of all nerves outside the CNS.

THE CRANIAL NERVES

The 12 pairs of cranial nerves, identified by Roman numerals, are:

- *I*— Olfactory nerve: sense of smell
- *II*— Optic nerve: sight
- *III*— Oculomotor nerve: contraction of eye muscles
- *IV*—Trochlear nerve: eye movement
- *V*—Trigeminal nerve: sensory nerve to face, chewing
- *VI*—Abducens nerve: eye movement
- *VII*—Facial nerve: facial expression, taste, secretions of salivary and lacrimal glands
- *VIII*—Vestibulocochlear (or auditory) nerve: hearing, balance
- *IX*— Glossopharyngeal nerve: taste, sensory fibers of pharynx and tongue, swallowing, secretions of parotid gland
- *X*—Vagus nerve: motor fibers to glands producing digestive juices, heart rate, muscles of speech, gastrointestinal motility, respiration, swallowing, coughing, vomiting reflex
- *XI*—Accessory (or spinal accessory) nerve: head and shoulder movement
- *XII*—Hypoglossal nerve: movement of the tongue

THE SPINAL NERVES

There are 31 pairs of spinal nerves: 8 cervical, 12 thoracic, 5 lumbar, 5 sacral, and 1 coccygeal. Spinal nerves have two roots: the dorsal root and the ventral root. Dorsal nerve fibers are sensory, and ventral nerve fibers are motor. Peripheral sensory nerve fibers in various areas of the body transmit impulses to the spinal nerves, which transmit impulses up the spinal cord to the brain. Motor impulses traveling from the brain and down the spinal cord leave by the ventral root and travel to areas of the body. Each spinal nerve root innervates a specific area or dermatome of body surface (Fig. 43–4). Knowledge of the distribution of dermatomes is useful for the nurse's assessment and evaluation.

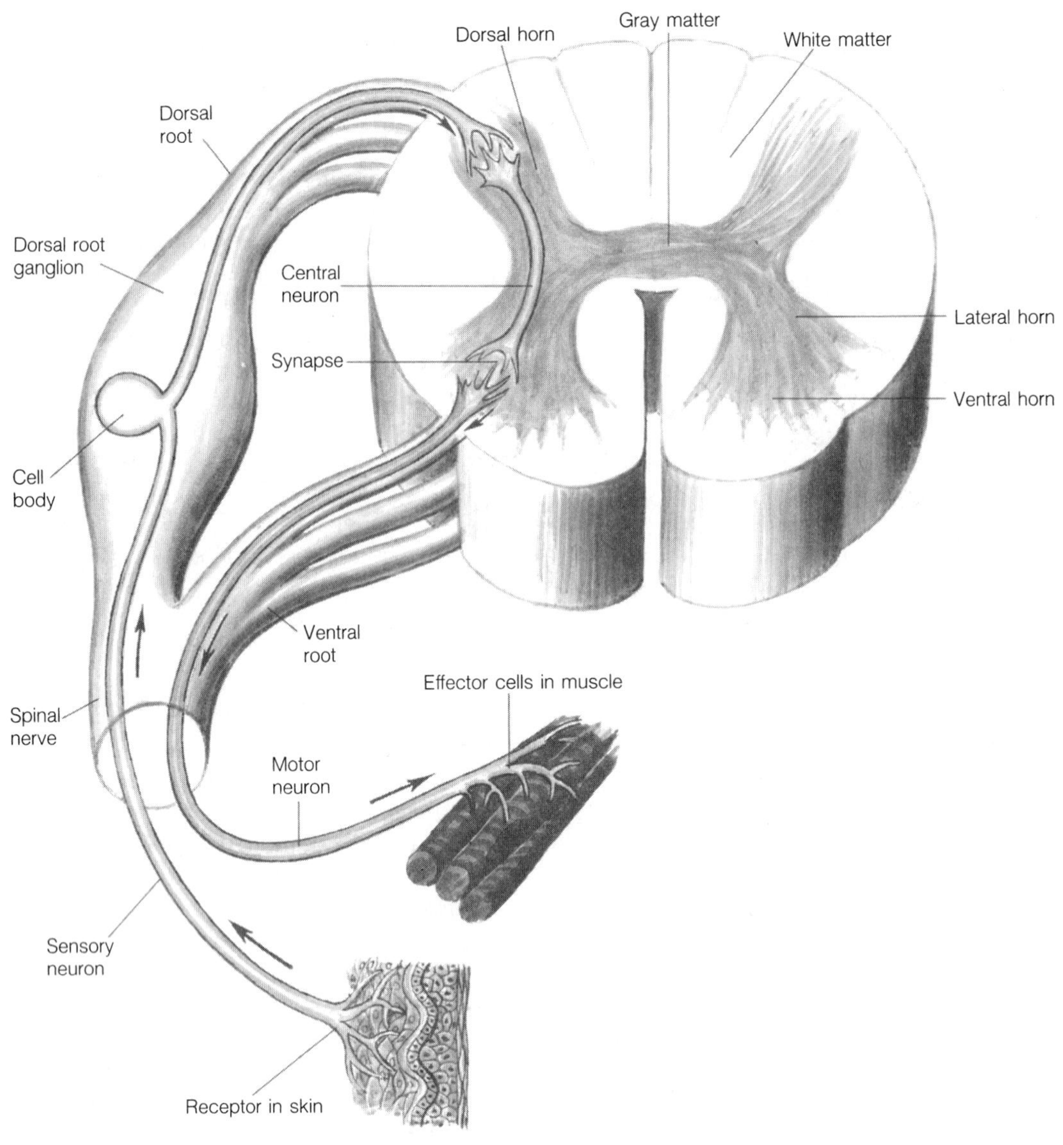

FIGURE 43-3. Reflex arc showing the pathway of impulses and cross section of the spinal cord.

AUTONOMIC NERVOUS SYSTEM

The autonomic nervous system consists of the **sympathetic nervous system** and the **parasympathetic nervous system.** It is concerned with functions essential to the survival of the organism.

The Sympathetic Nervous System

This division of the autonomic nervous system regulates the expenditure of energy. The neurotransmitters of the sympathetic nervous system, collectively known as catecholamines, are **epinephrine, norepinephrine,** and **dopamine.** The adrenal medulla produces and secretes epinephrine and norepinephrine. Norepinephrine is also produced at sympathetic nerve endings. Dopamine is a precursor (a substance that precedes another) of norepinephrine. Norepinephrine then becomes epinephrine. Stressful situations such as danger, intense emotion, and severe illness result in release of catecholamines.

The Parasympathetic Nervous System

This division of the autonomic nervous system works to conserve body energy and is partly responsible for slowing the heart rate, digesting food, and eliminating body wastes. **Acetylcholine** is a neurotransmitter that is released at nerve endings of parasympathetic nerve fibers, at some nerve endings in the sympathetic nervous system, and at nerve endings of skeletal muscles. Release of this neurotransmitter allows passage of a nerve impulse from the nerve fiber to the effector organ or structure, where acetylcholine is inactivated by the enzyme **acetylcholinesterase.**

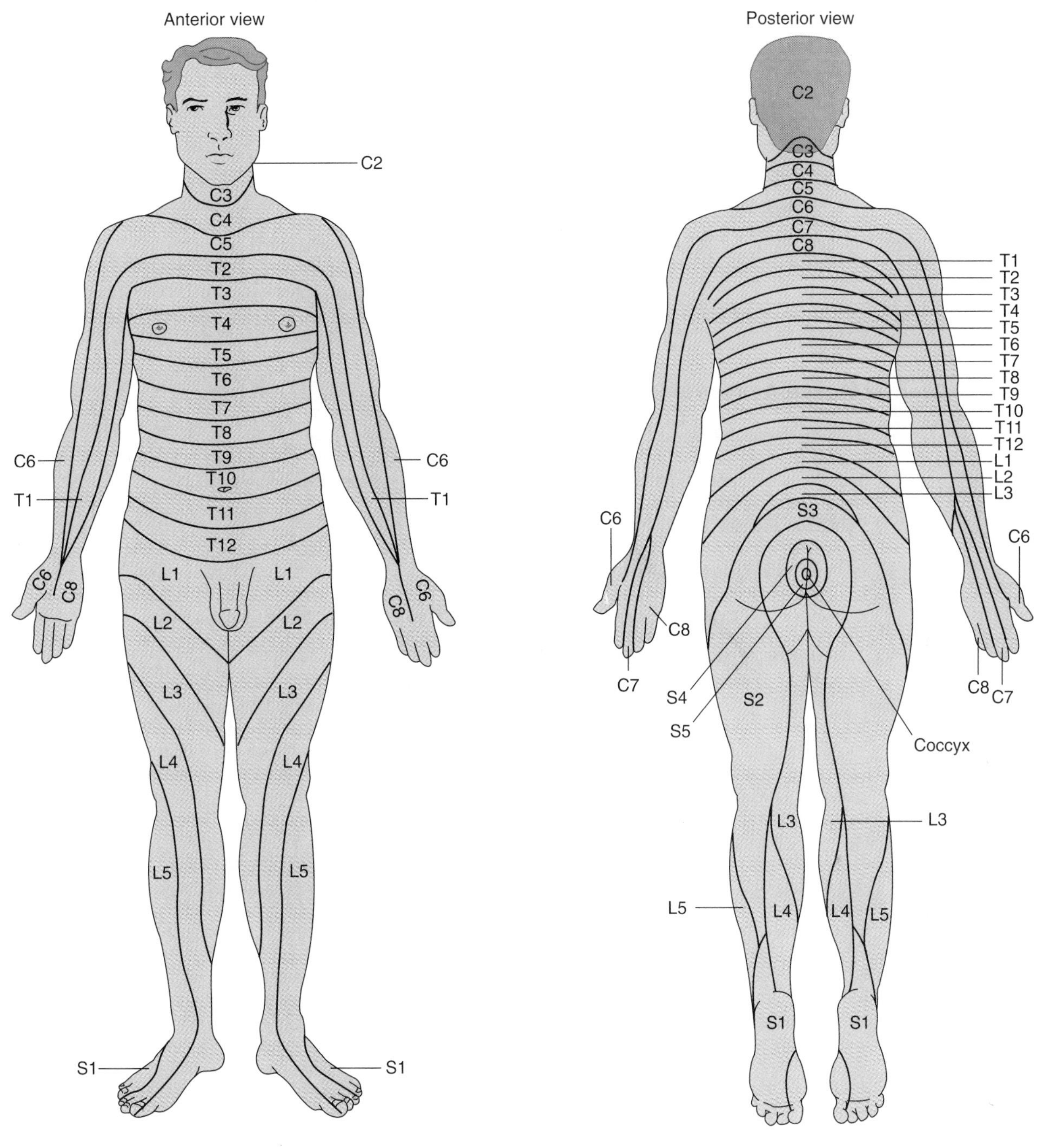

FIGURE 43-4. Anterior and posterior views of dermatomes.

Physical Assessment

A neurologic examination is performed to identify and locate disorders of the nervous system. The scope and extent of the neurologic examination often depends on the symptoms and the probable or actual diagnosis.

A thorough history is essential. The nurse explores all symptoms and asks questions to clarify or describe each symptom. The history must include a record of trauma (no matter how slight) to the head or body within the past 6 to 12 months, a drug history, an allergy history, and a family medical history. The nurse observes the client's speech pattern, mental status, intellectual functioning, reasoning ability, and movement or lack of movement of all extremities.

The physical examination consists of assessment of the cerebral, motor, and sensory areas. Intellectual function and the speech pattern are initially assessed during the history by noting responses to questions. Additional testing of intellectual function includes asking a variety of questions that require mental tasks (see mini mental status examination in Chap. 11).

Body posture is evaluated, and any abnormal position of the head, neck, trunk, or extremities noted. If head trauma has occurred, the ears and nose are examined for evidence of bleeding or other type of drainage. The head is carefully examined for bleeding, swelling, or wounds. The head is not moved or manipulated during this part of the assessment, especially if there is a recent history of trauma.

Cranial Nerves

Evaluation of all or some of the 12 cranial nerves is performed by the experienced examiner (Table 43–1).

Motor Function

Assessment of motor function includes muscle movement, size, tone, strength, and coordination. Large muscle areas are inspected for evidence of atrophy.

TABLE 43-1 **Cranial Nerve Assessment**

Cranial Nerve	Assessment Technique	Normal Finding(s)
Cranial nerve I Olfactory	Occlude each nostril separately and close the eyes. Present sources of familiar odors such as vinegar, lemon, coffee, ammonia.	Identifies odors correctly.
Cranial nerve II Optic	Cover each eye separately and test visual acuity using a Snellen chart (see Chap. 48) or newspaper.	Names letters or reads words accurately.
	The client and examiner cover an eye and the examiner moves an object from the periphery toward the nose from superior, inferior, medial, and lateral positions while both fix their gaze straight ahead; the opposite eye is then tested.	Client sees the object at the same time in the visual field as the examiner.
	Inspect the optic nerve with an ophthalmoscope.	The optic nerve appears round and lighter than the surrounding retina.
Cranial nerve III Oculomotor	In a darkened room, shine a light in each pupil; ask the client to look at a near and far object. (See Chap. 48).	Brisk pupil constriction in response to light; pupil dilation when looking far away
	Have the client follow an object that is moved in horizontal, vertical, and oblique directions (see Chap. 48).	Coordinated eye movement in all directions
Cranial nerve IV Trochlear	See assessment for motor function of oculomotor nerve.	Moves eyes inferiorly and medially.
Cranial nerve V Trigeminal	Observe for jaw symmetry when the client's mouth is opened.	Symmetrical appearance
	Instruct the client to clamp the jaws tightly together.	The muscles contract bilaterally.
	Stroke the forehead, cheeks, and jaw with a wisp of cotton, sharp object like a pin, cold and warm object, and a vibrating tuning fork.	Bilateral sensitivity and correct identification of sensory experience
	Touch each cornea with a wisp of cotton.	Client blinks.
	Tap the center of the chin with a reflex hammer when the client's mouth is slightly opened.	Sudden, slight closing of the jaw
Cranial nerve VI Abducens	See assessment for motor function of oculomotor nerve.	Moves eyes in lateral directions.
Cranial nerve VII Facial	Ask the client to wrinkle the forehead, smile, frown, raise the eyebrows, look at the ceiling, and whistle.	Symmetrical facial movement
	Instruct client to close eyelids and resist the examiner's efforts to open them.	Resists eye opening equally bilaterally.
	Apply sweet, sour, salty, bitter flavors to both sides of the anterior tongue.	Accurate identification
Cranial nerve VIII Vestibulocochlear	Test hearing acuity and perform the Rinne and Weber tests with a tuning fork (see Chap. 49).	Repeats whispered words correctly; sound is lateralized equally; sound is heard longer by air rather than bone conduction.
	Have the client stand with both feet close together and note for swaying with the eyes open and then shut.	Maintains balance or sways slightly.
Cranial nerve IX Glossopharyngeal	Touch the palate with a tongue blade.	Elicits a gag response.
	Ask the client to say, "ah."	Uvula remains in midline.
Cranial nerve X Vagus	Have the client say "la, la, la." Sensory functions are not routinely assessed.	Speaks clearly and distinctly; no hoarseness noted.
Cranial nerve XI Spinal-Accessory	Instruct client to shrug the shoulders as resistance is applied.	Raises shoulders.
Cranial nerve XII Hypoglossal	Tell the client to stick out the tongue.	Tongue remains in midline with no lateral deviation.

and opposing muscles are assessed for equality of size and strength. The client is asked to perform tasks such as:

- Pushing the palm or sole against the examiner's palm
- Picking up small and large objects between the thumb and forefinger
- Grasping objects firmly
- Resisting removal of an object from the fist or fingers

To assess gait, movement, and balance, the client is asked to walk away from the examiner, turn, and walk back. Other tests include climbing a small set of stairs, walking and turning abruptly, and walking heel to toe. In the Romberg test the client stands with feet close together and eyes closed. If the client sways and tends to fall, this is considered a positive Romberg test, indicating a problem with equilibrium. The examiner stands fairly close to the client during this test in case the client loses balance.

Tests that evaluate motor and cerebral function include the finger-to-nose test with eyes closed, writing words, and identifying common objects. The choice of tests depends on the original complaints and the findings of diagnostic tests.

Motor response in the comatose or unconscious client is evaluated by administering a painful stimulus to determine if the client makes an appropriate response by reaching toward or withdrawing from the stimulus (Fig. 43–5*A* and *B*). Those with impaired cerebral function manifest **decorticate posturing** (decorticate rigidity), **decerebrate posturing** (decerebrate rigidity), or **flaccidity** (Fig. 43–5*C*–*E*). Decerebrate posturing is more serious than decorticate posturing; flaccidity is an even more ominous sign.

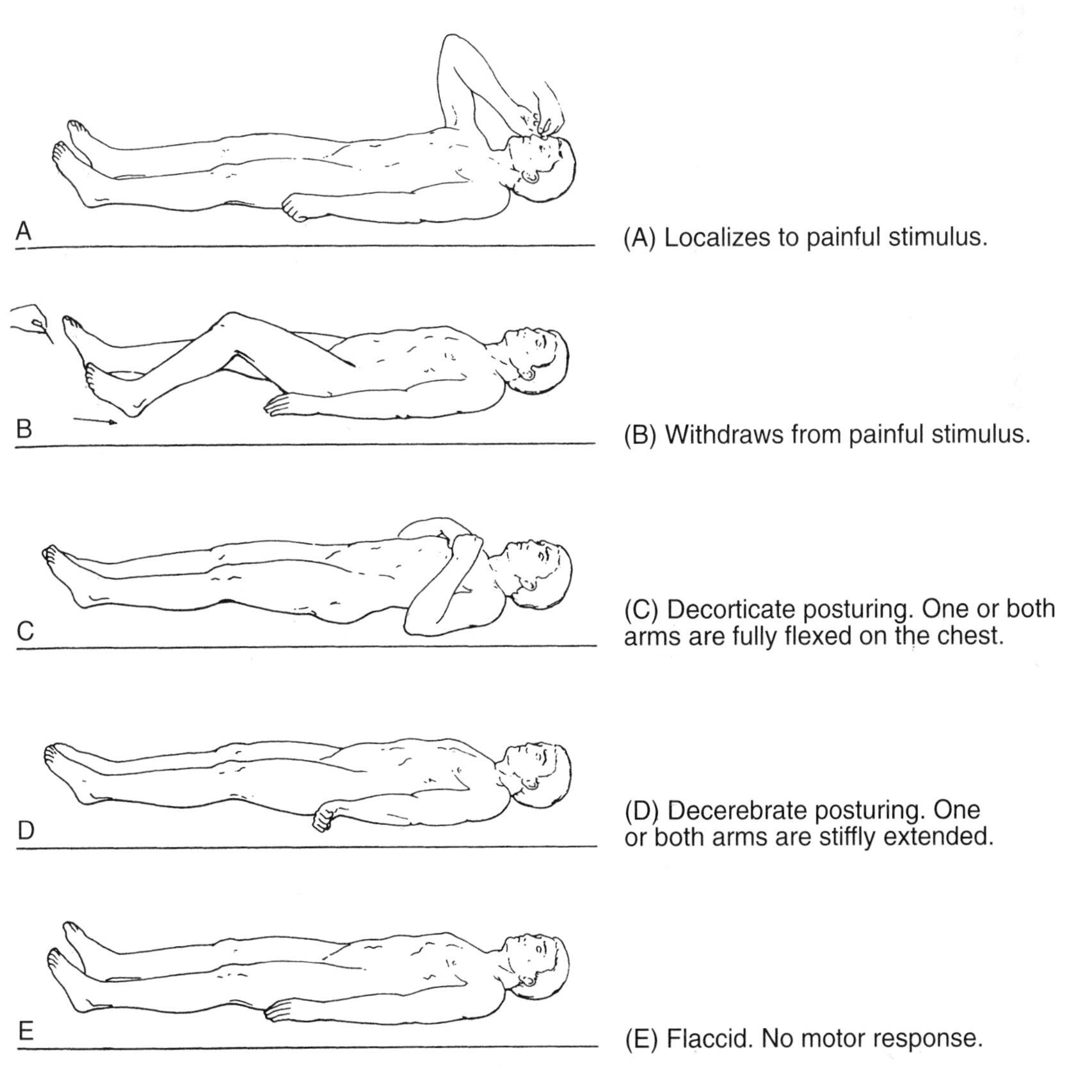

A
(A) Localizes to painful stimulus.
B
(B) Withdraws from painful stimulus.
C
(C) Decorticate posturing. One or both arms are fully flexed on the chest.
D
(D) Decerebrate posturing. One or both arms are stiffly extended.
E
(E) Flaccid. No motor response.

FIGURE 43-5. Responses to pain and posturing.

Sensory Function

The extremities are evaluated for sensitivity to heat, cold, touch, and pain. Various objects such as cotton balls, tubes filled with hot or cold water, and sharp objects (that do not pierce the skin) are used to check sensation in the extremities.

Level of Consciousness

Depending on the client's symptoms, it is often necessary to evaluate the level of consciousness (LOC). The following classification of LOC applies to altered consciousness from any cause. Sometimes it is difficult to differentiate between each of the levels; some clients show characteristics of two or more levels.

- *Conscious*: The client responds immediately, fully, and appropriately to visual, auditory, and other stimulation.
- *Somnolent or lethargic*: The client is drowsy or sleepy at inappropriate times but can be aroused only to fall asleep again. Responses to questions are delayed or inappropriate. Speech is incoherent. The client responds slowly to verbal commands. There is a response to painful stimuli.
- *Stuporous*: The client is aroused only by vigorous and continuous stimulation, usually by manipulation or by strong auditory or visual stimuli. Stimulation results in one- or two-word answers or in motor activity or purposeful behavior directed toward avoiding further stimulation.
- *Semicomatose*: The client is unresponsive except to superficial, relatively mild painful stimuli to which some purposeful motor response (movement) is made to evade stimulation. Spontaneous motion is uncommon, but the client may groan or mutter.
- *Comatose*: The client responds only to very painful stimuli by fragmentary, delayed reflex withdrawal; in deeper stages, all responsiveness is

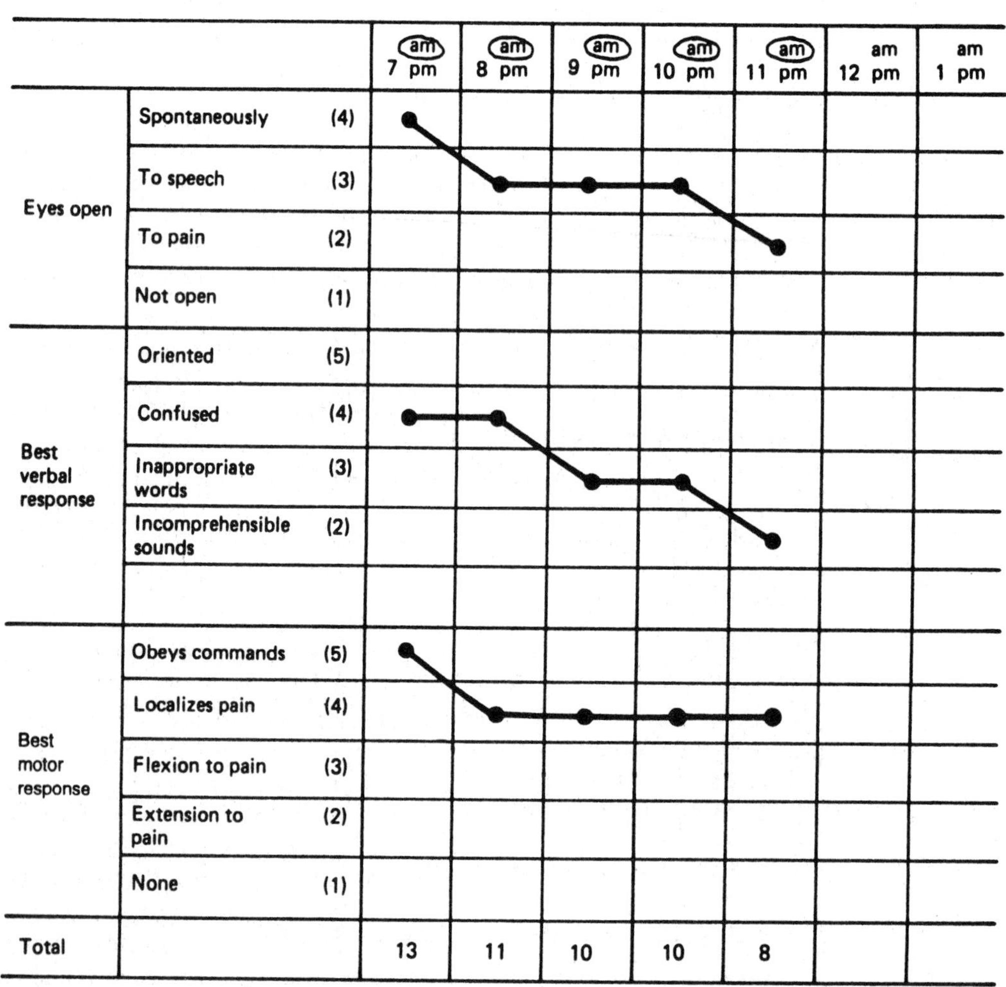

am 7 pm
am 8 pm
am 9 pm
am 10 pm
am 11 pm
am 12 pm
am 1 pm
Eyes open
Spontaneously (4)
To speech (3)
To pain (2)
Not open (1)
Best verbal response
Oriented (5)
Confused (4)
Inappropriate words (3)
Incomprehensible sounds (2)
Best motor response
Obeys commands (5)
Localizes pain (4)
Flexion to pain (3)
Extension to pain (2)
None (1)
Total
13
11
10
10
8

FIGURE 43-6. Example of a graphic record of hourly assessments using the Glasgow Coma Scale.

lost. There is no spontaneous movement, and the respiratory rate is irregular.

The LOC is assessed at frequent intervals after injury to the head or neck, cranial surgery, a cerebrovascular accident (acute phase), a ruptured cerebral aneurysm, and other neurologic disorders. This assessment is made hourly unless the physician orders otherwise or a change in the client's condition is noted.

The Glasgow Coma Scale (Fig. 43–6) is a measure of the LOC. It consists of three parts: eye opening response, best verbal response, and best motor response. To evaluate responses correctly, several verbal and motor responses are elicited, and the best response is recorded. The eye opening response is determined by talking to the client and calling his or her name. If no response is noted (eg, the eyes do not open spontaneously), a painful stimulus is introduced and the response noted. The verbal response is evaluated by a verbal reply to questions. The motor response is the ability of the client to follow commands, such as "wiggle your toes" or "move your left hand." If there is no response, a painful stimulus is introduced and the response noted. The responses are assigned numbers and the numbers are totaled. A normal response is 14. A score of 7 or less is considered coma. The evaluations are recorded on a graphic sheet. Connecting lines show an increase or decrease in the LOC.

The Rancho Los Amigos Scale (Box 43–1) is another tool for assessing LOC. Some rehabilitation centers prefer this scale because it is a more flexible assessment tool for identifying the client's status.

BOX 43-1 Rancho Los Amigos Scales

Level I No response to stimuli. Appears in deep sleep.
Level II Generalized response. First reaction may be to deep pain. Has delayed, inconsistent responses.
Level III Localized response. Inconsistent responses, but reacts in a more specific manner to stimulus. Might follow simple command "squeeze my hand."
Level IV Confused. Agitated. Reacts to own inner confusion, fear, disorientation. Excitable behavior, may be abusive.
Level V Nonagitated. Confused. Inappropriate. Usually disoriented. Follows tasks for 2 to 3 minutes, but easily distracted by environment, frustrated.
Level VI Confused appropriate. Follows simple directions consistently. Memory and attention increasing. Self-care tasks performed without help.
Level VII Automatic appropriate. If physically able, can carry out routine activities. Appears normal. Needs supervision for safety.
Level VIII Purposeful. Alert. Oriented. May have decreased abilities relative to premorbid state.

Pupils

The size and equality of the pupils and their reaction to light are an assessment of the third cranial (oculomotor) nerve (see Table 43–1). Pupil size (normal, pinpoint, dilated), equality (equal, unequal in size), and reaction to a bright light (normal, sluggish, no reaction, fixed) are noted (see Chap. 48). When the pupils are examined, any abnormal movement or position of one or both eyes is noted.

Unequal pupils (one pupil larger than the other), dilated or pinpoint pupils, and failure of the pupils to respond quickly to light are, in most instances, abnormal findings. *Any sudden change in pupil size, equality, or reaction to light is an important neurologic finding and is reported to the physician at once.*

Neck

The neck is examined for stiffness or abnormal position. The presence of rigidity is checked by moving the head and chin toward the chest. Do *not* perform this maneuver if a head or neck injury is suspected or known or trauma to any part of the body is evident.

Vital Signs

The blood pressure, pulse and respiratory rates, and temperature are closely monitored on all clients with a potential or actual neurologic disorder. The temperature often needs to be monitored every hour because CNS disorders can affect the temperature-regulating ability of the hypothalamus. A sudden increase or decrease in any of the vital signs indicates a change in the neurologic status, and the physician is notified immediately.

Diagnostic Tests

Imaging Procedures

Imaging procedures such as computed tomography (CT), magnetic resonance imaging (MRI), positron emission tomography (PET), and single photon emission computed tomography are used in the diagnosis of neurologic disorders. Imaging procedures are particularly useful in the diagnosis of neurologic disorders such as brain tumors, Alzheimer's disease, intracranial bleeding or hemorrhage, and cerebral infections. A radiopaque dye is used during a CT scan to emphasize or highlight a certain area. Use of a radiopaque dye decreases the safety of the procedure.

COMPUTED TOMOGRAPHY

Computed tomography scanning uses x-rays and computer analysis to produce three-dimensional views of thin cross sections, or "slices," of the body. A narrow x-ray beam rotates around the client and the results are analyzed by a computer. CT is extremely sensitive to differences in tissue densities, allowing differentiation between intracranial tumors, cysts, edema, and hemorrhage. The client is exposed to the same amount of radiation as a conventional x-ray.

MAGNETIC RESONANCE IMAGING

An MRI is based on the magnetic behavior of protons in body tissue. This imaging procedure uses radio frequency to produce images of tissues of high fat and water content such as soft tissue, veins, arteries, the brain, and spinal cord. Images are produced without contrast dye or radiation.

The client lies motionless on a stretcher enclosed in a tunnel containing a powerful magnet. The MRI lasts 15 to 90 minutes. Claustrophobia is commonly experienced. A call button and an intercom are available for two-way communication. The MRI cannot be used for clients with metal implants such as a hip or knee replacement or cardiac pacemaker because metal interferes with the magnetic field.

POSITRON EMISSION TOMOGRAPHY

Positron emission tomography uses radioactive substances to examine metabolic activity of body structures. The client either inhales or is injected with a radioactive substance with positively charged particles that combine with negatively charged particles found normally in the body. The energy emitted when these combine are converted into color-coded images indicating metabolic activity of the organ involved. The radioactive substances are short-lived resulting in minimal radiation exposure. PET is used less frequently than CT or MRI because the equipment is available only in major medical research centers.

Lumbar Puncture

Changes in CSF occur in many neurologic disorders. A lumbar puncture (spinal tap) is performed to obtain samples of CSF from the subarachnoid space for laboratory examination and to measure CSF pressure. Bacteriologic tests on specimens of CSF reveal the presence of pathogenic microorganisms. Strict aseptic technique is required during the procedure. The CSF is normally clear and colorless with a pressure of 80 to 180 mm H_2O; a pressure over 200 mm H_2O is considered abnormal. A lumbar puncture is also performed to inject a drug into the subarachnoid space (intrathecal injection), to administer a spinal anesthetic, to withdraw CSF for the relief of intracranial pressure, or to inject air, gas, or dye for a neurologic diagnostic procedure.

Sometimes a cisternal puncture is performed to remove CSF. The back of the neck is shaved, the skin washed with an antiseptic, and a needle inserted just below the occipital bone of the skull. This procedure is more commonly performed on children. Headache appears to occur less frequently with cisternal puncture than with lumbar puncture.

Contrast Studies

Contrast studies include cerebral angiogram, which detects distortion of cerebral arteries and veins, indicating an aneurysm, a tumor, or other vascular abnormality. A radiopaque dye is injected into the right or left carotid artery, the brachial artery, or the femoral artery. A rapid sequence of radiographs is taken as the dye circulates through the cerebral arteries and veins.

For a myelogram, a radiopaque substance is injected into the spinal canal by means of a lumbar puncture. Radiographs are taken to demonstrate abnormalities of the spinal canal such as tumors or a ruptured intervertebral disk.

Electroencephalogram

An electroencephalogram (EEG) records the electrical impulses generated by the brain. Electrodes are placed on the scalp and electrical activity is recorded on a graph.

Brain Scan

A brain scan identifies tumors, hematomas in or around the brain, cerebral abscesses, cerebral infarctions, or displaced ventricles. A radioactive material is injected before the procedure. The length of this procedure varies from a few minutes to 1 hour. CT scans and MRI are replacing this procedure.

Electromyography

Electromyography (EMG) studies the changes in the electrical potential of muscles and the nerves supplying the muscles. Needle electrodes are placed into one or more skeletal muscles and the results recorded on an oscilloscope. This test is useful in determining the presence of neuromuscular disorders.

Nerve Conduction Studies

Nerve conduction studies measure the speed with which nerve impulses travel along a peripheral nerve fiber when a specific nerve is electrically stimulated. This test aids diagnosis of nerve injury and compression or neurologic disorders affecting peripheral nerves.

Echoencephalography

An echoencephalogram is an ultrasound examination of the structures of the brain. This procedure is performed to detect abnormalities in the ventricles and the location of intracranial bleeding.

Nursing Management

The nurse determines the client's understanding of the diagnostic procedures or what questions remain. Because some contrast media contain iodine, the nurse checks the client's history for previous allergic reactions to radiographic dyes, allergies to iodine, or a seafood allergy. Focused assessments include baseline vital signs and neurologic data such as LOC, pupil response, and status of muscle strength in all four extremities. The assessment findings are used for comparison when monitoring the client's condition during and after diagnostic testing.

The nurse communicates assessment findings, obtains a signed consent form when indicated, prepares the client for the diagnostic test following agency policies, brings necessary equipment to the room before any bedside procedures, assists the physician and supports the client during a test performed on the nursing unit, monitors the client for adverse consequences, and promotes recovery following the test.

NURSING PROCESS
Care of the Client Undergoing Neurologic Testing

Assessment

In addition to the assessment factors discussed previously, chart the client's weight and vital signs before the procedure. Closely observe the client for any mental or physical deviations from the baseline assessment.

Diagnosis and Planning

Nursing care of clients undergoing diagnostic tests for a neurologic disorder includes, but is not limited to, the following:

Nursing Diagnoses and Collaborative Problems	Nursing Interventions
Knowledge Deficit related to unfamiliarity with diagnostic testing process **Goal:** The client will accurately describe the preparation, procedure, and after-care involved in the scheduled diagnostic test.	Clarify the physician's explanation. Provide answers to the client's questions. Describe the procedure to the client as well as what is required during the procedure, such as positions that are assumed or the need to lie still while the procedure is performed. Instruct the client on the preparation for the diagnostic test, which may include temporarily eliminating CNS depressants, such as barbiturates and minor tranquilizers, and CNS stimulants, such as caffeine for 24 to 48 hours in the case of an EEG. Explain that hair will be shampooed before an EEG to ensure that oil and hair products do not interfere with the testing process and results. Inform the client that a shampoo is required after an EEG to remove paste used to secure the electrodes to the scalp. Tell the client to expect some discomfort when undergoing a lumbar puncture, myelogram, EMG, and nerve conduction studies.
PC: Allergic Reaction to contrast dye **Goal:** An allergic reaction will be managed and minimized.	Report the allergy history to the physician and identify the information prominently on the client's chart. Attach an allergy band to the client's wrist when that is the agency's policy. Administer pretest antihistamine drugs according to the physician's medical order.

Monitor the client for severe hypotension, tachycardia, profuse diaphoresis, a sudden change in LOC, dyspnea, hives or itching, and notify the physician immediately.

Obtain the emergency cart that contains drugs and resuscitation equipment and follow instructions for administering oxygen, intravenous fluids, drugs, and airway management depending on the client's symptoms.

PC: Meningeal Irritation or CNS changes

Goal: CNS complications will be managed and minimized following diagnostic testing.

Observe closely for any neurologic abnormalities such as diminished LOC, weakness, numbness, paralysis in an extremity, unequal or unresponsive pupil reflexes, posturing, and speech disturbance.

Assess for changes in vital signs, restlessness, vomiting, and mental changes in orientation and thought processes.

Report the onset of a headache and sudden or severe pain in any area of the body to the physician immediately.

Inspect injection sites, especially those made during a lumbar puncture, for signs of a hematoma (collection of blood).

Position the client flat for at least 3 hours or as directed by the physician following a lumbar puncture or myelogram. Encourage a liberal fluid intake to restore the volume of CSF.

Keep the room dark and quiet after a lumbar puncture or myelogram and administer a prescribed analgesic if the client develops a headache.

Evaluation and Expected Outcomes

- The client demonstrates understanding of the procedure or diagnostic test.
- An allergic reaction, if it occurs, is controlled.
- Complications are avoided or minimized.

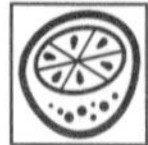

General Nutritional Considerations

Clients with an allergy to iodine cannot receive radiopaque dyes that contain this substance. A thorough allergy history is an essential part of the neurologic examination. Seafood allergies indicate an allergy to iodine.

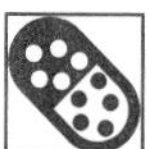

General Pharmacologic Considerations

When a client is receiving morphine or other narcotic depressants for pain, the response of the pupils to light is affected and the pupils are pinpoint in size. This is due to the drug and not a neurologic disorder.

The use of morphine, heroin, or other narcotic or CNS depressants shortly before a neurologic examination affects the results of a neurologic examination.

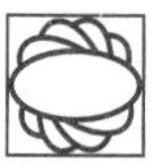

General Gerontologic Considerations

Diseases that occur with age (eg, dementia) often make it difficult to perform a neurologic assessment.

With age there is a decrease in brain weight and a decrease in the number of brain cells. Older adults experience short-term memory loss and a slower reaction time.

Pupillary response is more sluggish in the older adult. When cataracts are present, there may be no pupillary response.

The possibility of drug toxicity should always be considered when an elderly person has a change in mental status.

Older adults who have difficulty following directions during a neurologic examination or diagnostic procedure need brief instructions given one step at a time during the examination or procedure.

Obtain facts necessary for a health history from a family member or friend of an older adult who has difficulty remembering recent or past events, symptoms, drug and medical history, and other facts necessary for a history.

SUMMARY OF KEY CONCEPTS

- The nervous system consists of the brain, spinal cord, and peripheral nerves. It is responsible for coordinating many body functions and responding to changes in or stimuli from the internal and external environment.
- The nervous system is divided into the central nervous system and the peripheral nervous system. The central nervous system consists of the brain and spinal cord.
- The brain is divided into three parts: the cerebrum, cerebellum, and brain stem.
- The brain is protected by the rigid bones of the skull and covered by three membranes or meninges. Within the brain are four hollow structures called ventricles.
- The spinal cord is a passageway for ascending sensory and descending motor neurons. It also acts as a center of reflex action.
- The basic structure of the nervous system is the nerve cell or neuron.
- There are 12 pairs of cranial nerves and 31 pairs of spinal nerves.
- The autonomic nervous system consists of the sympathetic nervous system and the parasympathetic nervous

system. The sympathetic nervous system regulates the expenditure of energy when the organism is confronted with stressful situations. The parasympathetic nervous system works to conserve body energy.

Assessment of motor function includes muscle movement, size, tone, strength, and coordination. Large muscle areas are inspected for evidence of atrophy, and opposing muscles assessed for equality of size and strength. Assessment of sensory integrity includes evaluating the extremities for sensitivity to heat, cold, touch, and pain.

Diagnostic imaging procedures include computed tomography, magnetic resonance imaging, and positron emission tomography. Other diagnostic procedures include lumbar puncture, electroencephalogram, brain scan, electromyography, and echoencephalography.

The nurse assesses the client, reports abnormal findings, prepares the client for diagnostic testing, and monitors for complications.

CRITICAL THINKING EXERCISES

1. Discuss nursing assessments that are appropriate when managing the care of clients with neurologic disorders.
2. Name two potential complications of neurologic testing procedures and discuss how the nurse could prevent, manage, and minimize them.

Suggested Readings

Barker, E., & Moore, K. (1992, April). Neurological assessment. *RN, 55*, 28.

Barker, E., & Moore, K. (1992, May). Cranial nerve assessment. *RN, 55*, 62.

Crigger, N., & Forbes, W. (1997). Assessing neurologic function in older patients. *American Journal of Nursing, 97*(3), 37–40.

Darovic, G. (1997). Assessing pupillary responses. *Nursing, 27*(2), 49.

Fuller, J., & Schaller-Ayers, J. (1994). *Health assessment: A nursing approach* (2nd ed.). Philadelphia: J. B. Lippincott.

Lower, J. (1992). Rapid neuro assessment. *American Journal of Nursing, 92*(6), 38, 47.

Memmler,R. L., Cohen, B. J., & Wood, D. L. (1996). *The human body in health and disease* (8th ed.). Philadelphia: Lippincott-Raven.

Neal, L. (1997). Is anybody home? Basic neurologic assessment of the home care client. *Home Healthcare Nurse, 15*(3), 156–169.

Perry, S. H. (1997). Caring for Jason . . . one day at a time. *Nursing, 27*(10), 46–48.

Shpritz, D. W. (1995). Understanding neurological assessment. *Journal of Post-Anesthesia Nursing, 10*(4), 216–219.

Stewart, N. (1996). Neurological observations. *Professional Nurse, 11*(6), 377–378.

Woodward, S. (1997). Practical procedures for nurses. Neurological observations —2, pupil response. *Nursing Times, 93*(46), 2.

Wooton, C. (1996). The top 10 ways to detect deteriorating central neurologic status. *Journal of Trauma Nursing, 3*(1), 25–27.

Additional Resources

American Association of Neuroscience Nurses
www.aans.org

Chapter 44

Caring for Clients With Central and Peripheral Nervous System Disorders

KEY TERMS

Aura
Automatisms
Bradykinesia
Brudzinski's sign
Cheyne-Stokes respirations
Choreiform movements
Convulsion
Cushing's triad
Demyelinating disease
Diplopia
Epilepsy
Fasciculations
Foramen magnum
Kernig's sign
Neuralgia
Nuchal rigidity
Nystagmus
Opisthotonos
Papilledema
Parkinsonism
Photophobia
Preictal phase
Ptosis
Seizure

LEARNING OBJECTIVES

On completion of this chapter, the reader will:

- List at least four signs and symptoms of increased intracranial pressure and discuss the nursing care of the client with increased intracranial pressure.
- Name four infectious or inflammatory diseases that affect the central or peripheral nervous system.
- Discuss three neuromuscular disorders, the common problems confronting clients with a neuromuscular disorder, and the nursing management.
- Discuss the nursing management of clients with a cranial nerve disorder.
- List the signs and symptoms of Parkinson's disease.
- Name the drugs commonly prescribed for Parkinson's disease and discuss the purpose of drug therapy.
- Discuss the pathophysiology of seizure disorders and describe different types of seizures.
- Discuss the nursing management of clients with seizure disorders.

Acute disorders of the central and peripheral nervous system are potentially life-threatening. Chronic neurologic disorders, although not imminently fatal, have a profound effect on a person's quality of life. When any part of the central or peripheral nervous system is damaged, removed, or destroyed, a permanent neurologic deficit can occur.

Increased Intracranial Pressure

The cranium consists of (1) brain tissue, (2) blood, and (3) cerebrospinal fluid (CSF). If one or more of these increases significantly without a decrease in one or the other two, intracranial pressure becomes elevated.

ETIOLOGY AND PATHOPHYSIOLOGY

Many conditions result in IICP including brain tumors, head injury, and infectious and inflammatory disorders of the brain such as encephalitis. As pressure increases, cerebral blood flow decreases. This is followed by an increase in the $PaCO_2$ (carbon dioxide level in the blood) and a decrease in the blood pH and PaO_2 (oxygen level in the blood). These changes result in cerebral edema, which further increases the intracranial pressure (ICP).

If IICP goes unrecognized or untreated, the contents of the cranium become further compressed. The **foramen magnum** (an opening in the lower part of the skull through which the upper part of the spinal cord exits the cranium) provides the only exit for brain tissue. As pressure increases, the brain herniates through the foramen magnum (Fig. 44–1). The brain stem, which con-

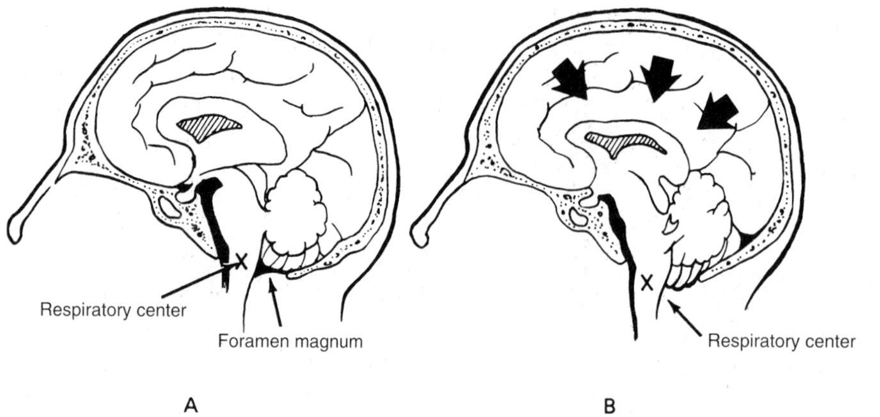

FIGURE 44-1. (*A*) Normal brain. (*B*) Herniation of the lower portion of the brain stem through the foramen magnum. Note the position of the respiratory center.

trols respiration, heart rate, and blood pressure, and is a passageway for descending and ascending nerve fibers, becomes compressed. As the condition progresses, vital functions ultimately may cease.

ASSESSMENT FINDINGS

Signs and Symptoms

The signs and symptoms of IICP (Box 44–1) develop rapidly or slowly. When IICP develops slowly, subtle changes can be overlooked.

Decreasing level of consciousness (LOC) is one of the earliest signs of IICP. Clients may slip from alert and oriented to lethargic, stuporous, semicomatose, and, finally, comatose (see Chap. 43). Confusion, restlessness, and periodic disorientation often accompany decreasing LOC.

A headache is another sign and symptom of IICP. Pain is typically intermittent and increases with activities that elevate the ICP such as coughing, sneezing, or straining at stool. Rest or elevation of the head relieves the pain. A constant headache is a grave sign.

Vomiting when associated with a neurologic condition also suggests increasing ICP. Emesis commonly occurs without any forewarning of nausea.

Papilledema (swelling of the optic nerve) is caused by interference with venous drainage from the eyeball and is observed when the eyes are examined with an ophthalmoscope. Pressure on the oculomotor nerve usually occurs with IICP and affects pupillary response to light. Normal pupil response to strong light is rapid constriction. In IICP the response is sluggish or nonexistent (fixed).

Changes in ICP also influence vital signs. Body temperature may rise or fall depending on the etiology of the IICP or because of its effect on the temperature regulating center. The pulse is increased initially but then decreases, systolic blood pressure rises, and pulse pressure (the difference between the systolic and diastolic measurement) widens, three signs called **Cushing's triad.** Cushing's triad occurs late in the development of IICP. The respiratory rate is irregular. Later **Cheyne-Stokes respirations** occur, evidenced by shallow, rapid breathing followed by a period of apnea.

Decorticate or decerebrate posturing (see Chap. 43) develops spontaneously or in response to a painful stimulus when the ICP is increased.

BOX 44-1 Signs of Increased Intracranial Pressure

- Altered level of consciousness
- Headache
- Vomiting
- Papilledema
- Change in vital signs
- Unequal pupils and abnormal response to light
- Posturing

Diagnostic Findings

Diagnostic tests that determine the underlying cause of IICP include skull radiography, computed tomography (CT), magnetic resonance imaging (MRI), lumbar puncture, and cerebral angiography.

MEDICAL AND SURGICAL MANAGEMENT

Immediate treatment is aimed at relieving the cause, if possible. Monitoring devices (Fig. 44–2) are inserted to measure ICP and in some cases to withdraw CSF. These devices are connected to a transducer and a monitor that display the pressure and a waveform to detect the status of ICP. Normal ICP in the ventricles is 1 to 15 mm Hg; moderate elevation ranges from 15 to 40 mm Hg; high levels exceed 40 mm Hg. Although the ICP varies, a rise of 2 mm Hg from a previous measurement is cause for concern.

Osmotic diuretics such as mannitol (Osmitrol), glycerin (Osmoglyn), or urea (Ureaphil), and cortico-

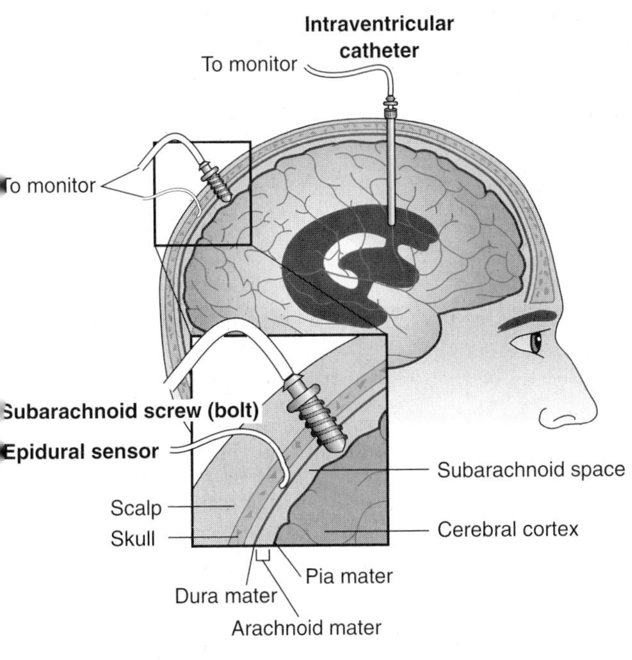

FIGURE 44-2. Technique for monitoring intracranial pressure.

steroids such as dexamethasone (Decadron) are given to reduce cerebral edema. Other treatment includes restriction of oral and intravenous (IV) fluids and hyperventilation therapy by means of mechanical ventilation. Hyperventilation produces vasoconstriction of the cerebral arteries followed by a decrease in cerebral blood volume and reduction in ICP.

Depending on the degree and cause of IICP, the physician may order the insertion of an indwelling catheter, a nasogastric tube for gastric decompression or to provide tube feedings, a stool softener to prevent straining at stool, and a histamine antagonist such as famotidine (Pepcid) to prevent stress ulcers. Persistent hyperthermia caused by altered functioning of the hypothalamus requires hypothermic measures such as a cooling blanket if the temperature does not respond to antipyretic drugs.

Emergency surgery is done to remove a blood clot if IICP is due to a head injury with bleeding above or below the dura. Surgery is also performed to relieve pressure caused by a brain tumor.

NURSING PROCESS
Care of the Client with Increased Intracranial Pressure

Assessment

The client with IICP requires intensive nursing care with frequent assessment and evaluation for changes in neurologic status. Because neurologic alterations are often subtle or unrelated to IICP, a change in a client's status is recorded and immediately reported to the physician. A neurologic assessment is done initially and at prescribed intervals thereafter. A neurologic flow sheet that includes the Glasgow Coma Scale or Ranchos Los Amigos Scale and ICP pressure measurements (see Chap. 43) is used to establish a data base and record ongoing assessments. Vital signs are monitored at 30-minute or hourly intervals.

Intake and output and daily weights are recorded to monitor the fluid and nutritional status of the client. Laboratory findings such as serum electrolyte levels and arterial blood gas measurements are analyzed to detect fluid, electrolyte, and acid–base complications, or to evaluate the effectiveness of medical management. The abdomen is auscultated to ensure that bowel sounds are present in all quadrants and palpated to determine if there is distention. Bowel elimination patterns are monitored.

Diagnosis and Planning

The plan of care for a client with IICP includes, but is not limited to, the following:

Nursing Diagnoses and Collaborative Problems	Nursing Interventions
Altered Tissue Perfusion (cerebral) related to IICP as evidenced by a decreased LOC, sluggish pupil response, papilledema, posturing	Keep the head of the bed slightly elevated and the head in midline (straight). For those with a basal skull fracture, keep the bed flat.
Goal: The ICP will be between 1 and 15 mm Hg and the Glasgow Coma Scale score will be greater than 8.	Limit movement, space essential nursing tasks, and reduce or eliminate environmental stimuli, such as loud noise and bright lights, and other factors that raise ICP (Box 44-2).
	Avoid extreme flexion of the hip because this position interferes with blood flow.
	Keep the client quiet. Change the client's position with assistance and the use of a turning sheet. Avoid range-of-motion (ROM) exercises unless ordered by the physician until ICP approaches normal.
	Administer reduced fluid volumes at an even rate over a 24-hour period. Give diuretics and corticosteroids as prescribed and note the client's response to therapy.

	Hyperventilate the mechanically ventilated client according to medical orders. Suction only when necessary. Give 100% oxygen before and after suctioning when it is required. Keep suctioning as brief as possible without exceeding 10 to 15 seconds per pass of the catheter. Notify the physician if the abdomen is distended or bowel sounds are absent. Administer prescribed stool softener to reduce the potential for the Valsalva maneuver. Ensure that a gastric tube used for decompression remains patent. Administer prescribed medications if vomiting and persistent coughing occur.
Risk for Ineffective Breathing Pattern and **Ineffective Airway Clearance** related to diminished LOC and herniation of the brain stem secondary to IICP **Goal:** The client's respiratory rate will be sufficient to maintain the SPO_2 above 90% and PO_2 above 80 mm Hg; the airway will be patent.	Attach a pulse oximeter to the finger, earlobe, bridge of the nose, or toe. Insert an oral airway if the client is comatose to prevent the tongue from occluding the airway. Administer prescribed oxygen. For the mechanically ventilated client, ensure that the ventilator is delivering the prescribed tidal volume at the rate that is ordered. Suction when necessary to clear tracheal secretions or to keep the endotracheal tube patent.
Risk for Altered Nutrition: Less than Body Requirements related to inability to consume food orally **Goal:** The client's body weight will remain within +2 lb of preadmission.	Administer nutritional supplements by gastric tube or total parenteral nutrition (TPN) via a central venous catheter as medically prescribed.
Risk for Aspiration related to diminished LOC, gastric distention, ineffective airway clearance **Goal:** The client's airway will be free of oral or gastric secretions.	Keep the mouth free of secretions by using an oral suction catheter or Yankeur suction tip. Check gastric residuals before each administration of formula or on a scheduled basis. Postpone tube feedings when the gastric residual exceeds safe limits. Ensure that a gastric tube used for decompression remains patent. Administer prescribed medications if vomiting occurs.
Risk for Infection related to impaired skin and tissue integrity secondary to surgery, invasive diagnostic or monitoring procedures, original head injury **Goal:** The client will be free of infection as evidenced by absence of fever, no purulent drainage from open areas of skin, white blood count within normal limits.	Keep wounds clean and dry. Use aseptic technique when handling any part of the intracranial monitoring device or when changing a dressing applied after surgery. Administer antibiotic therapy, if prescribed.
PC: Hyperglycemia related to corticosteroid therapy or administration of TPN **Goal:** Elevated blood sugar will be managed and minimized.	Monitor capillary blood glucose levels three times daily and at bedtime. Follow medical orders for administering insulin according to a sliding scale.
PC: Stress Ulcer related to hyperacidity secondary to stress response **Goal:** The potential for stress ulcers will be managed and minimized.	Check the pH of gastric secretions per shift. Report a pH of less than 3. Administer prescribed antagonists or antacids.
Risk for Impaired Skin Integrity related to low capillary blood flow secondary to pressure and inactivity **Goal:** The client's skin will remain intact.	Tilt the patient from side to side every 2 hours. Avoid friction by using a lift sheet. Use a pressure-relieving mattress or mechanical bed for clients whose position cannot be readily changed. Keep the skin clean and dry.
Self-Care Deficit (Total or specify type) related to diminished level of consciousness as manifested by inability to follow directions and impaired musculoskeletal function **Goal:** The client's basic needs will be met.	Give the client complete care including bathing, oral care, nutrition, and elimination until the ICP is normal and the client can resume these activities.
Impaired Verbal Communication related to decreased LOC or endotracheal intubation as evidenced by an inability to speak **Goal:** The client's needs will be communicated.	Look for grimacing or moaning that may indicate discomfort or other problems. Correct problems that may be causing discomfort such as a wrinkled sheet or an object pressing on the skin. If the client is alert but intubated, provide paper and pencil or a magic slate for communicating by writing.

Evaluation and Expected Outcomes

- The client's ICP returns to normal levels.
- The client's respirations are normal, airway is clear, and lungs are clear to auscultation.
- The client's nutritional needs are met with no evidence of aspiration.
- The client's temperature is normal with no sign of infection.
- Blood sugar is within normal range.

BOX 44-2 Activities That Increase Intracranial Pressure

- Coughing
- Range of motion exercises
- Sneezing
- Hip flexion of 90 degrees or greater
- Vomiting
- Suctioning
- Straining to have a bowel movement (Valsalva maneuver)
- Holding breath
- Digging heels into bed to help in repositioning
- Turning in bed without help

- The client can communicate needs to others when conscious.
- Gastric mucosa is intact.
- Skin integrity is maintained.
- ADLs are met.

For additional suggestions for nursing management of a client undergoing surgery or who develops a neurologic deficit, see Chapter 47.

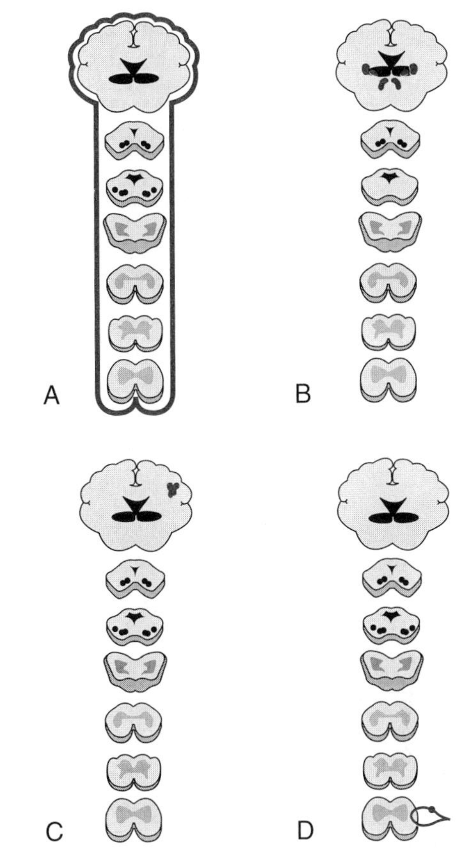

FIGURE 44-3. Sites of infectious and inflammatory disorders. (*A*) meningitis (*B*) encephalitis (*C*) Guillain-Barré syndrome (*D*) brain abscess.

Infectious and Inflammatory Disorders of the Nervous System

Four neurologic conditions are infectious or inflammatory in nature: meningitis, encephalitis, Guillain-Barré syndrome, and brain abscess (Fig. 44–3).

Meningitis

Meningitis is an inflammation of the meninges. The cerebral cortex is often affected. The client's condition rapidly becomes critical and death will occur without immediate intervention. Most adults with bacterial meningitis recover without permanent neurologic damage or dysfunction. When complications do occur, they usually are serious.

ETIOLOGY AND PATHOPHYSIOLOGY

The meningococcus, streptococcus, staphylococcus, and pneumococcus are the most common causative microorganisms of meningitis. They reach the meninges by way of the bloodstream or by direct extension from infected areas such as the middle ear and the paranasal sinuses. Meningococcal meningitis, a common and highly contagious form of bacterial meningitis, generally affects school-aged children and young adults. Viruses such as herpes simplex virus, mumps virus, and enteroviruses can cause viral meningitis, usually in children.

The inflammatory process can advance to cerebral edema, irreversible coma, seizure disorders, brain abscess, and neurologic changes. Vasculitis, inflammation of a blood vessel, may be present and cerebral blood flow may be decreased. Neurologic complications include damage to the cranial nerves that facilitate vision and hearing.

ASSESSMENT FINDINGS

Signs and Symptoms

Symptoms include fever, **nuchal rigidity** (pain and stiffness of the neck, inability to place the chin on the chest), nausea, vomiting, **photophobia** (aversion to light), headache, restlessness, irritability, and seizures. Severe irritation of the meninges causes **opisthotonos,** an extreme hyperextension of the head and arching of the back. A positive **Kernig's sign** (inability to extend the leg when the thigh is flexed on the abdomen) and a positive **Brudzinski's sign** (flexion of the neck produces flexion of the knees and hips) are seen (Fig. 44–4).

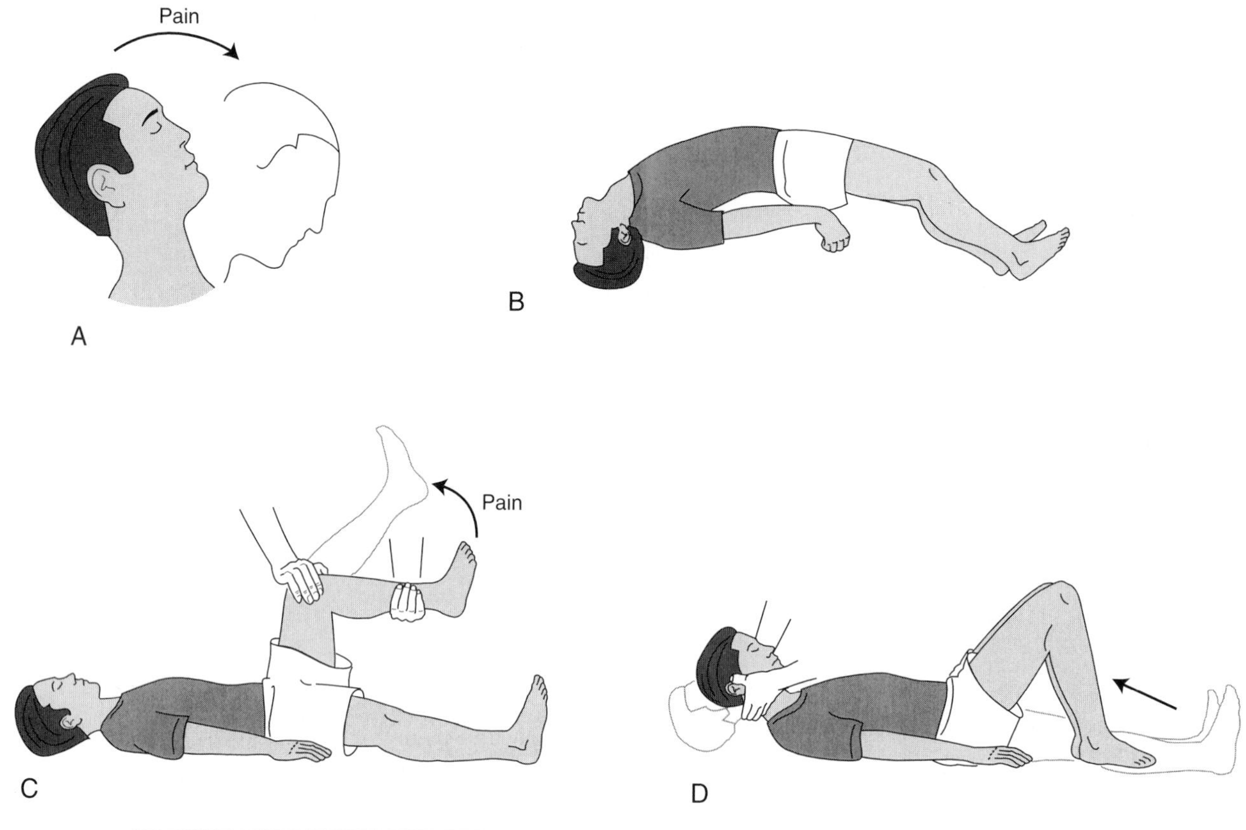

FIGURE 44-4. Signs of meningeal irritation. (*A*) nuchal rigidity, (*B*) opisthotonos, (*C*) Kernig's sign, (*D*) Brudzinski's sign.

The client with meningococcal meningitis may have multiple small-to-large petechiae on the body.

Diagnostic Findings

A lumbar puncture is done and samples of CSF obtained. If the meningitis is bacterial in origin, the CSF appears cloudy. The CSF pressure is elevated, glucose concentration is decreased, protein levels are elevated, and white and red blood cell counts are elevated. Culture and sensitivity studies are done to identify the specific bacterium that is causing meningitis. If meningitis is viral in origin, the results of culture and sensitivity studies are negative. A CT scan, blood culture, complete blood cell count, and other laboratory tests are used to rule out other possible disorders.

MEDICAL MANAGEMENT

Intravenous (IV) fluids and antimicrobial therapy are started immediately. The appropriate antibiotic is determined when the causative microorganism is identified from the results of the sensitivity tests. Drug therapy is continued after the acute phase of the illness to prevent recurrence of the infection. Anticonvulsants are necessary if seizures occur. People who have had recent contact with a person with meningococcal meningitis are placed on prophylactic oral rifampin (Rifidin). The local public health department is notified of all cases.

NURSING PROCESS
Care of the Client With a Neurologic Infectious or Inflammatory Disorder

Assessment

Obtain a medical and nursing history. Because the client is acutely ill, obtain the history from a family member.

Check vital signs and do a neurologic examination. Initiate an assessment flow sheet for ongoing comparisons. Observe the rate and characteristics of respirations. Auscultate the lungs every 4 to 8 hours. Determine the client's ability to swallow and clear the airway of secretions. Measure intake and output. Record bowel elimination. Ask the client to indicate the severity of a headache, when present. If seizures occur, note the duration of the seizure and physical manifestations, whether it involved only one side of the body or started in a particular location and spread elsewhere.

Diagnosis and Planning

Caring for a client with meningitis and other infectious or inflammatory neurologic disorders includes, but is not limited to, the following:

Nursing Diagnoses and Collaborative Problems	Nursing Interventions
Risk for Impaired Gas Exchange related to ineffective breathing, ineffective airway clearance, and aspiration	Keep an oral airway at the bedside and insert it immediately to maintain a patent airway.
	Administer oxygen as prescribed.
Goal: The client's blood gases will be within normal ranges, breathing will be sufficient to maintain an SPO_2 above 90%, the airway will be free of oral or gastric secretions.	Report respiratory difficulty, which may require emergency intubation.
	Elevate the head of the bed.
	Hyperoxygenate and hyperventilate before and after tracheal suctioning.
	Use caution when giving oral fluids, food, or medications to a lethargic client.
Hyperthermia related to fever-producing mechanisms secondary to microbial infection	Administer prescribed antipyretic drugs.
Goal: Body temperature will be controlled below 101°F (38.3°C).	Remove unnecessary clothing and blankets.
	Administer tepid sponge baths.
	Apply a cooling blanket beneath the client.
	Maintain adequate hydration.
Pain (headache) related to meningeal irritation, cerebral edema as manifested by client's description of head discomfort	Report a continuous headache or one that goes unrelieved.
Goal: The client's discomfort will be relieved or reduced to a tolerable level within 30 minutes of a nursing measure.	Give a prescribed mild analgesic that does not affect the size or reaction of the pupils.
	Facilitate rest and a reduction in environmental stimuli.
PC: Seizures related to meningeal irritation, high fever, or IICP	Raise and pad side rails with soft material.
Goal: Seizures will be managed and minimized.	Stay with the client if a seizure develops and call for assistance.
	Turn the client to the side, do not restrain the client's movements.
	Provide privacy.
	Insert a padded tongue blade in the mouth *only if the teeth are not tightly shut.*
	Suction the client's mouth and pharynx to clear secretions.
	Provide oxygen during and after the seizure.
	Reorient the client to the surroundings and provide rest following the seizure.
	Check for injuries.
	Administer prescribed anticonvulsant medications.

Evaluation and Expected Outcomes

- Adequate oxygenation is maintained.
- The client's temperature is normal and vital signs are stable.
- The client reports an absence of pain and headache.
- The client is protected during seizure activity.

If IICP develops, refer to the previous discussion for additional nursing management.

Encephalitis

Encephalitis is an infectious disease of the central nervous (CNS) system characterized by pathologic changes in both the white matter and the gray matter of the spinal cord and. brain.

ETIOLOGY AND PATHOPHYSIOLOGY

Bacteria, fungi, or viruses cause encephalitis. The disease can occur after a viral infection elsewhere in the body, such as measles, or after vaccination. Viruses identified as causing encephalitis include the St. Louis virus, Western equine virus, and Eastern equine virus. Some viruses are transmitted by ticks or mosquitoes. Poisoning by drugs and chemicals, such as lead, arsenic, or carbon monoxide, may closely resemble encephalitis clinically.

Severe, diffuse inflammation of the brain occurs. Extensive nerve cell destruction can develop. Cerebral edema, neurologic deficits such as paralysis and speech changes, IICP, respiratory failure, seizure disorders, and shock can occur.

ASSESSMENT FINDINGS

Signs and Symptoms

Sudden fever, severe headache, stiff neck, vomiting, and drowsiness signals the onset of viral encephalitis. Other symptoms include tremors, seizures, spastic or flaccid paralysis, irritability, and muscle weakness. Lethargy, delirium, or coma develop. Incontinence and visual disturbances such as photophobia, involuntary eye movements, and double or blurred vision occur.

Diagnostic Findings

A lumbar puncture is performed. CSF pressure is elevated, but the fluid is clear. In some types of encephalitis, serologic studies show a rise in viral antibodies. Electroencephalography (EEG) reveals slow waveforms.

MEDICAL MANAGEMENT

Because no specific antiviral measure has been developed, treatment of encephalitis is supportive.

NURSING MANAGEMENT

Monitor vital signs and LOC at frequent intervals; compare findings with previous assessments. If urinary retention or urinary incontinence develops, an indwelling urethral catheter is necessary. Measure fluid intake and output to detect signs of fluid volume deficit and electrolyte imbalances. Assess bowel elimination to determine if an enema or a stool softener is needed. Refer to the nursing process discussion on caring for a client with an infectious or imflammatory neurologic disorder for additional nursing management.

Guillain-Barré Syndrome

Guillain-Barré syndrome (acute postinfectious polyneuropathy, polyradiculoneuritis) affects the peripheral nerves and the spinal nerve roots. Most clients begin to show signs of recovery about 1 month after the progression of symptoms ceases. Recovery may be slow and take a year or more. Death can occur from complications of immobility, such as pneumonia and infection.

ETIOLOGY AND PATHOPHYSIOLOGY

Although the exact cause of the disorder is unknown, it is believed that Guillain-Barré syndrome is an autoimmune reaction (see Chap. 41) that follows a primary disorder, especially one that is infectious. Many clients have a history of a recent viral infection, particularly of the respiratory tract. Others have a history of recent surgery or recent vaccination. The syndrome also occurs in clients with malignant diseases and lupus erythematosus.

The affected nerves become inflamed and edematous. There is a loss of myelin. Mild to severe ascending muscle weakness or paralysis develops. Overactivity or underactivity of the sympathetic or parasympathetic nervous system is evidenced by blood pressure changes and changes in heart rate and rhythm.

ASSESSMENT FINDINGS

Signs and Symptoms

Although symptoms vary, weakness, numbness, and tingling in the arms and legs are often the first symptoms. The weakness is progressive and moves to upper areas of the body and affects the muscles of respiration. Muscle weakness may be followed by paralysis. If cranial nerve involvement develops, chewing, talking, and swallowing become difficult.

Diagnostic Findings

A lumbar puncture reveals elevated CSF protein levels and pressure. The results of electrophysiologic testing show a marked slowing in the conduction of nerve impulses. Additional neurologic tests are performed to rule out other possible CNS disorders that have similar symptoms.

MEDICAL MANAGEMENT

Plasmapheresis, removal of plasma from the blood and reinfusion of the cellular components with saline, has been shown to shorten the course of the disease if performed within the first 2 weeks. Otherwise, treatment is primarily supportive. If the respiratory muscles are involved, endotracheal intubation and mechanical ventilation become necessary. Difficulty chewing and swallowing necessitate the administration of intravenous fluids, gastric tube feedings, or total parenteral nutrition (TPN).

NURSING MANAGEMENT

Observe the client closely for signs of respiratory distress. Use a spirometer to evaluate the client's ventilation capacity. Check vital signs and lung sounds frequently to assess for pneumonia.

Because the client is incapacitated by immobility, provide meticulous skin care and change position every 2 hours. Give passive range-of-motion (ROM) exercises to prevent muscle atrophy. See the discussion of nursing diagnoses and collaborative problems that accompany the care of the client with meningitis.

Brain Abscess

A brain abscess is a collection of purulent material within the brain. If untreated it can be fatal.

ETIOLOGY AND PATHOPHYSIOLOGY

A brain abscess occurs from an infection in nearby structures such as the middle ear, sinuses, or teeth, or from an infection in other organs. A brain abscess can develop after intracranial surgery or head trauma. It can be secondary to such disorders as bacterial endocarditis, bacteremia, and pulmonary or abdominal infections.

The presence of a brain abscess produces neurologic changes according to the location in which it occurs. Because it occupies space in the cranium, IICP can develop. Complications include paralysis, mental deterioration, seizure disorder, and visual disturbances.

ASSESSMENT FINDINGS

Signs and Symptoms

Manifestations of a brain abscess include signs of IICP, fever, headache, and neurologic changes such as paralysis, seizures, muscle weakness, and lethargy.

Diagnostic Findings

Laboratory tests show an elevated white blood cell count. Analysis of CSF obtained by lumbar puncture helps to confirm the diagnosis, but this procedure has a risk of herniation of the brain stem. A CT scan, MRI, and skull radiographs are safer techniques for diagnosing and locating the abscess.

MEDICAL AND SURGICAL MANAGEMENT

Antimicrobial therapy is started once the diagnosis is confirmed. A craniotomy (see Chap. 46) typically is performed to drain the abscess. Cerebral edema and seizures are treated with drug therapy. Additional treatment includes control of fever, mechanical ventilation, IV fluids, and nutritional support.

NURSING MANAGEMENT

Assess the client frequently for changes in LOC, changes in sensory and motor functions, and signs of IICP. Monitor vital signs at frequent intervals. Measure fluid intake and output because overhydration can lead to cerebral edema. Refer to the interventions for specific nursing diagnoses and collaborative problems discussed in the nursing process section for meningitis.

Neuromuscular Disorders

A neuromuscular disorder involves the nervous system and indirectly affects the muscles. Some examples include: multiple sclerosis (MS), myasthenia gravis, and amyotrophic lateral sclerosis (ALS)—all of which are chronic and progressively debilitating.

Multiple Sclerosis

Multiple sclerosis (MS) is a chronic, progressive disease of the peripheral nerves. MS has its onset in young adult and early middle life. The highest incidence occurs about equally in men and women between ages 20 and 40. The disease is more common in northern temperate zones than in warm climates.

ETIOLOGY AND PATHOPHYSIOLOGY

The cause of MS is unknown, but it is considered an autoimmune disorder. It is characterized as a **demyelinating disease** because it causes permanent degeneration and destruction of myelin. Myelin acts as an insulator, enabling nerve impulses to pass along a nerve fiber. Loss of myelin and subsequent degeneration and atrophy of nerve axons interrupt transmission of impulses along these fibers.

Many clients experience gradual and continuous worsening of their symptoms. A few have the disease in a mild form and do not experience an increase in severity of symptoms. For some, the symptoms subside during early phases of the illness (remission), and the client seems healthy for several months or even years. With each reappearance (exacerbation), however, the symptoms become more severe and last longer. Infections and emotional upsets precipitate exacerbations. Some people live a long time with MS. Survival for 20 years after the diagnosis is not unusual.

As the disease progresses, many complications such as pressure ulcers, cachexia, deformities, and contractures develop. Pneumonia, brought about by limited activity, shallow breathing, and general debility, is often the immediate cause of death.

ASSESSMENT FINDINGS

Signs and Symptoms

Minor symptoms are often dismissed as a result of fatigue or strain. When they can no longer be ignored, people with MS report experiencing blurred vision, **diplopia** (double vision), **nystagmus** (involuntary movement of the eyeball), weakness, clumsiness, and numbness and tingling of an arm or a leg. An intention tremor and slurred, hesitant speech (scanning speech) may develop. Mood swings (emotional lability) are common.

Weakness of an arm or a leg progresses to ataxia (motor incoordination) or paraplegia (paralysis of both legs). Occasional bowel and bladder incontinence leads to total incontinence. Slight visual disturbances end in blindness. Intellectual functioning is impaired late in the course of the illness. Loss of memory, difficulty concentrating, and impaired judgment occur.

Diagnostic Findings

Early diagnosis is difficult because symptoms are vague and in some cases temporary. A lumbar puncture and CSF analysis reveal an increased white blood cell count. Electrophoresis of the CSF, a technique for electrically separating and identifying proteins, demonstrates abnormal immunoglobulin G bands, described as oligoclonal bands. The bands appear separated rather than homogeneous, which is the normal finding. A CT scan and MRI may or may not disclose lesions in the brain's white matter.

MEDICAL MANAGEMENT

There is no cure for MS nor any single treatment that relieves all of the symptoms. The primary aim of treatment is to keep the client functional as long as possible.

Drugs used to treat symptoms of the disorder include baclofen (Lioresal) and dantrolene (Dantrium) for muscle spasticity and rigidity, antibiotics for infection, and tranquilizers to alleviate mood swings. Oxybutynin (Ditropan) is used to treat urinary incontinence and bethanechol (Urecholine) to relieve urine retention. The anti-inflammatory action of corticosteroids relieve symptoms and hasten a period of remission.

NURSING PROCESS
The Client With a Neuromuscular Disorder

Assessment

Perform a thorough neurologic assessment on the client with MS or any of the neuromuscular disorders. Evaluate pulmonary function including respiratory rate, depth, and lung sounds to determine the status of the client's ability to ventilate adequately. Assess temperature on a regular basis to detect early signs of infection. The client's ability to chew and swallow effectively are noted. Observe for drooling, choking when swallowing liquids, and regurgitation of fluids through the nose. Note muscle strength and coordination as well as the client's response to physical activity. Measure intake and output to evaluate fluid status. Document elimination patterns. Analyze data with the initial baseline for comparisons. In addition, monitor the client's and caregivers' ability to cope with the progressively debilitating nature of the disorder.

Diagnosis and Planning

The plan of care for clients with MS or other neuromuscular disorders includes, but is not limited to, the following:

Nursing Diagnoses and Collaborative Problems	Nursing Interventions
Risk for Ineffective Breathing Pattern related to weakening of the muscles for respiration **Goal:** The client's ventilation will be sufficient to maintain the SPO_2 above 90% and PO_2 above 80 mm Hg.	Position the client in a Fowler's position and support the arms on pillows to facilitate maximum expansion of the chest. Eliminate foods that form intestinal gas or promote the expulsion of gas with a rectal tube to avoid pressure on the diaphragm. Encourage the client to deep breathe several times an hour. Notify the physician immediately if the client experiences inadequate ventilation.
Risk for Ineffective Airway Clearance related to weak or ineffective cough, **Impaired Swallowing, Risk for Altered Nutrition: Less than Body Requirements** and **Risk for Aspiration** related to muscular weakness **Goal:** The client's airway will be patent; the client's nutritional needs will be met.	Help the client to cough and raise respiratory secretions. Suction the oral cavity and airway. Offer liquids frequently in small amounts. Consult with the dietitian on techniques for modifying the texture and consistency of foods. Provide a period of rest before meals to conserve strength for chewing and swallowing. Help the client to sit upright when eating. Place food in the posterior of the mouth. Flex the chin toward the chest when swallowing to facilitate the passage of food into the esophagus. Feed the client slowly. Wait to place more food in the client's mouth until the previous bolus has been swallowed. Consult with the physician about the plan for tube feedings or TPN if the oral nutritional intake becomes inadequate or dangerous.
Impaired Physical Mobility, Self-Care Deficit (specify type), and **Risk for Impaired Skin Integrity** related to diminished muscle strength and inactivity **Goal:** The client's mobility and use of muscles will be utilized to the maximum extent possible; basic needs will be met; the skin will remain intact.	Encourage the client to participate in self-care. Provide periods of rest between bathing, shaving, oral care, eating, ambulating, toileting, and diversional activities. Complete whatever tasks the client is unable to perform. Change body position every 2 hours. Perform ROM every 8 hours. Use a foot board and trochanter rolls to promote a neutral body position. Consult with a physical or occupational therapist on techniques to facilitate the client's independence and self-care. Use pressure-relieving devices to prevent skin breakdown. Keep the bed dry and free of wrinkles. Wash and dry the skin well.
Constipation related to inactivity and abdominal muscle weakness; **Incontinence** (spec-	Consult with the physician about a regularly prescribed stool softener, bulk-forming

ify type, such as Total, Functional, or Reflex) related to neuromuscular degeneration **Goal:** The client's stool will be soft and bowel elimination will occur at least every 3 days; the client's urine elimination will be controlled.	laxative, or suppository to facilitate bowel elimination. Include soft fruit or fruit puree in the daily menu. Assist the client to move about as much as possible. Place the client on the toilet or a commode after a meal, especially after breakfast, or near the time of the client's usual bowel movement. Help the client select clothing that facilitates toileting. Assist the client with urinary control to the toilet at regular and frequent intervals. Use incontinence garments or consult with the physician when there is a need for an indwelling or external catheter.
Ineffective Individual Coping related to feelings of helplessness secondary to chronic illness **Goal:** The client will cope effectively with situational stressors.	Suggest joining a support group of people with a similar disorder or subscribing to the support group's newsletter. Encourage the client to ventilate his or her feelings. Provide opportunities in which the client can make choices among two or more alternatives. Facilitate the client's network of social support such as with family, neighbors, coworkers, church members, via personal visits, telephone conversations, cards, and letters. Provide diversional activities that foster feelings of personal accomplishment.
Risk for Caregiver Role Strain related to unrelenting responsibility for care of the client **Goal:** The primary caregiver will cope with long-term care of a family member.	Listen empathetically while the caregiver unburdens his or her feelings about caring for the client. Help the caregiver develop a list of surrogates that may provide periods of relief on a regular basis. Give the caregiver permission to meet his or her own needs. Identify community resources that are available and offer to facilitate a referral.

Evaluation and Expected Outcomes

- Respirations are of normal rate and depth.
- The client's airway is clear, respirations are normal.
- The client's nutrition is adequate to maintain body weight.
- The client regains mobility and attends to ADLs.
- The client's skin is intact with no area breakdown.
- The client's bowel elimination pattern is regular, urinary incontinence is controlled.
- The client demonstrates effective coping skills.
- The caregiver has periodic relief from responsibilities.

Myasthenia Gravis

Myasthenia gravis is a neuromuscular disorder characterized by severe weakness of one or more groups of skeletal muscles.

ETIOLOGY AND PATHOPHYSIOLOGY

Although the exact cause of the disease is unknown, it is believed to be an autoimmune disorder that develops when blood cells and thymus gland antibodies destroy the nerve ending receptor site of skeletal muscles. The symptoms develop because of the defect in nerve transmission resulting in extreme muscle weakness.

ASSESSMENT FINDINGS

Signs and Symptoms

Muscle weakness varies depending on the muscles affected. The most common manifestations are **ptosis** (drooping) of the eyelids (Fig. 44–5), difficulty chewing and swallowing, diplopia, voice weakness, masklike facial expression, and weakness of the extremities. The respiratory system is also affected. During a myasthenic crisis, the client experiences increased muscle

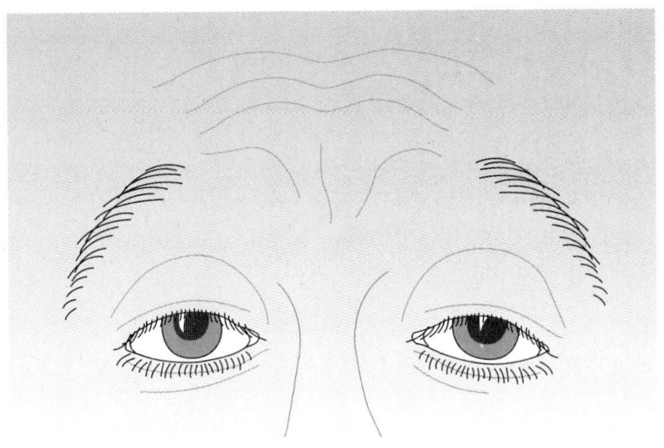

FIGURE 44-5. Ptosis of the eyelids.

weakness, respiratory distress, decreased tidal volume, and difficulty talking, swallowing, and chewing.

Diagnostic Findings

Diagnostic confirmation is made by IV administration of edrophonium (Tensilon), which relieves symptoms in a few seconds. Chest radiography may show a tumor of the thymus (thymoma). Electromyography measures the electrical potential of muscles.

MEDICAL AND SURGICAL MANAGEMENT

Treatment involves facilitating normal neurotransmission with administration of an anticholinesterase drug, such as pyridostigmine bromide (Mestinon) or ambenonium chloride (Mytelase). The therapeutic effect prolongs the action of acetylcholine, which sustains muscle contraction. The dose of the drug is adjusted according to the client's response to therapy.

Other treatments include surgical removal of the thymus gland, prednisone, and plasmapheresis for clients who do not respond to other methods of therapy. If myasthenic crisis with severe respiratory distress occurs, intubation and mechanical ventilation are required.

NURSING MANAGEMENT

Observe the effects of drug therapy, especially when first initiated or at times of stress. Medications must be given at the exact intervals ordered to maintain therapeutic blood levels and prevent a return of symptoms. Look for signs of drug overdose such as abdominal cramps, clenched jaws, and muscle rigidity, which indicate that the dose is excessive.

Review the nursing diagnoses and collaborative problems that accompany the previous discussion about caring for a client with MS. Many problems and interventions are similar.

Amyotrophic Lateral Sclerosis

Amyotrophic lateral sclerosis (ALS) is also known as Lou Gehrig's disease. It is a progressive, fatal neurologic disorder. The disease is more common in men than in women.

ETIOLOGY AND PATHOPHYSIOLOGY

The cause of ALS is unknown. The disease is characterized by degeneration of the motor neurons of the spinal cord and brain stem, which results in muscle weakness and wasting.

ASSESSMENT FINDINGS

Signs and Symptoms

Progressive muscle weakness and wasting of the arms, legs, and trunk develop. Episodes of muscle **fasciculations** (twitching) are experienced. If the brain stem is affected, speaking and swallowing become difficult. Periods of inappropriate laughter and crying are manifested. Respiratory failure and total paralysis are seen in the terminal stage of the disease.

Diagnostic Findings

The disorder is difficult to diagnose in the early stages because there are no specific diagnostic tests for this disease. Electromyography validates weakness in the affected muscles.

MEDICAL MANAGEMENT

There is no specific treatment, and in many cases, death occurs several years after diagnosis. The client is encouraged to remain active as long as possible. Death usually occurs from respiratory arrest or overwhelming respiratory infection. Mechanical ventilation is necessary when the muscles of respiration are affected.

NURSING MANAGEMENT

After a comprehensive assessment, develop a plan of care based on the identified problems of the client. Refer to the nursing diagnoses and collaborative problems that are discussed in relation to MS because they are common among all clients with a neuromuscular disease.

During the early stages of the disease, provide assistance with activities such as walking, bathing, shaving, and dressing. As the disease progresses, the client becomes totally dependent on the family or health care personnel for care. Additional information on caring for clients with a neurologic deficit is covered in Chapter 47. Review the nursing management of dying clients in Chapter 25 for the care of clients in the terminal phase of ALS.

Client and Family Teaching

If the client with a neuromuscular disorder is being cared for at home, teach family members required skills, such as suctioning techniques, how to administer tube feedings, and catheter care.

Develop a teaching plan that includes the following general areas:

- Medication schedule, adverse effects of medications
- Dietary and feeding suggestions
- Agencies that can help with or give home care
- Sources of financial assistance
- Exercises to prevent muscle atrophy

- Positioning and good skin care
- Techniques for preventing skin breakdown

Cranial Nerve Disorders

Trigeminal Neuralgia (Tic Douloureux)

Trigeminal neuralgia is a painful condition that involves the fifth cranial nerve, the trigeminal nerve, that has three major branches: mandibular, maxillary, and ophthalmic (Fig. 44–6). This sensory and motor nerve is important to chewing, facial movement, and sensation.

ETIOLOGY AND PATHOPHYSIOLOGY

The cause of the disorder is unknown. It has been suggested that it is related to compression of the trigeminal nerve root. For reasons not fully understood, **neuralgia** (nerve pain) is experienced in one or more branches of the trigeminal nerve. Certain trigger spots (or areas that provoke the pain) initiate an attack when there is the slightest stimulus (eg, vibration of music, a passing breeze, a temperature change). The forehead over the eyebrow is a common trigger spot when the ophthalmic branch of the nerve is affected.

ASSESSMENT FINDINGS

Signs and Symptoms

The pain is described as sudden, severe, and burning. It ends as quickly as it began, usually lasting a few seconds to several minutes. The cycle is repeated many times a day. During a spasm, the face twitches and the eyes tear.

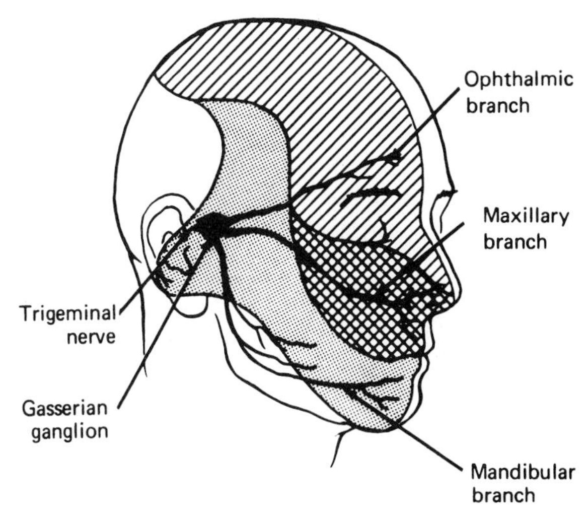

FIGURE 44-6. Areas innervated by the three branches of the trigeminal nerve. These are the areas that become painful in trigeminal neuralgia.

Diagnostic Findings

Skull radiography, MRI, or CT are performed to rule out other pathology, such as a brain tumor and intracranial bleeding. Ultimately the diagnosis is made on the basis of the symptoms.

MEDICAL MANAGEMENT

Medical treatment is primarily supportive and symptomatic rather than curative. Narcotic analgesics are necessary. Anticonvulsants such as phenytoin (Dilantin) and carbamazepine (Tegretol) are used to reduce pain but are not successful in all cases. The client is referred to a dentist because some cases of trigeminal neuralgia have been relieved by correction of dental deformities.

SURGICAL MANAGEMENT

If medical management is unsatisfactory, surgical intervention is an option. Surgical division of the sensory root of the trigeminal nerve provides permanent relief. Some permanent loss of sensation can occur. If the mandibular branch is severed, eating becomes a problem. The client may bite the tongue without realizing it, food gets caught in the mouth, and the jaw deviates toward the operative side. Until the client adjusts to the altered sensation, swallowing is difficult.

NURSING MANAGEMENT

Obtain a complete history, then carefully and gently examine the affected area. Document the location, pattern, and events associated with pain. Inspect the oral cavity for signs of injury. Obtain the client's weight and assess the client's ability to eat food.

The plan for nursing care includes, but is not limited to, the following:

Nursing Diagnoses and Collaborative Problems	Nursing Interventions
Pain related to nerve compression as evidenced by the client's description of localized discomfort **Goal:** The client's pain will be relieved or reduced to a tolerable level.	Use a scale from 1 to 10 to help the client quantify the severity and intensity of the pain both before and after implementing a nursing measure. Administer prescribed drugs. Observe and record the client's response. Avoid drafts in the room.

	Place a sign on the client's bed stating that the bed is not to be jarred or the face touched in any way.
	Advise the client to use protective measures such as shielding the face from wind and cold, avoiding shaving, and avoiding situations or activities that cause pain.

Client and Family Teaching

The client is instructed to:

- Inspect the mouth daily for breaks in the mucous membrane.
- Take small sips or bites of food and concentrate on chewing and swallowing if surgery has been performed.
- Chew on the opposite side.
- Avoid eating hot foods.
- Use mouth rinses after eating.
- Keep regular dental appointments because the warning pain of a cavity, abscess, or other dental problem may be mistaken for neuralgia.

Bell's Palsy

Bell's palsy involves the seventh cranial nerve, which is responsible for movement of the facial muscles.

ETIOLOGY AND PATHOPHYSIOLOGY

The cause of Bell's palsy is unknown, but a viral link is suspected. Inflammation occurs around the nerve, blocking motor impulses to facial muscles. As a result there is weakness and paralysis of facial muscles including the muscles of the eyelids on one side of the face. Most clients who recover begin to show improvement in a few weeks. Those whose paralysis is permanent fail to show improvement after 3 months or more.

ASSESSMENT FINDINGS

Signs and Symptoms

Symptoms develop in a few hours or during a period of 1 to 2 days. Facial pain, pain behind the ear, numbness, diminished blink reflex, ptosis of the eyelid, and tearing of the affected side occur. Speaking and chewing become difficult.

Diagnostic Findings

There are no specific diagnostic tests for this disorder, and the diagnosis is based on symptoms and visual examination of the face. In some instances it is necessary to rule out other neurologic problems such as brain tumor and stroke, which have comparable symptoms.

MEDICAL MANAGEMENT

Short-term prednisone (steroid) therapy is prescribed to reduce nerve inflammation and edema. Analgesics are prescribed for pain. Electrotherapy or a facial sling help to prevent atrophy of the facial muscles on the affected side.

NURSING MANAGEMENT

Once the diagnosis is confirmed, the client is assured that a more serious problem (eg, stroke, tumor) has not occurred. The care of a client with Bell's palsy includes, but is not limited, to:

Nursing Diagnoses and Collaborative Problems	Nursing Interventions
Risk for (Opthalmic) **Infection** related to diminished blink reflex **Goal:** The eye will remain free of infection as evidenced by the absence of redness and purulent drainage.	Cover the eye with an eyepatch to keep the eyelid closed. Apply a protective eye shield at night. Inspect the eye daily for signs of inflammation and infection. Irrigate the eye with normal saline, especially after surgery has been performed. Instill prescribed antibiotic ophthalmic ointment.
Altered Oral Mucous Membranes related to loss of sensation in the mouth, paralysis of chewing muscles as manifested by trauma to the cheeks, gums, teeth, or tongue **Goal:** The integrity of the oral cavity will be restored.	Provide supplies for oral hygiene before and after meals. Check the client's mouth after eating. Remove particles of food that remain by using mouth rinses, cotton-tipped applicators, or a pulsating oral irrigator. Ensure that food and beverages are not too hot to avoid burning oral mucous membranes. Encourage biannual dental examinations.
Impaired Verbal Communication related to facial paralysis, pain **Goal:** The client will communicate verbally.	Instruct the client to speak slowly and in short sentences. Provide a pad of paper and a pencil to facilitate communication during times of severe pain.

Client and Family Teaching

Instruct and demonstrate the instillation of ophthalmic ointment and application of an eye patch and eye shield. Show the client how to place the finger on the eyelid, draw it gently downward, and cover the eye to keep it closed. Explain that excessive tearing necessitates frequent changes of the eye patch.

Temporomandibular Joint Syndrome

Temporomandibular joint (TMJ) syndrome is a cluster of symptoms that are localized at and about the jaw.

ETIOLOGY AND PATHOPHYSIOLOGY

Causes of TMJ include degenerative arthritis of the mandibular joint, malocclusion of the teeth, and excessive movement of the jaw at the time of endotracheal intubation.

Temporomandibular joint syndrome results when the meniscus between the condyle of the mandible and the temporal bone becomes displaced, causing muscle spasm and compression of nerves and arteries in the area. The disorder can be confused with trigeminal neuralgia and migraine headache.

ASSSESSMENT FINDINGS

Signs and Symptoms

Symptoms include jaw pain, pronounced muscle spasm, and tenderness of the masseter and temporalis muscles. The localized discomfort is accompanied by headache, tinnitus (ringing in the ears), and ear pain. The client experiences clicking of the jaw when the joint is moved, or the jaw can lock, which interferes with opening the mouth.

Diagnostic Findings

Special dental radiographs often reveal evidence of joint displacement.

MEDICAL AND SURGICAL MANAGEMENT

Treatment is referred to a dentist who has experience with managing clients with TMJ. Analgesics are prescribed or recommended, and a custom-fitted mouth guard is worn during sleep. Transcutaneous electrical nerve stimulation (TENS), injection of a local anesthetic to relieve muscle spasm, and ice water oral irrigations are also used to reduce and relieve discomfort. Reconstructive surgery of the mandibular joint is available if conservative treatment is ineffective.

NURSING MANAGEMENT

Monitor the client's weight and ability to consume food. Obtain a nutritional consultation with the dietician if possible. Modify the diet to include soft food rather than those that are coarse or difficult to chew. Provide nutritional liquid supplements. Assist the client in acquiring skills to control pain, such as using a bite guard during sleep.

Extrapyramidal Disorders

Extrapyramidal disorders have their origin in the motor cortex and surrounding areas of the cerebellum and basal ganglia. Two common extrapyramidal disorders are Parkinson's disease and Huntington's disease. One of their primary characteristics is abnormal movement.

Parkinson's Disease

Parkinson's disease usually begins after the age of 50. It primarily affects the basal ganglia and connections in the substantia nigra and corpus striatum (Fig. 44–7). The term **parkinsonism** is used to describe the cluster of Parkinson-like symptoms that develop from a variety of etiologies.

ETIOLOGY AND PATHOPHYSIOLOGY

Parkinson's disease and parkinsonism results from a deficiency of the neurotransmitter dopamine. Depletion of dopamine in the affected areas of the brain upsets the balance between dopamine and acetylcholine, which results in movement disorders (Fig. 44–8).

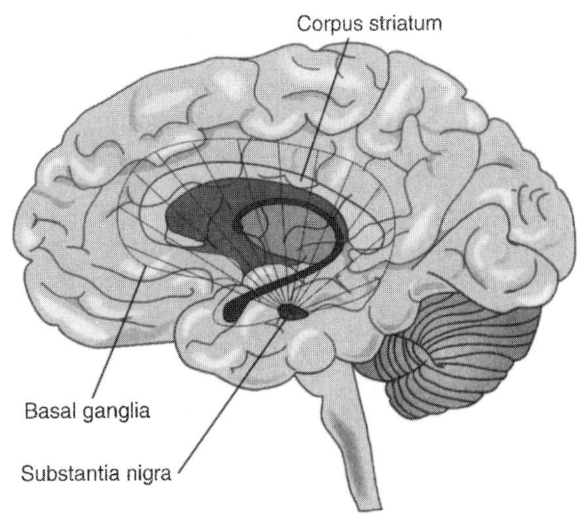

FIGURE 44-7. The loss of dopamine-producing nerve cells in the substantia nigra is thought to be responsible for the symptoms of parkinsonism.

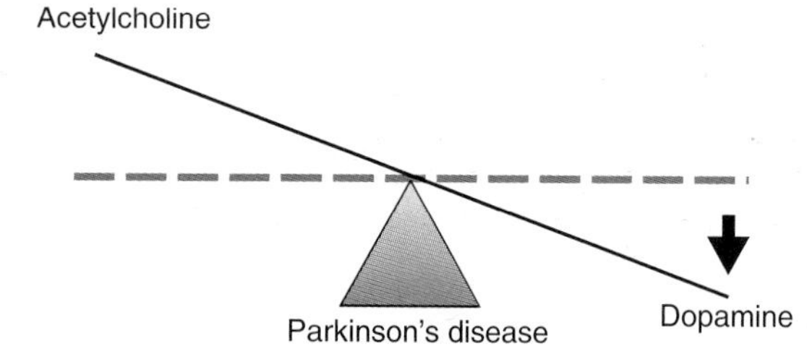

FIGURE 44-8. The normal balance of acetylcholine and dopamine is upset in Parkinson's disease.

In the majority of cases of Parkinson's disease, no cause can be found for dopamine depletion. The symptoms of parkinsonism are associated with exposure to environmental toxins such as insecticides and herbicides, self-administration of an illegal synthetic form of heroin known as MPTP, and as a sequela of head injuries and encephalitis. Phenothiazine, a category of antipsychotic drugs used to treat schizophrenia, also produces parkinsonism, but the symptoms are reversible when the drug is discontinued.

Manifestations of the disorder progress so slowly that years may lapse between the time of the first symptom and the time of diagnosis. The symptoms are initially unilateral but eventually, whether quickly or slowly, become bilateral.

ASSESSMENT FINDINGS

Signs and Symptoms

Early signs include stiffness referred to as rigidity and tremors of one or both hands described as "pill-rolling" (a rhythmic motion of the thumb against the fingers). The hand tremor is obvious at rest and typically decreases when movement is voluntary, for example, picking up an object.

Bradykinesia, slowness in performing spontaneous movements, develops. Clients have a masklike expression, stooped posture, monotonous speech, and difficulty swallowing saliva. Weight loss occurs. A shuffling gait is apparent and the person has difficulty turning or redirecting forward motion. Arms are rigid while walking (Fig. 44–9).

In late stages of the disease, the jaw, tongue, and larynx are affected; speech is slurred and chewing and swallowing become difficult. Rigidity can lead to contractures. Salivation increases, accompanied by drooling. In a small percentage of people, the eyes roll upward or downward and stay there involuntarily (oculogyric crises) for several hours or even a few days.

Diagnostic Findings

Diagnosis is based on typical symptoms and a neurologic examination. There are no specific tests for this disorder.

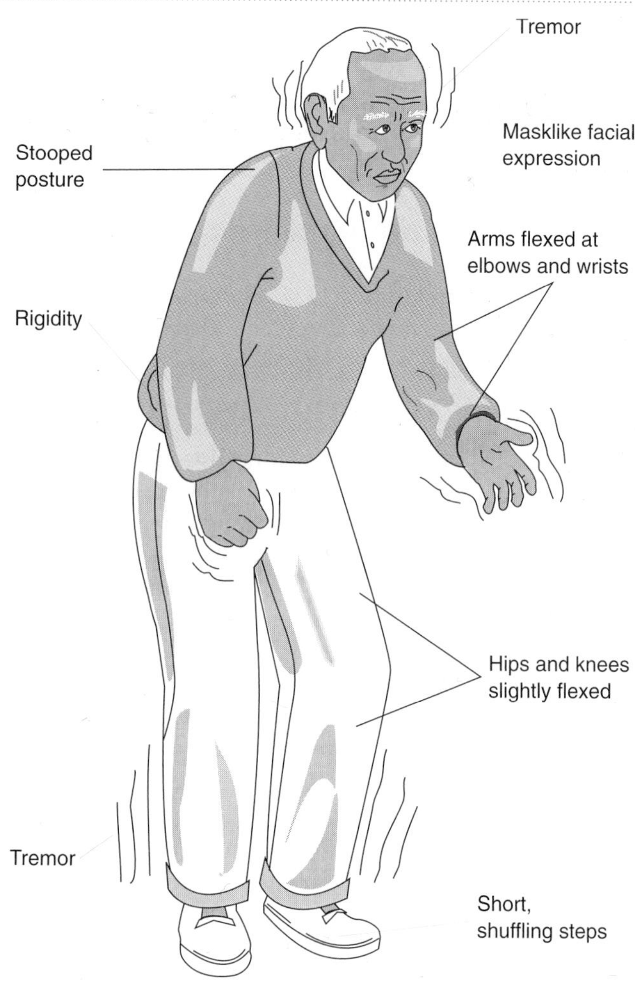

FIGURE 44-9. Typical manifestations of Parkinson's disease.

MEDICAL MANAGEMENT

Treatment is aimed at prolonging independence. Drugs such as segiline (Eldepryl), a drug with neuroprotective properties, dopaminergics such as levodopa (Larodopa) or levodopa-carbidopa (Sinemet), amantadine (Symmetrel), dopamine agonists such as bromocriptine (Parlodel), and anticholinergics such as benztropine (Cogentin) are prescribed (Table 44–1). The sequence of their use is based on the stage of the disorder and the dwindling effectiveness of the medication initially prescribed. Rehabilitation measures, such as physical therapy, occupational therapy, client and family education, and counseling, are used concurrently with drug therapy.

SURGICAL MANAGEMENT

Surgery (stereotaxic thalamotomy) is performed in selected cases. The procedure destroys part of the thalamus so that excessive muscle contraction is de-

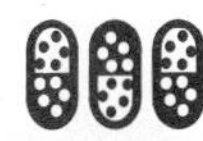

TABLE 44-1 **Drugs Used in Management of Parkinson's Disease**

Drug Category/ Drug Action	Side Effects	Nursing Considerations
Monoamine Oxidase B Inhibitor (MAOI)		
selegiline (Eldepryl) Increases dopaminergic activity, slows Parkinson's disease.	Dizziness, light-headedness, confusion, nausea, vomiting, diarrhea, dry mouth, palpitations	Narcotic analgesics must not be given with an MAOI. Administer twice daily with breakfast and lunch. Use ice chips and sugarless candy for dry mouth.
Dopaminergics		
levodopa (Larodopa, Sinemet) Dopamine replacement to decrease symptoms.	Nausea, vomiting, orthostatic hypotension, dry mouth, constipation, dizziness, cardiac arrhythmias, sleep disturbance	Do not give with MAOIs. Give with meals. Avoid multivitamins with pyridoxine.
Antiparkinsonism		
amantadine (Symmetrel) May increase dopamine release to relieve symptoms.	Mood changes, drowsiness, blurred vision, insomnia, nausea, orthostatic hypotension, urinary retention	Do not discontinue abruptly to avoid parkinsonian crisis. Report swelling of fingers, ankles, shortness of breath, difficulty urinating, tremors, slurred speech.
Anticholinergics		
benztropine (Cogentin) trihexphenidyl (Artane) Decrease rigidity, akinesia, tremor, and drooling.	Dry mouth, constipation, urinary retention, blurred vision, skin rash, flushing, increased temperature, decreased sweating	Dosage is decreased or discontinued if dry mouth interferes with eating. Client must use caution in hot weather. Give with meals. Avoid alcohol and sedatives.
Dopamine Agonists		
bromocriptine (Parlodel) Mimics effects of dopamine, may be effective when levodopa has decreased efficacy.	Hallucinations, confusion, dizziness, drowsiness, nausea, vomiting, constipation, hypotension, shortness of breath	Give with food. Dosage is tapered before discontinued. Monitor client's mental status.

creased. Some success has been reported with fetal tissue transplantation in which brain tissue containing the basal ganglia and dopamine-secreting cells is extracted from an aborted fetus and transplanted into the recipient's brain. This procedure is experimental and requires craniotomy. Another technique recently approved for use is the implantation of a brain pacemaker. The pacemaker blocks the tremor with tiny electrical shocks directed at the thalamus and produces immediate elimination of the tremor in approximately 65% of the people in whom it has been used.

NURSING MANAGEMENT

Clients with parkinsonism are admitted to the hospital because of the debilitating effects of the disease. On admission, assess the functional ability of the client before developing a plan of care. Evaluate the client's mental and emotional status as well. A sample plan of care for a client with an extrapyramidal disorder, like Parkinson's or Huntington's disease, is provided in Nursing Care Plan 44–1.

Determine the type of drugs and the time of day the client takes them. Levodopa is associated with periods of "break through" when the symptoms become exacerbated if a consistent level is not maintained. It is important, therefore, to administer the drugs closely to the schedule the client previously established at home. Drugs administered for parkinsonism are capable of causing a wide variety of adverse effects and careful observation of the client is required.

Safety measures to avoid aspiration and prevent falls and other complications are primary concerns for nursing care. The nurse works with the physical and occupational therapists to plan exercises that maintain mobility and joint flexibility. Provide necessary support to keep the client clean and well groomed.

NURSING CARE PLAN 44-1

Nursing Management of a Client With an Extrapyramidal Disorder

Nursing Diagnoses and Collaborative Problems	Nursing Management	Outcome Criteria
Impaired Physical Mobility and **Self-Care Deficit** (Total or specify areas) related to muscle rigidity, tremors, choreiform movements, dementia as evidenced by inability to complete all or some activities of daily living	Assist with walking and physical activity. Gradually increase the type and amount of activity to promote endurance. Minimize fatigue by providing periods of rest. Promote involvement in self-care activities within the client's ability to perform them. Avoid total dependence on others as long as possible. Allow ample time to perform activities of daily living. Modify clothing and self-care supplies to promote independence. Assist the client, but only when the client is unable to perform certain tasks.	The client is physically active and participates in activities of daily living.
Impaired Swallowing, Risk for Aspiration related to neuromuscular dysfunction as evidenced by coughing, choking, and stasis of food in the oral cavity, and **Altered Nutrition: Less than Body Requirements** related to difficulty chewing, swallowing, or holding utensils	Place in a sitting position. Keep suction equipment at the bedside and use it when the client chokes. Decrease environmental distractions so the client can focus attention on the tasks of chewing and swallowing. Cut food into small pieces. Incorporate foods with mashed potatoes to bind them together in a soft bolus so they are more easily swallowed. Thicken liquids with gelatin, cornstarch, applesauce, mashed bananas, or ice cream to provide a consistency that is easily manipulated by the tongue against the palate. Position the chin on the chest during swallowing to decrease the potential for food entering the airway. Stroke the throat as the client swallows or instruct the client to swallow several times in a row to ensure that the bolus moves to the esophagus. Modify utensils to enable the client to grasp and hold them.	The client swallows without aspiration. Nutritional intake is adequate.
Impaired Verbal Communication related to soft voice or inability to articulate words	Reduce environmental noise. Listen closely to what the client attempts to verbalize. Ask the client to speak slowly. Anticipate the client's needs.	Client communicates needs, feelings and ideas.
Anxiety and **Ineffective Individual Coping** related to awareness of diminishing physical and mental capacities as manifested by periods of agitation, frustration, emotional irritability, anger	Help the client to realistically determine what tasks are feasible and those that are not. Suggest taking a break when the client is unable to accomplish a task successfully. Offer support and encouragement when the client is successful. Help the client focus on his or her remaining strengths rather than deficits. Provide information on support groups with others with similar problems or disorders.	The client is relaxed and confident when performing tasks and managing self-care. The client accepts the gradual loss of physical or mental attributes and allows others to help without opposition.

continued

NURSING CARE PLAN 44-1
Continued

Nursing Diagnoses and Collaborative Problems	Nursing Management	Outcome Criteria
Risk for Loneliness related to depression, perceived potential for rejection secondary to altered physical appearance or cognitive function	Have the client identify persons whose company he or she enjoys and activities that they share in common. Encourage the client to interact with one or two of the designated people for short periods of time in a place where the client feels secure and comfortable, such as the client's residence. Encourage the client to participate in social activities outside the place of residence. Refer client to and encourage joining a support group.	The client maintains social contacts.

Huntington's Disease

Huntington's disease (Huntington's chorea, hereditary chorea) is a hereditary disorder of the CNS.

ETIOLOGY AND PATHOPHYSIOLOGY

This extrapyramidal disorder is transmitted genetically and inherited by either sex. The basal ganglia and portions of the cerebral cortex degenerate. In the early stages, the client is able to participate in most physical activities. As the disease progresses, hallucinations, delusions, impaired judgment, and increased intensity of abnormal movements develop.

ASSESSMENT FINDINGS

Signs and Symptoms

Symptoms occur slowly and include mental apathy and emotional disturbances, **choreiform movements** (uncontrollable writhing and twisting of the body), grimacing, difficulty chewing and swallowing, speech difficulty, intellectual decline, and loss of bowel and bladder control. Severe depression is common and can lead to suicide.

Diagnostic Findings

Diagnosis is based on symptoms as well as a family history of the disorder. Positron emission tomography shows CNS changes, but there is no specific diagnostic test for the disorder. Genetic testing can predict which offspring will develop the disease, but not all individuals choose to undergo testing.

MEDICAL MANAGEMENT

Treatment is supportive because there is no specific therapy or cure. Tranquilizers and antiparkinson drugs relieve the choreiform movements in some clients. No drugs are available that can halt the mental deterioration. Because this disorder is inherited, genetic counseling before a pregnancy is advised.

NURSING MANAGEMENT

Nursing management is aimed at meeting client and family needs, such as preventing complications as well as encouraging counseling. The scope of nursing care is determined by the stage of the disease. The client eventually becomes totally dependent on others.

Pneumonia, contractures, infections, aspiration of food or fluids, falls, and pressure ulcers are complications. The nurse prevents these complications by assessing the client frequently and updating the plan of care. See Nursing Care Plan 44–1 for additional nursing management.

Client and Family Teaching

Encourage the client to lead as normal a life as possible. Emphasize the importance of exercise and self-care, and explain the medical regimen to the client and family. Demonstrate to the client and family how to facilitate tasks such as using both hands to hold a drinking glass, using a straw to drink, and wearing slip-on shoes.

Seizure Disorders

The terms *seizure disorder* and *convulsive disorder* are used interchangeably, but they are not necessarliy synonymous. A **seizure** is a brief episode of abnormal electrical activity in the brain. A **convulsion,** one manifestation of a seizure, is characterized by spasmodic contractions of muscles. **Epilepsy** is a chronic recurrent pattern of seizures.

ETIOLOGY AND PATHOPHYSIOLOGY

Seizure disorders are classified as idiopathic (no known cause) or acquired. Causes of acquired seizures include high fever, electrolyte imbalances, uremia, hypoglycemia, hypoxia, brain tumor, and drug withdrawal. Once the cause is removed the seizures cease. The known causes of epilepsy include brain injury at birth, head injuries, and inborn errors of metabolism. In some people, the cause of epilepsy is never determined.

Seizures represent abnormal motor, sensory, or psychic activity. Each type of seizure disorder is characterized by a specific pattern of events. Box 44–3 lists the international classification of seizures.

The abnormal electrical activity occurs alone or in combination from discharges in one or more specific areas of the cerebral cortex of the brain. If the electrical discharges involve the entire brain, a generalized seizure occurs.

TYPES OF SEIZURES

Partial Seizures

Partial, or focal, seizures begin in a specific area of the cerebral cortex. A partial seizure can progress to a generalized seizure. There are two general types of partial seizures: those with elementary (or simple) symptoms and those with complex symptoms. A client who has a partial seizure with elementary symptoms usually does not lose consciousness and the seizure lasts less than 1 minute. Partial elementary seizures with motor symptoms are accompanied by uncontrolled jerking movements of a body part, such as a finger, mouth, hand, or foot. Partial elementary seizures with sensory symptoms are accompanied by hallucinatory sights, sounds, and odors, mumbling, and the use of nonsense words. The terms jacksonian, focal motor, and focal sensory describe partial elementary seizures.

A client who has a partial seizure with complex symptoms may have a variety of sensory or motor manifestations. These also last less than 1 minute. After the seizure the client is often confused. Complex partial seizures are manifested by automatic repetitive movements (**automatisms**) that are not appropriate such as lip smacking and picking at clothing or objects. The terms psychomotor and psychosensory are used to describe complex partial seizures.

BOX 44-3 International Classification of Seizures

I. Partial (Focal) Seizures

A. Partial seizures (no loss of consciousness)
   1. Motor symptoms
   2. Special sensory symptoms
   3. Autonomic symptoms
   4. Psychic symptoms

B. Complex partial seizures (with loss of consciousness)
   1. Begins as a partial seizure and progresses to complex partial with loss of consciousness.
   2. Loss of consciousness at onset of seizure

II. Generalized Seizures

A. Absence seizures
B. Myoclonic seizures
C. Clonic seizures
D. Tonic seizures
E. Tonic-clonic seizures
F. Atonic seizures

III. Unclassified Seizures

All seizures that do not fit into other classifications

Generalized Seizures

Generalized seizures involve the entire brain. Consciousness is lost, and the seizure may last from several seconds to several minutes. Types of generalized seizures include absence seizures, myoclonic seizures, and tonic-clonic seizures.

Absence Seizures

Absence seizures, formerly referred to as petit mal seizures, are more common in children. They are characterized by a brief loss of consciousness during which physical activity ceases. The person stares blankly, the eyelids flutter, the lips move, and slight movement of the head, arms, and legs occur. These seizures typically last for a few seconds, and the person seldom falls to the ground. Because of their brief duration and relative lack of prominent movements, these seizures often go unnoticed. People with absence seizures can have them many times a day.

Myoclonic Seizures

These seizures are characterized by sudden, excessive jerking of the arms, legs, or entire body. In some instances, the muscle activity is so severe that the client falls to the ground. These seizures are brief.

Tonic-Clonic Seizures

Formerly referred to as grand mal seizures, tonic-clonic seizures are characterized by a sequence of events that begins with a preictal (or prodromal) phase. The **preictal phase** is the time immediately before a seizure and consists of vague emotional changes, such as depression, anxiety, and nervousness. This phase lasts for minutes or hours and is followed by an **aura,** a sensation that occurs immediately before the seizure.

The aura is sensory (ie, a hallucinatory odor or sound) or a sensation of weakness or numbness. In clients who experience an aura, the aura is almost always the same.

The aura is followed by the epileptic cry, which is caused by spasm of the respiratory muscles and muscles of the throat and glottis. This cry immediately precedes loss of consciousness and the ensuing tonic and clonic phases of the seizure. In the tonic phase, the muscles contract rigidly; in the clonic phase, the muscles alternate between contraction and relaxation, resulting in jerking movements and thrashing of the arms and legs. The skin becomes cyanotic, and breathing is spasmodic. Saliva mixes with air, resulting in frothing at the mouth. The jaws are tightly clenched and biting of the tongue and inner cheek occurs. Urinary or fecal incontinence is common. The clonic phase lasts for 1 minute or more, gradually subsides, and is followed by the postictal phase. The manifestations of this phase include headache, fatigue, deep sleep, confusion, nausea, and muscle soreness. Many people fall into a deep sleep for several hours.

Status epilepticus is marked by a series of tonic-clonic seizures in which the client does not regain consciousness between seizures. If this extremely dangerous condition is not terminated, death can occur. Status epilepticus occurs spontaneously in acute neurologic disorders or for no known reason; it and be precipitated by the abrupt discontinuation of anticonvulsant medication.

Other Seizure Types

Atonic (loss of muscle tone) *seizures* affect the muscles. The person loses consciousness briefly and falls to the ground. Recovery is rapid. An *akinetic* (loss of movement) *seizure* is similar because muscle tone is lost briefly. The client may or may not fall and recovery is rapid.

ASSESSMENT FINDINGS

Signs and Symptoms

Unless the client is having a seizure, there are no physical signs. On physical examination there can be

TABLE 44-2 **Drugs for Controlling Seizures**

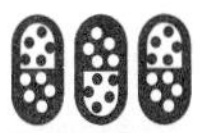

Drug Category/ Drug Action	Side Effects	Nursing Considerations
Anticonvulsants		
phenytoin (Dilantin) Stabilizes neuronal membranes; limits spread of seizure activity; controls grand mal seizures.	Nystagmus, rash, sedation, gingival hyperplasia, liver toxicity, pancytopenia	Evaluate regular serum levels. Evaluate liver function tests, complete blood count and differential. Assess skin daily. Give oral dose with food. Dose is tapered gradually; never discontinue abruptly. Instruct client to wear Medic Alert bracelet and have regular dental care.
carbamazepine (Tegretol) Controls partial seizures with complex symptoms, also grand mal seizures.	Dizziness, ataxia, nystagmus, rash, nausea, vomiting, liver toxicity, bone marrow suppression	Same as above
ethosuximide (Zarontin) Reduces frequency of attacks of absence (petit mal) seizures.	Drowsiness, rash, headache, nausea and vomiting	Same as above
valproic acid (Depakene, Depakote) Adjunct treatment for multiple seizure types.	Nausea and vomiting, drowsiness, diarrhea, liver toxicity	Avoid alcohol intake. Monitor bruising, bleeding gums. See above nursing considerations
Barbiturates		
phenobarbital (Luminal) Anticonvulsant activity	Sedation, rash, hyperactivity, ataxia, respiratory depression	Take oral dose at bedtime. Monitor vital signs, especially respiratory rate. Administer intramuscular dose in deep muscle mass. Dosage is tapered before drug is discontinued. Periodic laboratory tests are required.
Benzodiazepines		
diazepam (Valium) Skeletal muscle relaxation; adjunct anticonvulsant treatment.	Respiratory depression, hypotension, sedation	Monitor blood pressure, pulse and respiration. Evaluate liver, kidney function, and blood studies. Dose is tapered before drug is discontinued. Instruct client to wear Medic Alert bracelet.

an absence of signs. Identification of the type of seizure often depends on a witness's description of the client's actions during the seizure.

Diagnostic Findings

A neurologic examination and EEG are performed. Other laboratory or diagnostic studies, such as a CT scan, MRI, serology, and serum electrolyte levels are used to confirm the diagnosis and to determine the cause of the seizure disorder. When epilepsy is suspected, a series of EEGs is required if the first results are normal.

MEDICAL MANAGEMENT

Once a diagnosis of a seizure disorder is confirmed, one or more anticonvulsant drugs are used to control the seizures. Examples of anticonvulsants are phenytoin (Dilantin), phenobarbital, carbamazepine (Tegretol), ethosuximide (Zarontin), valproic acid (Depakene), felbamate (Felbatol), and fosphenytoin injection (Cerebyx) (Table 44–2). IV barbiturates or diazepam (Valium) are administered to terminate status epilepticus.

Drug therapy controls the seizures or reduces their frequency or severity. The dose is adjusted over a period of several weeks. The drug is changed or another drug is added to the regimen to obtain optimum control. Blood levels of some anticonvulsant drugs are monitored for accurate dose adjustment and to prevent toxicity (Table 44–3). Serum levels also identify clients who are not taking the drug as ordered.

SURGICAL MANAGEMENT

Seizures that are caused by brain tumor, brain abscess, or other disorders often require surgical intervention. Surgery for epilepsy is not considered unless the client does not respond to drug therapy and seizures are frequent and severe. The area of the brain in which abnormal electrical discharges are present is identified (mapped). The surgeon must consider if removal of the involved area would result in permanent neurologic dysfunction such as paralysis or loss of speech.

TABLE 44-3 **Anticonvulsant Drug Monitoring**

Drug	Therapeutic Level	Toxic Level
carbamazepine	5–12 μg/mL	>12 μg/mL
ethosuximide	40–100 μg/mL	>100 μg/mL
phenobarbital	10–30 μg/mL	>40 μg/mL
phenytoin	10–20 μg/mL	>30 μg/mL
valproic acid	50–100 μg/mL	>100 μg/mL

(From Pagana, K. D., Pagana, T. J. (1995). *Mosby's diagnostic and laboratory test reference* (2nd ed.). St. Louis: Mosby.)

BOX 44-4 Seizure Assessment Data

- Onset—sudden or preceded by an aura
- Duration of seizure
- Behavior immediately before and after
- Type of body movements
- Loss of consciousness, for how long
- Incontinence or not
- Seizure awareness afterward

NURSING PROCESS
The Client With a Seizure Disorder

Assessment

Obtain a complete history, including drug, allergy, and family history. Question the client regarding events or symptoms that occurred before and after the seizure. Obtain a description of the seizure from an observer. Include information about any past injury, previous treatment for a seizure disorder, and whether medication is taken as prescribed.

Clients with a seizure disorder are closely observed, especially when the seizures are frequent and severe. If the client's history is inconclusive and the type of seizure is unknown, it is important to provide a full, detailed description of the seizure (Box 44–4).

Diagnosis and Planning

The nursing management of a client with a seizure disorder includes, but is not limited to, the following:

Nursing Diagnoses and Collaborative Problems	Nursing Interventions
Risk for Injury related to uncontrolled movements, altered consciousness during seizure and **Risk for Altered Oral Mucous Membranes** related to oral injury during a seizure and side effects of phenytoin drug therapy **Goal:** The client will be free of injuries; the oral mucous membranes will remain unaltered.	Refer to the nursing management of seizures in the nursing process section on caring for a client with infectious and inflammatory disorders earlier in this chapter. Use padded head gear on clients with atonic or akinetic seizures. Pad side rails with soft material. Protect the client at the onset of the seizure by assisting the client to the floor or moving objects away from the client. Never forcibly restrain the client to prevent fractures. Inspect the oral cavity and teeth after a generalized

	seizure for signs of injury; report injuries to the physician.
	Apply ice to bleeding areas; if broken teeth are noted, notify the client's dentist.
	Promote oral hygiene after each meal and recommend dental checkups every 3 to 6 months to control gingival hyperplasia (overgrowth of gum tissue).
Anxiety related to fear of unpredictable seizure and social stigma as evidenced by uneasiness about resuming previous lifestyle activities with social acquaintances	Help the client understand the disorder and treatment options.
	Explain that a variety of drugs are available that can successfully reduce or control seizures.
Goal: The client will feel secure about resuming activities.	Encourage the client to share information about the disorder with others in an effort to educate them and eliminate the misconceptions that those with seizure disorders have subnormal intelligence.
	Suggest contacting the Epilepsy Foundation of America, which provides counseling, low-cost prescription services, and referrals to agencies for vocational rehabilitation, job opportunities, personal and genetic counseling, and sheltered workshops.

Evaluation and Expected Outcomes

- The client's seizures are controlled.
- The client remains safe from injury.
- The client's anxiety is reduced to a tolerable level on a scale of 0 to 10.

Client and Family Teaching

The client newly diagnosed with seizures needs information about the specific type of disorder, the medications needed to control the seizures, and the precautions, if any, to be taken. In addition, teach the client to:

- Take the medication daily as prescribed.
- Recognize adverse effects of the medication.
- Keep routine follow-up visits and laboratory appointments for blood level tests.
- Operate a motor vehicle or perform dangerous tasks only when seizures are controlled for at least 6 months.
- Wear a Medic Alert bracelet, tag, or other medical identification.
- Avoid situations known to trigger seizures such as repetitively flashing or blinking lights, stress, or lack of sleep.

Brain Tumors

A brain tumor is a growth of abnormal cells within the cranium. Brain tumors occur in all age groups. Some types are more common in people younger than 20 years of age, whereas others more frequently affect older people. About 50% of all brain tumors are malignant. A brain tumor, whether malignant or benign, can result in death.

ETIOLOGY AND PATHOPHYSIOLOGY

The cause of brain tumors remains unknown. A small percentage are congenital, such as hemangioblastomas. Genetics are associated with two types of brain tumors, astrocytoma, a tumor in the frontal lobe, and those associated with neurofibromatosis. Other causative factors include viral infection, exposure to radiation, head trauma, and immunosuppression. The brain also is the site of metastatic lesions from primary tumors, especially tumors of the lung and breast.

Tumors that arise from cerebral tissue, such as malignant gliomas and glioblastomas, and angiomas that involve cerebral blood vessels, expand within the confines of the skull and encroach on brain tissue that is vital for life. Extracerebral tumors, such as meningiomas (tumors of the meninges), press on the brain tissue from without.

ASSESSMENT FINDINGS

Signs and Symptoms

Because tumors take up space and block the flow and absorption of CSF, symptoms associated with IICP occur. The classic triad of headache, vomiting, and papilledema is common. Headache is most common early in the morning. It becomes increasingly severe and occurs with greater frequency as the tumor grows. Vomiting occurs without nausea or warning. Seizures also develop. Symptoms of disturbed neurologic function, such as speech difficulty, paralysis, and double vision, develop depending on the tumor's location.

When the ICP is greatly increased the brain stem is forced through the foramen magnum. The client is in grave danger because the vital centers that control respiration and heart rate are compressed. Respirations become deeper, labored, and noisy and then slow to only periodic. Unless the condition is relieved, the client dies of respiratory failure and cardiac arrest. Hyperthermia occurs as the temperature-regulating center in the brain is affected. Coma progressively deepens.

Diagnostic Findings

Diagnosis is confirmed with CT scan, MRI, brain scan, and cerebral angiography, which reveal the tumor's size and location.

MEDICAL MANAGEMENT

Treatment depends on several factors, including the tumor's location and type (primary or metastatic) and the client's age and physical condition. Brain tumors are treated by surgery, radiation therapy, chemotherapy, or a combination of these methods.

Metastatic tumors and some primary tumors are inoperable, and radiation therapy and chemotherapy are the only treatment choices. Clients who cannot withstand surgery, chemotherapy, or radiation therapy are kept as comfortable and free from pain as possible. Intra-arterial or intrathecal administration of antineoplastic drugs is used to destroy the tumor or slow tumor growth. Symptomatic drug therapy includes corticosteroids and osmotic diuretics to reduce cerebral edema, analgesics, anticonvulsants, and antibiotics.

Complications, such as IICP, paralysis, mental changes, infection, seizures, and prolonged immobility, are treated symptomatically.

SURGICAL MANAGEMENT

Surgery for an operable brain tumor involves a craniotomy (incision through the skull) or craniectomy (excision of part of the skull). A section of bone (bone flap) is removed to reach the brain (Fig. 44–10). After the tumor is removed, the dura is reapproximated (the cut edges are lined up and sewn together), the bone flap replaced, and the skin sutured. The bone flap is not reinserted when increasing ICP or tumor growth is expected.

The client's postoperative symptoms are determined by the location and function of any damaged or removed brain tissue. Brain tissue does not regenerate.

Another method of removing brain tumors uses a laser beam directed at the tumor site. This surgical technique enables the physician to reach tumors that were previously considered inoperable. Radioisotopes are also surgically inserted into the tumor. The cure rate for this procedure, however, is about the same as for external radiation therapy.

NURSING MANAGEMENT

Nursing management depends on the area of the brain affected, tumor type, treatment approach, and the client's signs and symptoms. If the tumor is inoperable or has expanded despite treatment, IICP is a major threat (refer to nursing care at the beginning of this chapter). See Chapter 46 for the care of the client undergoing intracranial surgery. Clients who receive chemotherapy and radiation are supported through the adverse effects associated with antineoplastic drug administration (see Chap. 19). Explain all treatment modalities to the client and family. Allow them time to ask questions and direct them to appropriate professionals to discuss treatment alternatives.

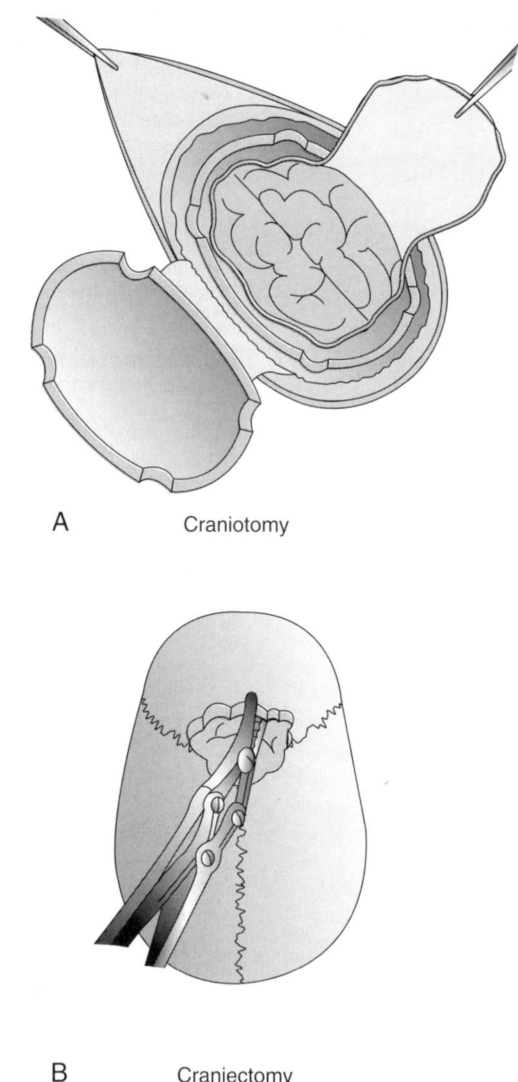

FIGURE 44-10. Neurosurgical techniques (*A*) Craniotomy (*B*) Craniectomy.

NURSING PROCESS
The Client With a Brain Tumor

Assessment

Identify affected areas following a thorough history and neurologic examination. Record additional assessments of the client's symptoms and general condition.

Diagnosis and Planning

The plan of care for a client with a brain tumor includes nursing diagnoses and collaborative problems added at various stages to correlate with the client's treatment, as well as the following:

Nursing Diagnoses and Collaborative Problems	Nursing Interventions
Pain related to IICP secondary to expansion of the tumor or sequela of surgery **Goal:** Pain will be controlled within the client's level of tolerance.	Assess and monitor characteristics of pain. Administer prescribed analgesia and monitor for respiratory depression. Give analgesia on a scheduled rather than an as needed basis. Advocate for patient-controlled analgesia or transdermal analgesic patch.
Altered Nutrition: Less than Body Requirements related to nausea and vomiting or altered LOC **Goal:** The client's nutritional and fluid needs are met as evidenced by maintenance of weight and intake above 2,000 mL.	Administer prescribed antiemetics before meals. Determine the client's food preferences and supply them. Serve small, frequent servings of food or nourishing beverages. Collaborate with the physician concerning gastric tube feedings or TPN if oral intake is inadequate.
Altered Oral Mucous Membranes related to fluid volume deficit, tissue damage secondary to chemotherapy or radiation as manifested by xerostomia (oral lesions) **Goal:** The oral mucous membranes will be pink, moist, and intact.	Relieve discomfort with a prescribed topical anesthetic. Provide meticulous mouth care. Offer mouth rinses frequently.
Anticipatory Grieving related to uncertain future, physical and social losses **Goal:** The client will express feelings while working through acceptance of the diagnosis.	Give the opportunity to express feelings privately. Remain with the client when emotions are overwhelming. Help clarify any and all questions the client may have. Reassure the client that he or she will not be abandoned and that comfort and preservation of dignity are priorities of nursing care. Assist the client to complete unfinished business however the client defines it. Refer the client and family to the local Hospice organization if the client is in the terminal stage

Evaluation and Expected Outcomes

- The client reports relief of pain.
- The client's intake is sufficient to maintain body weight.
- The client's oral mucosa is intact.
- The client and family progress through the grieving process.
- The client and family implement a plan for post-discharge care.

Client and Family Teaching

Before the client is discharged, evaluate the client's and family's emotional needs for immediate and long-term needs. Develop an individualized teaching plan that includes:

- Medication regimen
- Appointments for chemotherapy or radiation therapy
- Adverse effects of chemotherapy or radiation and techniques for managing them
- Nutritional support
- Home care considerations
- Rehabilitation (exercises, physical therapy)
- Referrals to support services for physical, emotional, and financial assistance

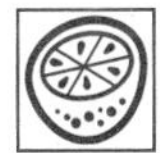

General Nutritional Considerations

General nutritional goals are to maintain healthy weight, prevent or correct malnutrition, reduce the risk of aspiration, and prevent constipation. Calories are adjusted to prevent weight gain (e.g., clients with multiple sclerosis) or weight loss (e.g., clients with Guillain-Barré syndrome); small frequent feedings of nutrient- and calorie-dense foods help maximize intake and reduce fatigue. Clients with muscle wasting benefit from an increased protein intake; commercial supplements (e.g., thickened liquids, fortified puddings, fortified gelatins) are tasty and easy options. Semi-solid foods like puddings and mashed potatoes are easier to swallow than thin liquids or a regular diet. Gastrostomy feedings are usually the best route for clients who require long-term enteral nutritional support. Foods high in fiber, such as whole wheat bread and cereals, bran cereal, and fiber fortified supplements, help prevent constipation when consumed with adequate fluids. Prunes and prune juice stimulate peristalsis.

Drug-nutrient interactions and side effects of drug therapy are minimized with diet modifications. Clients taking levodopa should avoid high intakes of protein (meat, fish, poultry, and dairy foods) and vitamin B_6 (legumes, sweet potatoes, avocado, fortified cereal, bran, wheat germ, pork, tuna), because they decrease its effectiveness. Limit daily sodium intake to 2000 mg in clients receiving corticosteroids; if hyperglycemia develops, a diabetic diet is used. Anticonvulsants impair vitamin D metabolism, leading to calcium imbalance, rickets, or osteomalacia if supplemental vitamin D is not given.

A high-fat diet, called the ketogenic diet, is used as part of treatment for seizures in children. The high fat content simulates starvation, except that the fat burned for energy comes from food, not stored body fat. Mild dehydration helps concentrate blood ketones; it is not known how or why ketosis affects seizure activity. Grams of fat to grams of protein and carbohydrate start with a 4:1 ratio; simulated starvation results in more efficient use of protein, so needs for growth can be met with 1.0 gm protein/kg of body weight. Fruits and vegetables are preferred as the major sources of carbohydrate because they are rich in other nutrients. The diet is inadequate in many vitamins and minerals, so carbohydrate-free supplements are needed. The diet is difficult to follow and unpalatable, but highly motivated families have overcome these obstacles and benefited from this low-risk, noninvasive therapy.

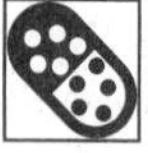

General Pharmacologic Considerations

Carbamazepine, a drug used in the treatment of trigeminal neuralgia, is taken with meals. The dose in gradually increased until relief is obtained. The effectiveness of carbamazepine may decrease over time.

Phenytoin, also used in the treatment of trigeminal neuralgia, requires periodic laboratory evaluation to detect bone marrow depression. This drug has also been implicated in birth defects and, therefore, must not be taken by pregnant women or those planning to become pregnant.

Phenytoin may discolor the urine pink or reddish-brown. This color change is not clinically significant.

Patients on anticonvulsant therapy should carry a Medic alert bracelet identifying the current medications and disease condition.

Abrupt withdrawal of any anticonvulsant drug may trigger status epilepticus (continuous seizure activity). The drug must gradually be withdrawn.

Corticosteroid administration may produce hyperglycemia, gastrointestinal bleeding, or gastric ulcer. The blood is checked for glucose every 4 hours and the stools are checked for blood. To decrease the risk for gastric ulcers, an antacid may be prescribed.

Narcotic analgesics depress the respiratory center and raise CSF pressure. Their use is contraindicated in clients with head trauma or increased ICP, unless administration is necessary.

In addition to Parkinsonism, tardive dyskinesia, characterized by rhythmic and involuntary movement of the tongue, jaw, neck, arm, and legs as well as grimacing, may be seen with the administration of the phenothiazines.

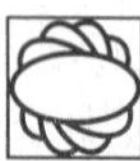

General Gerontologic Considerations

Older adults are more susceptible to the complications of prolonged bed rest and immobility and are watched closely for such problems as hypostatic pneumonia, pressure ulcers, contractures, and deformities.

Older adults may not exhibit the typical signs and symptoms of meningitis, but rather display a change in mental status, slight to no fever, and no nuchal rigidity or headache.

Mortality rates are high in the older adult with meningitis. Factors that contribute to increased mortality rate are the presence of chronic illness and delays in diagnosis (partly due to the atypical signs and symptoms).

The incidence of brain tumor decreases with age. Headache and papilledema are less common symptoms of a brain tumor in the older adult.

SUMMARY OF KEY CONCEPTS

- The signs of increased intracranial pressure include changes in level of consciousness, headache, vomiting, and sluggish pupil reaction to light.
- Nursing care of the client with increased intracranial pressure includes monitoring ICP levels and respirations, meeting nutritional needs, monitoring temperature and blood sugar levels, and assisting the patient to communicate.
- Infectious and inflammatory diseases affecting the central or peripheral nervous system include meningitis, encephalitis, Guillain-Barré syndrome, and brain abscess.
- Assessment findings associated with meningitis include nuchal rigidity, photophobia, a positive Kernig's sign, and a positive Brudzinski's sign.
- Chronic neuromuscular disorders include multiple sclerosis, myasthenia gravis, and amyotrophic lateral sclerosis.
- Nursing management of clients with neuromuscular disorders includes assisting with breathing, airway clearance, swallowing, aspiration, nutrition, communication, and coping.
- Cranial nerve disorders include trigeminal neuralgia and Bell's palsy.
- Nursing management of clients with cranial nerve disorders includes pain management, monitoring for infection, oral and mucosal care, and assistance with communication.
- Parkinson's disease primarily affects the motor nerves responsible for automatic movements. Symptoms include stiffness, "pill-rolling," tremors, masklike expression, stooped posture, monotonous speech, shuffling gait, and weight loss.
- Drug therapy for Parkinson's disease is aimed at prolonging independence. Drugs commonly prescribed include monoamine oxidase B inhibitor, dopaminergics, antiparkinsonisms, anticholinergics and dopamine agonists.
- Seizures are caused by abnormal motor, sensory, or psychic activity. Epilepsy is a permanent, recurrent seizure disorder. The nurse's primary goals for a client having a seizure are to protect the client from injury and to maintain a patent airway.
- Nursing management of the client with a seizure disorder includes injury prevention, care of oral mucosa, and anxiety alleviation.

- Symptoms associated with a brain tumor are related to increased intracranial pressure and the location of the tumor.

CRITICAL THINKING EXERCISES

1. When caring for a client with a seizure disorder, what nursing interventions are indicated?
2. What information can the nurse provide to a person who has recently been diagnosed with multiple sclerosis?
3. What discharge teaching is appropriate when discussing home care with the spouse of a client in the deteriorating stages of Parkinson's disease?

Suggested Readings

Campion, K., & Cole, A. (1997). Multiple sclerosis: The role of the nurse...part 2. *Nursing Times, 93*(11), 59–62.

Chiocca, E. M. (1995). Emergency! Meningococcal meningitis. *American Journal of Nursing, 95*(12), 25.

Davies, D. (1996). The cause of meningitis and meningococcal disease. *Nursing Times, 92*(6), :24–27.

Kernich, C. A., & Kaminskin, H. J. (1996). Myths and facts...about myasthenia gravis. *Nursing, 26*(7), 21.

Marcus, J. R. (1996). When GBS strikes: Insights from a nurse who's been there...Guillain-Barré syndrome. *Nursing, 26*(11), 32a–32b, 32d, 32f.

O'Donnell, L. (1996). An elusive weakness: Myasthenia gravis. *MEDSURG Nursing, 5*(1), 44–49.

Specht, D. M. (1995). Cerebral edema: Bringing the brain back down to size. *Nursing, 25*(11), 34–38, 45–46.

Tucker, S. M., Canobbio, M. M., Paquette, E. V., & Wells, M. F. (1996). *Patient care standards, collaborative practice planning guidelines* (6th ed.). St. Louis: Mosby.

Additional Resources

National Multiple Sclerosis Society
733 Third Avenue
New York, NY 10017
(800) Fight-MS
http://www.nmss.org/

Multiple Sclerosis Foundation
http://www.msfacts.org/

Myasthenia Gravis Foundation of America
230 Park Avenue
New York, NY 10007
(800) 541–5454
http://www.med.unc.edu/mgfa

National Parkinson Foundation
1501 NW Ninth Avenue
Bob Hope Road
Miami, FL 33136–9990
(800) 327–4545

Amyotrophic Lateral Sclerosis Association of America
21021 Ventura Boulevard
Suite 321
Woodland Hills, CA 91364
(800) 782–4747

Epilepsy Foundation of America
4351 Garden City Drive
Landover, MD
(800) 332–1000
http://www.efa.org/

Guillain-Barré Syndrome Foundation
P.O. Box 262
Wynnwood, PA 9096
(610) 667–0131

Chapter 45

Caring for Clients With Cerebrovascular Disorders

KEY TERMS

Aneurysm
Bruit
Cephalalgia
Cerebral infarction
Cerebrovascular accident
Collateral circulation
Endarterectomy
Expressive aphasia
Hemianopia
Hemiplegia
Receptive aphasia
Transient ischemic attack

LEARNING OBJECTIVES

On completion of this chapter, the reader will:

- Identify three types of headaches and discuss their characteristics.
- List three nursing techniques that supplement drug therapy in reducing or relieving headaches.
- Name three types of cerebrovascular disorders and their usual causes.
- Explain the significance of a transient ischemic attack.
- Discuss medical and surgical techniques used to reduce the potential for a cerebrovascular accident.
- Identify five manifestations of a cerebrovascular accident; discuss those that are unique to right-sided and left-sided infarctions.
- Identify at least five nursing diagnoses common to the care of a client with a cerebrovascular accident and interventions for managing them.
- Describe a cerebral aneurysm and the danger it presents.
- Discuss appropriate nursing interventions when caring for a client with a cerebral aneurysm.

Cerebrovascular disorders are major medical problems that affect adults. Some cerebrovascular disorders, such as a cerebrovascular accident (CVA) and transient ischemic attacks (TIAs), are life-threatening. Others, such as headaches, can disrupt an individual's lifestyle with tremendous discomfort and anxiety.

Headache

Aching in the head is referred to as **cephalalgia**. It is a symptom that accompanies many disorders such as meningitis, increased intracranial pressure (ICP), brain tumors, and sinusitis. When the duration of discomfort is relatively brief, a headache is considered transient and benign. Headaches fall generally into three categories: tension, migraine, and cluster headaches.

Tension Headache

Tension headache is the most common type of headache.

ETIOLOGY AND PATHOPHYSIOLOGY

Some causes of tension headache are emotional stress, eyestrain, and maintaining one position for a prolonged time. Pain is caused by contraction or strain of the muscles of the neck, head, or eyes.

ASSESSMENT FINDINGS

Signs and Symptoms

Symptoms vary from a mild ache to severe disabling pain.

Diagnostic Findings

Persistent headache requires tests such as computed tomographic (CT) scan, brain scan, head and neck radiographs, and angiography to rule out a brain tumor or intracerebral hemorrhage, cervical spondylitis, temporomandibular joint (TMJ) syndrome, or infected sinuses.

MEDICAL MANAGEMENT

Occasional headaches that result from fatigue or emotional stress are usually relieved by rest, a mild analgesic, and stress management techniques (see Chap. 11). Treatment for severe, recurrent headache starts with removing or correcting factors or situations that result in headache. Therapy involves prescription of glasses, drainage of an infected sinus, or psychotherapy.

NURSING PROCESS
Care of the Client with a Headache

Assessment

The nurse asks the client questions about the location, type of pain, and past history of the same type of headache because another disorder or problem may be occurring. Determine if the pain is in one area or over the entire head; factors that appear to bring on, worsen, or relieve the headache; how long the pain lasts; and symptoms such as tearing, nasal congestion, nausea, or vomiting.

Those with chronic headaches or headaches that result in a variety of symptoms require a complete medical and allergy history, as well as a record of frequency and description of the pain experienced during an attack. Vital signs are taken. A neurologic examination is indicated if the cause of the headache is unknown.

Diagnosis and Planning

The care of a client with a headache includes, but is not limited to, the following:

Nursing Diagnoses and Collaborative Problems	Nursing Interventions
Pain related to muscle tension, changes in cerebral blood flow, or vasculitis (inflammation of cerebral artery), or unknown etiology	Eliminate environmental factors that intensify the pain, such as bright light and noise.
Goal: The client's headache will be reduced or eliminated within 30 minutes of nursing intervention.	Administer a prescribed analgesic and note its effect. Offer a back massage to promote muscle relaxation. Apply warm (or cool) cloths to the forehead or back of the neck. Provide distraction with soft soothing music or suggest using a relaxation tape or one that provides guided imagery.

Evaluation and Expected Outcomes

- Pain is reduced or eliminated.
- The client demonstrates understanding of the medication regimen and possible side effects.
- The client identifies ways to modify behavior to minimize pain.

Migraine Headaches

Migraine headaches are generally recurrent and severe. Symptoms last for a day or more. More women than men experience migraine headaches, and there is a marked familial tendency for the disorder.

ETIOLOGY AND PATHOPHYSIOLOGY

The cause for migraines is not fully understood. The discomfort is believed to be due to vasodilation of intracranial blood vessels. The vasodilation is linked to elevated levels of an endogenous chemical (originating in the body) similar to bradykinin, a substance released during inflammatory responses. It has been noted that emotional stress, excess carbohydrates, iodine-rich foods, alcohol, chemical additives, and fatigue play a part in precipitating attacks. The cause and effect relationship between the headache and a specific precipitating event is not clear.

ASSESSMENT FINDINGS

Signs and Symptoms

Just before the headache begins, some individuals experience visual disturbances such as flashing lights or wavy lines or some other sensory experience. The headache usually starts on one side but it can involve the entire head before the attack is over. The pain is described as "throbbing" or "bursting." The headache is accompanied by nausea and vomiting, puffiness of the face, irritability, and fatigue.

Diagnostic Findings

The pattern of headache occurrence and the signs and symptoms are typical of migraine headaches. CT scan, angiography, brain scan, and radiographs are used to rule out other neurologic disorders.

MEDICAL MANAGEMENT

Rest and drug therapy (Table 45–1) are the mainstays of treatment for migraine headaches. Mild analgesics are generally ineffective. Antiemetics are also prescribed if nausea and vomiting become acute during an attack. Some individuals learn to shorten or abort migraines with biofeedback techniques (see Chap. 11).

NURSING MANAGEMENT

Reinforce the drug therapy regimen and instruct the client on self-administration. In most cases, stress the importance of taking medication as soon as symptoms of the migraine begin. Encourage the client to lie in bed in a dark room and keep noise and other stimuli to a minimum.

Cluster Headache

The term *cluster* is used to describe a certain type of headache in which the attacks are closely spaced and last for several days or weeks then cease for an extended period of time. Some believe that cluster headaches are a variant of migraine headache.

TABLE 45-1 **Drug Therapy for Treating Migraine Headaches**

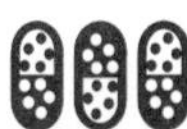

Drug Category/Drug Action	Side Effects	Nursing Considerations
Beta-Blockers		
propranolol (Inderal) Prevents vasodilation, drug of choice for prophylaxis.	Bradycardia, fatigue, lethargy, depression, gastrointestinal (GI) complaints, orthostatic hypotension	Do not discontinue drug abruptly. Give with food to facilitate absorption. Report difficulty breathing, slow pulse, confusion, depression.
Nonnarcotic Analgesics		
aspirin (ASA) Analgesic effect early in the attack	Bleeding disorder, GI distress	Monitor for overuse. Give with food to decrease GI upset. Report unusual bleeding.
acetaminophen (Tylenol) Analgesic effect early in the attack	GI, liver, renal effects	Monitor liver and renal function tests. Avoid with use of other over-the-counter preparations.
Nonsteroidal Anti-inflammatories (NSAIDs)		
ibuprofen (Advil) naproxen (Naprosyn) Analgesic for mild to moderate pain	Headache, dizziness, somnolence, nausea, GI upset, constipation	Better tolerated than ASA. Assess allergy to other NSAIDs. Give with food to reduce GI upset.
Narcotic Analgesics		
codeine (Codeine Phosphate) For severe headache unrelieved by nonnarcotics	Sedation, confusion, constipation	Addictive, use with caution. Report severe nausea, vomiting, palpitations, shortness of breath or difficulty breathing.
meperidine (Demerol) As above	Same as above	Never give to clients taking monoamine oxidase inhibitors. Reassure client that most people who receive opiates for medical reasons do not develop dependency. Avoid alcohol, antihistamines, sedatives, tranquilizers and over-the-counter drugs. Report severe nausea, vomiting, constipation, shortness of breath, or difficulty breathing.
butorphanol (Stadol) Relief of severe migraine headache pain (nasal spray)	Sedation, nausea, sweating, vertigo, lethargy, confusion	Very addictive, must be used cautiously. Report severe nausea, vomiting, palpitations, shortness of breath or difficulty breathing, nasal lesions or discomfort.

(*continued*)

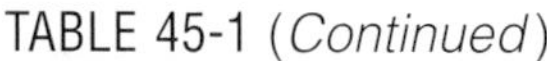

TABLE 45-1 (*Continued*)

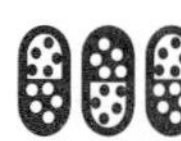

Drug Category/Drug Action	Side Effects	Nursing Considerations
Ergots		
ergotamine tartrate (Ergostat) Prevents or aborts vascular headaches such as migraine and cluster.	Nausea, ergotism: numbness and tingling of fingers and toes, muscle pain and weakness	Administer at first sign of attack. Need to premedicate with antiemetic. Use sparingly to prevent ergotism.
dihydroergotamine (DHE) Rapid control of vascular headaches, parenteral treatment for established headache.	Nausea and vomiting, ergotism: numbness, tingling of fingers and toes, muscle pain and weakness	Premedicate with antiemetic. Administer as soon as possible after first sign of attack. Use sparingly to prevent ergotism.
Antiemetics		
promethazine (Phenergan) Controls nausea early in attack.	Drowsiness, dizziness, confusion, hypotension, insomnia, vertigo	Give 15–30 min before meperidine or DHE. Avoid alcohol. Avoid sun exposure. Maintain fluid intake. Report sore throat, fever, unusual bleeding, rash, weakness.
prochlorperazine (Compazine) Control of severe nausea and vomiting	See above	See above
Other		
sumatriptan (Imitrex) Antimigraine agent for acute attacks	Dizziness, vertigo, weakness, myalgia, blood pressure alterations	Give as soon as possible after first sign of attack. Monitor blood pressure. Report chest pain or pressure, flushing, facial swelling.

ETIOLOGY AND PATHOPHYSIOLOGY

The cause of cluster headaches is unknown. The headaches can be triggered by vasodilating agents such as nitroglycerin and alcoholic beverages.

ASSESSMENT FINDINGS

Signs and Symptoms

The headache, usually on one side of the head, is accompanied by nasal congestion, tearing and redness of the eye on the affected side, and pain behind the eye. The pain is severe.

Diagnostic Findings

The diagnosis is made on the basis of the history the client provides, the signs and symptoms experienced, and by ruling out other neurovascular causes.

MEDICAL MANAGEMENT

Symptoms are controlled with the administration of an ergotamine derivative (eg, Ergostat) or methysergide (Sansert).

NURSING MANAGEMENT

Use nursing interventions for relieving pain as with any type of headache. Administer prescribed medications and note their effect.

Client and Family Teaching

Include the following:

- Follow the indications and dosage regimen for medication, and notify the physician of any adverse drug effects.
- Identify and avoid factors that precipitate or intensify an attack.
- Keep a record of the attacks, including activities before the attack, and environmental or emotional circumstances that appear to bring on the attack.
- Lie down in a darkened room, and avoid noise and movement when an attack occurs.

Cerebrovascular Disorders

Cerebral nerve cells are extremely sensitive to a lack of oxygen. If the brain is deprived of oxygenated blood for 3 to 7 minutes, nerves and brain cells begin to die. Cerebral nerve cell destruction is irreversible because they do not regenerate. Three million people in the United States experience oxygen deprivation to the brain caused by TIAs or prolonged interruption of blood flow as in a CVA. Many who survive have permanent disabilities.

Transient Ischemic Attacks

Transient ischemic attacks are brief, fleeting attacks of neurologic impairment. Symptoms last for a few moments to as long as a day, followed by complete recovery. A TIA is a warning that a CVA could occur in the future.

ETIOLOGY AND PATHOPHYSIOLOGY

Transient ischemic attacks result from impaired circulation in a specific area of the brain. The role of hypertension is not entirely clear, but it is thought to involve narrowing of cerebral vessels, which reduces the amount of blood traveling through them. Circulation is interrupted by atherosclerosis (build up of fatty plaque) within cerebral blood vessels or the release of small emboli (microemboli). During the ischemic period, motor and sensory functions are temporarily affected.

ASSESSMENT FINDINGS

Signs and Symptoms

Symptoms include temporary light-headedness, speech disturbances, visual loss in one eye, diplopia, variable changes in consciousness, and numbness, weakness, or paralysis on one side.

Diagnostic Findings

A neurologic examination during an attack reveals neurologic deficits. Auscultation of the carotid artery may reveal a **bruit** (abnormal sound caused by blood flowing over the rough surface of the carotid artery). Ultrasound examination of the carotid artery shows an irregular shape to the carotid artery lining caused by atherosclerotic plaques. A carotid arteriogram shows narrowing of the carotid artery. A CT scan or magnetic resonance imaging (MRI) is used to rule out other neurologic disorders with similar manifestations, such as a brain tumor.

MEDICAL AND SURGICAL MANAGEMENT

Antiplatelet and anticoagulant therapy with aspirin, dipyridamole (Persantine), ticlopidine (Ticlid), and warfarin (Coumadin) are prescribed. Hypertension is controlled with drug and diet therapy (see Chap. 34). If narrowing of the carotid artery by atherosclerotic plaques is the cause, a carotid **endarterectomy** (surgical removal of atherosclerotic plaque) is an option (Fig. 45–1). A balloon angioplasty, a procedure similar to a percutaneous coronary artery angioplasty (PTCA) described in Chapter 32, is performed to dilate the carotid artery and increase blood flow to the brain.

NURSING MANAGEMENT

Obtain a complete history of symptoms and a medical, drug, and allergy history. Although symptoms of a TIA usually are not permanent, perform a neurologic examination to identify the client's current status and form a baseline for future comparisons. Report subtle changes.

If the client undergoes carotid artery surgery, perform frequent neurologic checks to detect paralysis, confusion, facial asymmetry, or aphasia. Monitor the heart rhythm because arrhythmias (see Chap. 33) can alter blood flow to the brain as well. Observe the client closely for difficulty breathing or swallowing and hoarseness because neck swelling after surgery can occur. Keep an airway at the bedside and be prepared for endotracheal intubation or an emergency tracheostomy should an airway obstruction occur.

Client and Family Teaching

Teach the client to:

- Maintain hydration by drinking the equivalent of 8 glasses of fluid a day, unless contraindicated.
- Follow directions for drug therapy including medications for controlling hypertension.

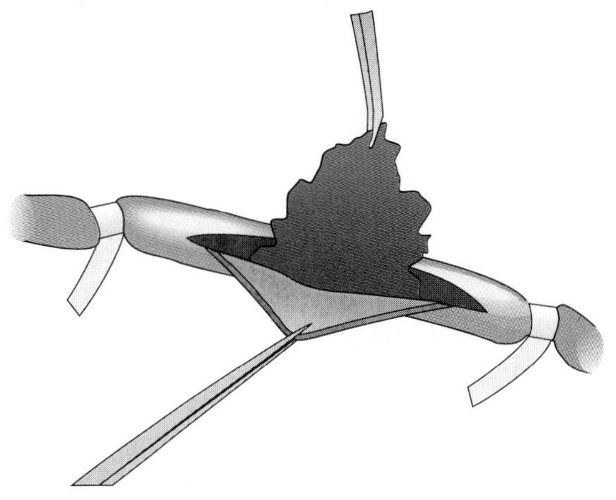

FIGURE 45-1. Carotid endarterectomy is a surgical technique for removing fatty plaque from within the inner arterial wall.

- Monitor for signs of excessive bruising or bleeding if antithrombotic drugs are prescribed.
- Keep appointments for laboratory tests and medical follow-up to monitor the effectiveness of therapy.
- Report any future instances of sensory or motor impairment or call 911 for emergency assistance.

Cerebrovascular Accident (Stroke)

A common cerebrovascular disorder is a **cerebrovascular accident** (*stroke*), sudden impairment of cerebral circulation caused by a partial or total blockage in one or more cerebral blood vessels. During the early stage, it is not possible to tell whether the neurologic deficits are temporary or permanent. Improvement in neurologic symptoms can occur for at least 6 months after a CVA. Permanent neurologic deficits have a profound physical, emotional, and financial effect on the client and the family.

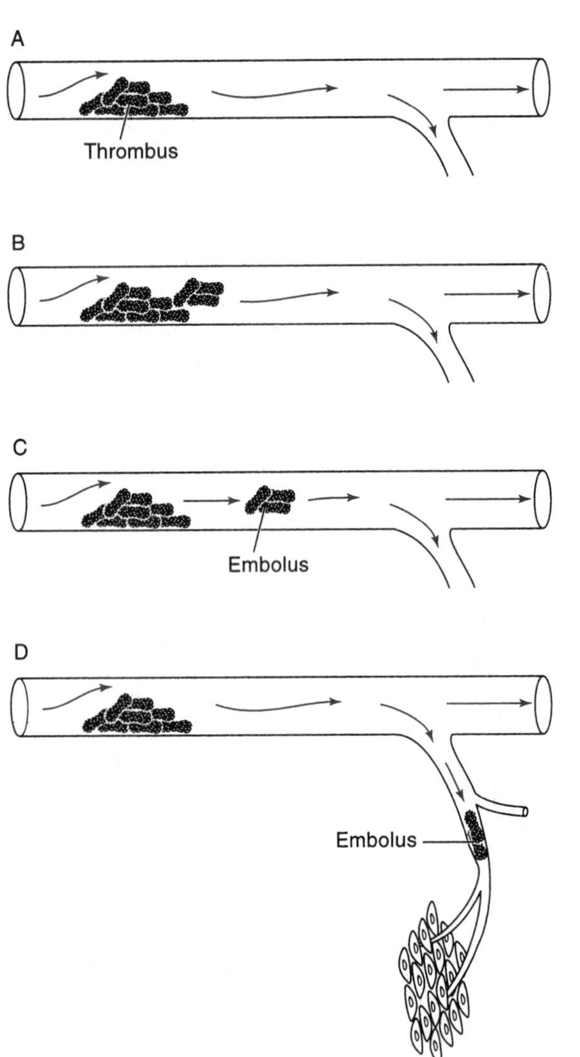

FIGURE 45-2. Evolving thrombotic CVA. (*A*) A thrombus forms in a vessel. (*B*) The force of the flowing blood over the clot helps to break off a piece from it. (*C*) The embolus is loose in the bloodstream and travels to any tissue fed by connecting blood vessels. (*D*) The embolus is pushed into a small terminal vessel, completely occluding it and causing anoxia of the tissue served by the occluded vessel.

ETIOLOGY AND PATHOPHYSIOLOGY

The most common causes of a CVA are thrombus formation in cerebral blood vessels (Fig. 45–2), emboli, and cerebral hemorrhage (Fig. 45–3). Atherosclerosis and arteriosclerosis of cerebral vessels contribute to the formation of a cerebral thrombus. Endocarditis, mitral valve disease, and atrial fibrillation are also common causes of emboli and subsequent CVA. Embolus formation is a potential risk after the insertion of a heart valve prosthesis. Common causes of cerebral hemorrhage are rupture of cerebral vessels (discussed later in this chapter), hemorrhagic disorders such as leukemia and aplastic anemia, severe hypertension, and brain tumors.

In some instances, one or more TIAs are experienced days, weeks, or years before a CVA occurs. There may be no warning, however, and the symptoms can occur suddenly. Blockage results in a decreased or absent blood flow to cerebral tissues supplied by the involved blood vessel. The lack of oxygen to cerebral tissues is followed shortly by death of brain tissue (**cerebral infarction**). Clinical manifestations are highly variable and depend on the area of the cerebral cortex and the hemisphere that is affected (Table 45–2),

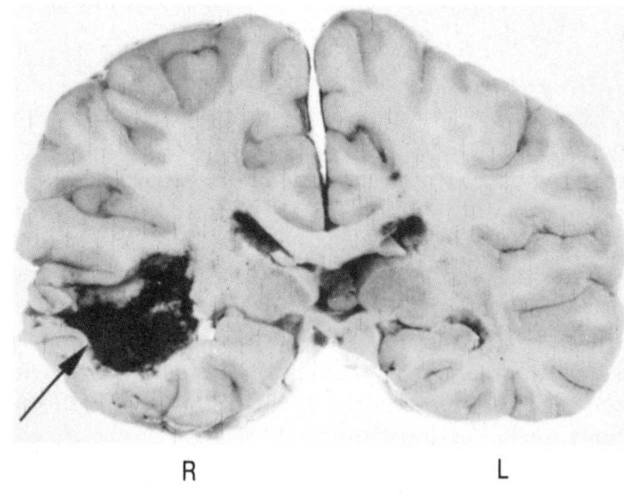

FIGURE 45-3. Postmortem specimen of a cerebral hemorrhage of the right temporal lobe. (Courtesy of P. S. Milley, MD. Photograph by D. Atkinson)

TABLE 45-2 **Comparison of Signs and Symptoms Associated With Right-Sided and Left-Sided Hemiplegia**

Right-Sided Hemiplegia (Stroke on Left Side of Brain)	Left-Sided Hemiplegia (Stroke on Right Side of Brain)
Expressive aphasia or Receptive aphasia or Global aphasia Intellectual impairment Slow and cautious behavior Defects in right visual fields	Spatial-perceptual defects Denial and the deficits of the affected side require special safety considerations Tendency for distractibility Impulsive behavior; unaware of deficits Poor judgment Defects in left visual fields

the degree of blockage (total, partial), and the presence or absence of adequate collateral circulation. **Collateral circulation** is circulation formed by smaller blood vessels branching off from or near larger occluded vessels.

ASSESSMENT FINDINGS

Signs and Symptoms

Immediately after a large cerebral hemorrhage, the client is unconscious. Breathing is noisy and labored. The cheek on the side of the CVA blows out on exhalation. The eyes deviate toward the affected side of the brain. The pulse is slow, full, and bounding. Initially, the blood pressure is elevated. The temperature is elevated during the acute phase and persists for several days.

Numbness, tingling, weakness, paralysis, speech impairment, memory impairment, severe headache, nausea, vomiting, changes in the level of consciousness (LOC), or blurred vision are examples of signs and symptoms associated with a CVA. The LOC ranges from lethargy and mental confusion to deep coma. Coma can persist for days or even weeks. The longer the coma, the poorer the prognosis and the less likely that consciousness will return.

A common neurologic result of a CVA in the motor area of the cerebrum is **hemiplegia** (paralysis on one side of the body). Hemiplegia below the level of the neck occurs on the side *opposite* the area of the brain that is affected because motor nerves cross over (decussate) at the level of the neck. For example, when the motor area on the right side of the brain incurs a CVA, hemiplegia exists on the right side of the head and the left side of the body. Immediately after the CVA, the affected side is flaccid. This progresses to spastic limbs. The arm is typically more severely affected than the leg.

Expressive aphasia, the inability to speak, or **receptive aphasia**, the inability to understand spoken and written language, can result. Hemianopia on the

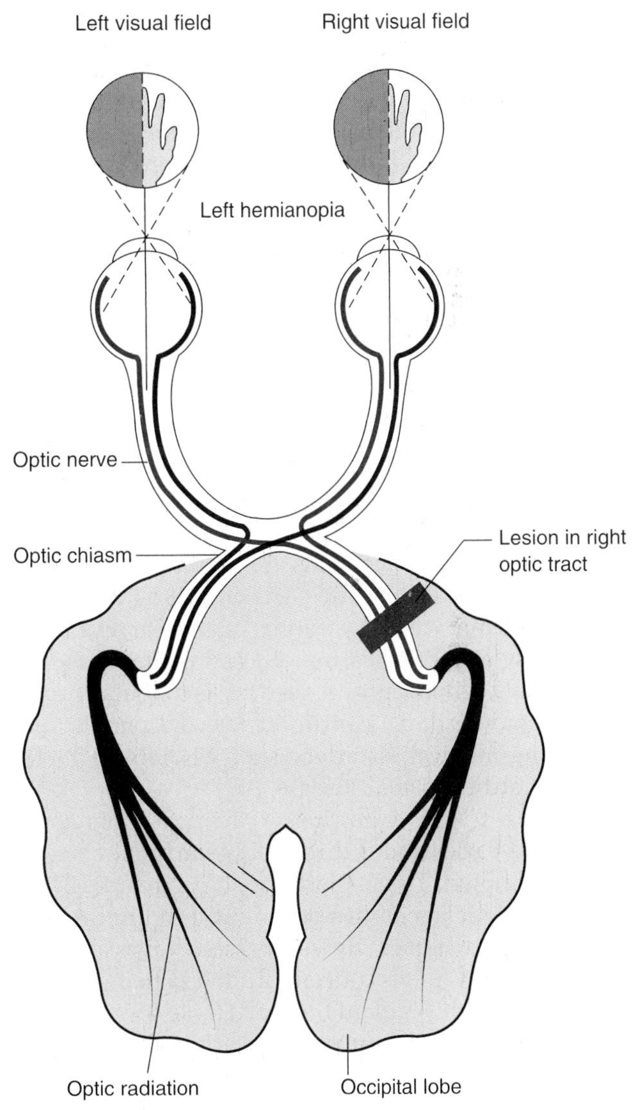

FIGURE 45-4. Hemianopia is a visual field defect in which a person experiences an inability to see the left or right half of an image. It develops when a stroke involves the visual pathway.

affected side is another potential consequence. **Hemianopia** is the ability to see only half of the normal visual field (Fig. 45–4). When looking straight ahead, the client cannot see anything to the right or left with either eye. This condition is caused by damage to the visual area of the cerebral cortex or its connections to the brain stem (optic radiations). This deficit, like other deficits that result from a CVA, may subside completely, partially, or not at all. Confusion and emotional lability are also characteristic symptoms of a CVA (see Table 45–2).

Diagnostic Findings

A CT scan or MRI differentiate a CVA from other disorders, such as a brain tumor or cerebral edema, and show the size and location of the infarcted area. Transcranial Doppler ultrasonography determines the size of intracranial vessels and the direction of blood flow and locates the obstructed cerebral vessel. Single photon emission tomography also determines cerebral blood flow. An electroencephalogram reveals reduced electrical activity in the involved area but is not a specific diagnostic test for a CVA. A lumbar puncture is often performed. If subarachnoid bleeding has occurred, the cerebrospinal fluid will be bloody. Cerebral angiography shows displacement or blockage of cerebral vessels.

MEDICAL AND SURGICAL MANAGEMENT

Cerebrovascular accidents are prevented by reducing certain risk factors such as: controlling hypertension, reducing weight, treating cardiac arrhythmias (especially atrial fibrillation), lowering blood cholesterol levels, giving prophylactic anticoagulant therapy (including daily aspirin) in selected people, and managing medical disorders, such as diabetes mellitus and cardiovascular disease.

When a CVA occurs, it is a medical emergency. Treatment varies and is directed toward relieving the cause, if known. Tissue plasminogen activator (TPA), a thrombolytic agent, has been found to limit neurologic deficits when given within 3 to 6 hours after the onset of the CVA. It is contraindicated in hemorrhagic CVAs, as is anticoagulant therapy (Table 45–3). An osmotic diuretic is administered during the first few days of the acute phase to treat cerebral edema. If atherosclerosis of the carotid artery is the cause, a carotid endarterectomy is considered. A ruptured cerebral aneurysm is treated surgically.

In many cases, treatment is supportive because medical or surgical interventions cannot repair damaged brain tissue. The best treatment available involves an intensive medical program aimed at rehabilitation and the prevention of future CVAs.

TABLE 45-3 **Inclusion and Exclusion Criteria for Therapy With Tissue Plasmogen Activator**

Inclusion Criteria	Exclusion Criteria
Clinical evidence of an ischemic attack Age >18 years Signed consent, if possible Onset of stroke within 3 hours of initiation of therapy (or from time client was last seen as "normal") Normal prothrombin and partial thromboplastin times	Stroke or serious head trauma in past 3 months Major surgery or invasive procedure within past 14 days Gastrointestinal or urinary bleeding within past 21 days Puncture of noncompressible artery or biopsy of internal organ within past 7 days Seizure preceding or during stroke History of intracranial hemorrhage or known history of cerebral vascular malformations Pericarditis, endocarditis, septic emboli, recent pregnancy, or active inflammatory bowel disease

NURSING PROCESS
The Client With a Cerebrovascular Accident

Assessment

When caring for a client with a stroke, obtain a medical, drug, and allergy history from the family or client if he or she is able to communicate. Monitor the vital signs and perform a neurologic assessment.

Assess the client's swallowing reflex. Initiate a record of intake and output. Keep a record of bowel and bladder elimination. Determine the client's ability to understand language. Check muscle strength in all extremities. Inspect the skin for impairment and the body for signs of injury if the client fell at the time of the CVA.

Diagnosis and Planning

Because the number and severity of symptoms vary with each client, nursing management is based on the problems identified during initial and ongoing assessments. The plan of care includes, but is not limited to, the following:

Nursing Diagnoses and Collaborative Problems	Nursing Interventions
Impaired Swallowing related to hemiplegia; **Risk for Aspiration** related to impaired swallowing; **Risk for Fluid Volume Deficit** related to impaired swallowing **Goal:** The client will swallow without aspiration; fluid intake will be at least 2,000 mL/24 hours.	Keep a suction machine at the bedside. Place thickened liquids or pureed food in the unaffected side of the mouth. Lower the chin to the chest when swallowing.

	Check the mouth for pocketed food before offering more. Collaborate with the physician concerning gastric or enteral tube feedings if oral intake is inadequate.
Total Incontinence; Bowel Incontinence or Colonic Constipation related to diminished level of consciousness, immobility **Goal:** The client's urinary and bowel elimination will be controlled.	Apply incontinence garments or place absorbent pads beneath the client. Collaborate with the physician concerning the insertion of an external or indwelling catheter. Administer a prescribed suppository or low volume enema to evacuate the lower bowel when necessary.
Self-Care Deficit related to unilateral use of hands; **Unilateral Neglect** related to hemianopia; **Impaired Physical Mobility** related to hemiplegia **Goal:** The client will resume activities of daily living; the client will identify and care for paralyzed body parts; the client will use paralyzed limbs to the fullest extent possible.	Approach and place objects within the client's field of vision. Help reintegrate weak side by reminding client to look at the paralyzed side. Set realistic goals to reduce frustration. Modify clothing and supplies and utensils to accommodate for the client's neurologic deficits. Attach a trapeze above the bed to facilitate position changes. Perform range of motion exercises at least once each shift. Position the client to avoid contractures. Use a foot board, trochanter roll at the hip, rolled cloth in the paralyzed hand. Support the affected arm with pillows or sling to prevent dangling and possible shoulder injury. Consult physical therapist regarding devices to assist ambulation such as a leg brace and a walker.
Risk for Impaired Skin Integrity related to pressure over bony prominences secondary to immobility Goal: The client's skin will remain intact.	Keep the skin clean and dry. Use a turning sheet and assistance when changing the client's position. Massage skin areas that blanch when pressure is relieved. Use pressure relieving devices or a therapeutic bed that alternately distributes the client's body weight.
Impaired Verbal Communication related to aphasia Goal: The client will make needs understood either verbally or nonverbally.	Ask questions requiring a "yes" or "no" and suggest the client respond by nodding the head. Advise speaking slowly if speech is difficult to understand. Have the client point to or write key words or phrases. Support and practice techniques used in speech therapy.
Risk for Ineffective Individual and Family Coping: Disabling related to diminished psychosocial resources to deal with multiple stressors **Goal:** The client and family will cope with illness and changes in lifestyle.	Listen and try to identify clues to the client's or family's future concerns. Acknowledge personal strengths. Refer to a discharge planner, social worker, or community social services for arranging extended care or home care.

Evaluation and Expected Outcomes

- Airway remains patent, and lungs are clear to auscultation.
- The client maintains an adequate intake of fluid and food.
- The client achieves normal bowel and urinary elimination.
- Performs ADLs alone or with assistance.
- Skin integrity is maintained.
- Communicates with others.
- Copes with illness and neurologic deficits.
- Family pursues a plan for postdischarge management.

Client and Family Teaching

Teach the client and family to administer medications as directed and inform them of potential side effects and adverse effects. Review aspiration precautions and suggest foods that are easily swallowed. Arrange a meeting with the family, speech pathologist and dietitian for clients with impaired swallowing. Instruct family members how to perform the Heimlich maneuver to clear the airway. Provide the family with community resources for special care devices such as a hospital bed, bedside commode, walker, or tripod cane. Review fall prevention tactics such as removing throw rugs, clutter, and electrical cords. Remind caregiver of the importance of having the client perform regular exercises and change position frequently. Instruct family in proper placement and care of any braces or splints designed to maintain extremities in proper anatomic position.

Cerebral Aneurysms

An **aneurysm** is an abnormal dilatation of a blood vessel wall. Most aneurysms occur in arteries where blood flow is under high pressure. Cerebral aneurysms generally occur in the circle of Willis (Fig. 45–5), a ring of arteries that supply the brain.

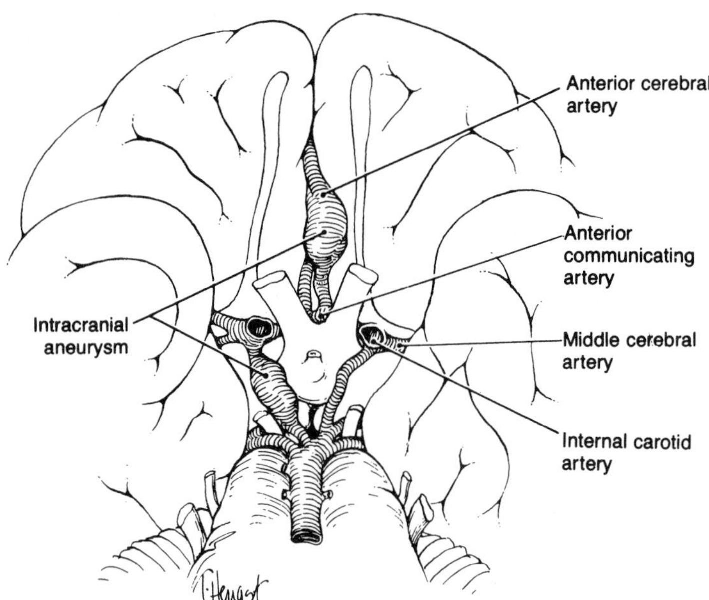

FIGURE 45-5. Intracranial aneurysm in the circle of Willis.

ETIOLOGY AND PATHOPHYSIOLOGY

Aneurysms develop at the site of a weakened area in the blood vessel wall. The defect is congenital or secondary to hypertension and atherosclerosis.

The presence of an aneurysm can affect cranial nerve function (see Chap. 43) as it presses on these structures. For many, there is no prior warning that an aneurysm exists. Berry aneurysms, a type of congenital cerebral aneurysm, can rupture at any time without prior symptoms. The sudden cerebral hemorrhage causes immediate neurologic changes due to rising ICP, interruption of oxygenated blood flow to the surrounding cells and tissues, and blood collecting within the subarachnoid space. Occasionally, there is a slow leakage of blood from an aneurysm, in which case, the symptoms are less severe.

ASSESSMENT FINDINGS

Signs and Symptoms

Symptoms include sudden and severe headache, dizziness, nausea, and vomiting, usually followed by a rapid loss of consciousness. If the ruptured aneurysm produces a slow leak, a stiff neck, headache, visual disturbances, and intermittent nausea develop.

Diagnostic Findings

Cerebral angiography can reveal an unruptured aneurysm. The procedure is done with caution because the added fluid pressure can increase the risk of rupturing the blood vessel, dislodge plaque-formed emboli, and cause ischemia due to vasospasm. A CT scan and MRI are safer to locate the site of the aneurysm and determine the amount of blood present in the subarachnoid space. A lumbar puncture reveals grossly bloody cerebrospinal fluid.

MEDICAL MANAGEMENT

Conservative management is attempted until a decision is made regarding surgical repair of the aneurysm. Some aneurysms are considered inoperable because of anatomic location and only medical treatment is possible.

Complete bed rest, the prevention of rebleeding at the rupture site, and treatment of complications are primary goals. Absolute bed rest in a quiet area, preferably a private room, is essential. Visitors are restricted except for family members. The head of the bed is elevated to reduce ICP and cerebral edema. Hypertension is treated with antihypertensive agents. Anticonvulsants are given to prevent seizures. Tranquilizers or barbiturates are used to keep the conscious client relaxed and quiet. Increased ICP is managed with osmotic diuretics and corticosteroids (see Chap. 44).

Mechanical ventilation is necessary to support respirations and provide oxygenation if the client is unconscious. Aminocaproic acid (Amicar) is used to delay lysis (breaking up) of the blood clot because lysis results in rebleeding.

SURGICAL MANAGEMENT

Surgical repair is attempted after the initial hemorrhage because the danger of further hemorrhage from the weakened sac is great. The operation is not without hazard; manipulation of the small cerebral vessels can result in increased vasospasm or thrombosis and cerebral infarction. The risks of surgery are less serious than the dangers of recurrent hemorrhage from the aneurysm. Surgical approaches with a craniotomy

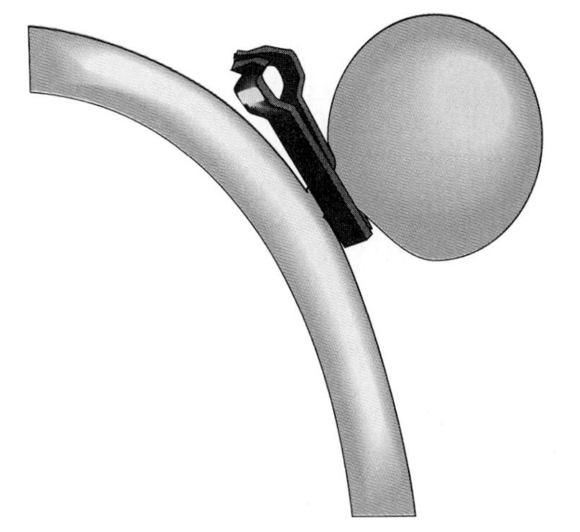

FIGURE 45-6. An aneurysm is clamped to prevent rupture. Wrapping the aneurysm with supportive material is another alternative.

include wrapping or clipping the aneurysm in an attempt to control further bleeding (Fig. 45–6).

An alternative to direct repair of the aneurysm by a craniotomy approach is ligation of or application of a clamp to one of the carotid arteries. This is an extracranial (outside the cranium) procedure, because the surgical approach is below the jaw. The purpose of this approach is to obstruct blood flow to the vessel that has an aneurysm, thus reducing the pressure in the aneurysm and preventing rupture or further bleeding. Collateral circulation in the cerebral vessels must be adequate for success.

NURSING PROCESS
The Client With an Aneurysm

Assessment

A neurologic examination is performed with care because the client must be kept as quiet as possible. Vital signs are obtained. If the client is conscious, the history is kept as brief as possible and focused primarily on current symptoms. A more complete history is obtained from the family.

Diagnosis and Planning

The care of a client with a cerebral aneurysm includes, but is not limited to, the following:

Nursing Diagnoses and Collaborative Problems	Nursing Interventions
PC: Increased Intracranial Pressure related to bleeding within the brain	Keep the client calm and inactive.
Goal: Increased intracranial pressure will be managed and minimized.	Perform neurologic assessments every 15 minutes to 1 hour or as ordered. Compare findings and report changes that indicate worsening status (see Chap. 43).
	Avoid any activities that cause a Valsalva maneuver such as coughing, straining at stool, rough position changes.
	Follow the physician's orders for fluid restrictions and drug therapy for reducing hypertension, the potential for seizures, and restlessness and anxiety.
	Elevate the client's head or follow the physician's directive for body position (some prefer that the client remain flat).
	Limit the visitors to the immediate family and suggest they take turns and stay briefly.
PC: Seizures related to increased intracranial pressure	Institute seizure precautions (see Chap. 44).
Goal: Seizures will be managed and minimized.	Implement anticonvulsant drug therapy as prescribed.
Pain (headache) related to increased intracranial pressure	Avoid narcotic analgesia, except codeine, which may interfere with pupil assessment and assessing LOC.
	Reduce environmental stimuli and use nursing interventions such as distraction, guided imagery, soothing music.
	Take care not to jar the bed or cause unnecessary activity.
Self-Care Deficit related to imposed rest	Perform only those activities of daily living for client that are absolutely necessary.
Goal: The client's basic needs will be met.	Provide a period of rest between necessary nursing tasks.
	Feed the client calorie dense foods in small amounts at frequent intervals.
Risk for Altered Tissue Perfusion and **Risk for Impaired Skin Integrity** related to enforced inactivity	Apply elastic stockings to lower extremities or use a pneumatic compression device to promote venous circulation as ordered.
Goal: The client's peripheral circulation will be maintained; the client's skin will remain intact.	Use pressure-relieving pads or a similar type of mattress.

Evaluation and Expected Outcomes

- Intracranial pressure is in normal range.
- No evidence of seizures.
- Pain is relieved.
- Self-care needs are met.

- Adequate circulation to tissues; no signs of skin breakdown.

For the client who undergoes a craniotomy, refer to Chapter 46.

Client and Family Teaching

Discharge teaching depends on the method of treatment and the recommendations of the physician. Usually, the nurse instructs clients to avoid:

- Heavy lifting
- Straining at stool
- Extreme emotional situations
- Other work related activities that could raise the blood pressure and increase ICP

When the client must restrict his or her lifestyle, the changes are likely to cause financial, physical, and social hardships for the client and family. Referrals to a social service worker, counselor, or social service agency are appropriate.

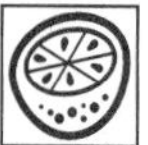

General Nutritional Considerations

When the client is able to resume an oral intake after a CVA, the diet is individualized according to the client's ability to chew and swallow. Semisolid and medium-consistency foods such as pudding, scrambled eggs, cooked cereals, and thickened liquids are easiest to swallow. Foods most likely to cause choking should be avoided: peanut butter, bread, tart foods, dry or crisp foods, and chewy meats. Progress the texture as swallowing ability improves.

Cold foods stimulate swallowing; avoid tepid foods, because they are more difficult to locate in the mouth, and extremely hot foods, which can cause overreaction.

Clients with decreased salivation benefit from the use of added gravies and sauces. Thinking of a specific food prior to eating stimulates salivation, as do eating dill pickles and sucking on lemon slices.

To minimize the volume of food needed, provide nutritionally dense foods such as thickened commercial beverages, fortified puddings, fortified cooked cereals, and scrambled eggs.

When a normal oral diet is resumed, encourage the client to eat "heart healthy"—less total fat and saturated fat and more fruits, vegetables, and whole grains. Encourage overweight clients to lose weight to reduce cardiac workload. Sodium restriction is appropriate for clients with hypertension.

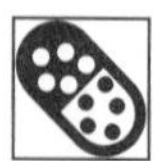

General Pharmacologic Considerations

Anticoagulant therapy with heparin is given parenterally or with an oral anticoagulant for some clients who have had a CVA.

If the client is receiving heparin, the dose is ordered after each clotting time determination.

If heparin is administered by the subcutaneous route, the site of injection *is not massaged before or after* the drug is given. There is no need to aspirate before injecting the heparin. The recommended site for subcutaneous injection is the abdomen. Injection sites are rotated and areas within 2 inches of the umbilicus are avoided.

Aspirin (1–1.3 g daily PO) may be given prophylactically for TIAs. Aspirin prolongs the bleeding time and inhibits platelet aggregation. If gastric upset occurs the drug may be given with food, with an antacid, or in an enterically coated form.

The most notable adverse effect of heparin is hemorrhage. Protamine sulfate is kept available if it becomes necessary to counteract the effects of heparin.

If the client is receiving an oral anticoagulant, the dose is adjusted according to laboratory findings. Optimum therapeutic results are obtained when prothrombin levels are 1½ to 2½ times the normal control value or the international normalized ratio (INR) value is 2.0 to 4.0.

Bleeding can occur at any time, even when the prothrombin level appears to be within safe limits. The client is observed for evidence of bleeding such as easy bruising, nosebleeds, excessive bleeding from small cuts, and blood in the urine or stool. The antidote for oral anticoagulants, parenteral vitamin K, is kept available.

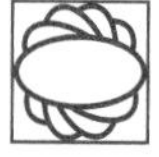

General Gerontologic Considerations

Older adults who experience a TIA may ignore the symptoms thinking that they are part of the normal aging process because symptoms usually subside after a short time.

One of the major risk factors for stroke is hypertension. At times the older adult with hypertension may become noncompliant with the medication regimen, thus increasing the risk of CVA. Client education is important to foster compliance.

The rehabilitation of the elderly client with a CVA is difficult and subject to more complications than with a younger adult. The family may be unable to provide the care needed in the home setting and the client may need to go to a rehabilitation or a nursing home for rehabilitation.

The older adult client is more susceptible to the complications of prolonged bed rest and inactivity. Because the rehabilitation period after a CVA is often prolonged, closely observe the elderly client for problems such as hypostatic pneumonia, pressure ulcers, and contractures.

Older clients with moderate to severe neurologic deficits may place a financial and physical burden on their spouse or children. The nurse must work closely with the family and social service agencies to help the family assume the care of their family member to the extent possible.

SUMMARY OF KEY CONCEPTS

- The three types of headaches are tension, migraine, and cluster.
- Tension headaches can be mild or severe and are caused by emotional stress, eye strain, sinusitis, or cervical neck strain.
- Migraine headaches are severe and accompanied by nausea and vomiting. They are caused by vasodilation of intracranial blood vessels.
- Cluster headaches occur in clusters or groups and last for several days. They can be triggered by vasodilating agents such as nitroglycerin or alcoholic beverages.
- Nursing techniques that may help to relieve headache pain by supplementary drug therapy include eliminating environmental factors that intensify pain, using back massage, applying warm or cool cloths, and using distraction.
- Cerebrovascular disorders include transient ischemic attacks (TIA), cerebrovascular disorder (stroke), and cerebral aneurysm.
- Cerebrovascular disorders are caused by oxygen deprivation to the brain.
- Transient ischemic attacks are fleeting attacks of impaired circulation to a specific area of the brain which deprives the tissue of adequate oxygen and may be a warning that a cerebrovascular accident could occur.
- Treatment of a cerebrovascular accident includes tissue plasminogen activator, anticoagulants, and carotid endarterectomy for blockage of the carotid artery.
- Manifestations of a cerebrovascular accident include paralysis on the side opposite to the damaged area of the brain. Right-sided hemiplegia includes expressive aphasia, intellectual impairment, slow and cautious behavior, and defects in the right visual fields; left-sided hemiplegia includes spatial-perceptual deficits, distractibility, impulsivity, poor judgment, and defects in the left visual fields.
- Nursing diagnoses following a cerebrovascular accident include *Impaired Swallowing, Risk for Aspiration, Risk for Fluid Volume Deficit, Bowel and Bladder Incontinence, Self-Care Deficits, Impaired Physical Mobility, Risk for Impaired Skin Integrity,* and *Risk for Ineffective Individual and Family Coping.*
- Cerebral aneurysms are due to weakening of the blood vessel wall. Usually there are no symptoms until the aneurysm ruptures, causing severe headache, dizziness, nausea and vomiting, followed by loss of consciousness.
- Nursing care of a client with a cerebral aneurysm is focused on maintaining strict bed rest to prevent further bleeding and to reduce increased intracranial pressure, facilitate pain relief, and reduce anxiety.

CRITICAL THINKING EXERCISES

1. What suggestions could you give a friend who has migraine headaches that could help reduce their severity?
2. What nursing interventions are appropriate to implement when caring for a client who has experienced a cerebrovascular accident?
3. When assigned to care for a client with a leaking cerebral aneurysm, what nursing interventions are appropriate for reducing the potential for a serious intracranial bleed?

Suggested Readings

Cochran, I., Flynn, C. A., Goetz, G., et al. (1994). Stroke care. *Nursing, 24*(6), 34–42.

Fowler, S., Durkee, C. M., & Webb, D. J. (1996). Rehabilitating stroke patients in the acute care setting. *Med-Surg Nursing, 5*(5), 327–332.

Hayn, M. A., & Fisher, T. R. (1997). Stroke rehab. *Nursing, 27*(3), 40–47.

Hydo, B. (1995). Designing an effective clinical pathway for stroke. *American Journal of Nursing, 95*(3), 44–51.

Keeping the circle of love alive. (1996). *Nursing, 26*(9), 50–53.

McLaren, C. (1996). Nutrition risks after a stroke. *Nursing Times, 92*(42), 64, 66, 68.

Moules, C. (1996). Communication difficulties...dysphasia. *Nursing Times, 92*(7), 32–33.

Mower, D. M. (1997). Brain attack. *Nursing, 27*(3), 34–37.

Nussbaum, E. (1996). Migraines. *American Journal of Nursing, 96*(10), 36–37.

What's new in drugs. (1996). Better use of warfarin means fewer CVAs. *RN, 59*(1), 71.

What's new in drugs. (1996). A breakthrough in the treatment of ischemic stroke. *RN, 59*(4), 74.

Additional Resources

American Council for Headache Education
19 Mantua Road
Mount Royal, NJ 08061
(609) 423–0258
http://www.achenet.org/

National Headache Foundation
428 West Saint James Place
2nd floor
Chicago, IL 60614–2750
http://www.headaches.org/

Headache Prevention Institute
800 West Long Lake Road
#135
Bloomfield Hills, MI 48302
(248) 258–6182
http://www.h-p-i.com/

National Stroke Association
96 Inverness Drive East
Suite 1
Englewood, CO 80112–5112
(303) 649–9299
http://www/stroke.org/

Stroke Support
http://members.aol.com/scmmlm/main.htm

Chapter 46

Caring for Clients With Head and Spinal Cord Trauma

KEY TERMS

Autonomic dysreflexia
Autoregulation
Battle's sign
Cerebral hematoma
Chemonucleolysis
Closed head injury
Concussion
Contrecoup injury
Contusion
Coup injury
Craniectomy
Cranioplasty
Craniotomy
Diskectomy
Epidural hematoma
Extramedullary
Halo sign
Infratentorial
Intracerebral hematoma
Intramedullary
Laminectomy
Open head injury
Otorrhea
Paraplegia
Paresthesia
Periorbital ecchymosis
Poikilothermia
Rhinorrhea
Spinal fusion
Spinal shock
Subdural hematoma
Supratentorial
Tentorium
Tetraplegia
Uncal herniation

LEARNING OBJECTIVES

On completion of this chapter, the reader will:

- Differentiate between a concussion and a contusion.
- Explain the differences between an epidural, subdural, and intracerebral hematoma.
- Discuss the nursing management of a client with a head injury.
- Discuss the nursing management of a client undergoing intracranial surgery.
- Explain the phenomenon of spinal shock and list four symptoms.
- Discuss autonomic dysreflexia and list at least five manifestations.
- Describe the nursing management of a client with a spinal cord injury.
- Name three conditions that cause pressure on spinal nerve roots.
- Identify three surgical procedures used to relieve spinal nerve root compression.
- Discuss the nursing management of a client with spinal nerve root compression.

Head and spinal cord trauma can result in permanent disability and dysfunction. Head injuries include lacerations, fractures of the skull, internal bleeding, and edema of the brain and surrounding tissues. The cervical and lumbar areas are common sites of spinal injury.

Head Injuries

Injury to the head can cause brain concussion, contusion, epidural or subdural hematoma, or skull fracture.

Concussion

A **concussion** results from a blow to the head that jars the brain.

ETIOLOGY AND PATHOPHYSIOLOGY

The injury is often a consequence of a fall, striking the head against a hard surface like a windshield, a collision between athletes, battering while boxing, or violence.

A concussion results in diffuse and microscopic injury to the brain. The force of the blow causes temporary neurologic impairment but no serious damage to cerebral tissue. Recovery is complete and usually occurs in a short time. In older adults, recovery may take longer.

ASSESSMENT FINDINGS

Signs and Symptoms

The injury may be accompanied by a brief lapse of consciousness. It is often followed by temporary disorientation, headache, blurred or double vision, irritability, and dizziness.

Diagnostic Findings

Skull radiography, computed tomography (CT), and magnetic resonance imaging (MRI) rule out a more serious head injury, such as skull fracture or intracranial bleeding.

MEDICAL MANAGEMENT

The client's activity is temporarily halted until the seriousness of the injury is determined. Mild analgesia (usually acetaminophen) relieves the headache. The client is observed for neurologic complications.

NURSING MANAGEMENT

Following a neurologic assessment, instruct the family to watch the client closely for signs of increased intracranial pressure (IICP) such as alterations in behavior, sleepiness, personality changes, vomiting, and speech or gait disturbances (see Chap. 43). If any of these symptoms occur, return the client to the physician or emergency department.

Contusion

A **contusion**, which is more serious than a concussion, results in gross structural injury to the brain.

ETIOLOGY AND PATHOPHYSIOLOGY

The brain is injured when the head is struck directly, a **coup injury**. Dual bruising can result if the force is strong enough to send the brain ricocheting to the opposite side of the skull, a **contrecoup injury** (Fig. 46–1).

Contusions result in bruising and possibly hemorrhage of superficial cerebral tissue. Edema develops at the site of injury or in areas opposite to the injury. A skull fracture can accompany a contusion.

ASSESSMENT FINDINGS

Signs and Symptoms

Signs and symptoms vary depending on the severity of the blow and the degree of head velocity. Clients exhibit hypotension, rapid and weak pulse, shallow respirations, loss of consciousness, and pale, clammy skin. While unconscious, the client generally responds to strong stimuli like pressure applied to the sternum. On awakening, the client often has temporary amnesia (loss of memory) for recent events. Permanent brain damage can cause impaired intellect, speech difficulty, seizures, paralysis, and impaired gait.

Diagnostic Findings

Skull radiography is performed to rule out or confirm skull fracture. CT or MRI detects bleeding or small hemorrhages in brain tissue, a shift in brain tissue, and edema at the injury site.

MEDICAL MANAGEMENT

The unstable client's vital functions are supported with drug therapy and mechanical ventilation if necessary.

NURSING MANAGEMENT

Observe the client closely for changes in level of consciousness (LOC), signs of IICP (see Chap. 44), neurologic changes, respiratory distress, and changes in vital signs. Immediately report a change in the client's neurologic status to the physician.

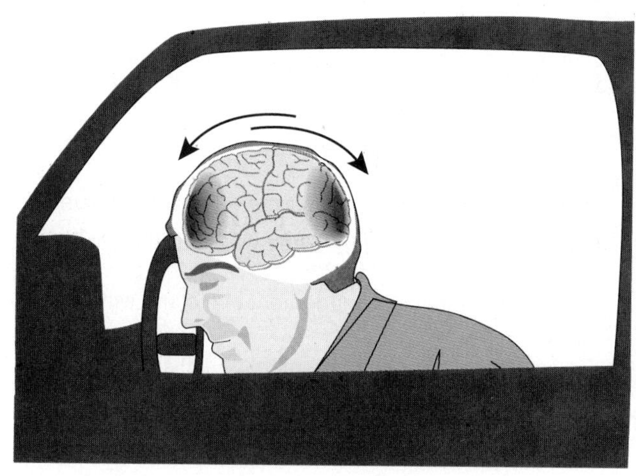

FIGURE 46-1. Coup and contrecoup injuries occur at the point of contact and when the brain rebounds from the opposite direction.

Client and Family Teaching

To reduce the potential for head injuries, both minor and life-threatening, advocate for:

- Using seatbelts for all passengers in an automobile
- Restraining infants in an approved car seat located in the rear seat of the automobile
- Wearing protective head gear while riding a bicycle or motorcycle, and participating in contact sports like hockey, baseball or softball
- Raising neck restraints on the backs of car seats
- Not driving under the influence of alcohol or drugs

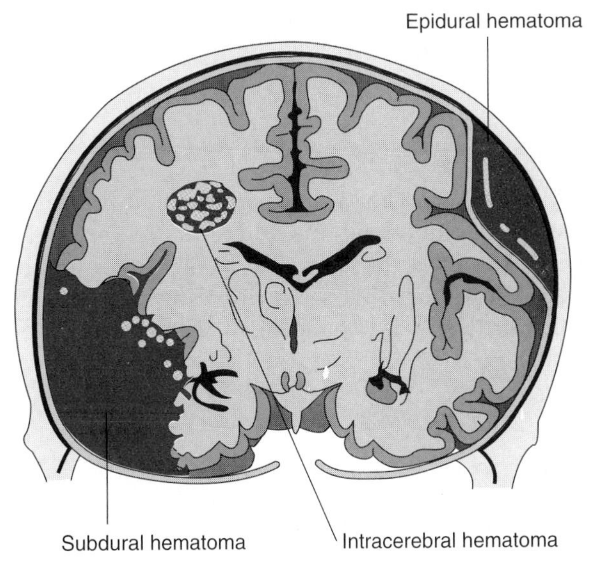

FIGURE 46-2. Hematomas can be located above the dura, below the dura, and within the brain itself.

Cerebral Hematomas

A **cerebral hematoma** is bleeding within the skull that forms an expanding lesion. Examples include: (1) epidural hematoma, (2) subdural hematoma, and (3) intracerebral hematoma (Fig. 46–2).

ETIOLOGY AND PATHOPHYSIOLOGY

Most hematomas are the result of head trauma or a cerebral vascular disorders. An **epidural hematoma** is caused by arterial bleeding and accumulation of blood *above* the dura. A **subdural hematoma** occurs as a result of venous bleeding and the accumulation of blood in the space *below* the dura. An **intracerebral hematoma** is bleeding *within* the brain that results from an open or closed head injury or from a cerebrovascular condition such as a ruptured cerebral aneurysm (see Chap. 45). Individuals at high risk for cerebral hematomas are those receiving anticoagulant therapy or those with an underlying bleeding disorder such as hemophilia, thrombocytopenia, leukemia, and aplastic anemia.

Bleeding increases the volume of brain contents and results in IICP. As the ICP increases, cerebral blood flow is disrupted and the brain becomes hypoxic. Unrelieved pressure causes the brain to shift to the lateral side **(uncal herniation)** or herniate downward through the foramen magnum. The vital centers for respiration, heart rate, and blood pressure are affected as well as cranial nerve functions. Death occurs if the symptoms are not recognized and the bleeding is not stopped.

ASSESSMENT FINDINGS

Signs and Symptoms

The rapidity and severity of neurologic changes (Table 46–1) depends on the location, the rate of

TABLE 46-1 **Differences in Cerebral Hematomas**

Type	Location	Signs and Symptoms
Epidural	Arterial blood collects between the skull and dura.	May be alert after initial unconsciousness, but then becomes more and more lethargic before lapsing into coma Headache, ipsilateral (same side of injury) pupil changes, and contralateral hemiparesis (weakness or paralysis on opposite side of injury)
Subdural	Venous blood collects between the dura and subarachnoid layers.	Progressive deterioration in LOC Ipsilateral pupil changes, decreased extraocular muscle movement, contralateral hemiparesis Periodic episodes of memory lapse, confusion, drowsiness, and personality changes
Intracerebral	Blood collects within the brain.	Classic signs of IICP; headache, vomiting, seizures, posturing, hyperthermia, irregular breathing

bleeding and size of hematoma, and ef fectiveness of **autoregulation**, the brain's ability to provide sufficient arterial blood flow despite rising ICP.

Diagnostic Findings

MRI and CT scans show densities that indicate the location of the hematoma and shifts in cerebral tissue. ICP monitoring (see Chap. 44) provides direct and continuous data for evaluating the extent to which the lesion is expanding or responding to treatment.

MEDICAL MANAGEMENT

Some subdural hematomas become walled off and absorbed by the body with no treatment. However, a rapid change in LOC and signs of uncontrolled IICP indicate a surgical emergency.

SURGICAL MANAGEMENT

Surgery consists of drilling holes (burr holes) in the skull to relieve pressure, removing the clot, and stopping the bleeding. If the source of bleeding cannot be located by means of burr holes, more invasive surgery is performed.

Intracranial surgery consists of three possible procedures: craniotomy, craniectomy, and cranioplasty. A **craniotomy** is the surgical opening of the skull to gain access to the structures beneath the cranial bones. It is done to remove a blood clot or a tumor, stop intracranial bleeding, or repair damaged brain tissues or blood vessels. A **craniectomy** is the removal of a portion of a cranial bone, and **cranioplasty** is the repair of a defect in a cranial bone. A metal or plastic plate or wire mesh is used to replace the area of removed bone or to reinforce a defect in a cranial bone.

One of two surgical approaches above or below the *tentorium,* a double fold of dura mater that separates the cerebrum from the cerebellum, is used. A **supratentorial** (above the tentorium) approach is made through a scalp incision where a particular lobe of the cerebrum requires surgical access. The **infratentorial** (below the tentorium) approach provides an opening to the midbrain and structures of the brainstem. The incision is made at the back of the head with the client in a sitting position.

In cranial surgery, several burr holes are first made in the skull. A saw is then used to cut a section of bone (bone flap). The bone flap is removed to provide a visual field for surgery. After surgery is completed, the bone flap usually is replaced. In some instances, such as with an inoperable tumor, the bone flap is not replaced, allowing the tumor to expand and, thus, preventing increased ICP.

Complications associated with intracranial surgery include cerebral edema, infection, shock, fluid and electrolyte imbalances, venous thrombosis (especially in the arms and legs), IICP, seizures, leakage of cerebrospinal fluid (CSF), and stress ulcers and hemorrhage.

NURSING MANAGEMENT

Regard a head injury, no matter how mild it appears, as an emergency. Obtain a history of the injury and perform a neurologic examination with particular attention to vital signs, LOC, presence or absence of movement in the arms and legs, pupil size, equality, and reaction to light for evidence of IICP. If the head injury is caused by trauma, examine the head for bleeding, abrasions, and lacerations. Evaluate the respiratory status with particular attention to the client's ability to maintain adequate oxygenation. Recognize and report changes immediately. Refer to Chapter 44 for a suggested plan of nursing care for a client with IICP that is treated medically.

Preoperative Nursing Management

Once the physician decides to perform surgery, the client is prepared. Shave the head in the area where burr holes will be drilled (this is sometimes deferred until the client is in the operating room). Take vital signs, making sure continuing neurologic assessments are recorded. Administer prescribed medications such as an anticonvulsant like phenytoin (Dilantin) to reduce the risk of seizures before and after surgery, an osmotic diuretic, and corticosteroids. Preoperative sedation is generally omitted. Restrict fluids to avoid intraoperative complications, reduce cerebral edema, and prevent postoperative vomiting. Insert an indwelling urethral catheter and intravenous line. Apply antiembolism stockings to prevent thrombophlebitis and deep vein thrombosis, which develop from prolonged immobility during neurosurgery. These stockings are removed and reapplied every 8 hours for several days after surgery or as long as the client is immobile.

Postoperative Nursing Care

After surgery, place the client in either a supine position or a side-lying position on the unaffected side. Postoperative assessments are performed at 15- to 30-minute intervals and include all areas of neurologic function. Edema around the eyes (periorbital edema) may make examination of the pupils difficult during the immediate postoperative period. Ecchymosis can also be present. Maintain a neurologic flow sheet to compare assessment findings.

Observe the client closely for IICP. Administer corticosteroids and restrict fluids as ordered to control cerebral edema and to increase cerebral perfusion.

NURSING PROCESS
Care of the Client Undergoing Intracranial Surgery

Assessment
A neurologic examination provides both a preoperative and a postoperative data base. The results of diagnostic test are reviewed.

Diagnosis and Planning
Nursing care for a client undergoing intracranial surgery includes, but is not limited to, the following:

Nursing Diagnoses and Collaborative Problems	Nursing Interventions
Risk for Ineffective Breathing related to depressive effects of anesthesia and compression of medulla secondary to edema of the brain **Goal:** The client's ventilation will be adequate to maintain the SPO_2 of 90% or greater and the PO_2 at 80 mm Hg or above.	Maintain a patent airway. Keep the head and neck positioned in midline. Maintain mechanical ventilation until the client can be safely weaned. Provide supplemental oxygen when mechanical ventilation is no longer necessary. Instruct to deep breathe or use an incentive spirometer at least 10 times an hour while awake. Elevate the head of the bed to maximize breathing and reduce ICP.
Risk for Altered Tissue Perfusion related to edema and bleeding within the cranium **Goal:** The client's ICP will be adequate to perfuse the brain as evidenced by absence of abnormal neurologic signs and symptoms.	Refer to Nursing Management of the client with IICP in Chapter 44.
Pain related to chemicals released from traumatized tissue **Goal:** The client's pain will be reduced to a tolerable level.	Reduce bright lights and noise. Administer prescribed analgesia. Assess for adverse effects on respiration or neurologic function.
Risk for Infection related to impaired skin integrity and suppression of the inflammatory response secondary to steroid drug therapy; **Risk for Hyperthermia** related to hypothalamic dysfunction or infection **Goal:** There will be no incisional infection as evidenced by absence of wound drainage, normal temperature and normal leukocyte count.	Check for drainage on dressing; notify surgeon if drainage appears straw colored, suggesting CSF, or purulent. Administer prophylactic antibiotics as prescribed. Follow principles of asepsis when assessing incision and changing dressings. Administer an antipyretic if body temperature becomes elevated above normal. Apply a cooling blanket to relieve a high fever.
Altered Thought Processes and **Risk for Injury** related to confusion, poor judgment, seizures **Goal:** The client will be oriented and injuries will not occur.	Orient the client at frequent intervals. Provide environmental cues such as a calendar with large numbers. Investigate contributing causes of restlessness such as a full bladder, pain, or nausea and intervene when appropriate. Share current events. Turn on newsworthy television or radio programs. Repeat explanations or answers to questions as needed. Locate the client near the nursing station and place a bed alarm that sounds if the client gets out of bed. Institute seizure precautions (see Chap. 44).
Risk for Ineffective Individual and Family Coping related to multiple stressors involving physical losses, lengthy rehabilitation, and compromised financial resources **Goal:** The client and family will cope with neurologic deficits, participate fully in rehabilitation, and seek assistance from social agencies.	Consult with the physician regarding the client's prognosis. Concur with the physician's explanations if the client or family raises questions. Keep the client and family informed of progress or changes as they occur. Accept the client's and family's behavior in dealing with stress in a nonjudgmental manner. Encourage independent problem solving and acknowledge positive outcomes. Refer the client and family to a social worker, discharge planner, or home health agency.

Evaluation and Expected Outcomes
- The airway is patent and respirations are normal.
- The client shows neurologic stability.

- The client reports absence from pain.
- The surgical site remains free of infection and fever.
- The client is oriented to person, place, and time.
- No injuries occur.
- The client and family effectively cope with the stress of surgery and possibility of long-term disability.

Client and Family Teaching

If the client is discharged directly to his or her home, it is essential to provide verbal and written instructions for the following:

- Signs that indicate intracranial bleeding and infection (swelling around the eye and face below the incision can be expected)
- Purposes for prescribed medications such as anticonvulsant medication, anti-inflammatory drugs, and medication to control gastric secretions; schedule for their administration; and side effects to report
- Sensory changes that can be expected such as hearing a "clicking" sound around the bone flap that disappears as healing takes place. Headaches are also common, but notify the surgeon if they are unrelieved by a mild analgesic like acetaminophen (Tylenol).
- Care for the surgical site as directed by the physician. Some recommendations include: keep the incision clean, avoid scrubbing it; secure remaining hair away from the incision; resume shampooing the hair when the staples or sutures are removed; and wear a hat when outside to avoid sunburn where the hair has been shaved.
- Safety precautions to maintain at home include assistance with ambulation and ensuring well lighted and clutter free rooms. Driving privileges are temporarily restricted until it is established that the risk for seizures is eliminated.
- Exercises that promote strength and endurance
- Techniques for ensuring bowel and bladder elimination (see Chap. 47)
- Feeding or nutritional suggestions
- Follow-up appointments for measuring anticonvulsant blood levels, electroencephalograms, and continued medical care and evaluation

Skull Fractures

A skull fracture is a break in the continuity of the cranium. The most common types are simple, depressed, or comminuted fractures (Table 46–2).

TABLE 46-2 **Types of Skull Fractures**

Type	Description
Simple	Linear crack without any displacement of the pieces.
Depressed	Broken bone is pushed inward toward the brain.
Comminuted	Bone is splintered into fragments.

ETIOLOGY AND PATHOPHYSIOLOGY

A skull fracture is caused by a blow to the head. The fracture can be associated with an **open head injury** in which the scalp, bony cranium, and dura mater (the outer meningeal layer) are exposed. There may be a **closed head injury** in which the fractured skull remains covered by an intact layer of scalp.

Open head injuries create a potential for infection due to exposure to the environment. They are less likely to produce rapid intracranial hypertension (IICP) because the opening provides some ability for the brain to expand as pressure increases.

Basilar skull fractures are located at the base of the skull. Trauma in this location is especially dangerous because it can cause edema of the brain near the origin of the spinal cord (foramen magnum), interfere with the circulation of CSF, injure the nerves that pass into the spinal cord, or create a pathway for infection between the brain and the middle ear (Fig. 46–3) that can result in meningitis.

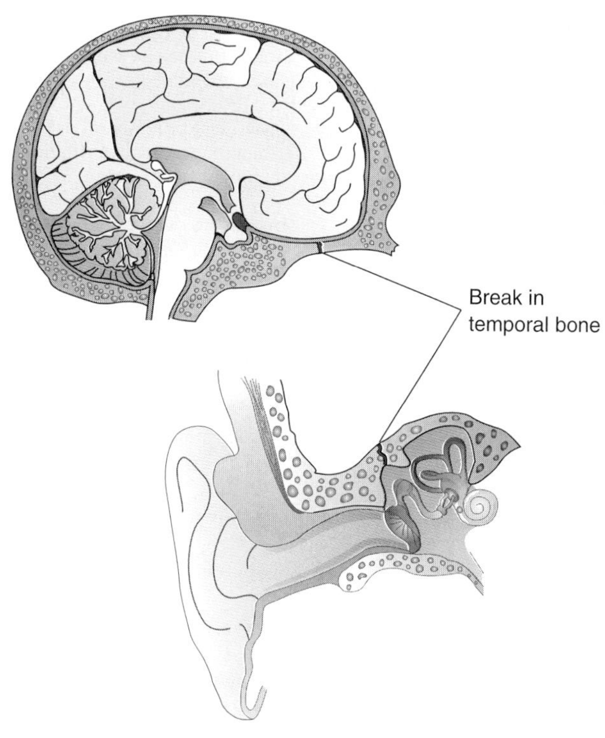

FIGURE 46-3. Basilar fracture in the temporal bone can cause CSF to leak from the nose or ear.

ASSESSMENT FINDINGS

Signs and Symptoms

Simple skull fractures produce few, if any, symptoms and heal without complications. The client may complain of a localized headache. A bump, bruise, or laceration may be found on the scalp.

Symptoms depend on the area of the brain that has been injured. For example, a large bone fragment that is pressing on the motor area can cause hemiparesis. In any type of skull fracture, shock can develop from the skull injury or from injury to some other area of the body.

Because basilar skull fractures tend to tear the dura, **rhinorrhea**, leaking of CSF from the nose, or **otorrhea**, leakage of CSF from the ear, may occur. In some cases **periorbital ecchymosis**, referred to as "raccoon eyes," or bruising of the mastoid process behind the ear, called **Battle's sign**, can be present (Fig. 46–4). Conjunctival hemorrhages can occur as well. Seizures may occur because of injury to the brain tissue. Epilepsy can develop as a sequela of head injury.

Diagnostic Findings

Skull radiographs, a CT scan, or MRI show brain tissue injuries such as a fracture line or embedded skull fragments (compound skull fracture), cerebral edema, or presence of a subdural or epidural hematoma.

MEDICAL AND SURGICAL MANAGEMENT

Simple skull fractures require bed rest and close observation for signs of IICP. If the scalp is lacerated, the wound is cleaned, debrided, and sutured.

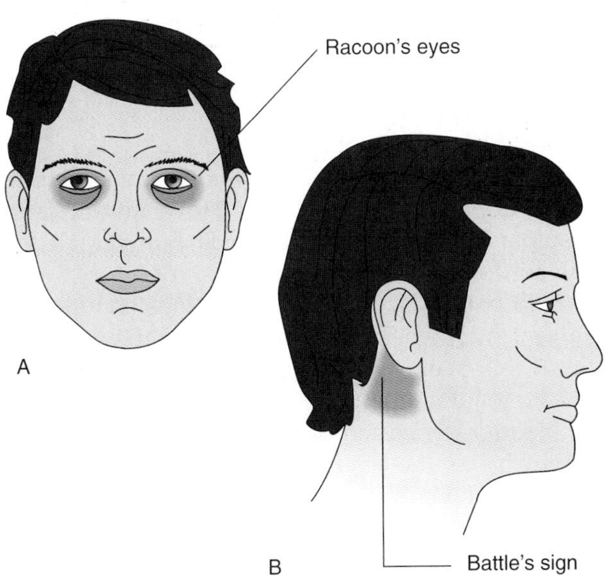

FIGURE 46-4. (*A*) Periorbital ecchymosis, called racoon's eyes, and (*B*) periauricular ecchymosis, called Battle's sign.

Depressed skull fractures require a craniotomy to remove bone fragments and control bleeding, elevation of the depressed fracture, and repair of damaged tissues. A piece of mesh is inserted to replace the bone fragments that are removed. Additional treatment includes antibiotics to control infection, an osmotic diuretic or corticosteroids to prevent or treat cerebral edema, and an anticonvulsant to prevent or treat seizures.

NURSING MANAGEMENT

Most clients are hospitalized for 24 hours or more after a significant head injury. Examine the client to identify signs of head trauma. Use methods described in Nursing Guidelines 46–1 to test drainage from the nose or ear. Look for a **halo sign** (Fig. 46–5) which indicates the presence of CSF in drainage. Allow the drainage to flow freely onto porous gauze; *never* plug the orifice tightly.

Assess the client neurologically, even if the injury appears mild. It is possible for a hematoma to accompany a skull fracture. Evaluate LOC, assess motor and sensory status, and check pupils hourly. Take vital signs every 15 to 30 minutes. Prepare for the possibility of seizures.

Refer to Chapter 44 for suggestions in the plan of nursing care for a client with IICP and implement nursing measures for clients undergoing surgical intervention (see previous discussion).

Spinal Cord Injuries

Spinal cord trauma is serious and sometimes fatal. The cervical and lumbar spines are the most common

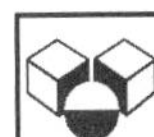

Nursing Guidelines 46-1

Detecting Cerebrospinal Fluid in Drainage

Method #1

- Wet a Dextrostick or Testape strip with drainage from the nose or ear.
- Observe if the color change indicates the presence of glucose.
- Use method #2 if the test is positive because blood also contains glucose and can result in false results.

Method #2

- Collect droplets of drainage on a white absorbent pad.
- Observe the wet area after a few minutes for a halo sign.
- Note if a yellow ring encircles a central ring that is red; the red ring indicates blood; the yellow ring is suggestive of CSF.

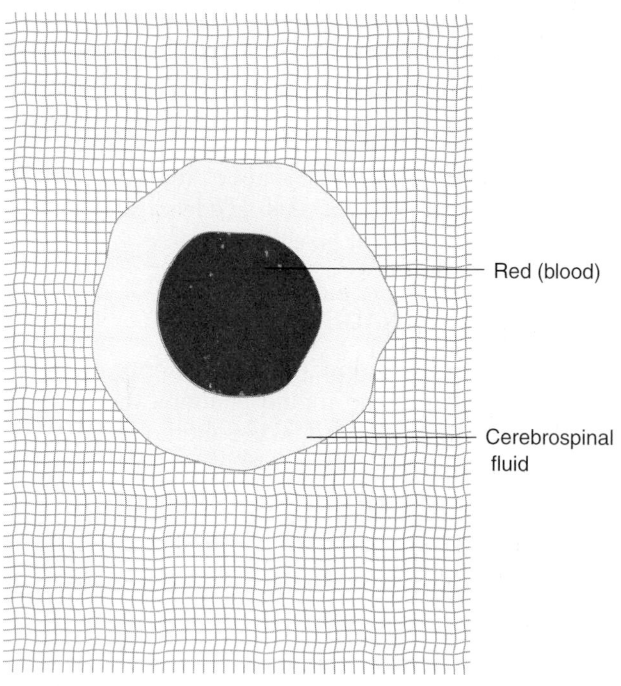

FIGURE 46-5. Halo sign. Clear drainage that separates from bloody drainage suggests the presence of CSF.

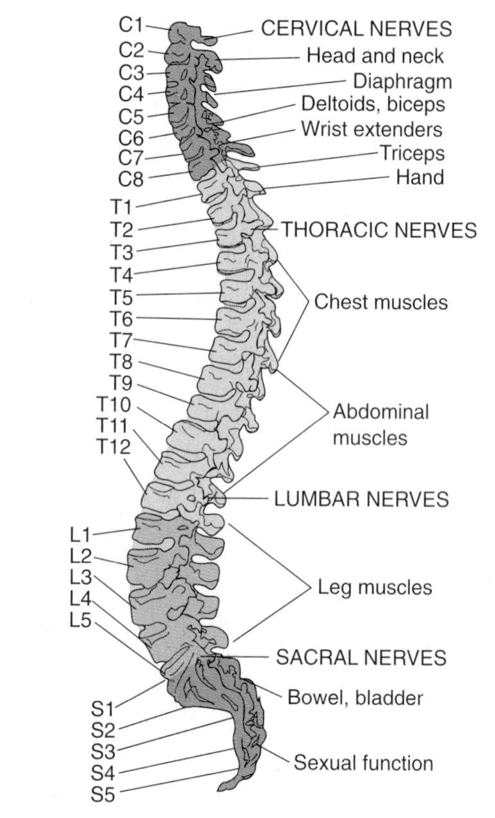

FIGURE 46-6. Structures affected by spinal nerves.

sites of injury. Emergency management at the time of injury is crucial because the spinal cord can be permanently damaged if the client is moved incorrectly.

ETIOLOGY AND PATHOPHYSIOLOGY

Common causes of spinal cord injury include accidents and violence. Vehicular accidents result in the most spinal cord injuries, followed by violence, falls, sports, and miscellaneous injuries.

Trauma to the back can fracture or collapse one or more vertebrae, resulting in a portion of bone injuring the spinal cord and interfering with the transmission of nerve impulses (Fig. 46–6). Even if there is no fracture, edema can lead to compression of the cord. Edema with subsequent cord compression can result in permanent cord damage.

Spinal cord injury can also lead to bleeding within the cord. Because the blood has no place to drain, it forms a hematoma that occupies space and compresses the nerve roots. An injury to the cord can also completely or partially sever spinal cord nerve fibers. When this kind of injury occurs, the client experiences a variety of motor and sensory dysfunction below the site of the injury to the cord (Table 46–3). **Tetraplegia**, a term that replaces quadriplegia, results in paralysis of all extremities when there is a high cervical spine injury. **Paraplegia**, paralysis of both legs, occurs with injuries at the thoracic level. When the tracts of the spinal nerves are severed, no effective nerve regeneration occurs. Muscle spasms occur spontaneously, but they are not evidence that the client is regaining motor function.

Respiratory arrest and spinal shock are immediate complications of spinal cord injury. Long-term complications include autonomic dysreflexia, pressure ulcers, contractures, respiratory and urinary tract infections, loss of calcium from the bones, and renal calculus formation.

Spinal Shock (Areflexia)

Spinal shock is a loss of sympathetic reflex activity below the level of injury within 30 to 60 minutes after the spinal injury. It is characterized by immediate loss of all cord functions below the point of injury. In addition to paralysis, other manifestations include pronounced hypotension, bradycardia, and warm, dry skin. If the level of injury is in the cervical or upper thoracic region, respiratory failure can occur. Bowel and bladder distention develop. The client does not perspire below the level of injury and, therefore, temperature control is impaired. The client manifests **poikilothermia**, body temperature of the environment. Spinal shock may persist for a week to months until the body readjusts to the damage imposed by the injury. Until then, vital functions require medical support.

TABLE 46-3 **Consequences of Spinal Cord Injuries**

Level of Injury	Common Motor Effects	Common Sensory Effects
C1, C2, C3	Paralysis below neck, breathing impaired, bowel and bladder incontinence, sexual dysfunction	No sensation below neck
C4, C5	Shoulder elevation possible, requires ventilation support	No sensation below clavicle
C6, C7, C8	Some elbow, upper arm, and wrist movement can do diaphragmatic breathing	Some sensation in arms and thumb; sensation in chest impaired
T1–T6	Paralysis below waist, control of hands, abdominal breathing	No sensation below midchest
T7–T12	Varying degrees of trunk and abdominal control	Varying degrees of sensation below the waist
L1–L2	Hip adduction impaired	No sensation below lower abdomen; some sensation in inner thighs
L3–L5	Knee and ankle movement impaired	No sensation below upper thighs
S1–S5	Varying degrees of bowel/bladder control and sexual function	No sensation in perineum

C, cervical; T, thoracic; L, lumbar; S, sacral.

Autonomic Dysreflexia (Hyperreflexia)

Autonomic dysreflexia is an exaggerated sympathetic nervous system response among those who have a spinal cord injury above the T6 level. It can occur suddenly at any time after spinal shock subsides. It is precipitated by a full bladder, abdominal distention, impacted feces, or any uncomfortable stimuli below the level of spinal injury. This acute emergency is characterized by:

- Severe hypertension
- Tachycardia
- Pounding headache
- Nausea
- Blurred vision
- Flushed skin
- Sweating
- Goosebumps (erection of pilomotor muscles in the skin)
- Nasal stuffiness
- Anxiety

Uncontrolled autonomic dysreflexia can lead to seizures, stroke, and death. Prevention is the best treatment, but additional measures such as antihypertensive drug therapy with phentolamine (Regitine), hydralazine (Apresoline), or diazoxide (Hyperstat), raising the client's head, and relieving the precipitating cause are necessary once it develops.

ASSESSMENT FINDINGS

Signs and Symptoms

The degree and location of the injury determine the symptoms that occur immediately after the injury. There is pain in the affected area, difficulty breathing, numbness, and paralysis. If the injury is high in the cervical region, respiratory failure and death occur because the diaphragm is paralyzed. When the cord is completely severed, function is permanently lost below the level of the injury. Some function is maintained if the damage to the cord is minimal.

Diagnostic Findings

A neurologic examination reveals the level of spinal cord injury. Radiography, myelography, MRI, and CT scan show evidence of fracture or compression of one or more vertebrae, edema, or a hematoma.

MEDICAL MANAGEMENT

Initially, the head and back are immobilized mechanically with a cervical collar and back support. An intravenous line is inserted to provide access to a vein if shock develops. Vital signs are stabilized. Corticosteroids may be given to reduce spinal cord edema.

After the client is stabilized, the injured portion of the spine is further immobilized using a cast or brace or surgical intervention. Traction with weights and pulleys is applied to provide correct vertebral alignment and to increase the space between the vertebrae. Additional weight is added over the next few days to increase the space between the vertebrae and to move them into correct alignment. A turning frame is used to change the client's position without altering the alignment of the spine (Fig. 46–7).

SURGICAL MANAGEMENT

Depending on the extent of the injury, it may be necessary to surgically remove bone fragments, re-

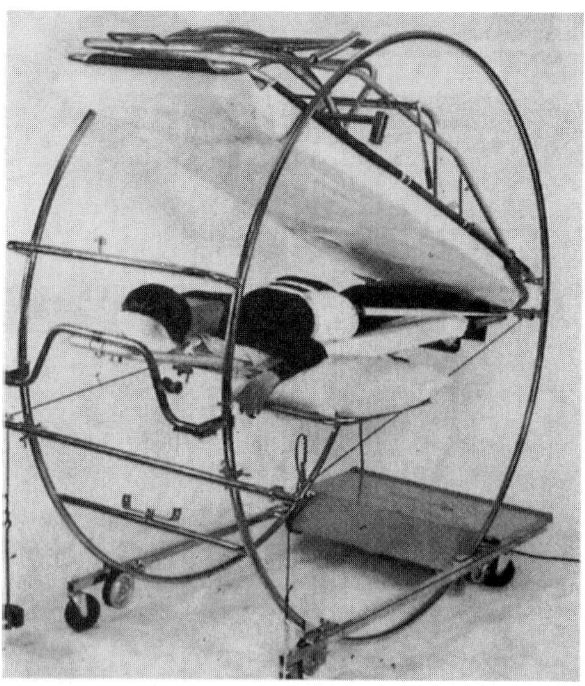

FIGURE 46-7. A circular bed facilitates turning a client who must remain immobile.

pair dislocated vertebrae, and stabilize the spine. The vertebrae are fused with bone obtained from the iliac crest or stabilized with a steel rod. External immobilization with a brace or cast is often necessary.

NURSING MANAGEMENT

Keep the body and head in alignment and limit all movement. Insert a urinary retention catheter if directed by the physician.

Assist with immobilization of the injured spine (Fig. 46–8). Burr holes in the skull are required for inserting the pointed ends of traction tongs or the halo traction apparatus (the Gardner-Wells traction does not require burr holes). When traction is applied, check to be sure that the weights hang free. *Never* lift or remove the weights or increase or decrease the amount of weight.

NURSING PROCESS
Care of the Client With Spinal Trauma

Assessment

On the client's arrival, obtain information about the injury and treatment given at the scene from the family, witnesses, or those who transported the client to the hospital.

Initiate a neurologic assessment flow sheet to provide a data base for future comparisons. Assess vital signs with particular attention to the client's respiratory status. During the acute phase, perform neurologic assessments at frequent intervals. Check for movement and sensation below the level of injury, look for progression of neurologic damage, and observe for signs of respiratory distress and spinal shock.

Diagnosis and Planning

Besides monitoring for and intervening if spinal shock and autonomic dysreflexia occur, the plan for nursing care includes, but is not limited to, the following:

Nursing Diagnoses and Collaborative Problems	Nursing Interventions
Ineffective Breathing Pattern, Ineffective Airway Clearance, and **Risk for Impaired Gas Exchange** related to paralysis of respiratory, chest, and abdominal muscles **Goal:** The client's breathing will remain adequate to maintain a SPO_2 of 90% or above; the airway will be clear.	Maintain a patent airway. Be prepared for endotracheal intubation and mechanical ventilation if respiratory failure ocurs. Administer oxygen as prescribed. Suction the airway to remove secretions.
Risk for Neuropathic Pain related to irritated nerve root and soft tissue injury **Goal:** Pain will be managed and minimized.	Administer prescribed analgesia IV to avoid injections into tissues where absorption is compromised. Assist the physician with nerve block procedures if analgesia is ineffective.
Impaired Physical Mobility and **Disuse Syndrome** related to loss of motor function **Goal:** The client's potential for mobility will be maintained; basic needs will be met.	Position the client to avoid joint contractures and foot drop. Maintain skin integrity with pressure relieving devices, massage of bony prominences, keep the skin clean and dry. Perform exercises identified by physical therapist. Apply leg braces when ambulation is possible. Control urine elimination and keep the bowel evacuated. Keep the client hydrated to reduce renal stone formation. Provide oral or enteral nutrition.
Anxiety and **Risk for Ineffective Individual Coping** related to prognosis of neurologic deficits **Goal:** The client's anxiety will be relieved and ability to cope will be supported.	Collaborate information on prognosis with the physician. Reiterate that it is difficult to determine the severity of deficits immediately after a spinal cord injury. Explain that the outcome is varied depending on each person's injury and resonse to rehabilitation. Be a good listener and offer encouragement as the client makes progress.

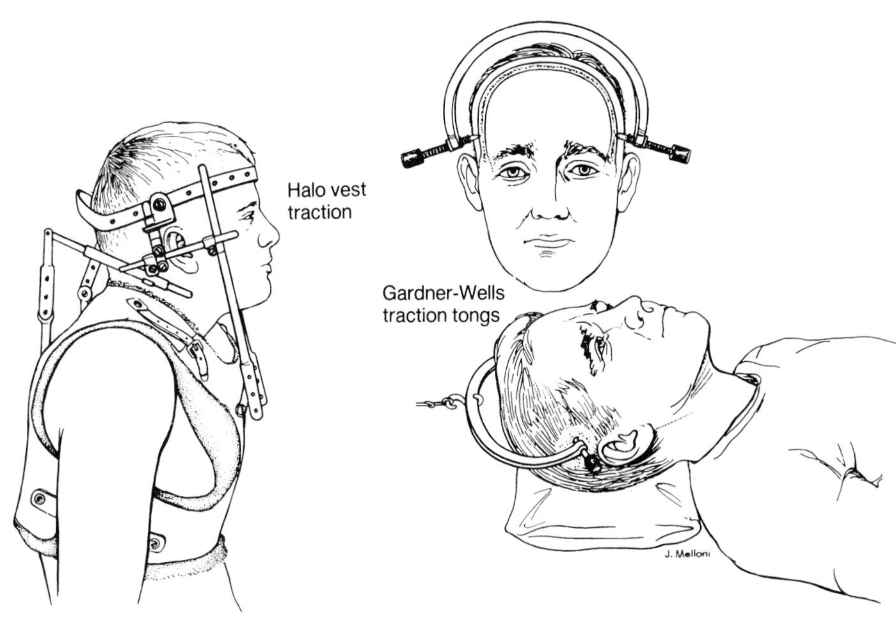

FIGURE 46-8. Halo vest traction and Garner-Wells traction stabilize the cervical spine.

The level of the cord injury, occurrence of complications, the client's motivation and perseverance, and intervention of the health care team influence the client's prognosis. Many paraplegics return home and live independently, and in some instances, resume work. A tetraplegic may return home but requires extensive physical care.

Evaluation and Expected Outcomes

- Spinal shock and dysreflexia are identified and treated.
- Breathing is adequate to maintain oxygenation.
- Pain is controlled.
- Complications from inactivity are prevented or reduced.
- The client begins to cope with the effects of the injury.
- The client and family demonstrate understanding of postdischarge home care.

Client and Family Teaching

The use of external stabilizing devices like the halo vest facilitate early discharge from the acute care facility. To ensure the client's safety and prevention of complications, use the information in Nursing Guidelines 46–2 for teaching purposes.

Spinal Nerve Root Compression

There are two basic types of spinal nerve root compression: **intramedullary** lesions that involve the spinal cord, or **extramedullary** lesions that involve the tissues that surround the spinal cord. The most common sites of nerve root compression are at the level of the three lower lumbar disks, but they also occur in the cervical spine.

ETIOLOGY AND PATHOPHYSIOLOGY

Pressure on spinal nerve roots is caused by trauma, herniated intervertebral disks, and tumors of the spinal cord and surrounding structures (Fig. 46–9). Stress due to poor body mechanics, age, or disease weakens an area in the vertebra, causing the spongy center of the vertebrae, the nucleus pulposus, to swell and herniate. A condition commonly known as a "slipped disk," the displacement puts pressure on the nearby nerves.

Pain along the distribution of the nerve root is common. Actions that increase pressure intensify the pain. Weakness and changes in sensation occur. The symptoms intensify with increasing nerve root compression.

ASSESSMENT FINDINGS

Signs and Symptoms

Symptoms vary depending on the cause of the compression and the level involved, but usually include weakness, paralysis, pain, and **paresthesia** (numbness, tingling). When the sciatic nerve is compressed by a herniated disk in the lumbar region, the client describes feeling pain down the buttocks and into the posterior thigh and leg. Physical assessment reveals weakness or paralysis of an arm or a leg. The client experiences pain when lying supine and lifting each leg without bending the knee. The pain increases when straining, coughing, or lifting a heavy object. Walking and sitting become difficult.

Diagnostic Findings

Spinal radiography, CT, MRI, myelography, and electromyography show displacement or herniation

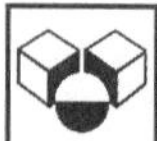

Nursing Guidelines 46-2

Instructing Clients in Halo Vest Management

Tell the client the following:

- Turn your whole body rather than try to turn your head; you will not be able to look down.
- Do not drive a car.
- Walk only on level surfaces until you become accustomed to the vest; avoid stairs, curbs, and uneven terrain unless assistance is available.
- Take care getting in and out of a vehicle so as to avoid bumping the halo and loosening the pins.
- Use a mirror to inspect the pin sites and as a guide while cleaning them.
- Clean the pin sites two to three times a day with cotton-tipped applicators saturated with hydrogen peroxide; remove loose crusts.
- Use a clean applicator after making a full circle around the pin site.
- Clip the hair that grows around the pin sites.
- Report pain, redness, drainage from the pin sites, fever, or tingling or pain in the neck to the physician.
- Never independently adjust the vest if it becomes tight or loose; consult the physician.
- Pad the vest if it causes pressure or friction.
- Take sponge baths to maintain hygiene; seek assistance for areas you are able to bathe such as around your anus.
- Use a dry shampoo or consult the physician on how to shampoo the hair without getting the vest wet.
- Use pillows for support and comfort when sleeping.
- Wear clothing that is loose fitting and has wide necklines for ease in dressing.
- Wear shoes with flat heels that are easy to slip on and off.

of an intervertebral disk, tumor, or bleeding around the nerve root.

MEDICAL MANAGEMENT

When a client has a herniated intervertebral disk, conservative therapy is tried first. Metastatic spinal cord tumors are also treated conservatively because removal is not feasible.

A herniated cervical disk is treated by immobilizing the cervical spine with a cervical collar or brace. Later, as inflammation subsides, the collar or brace is worn intermittently when walking or sitting. Bed rest with a firm mattress and bed board is used for clients with a lumbar herniated disk.

Skin traction, which can be applied in the home, is used to decrease severe muscle spasm as well as increase the distance between adjacent vertebrae, keep the vertebrae in correct alignment, and, in many instances, relieve pain. Treatment relieves symptoms for an extended period.

Hot moist packs are used to treat muscle spasm. Skeletal muscle relaxants, such as carisoprodol (Rela) and chlorzoxazone (Paraflex), help clients with a herniated intervertebral disk. Diazepam (Valium), a tranquilizer with skeletal muscle-relaxing action, is used for its twofold effect: to reduce anxiety associated with the pain of a herniated disk and to relax the skeletal muscle. Drugs such as aspirin, phenylbutazone (Butazolidin), and corticosteroids are used to treat inflammation. Reducing inflammation and muscle spasm helps ease pain, but additional analgesics are given to control pain. Clients with an inoperable spinal cord tumor are given analgesics to maintain comfort.

SURGICAL MANAGEMENT

If conservative therapy fails to relieve symptoms of a herniated disk with spinal nerve root compression, surgery is considered. Procedures for relieving spinal nerve root compression include:

- **Diskectomy**—removal of the ruptured disk
- **Laminectomy**—removal of the posterior arch of a vertebra to expose the spinal cord. The surgeon can remove whatever lesion is causing compression—a herniated disk, tumor, blood clot, bone spur, or broken bone fragment.
- Diskectomy with **spinal fusion**—removal of the ruptured disk followed by grafting a piece of bone taken from another area, such as the iliac crest, onto the vertebra to fuse the vertebral spinous process. Bone also may be obtained from a bone bank.
- **Chemonucleolysis**, injection of the enzyme chymopapain into the nucleus pulposus to shrink or dissolve the disc, which then relieves pressure on spinal nerve roots.

Spinal fusion stabilizes the vertebrae weakened by degenerative joint changes, such as osteoarthritis, and by laminectomy. It results in a firm union; mobility is lost, and the client must become accustomed to a permanent area of stiffness. When a portion of the lumbar spine is fused, the client usually does not feel the stiffness after a short time because motion increases in the joints above the fusion. Motion is more limited when the area of fusion is in the cervical spine. Spinal fusion also is performed for spinal cord tumors, fractures and dislocations of the spine, and Pott's disease (tuberculosis of the spine).

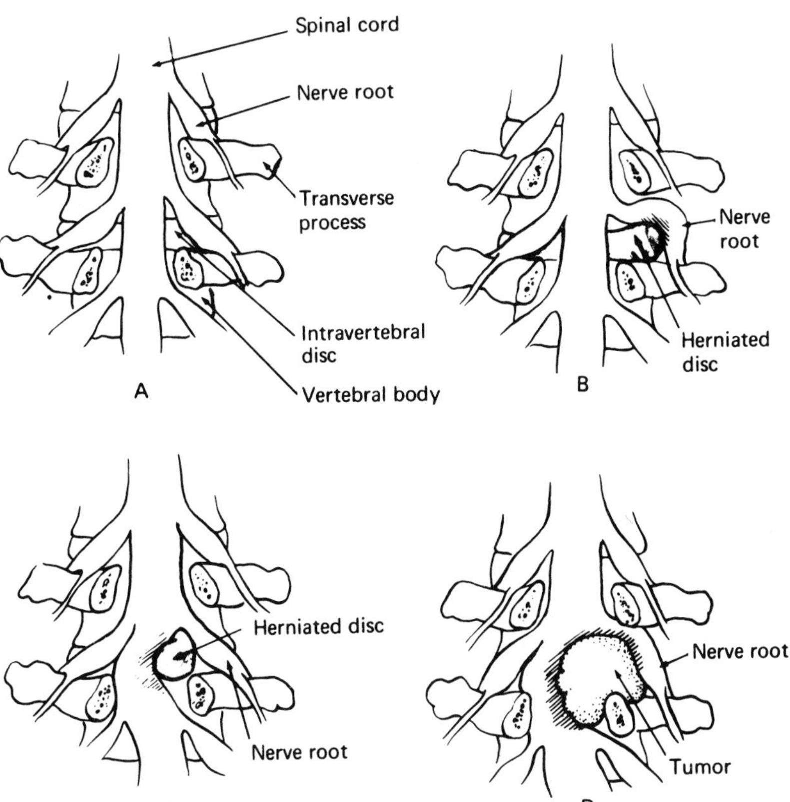

FIGURE 46-9. (*A*) Normal vertebral column. (*B*) Herniated disc pressing on spinal nerve root. (*C*) Herniated disk pressing on spinal cord. (*D*) Tumor compressing both the spinal cord and spinal nerve.

NURSING MANAGEMENT

Perform a neurologic examination and note any limitation of motion and the type of movement that causes pain. For clients being treated conservatively, the nursing care plan includes, but is not limited to, the following:

Nursing Diagnoses and Collaborative Problems	Nursing Interventions
Pain related to movement secondary to nerve root compression **Goal:** The client's pain will be relieved or reduced to a tolerable level.	Use a firm mattress or apply a bedboard. Maintain bed rest; place in Williams position with the knees and head slightly elevated to relieve lumbosacral pain. Apply traction following the guidelines in Box 46-1; for intermittent application support the weights and lower them gently to avoid a sudden and strong pull. Remind the client to roll from side to side without twisting the spine; when getting out of bed reinforce the use of proper body mechanics. Advise clients with cervical nerve root compression to avoid extreme hyperextension of the neck and side-to-side rotation of the head. Administer prescribed muscle relaxants and analgesics. Apply moist heat for no longer than 20 minutes, but repeat several times a day.

Periodically evaluate the client's response to conservative therapy. It is important to note the activities and positions that increase pain and the gain or loss

BOX 46-1 Maintaining Traction

For proper application and use of traction:
- The prescribed amount of weight must be used.
- Traction weights must hang above the floor.
- Ropes must move freely through the pulley grooves.
- The client's position must be in line with the pull of the traction apparatus.

in motion or sensation since the previous observation. Comparison of current symptoms with those first exhibited provides an evaluation of response to therapy. It is important to note a change in symptoms when the client is removed from traction.

Postoperative Nursing Management

Nursing interventions after spinal surgery include:

- Monitor vital signs.
- Perform hourly deep breathing exercises while awake, but avoid forced coughing because it increases pressure within the spinal canal.
- Examine the dressing for CSF leakage or bleeding.
- Assess neurovascular status (color, temperature, mobility, and sensation) in extremities below the area of surgery, which may be caused by edema or hemorrhage at the operative site.
- Report an inability to void or an output of less than 240 mL in 8 hours.
- Use a fracture bed pan.
- For unique nursing responsibilities for other types of spinal surgery, refer to Nursing Guidelines 46–3.

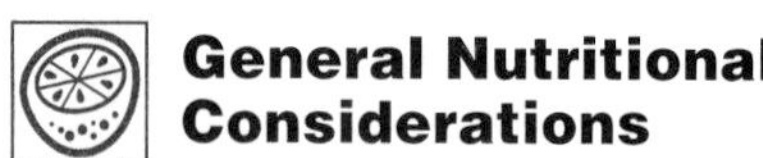

General Nutritional Considerations

Extended immobility accelerates calcium loss from bone leading to hypercalcemia. Symptoms include nausea, vomiting, anorexia, abdominal pain, constipation, polyuria, polydipsia, calcium renal stones, headache, and lethargy. Diet interventions help relieve symptoms but cannot prevent or treat the altered calcium metabolism. For instance, a high fluid intake of up to 3L/d helps keep the urine dilute to prevent the precipitation of calcium renal stones.

Thirst may not be a valid indicator of need in clients who are immobilized, and clients on a bladder rehabilitation program may be reluctant to drink liquids, fearing "accidents." Counsel the client on the importance of adequate fluid taken at regular, specified intervals. Likewise, assure clients participating in bowel training that a high-fiber diet (whole grains, legumes, fruits, vegetables) aids in normalizing bowel movements.

Tetraplegics and paraplegics have lower calorie requirements due to reduced energy expenditure; adjust calorie intake to avoid excessive weight gain. However, nutrient needs are stable or higher, depending on the development of complications. For instance, prolonged immobility promotes nitrogen excretion, resulting in a higher protein requirement. Clients with skin breakdown have increased requirements for protein (meat, milk, supplements), vitamin C (citrus fruit and juices, strawberries, "greens," tomatoes), and zinc (meat, seafood, milk, egg yolks, legumes, and whole grains) to promote healing.

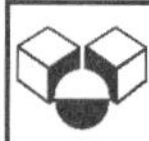

Nursing Guidelines 46-3

Nursing Care Following Specific Spinal Surgeries

Postcervical Diskectomy

- Keep a cervical collar in place at all times; do not remove without physician's order.
- Instruct to keep the neck straight in midline position until healing occurs.
- Support the head, neck, and upper shoulders when moving from a lying to sitting to standing position or when getting into and out of a chair.
- Observe for Horner's syndrome, a complication following anterior cervical diskectomy from cervical sympathetic nerve damage, manifested by lid ptosis (drooping), constricted pupil, regression of eye in the orbit, and lack of perspiration on one side of the face.

Postlumbar Laminectomy or Diskectomy with Spinal Fusion

- Logroll when turning every 2 hours; maintain alignment at all times.
- Caution the client to avoid turning self.
- Teach the client to avoid:
  Twisting or jerking the back
  Sitting during the first week
  Prolonged sitting thereafter; use a straight backed chair and do not slump.
  Bending from the waist; bend from the knees and hips.

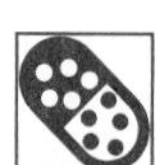

General Pharmacologic Considerations

An osmotic diuretic such as mannitol may be prescribed for the reduction of intracranial pressure after intracranial surgery. The mannitol vial is inspected prior to use. If the solution contains crystals, the container is warmed in hot water and shaken vigorously. The drug is not administered if crystals are present in the solution.

Because the respiratory depressant effects are less, codeine may be prescribed for postoperative pain after intracranial surgery.

Body temperature is monitored closely after intracranial surgery. Temperature elevation is relieved with an antipyretic and other measures because hyperthermia increases brain metabolism, resulting in brain damage.

Clients given a skeletal muscle relaxant or tranquilizer for a herniated intervertebral disk, back strain, or spasms of the back muscles may experience drowsiness and dizziness. They must be assisted with ambulatory activities.

Clients with impaired swallowing may have difficulty taking pills or capsules. Whenever possible, give medications in liquid form.

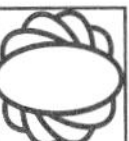

General Gerontologic Considerations

Elderly clients often respond less favorably to therapies for a neurologic deficit.

The elderly client has a tendency to drink less water and, therefore, may incur a chronic fluid volume deficit. Encourage fluid intake of 1,500 to 2,000 mL/d (if physical condition permits).

SUMMARY OF KEY CONCEPTS

- With a concussion, there is temporary loss of cerebral function with no damage to cerebral tissue. Recovery is complete in a short time.
- In a contusion, bruising and hemorrhage of superficial cerebral tissue occur. Cerebral edema can occur at the site of injury.
- An epidural hematoma is caused by arterial bleeding and occurs on top of the dura. This condition is a true surgical emergency. The nurse must make rapid neurologic observations to recognize changes in vital signs and level of consciousness and signs of increased intracranial pressure.
- A subdural hematoma occurs as a result of venous bleeding in the space below the dura. Bleeding is slower than that with an epidural hematoma.
- A simple skull fracture is a break in the continuity of the bone without displacement of bone. In a depressed skull fracture, the broken bone is pushed inward, injuring the underlying cerebral tissue. A basilar fracture causes edema of the brain near the origin of the spinal cord and can injure the nerves of the spinal cord.
- Nursing management of the client with a head injury involves neurologic examinations: level of consciousness, motor and sensory status, pupillary response, vital signs, seizure activity, signs of increased intracranial pressure; look for the halo sign on wound dressings.
- Craniotomy is the surgical opening of the skull to access the structures below the cranial bones. Craniectomy is the removal of a portion of the skull. Cranioplasty is the repair of a defect in the skull.
- Spinal cord trauma can lead to bleeding within the cord where it forms a hematoma that compresses the nerve roots. An injury to the cord can sever the spinal cord nerve fibers; complete severance results in permanent paralysis and loss of sensation below the site of the injury.
- Spinal shock is a sudden depression of reflex activity below the level of injury. Pronounced hypotension, bradycardia, decreased respiratory rate, decreased temperature, flaccid paralysis and warm, dry skin occur. If the level of injury is in the cervical or upper thoracic region, respiratory failure can occur.
- Autonomic dysreflexia is an acute emergency and is seen in clients with a cervical or high thoracic spinal cord injury, usually after spinal shock subsides. It is caused by a full bladder, paralytic ileus, or impacted fecal mass.
- Nursing management of the client with a spinal cord injury includes assistance with breathing, pain management, mobility, and coping.
- Procedures for relieving spinal nerve root compression include diskectomy, laminectomy, diskectomy with spinal fusion, and chemonucleolysis.
- Pressure on spinal nerve roots can be caused by trauma, a herniated intervertebral disk, and tumors of the spinal cord and surrounding structures.
- Nursing management of a client with spinal nerve root compression includes pain control, traction, and measures to combat effects of immobility.

CRITICAL THINKING EXERCISES

1. A man involved in a motor vehicle accident is brought to the emergency department. You are informed that he was not wearing a seat belt and struck his head on the steering wheel. What neurologic assessments would you make and why?
2. You are caring for a paraplegic client. What signs and symptoms suggest that the client is experiencing autonomic dysreflexia? What nursing measures are appropriate?

Suggested Readings

Bicycle helmets and safety. (1997). *Lippincott Health Promotion Letter, 2*(5), 5, 10.

Blank-Reid, C., & Reid, P. C. (1997). Action stat. Traumatic fall. *Nursing, 27*(5), 33.

Centers for Disease Control and Prevention. (1997). Sports-related recurrent brain injuries—United States. *International Journal of Trauma Nursing, 3*(3), 88–90.

Edwards, P. A. (1996). Health promotion through fitness for adolescents and young adults following spinal cord injury. *SCI Nursing, 13*(3), 69–73.

Grossman, S. (1997). How can nurses use limit setting to facilitate spinal cord patients' independence? *SCI Nursing, 14*(3), 105–107.

Huston, C. J., & Boelman, R. (1995). Emergency: Autonomic dysreflexia. *American Journal of Nursing, 95*(6), 55.

Johnson, C. C. (1995). After a brain injury: Clearing up the confusion. *Nursing, 25*(11), 39–45; quiz 47–48.

Johnson, L. H., & Roberts, S. L. (1996). Hope facilitating strategies for the family of the head injury patient. *Journal of Neuroscience Nursing, 28*(4), 259–266.

Mattice, C. (1995). Consult stat. Alert patients with a concussion to future problems...post-concussion syndrome. *RN, 58*(6), 58.

Miller, T. W., & Geraci, E. B. (1997). Head injury in the presence of alcohol intoxication. *International Journal of Trauma Nursing, 3*(2), 50–55.

Monti, E. J., Bender, C., & Kerr, M. E. (1995). Monitoring neuromuscular function. *Journal of Neuroscience Nursing, 27*(4), 252–257.

Quigley, P., & Veit, N. (1996). Interdisciplinary pain assessment of spinal cord injury patients. *SCI Nursing, 13*(3), 62–68.

Sexuality and the spinal cord injured. (1997). *Lamp, 54*(9), 5–6.

Additional Resources

National Association of the Physically Handicapped
4230 Emerick
Saginaw, MI 48603
(517)779-3060
http://www.saginawvalley.com/csdir/WWW0763.HTM

National Spinal Cord Injury Association
8300 Colesville Rd.
Silver Spring, MD 20910
(301)588-6959
http:www.erols.com/nscia

Chapter 47

Caring for Clients With Neurologic Deficits

KEY TERMS

Credé's maneuver
Cutaneous triggering
Neurologic deficit
Reflex incontinence

LEARNING OBJECTIVES

On completion of this chapter, the reader will:

- Define the term neurologic deficit.
- Describe three phases of a neurologic deficit.
- Give the primary aims of medical treatment of a neurologic deficit.
- Name six members of the health care team involved with the management of a client with a neurologic deficit.
- Discuss the nursing management of a client with a neurologic deficit.

The client with a neurologic deficit is faced with many problems. A **neurologic deficit** occurs when one or more functions of the central and peripheral nervous systems are decreased, impaired, or absent. Examples of neurologic deficits include paralysis, muscle weakness, impaired speech, inability to recognize objects, abnormal gait or difficulty walking, memory impairment, impaired swallowing, or abnormal bowel and bladder elimination. Often, more than one body system is affected. The client may be unable to walk, talk, do simple tasks like feeding and bathing, or recognize family members. Many members of the health care team are involved with the complex management of the client with a temporary or permanent neurologic deficit. These members include the physician, nurse, nursing assistant, social worker, physical therapist, occupational therapist, speech therapist, prosthetist, psychotherapist, dietitian, pharmacist, and vocational counselor. With intensive therapy and a coordinated approach by all members of the health team, many clients have the potential to return to normal or near normal function or successfully adapt to the changes in function.

Phases of a Neurologic Deficit

Neurologic deficits are divided into three phases: acute, recovery, and chronic. Not all individuals with a neurologic deficit experience all three phases. Some individuals' problems begin with an acute phase and move into a recovery phase, followed by a lifelong chronic phase. Other individuals' deficits begin with the chronic phase.

Acute Phase

The acute phase occurs after a sudden neurologic event, such as a cerebrovascular accident (CVA) or a head or spinal cord injury. During the acute phase, the client is usually critically ill. Many signs and symptoms may be present, such as altered level of consciousness (LOC), hypertension or hypotension, fever, difficulty breathing, or paralysis.

MEDICAL AND SURGICAL MANAGEMENT

The focus of management during the acute phase is to stabilize the client and prevent further neurologic damage. The client with a CVA may require management of hypertension or hypotension by means of drug therapy or respiratory support by means of mechanical ventilation. Clients with a head or spinal cord injury may require surgical intervention to stabilize the injured area or remove bone fragments, blood clots, or foreign objects. Sometimes, surgery may be postponed until the client is stabilized and the acute phase has passed. For others, surgery is performed during the acute phase as a lifesaving measure.

NURSING MANAGEMENT

Perform frequent and thorough neurologic assessments to evaluate the client's status, need for additional medical or surgical interventions, and response to treatment. Use the Glasgow Coma Scale (see Chap. 43) or other assessment tools to record observations. Report any changes immediately to the physician. Assess vital signs as often as necessary; maintain the blood pressure to ensure adequate cerebral oxygenation. Measure intake and output, and observe the client for signs of electrolyte imbalances and dehydration. Report a urinary output of less than 500 mL/day or urinary or bowel incontinence.

Beginning basic rehabilitation during the acute phase is an important nursing function. Measures such as position changes, prevention of skin breakdown and contractures are essential aspects of care during the early phase of rehabilitation. The nursing goal is to prevent complications that may interfere with the client's potential to recover function. (See Nursing Process: The Client With a Neurologic Deficit for additional nursing management.)

Recovery Phase

The recovery phase begins when the client's condition is stabilized. This phase may begin several days or weeks after the initial event and lasts weeks or months.

MEDICAL AND SURGICAL MANAGEMENT

Medical management during the recovery phase is aimed at keeping the client stable and preventing or treating complications, such as pneumonia, and further neurologic impairment.

NURSING MANAGEMENT

During recovery, a rehabilitation program is planned. A successful rehabilitation program includes all members of the health care team.

Rehabilitation is designed to meet the client's immediate and long-term needs and to create environmental changes that help the client adapt to the disability and fully use any remaining abilities. Even though deficits can be temporary, a prolonged period and enrollment in a rehabilitation program are often necessary before a client regains partial or full functions.

Members of the health care team recommend devices or procedures to prevent complications and enhance the client's remaining abilities. By means of continuous assessment and identification of the client's needs, the nurse plays an important role in rehabilitation. Devices that help a client walk, eat, groom, and perform other motor skills are recommended or devised to suit particular needs. Flotation pads for wheelchairs, walkers, sheepskin boots, and range-of-motion (ROM) exercises are examples of the many appliances and procedures used in rehabilitation. (See Nursing Process: The Client With a Neurologic Deficit for additional nursing management.)

Chronic Phase

For some clients, a neurologic deficit begins in the chronic phase, for example, the client with multiple sclerosis or Alzheimer's disease. In the chronic phase, the client shows little or no improvement, remains stationary, or becomes progressively worse. Physical and psychological rehabilitation is continued in the chronic phase to prevent complications such as pressure ulcers and muscle contractures.

MEDICAL AND SURGICAL MANAGEMENT

Medical management continues throughout the chronic phase of a neurologic deficit and uses a wide range of therapies and treatments, such as control of the blood pressure, physical therapy, dietary management, and the treatment of complications related to disuse and immobility. In some cases, surgery is performed to correct deformities or problems that have developed. Examples include muscle and skin grafts to close a pressure ulcer, surgery to correct a contracture deformity, or removal of a kidney stone (a complication of prolonged immobility).

NURSING MANAGEMENT

Clients in the chronic phase are often admitted to a hospital for treatment of complications. They also are transferred to a skilled nursing facility or long-term care facility when family members can no longer manage their care, or when the disease has become progressively worse so that skilled care is mandatory. Nursing management during the chronic phase focuses on the prevention of physical and psychological complications.

BOX 47-1 Additional Nursing Diagnoses for the Client With a Neurologic Deficit

- *Knowledge Deficit* (specify) related to cognitive limitation, lack of recall, misinterpretation of information
- *Impaired Memory* related to neurologic disturbances
- *Relocation Stress Syndrome* related to losses involved in decision to move, feeling of powerlessness
- *Altered Role Performance* related to change in ability to resume role
- *Caregiver Role Strain* related to complexity or amount of care needed
- *Chronic Confusion* related to cognitive changes
- *Powerlessness* related to inability to control situation, dependence on others
- *Hopelessness* related to feeling overwhelmed by prognosis
- *Ineffective Individual Coping* related to chronic stress
- *Diversional Activity Deficit* related to immobility, depression, withdrawal, inability to participate in social activities, monotonous environment
- *Individual, Ineffective Management of Therapeutic Regimen* related to insufficient knowledge of tests, treatments, home care management, other (specify)

NURSING PROCESS
The Client With a Neurologic Deficit

Assessment

To establish baseline data, obtain a thorough history including all symptoms and a medical and allergy history from the client or a family member. Perform a general neurologic assessment; note the extent of neurologic involvement and the physical capabilities and limitations. The initial assessment includes an evaluation of the airway, breathing, circulation, and LOC. Because neuromuscular and central nervous system disorders and spinal cord injury can affect bowel and bladder tone, auscultate the abdomen for bowel sounds and palpate the bladder for distention. Note ability to control bowel and bladder.

BOX 47-2 Family and Home Management Nursing Diagnoses

- *Impaired Home Maintenance Management* related to inability to care for self, inadequacies such as housing, care, financial resources (specify)
- *Impaired Adjustment* related to inability to accept the physical changes and impaired cognition
- *Impaired Social Interaction* related to aphasia, immobility
- *Social Isolation* related to immobility, lack of transportation, other (specify)
- *Altered Family Processes* related to changes in health status, disability of family member
- *Disabling Ineffective Family Coping* related to impaired ability to fulfill role responsibilities

Diagnosis and Planning

A multitude of nursing diagnoses are applicable for the client and family faced with a neurologic deficit (Boxes 47–1 and 47–2).

Nursing Diagnoses and Collaborative Problems	Nursing Interventions
Risk for Impaired Skin or Tissue Integrity related to immobility, incontinence, other factors (specify)	See Nursing Process: The Client With a Spinal Cord Injury in Chapter 46.
Goal: The client's skin will remain intact and free from infection.	Inspect all pressure points daily, keep skin clean and dry at all times. Massage bony prominences that blanch when pressure is relieved. Use a flotation mattress, sheepskin pads and other devices to relieve pressure when lying and sitting (Fig. 47-1).
	Change the client's position every 2 hours to prevent pressure ulcers
Risk for Disuse Syndrome related to musculoskeletal inactivity and neuromuscular impairment	Keep the extremities in alignment with pillows, trochanter rolls, and splints.

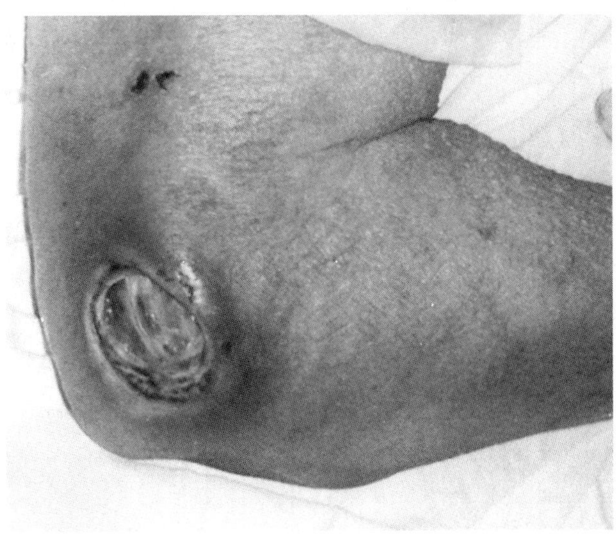

FIGURE 47-1. Pressure ulcer of the elbow in a client with a cerebrovascular accident cared for at home. This client was admitted to the hospital for treatment of multiple pressure ulcers. (Photograph by D. Atkinson)

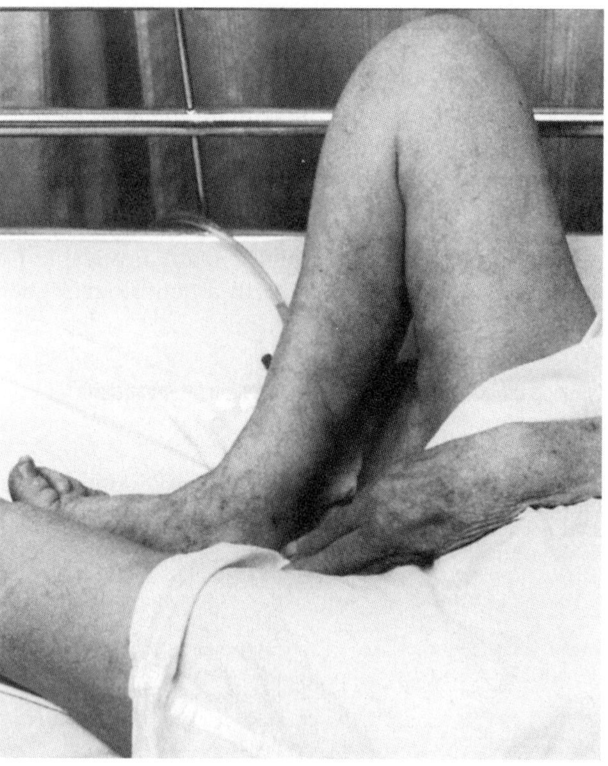

FIGURE 47-2. Contracture of the right leg in a client cared for at home after a cerebrovascular accident. (Photograph by D. Atkinson)

Goal: The client will maintain ROM in all joints.	Perform passive ROM exercises to the paralyzed extremity to prevent contractures. Contractures can result in permanent deformity (Fig. 47-2). Prevent footdrop with a footboard. Use elastic stockings to improve circulation; remove and reapply at least twice daily.
Constipation or Diarrhea (specify) related to prolonged immobility, tube feedings, decreased fluid intake, effect of disease or injury on the spinal cord nerves	Keep a daily record of all bowel movements. Avoid constipation by administering a stool softener and increased fluid intake. Institute a bowel training program (Nursing Guidelines 47-1).
Goal: The client will have regular bowel movements at least every 3 days.	Perform a digital examination of the rectum to assess for fecal impaction, a common cause of diarrhea. Add foods high in fiber to the diet. Give meticulous skin care when the client is incontinent. Discuss persistent diarrhea with physician. Inspect stool for a dark, tarry appearance and test for occult blood.
Urinary Incontinence or Retention related to effects of disease or injury on the nervous system or spinal cord nerves, loss of bladder tone.	Depending on the level of injury, an indwelling catheter or use of intermittent catheterization to empty the bladder may be needed on a permanent basis.
Goal: The client will void and/or the bladder will empty with no urinary retention.	Measure intake and output when the client has an indwelling urethral catheter, when the client takes fluids poorly, and when an indwelling urethral catheter is first removed. Palpate the lower abdomen for bladder distention. If distended, notify the physician. Use incontinence pads to absorb urine and keep the bedding dry. Give meticulous skin care when the client is incontinent of urine. Institute a bladder training program as soon as possible (Nursing Guidelines 47-2).
Impaired Physical Mobility related to muscle weakness, paralysis	Perform active or passive ROM exercises (Figs. 47-3 and 47-4) on the affected and unaffected extremities to prevent contractures and muscle atrophy. Encourage the client to perform ROM exercises independently.
Goal: The client is able to tolerate increased physical mobility as demonstrated by use of devices for mobility, and remains free of contractures.	Position paraplegic and tetraplegic clients in an upright posture at regular intervals.

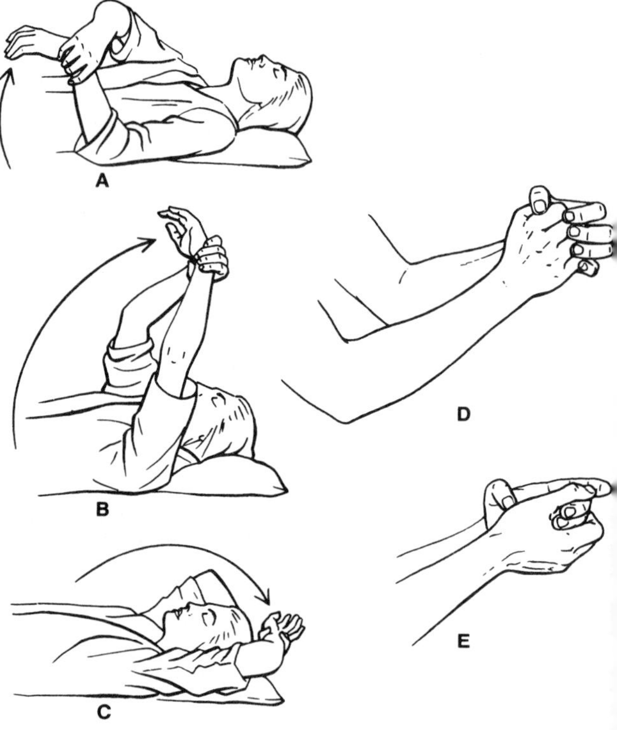

FIGURE 47-3. Exercises of the affected hand and arm that hemiplegic clients can learn to do themselves. (*A–C*) The affected arm is grasped at the wrist by the unaffected hand and is raised over the head. (*D* and *E*) The unaffected hand is slipped into the spastic hand, and each finger is extended slowly in turn.

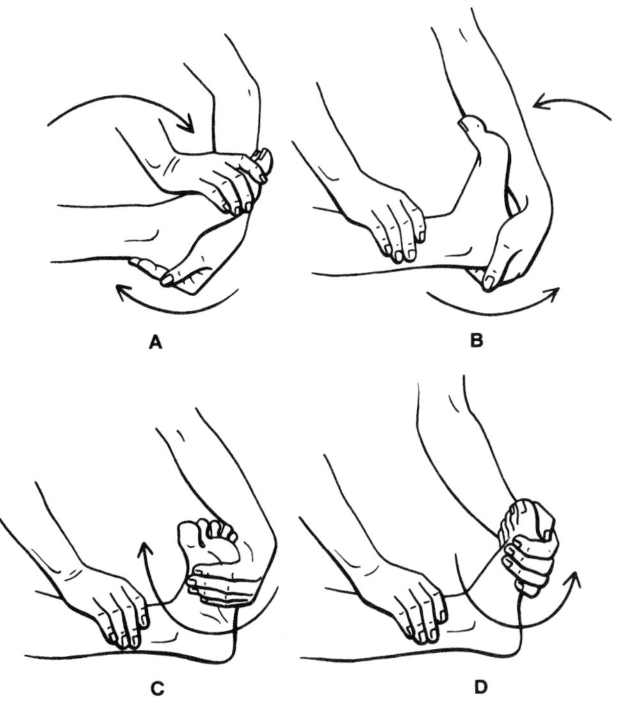

FIGURE 47-4. Range-of-motion exercises for the affected foot in hemiplegia. The motions should be conducted slowly and smoothly, with a momentary pause when spasticity causes resistance. As soon as the client has movement, these exercises can be done actively rather than passively.

	Apply an abdominal binder and elastic stockings before the client gets up to prevent dizziness and faintness.
	Suggest using parallel bars or a walker to support body weight (Fig. 47-5).
Risk for Altered Sexuality Patterns related to disturbance or loss of nerve supply to the genitalia **Goal:** The client will explore sexual alternatives.	Be alert to subtle references to sexual dysfunction or problem. Allow the client time to talk or ask questions. Convey acceptance and recommend that client and sexual partner speak with the physician or a sexual therapist. Explain to paralyzed males that spontaneous erections may occur when the bladder is full. However, because they are unpredictable and sometimes circumstantially inconvenient, offer information about penile implants (see Chap. 60). Inform paralyzed males that ejaculation is rare, which reduces the potential for fathering future children. Suggest to partners in which one is paralyzed that sexual activity is facilitated by having intercourse on a water bed to promote pelvic movement.

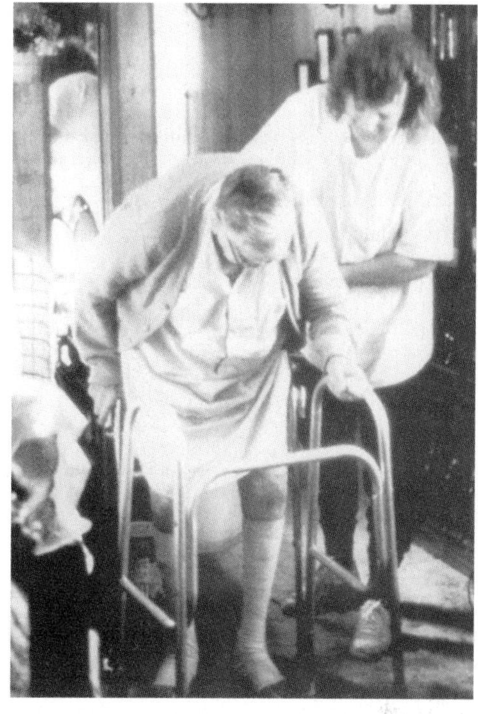

FIGURE 47-5. Ambulatory training in the physical therapy department is started as soon as the client is able to stand. (Photo courtesy of Visiting Nurse Association of Southwest Michigan)

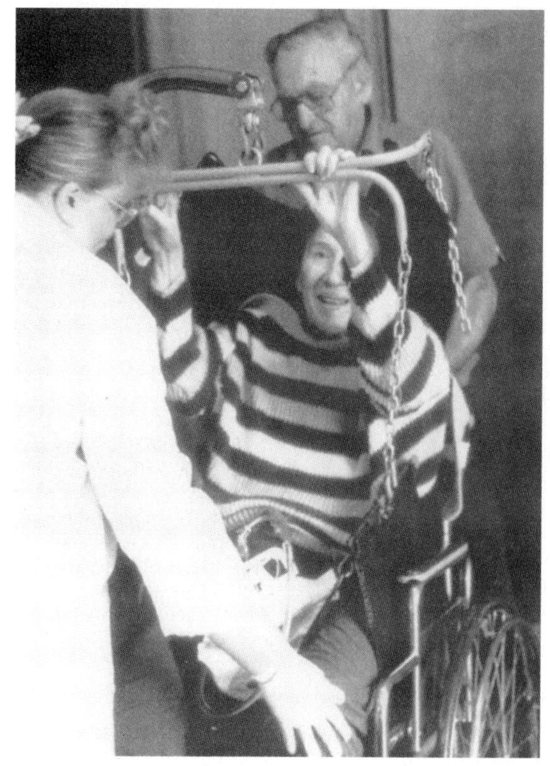

FIGURE 47-6. A Hoyer lift may be used to transfer a client to and from the bed, wheelchair, or shower. (Photo courtesy of Visiting Nurse Association of Southwest Michigan)

	Share that some couples use mutual masturbation or electronic vibrators during sexual activity.
	Instruct female clients that they are still fertile and may need contraception if a pregnancy is undesired.
Risk for Injury related to muscle weakness, paralysis, seizure disorder, loss of calcium from bone, other (specify) **Goal:** The client remains free from injury.	Use caution when moving and lifting a client who has been immobile. Use a Hoyer lift (Fig. 47-6) to safely transfer client. Prolonged immobility results in loss of calcium in the bone and increased susceptibility to fractures.
	Implement seizure precautions for clients with head injuries or brain tumors; see Nursing Process: The Client With a Seizure Disorder in Chapter 44, for more interventions.
Risk for Self-Concept Disturbance related to effects of disability on lifestyle **Goal:** The client will accept changes in body function, express feelings about the disability, and participate in rehabilitation.	Assess for signs of negative responses, such as refusal to discuss loss, lack of participation in care, and increased isolation. Consult health care team if such responses are observed.
	Convey respect, hope, and encourage verbalization of feelings.
	Help the client identify his or her positive attributes and strengths from past experiences.
	Identify ways to support the client's independence and role in the family. Discuss the client's support system.
Grieving related to loss of body function **Goal:** The client will progress through various stages of the grieving process in an adaptive manner.	Convey support and acceptance of client's feelings.
	Explain the grieving process as a natural progression of feelings leading to acceptance of the changes in lifestyle.
	Encourage the client to focus on positive strengths.
	Support grief work: explain denial; promote hope during depression; encourage adaptive outlets for anger; encourage decision making in all aspects of self care; focus on the present and future goals to promote the client's acceptance of the loss.

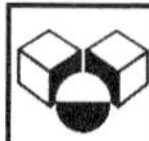

Nursing Guidelines 47-1

Implementing a Bowel Training Program

Some clients can achieve self-controlled emptying of the bowel provided they and those who care for them exert the persistent effort required to achieve this goal. Bowel control is typically easier to achieve than bladder control. For a bowel training program:

- Keep a record of bowel movements over a period of several weeks. This helps to determine the time of day the client is most likely to have a bowel movement.
- Encourage liquids throughout the day. Include foods that produce bulk, such as fresh fruits and vegetables, in the diet. Eliminate foods that cause loose stools.
- Assist the client to the bathroom at a certain time each day. The physical activity involved in getting out of bed often increases peristalsis and encourages defecation.
- Administer a low-volume enema or suppository each day at the same time to stimulate a bowel movement. Later, bowel function will become regulated so that the client can have a bowel movement at this time without these aids.

1. Tape the paralyzed client's buttocks together to keep a suppository in place. Remove the tape at the time the suppository is expected to work.
2. Give enemas slowly, about 1 to 2 oz followed by a waiting period to tetraplegic and paraplegic clients who are able to retain a sufficient amount of the enema solution.
3. Check the temperature of the enema solution immediately before administration. Insert the rectal tube gently, especially for clients who cannot feel because they are vulnerable to trauma.
4. Allow the client privacy and sufficient time to have a bowel movement.

Evaluation and Expected Outcomes

Expected outcomes vary, depending on the original goals and nursing diagnoses.

- No evidence of skin breakdown.
- Complications associated with inactivity and immobility do not develop.
- Defecation and urinary elimination are managed.
- The client is physically active, as demonstrated by use of trapeze, wheelchair, and other methods for mobility.
- The client continues sexual activities.
- No injuries occur.
- The client participates in decision-making regarding daily activities, social outlets, vocational options, and applicable therapies.
- The client and family accept disability.

Psychosocial Issues and Home Management

Leaving the inpatient setting where the daily, intensive support of the health care team is readily avail-

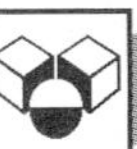

Nursing Guidelines 47-2

Implementing a Bladder Training Program

- Keep a record of the times the client voids over a period of several weeks to help establish patterns of voiding.
- Plan a schedule for voiding that is similar to the assessed voiding patterns.
- Encourage increased intake of fluids; people who remain relatively immobile for the rest of their lives are subject to bladder infections and calculus (stone) formation in the urinary tract.
- Advise the client to note any sensation (chilliness, lower abdominal discomfort, restlessness) that precedes voiding. This helps the client identify when there is a need to void.
- Encourage the client to void every 30 minutes to 2 hours while awake. If the client is able to use the bedpan or urinal, keep these readily available, and answer the call light promptly when assistance is required.
- Instruct the client to bend at the waist or press inward and downward over the bladder, a technique referred to as **Credé's maneuver.** This increases abdominal pressure and facilitates emptying the bladder.

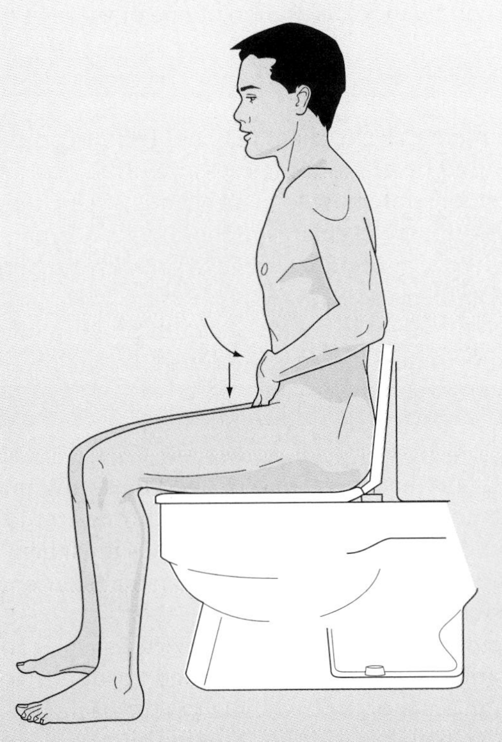

- Use other measures to stimulate voiding, such as running water and placing a hand in a basin of water.
- Propose that paralyzed clients with **reflex incontinence,** which occurs spontaneously when the bladder is full, lightly massage or tap the skin above the pubic area, a method known as **cutaneous triggering** that stimulates relaxation of the urinary sphincter.

able and returning home with a life-altering disability can be tremendously frightening. The client and family need additional support to adapt to a new lifestyle. Although many clients recover sufficiently to assume responsibility for some aspects of their own care, others do not. The burden of care often falls on the spouse who may have physical problems as well, or the adult children, who may not be available or willing to share this responsibility.

Financial resources are strained during a lengthy hospitalization and may continue after discharge. Adapting the home to accommodate a wheelchair or special bed can be costly. Wide doorways, ramps instead of stairs, special fixtures in the bathroom for bathing and toileting are examples of changes that are often necessary. The client may have been the major wage earner. Some clients are able to enter a training program that allows them to find employment outside the home, whereas others learn a skill that enables them to be employed at home. Others, because of age or extreme physical disability, are not able to be gainfully employed.

Nursing Management

Listen and be alert to subtle hints given by the client or family and ask questions to identify their problems and needs. Evaluate the client's ability to perform self-care, to resume his or her role in the family, and to call on a support system. Take appropriate steps to help the client and family attain and maintain a home life as near normal as possible. Assess the available facilities, the family support system, physical aids required (eg, a wheelchair, cane, or walker), and the amount of assistance required with activities of daily living when planning home care. Encourage the family to help plan for the client's return home, to ask questions about care, and to seek assistance from those agencies that can provide emotional, physical, and financial support.

COPING

Address each client in an individual manner. Offer reassurance and emotional support and display understanding of the multiple problems faced by the client. Many clients have difficulty coping with their disability. Crises such as being unable to move, having limited movement, being unable to attend to one's most basic needs, and having to totally depend on others for housing, clothing, mobility, and food creates strong emotional responses. Some clients eventually accept their disability; others do not. Offer encouragement and praise during rehabilitation and show personal interest and pleasure in each accomplishment, no matter how small, to help clients accept what they cannot or never will be able to do.

Give clients time to talk about their problems, fears, and concerns. Once needs are identified, encourage the client to set attainable goals, which may help maintain independence as long as possible. Work with the client and family to develop solutions and possible alternatives. This helps the client and family meet each problem as it arises, understand the limitations, establish goals, and work toward a solution.

With rehabilitation comes the client's awareness of progress or lack of progress. At times, improvement is slow and barely noticeable. A client often has difficulty coping. Discouragement, depression, withdrawal, and anger are not unusual. Suggest available support groups for those with neurologic deficits. Encourage contact with a support group for emotional, physical, and social support.

SOCIALIZATION

As soon as clients are able to respond to those around them, encourage socialization with others. At first, socialization can be limited to health team members and family. Encourage the family to talk to the client, discuss current events, and motivate the client to respond. Those with speech difficulties tend to become withdrawn and depressed. Encourage visitors to talk to the client, include the client in their conversations, and ask the client questions. Suggest to family members to use patience when trying to understand what the client is trying to communicate.

Occupational and recreational therapies are part of the rehabilitation program and require a team effort. In the beginning, occupational therapy is designed to help strengthen muscles that are under voluntary control. Later, certain tasks may be learned or relearned to help the client interact with others. Participation in these therapies increases socialization time and helps the client interact with others.

FAMILY PROCESSES

Recognize the family faces many disruptions because of the permanent disability of a family member. Lifestyles are altered, financial resources are strained, conflicts arise, and people must accept new responsibilities. Allow the family time to deal with and accept these changes. Provide a chance to talk and openly express their anger, fears, guilt, and helplessness. Although no single perfect solution to any problem exists, the following may help the family adjust to present and future changes:

- Include the family in the client's rehabilitation.
- Give encouragement and praise when a family member is able to help with a part of home care or shows interest in becoming involved in the client's care.
- Explain the purpose of each segment of rehabilitation (eg, ROM exercises, positioning).
- When the family expresses a desire to assume responsibility for certain procedures to be performed at home, teach each procedure or task slowly and give the family time to practice under supervision.
- Prepare a list of public or private agencies that may assist with home care, transportation, and financial and emotional support.

CLIENT AND FAMILY TEACHING

Develop a teaching plan for home care management that incorporates the therapies prescribed by the physician and other members of the team. The client and family usually have many questions. Begin teaching long before discharge so that the client and family have sufficient time to learn and understand home care management. The individualized teaching plan will include discussion of one or more of the following:

Skin Care

- Explain that the client may not feel discomfort caused by a beginning pressure ulcer.
- Demonstrate how to inspect and care for the skin.
- Recommend a change in the client's position at least every 2 hours to relieve pressure on bony prominences.
- Tell the client to contact a health care provider immediately if skin is reddened, warm, or disrupted.

Maintaining Body Alignment

- Explain the importance of good body alignment.
- Demonstrate how to put joints through a full ROM. Explain that ROM exercises must be performed several times per day or as ordered by the physician or physical therapist.
- Demonstrate how various devices, such as rolled blankets or pillows, can be used to support or align areas of the body, such as the back, hips, and legs. Explain the use of a footboard or other type of device to prevent footdrop.

Nutrition and Fluids

- Discuss the importance of a high fluid intake to prevent urinary tract complications. Recommend taking fluids at frequent intervals.
- Discuss the importance of a balanced diet in maintaining optimal health.

- Emphasize that small meals and interval snacks may be better tolerated than three large meals.
- Explain that the client who must be fed needs time to chew the food and take fluids.

Bowel and Bladder

- Stress the importance of continuing a bowel and bladder training program.
- Demonstrate clean technique, which must be used when irrigating, changing, or inserting catheters at home.
- Advise inspecting the urine for cloudiness (which may or may not indicate a urinary tract infection), blood, and offensive odor.
- Recommend contacting the physician if chills and fever occur or if the urine is bloody, cloudy, or has an offensive odor.
- Describe skin care of the genitalia and perineum. Emphasize and demonstrate the special care that must be given to the anal area and the genitalia after defecation. If an external sheath is used for the male client, demonstrate its application and how to clean the penis daily to remove urine and dried secretions.

Activity

- Stress the importance of social contacts, hobbies, and changes in the daily routine to relieve boredom.
- Emphasize the importance of avoiding fatigue and exposure to infection.
- Discuss the importance of having the client take deep breaths every 1 or 2 hours while awake and to cough to raise secretions.

Therapies, Community Services, and Equipment

- Discuss the importance of working with the therapists and of following their advice about performance or practice of the therapies.
- Make the client and family aware of services available for home care.
- Discuss and list the specific types of equipment that will be necessary for home care.
- Provide the names of agencies or retail stores from which the equipment may be purchased, rented, or borrowed.
- Recommend a consultation with a social service worker for information regarding financial assistance or the availability of loan closets that allow people who need certain types of equipment to borrow these materials.

General Nutritional Considerations

Clients on a bladder rehabilitation program may be reluctant to drink liquids, fearing "accidents." Counsel the client on the importance of adequate fluid to maintain normal urine output and to help prevent the formation of renal stones. Participants in bowel training programs may avoid dietary fiber to decrease stools. Assure the client that adding fiber will aid in normalizing bowel movements.

Paraplegics and quadriplegics have decreased energy expenditures and, therefore, need to consume fewer calories to avoid excessive weight gain. Most nutrient requirements are not lowered. It is important that the diet contain nutrient-dense foods to be nutritionally adequate.

To help prevent or heal pressure ulcers, the diet should be high in protein (meat, fish, poultry, dairy products, eggs, commercial supplements), vitamin C (citrus fruits and juices, strawberries, "greens," broccoli, tomatoes), and zinc (meat, seafood, milk, egg yolks, legumes, and whole grains).

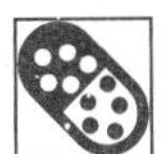

General Pharmacologic Considerations

Examples of suppositories used for a bowel training program are glycerin suppositories, which soften the stool in the lower rectum, and bisacodyl (Dulcolax), which stimulates peristalsis in the terminal section of the large colon. Enemas used in a bowel training program may be plain water, glycerin, and Fleet brand enema.

Clients with impaired swallowing often have difficulty taking pills or capsules. Whenever possible, medications are given in liquid form.

If a client must take solid medications at home, advise the family to check with their physician or pharmacist before crushing or breaking tablets or opening capsules; some medications must not be crushed or opened.

General Gerontologic Considerations

The older adult with a neurologic deficit may lack an adequate support system once he or she is discharged from the hospital. Involve social services and other agencies to assist the client and the caregiver with the rehabilitation process.

Functional problems that occur with age may complicate the recovery for a client with a neurologic deficit. For example, an age-related delay in the relaxation of the internal bladder sphincter can make bladder training more difficult.

Older adults cannot perform activities as fast or answer as quickly as younger adults. Therefore, they may become frustrated, irritable, or depressed when unable to respond quickly. To prevent feelings of frustration and depression, allow extra time for the older adult to answer questions, perform activities, and so forth.

At regular intervals, palpate the bladder of an older adult for distention. A behavior change or irritability may be the only sign of urinary retention in an older adult with a neurologic deficit.

SUMMARY OF KEY CONCEPTS

- A neurologic deficit has occurred when one or more functions of the central and peripheral nervous systems are decreased, impaired, or absent.
- Neurologic deficits may be arbitrarily divided into three phases: the acute, the recovery, and the chronic. Not all those with a neurologic deficit have all three phases. Some begin with an acute phase and move into a recovery phase, and then a lifelong chronic phase. Others begin with and continue in a chronic phase.
- The acute phase is usually seen in those who have had a sudden onset of a neurologic deficit, such as a CVA or a head or spinal cord injury. During the acute phase, the client is usually critically ill.
- The recovery phase begins when the acute phase is over and the client's condition is stabilized and may begin several days or weeks after the acute phase.
- In some clients, a neurologic deficit begins in the chronic phase, for example, the client with multiple sclerosis. In the chronic phase, the client shows little or no further evidence of improvement, and the neurologic deficit remains stationary or may become progressively worse.
- The primary aims of medical treatment of a neurologic deficit involves the use of drugs and various types of therapies to treat the original disorder, prevent and treat complications, and restore maximum sensory and motor function. Surgery may be necessary to rectify or treat the original cause or a complication of the deficit.
- Members of the health care team involved with the management of the client with a temporary or permanent neurologic deficit include the physician, nurse, nurse assistant, physical therapist, occupational therapist, speech therapist, prosthetist, psychotherapist, dietitian, pharmacist, vocational counselor, and social worker.
- Nursing management of a client with a neurologic deficit includes providing skin care to prevent breakdown and infection; assisting with ROM exercises; promoting regular bowel movements, bladder emptying, physical activity, and sexual health; and preventing injury.

CRITICAL THINKING EXERCISES

1. Discuss methods that help a client achieve success in a bowel and bladder training program.
2. A client had a CVA 6 months ago and has paralysis on his right side. He is unable to speak and shows signs of mental changes due to his CVA. He now appears agitated and is making motions with his left hand to various areas of his body, mainly his abdomen. What assessments could you make to determine the possible cause of his agitation?
3. A 22-year-old client had a spinal cord injury at T-11 and is a paraplegic. His depression and withdrawal are mentioned at a team conference. What other members of the health care team and services may be helpful in this client's care?
4. A client has multiple sclerosis. Within the past year, she has required a wheelchair and has limited use of her arms. She is admitted for a skin graft to a sacral pressure ulcer. What suggestions can you include in a plan of care to help her perform as much self-care as possible?

Suggested Readings

Brillhart, B., & Johnson, K. (1997). Motivation and the coping process of adults with disabilities: A qualitative study. *Rehabilitation Nursing, 22*(5), 249–252, 255–256.

Campion, K. (1996). Living with multiple sclerosis. *Community Nurse, 2*(9), 27–29.

Christensen, J. M., Martin, B. C., & Cook, E. A. (1997). Identifying denial in stroke patients. *Clinical Nursing Research, 6*(1), 105–118.

Donohoe, K. M., O'Brien, R. A., & Wineman, N. M. (1996). Are alternative long-term-care programs needed for adults with chronic progressive disability? *Journal of Neuroscience Nursing, 28*(6), 373–380.

Eliopoulos, C. (1997). *Gerontological nursing* (3rd ed.). Philadelphia: Lippincott-Raven.

Gauwitz, D. F. (1995). How to protect the dysphagic stroke patient. *American Journal of Nursing, 95*(8), 34–38.

Hickey, J. V. (1992). *The clinical practice of neurological and neurosurgical nursing* (3rd ed.). Philadelphia: J. B. Lippincott.

Johnson, J., McDivitt, L., & Pearson, V. (1997). Stroke rehabilitation: Assessing stroke survivors' long-term learning needs. *Rehabilitation Nursing, 22*(5), 243–248.

Kirk, P. M., Thomas, P., Bourjaily, J., Temple, R., & King, R. B. (1997). Long-term follow-up of bowel management after spinal cord injury. *SCI Nursing, 14*(2), 56–63.

Krause, T. M. (1997). Case management through a multidisciplinary spinal evaluation. *Orthopedic Nursing, 16*(2 Suppl.), 46–50.

Pieper, B., & Weiland, M. (1997). Pressure ulcer prevention within 72 hours of admission in a rehabilitation setting. *Ostomy Wound Management, 43*(8), 14–18, 20, 22, passim.

Perry, S. H. (1997). Caring for Jason—one day at a time. *Nursing 27*(11), 46–48.

Shaw, F. (1998). Continence—it's never too late. *Nursing Times, 94*(6), 68–70, 72.

Stuifbergen, A. K., & Rogers, S. (1997). Health promotion: An essential component of rehabilitation for persons with chronic disabling conditions. *Advances in Nursing Science, 19*(4), 1–20.

Timby, B. K. (1996). *Fundamental skills and concepts in patient care* (5th ed.). Philadelphia: J. B. Lippincott.

Vanetzian, E. (1997). Learning readiness for patient teaching in stroke rehabilitation. *Journal of Advanced Nursing, 26*(3), 589–594.

Vernon, S., & Bleakley, S. (1997). A successful bladder retraining program. *Nursing Times, 93*(38), 50–51.

Additional Resources

National Association of the Physically Handicapped
76 Elm Street
London, OH 431140
(614) 852–1164

Association for Rehabilitation Nurses
2506 Gross Point Road
Evanston, IL 60201
(847) 475–7300

National Association of Rehabilitation Facilities
5530 Wisconsin Avenue
Suite 955
Washington, DC 20015
(301) 654–5882

National Rehabilitation Association
633 South Washington Street
Alexandria, VA 22314
(703) 836–0850

P.R.I.D.E. Foundation (Promote Real Independence for the Disabled and Elderly)
1159 Poquonnock Road
Groton, CT 06340
(203) 447–7433

Information Center for Individuals with Disabilities
20 Park Plaza
Room 330
Boston, MA 02116
(617) 727–5540

11

Caring for Clients With Sensory Disorders

Chapter 48

Caring for Clients With Eye Disorders

KEY TERMS

Accommodation
Anterior chamber
Astigmatism
Cataract
Central vision
Conjunctivitis
Corneal transplantation
Corneal trephine
Diplopia
Emmetropia
Endophthalmitis
Enucleation
Glaucoma
Hordeolum
Hyperopia
Intraocular lens implant
Iridectomy
Keratitis
Keratoplasty
Myopia
Nystagmus
Ophthalmoscopy
Photophobia
Posterior chamber
Presbyopia
Refraction
Renal detachment
Tonometry
Trabeculoplasty
Uveitis
Visual acuity
Visual field examination
Visually impaired

LEARNING OBJECTIVES

On completion of this chapter, the reader will:

- Describe the basic anatomy and physiology of the eyes.
- Name and explain the four types of refractive errors.
- Differentiate between the terms blindness and visually impaired.
- List at least four nursing interventions appropriate when caring for a blind client.
- Discuss the nursing management of clients with eye trauma.
- Describe the technique for instilling ophthalmic medications.
- List seven infectious and inflammatory eye disorders and explain how they are acquired.
- Describe the visual change that results from delayed or unsuccessful treatment of macular degeneration.
- Differentiate between open-angle and angle-closure glaucoma.
- Name at least three categories of medications used to control intraocular pressure, and explain their mechanisms of action.
- Name a category of drugs that is contraindicated for clients with glaucoma.
- List three activities glaucoma clients should avoid because they elevate intraocular pressure.
- List three methods for improving vision after a cataract is removed.
- Discuss five postoperative measures that help prevent complications after a cataract extraction.
- Give two classic symptoms associated with a retinal detachment.
- Discuss the care and cleaning of an eye prosthesis.

Anatomy and Physiology

The eyeballs are globes located in a protective bony cavity of the skull. Fat and muscle protect the posterior, superior, inferior, and lateral aspects of each eyeball. The eyelids, eyelashes, and tears protect the exposed surface of the eye. The eyes (Fig. 48–1) are divided into the **anterior chamber**, which includes the structures of the cornea to the lens, and the **posterior chamber**, which contains the structures beyond the lens.

The cornea, the aqueous humor, the lens, and the vitreous body constitute the structures and media through which light passes for **refraction**, the bending of light rays to focus on the retina. The retina converts light to electrical energy that is then transmitted along the optic nerve to the occipital area of the brain where the image is perceived.

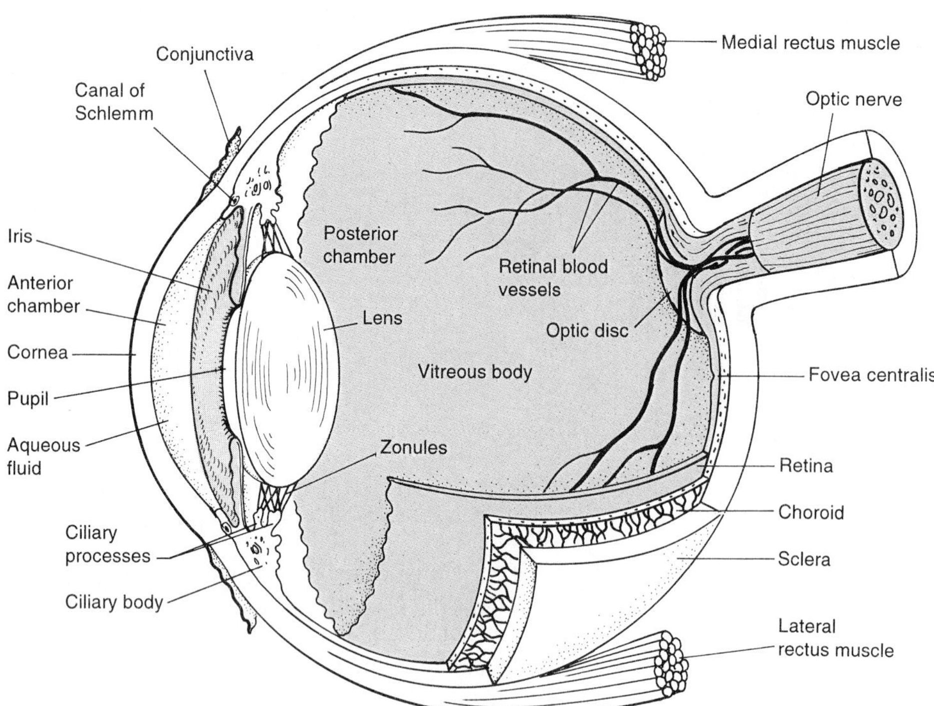

FIGURE 48-1. Transverse section of the eyeball. The cornea, aqueous humor, lens, and vitreous body are the refractive media.

The eyelids provide protection and adjust the amount of light entering the eye. They are lined with a sensitive mucous membrane called the *conjunctiva*. The eyelashes trap foreign debris. Periodic blinking clears dust and particles from the surface of the eyes.

Tears, composed of water, sodium chloride, and lysozyme, an antibacterial enzyme, are produced by *lacrimal* (tear) *glands* found beneath the bony orbital ridge. They flow across the eyes, continually bathing and lubricating the surface, and drain into the *nasolacrimal ducts*, tiny openings at the junction of the upper and lower lids, and then into the nose (Fig. 48–2).

Sclera, Choroid, and Retina

The layers of the eye are (1) the sclera, (2) choroid, and (3) retina. The *sclera* is the white outermost layer of the eye composed of tough connective tissue. The sclera protects structures within the eye. It connects directly to the dura mater that covers the brain. The optic nerve and retinal blood vessels enter the inner eye from an opening in the back of the sclera.

The middle layer, the *choroid*, contains blood vessels and darkly pigmented cells that prevent light from scattering inside the eye. The choroid gives rise to the *ciliary body*, which is composed of *ciliary processes* and the *ciliary muscle*. The ciliary processes produce *aqueous fluid*, a nutrient-rich liquid that nourishes eye structures. The ciliary muscle helps change the shape of the lens when adjusting to near or far vision.

The *retina*, the innermost layer of the eye, is composed of a pigmented outer layer and an inner neurosensory layer. The neurosensory layer is stimulated by light. It contains nerve cells called *rods*, which function in dim light, and *cones*, which function in bright light and are sensitive to color. The nerve cells of the retina are an extension of the optic nerve.

The *macula* and its yellow core called the *fovea centralis* lie in the center of the retina. It is easily identi-

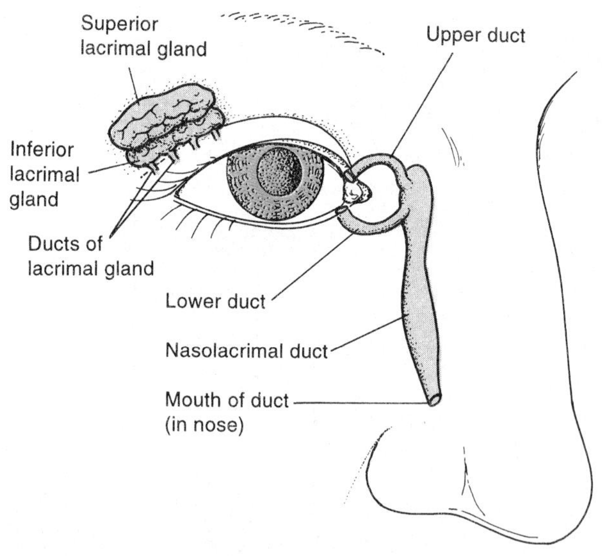

FIGURE 48-2. Lacrimal apparatus.

fied because there are no blood vessels radiating from it as there are in the *optic disc*, the anterior surface of the optic nerve (Fig. 48–3). The macula is the area of the eye that provides **central vision**, the ability to discriminate letters, words, and the details of any image. If the macula degenerates or is damaged, only the ability to see movement and gross objects in the peripheral fields of vision remains.

Cornea

The *cornea* is a transparent continuation of the sclera. Light passes undistorted through the aqueous fluid to the lens. The cornea contains no blood vessels but is nourished by aqueous fluid.

Iris and Pupil

The *iris* is the colored part of the eye. The iris controls light that reaches the retina. Circular and radial muscles in the iris contract in bright light and dilate in dim light. These muscles also are influenced by the autonomic nervous system and drugs such as atropine, which dilates the pupil, and pilocarpine, which constricts it.

The *pupil*, the black circle within the center of the iris, is not an actual structure. It is an opening that reflects the dark inner chamber of the eye.

Lens

The *lens* is a small, transparent, elastic structure that lies behind the iris. It is enclosed in a membrane called a capsule. The lens changes shape, called **accommodation**, when the ciliary muscles contract or relax to focus an image onto the macula. Aging results in loss of lens elasticity and makes the use of reading glasses for near vision necessary. When the lens becomes opaque, as when a cataract forms, light is blocked from reaching the macula and the visual image becomes blurred or cloudy.

Aqueous Fluid and Vitreous Body

Aqueous fluid is a watery substance that fills the anterior chamber of the eye. It maintains ocular pressure and nourishes the cornea, lens, and *vitreous body*. The vitreous body is a gelatinous substance in the posterior chamber of the eye that gives shape to the eye. Both substances are transparent, thus allowing light to pass through from the cornea and lens to the retina.

Schlemm's Canal

Schlemm's canal is a circular ring with multiple channels. Aqueous fluid moves through a filter, called the *trabecular meshwork*, and exits the eye through Schlemm's canal. This drainage system provides for outflow of aqueous fluid to the anterior ciliary veins that empty into the systemic circulation. Closure or blockage of any component within the system results in increased *intraocular pressure* (IOP; pressure within the eye).

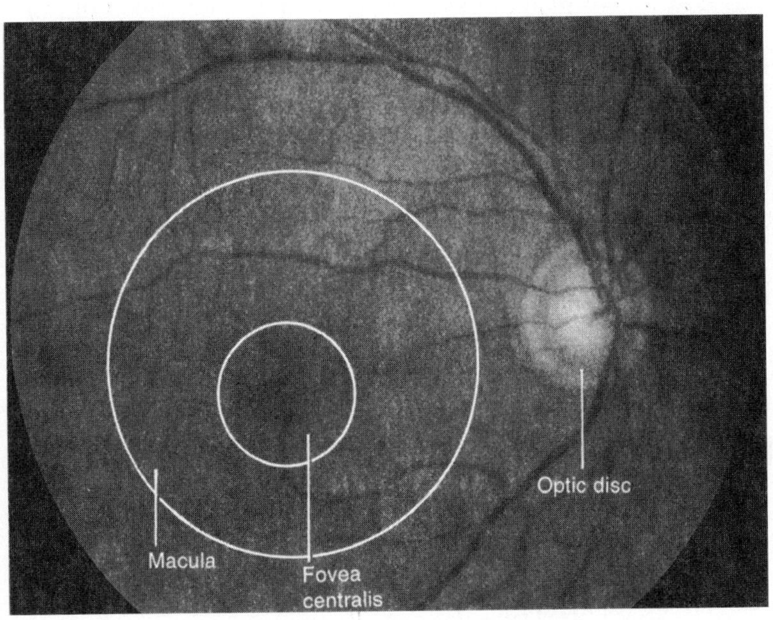

FIGURE 48-3. Within the anterior of the eye, the macula, fovea centralis, and optic disc can be seen.

Assessment

Vision Specialists

People with eye disorders use the services of a variety of professionals. An *ophthalmologist* is a physician who specializes in the medical and surgical treatment of eye diseases, including the prescription of corrective lenses. *Optometrists* are not physicians but test vision, prescribe, and fit corrective lenses. In some states they also do diagnostic tests. An *optician* takes the lens prescription written by an ophthalmologist or optometrist and makes eyeglasses or contact lenses that correct the client's vision. The optician ensures proper fit of corrective lenses.

Ophthalmoscopy

Ophthalmoscopy is the examination of the *fundus* or interior of the eye. This examination is done with a *direct ophthalmoscope*, an instrument that illuminates the internal surface of the eyes and allows the examiner to see the retina, retinal blood vessels, and the *optic disc* under magnification (Fig. 48–4).

Visual Screening Tests

The *Snellen eye chart* (Fig. 48–5) is a simple screening tool for determining **visual acuity**, the ability to see far images clearly. With the chart 20 feet away, the client is asked to identify letters of decreasing size.

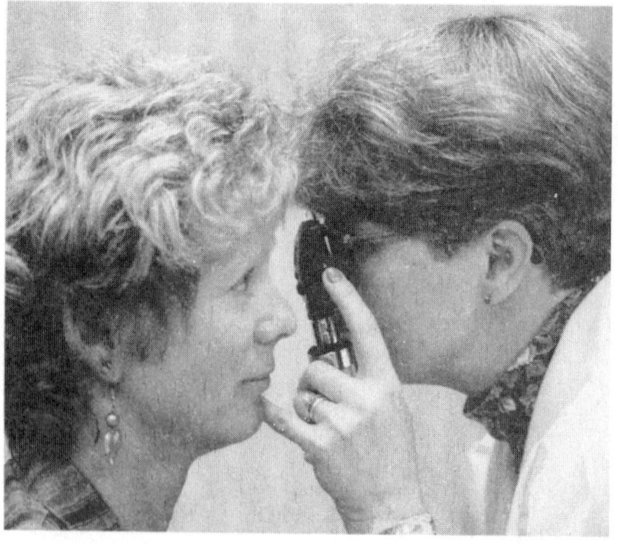

FIGURE 48-4. A nurse examines the interior of the eye with a direct ophthalmoscope.

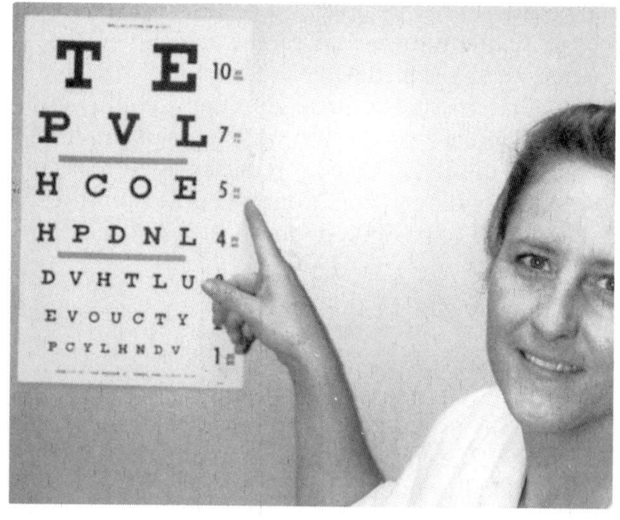

FIGURE 48-5. The Snellen chart is used to assess far vision.

Results are expressed as a fraction that compares the client's vision with standard norms. If a client has 20/20 vision, it means that the person sees letters at 20 feet that others see clearly and accurately at 20 feet; a person with 20/40 vision sees letters at 20 feet that most others can read at 40 feet and so on. If the client is unable to identify even the largest letters on the chart, he or she is asked to count the number of fingers held up by the examiner. If the finger count is inaccurate, the client's ability to distinguish light from dark is tested. Visual acuity also is measured with a computerized refractor that records the strength and type of lenses necessary to correct the client's visual problem.

A *Jaeger chart* evaluates near vision. It contains words, numbers and letters in various sizes of print. The client is instructed to hold the Jaeger chart approximately 14 inches away and read the smallest print that he or she can see comfortably. The size of the print the client reads indicates the quality of the client's near vision.

Color vision is assessed with *Ishihara plates*. The client is given a series of cards on which the pattern of a number is embedded within a circle of colored dots. The numbers are in colors that color blind individuals commonly cannot see. Individuals with normal vision readily identify the numbers.

Nursing Assessment

The nurse in the acute care, outpatient, or home setting performs a basic assessment of ocular health by obtaining:

- The client's description of vision changes, any visual or eye discomfort
- Use of glasses or contacts
- Use of prescription and nonprescription eye medication
- Previous eye trauma, ophthalmic and medical diseases, and surgery
- Family history of inherited eye diseases such as glaucoma
- Allergy history associated with seasonal **conjunctivitis** (inflammation of the conjunctiva) that often accompanies hay fever

After the interview, inspect the eyes for symmetry. Observe the lid margins for signs of inflammation, exudate, or loss of eyelashes.

Determine the pupil size, and their change and response to light. Normal pupils are round, of equal size, and constrict simultaneously when stimulated (Fig. 48–6). Check extraocular muscles by asking the client to keep his or her head still while following an object moved up, down, left, and right (Fig. 48–7).

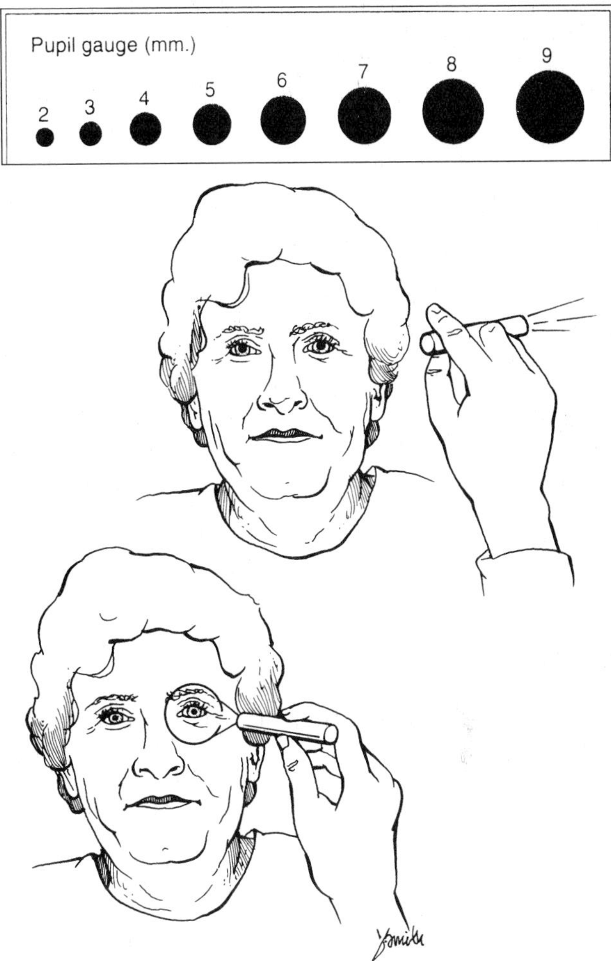

FIGURE 48-6. Assessing pupil response to light.

Diagnostic Studies

Retinoscopy

Use of a *retinoscope* and trial lenses determines the focusing power of each eye. A retinoscope is hand-held instrument that produces a line of light. The light appears distorted in the eyes of individuals with refractive errors. Trial lenses of varying refractive power are then placed in front of the eye until the light streak does not deviate in any direction.

Tonometry

Tonometry measures IOP. It is done by using a tonometer to indent the surface of the eye. The force that produces indentation is measured and converted to a pressure reading.

There are various methods for performing tonometry (Fig. 48–8). Applanation tonometry provides the greatest accuracy, but the hand-held Schiotz tonometer has the advantage of being small and portable. Before either is used, a local anesthetic solution, such as tetracaine or benoxinate with fluorescein (Fluress), is instilled in the eye. Anesthesia begins almost immediately and lasts a few minutes. The client does not feel the tonometer while the eye is anesthetized. A noncontact tonometer, although not as accurate, blows a puff of air against the cornea and no local anesthetic is required.

Visual Field Examination

A **visual field examination** measures peripheral vision and detects gaps in the visual field. The client fixes his or her gaze on a stationary point straight ahead. A light or white object is moved from a point on the side where it cannot be seen toward the center. The client indicates the point at which the stimulus is seen without directly looking at it. Certain disorders, such as glaucoma, a stroke, brain tumor, or retinal detachment, are associated with changes in the visual field.

Slit Lamp Examination

A *slit lamp* is a microscope that magnifies the surface of the eye. A beam of light, narrowed to a slit, is directed at the cornea, facilitating an examination of structures and fluid in the anterior segment of the eye. This examination is used to identify disorders such as corneal abrasions, iritis, conjunctivitis, and cataracts.

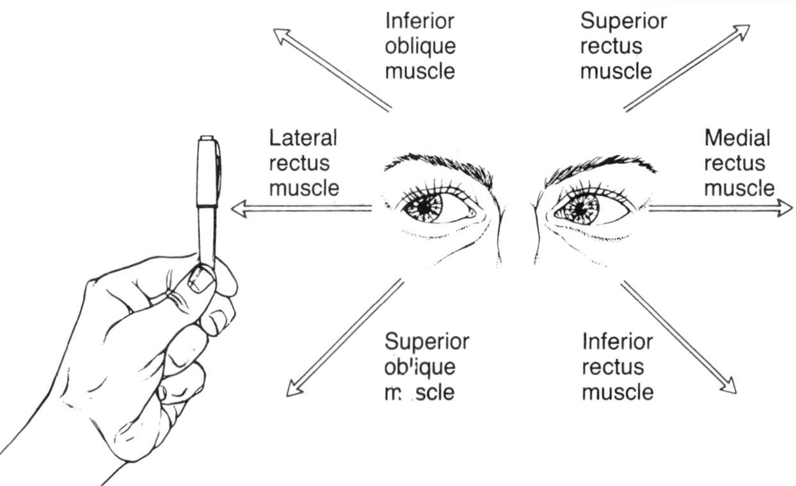

FIGURE 48-7. Assessing extraocular movements.

Retinal Angiography

Retinal angiography is used to detect vascular changes and blood flow through the retinal vessels. Sodium fluorescein, a water-soluble dye, is injected into a peripheral vein. The examiner uses a special camera to photograph the appearance and distribution of the dye in the retinal arteries, capillaries, and veins at 1-second intervals. The photographs provide a record of vascular filling and emptying defects. Many conditions affect retinal circulation, such as diabetes mellitus, hypertension, drug toxicity, tumors, and acquired immunodeficiency syndrome. Intravenous fluorescein causes skin to yellow slightly for 6 to 8 hours. The urine also turns bright yellow, but the color becomes less noticeable over the following 24 to 36 hours as the dye is excreted.

Ultrasonography

Ultrasonography is used when pathologic changes such as an opaque lens, cloudy cornea, or bloody vitreous make it difficult to look directly within the posterior of the eye. Using sound waves, the contour and shape of contents within the eye are imaged and recorded. After instillation of anesthetic ophthalmic drops, an ultrasound probe is placed on the cornea and a recording is made on an oscilloscope (Fig. 48–9). This technique is helpful in detecting eye le-

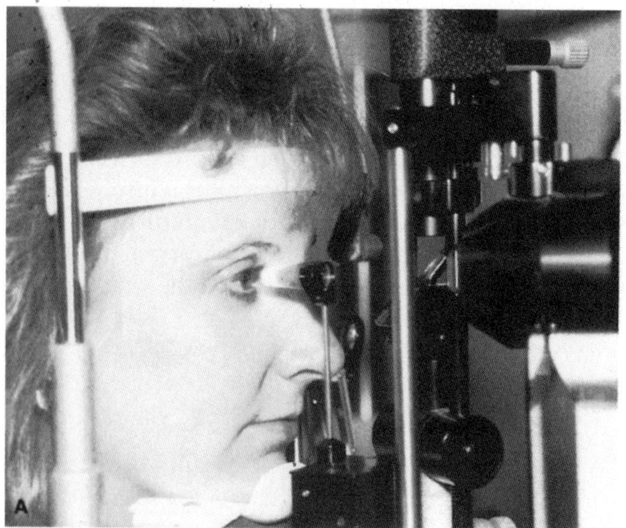

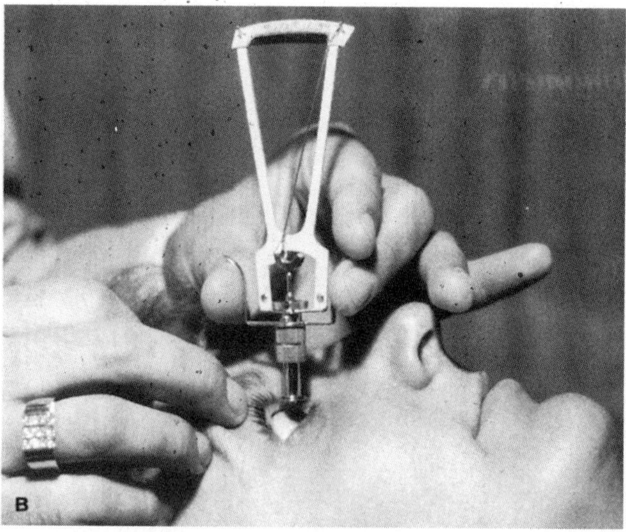

FIGURE 48-8. Intraocular pressure measured (*A*) with the Goldman applanation tonometer and (*B*) with the Schiotz tonometer.

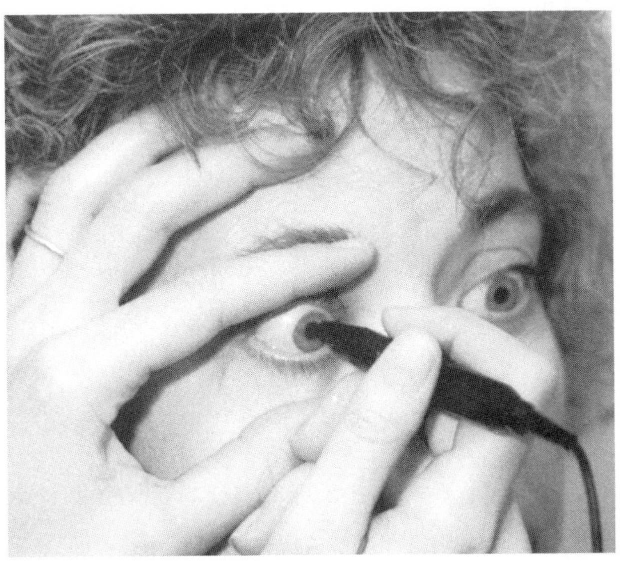

FIGURE 48-9. A transducer probe is placed on the cornea when performing an A-scan.

sions and measuring for an intraocular lens implant before extracting a cataract.

Impaired Vision

Refractive Errors

Emmetropia, or normal vision, means that light rays are bent to focus images precisely on the retina. In refractive errors, vision is impaired because light rays are not sharply focused on the retina (Fig. 48–10). Refractive errors include myopia, hyperopia, presbyopia, and astigmatism.

Myopia is nearsightedness. People who are myopic hold things close to their eyes to see them well. **Hyperopia** is farsightedness. People who are hyperopic see objects that are far away better than objects that are close. **Presbyopia** is associated with aging and results in difficulty with near vision. People with presbyopia hold reading material or handwork at a distance to see it more clearly. **Astigmatism** is visual distortion caused by an irregularly shaped cornea. Many people have both astigmatism and myopia or hyperopia.

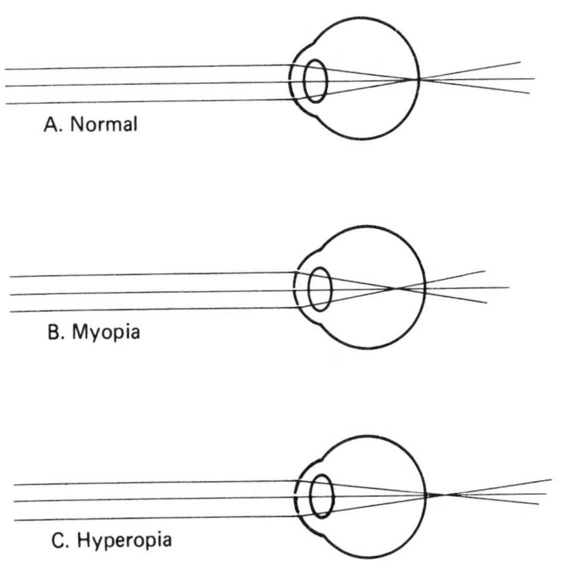

FIGURE 48-10. Ocular focusing of parallel light rays.

ETIOLOGY AND PATHOPHYSIOLOGY

Refractive errors such as myopia, hyperopia, and astigmatism are inherited or occur because of surgically treating disorders of the cornea or lens. Presbyopia occurs because of degenerative changes.

Myopia occurs in people with elongated eyeballs. Because of the excessive length of the eye, light rays focus in the vitreous body before they reach the retina. Hyperopia results when the eyeball is shorter than normal, causing the light rays to focus at a theoretical point behind the retina (see Fig. 48–10). Astigmatism results from unequal curvatures in the shape of the cornea. Presbyopia is caused by the gradual loss of elasticity of the lens, which leads to decreased ability to accommodate, or focus, for near vision. The loss of accommodation progresses gradually.

ASSESSMENT FINDINGS

Signs and Symptoms

People with refractive errors experience blurred vision. Some seek help for recurrent headaches caused by straining to see clearly.

Diagnostic Findings

Refractive errors are detected with the Snellen and Jaeger charts. During retinoscopy, the vision of myopes improves when concave-shaped trial lenses correct the focusing power of the eyes. Hyperopes experience improvement when convex-shaped lenses are used. The amount of power needed to improve visual acuity indicates the degree of refractive error. The refractive error is not always the same in both eyes.

MEDICAL MANAGEMENT

Refractive errors are usually corrected with eyeglasses or contact lenses. The lenses bend light rays to compensate for the refractive error. Not everyone can wear contact lenses; people with a history of recurrent eye infections, low tear production, or severe allergic reactions are more likely to have trouble with them.

SURGICAL MANAGEMENT

Incisional radial keratotomy (RK) is a surgical procedure used to correct refractive disorders. Under local anesthesia, the cornea is reshaped by making incisions. It is made flatter for clients with myopia and more cone-shaped for clients with hyperopia, enabling light rays to converge directly at the back of the retina. This procedure is not always successful. Complications include infection and increased glare from microscarring of the cornea. Some clients report a worsening of their vision after surgery. When successful, clients no longer need to wear corrective lenses. A similar procedure is performed using laser surgery.

NURSING MANAGEMENT

Nurses, especially those in pediatric offices, industrial sites, community school systems, and public health clinics, perform screening examinations and refer clients to diagnosticians. Nurses are instrumental in teaching clients how to care for their corrective lenses and remove and clean contact lenses (Nursing Guidelines 48–1).

Blindness

Blindness is a legal term for visual acuity of 20/200 or less even with corrective lenses. The term **visually impaired** is used to describe visual acuity between 20/70 and 20/200 in the better eye with the use of glasses. Many who are considered blind perceive light and motion. People with severe loss of visual field also are referred to as blind. Blindness can be congenital or caused by injury, a high fever that damages the optic nerve, or disorders such as cataracts, glaucoma, retinal detachment, and tumors.

MEDICAL MANAGEMENT

Vision is improved to its maximum extent with corrective lenses. Clients who are severely visually impaired or blind are referred to a rehabilitation center or other resource for supportive services. Blind or nearly blind clients are taught skills for independent living, how to use a cane for mobility, and how to read and write *Braille*, a system that uses raised dots to form letters of the alphabet and numbers. Some individuals use trained guide dogs.

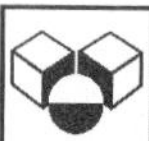

Nursing Guidelines 48-1

The Care of Eyeglasses and Contact Lenses

For Eyeglasses

- Clean eyeglasses daily or more often if needed with warm water and soap or detergent, or use a commercial glass cleaner.
- Rinse the glasses well and dry them with a soft, clean cloth.
- Do not use paper tissues because the wood pulp from which they are made can scratch the lenses.

For Contact Lenses

- Use a container that identifies the compartments for the right and left lens.
- Remove a soft lens by sliding it onto the sclera and grasping it between the thumb and forefinger.

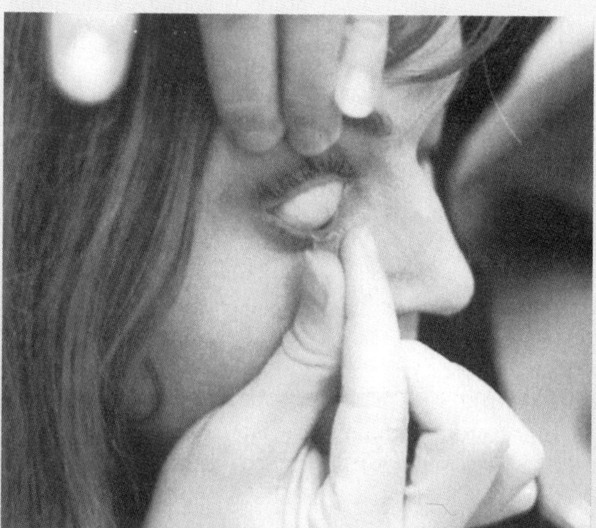

Removing a soft contact lens.

- Remove a hard lens by stretching the eyelid at the outer margin and blinking. Clients who cannot master this technique can remove the lens with a suction cup.
- Pour a small amount of cleaning solution into the palm, and rub the solution over the contact lens for 30 seconds on each side.
- Rinse and store the lens in a soaking solution.
- When replacing the lenses, wash hands and rinse the lens in normal saline solution.
- Drop wetting solution within the cup of a hard lens.
- Position the lens on the tip of the index finger and place the lens to the eye.
- To position a hard lens, gently close the eyelids or move the lens by manipulating it beneath the closed lid. To help center a soft lens, blink after its insertion.
- Wash soaking containers for hard lenses daily and allow them to drain dry. Once a day, usually in the evening, sterilize soft lenses in a heating unit. Also clean soft lenses weekly with an enzyme to remove protein deposits.

NURSING MANAGEMENT

Grief is a normal response to being newly blind or to having severely compromised vision. Anger or sadness are typical reactions as clients face the impact of their disability. The nurse helps and supports clients during depression. It is therapeutic to acknowledge the grief rather than attempt to cheer clients. Another helpful approach is to express confidence that the client has the inner resources to deal with the adversity.

One of the nurse's most important roles is to help the visually impaired client achieve independence. Whether the condition is temporary because both eyes are patched or permanent, the following measures are appropriate:

- Introduce yourself each time you enter the room because many voices sound similar.
- Call the client by name during group conversations because the blind client cannot see to whom questions or comments are directed.
- Speak before touching the client.
- Tell the client when you are leaving the room.

In addition, the care of a client who is blind or whose vision is severely impaired includes, but is not limited to, the following:

Nursing Diagnoses and Collaborative Problems	Nursing Interventions
Self-Care Deficit (specify areas) related to impaired vision **Goal:** The client will independently complete activities of daily living.	Ask the client's preference for where hygiene articles and other objects needed for self-care are stored. Keep personal care items in the same location at all times. Move food items from the tray to a larger surface area to facilitate locating food and eating utensils without accidental spilling or dropping. At mealtime, describe where food is on the plate using the positions on the face of a clock. Offer to open containers, butter bread, etc., to facilitate independence.
Risk for Injury related to compromised vision **Goal:** The client will remain free of trauma throughout care.	Orient the client to the physical environment. Indicate the location of the signal cord for obtaining nursing assistance. Keep doors fully opened rather than ajar. Help the client to feel where the door to the bathroom is located. Remove chairs or objects that are in the client's walking pathway. Instruct the client to grasp the nurse's elbow and walk slightly behind and to the side of the nurse when ambulating.
Risk for Impaired Home Maintenance Management related to unfinished rehabilitation, lack of assistance, and other factors (specify) **Goal:** The client will resume independent living.	Discuss the client's network of support who can help with shopping, banking, and transportation. Offer a home health nursing referral for the purpose of assessing the client's needs for a home aide that can help with household tasks.
Situational Low Self-Esteem related to impaired adjustment to loss of vision **Goal:** The client will redevelop a positive self-image.	Call attention to tasks the client successfully performs without assistance if the client focuses on self-pity. Help the client clarify those activities that are essential and then develop a plan for mastering each one. Review progress to nurture self-confidence, self-reliance, and improved self-image.
Altered Family Processes related to conflict in reversed roles **Goal:** The family will remain cohesive and supportive.	Encourage client and family members to verbalize their feelings. Promote a discussion of other life changes that were difficult but to which they eventually adjusted. Have each person share a list of inner strengths of the other to promote insight that regardless of roles, what each brings to the relationship remains unchanged.
Diversional Activity Deficit related to transition from sighted to nonsighted **Goal:** The client will develop interests in activities that contribute to the enjoyment and enrichment of life.	Refer the partially sighted client to the public library where large print editions of books and magazines are available, as well as "talking books" (recordings of printed books). Suggest that the partially sighted client use a magnifying lens to read. Contact or refer clients who can read Braille to special agencies (see Additional Resources at the end of this chapter) for books, Braille typewriters, and other assistive devices. Inform the client that optical scanners that use synthesized voice are available to "read" printed materials.

Tell the client that telephone companies exempt visually impaired customers from directory assistance charges and offer a "talking" yellow pages information service.

Instruct the client that laws prohibit the exclusion of patrons with guide dogs from public restaurants, public transportation, schools, and places for entertainment.

Eye Trauma

Trauma or injury to the eye and surrounding structures can result in a decrease or total loss of vision.

ETIOLOGY AND PATHOPHYSIOLOGY

Children and adults are subject to eye injuries from wind, sun, chemical sprays, direct blows to the eye, lacerations, and penetrating objects, such as fish hooks and bits of metal or wood. Cell and tissue injury cause an inflammatory response. Secondary infections may follow the initial injury. When trauma involves the cornea, scar tissue may affect the refraction of light. If the capsule that contains the lens is damaged, aqueous fluid and vitreous penetrate the lens, causing it to become an opaque cataract. Penetrating trauma can lead to **endophthalmitis**, a condition in which all three layers of the eye and the vitreous are inflamed; removal of the eye may be necessary.

ASSESSMENT FINDINGS

Signs and Symptoms

The injured eye is painful or described as feeling "gritty." There is tearing, and the client usually tries to relieve discomfort by squeezing the eyelids closed. The effort helps to control eye movement and reduces the light entering the eye. Vision may be blurred. If the bony orbit is fractured, the eyes may appear asymmetric and the client has **diplopia** (double vision).

A blow to or near the eye results in swelling and bleeding into soft tissues with ultimate discoloration (black eye) of the area. On inspection, hemorrhage may be observed in the subconjunctival tissue. The eye may appear to recede within the orbit, and there may be a change in the normal size or shape of the iris or pupil. Adjacent lid structures may be lacerated, bloody, and swollen (Fig. 48–11). Shining a penlight obliquely across the eye detects an obvious or obscured foreign body. Sometimes the upper lid must be everted to detect an object trapped beneath (Fig. 48–12). If treatment has been delayed, there may be

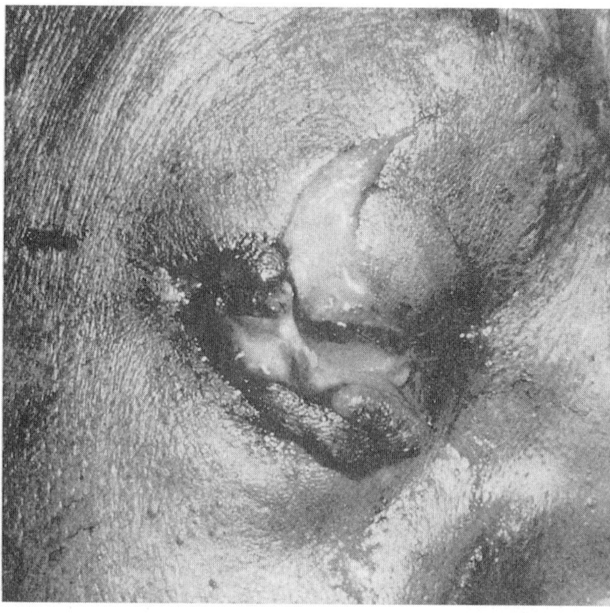

FIGURE 48-11. Severe eye lacerations. (Courtesy of Kalamazoo Ophthalmology, PC)

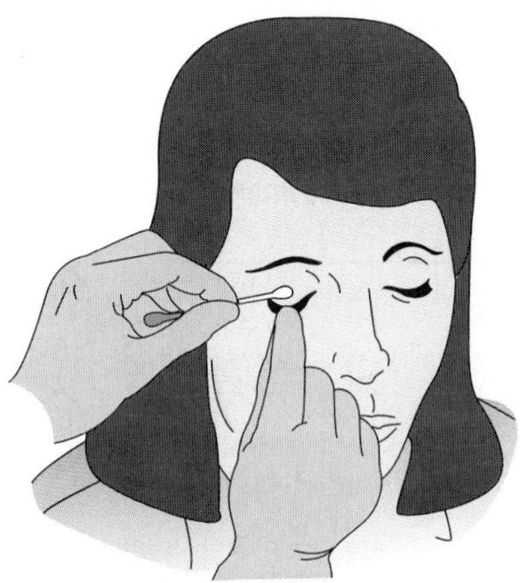

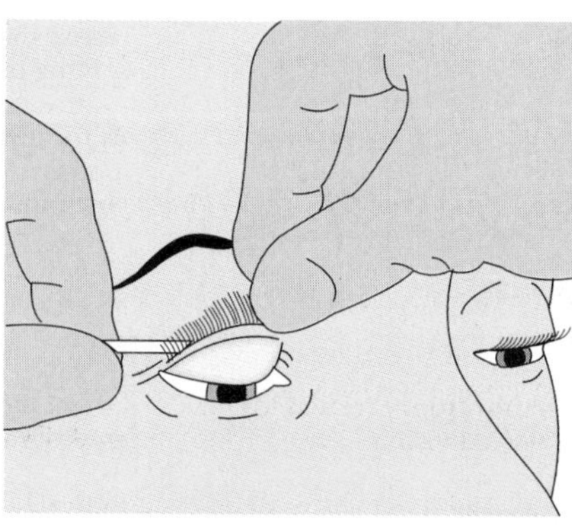

FIGURE 48-12. To evert the eyelid, the client looks down, and the eyelash is grasped and pulled up as a cotton-tipped applicator is pressed gently above the eyelid fold. The eyelid resumes its normal position when the client looks upward or the eyelash is pulled gently forward.

purulent drainage within the conjunctival sac. A rust ring is seen in retained foreign bodies that contain iron.

Diagnostic Findings

Staining the surface with fluorescein dye identifies a minute foreign body or abrasion to the cornea. A slit lamp examination provides magnification and light to visualize structures within the anterior and posterior segments. Radiography and computed tomography (CT) help find a penetrating foreign body. A radiograph confirms an orbital fracture.

MEDICAL AND SURGICAL MANAGEMENT

After emergency first aid is performed, the eye is anesthetized to ease examination. Antibiotic ointment or drops are instilled, and the eye is patched. Clients with blunt trauma are hospitalized to reduce the danger of intraocular complications. To repair a laceration of the eyelid, the physician injects a local anesthetic and the lid margins are approximated with sutures. A cut on the eyeball, especially the cornea, is serious and requires immediate treatment. Surgery is performed if internal eye structures are damaged.

NURSING MANAGEMENT

The nurse prevents eye trauma by recommending the use of glasses with shatter-resistant lenses or safety goggles while working with substances that can injure the eyes. When eye trauma occurs, a brief history of the type or cause of injury is obtained from the client or a family member. If eye pain is severe, or if the client is unable or unwilling to permit an initial examination, both eyes are loosely patched and the client is referred immediately for medical treatment. If a foreign body is present, pressure on the eye may push the object into the tissues of the eyeball.

NURSING PROCESS

The Care of the Client With Eye Trauma

Assessment

If the trauma does not involve gross injury, the eye is gently inspected. The room is darkened and a penlight is directed at the eye to inspect for the presence of a foreign body. If none is seen, the lower lid is everted and the client instructed to look up. The inferior conjunctival sac is inspected using direct vision or magnification. If this fails to locate a foreign body, the upper lid is everted and the client is directed to look down. If possible, a gross vision assessment is performed.

Diagnosis and Planning

The care of a client with eye trauma includes, but is not limited to, the following:

Nursing Diagnoses and Collaborative Problems	Nursing Interventions
Pain related to trauma of the eye or surrounding structures **Goal:** The client's eye discomfort will be reduced to a tolerable level.	Implement emergency measures, such as irrigating the eye, dimming bright lights, closing and patching both eyes. Instill anesthetic eye drops under the direction or standing orders of a physician. Apply cool compresses or an ice pack for the first 24 hours followed thereafter by warm compresses to reduce swelling.
Impaired Tissue Integrity related to physical or chemical injury to the epithelium **Goal:** The tissue of the eye will not be permanently damaged.	For a chemical splash, take the client to the nearest sink or water fountain, instruct the person to hold the eyes open, and flush the eyes with running water. Tilt the client's head to the side, and direct the flow of solution from the nasal area outward so that the solution does not flow into the other eye. Continue flushing the eye(s) for 10 to 15 minutes. After the irrigation, instill an antibiotic if prescribed and apply an eye pad. Instruct the client to close the eye while the eye pad is applied over the lid, and secure the pad with tape.
Risk for Infection related to disruption of corneal and conjunctival tissue **Goal:** The client will not acquire a secondary ophthalmic infection.	Wash hands before examining the eyes or performing any procedures about the face. Use sterile solutions to irrigate the eye, in nonemergency situations. Instill antibiotic ointment or drops as prescribed to prevent infection. Do not use a container of ophthalmic medication for any one other than the client. Avoid contaminating the medication dropper or tube by holding the tip above the eye and adjacent tissue. Change gauze eye dressings on a regular basis using aseptic technique.

Evaluation and Expected Outcomes

- Pain is reduced or eliminated.
- Trauma is minimized by immediate first aid measures.
- No purulent exudate is noted.

Client and Family Teaching

Include the following instructions for home care and instilling eye medications:

- Wash hands thoroughly.
- Wipe the lids and lashes in a direction away from the nose with a moistened, soft gauze pad, paper tissue, or cotton ball. Use a separate item for each wipe.
- Pull the tissue near the cheek downward, forming a sac within the lower lid (Fig. 48–13).
- Tilt the head slightly backward and toward the eye in which the medication is to be instilled.
- Do not allow the tip of the container to touch the eye.
- Instill the prescribed number of drops into the conjunctival pocket, or apply a thin ribbon of ointment directly into the conjunctival pocket, beginning at the inner corner and moving outward.
- Close the eye gently.
- Wipe away excess medication that falls into the skin.
- Secure dressing to the face with tape and use an eye shield for additional protection, especially at night.
- Do not rub the eye and visit an ophthalmologist or return to the emergency department if it is not completely comfortable within a short time.
- Keep all follow-up visits to check the condition of the eye and surrounding structures.

Infectious and Inflammatory Eye Disorders

Conjunctivitis

Conjunctivitis is an inflammation of the conjunctiva. It commonly is called "pinkeye." Some forms are highly contagious.

ETIOLOGY AND PATHOPHYSIOLOGY

Conjunctivitis results from a bacterial, viral, or rickettsial infection. The microorganisms are most often introduced by air transmission, direct contact with sources on the fingers, a contaminated face towel or washcloth, or transmission from infected lesions near the eye. Allergic reactions, trauma from chemicals, or foreign bodies in the eye also cause conjunctivitis. A local inflammatory response follows damage to the tissue. Untreated conjunctivitis, especially when caused by *Neisseria gonorrhoeae* and *Chlamydia trachomatis*, can lead to blindness.

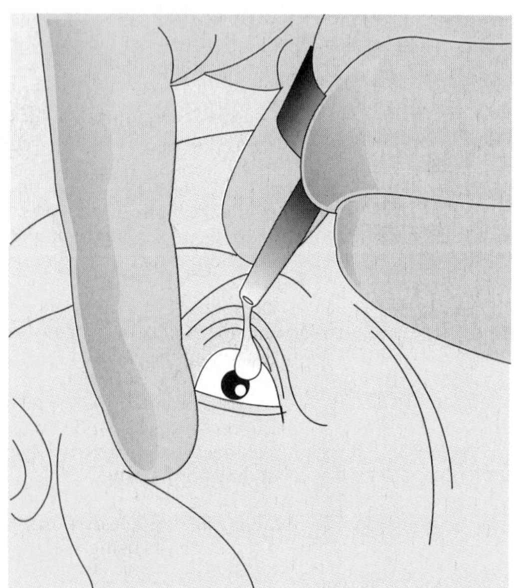

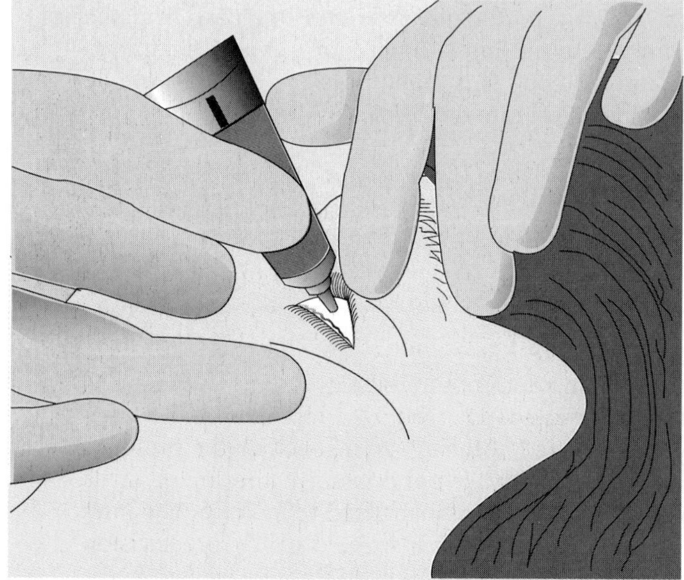

FIGURE 48-13. (*A*) When eyedrops are instilled, the client looks up. The lower lid is pulled down, and the drop is placed just inside the conjunctival sac. (*B*) Eye ointment is applied as a thin ribbon onto the margin of the lower lid.

ASSESSMENT FINDINGS

Signs and Symptoms

Symptoms include redness, excessive tearing, swelling, pain, burning or itching, and possibly, purulent drainage from one or both eyes. In infections from the herpes simplex virus, lesions appear on or near the lid margins. In severe cases, lymph nodes in the neck or throat area are enlarged.

Diagnostic Findings

Although cultures identify the causative microorganism, more often than not, the disorder is diagnosed by visual inspection and a history of exposure to someone with similar symptoms.

MEDICAL MANAGEMENT

Treatment includes antibiotic or antiviral ointment or drops. Warm soaks or sterile saline irrigations are used to remove purulent drainage, reduce swelling, and relieve pain or itching. If an allergen causes the conjunctivitis, antihistamines and decongestants are prescribed.

NURSING MANAGEMENT

The nurse cleans the eye and instills or applies the prescribed medication. Health teaching is provided so that the client can assume the necessary care independently. Because many forms of this condition are infectious, the nurse identifies methods for preventing its spread.

Uveitis

Uveitis is an inflammation of the uveal tract, which consists of the iris, ciliary body, and choroid.

ETIOLOGY AND PATHOPHYSIOLOGY

The cause of uveitis is unknown, but it definitely produces inflammatory changes. Pathogens are seldom identified. Although the disorder occurs randomly, it is detected with some frequency among clients with juvenile rheumatoid arthritis, ankylosing spondylitis, tuberculosis, toxoplasmosis, histoplasmosis, and herpes zoster infection. Because some of these diseases are autoimmune disorders, uveitis may be an atypical antigen antibody phenomenon (see Chap. 41). Complications such as glaucoma, cataracts, and retinal detachment are known to occur secondary to uveitis.

ASSESSMENT FINDINGS

Signs and Symptoms

Symptoms include blurred vision and **photophobia,** a sensitivity to light. Eye pain is experienced in varying degrees. The eye appears red and congested; the pupil reacts poorly to light.

Diagnostic Findings

Uveitis is confirmed by its clinical appearance during slit lamp examination. Skin tests for primary disorders, such as tuberculosis, are performed to confirm or rule out this etiology.

MEDICAL MANAGEMENT

Treatment includes oral and topical corticosteroids, mydriatic (dilating) eye drops such as atropine, and antibiotic eye drops. Analgesics are prescribed for pain. Sunglasses reduce the discomfort of photophobia.

NURSING MANAGEMENT

The nurse instructs the client on the medication regimen and drug administration technique and stresses compliance with therapy. Failure to follow the medication regimen can result in serious complications. The nurse also emphasizes the importance of close follow-up during treatment.

Keratitis and Corneal Ulcer

Keratitis is an inflammation of the cornea. A *corneal ulcer* is an erosion in the corneal tissue.

ETIOLOGY AND PATHOPHYSIOLOGY

Trauma to the cornea (eg, wearing hard contact lenses for an extended period) and infectious agents (eg, bacteria, fungi, viruses) cause keratitis. Secondary infections are common once the epithelium is damaged. Most clients experience severe pain because of the abundance of nerve endings in the cornea. Inflammation and disruption of the tissue interfere with the transparency and smoothness of the cornea, temporarily impairing vision. When and if scar tissue forms, visual impairment is permanent. The degree of visual change depends on the size and density of the corneal scar tissue.

ASSESSMENT FINDINGS

Signs and Symptoms

Keratitis is associated with localized pain or sensation that a foreign body is present. Blinking increases the discomfort. Photophobia, blurred vision, tearing, purulent discharge, and redness develop.

Diagnostic Findings

In addition to flashlight illumination and slit lamp examination, fluorescein drops or strips provide evidence of corneal tissue erosion.

MEDICAL AND SURGICAL MANAGEMENT

Treatment is begun promptly to avoid permanent loss of vision. Keratitis is treated with topical anesthetics, mydriatics, and local and systemic antibiotics. Dark glasses are recommended to relieve photophobia. Treatment in the early stages of a corneal ulcer is the same as for keratitis. Once corneal scar tissue has formed, the only treatment is **corneal transplantation** (**keratoplasty**).

NURSING MANAGEMENT

The nurse removes exudate that harbors microbes and instills antibiotic eye medication. Aseptic principles are followed to avoid transferring microorganisms to the injured corneal tissues. The client who wears contact lenses is advised to stop wearing them temporarily.

Blepharitis

Blepharitis is an inflammation of the lid margins.

ETIOLOGY AND PATHOPHYSIOLOGY

One form of blepharitis is associated with hypersecretion from sebaceous glands, which causes greasy scales to form. This type often occurs in conjunction with dandruff of the scalp or seborrheic dermatitis found about the ears and eyebrows. Infectious agents such as staphylococci cause other cases. Some infections are combinations of both. Blepharitis can coexist with conjunctivitis and lead to the development of hordeola and chalazions, which are discussed later.

ASSESSMENT FINDINGS

Signs and Symptoms

The lid margins appear inflamed. Patchy flakes cling to the eyelashes and are readily visible about the lids. Eyelashes may be missing. Purulent drainage may be present.

Diagnostic Findings

The condition is definitively diagnosed by scraping the lid margins and examining the scales microscopically, although that is not generally necessary.

MEDICAL MANAGEMENT

A topical antibiotic ointment is prescribed. The condition also improves with cleaning of the eyelids once or twice daily. Because seborrhea (excessive oiliness of the skin) of the face and scalp is associated with blepharitis, frequent washing of the face and hair is recommended.

NURSING MANAGEMENT

The nurse reinforces the instructions for conscientious performance of hygiene measures. Many clients become discouraged because the condition takes some time to improve. Noncompliance contributes to the chronicity of the condition.

Hordeolum (Sty)

A **hordeolum** or *sty* is an inflammation and infection of the Zeis or Moll gland, a type of oil gland at the edge of the eyelid.

ETIOLOGY AND PATHOPHYSIOLOGY

Staphylococcus aureus is the most common causative pathogen. The microorganisms multiply within the oil gland, which initiates an inflammatory response. A collection of purulent exudate accompanies the inflammation in the channel of the gland. As debris accumulates, it causes swelling and localized discomfort. Sties are common in clients with diabetes mellitus because their glucose-rich blood readily supports microbial growth.

ASSESSMENT FINDINGS

Signs and Symptoms

A sty appears as a tender, swollen, red pustule in the internal or external tissue of the eyelid.

Diagnostic Findings

A culture of the exudate, although seldom done, identifies bacterial pathogens.

MEDICAL AND SURGICAL MANAGEMENT

Treatment of sty includes warm soaks of the area and a topical antibiotic. Severe cases require incision and drainage.

NURSING MANAGEMENT

The nurse assures the client that treatment provides relief from pain and discomfort. The nurse explains how to avoid transferring microorganisms from the sty to areas of the body by cleaning the unaffected eye first and changing the washcloth, towel, and water after contact with the affected eye. The nurse instructs the client to use separate fresh tissues, cotton balls, or gauze for each wiping stroke when cleaning exudate from the eye.

Chalazion

A *chalazion* is a cyst of one or more meibomian glands, a type of sebaceous gland in the inner surface of the eyelid at the junction of the conjunctiva and lid margin.

ETIOLOGY AND PATHOPHYSIOLOGY

A chalazion forms when the meibomian gland becomes obstructed and the release of sebaceous secretions is blocked. Consequently, the meibomian gland becomes inflamed and enlarged.

ASSESSMENT FINDINGS

Signs and Symptoms

A chalazion appears similar to a sty, but the swelling in the upper or lower eyelid is not tender. As the chalazion matures, it feels hard. The enlargement within the eyelid causes clients to feel self-conscious about their appearance and affects their visual acuity.

Diagnostic Findings

If a chalazion grows large enough to obscure the pupil or compress corneal tissue, the distortion of vision is similar to that caused by astigmatism.

MEDICAL AND SURGICAL MANAGEMENT

Treatment of a chalazion is not necessary if the cyst is small and does not interfere with vision. Warm soaks and massage of the surrounding area are prescribed to promote spontaneous drainage. If the cyst is firm, becomes infected, or interferes with closure of the eyelid, it is surgically excised.

NURSING MANAGEMENT

The nurse prepares the patient for examination and treatment by a physician. Instructions are provided on methods for carrying out the treatment measures.

Client and Family Teaching

Some points to include when teaching clients with infectious and inflammatory eye disorders include:

- Comply with the full course of prescribed drugs to achieve satisfactory results.
- Wash hands thoroughly before cleaning the eyelids, instilling eye drops, or applying eye ointment.
- Do not rub the eyes, and keep hands away from the eyes.
- Use a separate washcloth or towel if the disorder is infectious.
- Do not use nonprescription eye products during or after treatment unless approved by the physician.
- Eliminate the use of eye cosmetics or use hypoallergenic products and replace them frequently to avoid harboring microorganisms.
- Keep all follow-up appointments.

Macular Degeneration

Macular degeneration is the breakdown of or damage to the macula, the point on the retina where light rays converge for the most acute visual perception. The disorder usually occurs in both eyes, but the vision in one eye tends to deteriorate more rapidly.

ETIOLOGY AND PATHOPHYSIOLOGY

Macular degeneration is more common in aging adults. The underlying problem seems to stem from an opening between one of the membranous layers of the retina and the choroid. Serous fluid seeps within the separation, like a blister, and elevates an area of the retina. One or more blood vessels grow into the defect and produce a subretinal hemorrhage. After the bleed, scar tissue forms. The damage almost always is confined to the macular area.

ASSESSMENT FINDINGS

Signs and Symptoms

Blurred or distorted vision is the first symptom of macular degeneration. Other symptoms include color vision disturbance (colors become dim), difficulty reading and doing close work, and distortion of objects (especially those with lines). When the macula becomes irreparably damaged, clients compare their vision to a target in which the bull's eye area of the image is absent (Fig. 48–14). The peripheral field, or side vision, is unaffected, but the client cannot see images by looking at them directly.

Diagnostic Findings

Fluorescein angiography shows pooling of the dye within the blister area.

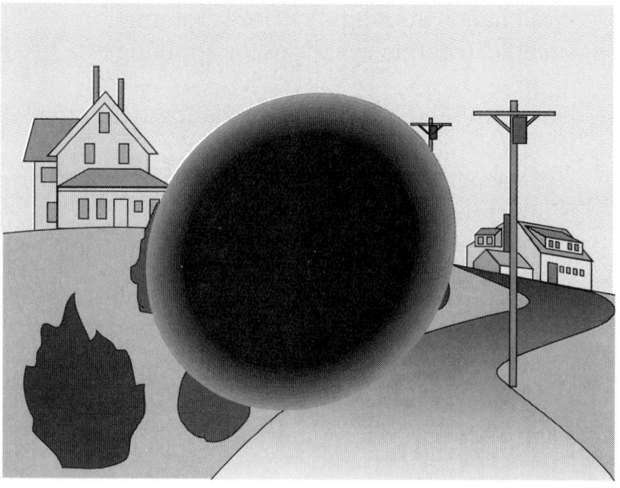

FIGURE 48-14. Loss of central vision from macular degeneration.

MEDICAL MANAGEMENT

A laser procedure called *photocoagulation* is done to seal the serous leak and destroy the encroachment of blood vessels in the area. It must be done early to prevent progression of the disorder. For many clients, the diagnosis is made too late and laser treatment is no longer an option. The client is then provided with suggestions for coping with the visual impairment. Aids, such as magnifying glasses, may be of value, and high-intensity reading lamps have helped some people. The ophthalmologist may refer the client to a specialized center for evaluation and selection of assistive devices.

NURSING MANAGEMENT

The nurse helps the client cope with loss of vision. For additional nursing management of the client with permanent visual impairment, review the information that accompanies the previous discussion of blindness.

Glaucoma

Glaucoma, the second most common cause of blindness in the United States, is due to an imbalance between the production and drainage of aqueous fluid. When the drainage system is obstructed, the anterior chamber becomes congested with fluid and IOP rises.

Glaucoma is classified as either open-angle or angle-closure. *Open-angle glaucoma*, formerly called chronic or simple glaucoma, is the most common form. Its onset is slow, and the client may not experience noticeable symptoms for several years. *Angle-closure glaucoma* is less common, but acute angle closure requires immediate recognition and treatment to prevent blindness.

ETIOLOGY AND PATHOPHYSIOLOGY

Glaucoma occurs congenitally; secondarily to other eye disorders such as ocular trauma, ophthalmic infections, and cataract surgery; or as a primary disease among adults after the age of 40. It is more prevalent among those who have a family history of the disorder. The incidence is higher among African Americans, who are four to eight times more likely to develop blindness from glaucoma than are other ethnic groups.

Open-angle glaucoma occurs when structures in the drainage system (ie, trabecular meshwork and Schlemm's canal) degenerate and the exit channels for aqueous fluid become blocked. As the IOP rises, it causes edema of the cornea, atrophy of nerve fibers in the peripheral areas of the retina, and degeneration of the optic nerve.

Angle-closure glaucoma occurs among people who have an anatomically narrow angle at the junction where the iris meets the cornea (Fig. 48–15). This

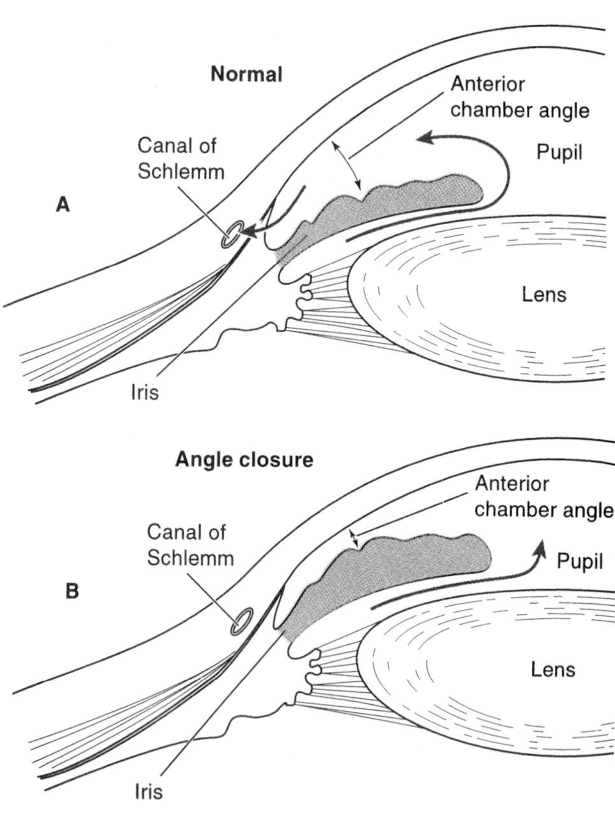

FIGURE 48-15. In the normal eye (*A*), the pathway to the canal of Schlemm is wide and unobstructed. In angle closure glaucoma (*B*), the movement of fluid is impaired because of the narrowed approach to the canal of Schlemm.

deviation makes them vulnerable to angle closure when nearby structures protrude into the anterior chamber and occlude the drainage pathway. For example, an attack can be precipitated when the iris thickens in response to a mydriatic drug, by pupil dilation while sitting in the dark, or when the lens enlarges with age and bulges forward. A delay in treatment may result in partial or total loss of vision in the affected eye.

ASSESSMENT FINDINGS

Signs and Symptoms

Many clients experience no symptoms with open-angle glaucoma and the condition may not be discovered until the client has a routine ophthalmologic examination. When symptoms do occur, they often are ignored because they are not dramatic. Clients may complain of eye discomfort, occasional and temporary blurred vision, the appearance of halos around lights, reduced peripheral vision, and the feeling that their eyeglass prescription needs to be changed (Fig. 48–16). Clients with acute angle-closure glaucoma become symptomatic quite suddenly. The eyes are rock hard, painful, and sightless. Nausea and vomiting may occur. The conjunctiva is red; the cornea becomes cloudy and commonly is described as appearing "steamy." The attack is self-limiting, but with each subsequent attack, vision becomes more impaired.

Diagnostic Findings

The optic disc, when visualized directly with an ophthalmoscope or with retinal angiographic photographs, shows a cupping effect (widening and deepening of the optic disc). When the anterior chamber of the eye of a client with angle-closure glaucoma is inspected with a penlight or slit lamp, the angle between the iris and cornea is found to be narrow. Tonometry reveals elevated IOP and reduced aqueous outflow. The visual field examination demonstrates a loss of peripheral vision; nasal and superior areas are usually impaired first.

MEDICAL MANAGEMENT

Clients with either type of glaucoma are treated initially with medications (Table 48–1). IOP can be controlled with miotics such as carbachol (Miostat) and pilocarpine (Pilocar), which constrict the pupil. Miotics pull the iris away from the drainage channels so that the aqueous fluid can escape. Other eye medications that are used for lowering IOP include echothiophate iodide (Phospholine Iodide), epinephrine, dipivefrin (Propine), and timolol maleate (Timoptic). Acetazolamide (Diamox) and methazolamide (Neptazane), which are carbonic anhydrase inhibitors, are given to slow the production of aqueous fluid. In an acute attack of angle-closure glaucoma, analgesics are given to relieve pain and the client is kept at complete rest.

SURGICAL MANAGEMENT

When compliance is poor (eg, client fails to instill eye drops as directed) or drug therapy is no longer effective, or if the client develops severe adverse reactions to the medication, more aggressive treatment becomes necessary to preserve vision. One of several procedures that create accessory drainage channels can be performed. These procedures include laser or surgical **iridectomy**, laser **trabeculoplasty**, and **corneal trephine**.

Laser iridectomy, in which holes are burned into the iris to increase areas for drainage, is performed first. If this procedure is unsuccessful, it is followed by a standard surgical iridectomy in which a section of the iris is removed. Either a peripheral or sector iridectomy is used. In a peripheral iridectomy, a small section of iris is removed at the outer margin of the iris. In a sector or keyhole iridectomy, a larger segment of the iris is removed in the direction of the pupil (Fig. 48–17). A laser trabeculoplasty is an alternative to a surgical iridectomy. In this procedure, the laser beam is directed at the trabecular network, which lies near Schlemm's canal, creating multiple openings for drainage. A *corneal trephine* is similar to a

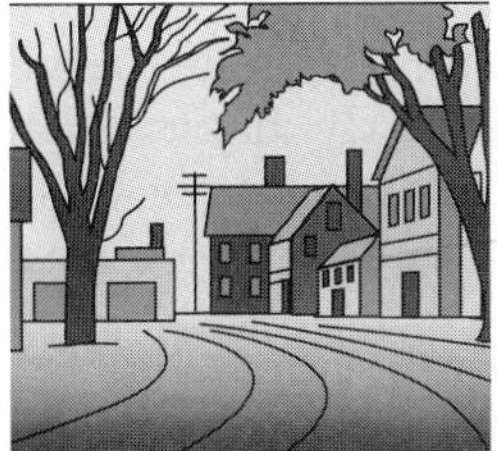
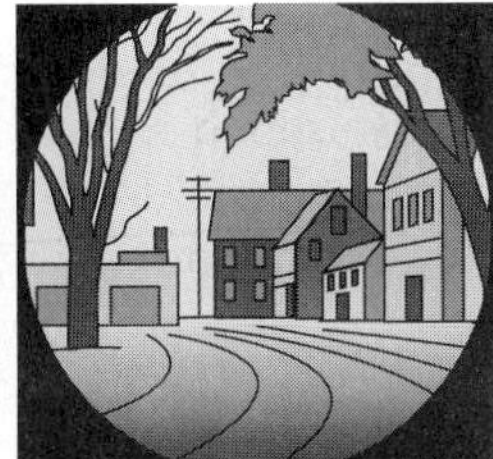
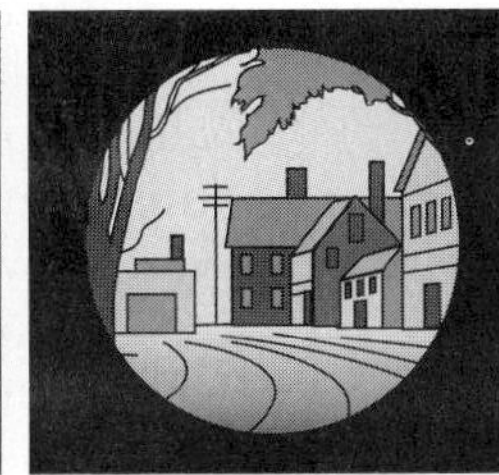
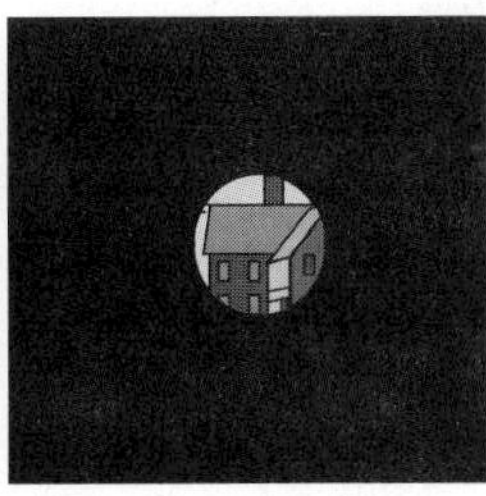

FIGURE 48-16. Gradual loss of vision from glaucoma.

TABLE 48-1 **Drug Therapy for Glaucoma**

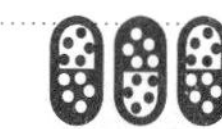

Drug Category/Drug Action	Side Effects	Nursing Considerations
Adrenergics		
dipivefrin solution (Propine) Decreases production of aqueous fluid and increases its outflow.	Headache, brow ache, stinging when instilled	Tell client that side effects will subside. Administer miotics first. Tell client to avoid blinking for 30 seconds after instillation and to apply gentle pressure to the inner corner of the eye for 1 minute (to decrease systemic absorption). Wait 5 minutes before giving other eye drops.
Beta-adrenergic Blockers		
timolol maleate (Timoptic) Decreases production of aqueous fluid; possibly increases its outlow.	Ocular irritation, change in refraction, diplopia, ptosis bradycardia, bronchospasm in sensitive persons	Contraindicated in severe bronchial asthma, use cautiously with cardiac disease. Administer properly to avoid systemic absorption (see above).
Cholinergics		
pilocarpine hydrochloride (Pilocar) Increases outflow of aqueous fluid	Blurry vision, brow pain, bronchial spasm, pupil constriction (miosis)	Inform client that vision will be blurry temporarily. Inform client not to exceed recommended dosage and to gently compress inner corner of eye to prevent systemic absorption.
Anticholinesterase		
isoflurophate (Floropryl) Increases outflow of aqueous fluid.	Headache, eye pain, blurry vision, bronchial constriction, salivation, sweating, diarrhea, muscle weakness	Administer at bedtime if blurred vision occurs with instillation. Tell client to adhere to recommended dose and to report any side effects.

trabeculoplasty in that it produces a small hole at the junction of the cornea and sclera to provide an outlet for aqueous fluid. The opening is then covered by a flap of the conjunctiva.

NURSING MANAGEMENT

Determine the client's history of symptoms, if the client is already on medication, the medications that have been prescribed, and whether the client is adhering to the prescribed medication schedule. Ask when the client was first diagnosed with glaucoma.

Acute angle closure glaucoma is an emergency; refer the client for medical treatment immediately because vision can be permanently lost in 1 to 2 days. Severe pain requires analgesics. To promote the maximum effect from analgesic drug therapy, limit sensory stimulation, such as loud noise, activity, and movement. Inform the physician immediately if the client states that the pain has worsened despite treatment. While clients are incapacitated by their pain or if the disease results in loss of vision, the nurse assists with meeting basic needs. Never administer mydriatics to clients with glaucoma. Consult the physician if drugs with anticholinergic properties, such as atropine sulfate, are prescribed because dilation of the pupil can further obstruct drainage of aqueous fluid, raise IOP, and damage whatever vision remains.

Client and Family Teaching

Because glaucoma tends to run in families, advise adults to be examined regularly. Early diagnosis and treatment are essential for preventing loss of vision. Clients who are already diagnosed with glaucoma are encouraged to maintain close follow-up and comply with the medication regimen. Explain drug instillation techniques. Besides eye drops, some clients insert an ocular therapeutic system under the upper lid. An *ocular therapeutic system* is a small, thin

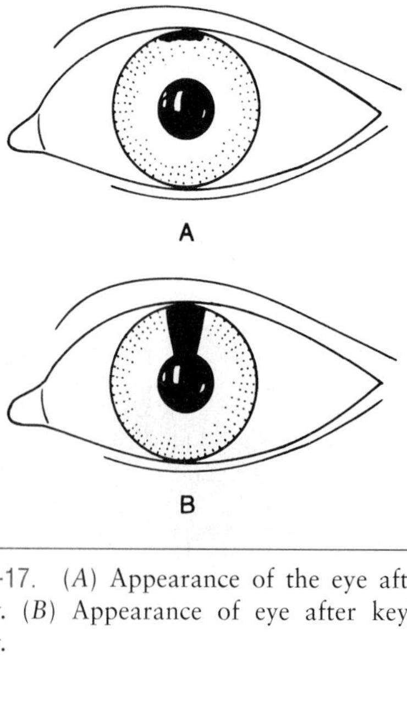

A

B

FIGURE 48-17. (*A*) Appearance of the eye after peripheral iridectomy. (*B*) Appearance of eye after keyhole (sector) iridectomy.

film that contains eye medication. The film, which is replaced weekly, continuously releases the medication and eliminates the need for frequent eye drop instillation.

If a client has difficulty remembering when to take the medication, recommend a watch with a timer. For the client who does not understand the chronic and progressive nature of the disease, stress that glaucoma has no cure but can be controlled and that blindness caused by glaucoma is usually preventable.

Other general instructions include:

- Obtain assistance from a family member, relative, or friend if you have trouble instilling eye drops.
- Avoid all drugs that contain atropine. Check with physician or pharmacist before using any nonprescription drug; preparations for cold or allergy symptoms may contain an atropine-like drug.
- Maintain regular bowel habits; straining at stool can raise IOP.
- Avoid heavy lifting and emotional upsets (especially crying) because they increase IOP.
- Limit activities that strain or tire the eyes.
- Keep an extra supply of prescribed drugs on hand for vacations, holidays, or in case some is lost or spilled.
- Seek medical attention *immediately* if pain or a visual disturbance occurs.
- Tell all physicians that you have this disorder and the treatment prescribed by the ophthalmologist. Carry identification stating that you have glaucoma in case of illness or injury.

Cataracts

A **cataract** is a condition in which the lens of the eye becomes opaque. One or both eyes may be affected.

ETIOLOGY AND PATHOPHYSIOLOGY

Cataracts are congenitally acquired, caused by injury to the lens, secondary to other eye diseases, or due to the aging process. When cataracts occur in response to injury, they usually develop quickly. Most cataracts are caused by degenerative changes associated with aging and develop slowly. A high incidence of cataracts occurs among people with diabetes and those with a family history. Prolonged exposure to ultraviolet rays (eg, sunlight, tanning lamps), radiation, or certain drugs (eg, corticosteroids) has been associated with cataract formation. In all cases, vision decreases because light no longer has a transparent pathway to the retina.

ASSESSMENT FINDINGS

Signs and Symptoms

One of the earliest symptoms is seeing a halo around lights. Other symptoms include difficulty reading, changes in color vision, glaring of objects in bright light, and distortion of objects. As the cataract worsens, visual acuity is so severely reduced that the client can only read the largest letter on a Snellen chart, count fingers, and distinguish movement. On inspection, a white or gray spot is visible behind the pupil.

Diagnostic Findings

Under ophthalmoscopic and slit lamp examination, the lens appears in varying stages of opacity. Some lenses are so cloudy that the examiner cannot see through the cataract to the posterior of the eye. Tonometry determines whether the cataract is raising the IOP.

SURGICAL MANAGEMENT

Cataracts cannot be treated medically and are surgically removed. Surgery often is performed under local anesthesia. A tranquilizer is given before and during surgery to relax the client. Sometimes general anesthesia is used and has certain advantages, especially with an apprehensive client.

The lens is removed by *intracapsular extraction* (removal of the lens within its capsule) or *extracapsular extraction* (removal of the lens, leaving the posterior portion of its capsule in position).

Phacoemulsification, which uses ultrasound to break the lens into minute particles that are then removed by aspiration, is a technique that may accompany the extracapsular method. When phacoemulsification is used, a smaller incision is required and most clients return to full activity sooner than after the other methods.

After surgery, vision is restored with one of three methods: corrective eyeglasses, a contact lens, or an **intraocular lens** (IOL) **implant**. When cataract eyeglasses are prescribed, the correcting lens for the *aphakic eye* (the eye without a lens) causes the client to see objects about one-third larger than normal. These lenses also distort peripheral vision, and the client must learn to turn his or her head to see objects that are not in the center of vision. If only one lens is removed, the client must use one eye or the other to avoid seeing a distorted image. A coating usually is applied to the eyeglasses so that only the aphakic eye with a corrective lens is used.

A contact lens can also restore vision after cataract extraction. Advantages of the contact lens are that peripheral vision is not lost and objects appear about their actual size. A disadvantage is that the lens must be removed at night, cleaned and reinserted daily, which can be difficult for an older client who has poor manual dexterity or a cataract in the other eye.

A third method for improving vision is the insertion of an IOL at the time of cataract surgery. IOLs most commonly are inserted behind the iris (Fig. 48–18). Candidates for IOLs are those who are age 60 or older and at risk for experiencing difficulty with a contact lens or cataract glasses. Ultrasonography is performed before surgery to determine the size and prescription of the IOL. When an IOL is implanted, vision is blurred for a week or more. Reading glasses are still required for optimum vision.

Complications after cataract surgery include infection, loss of vitreous, intraocular hemorrhage, retinal detachment, clouding of the lens capsule, and displacement of the IOL implant. Loss of vitreous is serious because the vitreous body does not regenerate. Its loss, as well as hemorrhage, seriously damages the eye.

NURSING MANAGEMENT

If outpatient surgery is planned, the nurse explains and provides a written list of preoperative preparations that the client is to perform. The nurse is responsible for providing preoperative and postoperative care of the surgical client as well as discharge instructions (Nursing Care Plan 48–1). In addition, the following measures are taken postoperatively to prevent complications and to keep the IOP from rising:

- Avoid coughing or sneezing.
- Give antiemetics if nausea occurs.
- Patch both eyes and give dilating drugs to keep the client from squinting.
- Tell the client to avoid lying on the operative side, bending, and lifting.
- Administer stool softeners to prevent straining.

Positioning depends on the type of cataract surgery performed. If an air bubble is instilled in the eye to occupy the space where the lens is removed, the client may have the head elevated slightly and is not permitted to lie flat because this would push the iris toward the anterior chamber and obstruct the flow of aqueous fluid. Intense pain in the eye or near the brow is an indication of intraocular hemorrhage or rising IOP and is reported immediately.

Retinal Detachment

In **retinal detachment**, the sensory layer becomes separated from the pigmented layer of the retina.

ETIOLOGY AND PATHOPHYSIOLOGY

Retinal separation is associated with a hole or tear in the retina that is caused by stretching or degenerative changes. Retinal detachment may follow a sudden blow, a penetrating injury, or eye surgery. Tumors, hemorrhage in front of or behind the retina, and loss of vitreous fluid are particularly likely to lead to retinal detachment. This condition may also be a complication of other disorders, such as advanced diabetic changes in the retina. In many instances, the cause of retinal detachment is unknown. Retinal separation is more common after age 40.

The separation of the two layers of the retina deprives the sensory layer of its blood supply. Vision is lost in the affected area because the sensory layer can

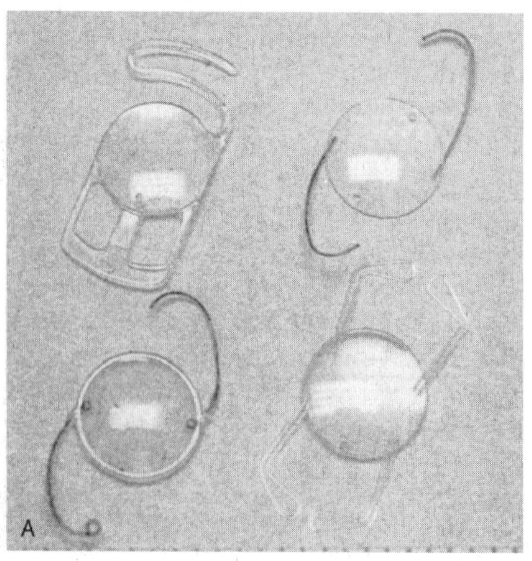

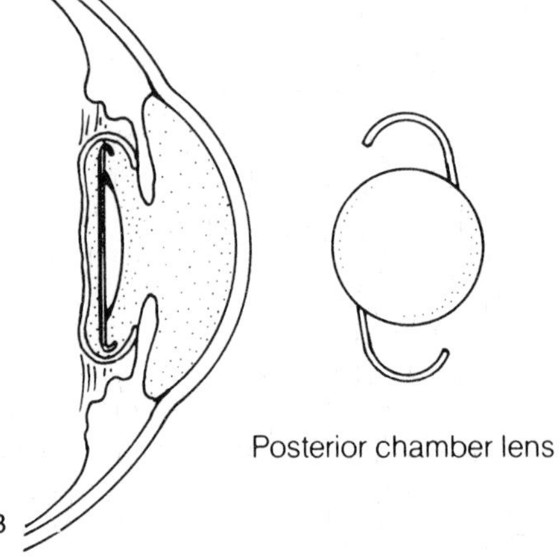

FIGURE 48-18. (*A*) Intraocular implants are designed to be held in place by various wing-like attachments that center and support the lens. (*B*) The intraocular lens implant is placed within the lens capsule after cataract extraction.

NURSING CARE PLAN 48-1

Postoperative Management of the Client Undergoing Eye Surgery

Potential Problems and Nursing Diagnoses	Nursing Management	Outcome Criteria
PC: Ophthalmic Hemorrhage or **Increased Intraocular Pressure**	Report sudden or intense pain immediately. Instruct the client to avoid coughing, vomiting, straining at stool, bending forward, or lifting anything over 5 lb.	Bleeding and IOP are managed and minimized.
Pain related to surgery	Acknowledge the discomfort and administer a prescribed analgesic that is appropriate for the level of pain. Keep room lights dim and aggravating noise to a minimum. Clean the eyelids when, and if, allowed. Provide dark glasses if light causes discomfort.	Pain is reduced or eliminated.
Risk for Infection related to impaired tissue integrity	Perform conscientious handwashing before an eye assessment or treatment procedure. Follow principles of asepsis when cleaning the eye or applying a new dressing. Keep the tips of all medication applicators free of contamination.	The incised tissue heals without evidence of infection.
Risk for Injury related to compromised vision	Raise the side rails and identify the location of the signal device. Use a night light or dim light in the room after sundown. Reorient the confused client. Ask a family member to sit at the bedside if confusion persists. Apply a shield over the patched eye for additional protection. Assist the client when ambulating and clear the pathway.	The client's safety is maintained.

no longer receive visual stimuli. Vitreous fluid moves between the separated layers of the retina, holding the layers apart and causing further separation.

ASSESSMENT FINDINGS

Signs and Symptoms

Many clients notice definite gaps in their vision or blind spots. They describe the sensation that a curtain is being drawn over their field of vision and they often see flashes of light. Seeing spots or moving particles, called floaters, is common. Complete loss of vision may occur in the affected eye. The condition is not painful, but clients usually are extremely apprehensive.

Diagnostic Findings

When the retina is inspected with an ophthalmoscope, the tissue appears gray in the detached area.

MEDICAL MANAGEMENT

In a few select cases, an office procedure called *pneumatic retinopexy* is performed. Before the procedure, the client must recline for about 16 hours to allow the separated retina to fall back toward the choroid. Then 0.5 to 1 cc of gas is injected intraocularly into the posterior area of the eye. The gas compresses the retina and holds it in place. To ensure success from the procedure, the client must again assume a restricted position, sometimes up to 8 hours each day for 3 weeks. If pneumatic retinopexy is not appropriate, the physician usually recommends prompt admission to the hospital for surgery.

SURGICAL MANAGEMENT

Surgical interventions for retinal reattachment include cryosurgery, electrodiathermy, laser reattachment, and scleral buckling. The amount of sight regained depends on the extent of the detachment and the success of the surgery.

Cryosurgery involves the application of a supercooled probe to the sclera. The sclera, choroid, and retina then adhere to one another as a result of scar tissue formation.

With *electrodiathermy,* an electrode needle is inserted into the sclera so that the fluid that has collected underneath the retina can escape. The retina ultimately adheres to the choroid. This method seldom is used.

Laser reattachment involves focusing a laser beam on the damaged area of the retina and causing a small burn. The exudate that forms between the retina and choroid results in adhesion of the retina to the choroid. Laser therapy can only be used when the retinal separation involves a small area.

Scleral buckling is a surgical procedure that shortens the sclera, thus allowing contact between the choroid and retina. A section of the sclera is exposed, opened, and retracted from the choroid. A laser beam or cryosurgery probe is then used to produce adhesion of the retina and choroid. A small silicone patch is placed between the sclera and choroid, and the sclera is pulled over the patch and sutured. The inward displacement of the choroid allows for reattachment of the retina to the choroid.

Preoperatively, the client is kept on complete bed rest with the affected eye dependent until surgery is performed. Sedation may be ordered. The eyes are patched and covered with an eye shield. Mydriatic eye drops are instilled to dilate the pupil and facilitate further examination of the retina.

NURSING MANAGEMENT

Anyone with sudden loss of vision is referred immediately for examination by a physician. If surgery is performed, the client usually is kept on complete bed rest for several days with the head immobilized. The client is not turned or moved without orders. If an air bubble is instilled to promote contact between the retina and choroid, the client is positioned with the face parallel to the floor so that the bubble floats to the posterior of the eye. If floaters are still seen after the eye heals, the nurse can tell the client that they eventually become absorbed or settle to the inferior floor of the eye, out of the line of vision. For additional postoperative nursing management, see Nursing Care Plan 48–1.

Enucleation

Enucleation is the surgical removal of an eye. Enucleation is necessary when the eye is destroyed by injury or disease, if a malignant tumor develops (rare), or to relieve pain if the eye is severely damaged and sightless. Sometimes only the contents of the eyeball are removed and the sclera is left in place. At other times, the entire eyeball is removed as well as tissues in the bony orbit.

When enucleation is performed, a metal or plastic ball is buried in the capsule of connective tissue from which the eyeball is removed (Fig. 48–19). A pressure dressing is applied to control hemorrhage, a complication of enucleation. After the tissues have healed, a shell-shaped prosthesis is placed over the buried ball. The shell is painted to match the client's remaining eye. The shell is the only portion that is removed for cleaning.

NURSING MANAGEMENT

The client is observed postoperatively for signs and symptoms of bleeding or infection. The client usually is allowed out of bed the day after surgery. When healing is complete, in about 2 to 4 weeks, the client is taught how to insert and remove the prosthetic shell. The prosthesis typically is removed before going to bed and inserted the next morning. Clients are instructed to hold their heads over a soft surface, such as a bed or padded table, when removing or inserting the prosthesis to avoid damage if it is dropped. The shell is cleaned after removal and kept in safe place where it will not become scratched or broken.

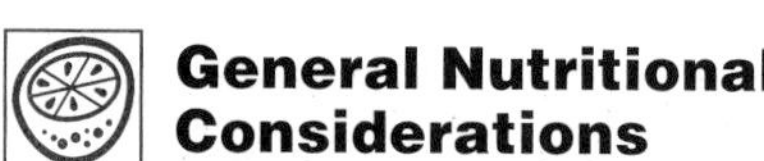

General Nutritional Considerations

Several studies suggest that carotenoids other than beta-carotene, particularly those found in green leafy vegeta-

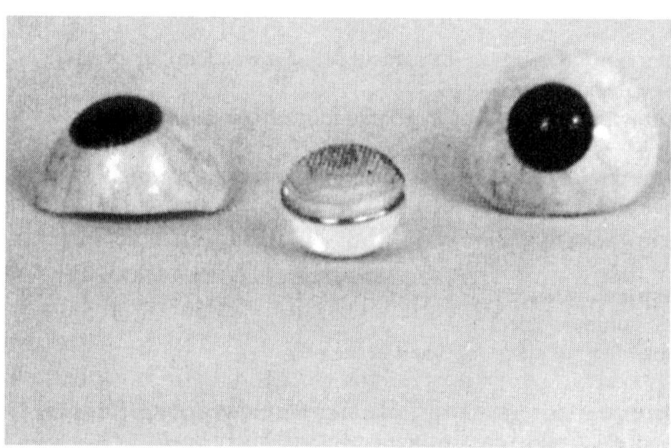

FIGURE 48-19. Front and side views of an artificial eye. The round implant in the center is positioned permanently within the bony orbit from which the natural eye has been removed. Only the cosmetic shell is removed for cleaning. (Courtesy of Ken Timby.)

bles, may protect against macular degeneration. It is theorized that luten and zeaxanthin, carotenoids that form the yellow pigment in the macula, may protect the eye against damage by filtering out visible blue light. One study showed that people who ate spinach or collard greens two to four times per week had half the risk of macular degeneration as people who ate them less than once per month.

Studies have shown that vitamins A and C are essential for preventing cataracts. Clinical trials are underway to determine if zinc can reduce the risk of cataracts and macular degeneration.

Advise clients who have cataract surgery to eat soft foods that are easily chewed until healing is complete to avoid tearing from excessive facial movements.

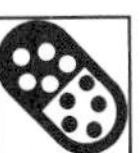

General Pharmacologic Considerations

Although many nonprescription ophthalmic preparations are available for dry eyes and irritation, an ophthalmologist should assess and treat all eye complaints to detect any underlying pathology.

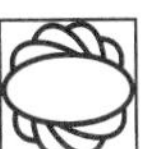

General Gerontologic Considerations

Older adults need to use their glasses or contact lenses when explanations are provided about test procedures.

Teaching aids with large-sized letters are helpful for older clients who are experiencing lens changes associated with aging.

Visual changes can result in accidents and injuries to the older client. It is important to assist older adults with visual deficits with their activities of daily living.

To ensure the safety of older adults with visual impairments, the room is kept dimly lighted at night. Objects, chairs, and footstools are placed away from areas where the client walks, and assistance is given whenever the client is out of bed.

Visual impairment curtails favorite activities such as reading, watching television, and engaging in hobbies or other forms of recreation, resulting in depression and withdrawal.

SUMMARY OF KEY CONCEPTS

- The eye is the sense organ for sight. Images enter on light waves through the eye. Nerve cells in the retina transmit the image via the optic nerve to the brain.
- When assessing the eyes, compare their external appearance. The interior of the eye is examined using an ophthalmoscope. The client is asked to describe visual problems and identify medical conditions that affect vision. Near vision, far vision, and color perception are evaluated using basic screening tests.
- More detailed diagnostic information is obtained using refractometry, tonometry, visual field assessment, slit lamp examination, retinal angiography, or ultrasonography.
- Professionals who provide eye care services include ophthalmologists, physicians who treat eye disorders; optometrists, nonphysicians who test vision, prescribe, and fit corrective lenses; and opticians who make eyeglasses or contact lenses.
- Corrective eyeglasses and contact lenses are prescribed to improve refractive errors, those conditions in which vision is less than perfect because light rays that transmit images are not sharply focused on the retina.
- Refractive errors include myopia or nearsightedness; hyperopia or farsightedness; presbyopia, difficulty with near-vision that occurs with aging; and astigmatism, an irregularly shaped cornea.
- Blindness is a legal term that indicates central visual acuity of 20/200 in the better eye with the use of glasses.
- When caring for a blind client or one with low vision, it is appropriate for the nurse to (1) speak before touching the client, (2) keep doors fully open, (3) describe where food is located using the positions on the face of a clock, and (4) instruct the client to grasp the nurse's elbow and walk slightly behind to the side of the nurse when ambulating.
- When caring for clients with eye trauma, the nurse obtains essential information about the injury, inspects the eye if possible, flushes the eye with copious amounts of water if there is a chemical splash, or loosely patches both eyes and refers the client to a physician.
- To instill eye medication, the nurse pulls the lower lid downward, instills eye drops into the lower conjunctival pocket or applies a thin ribbon of ointment along the inner to outer eyelid.
- Infectious and inflammatory eye disorders include endophthalmitis, conjunctivitis, uveitis, keratitis, blepharitis, hordeolum, and chalazion.
- Macular degeneration is the breakdown of or damage to the macula, which causes a loss of central vision.
- The two types of glaucoma are open-angle glaucoma and angle-closure glaucoma; both involve elevated intraocular pressure.
- Intraocular pressure is controlled with miotics, drugs that constrict the pupil, beta-adrenergic blocking agents, and carbonic anhydrase inhibitors that reduce the production of aqueous fluid.
- Mydriatics, drugs that dilate the pupil (eg, atropine), are contraindicated for clients with glaucoma.
- Glaucoma is controlled surgically with laser or surgical iridectomy, laser trabeculoplasty, and corneal trephine.
- The client must avoid straining to have bowel movements, heavy lifting, emotional upsets, and crying to prevent elevated intraocular pressure.
- A cataract is an opaque lens of the eye.
- Removal of a cataract restores vision with an alternative lens such as eyeglasses, a contact lens, or intraocular lens implant.
- Following a cataract extraction, clients must avoid coughing, sneezing, vomiting, squinting, lying on the operative side, bending over, heavy lifting, and straining to have a bowel movement.

- Clients with retinal detachments experience a loss in their visual field with flashes of light or floating particles.
- A detached retina is reattached using one of five techniques: pneumatic retinopexy, cryosurgery, electrodiathermy, laser reattachment, and scleral buckling.
- An entire eye is enucleated (removed) for the following reasons: injury or disease, a malignant tumor, and pain relief if the eye is severely damaged and sightless.
- A metal or plastic ball is permanently inserted within the empty eye socket; a natural-appearing shell is fitted beneath the eyelid. The shell is removed and cleaned nightly.

CRITICAL THINKING EXERCISES

1. If a client reports having difficulty seeing, what additional data are important to obtain?
2. Explain the meaning of 20/200 visual acuity.
3. Describe techniques for performing an examination of the eyes.
4. Describe nursing measures that are appropriate if a person experiences trauma to the eye.
5. Discuss preventive measures for an infectious eye disorder.
6. What advice is appropriate for someone who has a family history of glaucoma?
7. Explain the pre- and postoperative management of a client undergoing a cataract extraction.

Suggested Readings

Alexander, C., Hart, E., & Kopp, K. (1996). An alternate vision. *Nursing Times, 92*(1), 40–41.

Cooper, J. (1996). Improving compliance with glaucoma eye-drop treatment. *Nursing Times, 92*(32), 36–37.

McConnell, E. A. (1996). Clinical do's and don'ts. Caring for a patient who has a vision impairment. *Nursing, 26*(5), 28.

Elfervis, L. S. (1997). Age-related macular degeneration. *Insight, 22*(3), 88–91; quiz 92–93.

Gandham, S. B. (1997). New topical medications in the treatment of glaucoma. *Journal of Ophthalmic Nursing Technology, 16*(6) 290–291.

Hu, M. (1997). Preventing conjunctivitis in nursing homes. *Professional Nurse, 12*(12), 875–877.

Hunt, L. (1997). Visual field screening for glaucoma. *Insight, 22*(2), 65–66.

Kearney, K. M. (1997). Emergency! Retinal detachment. *American Journal of Nursing, 97*(8), 50.

Martin, S., & Barr, O. (1997). Preventing complications in people who wear contact lenses. *British Journal of Nursing, 6*(11), 614–619.

Needham, Y. (1997). Glaucoma. *Professional Nurse, 12*(11), 798–802.

Rose, K. E. (1997). Caring for patients with cataract. *Nursing Standards, 11*(52), 49–53; quiz 54–55.

Tomsak, R. L. (1997). An approach to acquired visual loss in adults. *Journal of Ophthalmic Nursing Technology, 16*(5), 229–234; quiz 256–257.

Vader, L. (1997). Vision and vision loss. *Insight, 22*(1), 13–19; quiz 20–21.

West, G. (1997). Detecting and treating eye problems in later life. *Community Nurse, 3*(5), 24, 27.

Additional Resources

American Academy of Ophthalmology
P.O. Box 7424
San Francisco, CA 94120–7424
(415) 561–8500
http://www.eyenet.org/public/pi/

American Federation for the Blind
15 West 16th Street
New York, NY 10011

Contact Lens Society of America
441 Carlisle Drive
Reston, VA 20170
(703) 437–0727
http://www.onlinenet.com/clsa

Prevent Blindness America
http://www.prevent-blindness.org/index.html

National Eye Institute
c/o National Institute of Health
Bethesda, MD 21230–4998
http://www/nei.nih.gov/

Chapter 49

Caring for Clients With Ear Disorders

KEY TERMS

- Audiometry
- Caloric stimulation test
- Cochlear implant
- Conductive hearing loss
- Decibels
- Electronystagmography
- Labyrinthitis
- Mastoiditis
- Mastoidectomy
- Meniere's disease
- Myringoplasty
- Myringotomy
- Nystagmus
- Otitis externa
- Otitis media
- Otosclerosis
- Otoscope
- Rinne test
- Romberg test
- Sensorineural hearing loss
- Sign language
- Speech reading
- Stapedectomy
- Tinnitus
- Tuning fork
- Weber test

LEARNING OBJECTIVES

On completion of this chapter, the reader will:

- Describe the anatomy and physiology of the ear.
- List five types of hearing impairment and the acuity levels for each.
- Name two techniques the hearing impaired use to communicate with others.
- Give three examples of support services available for the hearing impaired.
- Discuss the role of the nurse in caring for clients with a hearing loss.
- Name three conditions that involve the external ear.
- Explain the technique for straightening the ear canal of adults to facilitate inspection and the administration of medication.
- Discuss methods for preventing or treating disorders of the external ear.
- Name two conditions that affect the middle ear.
- Describe nursing interventions appropriate for managing the care of a client with ear surgery.
- Explain the pathophysiology of Meniere's disease, and name three consequences of this inner ear disorder.
- Discuss the nursing management of clients with Meniere's disease.

Ear disorders occur throughout the life cycle. Many ear disorders result in hearing loss, a common sensory deficit among older adults. Hearing aids can compensate for some but not all forms of hearing loss. Nurses play a pivotal role in preventing hearing loss by reducing the severity and frequency of ear infections among children and advocating for measures that reduce exposure to loud noise.

Anatomy and Physiology

The ear (Fig. 49–1) is divided into three areas: the outer, middle, and inner sections. Sound is perceived because of a chain reaction involving all three areas of the ear. The inner ear also helps maintain balance.

Outer Ear

The outer ear, or *auricle,* consists of the *pinna,* the fleshy external projection of the ear, and the *external acoustic meatus,* a 1-inch canal that extends to the *tympanic membrane,* or eardrum. The outer ear collects sound waves and directs them inward. The external acoustic meatus contains the glands that produce *cerumen,* a waxy substance that lubricates the ear canal, protects the eardrum, and helps prevent external ear infections. Chewing and talking help to move cerumen to the outer area of the external acoustic meatus where it is easily washed away.

Middle Ear

The middle ear is a small, air-filled cavity in the temporal bone. The *eustachian tube* extends from the floor of the middle ear to the pharynx and is lined with mucous membrane. It equalizes air pressure in the middle ear. A chain of three small bones, the *malleus,*

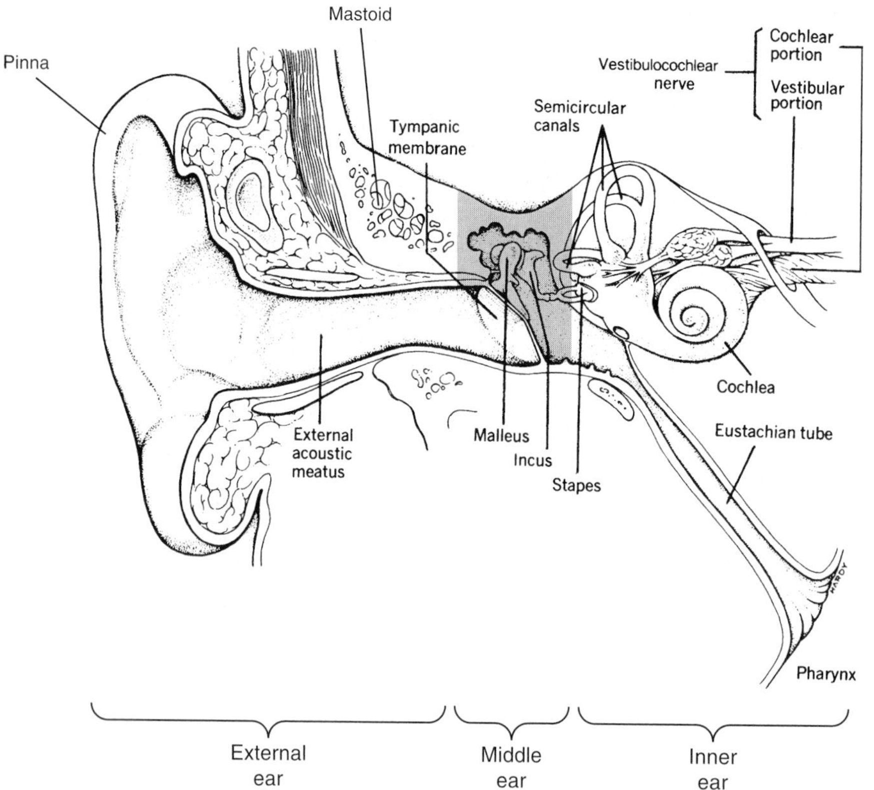

FIGURE 49-1. Diagram of the ear, showing the external, middle, and internal subdivisions.

the *incus*, and the *stapes*, stretches across the middle ear cavity from the tympanic membrane to the *oval window*. They move when struck by sound waves transmitted from the outer ear. When these bones are set in motion, the footplate of the stapes, which is very flexible, strikes the oval window, agitating the fluid in the inner ear.

Inner Ear

The inner ear, or *labyrinth*, consists of a series of cavities and canals that contain fluid. It has three sections: the *vestibule*, which lies just beyond the oval window; the *cochlea*, which provides for hearing; and the *semicircular canals*, which promote balance.

The fluid motion created by the vibrating stapes excites the nerve endings in the sensitive sound receptors of the *organ of Corti* located in the cochlea. The impulses are then converted to nerve impulses and transmitted along the cochlear nerve to the brain where sound is perceived.

Nerve receptors for balance are found both in the vestibule and semicircular canals. They transmit information about motion via the vestibular nerve, which joins with the cochlear nerve to form the eighth cranial nerve, the vestibulocochlear nerve (formally called the auditory or acoustic nerve).

Assessment

Although many ear disorders are assessed and treated by family practice physicians, some are referred to *otolaryngologists*, physicians who specialize in the diagnosis and treatment of ear, nose, and throat disorders. An *audiologist* is a paraprofessional with special training in performing hearing tests, measuring hearing loss, and recommending methods for improving the perception of sound. Box 49–1 outlines the nursing assessment.

Basic Hearing Acuity Test

Hearing acuity is grossly assessed by standing 1 to 2 feet beside one of the client's ears, then the other, and whispering a number, which the client is asked to repeat. Several numbers are provided to ensure valid test results. Another technique is to sit beside the client and bring a ticking watch toward the ear. The client should perceive the sound at the same time as the nurse, who is assumed to have normal hearing.

Otoscopic Examination

An otoscopic examination involves inspecting the external acoustic canal and tympanic membrane using

BOX 49-1 Nursing Assessment of the Ear and Basic Hearing Acuity

- Obtain the client's appraisal of his or her hearing including whether or not the client experiences tinnitus.
- Observe for actions that suggest a hearing problem such as leaning forward, turning the head, or cupping a hand to the ear to hear better.
- Document the use of a hearing aid.
- Ask the client about allergies, a history of upper respiratory and middle ear infections, high fevers, or exposure to loud sounds, because these can all cause hearing loss.
- Inspect the external ear for signs of infection, such as swelling, redness, drainage, or evidence of trauma.
- Shine a penlight into the ear to grossly inspect the ear canal; straighten the ear canal by gently pulling the ear up and back for an adult and downward and backward for small children.

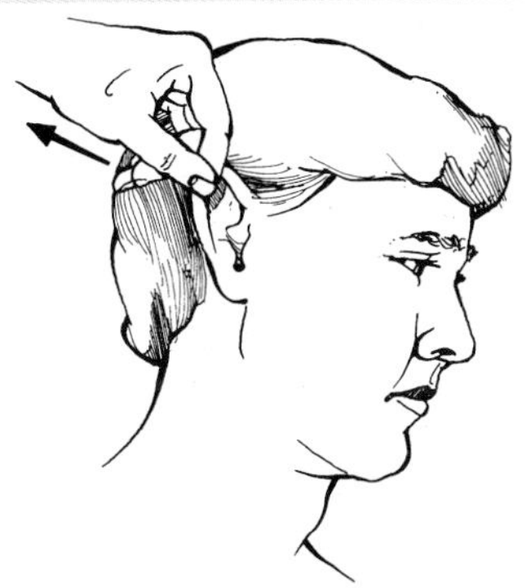

An adult's ear is pulled up and back.

- Palpate the areas in front of and behind the ear lobe for tenderness and swelling.
- Perform a basic hearing acuity test.

an **otoscope**, a hand-held instrument with a light, lens, and optional speculum for inserting into the client's ear (Fig. 49–2). If normal, the canal appears smooth and empty. The normal tympanic membrane is intact, looks pearly gray, and transmits light. Excessive cerumen interferes with inspection.

Tuning Fork Tests

A **tuning fork** is an instrument that produces sound in the same range as human speech. It is used to screen for conductive or sensorineural hearing loss. A **conductive hearing loss** involves interference in the transmission of sound waves to the inner ear. **Sensorineural hearing loss** is the result of nerve impairment.

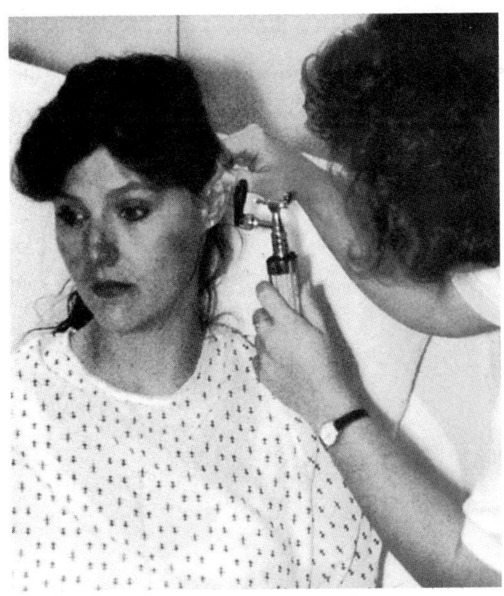

FIGURE 49-2. The nurse is inspecting the external ear with an otoscope.

The Rinne test and Weber test identify types of hearing loss. For the **Rinne test** (Fig. 49–3), the tuning fork is struck, placed on the mastoid process behind the ear, and held there until the client indicates the sound has stopped. Immediately after that, the still vibrating tuning fork is held beside the ear and the client again says when the sound stops. Normally, air conduction beside the ear measures twice as long as by bone conduction through the mastoid. The **Weber test** is performed by striking the tuning fork and placing its stem in the midline of the client's skull or center of the forehead (Fig. 49–4). A person with normal hearing perceives the sound equally well in both ears. If the sound seems lateralized to one ear, it suggests a conduction hearing loss in that ear or a sensorineural loss in the opposite ear.

Romberg Test

The **Romberg test** is used to evaluate a person's ability to sustain balance. The client stands with feet together and both arms extended. The client closes his or her eyes. Swaying, losing balance, or arm drifting are abnormal responses. Because central nervous system lesions cause similar abnormal results, additional testing is needed to confirm an inner ear dysfunction.

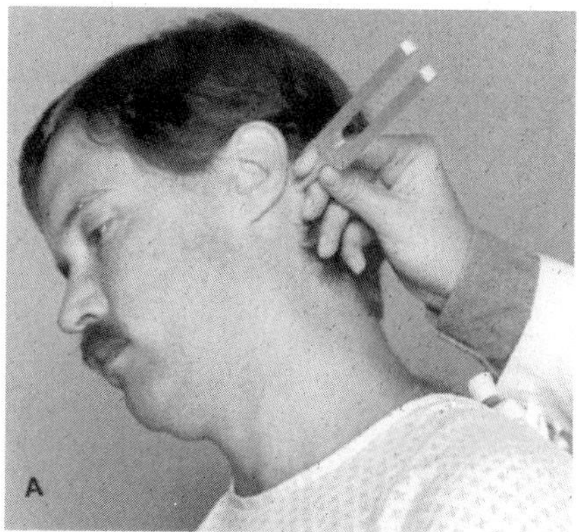

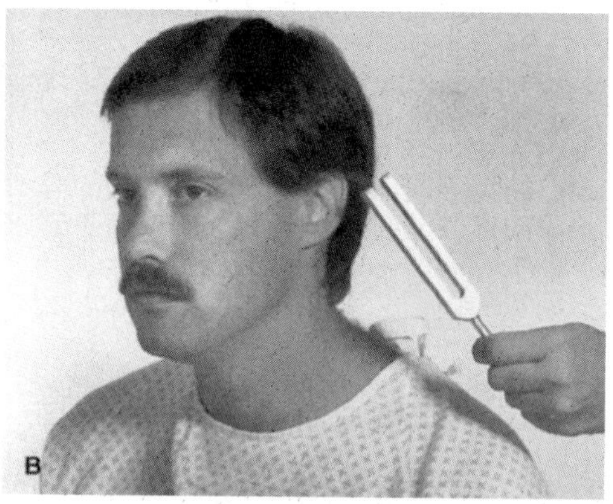

FIGURE 49-3. The Rinne test is performed by (*A*) striking a tuning fork and placing it on the mastoid bone, and then (*B*) holding it beside the ear.

Diagnostic Studies

Audiometry

Audiometry is done by an audiologist. Audiometric testing measures hearing acuity precisely. During the test, controlled intensities of sound, measured in **decibels** (dB), are projected to one ear at a time through a headset. The client indicates when the sound is heard. The lowest level of sound that normal individuals can first perceive is 20 dB; painful sounds occur at 120 dB. Hearing acuity is determined by measuring the intensity at which a person first perceives sound.

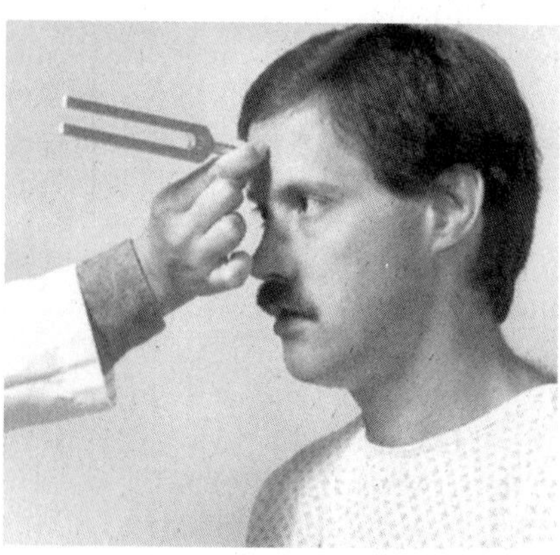

FIGURE 49-4. When a vibrating tuning fork is placed against the center of the head or middle of the forehead, the person with a conductive hearing loss will hear the sounds louder in the more affected ear; to the person with sensorineural hearing loss, the tone sounds louder in the less affected ear.

Caloric Stimulation Test

A **caloric stimulation test** assesses vestibular reflexes of the inner ear that control balance. Warm (40°C) or cool (25°C) water or air is instilled into the external meatus of each ear separately. The fluid alters the temperature of the temporal bone and creates convection currents in the fluid of the inner ear that simulate movement of the head. **Nystagmus**, a quivering movement of the eyes, is the expected response. Slight dizziness may also be experienced. A diminished response in one eye is significant for an inner ear disorder such as Meniere's disease (discussed later).

Electronystagmography

Electronystagmography is a more precise method for evaluating vestibular function, the mechanisms that facilitate maintaining balance. It is performed in conjunction with caloric stimulation. When the fluid is instilled within the ear, a machine records the duration and velocity of the eye movements with electrodes attached superiorly, inferiorly, and laterally about the eyes.

Hearing Impairment

Hearing impairment is described as mild, moderate, severe, or profound, depending on the intensity of sound required for a person to hear it (Table 49–1). Diminished hearing is due to a conductive or sensorineural loss or a combination of the two. Conductive hearing loss occurs from conditions such as an accumulation of cerumen in the external acoustic

TABLE 49-1 **Hearing Acuity**

Hearing Range	Decibels (dB)	Without a Hearing Aid	With a Hearing Aid
Normal	20–120	Can hear faint to painful sounds	Unnecessary
Mild impairment	40–120	Unable to hear unvoiced consonants such as "s" and "f"	Helpful, but not necessarily worth the expense
Moderate impairment	60–120	Unable to hear conversational volume unless others talk loudly	Beneficial for restoring ability to hear normal conversations
Severe impairment	70–120	Misses a majority of conversational content	Amplifies 40 dB sounds to 75 dB, but also amplifies nonspeech and background noise
Profound impairment	90–120	Depends heavily on speech reading	Helps hearing vowels, but amplified speech and background noise are painful
Total deafness	120	Hears only painfully loud sounds or vibrations created by loud sounds	Not useful for understanding speech

meatus or failure of the tiny ear bones to vibrate. Sensorineural hearing loss includes such etiologies as arteriosclerosis, a tumor of the vestibulocochlear nerve, infections, and drug toxicity. Clients with a hearing impairment often have **tinnitus,** hearing buzzing, whistling, or ringing noises in one or both ears.

Hearing loss seriously impairs one's ability to protect oneself and to communicate with others. The age at which hearing loss occurs plus the severity of the impairment have extensive consequences. For example, hearing loss during the first 3 years of life, the most critical period learning to make sounds, affects language acquisition at the word, phrase, and sentence levels. If uncorrected, hearing deficits can lead to depression and social isolation.

MEDICAL MANAGEMENT

Besides treating the cause of the hearing loss, medical management includes a recommendation for a hearing aid, a battery-operated device that fits in the external ear and amplifies sound. Clients with a conductive hearing loss benefit more from the use of a hearing aid because the structures that convert sound into energy and facilitate perception of sound within the brain continue to function.

SUPPORTIVE SERVICES AND PRODUCTS

Some clients with hearing deficits learn **sign language** (Fig. 49–5), a method for communication that

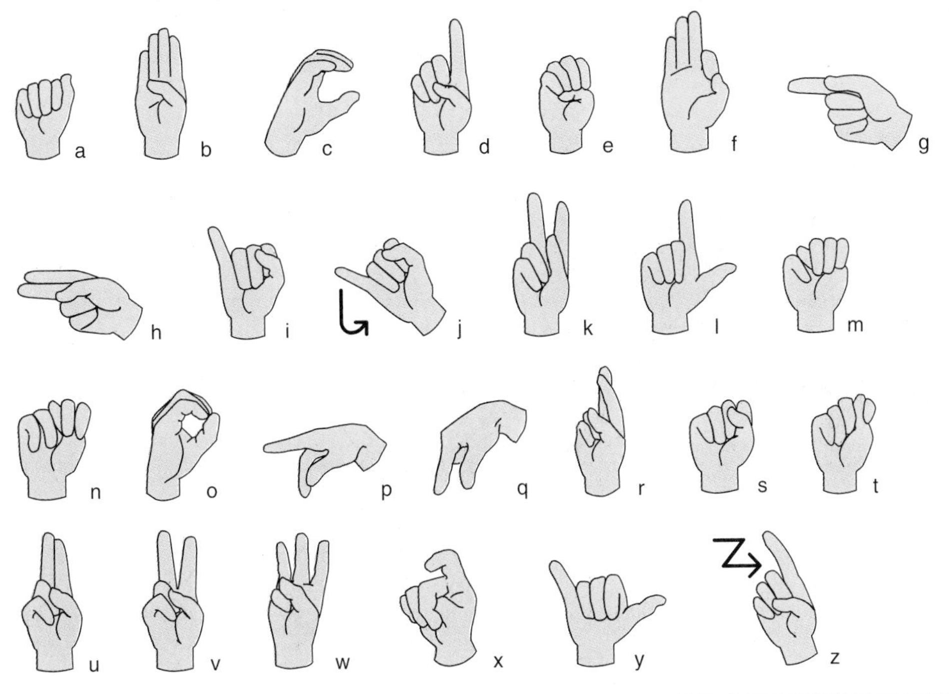

FIGURE 49-5. The alphabet in sign language.

uses a hand-spelled alphabet and word symbols, and **speech reading**, also called lip reading.

Many technologic devices have been developed to promote communication. Some television programs are transmitted using closed-caption inserts in which the dialogue is printed on the bottom of the screen or a person who simultaneously signs is displayed in a corner of the screen. Some theaters provide headsets that amplify actors' voices to individual patrons. Telephones can be adapted with a hearing amplifier that increases sound from incoming callers. Another device for people with severe hearing impairment is a telecommunication device for the deaf (TODD). This device is a combination special typewriter and telephone used to call someone else with a TODD. A TODD business directory is available, or the TODD user can call a relay center and the center will communicate for the TODD user. Computer modems also facilitate communication.

Many other products allow the hearing impaired to perceive (rather than hear) sound. For example, light-activated alarms in smoke detectors, alarm clocks, doorbells, and telephones flash a light when sound is produced. Hearing dogs, like guide dogs for the blind, are specially trained to warn their owners when certain sounds occur.

SURGICAL MANAGEMENT

Sensorineural hearing loss is usually irreversible. It is somewhat improved with a **cochlear implant**, a device that is surgically placed in the inner ear and connected to a receiver in the bone behind the ear (Fig. 49–6). Even with a cochlear implant, clients frequently have difficulty understanding and learning speech.

NURSING MANAGEMENT

The nurse observes for signs of hearing impairment such as leaning forward, turning and cupping the ear to hear better, and asking that words be repeated. Gross hearing is assessed using the techniques described earlier. The clarity of the client's speech also is determined. The nurse refers a client for the diagnosis and subsequent treatment of a hearing impairment and speech therapy. Many people reject the area that their hearing is impaired. Some consider it a sign of aging and deterioration. If the client fears that wearing a hearing aid is a stigma, the nurse describes the various types of hearing aids that are available, some of which fit almost unnoticeably within the ear (Fig. 49–7). The importance of avoiding the purchase of a hearing aid from a mail order catalogue or a company salesman is stressed.

If a hearing impairment exists, the nurse obtains information about its severity and the methods used to understand the speech of others. When a client hears poorly, the nurse determines the communication method the client prefers: speech reading, signing, writing, or typing. Suggestions for oral communication are listed in Nursing Guidelines 49–1. If the client uses a hearing aid, the nurse safeguards the instrument, assists the client with its insertion, and helps maintain its function.

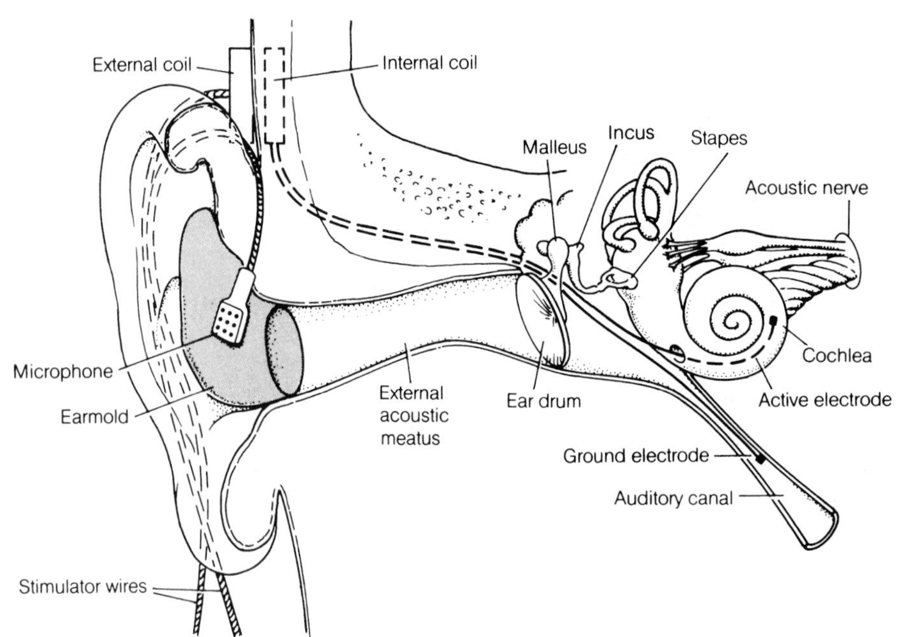

FIGURE 49-6. With a cochlear implant, sound is passed from the external transmitter to the inner coil by magnetic conduction and is then carried over an electrode to the cochlea.

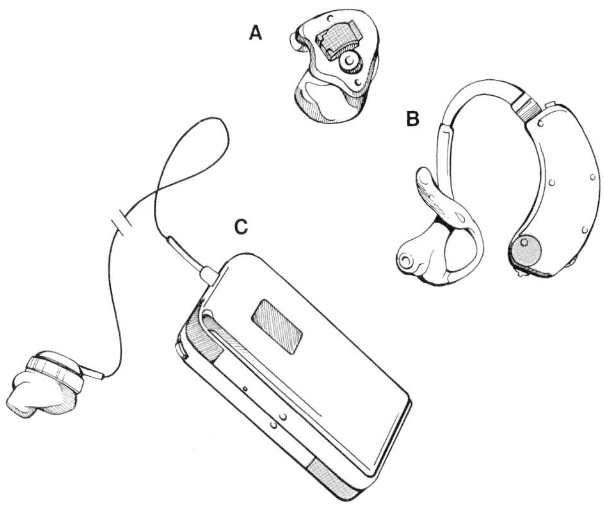

FIGURE 49-7. Examples of hearing aids: *(A)* in-the-ear, *(B)* behind-the-ear, and *(C)* body aid.

To protect their self-esteem, some clients with a hearing impairment nod their heads as if they are following the conversation or laugh along with others to conceal the fact that they do not understand what has been said. The nurse encourages clients with a hearing loss to be forthright and inform others about the hearing deficit. In addition, assistive hearing devices and aids for communication discussed earlier are identified. Clients are advised to maintain previously established relationships because genuine friendships are not likely to be affected by a physical impairment.

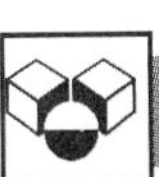

Nursing Guidelines 49-1

Communicating With People With A Hearing Loss

- Eliminate background noise as much as possible.
- Stand or sit on the side of the client's better ear.
- Ensure that there is adequate natural or artificial light.
- Get the client's attention.
- Face the client.
- Speak clearly and at a normal pace without exaggerating pronunciations.
- Do not shout, but avoid dropping conversational volume at the end of a sentence.
- Promote a clear image of your mouth; do not chew gum or cover your mouth.
- Use gestures and facial expressions to enhance what is being said orally.
- Rephrase whatever the client does not understand.
- Remain patient, positive, and relaxed.
- Provide paper and pencil if the client communicates by sign language or has speech that is difficult to understand.
- Use a support person who can communicate by signing.

(Adapted from Self Help for the Hard of Hearing People, Inc. (SHHH), 7910 Woodmont Avenue, Bethesda, MD 20814)

Client and Family Teaching

Use illustrations, pamphlets and written directions to aid teaching. Include a family member. Ask the client to repeat information and demonstrate technical skills. Initiate a referral to a community agency to evaluate if and how well the client is performing self-care after discharge.

Disorders of the External Ear

Various disorders such as impacted cerumen, injury from foreign objects, or otitis externa affect the external acoustic meatus. If these disorders are not treated carefully and adequately, they may spread to the middle ear.

Impacted Cerumen

Impacted cerumen is accumulated ear wax that obstructs the external acoustic meatus.

ETIOLOGY AND PATHOPHYSIOLOGY

Impacted cerumen is more common among people who have an excessive amount of thick or dry cerumen. Both qualities interfere with drainage toward the proximal end of the meatus where cerumen normally leaves the ear during regular shampooing and showering. The trapped cerumen interferes with the transmission of sounds carried on air waves.

ASSESSMENT FINDINGS

Signs and Symptoms

The client reports having a sense of fullness in the ears and diminished hearing. The client asks that words be repeated, misinterprets questions, or raises the volume on the television or radio. Visual inspection with an otoscope shows an orange-brown accumulation of cerumen in the distal end of the external acoustic meatus.

Diagnostic Findings

Audiometric, Rinne, and Weber tests reveal conductive hearing loss.

MEDICAL MANAGEMENT

Dried cerumen is hydrated by instilling 1 or 2 drops of peroxide, warm glycerin, or mineral oil, or it is softened with commercial agents, such as carbamide peroxide (Debrox) and triethanolamine (Cerumenex). Cerumen is removed mechanically by irrigating the ear if the eardrum is intact or using an instrument called a cerumen spoon.

NURSING MANAGEMENT

The nurse inspects the ears and implements measures to remove excessive cerumen. Ear drops are warmed by holding the container in the hand for a few moments or placing it in warm water. If irrigation or instillation of liquids is ordered, the liquid is warmed to body temperature. Cold or hot liquids cause dizziness, and the potential for injury exists if the liquid is hot. The nurse avoids inserting the irrigating syringe too deeply so as to close off the auditory canal. The flow is directed toward the roof of the canal rather than the eardrum.

Foreign Objects

ETIOLOGY AND PATHOPHYSIOLOGY

Foreign objects find their way into the ear either by accident or by deliberate insertion. Sharp objects can scratch the skin or cause blunt penetration of the eardrum. Insect stings cause local inflammation of the tissue.

ASSESSMENT FINDINGS

Signs and Symptoms

The client describes discomfort, diminished hearing, feeling movement, or hearing a buzzing sound. On gross inspection, there is evidence of abrasion from trauma or an insect, or an object is seen. Inspection with a penlight or otoscope reveals swelling and redness within the auditory canal.

MEDICAL MANAGEMENT

Mineral oil is instilled into the ear to smother an insect. Solid objects are removed with a small forceps.

NURSING MANAGEMENT

The nurse instructs clients to clean the ears with a face cloth rather than inserting objects into the ears. A hat with earflaps or a scarf is recommended when venturing into the woods or other areas where there is a high insect population.

Otitis Externa

Otitis externa is an inflammation of the tissue within the outer ear.

ETIOLOGY AND PATHOPHYSIOLOGY

Inflammation is generally caused by an overgrowth of pathogens. The microorganisms tend to follow trauma to the lining of the ear, or their growth is supported by retained moisture from swimming. Another possibility is that a hair follicle becomes infected, causing a furuncle or an abscess to develop.

ASSESSMENT FINDINGS

Signs and Symptoms

The tissue in the external ear looks red. Sometimes it is difficult to see the tympanic membrane because of swelling. Clients describe discomfort that increases with manipulation during the examination. Hearing is reduced because of swelling. In severe infections, a fever develops and the lymph nodes behind the ear enlarge.

Diagnostic Findings

Otoscopic examination reveals diffuse or confined inflammation, swelling, and pus. A culture of drainage identifies the specific pathogen.

MEDICAL MANAGEMENT

Treatment includes warm soaks, analgesics, and antibiotic ear medication.

NURSING MANAGEMENT

The nurse instructs the client on carrying out the medical treatment and provides health teaching to prevent recurrence. For example, swimmers are advised to wear soft plastic ear plugs to prevent trapping water within the ear. If chewing produces or potentiates discomfort, the nurse encourages the client to temporarily eat soft foods or consume nourishing liquids. Above all, the client is advised to avoid the use of nonprescription remedies unless they have been approved by the physician and to contact the physician if symptoms are not relieved in a few days.

Disorders of the Middle Ear

Otitis Media

Otitis media is an inflammation or infection in the middle ear. Clients may have acute or chronic forms of either serous otitis media, also known as secretory or nonsuppurative, or the purulent or suppurative type. Although otitis media is more common among young children, adults can and do develop middle ear infections.

ETIOLOGY AND PATHOPHYSIOLOGY

Serous otitis media, a collection of pathogen-free fluid behind the tympanic membrane, results from irritation associated with respiratory allergies and enlarged adenoids. Purulent otitis media usually results from the spread of microorganisms from the eustachian tube to the middle ear during upper respiratory infections.

When fluid or pus collects in the middle ear, pressure increases, which causes the eardrum to bulge and spontaneously rupture in some cases. Rupture results in a jagged tear of tissue that heals slowly and sometimes incompletely. Scarring interferes with the vibration of the eardrum, causing diminished hearing. Clients with perforated eardrums are prone to repeated infections.

Other potentially serious complications can occur. Because the middle ear connects with the mastoid process, a part of the temporal bone, pathogens that are unresponsive to antibiotic therapy can spread, causing **mastoiditis**, or they can travel deeper within the inner ear, causing **labyrnthitis**. Infection also may extend to the meninges, causing meningitis, or brain abscess may result from its extension to the brain. If septicemia occurs, the infection can spread to the large veins at the base of the brain and cause lateral sinus thrombosis. Facial nerve damage and facial paralysis may result from the infection. With prompt and adequate treatment, complications are rare.

ASSESSMENT FINDINGS

Signs and Symptoms

The client often describes a history of having had a recent upper respiratory infection or seasonal allergies. Signs and symptoms vary widely depending on the type and severity of the inflammation, but may include a fever, tinnitus, malaise, severe earache, and diminished hearing. Tenderness behind the ear indicates mastoiditis. The eardrum looks red and bulging. Pressure within the middle ear or dysfunction of inner ear structures can cause nausea, vomiting, and dizziness. If the tympanic membrane perforates, fluid drains into the external acoustic canal and pain is relieved.

Diagnostic Findings

The white blood cell count shows an elevated number of neutrophils and eosinophils. If the eardrum has ruptured and drainage is present, the cultured drainage reveals a specific infectious microorganism.

MEDICAL AND SURGICAL MANAGEMENT

Prompt treatment usually prevents rupture of the eardrum. In some cases, the fluid is aspirated by needle. Antibiotics are given to control the infection. The overuse of antibiotics, however, has created another problem: microorganisms are becoming resistant and, for some infections, the available antibiotics are of limited benefit.

To reduce the consequences of spontaneous rupture of the eardrum, subsequent scarring, and hearing loss, the physician performs a **myringotomy**, an incisional opening of the eardrum. The incised opening facilitates drainage of the purulent material, eases the pressure, and relieves the throbbing pain. The incision heals readily with little scarring.

Plastic surgery (**myringoplasty**) usually is successful in repairing the perforated eardrum. In one technique, the edges of the perforation are cauterized and a patch of blood-soaked absorbable gelatin sponge (Gelfoam) is used as a scaffolding over which new tissue grows until it has filled in the defect. Chronic infections are prevented if the eardrum is repaired. In the case of mastoiditis, a **mastoidectomy** is performed to remove the diseased tissue. With early and effective antibiotic therapy, mastoiditis is rare.

NURSING MANAGEMENT

After myringotomy, the discharge from the ear is bloody and then purulent. To remove the drainage, the external ear is wiped repeatedly with a dry sterile cotton applicator. An alternative is to insert a loose (not tightly packed) cotton pledget within the external ear to collect drainage. The cotton is changed when it becomes moist.

Otosclerosis

Otosclerosis is the result of a bony overgrowth of the stapes and a common cause of hearing impairment among adults. Fixation of the stapes occurs gradually over a period of many years.

ETIOLOGY AND PATHOPHYSIOLOGY

The underlying cause of otosclerosis is unknown. The condition, which is more common in women than in men, usually becomes apparent in the second and third decades of life. It seems to be accelerated during pregnancy. Most clients have a family history of the disease, which indicates a possible hereditary relationship.

Otosclerosis interferes with the vibration of the stapes and the transmission of sound to the inner ear. Although hearing loss in otosclerosis is of the conductive type, when and if progression of the disease involves the cochlea of the inner ear, a mixed type of hearing loss develops.

ASSESSMENT FINDINGS

Signs and Symptoms

A progressive, bilateral loss of hearing is the most characteristic symptom. The client notices the hearing loss when it begins to interfere with the ability to follow conversation. There is particular difficulty hearing others when they speak in soft, low tones, but hearing is adequate when the sound is loud enough. Tinnitus appears as the loss of hearing progresses. It is especially noticeable at night, when surroundings are quiet, and can be quite distressing to the client.

The eardrum appears pinkish orange from structural changes within the middle ear. When the Rinne test is performed, the sound is heard best when the tuning fork is applied behind the ear. The sound lateralizes to the more affected ear when the Weber test is performed.

Diagnostic Findings

Audiometric tests reveal the type and severity of hearing loss. A computed tomography (CT) scan demonstrates the location and extent of excessive bone growth.

MEDICAL AND SURGICAL MANAGEMENT

Although otosclerosis has no cure, a hearing aid helps. The level of restored hearing depends greatly on the severity of the sensorineural involvement. The outcome is best when the hearing loss is purely conductive. If the surgical treatment is selected, a **stapedectomy** is performed on the ear most affected. In this procedure, all or part of the stapes is removed and a prosthesis is inserted that can vibrate the oval window (Fig. 49–8). Once the stapes is freed or replaced, the client experiences an immediate, dramatic improvement in hearing. Hearing temporarily diminishes postoperatively because of swelling, but eventually returns. Complications include dislodgment of the prosthesis and continued hearing loss, infection, dizziness, and facial nerve damage. Depending on the outcome of surgery, the procedure may be repeated for the opposite ear.

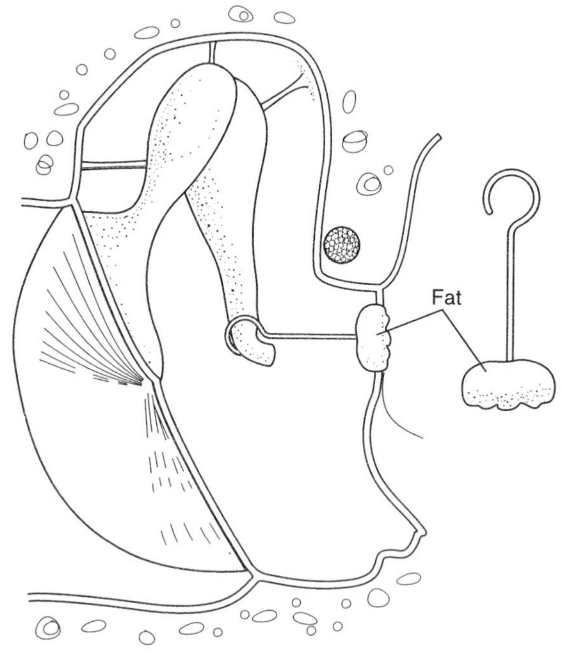

FIGURE 49-8. A wire prosthetic stapes is positioned within the middle ear.

NURSING MANAGEMENT

The nurse uses selected alternatives for communicating with the client as identified earlier in Nursing Guidelines 49–1 and provides the preoperative client with an explanation of what can be expected in the immediate postoperative period. The nurse tells the client that activity is restricted for 24 hours or more after surgery and that hearing may be temporarily the same as or worse than before surgery.

Postoperatively, the client is positioned with the operative ear upward. Care is taken to prevent dislodgment of the prosthesis as a result of coughing, sneezing, or vomiting. Nausea and dizziness are common problems. Facial nerve function is assessed by checking symmetry when the client smiles or frowns. The postoperative plan of care includes, but is not limited to, the following:

Nursing Diagnoses and Collaborative Problems	Nursing Interventions
Altered Comfort (pain, nausea, vertigo) related to tissue disruption	Administer prescribed analgesic and assess again in 30 minutes.
Goal: The client will experience relief of discomfort to at least a tolerable level.	Give an antiemetic for nausea or vomiting.

	Reinforce a positive outcome from medications to support the client's belief system and hasten beneficial effects.
	Provide small, frequent sips of fluid or light food to prevent nausea.
	Limit head movement and avoid jarring the bed to minimize pain, dizziness, and nausea.
Risk for Infection related to impaired tissue integrity secondary to the surgical incision	Adhere strictly to aseptic principles when changing a dressing or cleaning the ear.
Goal: The client will remain free of a secondary infection.	Administer prescribed antibiotics.
	Instruct the client to keep his or her hands away from the dressing or packing.
	Keep the external ear and surrounding skin meticulously clean and free of purulent drainage.
Risk for Injury related to vertigo	Use the side rails and handrails for support when preparing to ambulate.
Goal: The client will be free of injury.	Walk with the client who is dizzy.

Client and Family Teaching

The prescribed medical regimen and restrictions are discussed with the client or a family member. One or more of the following are included in a teaching plan:

- Avoid blowing the nose because this action can dislodge the prosthesis.
- Avoid high altitudes or flying.
- Do not lift heavy objects, strain when defecating, or bend over at the waist; these activities increase pressure in the middle ear.
- Do not get water in the ear. Avoid swimming, showering, and washing the hair until approved by the physician.
- Follow the physician's instructions for keeping the ear clean.
- Stay away from people with respiratory infections. If a head cold occurs, contact the physician immediately.
- Notify the physician immediately if severe pain, excessive drainage, a sudden loss of hearing, or fever occurs.
- Adhere to the restriction of activities recommended by the physician until told otherwise.

Disorders of the Inner Ear

Meniere's Disease

Meniere's disease is a term given to the episodic symptoms created by fluctuations in the production or reabsorption of fluid in the inner ear. It is typically unilateral, appears during middle age, and is more common in men than in women. In women, it seems to be influenced by reproductive hormones.

ETIOLOGY AND PATHOPHYSIOLOGY

The cause of the excessive production of fluid is unknown; however, allergies are implicated in some instances. When the fluid accumulates, it dilates the cochlear duct, which diminishes hearing. Equilibrium also is affected as the vestibular system becomes damaged. Tinnitus occurs. At times, the client is symptom free except for permanent, residual hearing loss as the number of attacks increase. Occasionally clients recover spontaneously, which leads some to suspect a psychobiologic connection.

ASSESSMENT FINDINGS

Signs and Symptoms

The client periodically experiences severe vertigo, tinnitus, and progressive hearing loss. Nausea and vomiting accompany the vertigo. Nystagmus of the eyes is observed. Some clients experience preattack symptoms of headache and a full feeling within the ear.

An attack lasts from a few minutes to weeks and can occur with alarming suddenness. Some clients are reluctant to leave their homes for fear they will have an attack in public. Continued employment becomes impossible for some clients.

DIAGNOSTIC FINDINGS

A caloric stimulation test and electronystagmography demonstrate a difference in eye movement response. A CT scan or magnetic resonance imaging rules out other possible causes of the symptoms, such as a tumor that involves the vestibulocochlear nerve. Audiometry identifies the type and magnitude of the hearing deficit.

MEDICAL AND SURGICAL MANAGEMENT

Treatment is aimed at reducing the production of fluid within the inner ear, facilitating its drainage, and treating the symptoms that accompany the attack. A low-sodium diet lessens edema. Treatment of the allergy or avoidance of the allergen is recommended. Antihistamines are also used. Smoking is contraindicated to prevent vasoconstriction, which interferes with fluid drainage. Nicotinic acid is beneficial for producing vasodilation. An antiemetic and tranquilizer are prescribed during an attack. Bed rest is usually necessary while the client is symptomatic.

If clients become extremely incapacitated, surgery becomes an option. In one type of surgery, the labyrinth is destroyed by ultrasonic waves, thus relieving symptoms but causing permanent deafness in the affected ear. Another type of surgery establishes permanent drainage for the fluid from the inner ear into the subarachnoid space to preserve whatever hearing remains.

NURSING MANAGEMENT

Obtain a history of symptoms, the length of time they have been present, and complete medical, drug, and allergy histories. Gross hearing is assessed, and the Weber and Rinne tests are performed.

The client with Meniere's disease requires a great deal of emotional support because of the unpredictability of the attacks and the resulting impairments that they cause. During an attack, the nurse administers drugs, limits movement, and promotes the client's safety. The nurse assists the client with activities of daily living because the least amount of motion can produce severe vertigo.

The nurse is available, empathic, and responsive to the client. Trust and confidence develop when the client does not feel abandoned or required to convince caregivers of the necessity for attention. Clients are comforted when the nurse acknowledges that dealing with temporary or permanent hearing loss is a challenge.

Client and Family Teaching

If a low-sodium diet is recommended, a list of foods to avoid or diet instruction is provided by the dietitian. If an allergy is suspected as the cause of the disorder, advise the client to take the prescribed antihistamines as directed and to avoid known allergens. If a hearing aid is recommended, refer the client to an audiologist for instructions on its use and care.

General Pharmacologic Considerations

Nonprescription preparations are available for softening hardened cerumen. Refer the client to a physician if hearing remains diminished.

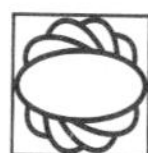

General Gerontologic Considerations

Older clients form drier cerumen and experience an increased incidence of impaction within the external acoustic meatus.

Hearing loss is common as adults age. Options in the style of prescribed hearing aid are limited by the client's ability to care and maintain it.

The older adult with a hearing impairment may become disoriented and confused in strange surroundings. Frequent contact and reorientation prevent confusion.

SUMMARY OF KEY CONCEPTS

- The ear consists of the outer, middle, and inner sections. A chain reaction involving all three areas results in the hearing of sounds.
- Hearing impairment may be mild, moderate, severe, profound, or total. The acuity level increases for each classification.
- Hearing-impaired people may communicate using speech reading, signing, or writing.
- Nursing care of the client with hearing loss involves assessing the severity of loss and preferred methods of communication, promoting self esteem, and referring to a community agency.
- Clients with ear and hearing disorders are referred to otolaryngologists and audiologists.
- Three conditions that commonly affect the external (outer) ear include impacted cerumen, foreign objects, and otitis externa.
- To facilitate inspection of the ear canal and administration of medications, the nurse pulls the pinna of the ear upward and backward on adults and the earlobe downward and backward on small children.
- Disorders of the external ear are prevented or treated by washing and drying the external ears at the time of bathing, using nonprescription medications that soften cerumen, gently irrigating substances from the ear, keeping the ears covered where there are insects, and using ear plugs to reduce the potential for trapped water within the ear.
- Two conditions that affect the middle ear are otitis media and otosclerosis. Otitis media is aggressively treated because serious complications such as mastoiditis, labyrnthitis, meningitis, brain abscess, septicemia, and facial nerve damage can occur.
- When otitis media develops, a myringotomy is performed for four reasons: (1) to facilitate drainage of purulent material, (2) to ease pressure within the middle ear, (3) to relieve pain, and (4) to promote healing with minimal scar formation.
- When caring for a client undergoing ear surgery, the nurse promotes effective communication, explains the pre- and postoperative routine, which includes lying with the operative ear up after surgery and avoiding coughing, sneezing, and vomiting.

- Meniere's disease is a disorder of the inner ear that is caused by an excessive production or slow reabsorption of fluid within the inner ear. The fluid buildup causes dizziness, which can be accompanied by nausea and vomiting. Tinnitus and progressive hearing loss occur with each subsequent attack of symptoms.
- The nurse caring for a client with Meniere's disease provides physical care and emotional support while the client is incapacitated by the symptoms.

CRITICAL THINKING EXERCISES

1. Discuss the problems associated with hearing loss that are unique and similar among disorders of the external, middle, and internal ear.
2. Describe techniques that promote communication when interacting with clients who have a hearing loss.

Suggested Readings

Chan, E. A talent for listening. (1997). *Nursing Times, 93*(51), 36–37.

Curry, M. D., Daniel, H. J., & Andrews, A. W. (1997). A community-based nursing approach to the prevention of otitis media. *Journal of Community Health Nursing, 14*(2), 81–110.

Jupiter,. T., & Spivy, V. (1997). Perception of hearing loss and hearing handicap on hearing aid use by nursing home residents. *Geriatric Nursing, 18*(5), 201–207; quiz 207–208.

Larsen, P. D., Martin, J. L., & Hazen, S. E. (1997). Assessment and management of sensory loss in elderly patients. *AORN Journal, 65*(2), 432–437.

Lusk, S. L. (1997). Noise exposures. Effects on hearing and prevention of noise induced hearing loss. *AAOHN Journal, 45*(8), 397–408; quiz 409–410.

McConnell, E. A. (1998). Communicating with a hearing-impaired patient. *Nursing, 28*(1), 32.

Now hear this! (1997). *Lippincott Health Promotion Letter, 2*(4), 3.

Shelp, S. G. (1997). Your patient is deaf, now what? *RN, 60*(2), 37–40.

Tolson, D. (1997). Age-related hearing loss: A case for nursing intervention. *Journal of Advanced Nursing, 26*(6), 1150–1157.

Tolson, D., & McIntosh, J. (1997). Listening in the care environment—Chaos or clarity for the hearing-impaired elderly person. *International Journal of Nursing Studies, 34*(3), 173–182.

Waddington, C., Goodlett, A., & McKennis, A. T. (1997). Treatment of conductive hearing loss with ossicular chain reconstruction procedures. *AORN Journal, 65*(3), 511–515, 518, 521 passim.

Additional Resources

American Speech-Language-Hearing Association
http://www/asha. org/

Animated American Sign Language Dictionary
5451 Woodland Lane, SW
Fort Lauderdale, FL 33312
http://www.feist.com~randys/index_nf/html

Association of Disability Advocates
5451 Woodland Lane, SW
Fort Lauderdale, FL 53312
http://www/incanect.net/fpa/index.htm

Better Hearing Institute
c/o National Institute of Health
Bethesda, MD 22130–4998
http://www/nei.nih.gov/

Gallaudet College for the Deaf
800 Florida Avenue, NE
Washington, DC 20002–3695

National Association of the Deaf
Woodland Executive Center
Suite 1
1218 Reidville Road
Spartanburg, SC 29306
(800) 237–6213 (voice)
(800) 237–6819 (TTY)

National Institute on Deafness and Other Communication Disorders
National Institute of Health
Bethesda, MD 20892
http://www.nih.gov/nidcd

Self-Help for Hard of Hearing People (SHHH)
7910 Woodmont Avenue
Suite 1200
Bethesda, MD 20814
(301) 657–2248
http://www.shhh.org

12

Caring for Clients With Gastrointestinal Disorders

Chapter 50

Introduction to the Gastrointestinal System and Accessory Structures

KEY TERMS

Barium enema
Barium swallow
Cholangiography
Cholecystography
Colonoscopy
Endoscopic retrograde cholangiopancreatography
Enteroclysis
Esophagogastroduodenoscopy
Flexible sigmoidoscopy
Lower gastrointestinal series
Panendoscopy
Percutaneous liver biopsy
Peristalsis
Proctosigmoidoscopy
PY test
Small bowel enteroscopy
Upper gastrointestinal series

LEARNING OBJECTIVES

On completion of this chapter, the reader will:

- Identify major organs and structures that contribute to the function of the gastrointestinal system.
- Discuss three areas of information that are important to ascertain about the client's health complaint.
- List facts in the client's history that provide pertinent data about the present illness.
- Discuss at least 10 physical assessments that provide information about the function of the gastrointestinal tract and accessory organs.
- List eight common diagnostic tests performed on clients with gastrointestinal disorders.
- Discuss the nursing process and management of clients undergoing diagnostic testing for a gastrointestinal disorder.

The gastrointestinal (GI) system is arbitrarily divided into two sections: the upper GI tract and the lower GI tract (Fig. 50–1). The upper GI tract begins at the mouth and ends at the jejunum. The lower GI tract begins at the ileum and ends at the anus. The accessory structures of the GI tract include the liver, gallbladder, peritoneum, and pancreas. The primary functions of the GI tract are ingestion and digestion of food, absorption of nutrients, and elimination of solid waste. Table 50–1 lists secretions that aid in digestion.

Anatomy and Physiology

Mouth

Food normally enters the GI system at the mouth, where it is chewed (masticated) before swallowing. Food that contains starch undergoes partial digestion when mixed with the enzyme *salivary amylase*, which is secreted by the *salivary glands*.

Esophagus

The *esophagus* begins at the base of the pharynx and ends at the opening to the stomach. This muscular, tubular structure transports food to the stomach by wavelike contractions of smooth muscle known as **peristalsis.**

Stomach

The opening between the esophagus and the stomach is called the *cardiac sphincter*; that between the stom-

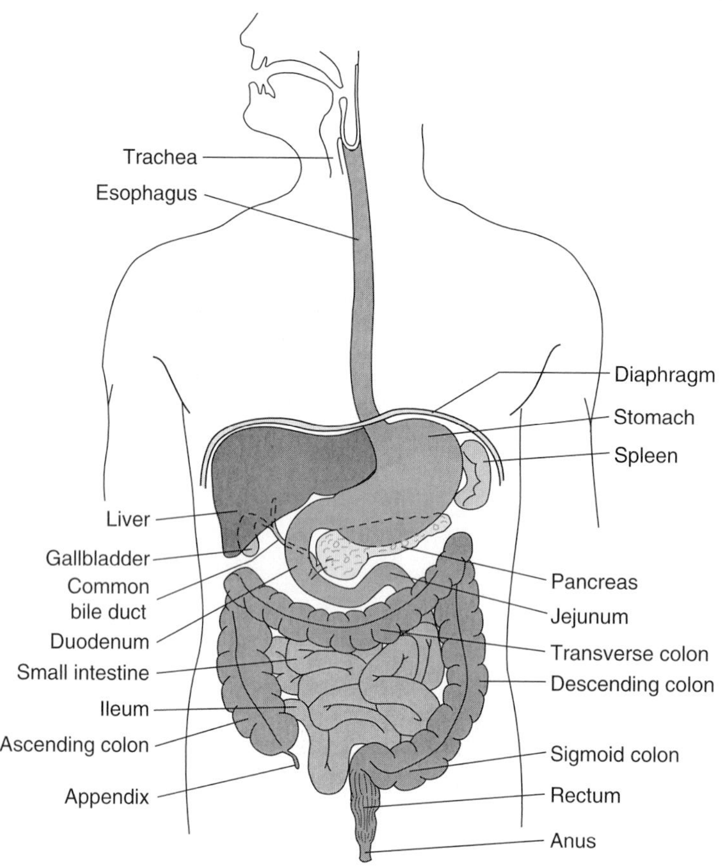

FIGURE 50-1. The upper GI tract begins at the mouth and ends at the jejunum. The lower GI tract begins at the ilium and ends at the anus. The accessory structures of the GI tract include the liver, gallbladder, peritoneum and pancreas.

ach and the duodenum is called the *pyloric sphincter*. Both sphincters are circular bands of muscle fibers. When contracted these sphincters keep stomach contents enclosed (or confined). When the pyloric sphincter relaxes, stomach contents flow to the duodenum.

The stomach temporarily holds ingested food and prepares it by mechanical and chemical action to pass in semiliquid form into the small intestine. Gastric secretions that contain digestive enzymes are released continuously but increase when food is eaten. Gastric secretions are acidic due to the presence of hydrochloric acid. The contractions of the stomach mix the food with the gastric secretions and move the mixture of semiliquid food called *chyme* to the small intestine by peristalsis. The length of time required for the stomach to empty depends on the amount and composition of food. Fats, for example, delay stomach emptying.

TABLE 50-1 **Chief Digestive Secretions**

GI Structure	Secretion	Action
Salivary glands	Salivary amylase	Begins starch digestion
Stomach	Hydrochloric acid (HCl)	Breaks down proteins
	Pepsin	Begins protein digestion
Small intestine	Peptidases	Converts peptides to amino acids
	Lactase, maltase, sucrase	Converts disaccharides to monosaccharides
Pancreas	Sodium bicarbonate	Neutralizes HCl
	Amylase	Breaks down starch
	Trypsin	Converts protein to amino acids
	Lipases	Converts fats to fatty acids and glycerol
Liver	Bile	Emulsifies fats

Adapted from Memmler, R. L., Cohen, B. J., & Wood, D. L. (1996). *The human body in health and disease* (8th ed.). Philadelphia: JB Lippincott.

Small Intestine

The small intestine is divided into three portions: the *duodenum*, the *jejunum*, and the *ileum*. The duodenum, which is about 10 inches long, is the first region of the small intestine and is the site where bile and pancreatic enzymes enter. These secretions continue to promote the chemical breakdown of food and transform the chyme to an alkaline state. The mixture, which is semiliquid at this point, is mechanically propelled by peristalsis into the jejunum and ileum. The jejunum and ileum have a combined length of approximately 23 feet.

The primary function of the small intestine is to absorb nutrients from the chyme. Absorption of different nutrients occurs at different sites in the small intestine. The duodenum is the primary site of iron and calcium absorption, and the jejunum is the site of absorption of fats, proteins, and carbohydrates. The ileum absorbs vitamin B_{12} and bile acids. When a part of the small intestine is diseased or removed surgically, absorption in that area is diminished or lost altogether.

The *ileocecal valve*, which lies at the distal end of the small intestine, regulates the flow of intestinal contents, which are liquid at this point, into the large intestine. This valve also prevents the reflux of bacteria from the large intestine, thus preserving the relative sterility of the small intestine.

Large Intestine

The large intestine receives waste matter from the small intestine and propels it toward the *anus*, the opening from the body for elimination. The cecum, colon, rectum, and anal canal make up the structures within the large intestine through which fecal material passes. The large intestine is approximately 4 to 5 feet long and approximately 2 inches in diameter. The large intestine absorbs water, some electrolytes, and bile acids. When the large intestine is diseased or surgically removed, these functions are diminished or lost. This may result in passage of loose stools, with potential for fluid and electrolyte imbalance. Passage of liquid stool, which contains a large amount of bile salts, makes the client especially vulnerable to skin breakdown in the perirectal area. If stool remains in the large intestine too long, constipation results. Then, straining to evacuate hard solid stool may disrupt skin integrity as well.

The *cecum* is a pouchlike structure at the beginning of the large intestine. At the tip of the cecum is a narrow blind tube called the *appendix*, which has no known function in humans.

The *colon* is divided into the *ascending, transverse, descending*, and *sigmoid* colons and *rectum*. Within the colon, the unabsorbed material that becomes fecal matter is composed of water, food residues, microorganisms, digestive secretions, and mucus. Water is absorbed as the mixture moves through the colon. By the time the mixture reaches the descending and sigmoid colon, the portion of the bowel adjacent to the rectum, it has become a formed mass.

Fecal matter is held within the *rectum* and retained there through the contraction of the internal and external anal sphincters. As the fecal mass accumulates, it distends the rectal wall, creating the urge to defecate. When the external anal sphincter relaxes, the fecal matter is expelled through the anus.

Accessory Structures

PERITONEUM

The abdominal organs are enclosed within the *peritoneum*, which is a membrane that lines the inner abdomen. The membrane, which encloses the viscera and the serous fluid that it secretes, allows the abdominal organs to move about without creating friction. The walls of the digestive organs normally prevent the gastric and intestinal contents from escaping into the peritoneal cavity. Any perforation that allows material to seep out of the digestive tract is serious because the microorganisms and enzymes can cause a severe inflammation and infection of the surrounding tissue called *peritonitis*.

LIVER

The *liver*, the largest glandular organ in the body, weighs between 1 and 1.5 kg (2–3 lb). It is located in the right upper abdomen just under the diaphragm, which separates it from the right lung. The liver is involved in a multitude of vital, complex metabolic activities. It forms and releases bile; processes vitamins, proteins, fats, and carbohydrates; stores glycogen; plays a role in blood coagulation; metabolizes and biotransforms many chemicals (including drugs), bacteria, and foreign matter; and forms antibodies and immunizing substances (gamma globulin). See Chapter 54 for more information.

GALLBLADDER

The *gallbladder* is attached to the midportion of the undersurface of the liver. It normally has a thin wall and holds about 60 mL of bile. The liver forms about 1 liter of bile each day but on reaching the gallbladder from the *common hepatic duct*, water and minerals are absorbed from the bile to form a more concentrated product. Gallbladder contraction triggered by ingested food, especially fats, causes bile to be released first through the *cystic duct* and then the *common bile duct* into the duodenum where it aids in the absorption of fats, fat-soluble vitamins, iron, and calcium. Bile also activates the pancreas to release its digestive enzymes, as well as an alkaline fluid that neutralizes stomach acids that reach the duodenum.

PANCREAS

The *pancreas* is both an *exocrine gland*, one that releases secretions into a duct or channel, and an *endocrine gland*, one that releases substances directly into the bloodstream. As an endocrine organ, it produces the hormones insulin and glucagon (see Chap. 57). As an exocrine organ, it produces a variety of protein-, fat-, and carbohydrate-digesting enzymes. At the appropriate time for digestion, the pancreatic enzymes are released in inactive forms and transported to the duodenum where they are activated.

Assessment of a Client With a Gastrointestinal Disorder

Many conditions can disrupt the normal function of the GI system. In addition to disorders of the GI tract and accessory organs, many disorders involving other organ systems can affect GI function. As a result, the client with a GI disorder may experience a wide variety of health problems that involve disturbances of ingestion, digestion, absorption, and elimination. Accurate recording of the client's health history, physical assessment findings, and outcomes of diagnostic tests help the health care team to diagnose and treat GI disorders.

Health History

The objective of the history is to identify the specific problem the client is experiencing and its possible cause. The history includes the client's chief complaint; a focus assessment of current nutritional, metabolic, and elimination patterns; and past history.

Gather as much data as possible about why the client has sought treatment and a description of the client's current symptoms. This includes the length of time the symptoms have been present, and what appears to cause or be related to the symptoms. Ask pertinent questions—Which types of food produce distress? When are symptoms most likely to occur? Also determine what measures, if any, the client uses to relieve the symptoms and what are the results.

During GI assessment, focus on *nutritional, metabolic*, and *elimination patterns*, including:

- Quality of the client's appetite
- Problems associated with chewing or swallowing foods
- What and how much the client eats each day
- Discomfort before, during, or after food consumption
- Nutritional supplements, if any, used by the client (eg, vitamins, herbs, home remedies)
- Weight gain or loss
- Bowel elimination patterns (usual consistency and color of stools, visible blood, stool frequency, effort or pain with passage of stool)

After obtaining a current health history, obtain a history of all past medical and surgical disorders and the treatment of each. Compile a family history of illnesses and causes of death. Family history of digestive disorders is especially important because several such as colorectal cancer, have a hereditary link. Explore the client's work history to evaluate the possibility of exposure to environmental toxic wastes or radioactive materials.

Obtain a complete allergy history, including adverse reactions to foods, because food allergies can result in various GI symptoms. List prescription and nonprescription drugs, especially those affecting GI function. Include the name of the drug, the dose, the frequency, and the reason for taking the drug.

Physical Assessment

GENERAL APPEARANCE

Assess the client's overall physical condition and measure the client's weight, height, and vital signs. Evaluate general appearance with regard to age and body size.

SKIN

Using natural sunlight or bright artificial light, inspect the skin for any abnormal color, such as a yellowish tint indicating jaundice. In very dark-skinned clients, inspect the hard palate, gums, conjunctiva, and surrounding tissues for jaundice. If the skin is jaundiced, inspect the sclerae to see if they are yellow. Keep in mind that the sclerae of some African Americans have a yellow cast from carotene and fatty deposits. Inspect the skin of the face and abdomen for other abnormalities, such as *spider angiomas* (superficial red discolorations consisting of blood vessels that assume a spider-shaped pattern), distended abdominal veins, and scars.

MOUTH

Examine the lips for sores, cracks, lesions, or other abnormalities. Use a tongue blade and a flashlight to inspect the mouth for inflammation, sores, swellings, or discolorations. Assess the quality of oral care. Look for missing teeth and partial plates, bridges, or dentures. If the client has dentures, ask if they fit well and whether regular food can be eaten. If the client can eat only soft foods, communicate this information to the physician and dietary department.

ABDOMEN

Continue the physical assessment by having the client lie supine for an abdominal examination. Abdominal areas are typically described in quadrants (right upper, right lower, left upper, and left lower quadrants), with the umbilicus as the center point for both horizontal and vertical divisions. Observe the contour of the abdomen noting whether it is flat, round, concave, or distended. Observe the effort associated with breathing because distention causes dyspnea due to upward pressure on the diaphragm. Auscultate the abdomen before palpation because palpation disrupts normal bowel sounds. Using a stethoscope, listen over each quadrant for bowel sounds, which sound like gurgles. Describe the location, quality pitch, and frequency of bowel sounds, which are generally heard every 5 to 30 seconds. Listen a full 5 minutes over each quadrant to confirm absence of bowel sounds. Measure abdominal girth at the widest point (usually at the umbilicus). Using a pen, mark the measurement location on the client's abdomen to ensure that additional examiners use the same reference point.

Next, palpate the abdomen to determine if it is soft or firm and to detect masses and areas of pain or tenderness. If the client reports tenderness, probe the lower liver margin. If it is enlarged, the liver is felt below the right lower rib cage. Pain or discomfort in this area suggests a liver disorder, gallbladder or intestinal disease, or a pancreatic disorder.

Percuss the abdomen to elicit changes in sounds from dullness over an area where there is a solid mass, such as the liver, to resonance over less dense structures or those filled with air.

ANUS

Using gloves, examine the anal area for external hemorrhoids, skin tags, or fissures (small tears in the anal opening). Inspect the skin surrounding the anus for breaks, lesions, rash, inflammation, and drainage. If and when stool passes, examine its characteristics. The shape, color, and consistency of stool are usually helpful in the differential diagnosis of GI disorders.

Diagnostic Studies

The diagnostic tests commonly used in GI disorders include radiographic studies, magnetic resonance imaging (MRI), computed tomographic (CT) scan, ultrasonography, endoscopy (with or without biopsy), nuclear imaging, percutaneous liver biopsy, and various laboratory tests.

RADIOGRAPHY

Radiographic studies are used to identify the location and structural appearance of organs or other space occupying masses, such as air, fluid, tumors, or foreign objects within the abdomen, chest, or GI system. Radiographic studies involve radiation in the form of radiopaque contrast media. One kind of radiographic study, fluoroscopy, is used to observe the shape and contour of empty organs and how these hollow structures fill with and evacuate radiopaque dye (contrast medium).

Barium Swallow or Upper Gastrointestinal Series

Sometimes the terms **barium swallow** and **upper gastrointestinal series** are used interchangeably. Strictly speaking, a barium swallow is the fluoroscopic observation of the client actually swallowing a flavored barium solution and its progress down the esophagus, whereas an upper GI series helps identify swallowing abnormalities, such as incoordination of swallowing, oral aspiration, and structural abnormalities of the upper GI tract.

An upper GI series also includes a radiographic observation of the barium moving into the stomach and the first part of the small intestine. Structural abnormalities in the esophagus may include tumors, strictures, varices, and hiatal hernia. Structural abnormalities below the esophagus include gastric tumors, peptic ulcers, and numerous gastric disorders (see Chap. 51). The examination may take as few as 20 minutes if only a barium swallow is performed. If stomach filling and emptying need to be observed, the test may take about 1 hour.

NURSING MANAGEMENT. Once any test using barium is completed, encourage the client to drink fluids liberally to dilute the barium and promote its elimination from the GI tract. Barium is very constipating. Advise the client that stools will appear white, streaky, or clay colored from the barium. Wait to obtain stool specimens until the barium is fully excreted. In some cases, a laxative is ordered. In all cases, failure to have a bowel movement within a reasonable time is reported to the physician because the retained barium may cause a bowel obstruction.

Small Bowel Series

Small bowel radiography tracks the movement of swallowed barium or other contrast media through the small intestine. It is used to identify disorders such as tumors, inflammation, or obstruction in the jejunum or ileum. It is performed like an upper GI, but the client swallows more barium for the small intestine to be well visualized. If the health care provider suspects an obstruction or fistula (a leaking channel between two structures), a water-soluble contrast medium such as methylglucamine diatrizoate (Gastrografin) is substituted for the barium. The test is longer to complete because it takes 5 to 6 hours for the contrast medium to reach the lower portion of the small intestine. When a small bowel series fails to detect subtle small bowel disease, *enteroclysis* may be indicated.

Enteroclysis

Also known as a small bowel enema, **enteroclysis** requires nasal or oral placement of a flexible feeding tube. The tip of the tube is positioned in the proximal jejunum, and barium is injected through the tube. X-ray films are taken of the various sections of the small intestine. If sedation is administered to ensure the client's comfort, the client is monitored accordingly (see Chap. 24).

Barium Enema or Lower Gastrointestinal Series

A **barium enema** or **lower gastrointestinal series** is used to identify polyps, tumors, strictures, and other lesions of the colon. A lower GI series is performed in the radiology department. One to 1.5 liters of barium solution is administered to the client by rectal instillation. The rectum, sigmoid colon, and descending colon are fluoroscopically observed during filling, facilitated by multiple position changes. The barium must be retained during this test, which may take up to 30 minutes. During this time, the client may experience abdominal cramping and a strong urge to defecate. Reassure clients that most people can retain the instilled barium throughout the test. Radiographs are taken again after the barium is expelled. In some cases, air is instilled to compress the barium residue against the wall of the lower intestine to aid in detecting mucosal defects. Stool specimens are not collected until the barium has been expelled completely.

NURSING MANAGEMENT. The diet may be limited the night before or for several days prior to the diagnostic examination to reduce the formation of stool. A laxative is administered the night before the lower GI study. Fluids are not generally restricted and it is usually unnecessary to withhold oral medications. Up to three cleansing enemas may be given before the procedure until the evacuated solution appears clear. After the radiographic examination, eating can be resumed. Rest and a generous fluid intake is encouraged. The passage of stool is monitored and the client is informed that the feces will appear white as the barium continues to be eliminated.

Oral Cholecystography or Gallbladder Series

Oral **cholecystography** identifies stones in the gallbladder or common bile duct and tumors or other obstructions of the gallbladder. The test also determines the ability of the gallbladder to concentrate and store a dyelike, iodine-based, radiopaque contrast medium. After the dye is absorbed, it goes to the liver, is excreted into the bile, and passes into the gallbladder, making it radiographically visible. Radiography of the gallbladder should be performed before other GI examinations in which barium is used because residual barium tends to obscure the image of the gallbladder and its ducts.

NURSING MANAGEMENT. To prepare for this test the client swallows six dye tablets—one every 5 minutes after the evening meal with a total of 250 mL of water or more. Then the client avoids eating or drinking anything else until the test. The tablets may cause nausea and vomiting, in which case the physician is notified so that more tablets can be administered or the test rescheduled. Once the initial radiographs are obtained, a fatty test meal is given and additional radiographs are taken to determine the gallbladder's ability to empty.

Cholangiography

Cholangiography determines the patency of the ducts from the liver and gallbladder. It is performed in the radiology department or during surgery. It is used when the gallbladder is not distinctly visualized with an oral cholecystogram, when vomiting has interfered with the retention of the oral dye, or intraoperatively or postoperatively to determine the status of the ductal system.

The dye for cholangiography is usually instilled intravenously (IV). However, it may be infused through a T-tube surgically placed within the common bile duct, a cannula advanced through the skin at a site below the rib margin, or an endoscope inserted through the upper GI tract into the *sphincter of Oddi* where the common bile duct empties into the duodenum.

NURSING MANAGEMENT. A signed consent form is required. A sensitivity to iodine must be reported. The bowel may be cleansed to promote clear radiographic images. Food and fluids may be restricted for several hours before the examination. The client is informed that a warm sensation and nausea may be experienced when the dye is instilled. Afterward, the client may eat and is encouraged to drink extra fluids to promote dye excretion.

Radionuclide Imaging

A radionuclide is a natural or synthetic element, such as technetium, that is radioactive. Once the substance is injected IV or ingested orally, a body organ may be examined by passing the **radionuclide imaging** scanner over the structure. This test is helpful in demonstrating the size of the organ, as well as defects or lesions such as tumors. Radionuclide imaging is used to detect lesions of the liver or pancreas and to evaluate gastric emptying. Specialized radionuclide studies are carried out to identify sites of bleeding or inflammation in the GI tract. Radionuclides have rather short half-lives, lasting a few hours to days during which they emit radiation. However, the amount of radiation is generally less than with diagnostic radiography.

NURSING MANAGEMENT. An allergy history is important to obtain since some clients may be sensitive to the particular radionuclide that may be used. An accurate weight is obtained because the dose of the radionuclide is usually individualized for each client. Female clients are questioned as to the possibility that they are pregnant because radiation can affect the fetus. Breast milk may be pumped and discarded temporarily if a female client is breastfeeding.

NONRADIOGRAPHIC IMAGING

Several imaging tests, such as computed tomography (CT), magnetic resonance imaging (MRI), and ultrasonography, do not rely on radioactive substances for visualization.

Computed Tomography

Computed tomography may be performed to detect structural abnormalities of the GI tract. It helps detect metastatic lesions that might not be apparent on GI radiographs. A CT scan may or may not be performed using a radiopaque contrast medium. Oral barium sulfate or calcium phosphate may be given to provide contrast for the hollow GI organs examined by CT scan.

NURSING MANAGEMENT. Before the test, the bowel may be cleaned to reduce stool and gas. Sometimes the client drinks fluids to expand the stomach, and drugs may be administered to decrease peristalsis or improve gastric motility.

Magnetic Resonance Imaging

Magnetic resonance imaging uses magnetic energy rather than radiation to visualize soft tissue structures.

NURSING MANGEMENT. Before MRI, the client removes any metal objects, credit cards, wristwatch, jewelry, and the like. Clients with internal metal devices or wounds closed with surgical staples, therefore, are excluded from testing. IV fluids, if required, are infused by gravity during an MRI because the changes in electrical charges during the test can affect mechanical infusers or pumps. Inform clients that the scanner, a narrow tunnel-like machine in which they are enclosed during the test, makes loud repetitive noises while the test is in progress. Clients who tend to be claustrophobic (fear of enclosed spaces) may need sedation because it is imperative that they lie still, not move, and not panic during the test.

Ultrasonography

In ultrasonography (also called ultrasound), high-frequency sound waves are directed through the body where they bounce off nearby structures, for example, the liver and pancreas. The returning sound waves are then interpreted and recorded electronically. Ultrasonography, which shows the size and location of organs and outlines structures and abnormalities, helps detect cholecystitis, cholelithiasis, pyloric stenosis, and some disorders of the biliary system (see Chaps. 51 and 54). It may be useful in detecting changes caused by appendicitis.

NURSING MANAGEMENT. Although the client can drink water before an ultrasound test, discourage drinking through a straw, smoking, or chewing gum. These activities are accompanied by swallowing air that thereby distorts sound wave transmission.

GASTROINTESTINAL TESTS

Percutaneous Liver Biopsy

In a procedure called **percutaneous liver biopsy,** the physician obtains a small core of liver tissue by placing a needle through the client's lateral abdominal wall. The tissue is examined microscopically to detect changes suggesting an infectious process or a benign, malignant, or metastatic lesion. The procedure is performed at the bedside or in the radiology department. Ultrasound or CT scan is performed before or during the biopsy to identify an appropriate puncture site. The client usually receives a sedative and anesthetic to promote comfort and cooperation.

NURSING MANAGEMENT. After ensuring that the biopsy equipment is assembled and in order, the nurse assists the client into a supine position with a rolled towel beneath the right lower ribs. Before the physician inserts the needle, instruct the client to take a deep breath and hold it to keep the liver as near to the abdominal wall as possible. After specimen cells are obtained, they are placed in a preservative, labeled, and delivered to the laboratory.

GASTROINTESTINAL ENDOSCOPY

Gastrointestinal endoscopy is the direct visual examination of the lumen of the GI tract, using a flexible fiberoptic instrument passed through one of the body openings or skin. It facilitates evaluation of the appearance and integrity of the GI mucosa and detects lesions. It provides access for therapeutic procedures. Diagnostic procedures include obtaining biopsies of the mucosa, obtaining samples of fluids found in the GI tract, and injecting dyes for radiographic purposes. Therapeutic procedures include inserting tubes and drains, electrocautery, and injecting medications. Among the variations of GI endoscopy are **proctosigmoidoscopy**, **esophagogastroduodenoscopy (EGD)**, **small bowel enteroscopy**, **colonoscopy**, **flexible sigmoidoscopy**, **panendoscopy**, and **endoscopic retrograde cholangiopancreatography** (ERCP). See Box 50–1.

NURSING MANAGEMENT. During an endoscopic procedure, the nurse monitors respiration and vital signs. After the procedure, the nurse watches for complications (fever, abdominal distention, abdominal or chest pain, vomiting blood, or bright red rectal bleeding) and makes sure the client receives food and fluid once the gag reflex returns and aspiration is less likely. To relieve a sore throat after upper GI endoscopy, the nurse may offer saline gargles, ice chips, or cool fluids.

LABORATORY TESTS

Depending on the suspected or confirmed diagnosis, various blood and urine tests may be ordered. Examples of laboratory tests are a complete blood count; urinalysis; serum bilirubin; cholesterol; serum ammonia level; prothrombin time; protein elec-

BOX 50-1 Common Gastrointestinal Endoscopic Procedures

Esophagogastroduodenoscopy (EGD)
Examination of the esophagus, stomach, and duodenum via an endoscope advanced orally to inspect, treat, or obtain specimens from any one or all of the upper GI structures

Colonoscopy
Examination of the entire large intestine with a flexible, fiberoptic colonoscope. The colonoscope is advanced anally from the rectum to the cecum allowing visualization of the rectum, sigmoid, and descending colon. The distal portion of the small intestine, the terminal ileum, may be inspected as well. Air may be instilled to promote visualization within the folds of the intestinal mucosa. Clients are sedated briefly (and monitored accordingly) with IV medication during the procedure.

Proctosigmoidoscopy
Examination of the rectum and sigmoid colon using a rigid endoscope inserted anally about 10 inches. To facilitate examination, the client must lie in a knee chest position. The test is brief and no sedation is needed.

Endoscopic retrograde cholangiopancreatography (ERCP)
Combined endoscopic and radiographic examination using radiopaque contrast medium instilled in the biliary tree to visualization the biliary and pancreatic ducts

Peritoneoscopy
Examination of GI structures via an endoscope inserted percutaneously through a small incision in the abdominal wall with the patient receiving a local, spinal, or general anesthetic. Also called laparoscopy.

Small Bowel Enteroscopy
Endoscopic examination and visualization of the lumen of the small bowel

Panendoscopy
Examination of both the upper and lower GI tracts

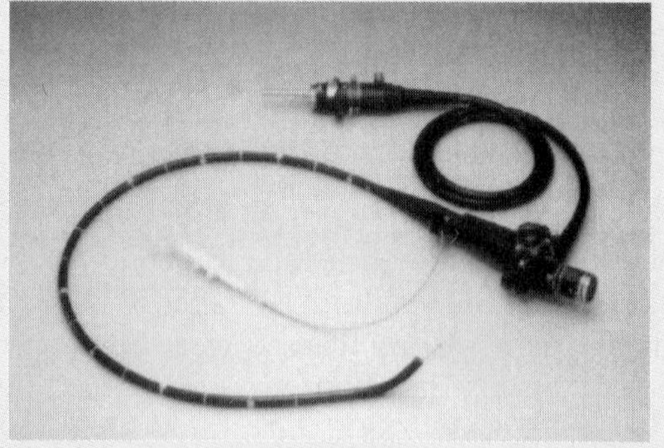

Flexible fiberoptic endoscope (Courtesy of Olympus America, Inc.).

trophoresis; and enzymes, such as amylase, lipase, aspartate aminotransferase, and lactic acid dehydrogenase; and tumor marker blood studies, such as carcinoembryonic antigen (CEA) and alpha-fetoprotein (AFT).

PY Test

The **PY test** uses ^{14}C-urea capsules to detect *Helicobacter pylori*, the bacteria associated with peptic ulcer disease (Fig. 50–2). If gastric urease, an enzyme not normally present in human cells, is identified in the balloon air, the client most likely has an *H. pylori* infection. This breath analysis is 90% accurate.

NURSING MANAGEMENT. Clients must avoid antibiotics or bismuth for 1 month, proton pump inhibitors and sucralfate for 2 weeks, and food and fluids for 6 hours before the test. To ensure accurate test results, advise the client not to handle or chew the test capsule; instead, swallow it intact.

Gastrointestinal Breath Test

This test involves collecting a breath sample before and at intervals after the ingestion of a carbohydrate solution. The two major gases in expired air are hydrogen and carbon dioxide. Elevated levels of hydrogen in the expired breath sample indicate carbohydrate malabsorption. The type of solution used for the test depends on the suspected type of malabsorption. Lactose malabsorption (lactose intolerance) is one of the more common disorders investigated using this technique.

Stool Analysis

Stool specimens are collected to identify white blood cells (indicating inflammation), red blood cells (indicating GI blood loss), and fat (indicating malabsorption). Stool specimens are also collected to identify infection. Bacterial infections (ie, salmonella, shigella, campylobacter) are detected through routine culture. Diagnosis of parasitic infections (ie giardia, cryptosporidium) requires placing the specimen in a specific preservative to detect parasites and their ova.

NURSING MANAGEMENT. It is best to deliver stool analysis specimens that require examination for microorganisms to the laboratory while they are fresh and warm. Only a small amount of stool needs to be collected and it is always placed in a covered container. Eating red meat or other foods containing peroxidase within the previous 3 days may produce a false-positive result when testing for occult blood. Box 50–2 lists substances to avoid.

BOX 50-2 Substances to Avoid Before Stool Analysis for Occult Blood

- Alcohol
- Aspirin
- Ascorbic acid (vitamin C)
- Bananas
- Broccoli
- Fish
- Horseradish
- Cantaloupe
- Cauliflower
- Grapes
- Meat
- Mushrooms
- Parsnips
- Turnips
- Steroids
- Nonsteroidal anti-inflammatory drugs, such as ibuprofen (Advil, Motrin)

Nursing Management

Although some clients undergo GI test procedures as outpatients, others have these tests during hospital-

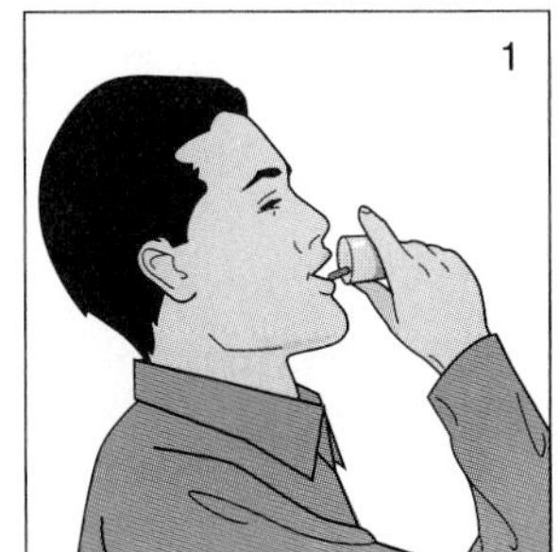

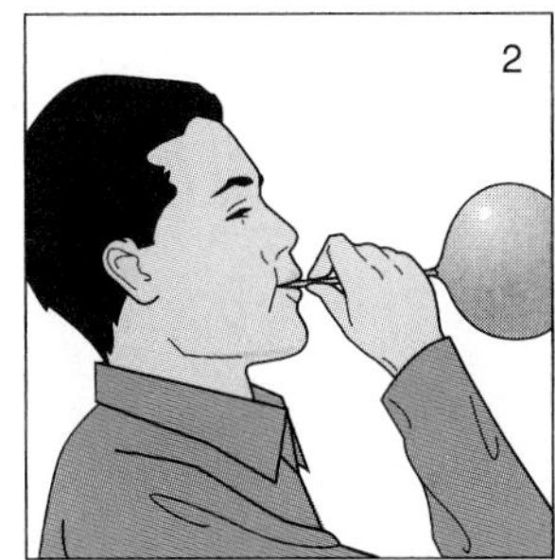

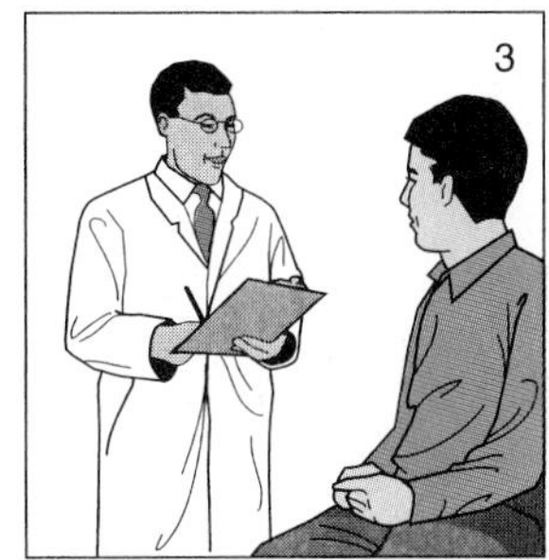

FIGURE 50-2. The breath test that indicates *Helicobacter pylori* is performed in three easy steps: (1) The client takes a ^{14}C-urea capsule and waits about 10 minutes. (2) The client blows up a balloon. (3) The client waits while the air in the balloon is analyzed for the presence of gastric urease.

ization. In either case, thorough initial assessment is needed.

In addition to a careful and thorough assessment, the client's informed consent for the test must be recorded before most GI testing. The client and family members need teaching and reassurance about the test's purpose and procedure. They also need to know about care measures to be implemented after the test.

NURSING PROCESS
The Client Undergoing Diagnostic Testing for a Gastrointestinal Disorder

Assessment

The nurse interviews the client to determine past familiarity with the test or similar procedure and encourages discussion of previous experiences or current expectations. If the client is responsible for self-preparation before the test, the nurse explores the client's compliance.

The nurse reviews the client's history and explores any data on prior hypersensitivity or allergy to testing substances, in particular elements in a radionuclide or iodine-based contrast medium (dye) signaled by allergy to seafood. The nurse labels an allergic client's chart and applies a special band or tag to the client's identification bracelet. Vital signs are taken and the client is weighed. Other essential baseline data are recorded for later comparison and to identify serious reportable changes or complications, such as rectal bleeding.

Diagnosis and Planning

Nursing care includes, but is not limited to, the following:

Nursing Diagnoses and Collaborative Problems	Nursing Interventions
Anxiety related to ignorance of test procedure or possible test findings **Goal:** The client's anxiety will be alleviated or put in perspective.	Identify test date, location, and time. Go over test preparations according to protocol. Provide printed guidelines for reference. Encourage client to express fears. Discuss the client's perceptions of the test and explain what to expect during and after testing. Respect client's individuality; remain nonjudgmental and supportive. Treat client with dignity; be available to answer questions and give care.
Pain related to test procedure **Goal:** The client's discomfort will be eliminated or reduced to a tolerable level.	Advise client to expect some discomfort. Use pillows, blankets, to relieve discomfort if client has physical problem that causes pain (eg, arthritis). Reassure client that examination table is constructed to facilitate positioning. Provide time to use restroom before and after test if possible. Have client inform test personnel of pressure or cramping that occurs with the instillation of test fluids. If possible, slow or interrupt instillation.
Risk for Fluid Volume Deficit related to fluid restriction or to loss associated with diarrhea or vomiting, or both **Goal:** The client's fluid volume will be maintained.	Weigh client and observe the color and amount of urine. Monitor the pulse rate and blood pressure. Report dizziness or confusion. Administer fluids as soon as safely permitted. After testing is complete, match fluid intake to fluid output; encourage liberal intake.
Risk for Constipation related to barium retention **Goals:** The client's regular bowel elimination pattern will resume within 2–3 days.	Encourage client to drink at least 2,000 mL of fluid/24 h after tests using barium. Check the post-test orders to determine whether a laxative or enema is prescribed. Monitor stool passage and observe that barium is excreted as light-colored or white-streaked stool. Report diminished or hyperactive bowel sounds.

Evaluation and Expected Outcomes

- The client reports minimal anxiety and pain.
- Fluid balance is maintained.
- Regular bowel elimination patterns resume.

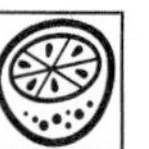

General Nutritional Considerations

Observe for weight loss or failure to gain weight in clients with GI problems. Many GI tests require at least an 8-hour fast beforehand. Repeated or multiple tests performed over a period of days can compound potential or existing nutritional problems.

Encourage adequate fluid intake to promote dilution and elimination of dyes and other test substances.

If the client receives a local anesthetic that suppresses the gag reflex, withhold food and fluids until the reflex returns.

Observe for subsequent signs and symptoms of intolerance in clients whose test required ingesting a special solution, such as a carbohydrate solution. For instance, clients tested for lactose intolerance may experience cramping, abdominal distention, and diarrhea.

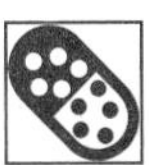

General Pharmacologic Considerations

Depending on the test procedure, the client's medication regimen, and physician's orders, some, all, or none of the client's medications may be withheld before and during testing.

For certain diagnostic tests of the GI tract, the bowel may be cleaned or the client may receive various cleansing medications orally so that internal structures can be visualized clearly. In such cases, the client may take cleansing preparations orally or by enema.

Polyethylene glycol/electrolyte (GoLYTELY, Colyte) is used for bowel cleansing in preparation for GI diagnostic examination. The solution is reconstituted with water and the client instructed to drink 240 mL every 10 minutes until 4 liters is consumed or fecal elimination is clear. Allow the client to drink only clear liquids after administration of the solution begins.

Before biopsy procedures, clients at risk for serious bleeding may receive precautionary vitamin K, which promotes blood clotting. If sedative, IV medications or dyes, or general anesthetics are administered, the client is monitored appropriately.

Emergency medications are kept stocked and oxygen must be readily available in case the client experiences an adverse reaction to the dye or drugs administered during the test.

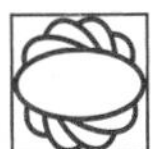

General Gerontologic Considerations

Fluid balance for clients, especially older adults, is precarious given the fluid restrictions and multiple enemas or laxatives required for GI tests.

Older adults are at higher risk for dehydration when undergoing a lower GI series or endoscopic examinations of the bowel because they tend to have less physiologic reserve to compensate for fluid loss. The potential for fluid deficit also may be compounded by a history of vomiting or diarrhea or diuretic therapy.

The older adult usually has less control of the rectal sphincter than a younger adult due to changes in nerve innervation, a diminished awareness of the filling reflex, and decreased muscle tone.

To prevent or detect fluid volume deficit, weigh the client and observe the color and amount of urine. Monitor the pulse rate and blood pressure. Report dizziness or confusion, concentrated urine, or a scanty amount of urine.

Explain the diagnostic examination to the older adult in simple language, allowing ample time to answer questions. Repeated explanations and assurances may be necessary to ease the older adult's anxiety.

After the diagnostic test, the older adult may experience dizziness or confusion due to the stress of the examination or from enduring 6 to 8 hours without food or fluids. Provide nourishment as soon as possible after the examination and give assistance with ambulation when necessary.

SUMMARY OF KEY CONCEPTS

- The GI system is composed of the mouth, esophagus, stomach, small intestine, large intestine, rectum, and anal canal. These structures as a whole play a role in food ingestion, digestion, absorption, and elimination. The liver, gallbladder, and pancreas also aid the GI organs in breaking down nutrients.
- During the initial assessment interview, the nurse determines the client's chief health complaint and obtains a description of all current symptoms, the length of time they have been present, and any cause-and-effect relationships the client may have observed.
- A thorough physical assessment of the GI system includes the client's weight and vital signs. Besides observing the client's overall general appearance, the nurse inspects the mouth, teeth, tongue, and mucosa and also the color of the skin and sclera. The location and cause of scars and any skin lesions are identified. The abdomen is auscultated and lightly palpated. If the client's condition warrants, deep palpation is performed to detect liver enlargement. Percussion may help assess the density of underlying tissue. The appearance of the anus is inspected and the characteristics of stool are observed whenever possible.
- The diagnostic tests commonly used in GI disorders include radiographic studies, magnetic resonance imaging, computed tomography, ultrasonography, endoscopy, radionuclide imaging, biopsy, and laboratory tests, such as the PY test and stool analyses.
- Diagnostic tests for detecting GI disorders may require fasting or a special diet, such as a liquid or low-residue diet, before the test. Dietary restrictions are reviewed with the client and the importance of following the recommendations is stressed.
- Once test procedures are complete, make food and beverages available as soon as they can be safely ingested.
- Keep emergency resuscitative equipment and medications on standby to be used in case of allergic reactions.
- Monitor all clients—but especially older ones—for fluid volume deficit.

CRITICAL THINKING EXERCISES

1. You have two clients who will be having GI tests. One is undergoing a lower GI series and the other is scheduled for a colonoscopy. Discuss the similarities and differences of these tests.

2. A client for whom you are caring becomes hypotensive after a liver biopsy. Determine additional data you need to assess before reporting the finding to the physician.

Suggested Readings

Bates, B. (1995) A guide to physical examination and history taking (6th ed.). Philadelphia: J. B. Lippincott.

Cave, D. R. (1996, January 15). Management of *Helicobacter pylori* infection in ulcer disease. *Hospital Practice,* 63–75.

Holmes, S. (1996). Percutaneous endoscopic gastrostomy: A review. *Nursing Times, 92*(17), 34–35.

Hughes, M. (1996). Key issues in the introduction of nurse endoscopy. *Nursing Times, 92*(8), 38–39.

Langan, J. C. (1998). Abdominal assessment in the home: From A to Z. *Home Healthcare Nurse, 16*(1), 50–57.

Womack, C., & Thomas, J. D. (1996). Easing the way through an MRI. *RN, 59*(10), 34–36.

Chapter 51

Caring for Clients With Disorders of the Upper Gastrointestinal Tract

KEY TERMS

Diverticulum
Dumping syndrome
Dyspepsia
Esophagitis
Fundoplication
Gastrectomy
Gastric decompression
Gastritis
Gastroduodenostomy (Billroth I)
Gastroesophageal reflux
Gastrojejunostomy (Billroth II)
Gastrostomy
Hiatal hernia (diaphragmatic hernia)
Nasoenteric
Nasogastric
Odynophagia
Peptic ulcer
Percutaneous endoscopic gastrostomy (PEG)
Pyloroplasty
Stoma
Vagotomy

LEARNING OBJECTIVES

On completion of this chapter, the reader will:

- Discuss the assessment findings, diagnosis, and treatment of cancer of the oral cavity, gastroesophageal reflux, esophageal diverticula, hiatal hernia, cancer of the esophagus, gastritis, peptic ulcer disease, and cancer of the stomach.
- Describe the nursing management of a client with a nasogastric or gastrointestinal tube or gastrostomy.
- List suggestions for relieving upper GI discomfort.
- Discuss the nursing management of clients undergoing gastric surgery.

Digestion begins in the mouth and continues in the stomach and small intestine. The nurse is commonly responsible for managing the care of clients with disorders affecting the upper gastrointestinal (GI) tract, which carries on such functions as eating and digestion (see Fig. 50–1 for an illustration of the upper GI tract). These problems and their treatment approaches are typically addressed in the nursing care plans of clients who have disorders of the upper GI tract.

Disorders That Affect Eating

Anorexia

Simple anorexia, or lack of an appetite, is a common symptom of many diseases. If the symptom is prolonged, serious consequences, such as malnutrition, may occur.

ETIOLOGY AND PATHOPHYSIOLOGY

The appetite center is located in the hypothalamus. The area that stimulates or suppresses the appetite may be influenced by pleasant or noxious food odors, the effects of a drug, emotional stress, fear, psychological problems, and illnesses.

Brief periods of anorexia are not life-threatening but can cause temporary malnutrition. During periods when consumption of food is reduced, most have a sufficient reserve of stored glycogen that can be converted to glucose for energy through the process of *gluconeogenesis*. Hormones such as glucagon, glucocorticoid hormones from the adrenal cortex, and thyroid hormones stimulate the liver to carry out this process. Stores of fat-soluble vitamins are used. Electrolytes are temporarily balanced through selective reabsorption by the kidneys.

ASSESSMENT FINDINGS

Signs and Symptoms

Hunger is generally absent and clients describe having no desire for food. Some eat a small amount only because they feel they should or because they are coerced by others. Varying amounts of weight loss occur depending on the length of anorexia and reduced food intake. Eventually the client may show signs of hypovitaminosis (vitamin deficiency) especially of water-soluble vitamins, which the body does not store. The client may have dry skin, brittle hair, sore mouth, bleeding gums, and easy bruising. Wound healing may be poor and mental state may deteriorate. Bones soften and taste and smell diminish with mineral deficiencies. The client is likely to feel weak and tired. Reduced stool volume, bowel irregularity, or constipation can occur.

Diagnostic Findings

Depending on the chronicity of the anorexia, the hemoglobin and blood cell counts may be reduced. The red blood cells may become abnormally enlarged. Serum albumin, electrolytes, and blood protein levels may be low. As a result, cardiac arrhythmias may occur. A deficiency of potassium, for example, will appear as a tall, peaked T wave on an electrocardiogram (ECG).

MEDICAL AND SURGICAL MANAGEMENT

Management of the client with anorexia depends on its cause. Short-term anorexia usually requires no medical intervention. Persistent anorexia may require a variety of approaches, such as a high-calorie diet, high-calorie supplemental feedings, tube feedings, total parenteral nutrition (TPN), and psychiatric treatment.

NURSING MANAGEMENT

To maintain sufficient nutrition and sustain normal body weight the client must eat food in adequate quantity. In assisting the client to meet this goal, monitor weight daily. Obtain a complete medical and allergy (drugs and food) history from the client or a family member and compile a dietary history, including a description of the client's eating patterns and food preferences. For more information see the Nursing Guidelines 51–1.

Additional nursing measures depend on problems that result from anorexia. In the case of altered bowel patterns (either diarrhea or constipation) from reduced bulk secondary to liquid supplements, potential interventions include keeping a record of bowel movements, consulting with the physician and dietitian about changing the type of supplement if diarrhea develops, substituting formula containing fiber to add bulk to the stools, diluting the formula temporarily until the client adjusts to the concentrated contents, increasing dietary fiber and administering a prescribed stool softener to promote the ease and frequency of bowel elimination.

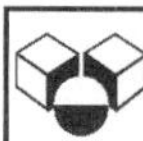

Nursing Guidelines 51-1

Managing Care of the Client With Anorexia

- Provide foods at mealtimes that the client likes.
- Offer between-meal snacks such as nourishing beverages (egg nog, milk shakes, and commercial concentrates such as Ensure or Instant Breakfast).
- While the client is hospitalized, encourage family members to bring favorite foods that can be refrigerated or reheated.
- Conduct a daily caloric count if necessary to determine total caloric intake and the amount of vitamins, minerals, fats, proteins, and carbohydrates in the client's diet.
- Keep serving sizes and containers small to avoid overwhelming the client.
- Serve and keep hot foods hot and cold foods cold.
- Encourage eating in the company of others.
- Formulate a nutritional plan with the client and dietitian that promotes weight gain (approximately 600 calories per meal).
- If necessary, arrange for supplementation based on documented deficiencies in the client's intake.
- Consult the physician and dietitian in cases of prolonged anorexia.

Nausea and Vomiting

Nausea and vomiting are common problems that often coexist. If the symptoms are prolonged, weakness, weight loss, nutritional deficiency, dehydration and electrolyte and acid–base imbalances may result.

ETIOLOGY AND PATHOPHYSIOLOGY

Some of the more common causes of nausea and vomiting include drugs, infections of the GI tract, intestinal obstruction, systemic infections, lesions of the central nervous system, food poisoning, emotional stress, early pregnancy, and uremia. Nausea generally precedes vomiting and is usually produced by distention of the duodenum. Nausea is accompanied by increased salivation and peripheral vasoconstriction causing cold, clammy skin and tachycardia. The vomiting center, located in the medulla, is particularly sensitive to parasympathetic neurotransmitters released in response to gastric irritation. The Valsalva maneuver, which accompanies the forceful expulsion of stomach contents, causes dizziness, hypotension, and bradycardia.

ASSESSMENT FINDINGS

Signs and Symptoms

The client describes an unpleasant feeling, identified as nausea. It is generally associated with a loss of appetite and refusal to eat. During vomiting the client is observed to retch while evacuating stomach contents. The process occurs once or several times in succession.

The client who has experienced excessive fluid loss (dehydration) may complain of excessive thirst and may report decreased or absent urine production. The client's eyes and oral mucosa will appear dry or dull, and fluid loss may be reflected in poor skin turgor (see Chap. 21).

The client's history may include ingestion of noxious substances, such as excessive amounts of alcohol, presumably contaminated food, or drugs that commonly cause GI side effects. Exposure to other individuals with similar symptoms suggests a bacterial or viral cause.

When vomiting is secondary to intestinal obstruction, the abdomen is distended, tender, and firm to touch. Bowel sounds may be absent or hypoactive.

Diagnostic Findings

If vomiting is prolonged, serum electrolyte levels of sodium and chloride may be low; bicarbonate levels may rise to compensate for the loss of chloride and accumulation of metabolic acids. Hematocrit, if high, is secondary to hemoconcentration in the presence of dehydration.

MEDICAL AND SURGICAL MANAGEMENT

Sometimes nausea and vomiting are short lived and do not require medical intervention. In some instances, intravenous (IV) fluids, electrolyte replacement, and drug therapy are necessary.

Elimination of the cause includes a variety of interventions ranging from stopping a drug to surgical intervention for intestinal obstruction. Symptomatic relief may be achieved by administering an antiemetic agent (Table 51–1), providing IV fluid and electrolyte replacement, and temporarily restricting the intake of food until the cause can be eliminated.

NURSING MANAGEMENT

Obtain a complete medical, dietary, drug, and allergy history. Compile a list of symptoms that occur before as well as along with the nausea and vomiting, the length of time the problem has been present, and information about the frequency, color, and amount vomited material. Because the cause may be unknown, a list of foods eaten in the past 24 hours and where the food was eaten also is obtained. Assess the client's general appearance, weight, and vital signs. Document intake and output and assess for signs of fluid volume deficit (see Chap. 21).

Ensure client comfort by providing frequent mouth care, administering antiemetic medications as prescribed and monitoring their effects, emptying the emesis basin promptly, changing bed linens as needed, and airing the room to rid it of unpleasant odors.

Additional care of clients who experience nausea and vomiting includes, but is not limited to, the following:

Nursing Diagnoses and Collaborative Problems	Nursing Interventions
Fluid Volume Deficit related to prolonged vomiting and decreased intake of oral fluids	Offer clear fluids in small amounts, which may be better tolerated.
Goal: Fluid balance will be restored as evidenced by intake of 1500–3000 mL/day with similar fluid loss.	Recommend commercial over-the-counter beverages (GatorAde) or replacement solutions for infants and small children (Pedialyte or Ricelyte).
	Inform physician of urine output below 500 mL/day or abnormally low serum electrolyte levels.
	Monitor weight and nutritional status and alert appropriate caregivers if hydration problems do not resolve in reasonable time.
Altered Nutrition: Less than Body Requirements related to nausea and vomiting	Administer prescribed parenteral nutrition or IV fluids to which additional nutrients and electrolytes may be added.
Goal: The client's nutritional status will be adequate as evidenced by maintenance of weight and normal laboratory test values.	Provide small initial amounts of clear liquids, then full liquids, and progress to soft bland foods, such as creamed soups with crackers or dry toast once the client can tolerate food.

Cancer of the Oral Cavity

Cancer cells undergo changes in structure and appearance. They multiply, eventually forming a colony of abnormal and dysfunctional cells (see Chap. 19).

TABLE 51-1 **Antiemetic Medications Used to Treat Nausea and Vomiting**

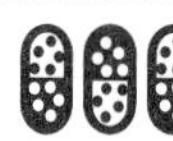

Drug Category/Drug Action	Side Effects	Nursing Considerations
Serotonin Receptor Antagonist		
ondanestron (Zofran) Blocks receptors for $5HT_3$, which affects the neural pathways involved in nausea and vomiting.	Headache, dizziness (low blood pressure), myalgia (muscle aches and pains), malaise, fatigue, drowsiness	Review client's allergy history before administering medication. Provide oral drug form q8h around the clock for 1 to 2 days after chemotherapy or radiation to prevent nausea and vomiting. Caution client about side effects that may make activities such as driving a car or operating other machinery hazardous.
Phenothiazine		
prochlorperazine (Compazine) Inhibits the chemoreceptor trigger zone (CTZ) and vomiting center in the brain.	Drowsiness, hypotension, changes in heart rhythms, photophobia, blurred vision, dry mouth, discolored urine	Tell client that this drug is for short-term control of nausea and vomiting and should be used exactly as directed. Explain side effects and advise client not to save any medicine for a later date or give any to anyone else. Monitor older clients because effects of drug may lead more rapidly to dehydration than in younger clients.
Antihistamines		
hydroxyzine (Atarax, Vistaril) Blocks H_1 receptors, decreasing stimulation of the CTZ and vomiting center.	Drowsiness, tremor, dry mouth, hypersensitivity reaction (includes difficulty breathing), tremors, loss of coordination, sore muscles, or muscle spasms	Take full health history to help determine underlying cause of nausea and vomiting. Give by deep intramuscular injection in volume prescribed to control vomiting. Report breathing problems, tremors, muscle problems and incoordination.
promethazine (Anergan, Phenergan) Blocks H_1 receptors, decreasing stimulation of the CTZ and vomiting center.	Dizziness, drowsiness, poor coordination, confusion, restlessness, excitation, epigastric distress, thickened bronchial secretions, urinary frequency, dysuria	Take drug and health history. Because this drug interacts with several others, review potential for drug interactions; for example, do not administer medication if client is taking monoamine oxidase inhibitor. Do not give to a client with a lower respiratory tract disorder. Advise client to avoid drinking alcohol when taking this medication.
dimenhydrinate (Dramamine) Inhibits vestibular stimulation in the ear, thereby relieving motion sickness.	Drowsiness, confusion, nervousness, restlessness, headache, dizziness, vertigo, tingling, heaviness and weakness of hands, epigastric discomfort, low blood pressure, nasal stuffiness, chest tightness, rash, photosensitivity	Advise client not to take if pregnant or lactating. Review client history for glaucoma, peptic ulcer, bronchial asthma, heart problems because drug may pose a danger. Urge client to avoid alcohol because serious sedation could result. Advise client to report breathing problems, tremors, loss of coordination, visual disturbances or hallucination, and irregular heartbeat.

When the oral cavity is affected, cells within the lips, mouth, or the pharynx undergo malignant changes. When cancers of the oral cavity are detected early, the rate of cure is fairly good.

ETIOLOGY AND PATHOPHYSIOLOGY

Smoking, chewing tobacco, and drinking alcohol in excess are linked to the development of oral cancers. Lip cancer is associated with pipe smoking and prolonged exposure to the wind and sun. As cancer cells in the oral cavity increase, the mass may distort a client's appearance, exert pressure on surrounding tissue making it difficult to *masticate* (chew), and cause local pain. In turn, the client may experience *dysphagia* (difficulty swallowing). Untreated, these cancerous growths may extend into nearby tissue, such as the middle ear or nasal sinuses; infiltrate regional lymph nodes; or invade large blood vessels, such as the carotid arteries, which are near the oral cavity. Serious hemorrhage ("carotid blowout") and death may result when an artery is invaded and becomes ulcerated by cancer cells or when necrosis follows radiation therapy.

ASSESSMENT FINDINGS

Signs and Symptoms

The early stage of oral cancer is characteristically symptom free. The client usually becomes concerned by a lesion, lump, or other abnormality of the lips or mouth. Other changes, such as pain, soreness, and bleeding occur later. If a lesion is on the tongue, the client commonly experiences difficulty in eating or tasting food. Pain, numbness, and a loss of feeling also follow. Dentists and oral hygienists may be the first to notice changes in mouth tissues, such as *leukoplakia*, a white patch on the tongue or inner cheek that may become cancerous.

Diagnostic Findings

A biopsy of the lesion discloses malignant cells, which confirms the diagnosis of oral cancer.

MEDICAL AND SURGICAL MANAGEMENT

Treatment depends on the location and type of tumor, the extent (or stage) of involvement, and the client's physical condition. If hemorrhage occurs, transfusions are given to replace lost blood. Ligation of the bleeding vessel is usually necessary. Drugs such as antianxiety agents are prescribed to relieve the client's apprehension.

Most oral cancers are treated surgically by tumor excision alone or with follow-up radiation therapy. Chemotherapy is not generally beneficial for primary tumors. Surgical excision may result in complete cure, provided that it is performed early. A neck dissection is performed if the cancer has spread to the lymph nodes about the jaw or below the ears. Cancer of the tongue generally involves radical surgery to remove part or all of the tongue. Excision of the tumor from parts of the jaw or palate is disfiguring.

For clients with advanced disease, treatment is only palliative. Chemotherapy or radiation therapy is used to relieve pain and temporarily decrease tumor size. A tracheostomy and tube feedings are instituted to maintain an adequate airway and to provide nourishment.

NURSING MANAGEMENT

The general nursing management of the client with an oral cancer is much the same as for any client with cancer (see Chap. 19). The focus of attention, however, is on maintaining a patent airway, promoting adequate fluid and food intake, and supporting communication impaired by the tumor or treatment. To review care of the client needing airway management refer to Chapter 27 and the discussion on endotracheal intubation and tracheostomy care.

Communication problems are usually addressed in collaboration with a speech pathologist. Meanwhile, be patient when the client chooses to communicate by speaking. Clarify or repeat what the client has said if the client's speech can be misunderstood. Substitute written forms for communicating if speech is impaired. Offer the client pencil and paper, a Magic Slate, an alphabet board, or suggest using hand signals.

The client returning from the operating room after oral surgery should be positioned flat, either on the abdomen or side, with the head turned to the side to facilitate drainage from the mouth. After recovery from the anesthetic, the client is positioned with the head of the bed elevated. This makes it easier for the client to breathe deeply and cough up secretions. It also controls edema in the operative area.

After oral surgery, keep equipment for suctioning, administration of oxygen, and tracheostomy supplies at the client's bedside. If the client does not have a tracheostomy, keep a tracheostomy tray nearby for emergency use because respiratory distress or an airway obstruction may require immediate attention. If the client has a tracheostomy, suction secretions from the cannula and clean it on a regular basis.

Wait to irrigate the client's mouth until he or she is awake and alert. When and if a mouth irrigation is carried out, turn the client's head to the side to allow the solution to run in gently and flow out into an emesis basin. Instill only a small amount of solution and wait for drainage to occur before administering more. Suction the client's mouth as necessary to remove secretions, blood, or irrigating solution.

Wait to give oral liquids or foods until a written order exists. Carefully observe the client's ability to swallow small amounts of liquid. In cases of coughing or other difficulty, suction the liquid from the mouth immediately.

Administer prescribed antiemetics if nausea or vomiting is experienced. Maintain patency of the gastric tube, if one is present. Discourage the use of a straw to avoid distending the stomach with swallowed air.

The client's emotional response to radical oral surgery is a real and difficult problem. Extensive surgery of the mouth and adjacent structures is not only disfiguring but also incapacitating. It interferes with communication, eating, and the control of saliva. Although the extent of surgery is explained before the operation, many clients and their families are unable to grasp the full impact of this type of surgery. The first time family members or clients see the effects of surgery is usually a traumatic experience. The nurse needs to promote effective coping and therapeutic grieving at this time. The client's response may range from crying or extreme sadness and avoiding contact with others to refusing to talk about the surgery or changes in appearance. Allow the client time to mourn, accept, and adjust to losses. To facilitate adaptation, give the client opportunities to ventilate feelings. Watch severely depressed clients closely. Refer any who may seem suicidal for psychological evaluation and counseling.

Nutritional management is a particular challenge when caring for clients with oral cancer. If the client can take oral nourishment, a nutritional consultation may be necessary to modify the diet according to the client's ability to chew and swallow. Because oral tissues are sensitive, hot and cold liquids and spicy foods are avoided. Typically the physician is consulted about prescribing a topical anesthetic or mouthwash containing lidocaine (Xylocaine) to numb the tissues or a systemic analgesic to relieve pain. Providing nourishment by a route other than the mouth may be necessary.

Gastrointestinal Intubation for Feeding

At some time during the care of the client with oral cancer, as well as when caring for others with GI disorders, the nurse may have to incorporate the insertion and management of GI tubes (**nasogastric**, orogastric, **nasoenteric**, or gastrostomy tubes) into the plan of care.

Gastrointestinal intubation is the insertion of a tube for providing nutrition or for **gastric decompression** (see Clinical Procedure 51–1). GI tubes are advanced to the upper GI tract by way of the mouth or nose, or they are introduced directly into the stomach or small intestine through the abdominal wall. A gastric tube lies in the stomach; an intestinal tube extends past the pylorus. When placed directly into the upper GI tract via an incision in the abdominal wall the tube is referred to as a gastrostomy tube.

During tube feeding the nurse's role is to ensure that the client's lungs remain free of liquid substances, the client does not acquire an infection, and that intake and output will be appropriate for age and size. Additional objectives include adequate nutrition, appropriate stooling patterns (amount, consistency, and frequency), and preservation of intact skin and nasal mucosa. Efforts to keep the mucous membranes moist are also important. Mucous membranes tend to dry from mouth breathing and restriction of

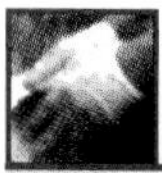

Clinical Procedure 51-1
Inserting a Nasogastric Tube

PURPOSE	EQUIPMENT
• To provide nutrition, initiate gastric decompression, or to administer medication	• Nasogastric tube (size and type selected according to reason for placement and client size) • Large syringe (50 to 60 mL) • Water-soluble lubricant • Stethoscope • Emesis basin • Tape • Gloves • Towel and tissues

Nursing Action	Rationale
ASSESSMENT	
Check the medical orders.	Integrates activities with medical treatment
Explain the procedure to the client.	Allows assessment of the client's learning needs and provides an opportunity for teaching
Inspect both nostrils.	Determines which nostril is wider or straighter or if client has a deviated septum
Inspect the tube to be inserted for cracks, breaks, or kinks.	Ensures that the tube is free of defects, which may hamper proper function
PLANNING	
Assemble the necessary equipment in one place.	Prevents unnecessary delays in the plan of care
Check the expiration date on the tubing package and read the manufacturer's instructions.	Prevents use of equipment that may be contaminated and reacquaints the nurse with details specific to placing the selected tube
Provide for the client's privacy.	Decreases client anxiety

continued

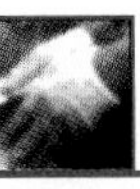

Clinical Procedure 51-1
Continued

Nursing Action	Rationale
IMPLEMENTATION	
Match the client's identification tag to the name on the order sheet.	Prevents errors
Wash your hands and put on gloves.	Reduces transmission of microorganisms (from the nurse to client and vice versa)
Measure tube for placement in the stomach: 1. Place the tip of the tube next to the client's *n*ose, extend the tube to the client's *e*arlobe, and continue to the *x*iphoid process (the NEX measurement). 2. Place a small piece of tape on the tube where it meets the xiphoid process. Measure tube for placement in the duodenum: 3. Add 9 inches to the above measurement.	Allows for proper placement 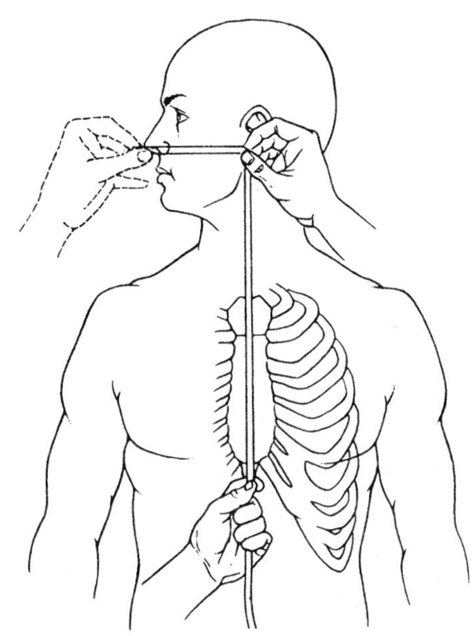 *Obtaining the NEX measurement.*
Coat the distal 4 to 6 inches of the tube with water-soluble lubricant. (Some small-diameter feeding tubes have lubricant bonded to the surface of the tube. Activate this lubricant by placing the tip of the tube in water after consulting the manufacturer's instructions.)	Eases tube insertion, adding to client comfort
Instruct the client to blow nose.	Clears the nasal passages
Put a towel over the client's gown and place an emesis basin and tissues within client's reach.	Prevents embarrassment and soiling of the gown should vomiting occur.

continued

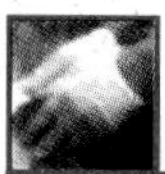

Clinical Procedure 51-1
Continued

Nursing Action	Rationale
Help the client into a high Fowler's position with the neck hyperextended.	Eases tube passage 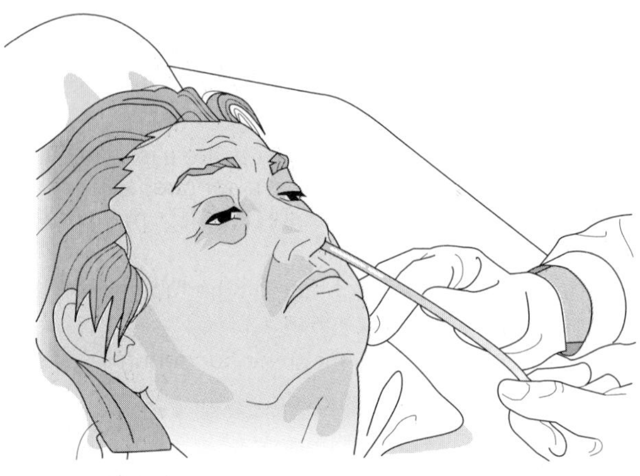 *Inserting the tube.*
Place the tip of the tube in the client's nostril. Advance the tube along the floor of the nostril while aiming the tip of the tube toward the earlobe.	Allows passage of the tube into the nasopharynx
Provide verbal reassurance that nasal irritation will resolve as the tube passes.	Reduces client anxiety
Ask the client to lower his or her chin to the chest and to swallow. Provide sips of water, if allowed.	Facilitates passage of the tube into the esophagus
Provide verbal reassurance that gagging will subside as the tube is advanced and that by swallowing, the client will help speed the procedure.	Reduces client anxiety and facilitates tube passage into the stomach
Slowly advance the tube until the tape mark appears at the entrance to the nostril.	Slow advancement of the tube helps to prevent the tube from coiling in the esophagus
Immediately remove the tube if the client turns blue (cyanotic), cannot speak, coughs, or begins wheezing.	These symptoms indicate that the tube may be misplaced in the client's trachea and obstructing the airway

continued

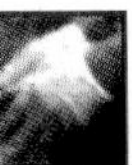

Clinical Procedure 51-1
Continued

Nursing Action	Rationale
Check for proper placement (a radiograph may be ordered to verify placement): 1. Draw back on a syringe; observe for gastric secretions. 2. Inject a small amount of air into the distal end of the tube, and auscultate with stethoscope just below the xiphoid for a "whooshing" or gurgling sound.	Ensures that the tip of the tube is in the correct location 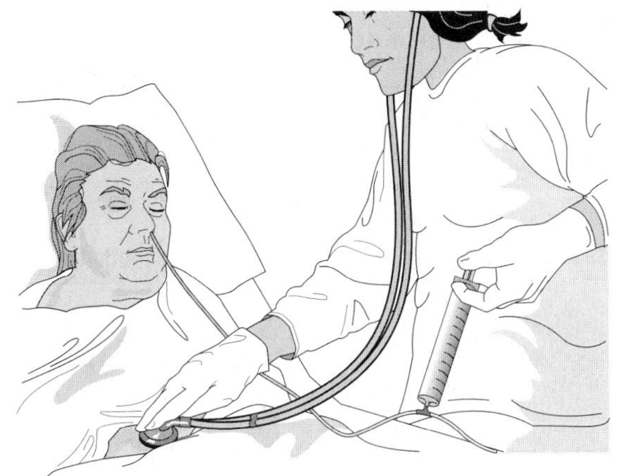 *Assessing placement.*
Secure the tube to the client's nares or under the nose with tape.	Prevents accidental removal or migration of the tube
Initiate feeding or gastric suction as ordered depending on the client's needs.	Provides for decompression or feeding
Document the time the procedure was performed, type of tube placed, results of the procedure, and client tolerance.	Provides a record of nursing activity and the client's response

oral fluids. Discomfort from dryness and unpleasant tastes and odors may be relieved with frequent mouth care. Ice chips and analgesic throat lozenges, gargles, or sprays may be helpful if the client's mouth and throat become sore. Always give mouth care after the tube is removed, and advise the client that a sore throat (an aftereffect of intubation) may persist for several days.

The client is at risk not only for dry mouth but also fluid volume deficit resulting from insufficient fluid intake. The nurse must be aware of the client's normal fluid needs and whether the formula alone can meet those needs. Observe for signs and symptoms of dehydration, for example, urine output of less than 500 mL daily. Then administer formula and additional water as ordered.

While ensuring adequate hydration, the nurse also needs to protect the client from infections that stem from microbes within the tube feeding formula. Signs and symptoms of infection include diarrhea, fever, or abnormal white blood cell count. Interventions to prevent infection include:

- Washing hands before handling equipment
- Keeping feeding formula refrigerated or unopened until ready to use

- Warming bolus or intermittent feeding formula to room temperature just before administering
- Hanging continuous formula-feeding containers with only the volume for 4 to 6 hours
- Flushing the tubing with water before adding more formula and after a bolus or intermittent feeding or medications are given
- Discarding any premixed formula after 24 hours
- Washing the syringe or container used for bolus and intermittent feedings after each use
- Replacing the infusion container for a continuous tube feeding every 24 hours or as directed by agency policy

When caring for a client receiving tube feedings, the plan of care includes, but is not limited to, the following:

Nursing Diagnoses and Collaborative Problems	Nursing Interventions
Risk for Aspiration related to client's inability to protect the airway during episodes of vomiting **Goal:** Lung sounds will be clear and client will not vomit.	Prevent vomiting by checking tube position and gastric residual volume before instilling formula.
	Place client in a semi-Fowler's position during feeding and for at least 30 minutes after a bolus or intermittent feeding.
	Clamp the feeding tube after a bolus or intermittent feeding.
	If the client vomits despite precautions, perform oral and pharyngeal suctioning as ordered and assess for respiratory distress.
	Prevent aspiration of any draining liquid during tube removal by instilling a small amount of air to clear secretions and formula from the tube, pinching the tube closed, and instructing the client to hold his or her breath until the tube is out of the nose.
Altered Nutrition: Less than Body Requirements related to inadequate or inappropriate tube feeding formula, malabsorption, or malfunction of the feeding device **Goal:** Client's nutrition will be adequate as evidenced by stable body weight.	Always refeed any gastric residual because it contains formula and digestive enzymes.
	Administer a GI motility agent such as cisapride (Propulsid), or metoclopramide (Reglan) if prescribed to promote gastric emptying and appropriate absorption of formula.
	Monitor the client's weight daily and report trends in weight loss or failure to gain. Consult physician and dietitian about changing to a higher calorie formula or one that better meets the client's metabolic needs.
Diarrhea or Constipation related to hypertonic liquid formula, lactose intolerance, gastroenteritis, lack of dietary fiber, fluid volume deficit, or other factors (specify) **Goal:** Bowel elimination patterns will be regular; stool will be formed.	Check the agency's policy or consult with the physician about diluting the formula or giving it at a slow rate at the beginning of therapy to help prevent diarrhea. Increase the concentration and rate according to the client's response.
	Consider lactose-free formulas for clients in whom lactose intolerance is suspected.
	Consider adding water or a high-fiber formula to relieve constipation.
	Consult with the physician and dietitian about the formula changes needed to restore normal bowel elimination.

Gastrointestinal Intubation for Decompression

The nasal route is the preferred route for passing a tube when the client's nose is intact and free from injury. The type of tube selected depends on the reason for placing the tube (Box 51–1). In general, smaller tubes are used for feeding because they tend to be more easily tolerated by clients; larger tubes are used for decompression because they allow for evacuation of large pieces of debris or blood clots from the upper GI tract.

BOX 51-1 Uses of Gastrointestinal (GI) Tubes

Gastrointestinal tubes come in several types depending on their uses. Among common GI tubes used for decompression are the Levin tube and the Salem sump. Narrower, more flexible tubes, such as Keofeed, Dubbhoff gastrostomy, jejunostomy, and others, are made of polyurethane or silicone and are used for administering liquid nourishment.

Feeding tubes are longer than Levin tubes and terminate in the upper, small intestine. The advantages to their use include ease of insertion, more comfort for the client, reduced potential for vomiting and aspiration because the formula is instilled below the pylorus, and extended use because they may remain in the same nostril for up to 4 weeks. The disadvantage is that distal location is difficult to assess without a chest or abdominal radiograph.

continued

BOX 51-1 *Continued*

Use and Maintenance

As a rule, GI tubes used for feeding are advanced in clients who have the ability to absorb nutrients through the GI tract but who cannot ingest food orally or cannot ingest sufficient quantities of food to provide adequate nutrition. Indications for insertion of a feeding tube include cancers of the oral cavity and esophagus, inability to swallow, history of aspirating orally ingested foods, malnutrition (such as that associated with cystic fibrosis), and provision of postoperative nutrition.

Feeding Methods

Liquid nourishment is administered by bolus, intermittent, cyclic, or continuous methods. Depending on institutional policy and individual feeding orders, the feeding tube is flushed with water at various intervals to ensure patency. A wide variety of tube feeding formulas are available to suit client's different nutritional needs. Nursing observation of the client's tolerance of the feeding is essential to determine which tube and formula are best for the individual client.

Bolus Tube Feedings

- Allows introduction of 250 to 400 mL formula through the tube in a short amount of time (usually 15–30 minutes).
- Administered by syringe or gravity flow system attached to the distal end of the feeding tube.

Intermittent Tube Feedings

- Allows delivery of between 250 and 400 mL formula over 30 to 60 minutes.
- Delivered by gravity flow system or an electronic feeding pump.

Continuous Tube Feedings

- Allows formula to be administered at lower rates—usually 1.5 mL/min over a longer time (usually 12–24 hours).
- Delivered by gravity flow system or an electronic feeding pump.

Cyclic Tube Feedings

- Allows formula to be administered continuously for 8 to 12 hours during sleep followed by a 16- to 12-hour pause.
- Ensures adequate nutrition during weaning from tube to oral feeding.
- Alternated with oral food intake until client can take most nutrition orally.

The larger GI tube is used to relieve abdominal distention caused by problems after surgery, by episodes of acute upper GI bleeding, by symptoms associated with intestinal obstruction, or for diagnostic purposes. It is inserted similarly to a feeding tube.

Some tubes, such as a gastric sump tube, have a double lumen, one of which serves as a vent, allowing a small amount of air to be drawn in when the tube is connected to suction. Sump tubes decrease the possibility of the stomach wall adhering to and obstructing the tube openings during gastric decompression. A common problem associated with vented tubes is leakage from the vent lumen. This may be prevented by keeping the vent above the level of the client's stomach. In many cases, decompression tubes may be connected to a source of suction, which is discussed in the Nursing Guidelines 51–2.

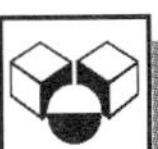

Nursing Guidelines 51-2

Managing the Care of a Client Needing Suction and Decompression

- Locate the suction source, usually a wall outlet or portable machine.
- Adjust the suction level on the wall outlet or portable machine to provide the amount and frequency of suction specified by the physician.
- Select intermittent high, low, or continuous suction when using a Salem sump tube; select low intermittent suction when using a Levin because the single lumen may adhere to the lining of the stomach during continuous suction. (If the tube is used only to obtain specimens for diagnostic purposes, manual suction may be achieved by attaching a syringe to the end of the tube and drawing back on the plunger.)

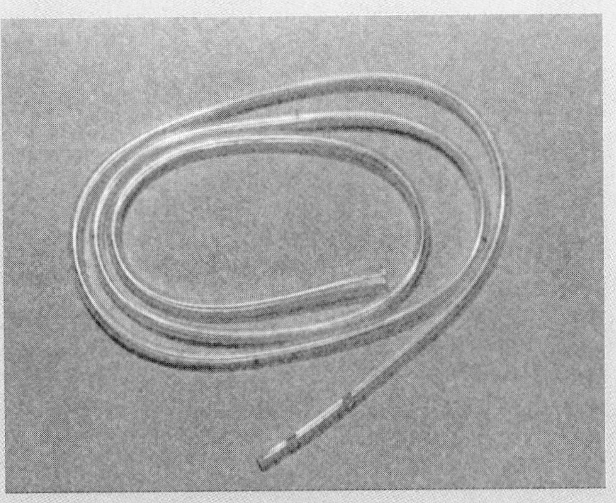

Levin tube. (Courtesy of Ken Timby.)

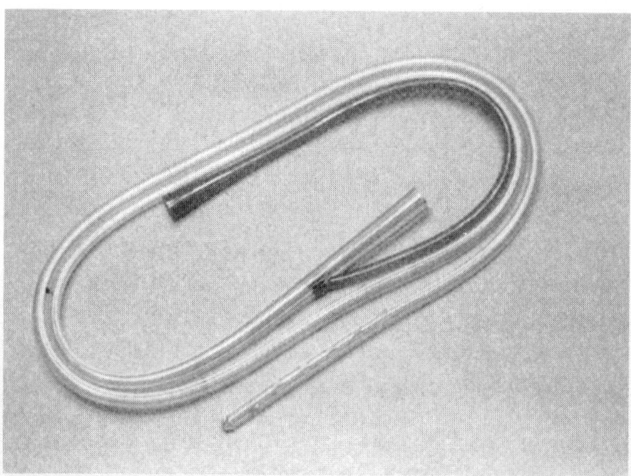

Vented Salem sump tube. (Courtesy of Ken Timby.)

- Insert the gastric decompression tube in accord with accepted standards and connect it to the suction.

Maintain Safe Suction

- Observe the amount and quality of the gastric contents being suctioned and the client's response.
- Monitor the procedure frequently because abdominal or gastric distention caused by suction failure may have serious consequences, such as strain on surgical sutures or vomiting around the tube.
- Check equipment frequently to make sure it is operating properly. If the suction is not operating satisfactorily, obtain another suction machine.

Maintain Tube Patency

- If the decompression tube is occluded, irrigate or replace it.
- First review the client's chart. The physician may order irrigation on an as needed basis.
- When irrigating the tube, use normal saline solution to prevent disturbance of electrolyte balance. Also use a large syringe to instill the irrigant into the distal end of the tube.
- After the fluid is instilled, remove it by gently pulling back on the plunger.
- Document the amount of solution used and the amount of fluid returned on the client's intake and output record.

Ensure Client Comfort

- Provide ice chips sparingly because water pulls electrolytes into the gastric secretions, which are then removed by suction, increasing the risk for an electrolyte disturbance.

Gastrostomy Tubes for Long-Term Feeding

A client with a **gastrostomy** has a transabdominal opening into the stomach. The gastrostomy provides long-term access for administering fluids and liquid nourishment. Creating a gastrostomy is a relatively minor procedure that can be performed surgically or endoscopically.

A surgical gastrostomy involves an external **stoma** and the feeding tube is placed through this opening. When a **percutaneous endoscopic gastrostomy** (PEG) is performed, an endoscope is introduced orally into the stomach so that the surgeon can see the correct location for the tube. The procedure can be performed in the endoscopy suite or at the bedside with the client needing a minimal amount of sedation (Fig. 51–1).

Because of the reduced risks, endoscopic placement is preferred to a surgical laparotomy unless the client has ascites, is morbidly obese, or has had previous gastric surgery. If the client's condition eventually improves, the gastrostomy tube is removed and the opening will close over time. On rare occasions the gastrostomy opening may require surgical closure.

Gastric feedings are administered by bolus, intermittent, or continuous methods, using the same techniques described previously. Bolus feedings are not given through tubes inserted below the pylorus because this causes abdominal cramping and diarrhea. Intermittent or continuous feedings simulate the normal passage of food into the small intestine and are generally well tolerated.

Gastrostomy feeding devices may be skin level devices (known as "buttons," appearing much like the air delivery/release button on inflatable toys) or tubes. Some gastrostomy tubes have a double lumen to allow infusion of two different fluids at once, for example, administration of medications and delivery of feeding formula without interruption. For stabilization most gastrostomy tubes have an external bumper and a firm internal bumper or an inflatable balloon. The advantage of the firm internal bumper is that it is difficult to accidentally dislodge. The disadvantage is that it may be difficult or painful to remove when replacement is desired. The advantage of the balloon-style internal bumper is that it is relatively painless and easy to replace. Disadvantages include relative ease of accidental dislodgment gradual loss of fluid from the inflated balloon resulting in leakage. The volume of fluid placed in the balloon is measured regularly and replaced as necessary.

Before a PEG tube is inserted, the nurse should weigh the client, assess vital signs, auscultate bowel sounds, and offer the client an opportunity to empty the bladder. Other nursing activities include determining the client's perception of the procedure, clarifying information, and checking that the proper consent forms are signed and in order. The skin is prepared and other ordered preprocedural activities, such as inserting an IV line and administering sedatives, are carried out.

Continue monitoring vital signs. Observe breathing characteristics. Inspect the skin and dressing. Examine the appearance and volume of the secre-

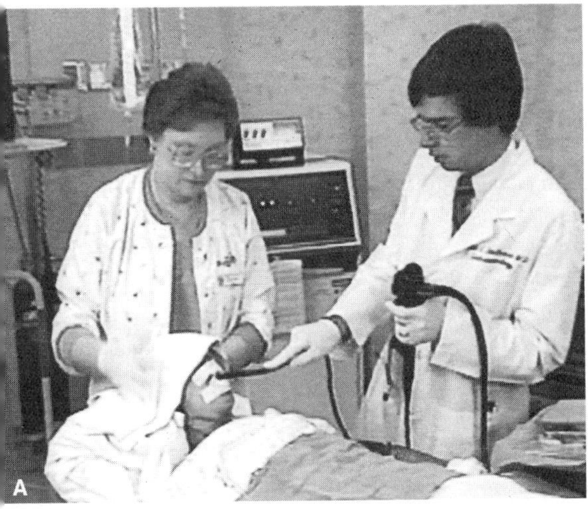

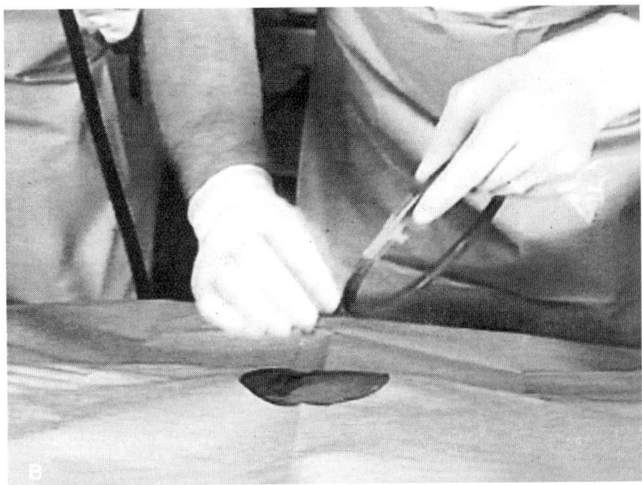

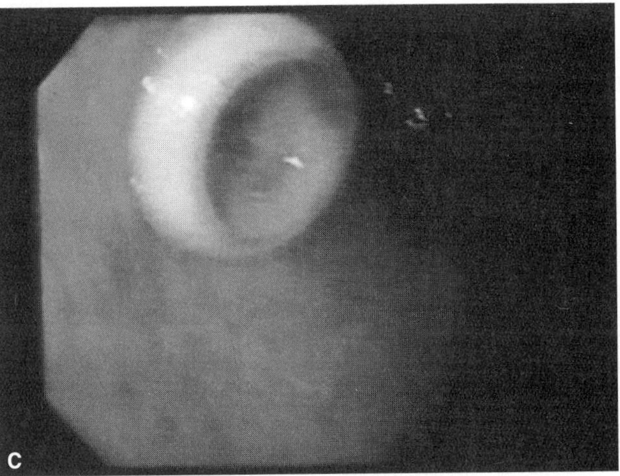

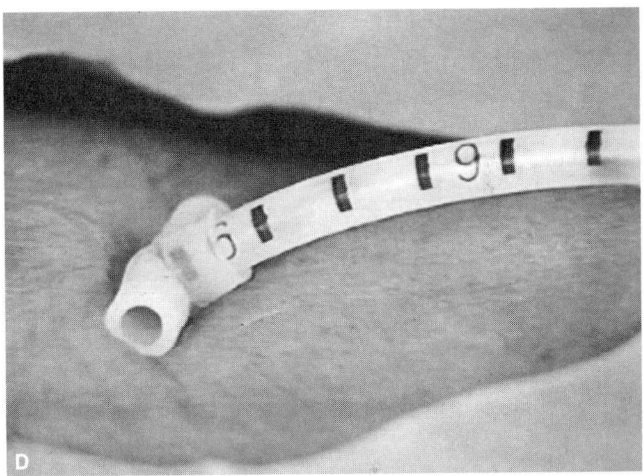

FIGURE 51-1. Percutaneous endoscopic gastrostomy (PEG) placement. To place a PEG tube endoscopically, the surgeon introduces an endoscope orally (*A*) into the stomach and identifies an appropriate site for the tube. Next a small incision is made through the skin of the abdomen and a trochar is advanced through the incision. A guidewire is threaded through the trochar (*B*), grasped with an instrument that is passed through the endoscope, and brought out through the client's mouth. The surgeon removes the endoscope and gently pushes the PEG tube over the guidewire advancing it through the client's mouth and esophagus to the stomach. When the proximal portion of the tube known as the "bumper" is against the interior wall of the stomach (C), the surgeon then secures the tube with another bumper type device (*D*) over the skin of the abdominal incision. (Photos courtesy of Bard Interventional Products Billerica, MA.)

tions during the first 24 hours when the gastrostomy tube may be temporarily attached to gravity drainage. Auscultate bowel sounds and palpate the abdomen lightly for signs of distention and tenderness. Inspect the oral mucosa for excessive dryness. Note the client's tolerance of the instilled formula when tube feeding is initiated. Promptly report abdominal distention, vomiting, fever, and severe pain to the physician. Monitor the characteristics and pattern of bowel elimination and trends in daily weight. In case the gastrostomy tube falls out, insert a clean Foley catheter, inflate the balloon, and clamp it to keep the stoma from sealing. Notify the physician so a new feeding device can be inserted as soon as possible. Leave the Foley catheter in place until a more appropriate device is available. Feedings can be administered through the Foley catheter until it is replaced.

A discussion of ongoing nursing management responsibilities appears in the Nursing Care Plan.

NURSING CARE PLAN 51-1
Managing the Care of a Client Undergoing Percutaneous Endoscopic Gastrostomy

Potential Problems and Nursing Diagnoses	Nursing Management	Outcome Criteria
Risk for Ineffective Breathing Patterns related to sedative medications administered during the procedure	Monitor respiratory rate and effort until vital signs and level of consciousness revert to preprocedural baseline. Continuously monitor oxygenation with pulse oximetry until baseline measurements are reached.	Client demonstrates respiratory status equal to the preprocedural assessment.
Pain related to tissue injury	Administer analgesic medications as prescribed. Tell client to ask for assistance when performing activity that requires using abdominal muscles, such as changing from a lying to a sitting position. Avoid excessive pressure on the gastrostomy site from clothing or bed linens. Show the client how to use a pillow to provide splinting when coughing. Encourage ambulation as tolerated to help to eliminate air remaining in the GI tract. Report severe pain, abdominal distention, and fever because these symptoms may indicate that a complication has occurred.	Client reports absence or reduction of pain.
Risk for Infection secondary to abdominal incision and potential for impaired skin integrity	Change dressing over gastrostomy site daily and as needed if the dressing becomes loose, wet, or soiled. Secure the dressing with paper or hypoallergenic tape. Inspect the gastrostomy site with each dressing change for signs of trauma (bleeding, bruising, edema) and infection (redness, swelling, tenderness, purulent discharge). Report abnormal findings to the physician. Clean the gastrostomy site thoroughly with each dressing change. • Lift the external bumper to expose the exit and clean the skin with povidone iodine (Betadine) or a prescribed antiseptic. • Depress the skin at the tube insertion site and look for the backflow of gastric drainage or formula that would irritate the skin and that should be scant or absent after a week. • Apply an antiseptic ointment to the insertion site or use karaya powder or skin protectant paste if the skin appears excoriated (red and sore). • Rotate the bumper approximately 90 degrees and reposition is so that it fits firmly, but not tightly, next to the skin. • After the site heals, clean the skin as prescribed by the physician or institutional policy. Pat dry. Eventually the site may be left open to air, allowing the area to dry. Clean any dried secretions from the site. When the site heals fully, a dressing is usually not necessary. • Stabilize a free bumperless tube by enclosing it within a baby bottle nipple that has been slit from the base to its excised tip and taped to the skin or skin protectant wafer. Keep the end of the catheter clamped to prevent the reflux of gastric contents unless the client is being fed.	The gastrostomy site remains free of infection and the skin at the tube insertion site is intact with no redness and no burning.

continued

NURSING CARE PLAN 51-1

Continued

Potential Problems and Nursing Diagnoses	Nursing Management	Outcome Criteria
Risk for Altered Nutrition: Less than Body Requirements related to occluded or dislodged tube or inappropriate tube feeding formula, malabsorption, or malfunction of the feeding device	Administer feeding formula according to standard practices: • Give bolus feeding through a gastrostomy tube using a large syringe (50–60 mL) over 15 to 30 minutes. • Hold the syringe perpendicular to the abdomen and 3 to 6 inches above it. Instill 30 to 60 mL of tap water into the syringe. Begin adding the formula if water instillation proceeds without difficulty. Tilt the syringe so that air bubbles can escape. • Instill intermittent feedings over at least 45 minutes, but no longer than 1 hour. Intermittent and continuous feedings stimulate normal passage of food into the small intestine and are usually well tolerated. Consult with the physician about modifying the volume of each feeding but administering them more frequently to deliver the total amount ordered. • Administer drugs prescribed to assist gastric emptying as prescribed. • Pulverize solid medications, if allowed, and mix them with a generous amount of water. • Flush formula and medications with 30 to 60 mL fluid to maintain a patent tube. • Inform the physician if the tube becomes obstructed, appears to be cracked from age and manipulation, or becomes dislodged. (To unclog an obstructed tube, use carbonated soft drink, a solution containing meat tenderizer, or Viokase, a pancreatic enzyme. Consult with the physician first.) • Plan to remove the gastrostomy tube and insert another one if an obstructed tube cannot be cleared. • When possible, encourage the client to join others during mealtime. The sensory stimulation of social interaction and the sight and smell of food promotes salivation, peristalsis, and gastric motility.	Client maintains stable body weight.
Knowledge Deficit regarding self-care after gastrostomy tube placement	Educate client and significant others regarding self-care. Include the following: • When it is safe to bathe or shower • How to care for the gastrostomy site (dressing changes, securing the tube to prevent accidental removal, cleaning the site) • Signs and symptoms of infection • How to administer nourishment through the tube • How to prepare and store prescribed formula • How to clean, store, and maintain associated equipment (tubing, bags, pumps) • Signs and symptoms of feeding intolerance	Client and significant others will demonstrate how to care for the gastrostomy site and administer feedings properly.
Risk for Altered Oral Mucous Membrane related to reduced salivation	Offer small sips of water or other beverages if allowed even though the gastrostomy is the main route for nourishment and hydration. Provide oral hygiene frequently or encourage the client to perform this independently. Suggest sucking on sugar-free candy or chewing gum to promote salivation.	Client's oral mucous membranes are moist and intact.

continued

NURSING CARE PLAN 51-1
Continued

Potential Problems and Nursing Diagnoses	Nursing Management	Outcome Criteria
Ineffective Individual Coping related to inability to eat normally	Acknowledge the client's feelings and encourage the expression of these feelings. Promote contact with the client's support system. Convey confidence that the client has the inner strength to handle adversity based on prior successes.	Client reports ability to cope effectively, expresses concerns and feels motivated to overcome physical problems.
Body Image Disturbance related to transabdominal tubing	Encourage the client to participate in usual social activities if possible. Provide reassurance that with the PEG tube closed, the client can dress comfortably, move about, and appear normal to others.	Client reports feeling positive about self and the changes necessary for nutrition.

Disorders of the Esophagus

Various disorders can affect the esophagus, among them gastroesophageal reflux disease (GERD), esophageal diverticulum, hiatal hernia, esophageal varices, and cancer.

Gastroesophageal Reflux Disease (GERD)

Gastroesophageal reflux is a common disorder that develops when gastric contents flow in an upward direction, into the esophagus. All adults and children normally have some degree of reflux, especially after eating. Gastroesophageal reflux is only considered a disease process when it is excessive or causes undesirable symptoms, such as pain or respiratory distress.

ETIOLOGY AND PATHOPHYSIOLOGY

Gastroesophageal reflux is caused by an inability of the cardiac sphincter to close fully, allowing the contents of the stomach to flow freely into the esophagus. Obesity and pregnancy increase susceptibility to reflux due to upward pressure on the diaphragm from increased abdominal girth.

ASSESSMENT FINDINGS

Signs and Symptoms

The most common symptoms associated with gastroesophageal reflux are epigastric pain or discomfort (**dyspepsia**) and regurgitation. Other symptoms include difficulty swallowing (dysphagia), painful swallowing (**odynophagia**), inflammation of the lining of the esophagus (**esophagitis**), aspiration pneumonia, and respiratory distress. Clients with reflux esophagitis may bleed—manifested by vomited blood (*hematemesis*) or tarry stools (*melena*). Sometimes *occult* (hidden) *bleeding* for long periods produces iron deficiency anemia. Because the esophagus is anatomically close to the heart, clients with epigastric pain may report thinking they are having a heart attack. Until a myocardial infarction is ruled out as a cause for the discomfort, it is considered a potential diagnosis.

Diagnostic Findings

Barium swallow findings show inflammation in the esophagus or stricture formation from chronic esophagitis. Upper endoscopy with biopsy confirms esophagitis. Stools may test positive for blood.

MEDICAL AND SURGICAL MANAGEMENT

Medications used to control esophageal reflux are discussed in Table 51–2. The most common surgical procedure performed for GERD reflux is a **fundoplication**, a laparoscopic procedure that tightens the cardiac sphincter by wrapping the gastric fundus around the lower esophagus and suturing it into place.

NURSING MANAGEMENT

Educate the client with GERD about diet and lifestyle changes needed to reduce the reflux symptoms. Mild symptoms are controlled by dietary management—avoiding foods and beverages that lower

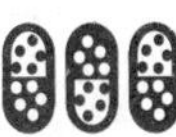

TABLE 51-2 **Medications Used to Treat Problems in the Upper GI Tract**

Drug Category/Drug Action	Side Effects	Nursing Considerations
Antacids		
calcium carbonate (Tums)	Constipation, hypercalcemia, hypophosphatemia	Avoid using in large amounts over prolonged time. May be used as a calcium supplement.
aluminum hydroxide (Alternagel, Gaviscon)	Constipation, indigestion	Do not administer to clients who are on sodium-restricted diet. Do not administer with tetracycline.
aluminum hydroxide with magnesium hydroxide (Maalox, Mylanta)	Hypermagnesemia, hypophosphatemia	Observe for CNS depression and other symptoms of hypermagnesemia, especially in clients with renal failure.
Neutralize gastric acid to relieve heartburn, sour stomach.		
Histamine-2 Antagonists		
cimetidine (Tagamet)	Blood abnormalities (agranulocytosis, neutropenia, thrombocytopenia), diarrhea, dizziness, sleepiness, headache, confusion, increased plasma creatinine level, cardiac rhythm disturbances, impotence (reversible), rash	Give drug at mealtimes and bedtime. Urge client to report sore throat, fever, unusual bruising or bleeding, dizziness.
ranitidine (Zantac)	Headache, GI disturbance, insomnia, nausea and vomiting, rash, blood abnormalities, impotence	Give drug with meals and at bedtime. Encourage regular checkups. Urge client to report sore throat, fever, unusual bruising, bleeding, dizziness, severe headache, muscle or joint pain.
famotidine (Pepcid)	Headache, dizziness, diarrhea, constipation, muscle cramps, sexual impotence	Give drug with meals and at bedtime. Encourage regular checkups. Advise client to report sore throat, fever, unusual bruising, bleeding, dizziness, severe headache, muscle or joint pain.
Suppress gastric acid by blocking H_2 receptors.		
Antiulcer Agents		
sucralfate (Carafate)	Dizziness, sleeplessness, vertigo, constipation, gastric discomfort, dry mouth, rash, back pain	Give drug on an empty stomach 1 h before or 2 h after meals and at bedtime. Do not give at the same time as antacid or H_2 antagonist. Advise client to report severe gastric pain.
Protect ulcers from acid and pepsin.		
Proton Pump Inhibitors		
omeprazole (Prilosec)	Headache, fatigue, dizziness, depression, abdominal pain, cramps, gas, nausea, diarrhea, flulike symptoms, rash, arthralgia	Give before meals to prevent stomach upset. Instruct client to swallow capsule whole without breaking, opening, or crushing contents. Caution client not to drive car or operate machinery if side effects are severe.
lanisoprazole (Prevacid)	Diarrhea, abdominal pain, nausea, vomiting, constipation, dry mouth, headache, dizziness, vertigo, insomnia, upper respiratory symptoms (reversible), rash	Give drug before meals. Arrange for client to be medically monitored while taking drug. Advise client to report worsening symptoms, severe headache, fever, chills.
Suppress gastric acid by blocking enzymes associated with the final step of acid production.		
Gastrointestinal Motility Agents		
metoclopramide (Reglan)	Restlessness, drowsiness, fatigue, extrapyramidal symptoms, parkinson-like reactions, nausea, diarrhea	Instruct client not to use alcohol or sleeping pills with this drug because resulting sedation may be dangerous. Advise client to report severe depression or diarrhea and involuntary tremors or tics of the face, eyes, arms, and legs.
cisapride (Propulsid)	Headache, abdominal pain, diarrhea, constipation, nausea, vomiting, serious cardiac arrhythmias resulting from potential drug interactions, runny nose	Assess history of medication and gallbladder disease, GI bleeding or obstruction, pregnancy or lactation. Give 15 minutes before each meal and at bedtime. Instruct client not to use alcohol or sleeping pills with this drug because resulting sedation may be dangerous.
Stimulate upper GI tract and speed gastric emptying without stimulating gastric acid release.		

(continued)

TABLE 51-2 *(Continued)*

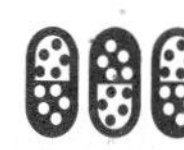

Drug Category/Drug Action	Side Effects	Nursing Considerations
Anticholinergics		
atropine sulfate (Atropine)	Blurred vision, dilated pupils, cycloplegia, dizziness, nervousness, insomnia, dry mouth, increased intraocular pressure, palpitations, heart rhythm changes, life-threatening paralytic ileus, urinary retention, intolerance to heat	Assess for health conditions that may contraindicate therapy. Give 30 minutes before meals. Be sure client has adequate fluid intake. Keep room temperature cool but comfortable. Tell client to report eye pain, abnormal heartbeats, difficulty swallowing, breathing problems, and so forth.
dicyclomine HCl (Bentyl)	Constipation, dry mouth, blurred vision, sensitivity to light, difficulty urinating, irregular heartbeat, intolerance to heat	Ensure adequate fluids. Keep room temperature stable to prevent problems resulting from intolerance to heat. Tell client to report eye pain, abnormal heartbeats, difficulty swallowing, breathing problems, and so forth.
propantheline bromide (Pro-Banthine [Can])	Constipation, dry mouth, blurred vision, sensitivity to light, difficulty urinating, irregular heartbeat, intolerance to heat.	Assess for health conditions that contraindicate therapy (glaucoma, bronchial asthma).
Relax smooth muscles of GI tract and inhibit gastric secretions.		

pressure in the cardiac sphincter, such as alcohol, peppermint, licorice, and caffeine. Additional measures include weight loss and avoiding tight-fitting garments, elevating the head of the bed, stopping smoking, and avoiding food and drink for several hours before bedtime. Advise pregnant clients that the symptoms usually resolve after delivery. Teach the client how to self-administer medications to control reflux. Emphasize strict compliance with drug therapy to reduce symptoms. Teach the client about the importance of controlling severe reflux disease to prevent possible complications, such as esophageal stricture formation and esophageal cancer. Closely observe for abdominal distention and nausea in postoperative clients because they cannot belch or vomit following fundoplication.

Esophageal Diverticulum

A **diverticulum** is a sac or pouch in one or more layers of the wall of an organ or structure. Esophageal diverticula (plural) are found at the junction of the pharynx and the esophagus or in the middle or lower portion of the esophagus.

ETIOLOGY AND PATHOPHYSIOLOGY

Diverticula form as a consequence of a congenital or acquired weakness of the esophageal wall. The diverticula trap food and secretions, which then narrows the lumen, interferes with the passage of food into the stomach, and exerts pressure on the trachea. The trapped food decomposes within the esophagus causing esophagitis or ulceration in the mucosa.

ASSESSMENT FINDINGS

Signs and Symptoms

The client has foul breath and experiences difficulty or pain when swallowing, belching, regurgitating, or coughing. Gurgling sounds may be heard when auscultating the mid-upper chest.

Diagnostic Findings

Barium swallow and endoscopic examination reveal the structural abnormalities within the esophagus.

MEDICAL AND SURGICAL MANAGEMENT

For mild symptoms, treatment usually includes a bland, soft, semisoft, or liquid diet to facilitate passage of food. Small meals eaten four to six times a day are recommended.

Clients with more severe symptoms may require surgical excision of the diverticulum. If the diverticulum is at the lower esophagus, it is repaired through a thoracic (chest) approach. The surgical approach for an esophageal diverticulum at the junction of the pharynx and esophagus usually is above the clavicle (collarbone).

NURSING MANAGEMENT

Explain that oral hygiene will not alter the foul breath. Provide instructions for dietary modifications or arrange a consultation with a dietitian. For additional nursing management see the discussion that accompanies nursing management of hiatal hernia and that which accompanies the care of a client undergoing upper GI surgery.

Hiatal Hernia

A **hiatal** or **diaphragmatic hernia** is a protrusion of part of the stomach into the esophagus. There are two types of hiatal hernia: the paraesophageal type (Fig. 51–2), which is an upward displacement of the fundus and greater curvature of the stomach through the diaphragm, and the sliding type, in which the junction of the stomach and the esophagus and part of the stomach slide up through the weakened portion of the diaphragm.

ETIOLOGY AND PATHOPHYSIOLOGY

A hiatal hernia is caused by a defect in the diaphragm at the point where the esophagus passes through. This condition results from a congenital weakness in the muscle or from trauma. Factors that increase intra-abdominal pressure, such as multiple pregnancies or obesity, contribute to hiatal hernia as do the loss of muscle strength and tone that occurs with aging. The condition is particularly common in women.

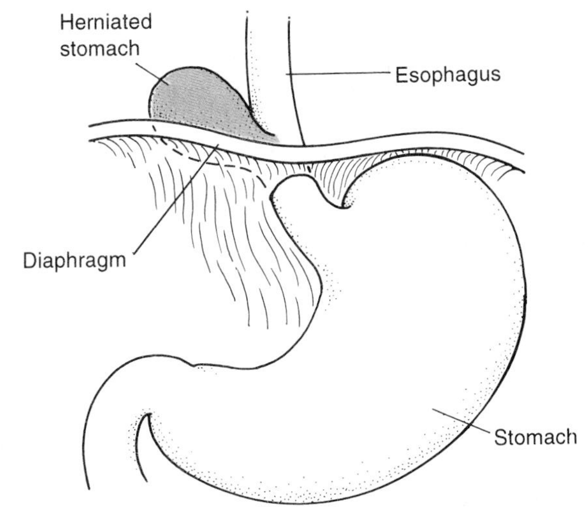

FIGURE 51-2. Hiatal hernia in which a portion of the stomach protrudes through the diaphragm into the chest cavity.

When the upper portion of the stomach slips from its usual position and becomes trapped, gastroesophageal reflux occurs.

ASSESSMENT FINDINGS

Signs and Symptoms

The client describes having heartburn, belching, and a feeling of substernal or epigastric pressure or pain after eating and when lying down. If scars form, swallowing becomes difficult. As food distends the esophagus, vomiting may occur.

Diagnostic Findings

A barium swallow confirms the diagnosis by outlining the abnormal positioning of the stomach. An esophagoscopy shows the extent of irritation and scarring occurring within the esophagus.

MEDICAL AND SURGICAL MANAGEMENT

Medical management of the client with hiatal hernia is the same as that for the client with GERD. The narrowed esophagus is stretched endoscopically, but the procedure may need to be repeated often. Clients who do not respond to a rigid medical regimen are treated surgically. Surgical treatment involves restoring the stomach to its proper position and repairing the defect in the diaphragm.

NURSING MANAGEMENT

For clients who undergo thoracic surgery to repair a hiatal hernia, nursing care is the same as for a client who had chest surgery (see Chap. 27). Regardless of the surgical approach, postoperative care will likely involve intubation for gastric decompression to prevent distention of the stomach and avoid pressure on the surgical repair (see Nursing Guidelines 51–2).

When managing nonsurgical care of clients with hiatal hernia or other esophageal disorders the plan of nursing care includes, but is not limited to, the following:

Nursing Diagnosis and Collaborative Problems	Nursing Interventions
Altered Nutrition: Less than Body Requirements, related to swallowing difficulties **Goal:** The client will consume nutrients according to metabolic needs.	Suggest the client eat frequent small, high-calorie, well balanced meals to meet metabolic requirements but avoid the overload that causes dysphagia.
Pain related to pressure or reflux of gastric secretions	Teach the client comfort measures:

Goal: The client will experience relief from epigastric discomfort.

- Eat small meals of nonirritating foods.
- Remain upright for at least 2 hours after meals.
- Avoid meals or snacks before bedtime.
- Raise the head of the bed 3 or 4 inches for sleeping.
- Avoid activities that incorporate Valsalva's maneuver (lifting heavy objects or straining during bowel movement), which can raise intra-abdominal pressure to such heights that the stomach becomes wedged above the diaphragm.
- Take medications exactly as prescribed to reduce gastric acidity and relieve pain.

Esophageal Varices

Esophageal varices are generally caused by cirrhosis of the liver; both are discussed in Chapter 54.

Cancer of the Esophagus

Esophageal malignant cell changes occur more often in men than in women, usually in the fourth or fifth decade of life. The tumor generally is a squamous cell carcinoma.

ETIOLOGY AND PATHOPHYSIOLOGY

A strong correlation exists among esophageal cancer, alcohol abuse, and cigarette smoking. As the cancer advances, the mass occupies space and interferes with swallowing. If the tumor grows unchecked, it may obstruct passage of food into the stomach, promoting the possibility for aspiration. Or the tumor may ulcerate, leading to occult or frank blood loss.

ASSESSMENT FINDINGS

Signs and Symptoms

Symptoms usually develop slowly. Beginning symptoms are mild, with vague feelings of discomfort and difficulty in swallowing some foods. Weight loss accompanies progressive dysphagia. As the disease progresses, solid foods become almost impossible to swallow, and the client resorts to liquids. By the time swallowing difficulty is pronounced, the cancer may have invaded surrounding tissues and lymphatics. When the tumor expands, the client experiences back pain and respiratory distress. Pain is a late symptom.

Diagnostic Findings

A barium swallow demonstrates a filling defect caused by a space-occupying mass. A biopsy of tissue removed during esophagoscopy reveals malignant cells.

MEDICAL AND SURGICAL MANAGEMENT

Clients who are not candidates for surgery are treated with palliative measures and, possibly, endoscopic laser surgery to destroy some of the tumor. Esophageal dilatation may be used to enlarge the obstructed area, or a prosthesis (stent placement) is inserted at the tumor site to widen the narrowed area. A prosthesis is inserted also when a fistula forms at the tumor site.

When surgery is a curative option, the kind of surgery depends on the tumor location as well as the extent of the lesion and evidence of metastasis. If the tumor is in the lower third of the esophagus, the surgeon removes the affected area and attaches the remaining two-thirds to the stomach. If the tumor is in the upper two-thirds of the esophagus, the surgeon removes the affected area and replaces that portion of esophagus with a section of jejunum or colon.

NURSING MANAGEMENT

When caring for a client who has an esophageal obstruction or whose nutritional needs cannot be met orally, review nursing care of a client receiving nourishment through a tube, either a GI tube or a gastrostomy tube (see Nursing Care Plan 51–1).

Consult with the dietitian before instituting measures for weight reduction or gain as ordered. Keep in mind that a major nursing goal is adequate or improved nutrition and eventually stable weight. Provide small, frequent meals for the client with esophageal reflux. Confer with the dietitian about modifying the texture of food or giving a high-calorie, high-protein semiliquid diet to clients with a swallowing problem. Have the client refrain from consuming foods that contain a lot of air or gas, such as soufflés and carbonated drinks. To reduce bloating, advise the client to avoid drinking from straws or from narrow-necked bottles to reduce the volume of air trapped in the esophagus or stomach. Supplement the diet with liquid nourishment between meals.

The nutritional needs of the client with inoperable cancer of the esophagus are met with nasogastric or gastrostomy tube feedings or TPN. In such cases essential nursing management involves caring for the skin at the tube insertion site, preventing infection, administering nourishment, maintaining tube patency, and preparing the client or family for self-care or home care after discharge.

Clients who return from esophageal or gastric surgery need to be turned and perform deep breathing and coughing every 2 hours. They need to know how to support the surgical incision for coughing and deep breathing as well. An incentive spirometer may be used to motivate the client and provide immediate feedback on respiratory efficiency. Encourage ventilation and coughing when the client is experiencing a reduction in pain. Provide oral liquids, if allowed, to thin secretions. Then encourage the client to ambulate to mobilize secretions, increase the depth of respiration, and promote the expulsion of intestinal gas. To avoid gastric distention, wait to provide oral nourishment until bowel sounds resume and are active. To minimize dyspnea, give frequent, small meals and do not allow the client to lie down immediately after eating.

Client and Family Teaching

Explain the rationale underlying the prescribed treatment. Stress the importance of adhering to the therapeutic regimen. Review the essentials of dietary modifications. Instruct the client on the purpose, administration, schedule, precautions, and side effects of prescribed medications. Emphasize the need for continued medical follow-up. Also advise the client to inform the physician immediately of worsening symptoms, steady weight loss, difficulty swallowing soft foods, abnormal bleeding, or other new problems.

Gastric Disorders

Among the most serious gastric disorders are gastritis, peptic ulcer disease, and cancer of the stomach.

Gastritis

Gastritis is the inflammation of the stomach lining (gastric mucosa). The disorder may be acute or chronic.

ETIOLOGY AND PATHOPHYSIOLOGY

The causes of gastritis include dietary indiscretions; reflux of duodenal contents; drugs, such as aspirin, steroids, nonsteroidal anti-inflammatory drugs (NSAIDs), alcohol, and caffeine; ingestion of poisons or corrosive substances; food allergies; infection; and gastric ischemia secondary to vasoconstriction caused by a stress response. Gastric secretions are highly acidic. *Parietal cells* in the stomach increase acid production (hydrochloric acid) in response to seeing, smelling, and eating food. These cells also are chemically stimulated by histamine and acetylcholine, which are released from the parasympathetic vagus nerve. An increasing acid level, triggers the conversion of pepsinogen to pepsin, creating a chemical mixture strong enough to digest the stomach wall. However, because the stomach lining is protectively coated with mucus, pepsin normally has little effect.

Prostaglandin E, a lipid compound secreted within the stomach, seems to promote mucous production. This mucus contains buffering substances and mechanically bars penetration by stomach acids. However, the submucosal layers of the stomach can become inflamed when the mucous layer is reduced or penetrated by irritating substances. As a consequence, the client experiences epigastric discomfort, often described as "heartburn." The mucus-producing cells generally heal and regenerate in 3 to 5 days. Chronic irritation leads to ulceration.

ASSESSMENT FINDINGS

Signs and Symptoms

Usually the client complains of epigastric fullness, pressure, pain, anorexia, nausea, and vomiting. When gastritis is caused by a bacterial or viral infection, the client may experience vomiting, diarrhea, fever, and abdominal pain. Drugs, poisons, toxic substances, and corrosives can cause gastric bleeding. Clients may describe seeing blood in emesis or note a darkening of their stool color. Chronic gastritis may give rise to no symptoms or symptoms similar to mild indigestion.

Diagnostic Findings

A complete blood count may reveal anemia from chronic blood loss. Stool testing for occult blood often detects red blood cells in the stool. In difficult cases, gastroscopy may be performed to visualize the mucosa and obtain specimens, which are examined for pathogens or cellular abnormalities.

MEDICAL AND SURGICAL MANAGEMENT

Treatment depends on the cause of gastritis and the symptoms experienced by the client. Ingestion of poisons requires emergency treatment. In acute cases, eating is restricted and IV fluids are given to correct dehydration and electrolyte imbalances, particularly if vomiting is severe. Drugs are prescribed to control nausea and vomiting, and antibiotics may be prescribed to inhibit or destroy infection.

Usually, chronic gastritis is treated by avoiding irritating substances such as spicy foods, alcohol, and caffeine. Various drugs, such as antacids and short-term histamine antagonist agents, are prescribed.

NURSING MANAGEMENT

Monitor the client's symptoms. Evaluate the response to dietary modifications and prescribed medications. Observe the color and characteristics of any vomitus or stool that the client passes. In addition, teach the client about diet, drug therapy, and the need for continued medical follow-up. For complications such as ulcer formation, refer to the nursing management discussion of peptic ulcer disease.

Peptic Ulcer Disease

A **peptic ulcer** is a circumscribed loss of tissue in an area of the GI tract that is in contact with hydrochloric acid and pepsin. Most peptic ulcers occur in the duodenum; however, they may occur at the lower end of the esophagus, in the stomach, or in the jejunum after the client has had surgery at the spot where the stomach and the jejunum were sutured. Gastric ulcers are more likely to recur and have the highest incidence for undergoing malignant changes. Men are affected more frequently than women. The highest incidence occurs during middle life, but the condition can occur at any age.

ETIOLOGY AND PATHOPHYSIOLOGY

Peptic ulcers occur when there is a disruption in the normal balance between factors that promote mucosal injury (gastric acid, pepsin, bile acid, ingested substances) and factors that protect the mucosa (intact epithelium, mucus, and bicarbonate secretion). Risk factors for gastric ulcers include *Helicobacter pylori* infection, cigarette smoking, family history, and chronic use of aspirin or NSAIDs.

Various irritants can disrupt the gastric mucosa and in recent years, a link between the bacteria *H. pylori* and peptic ulcer disease has been identified. The transmission of this bacteria is thought to be via fecal-oral or oral-oral pathways. *H. pylori*, a gram-negative microorganism, is present in the gastric or duodenal mucosa of 80% to 90% of clients with peptic ulcers. This bacteria, which shelters itself in the bicarbonate-rich mucus, is a factor in chronic gastritis and peptic ulcer disease. The mechanism by which this microorganism makes the mucosa more susceptible to erosion is not yet completely understood. What is known is that *H. pylori* secretes an enzyme that theoretically depletes gastric mucus, making it more vulnerable to injury.

Ulcers occur when there is prolonged hyperacidity or chronic reduction in mucus. Once the mucosal layer has been penetrated by gastric acid, the acid begins to digest the stomach wall. Histamine, released from the injured cells, adds insult to injury by triggering hypersecretion of more hydrochloric acid and pepsin. The body responds with the inflammatory process. Capillary permeability is increased; the mucosa swells and bleeds easily.

Because food dilutes the acid in the stomach, individuals with an ulcer experience more discomfort when the stomach is empty than after eating food. Unless the process is controlled, the erosion can lead to an obstruction from scar formation or penetrate the entire thickness of the stomach wall, spilling gastric contents into the peritoneal cavity, a process that may be accompanied by hemorrhage.

In a few cases, acute ischemia leads to ulcer formation. Decreased blood flow interferes with the ability of mucosal cells to survive and function. The sudden drop in mucus production makes the stomach vulnerable. This phenomenon occurs in critically ill clients who have had, for example, cardiac or respiratory arrest, severe burns, or multiple trauma. Their unstable medical condition is compounded by anxiety and fear. The diminished circulation of blood combined with vasoconstriction from sympathetic nervous system stimulation leads to what has been termed *stress ulcers*.

Aging and chronic stomach inflammation as in recurrent gastric ulcers, cancer of the stomach, or a long history of alcoholism, lead to atrophy of the glandular epithelium of the stomach. The ability of the parietal cells to secrete hydrochloric acid and the intrinsic factor is decreased. This explains the correlation of *hypochlorhydria* (reduced gastric acidity) or *achlorhydria* (absence of hydrochloric acid) and pernicious anemia that occurs in clients who fit this profile.

ASSESSMENT FINDINGS

Signs and Symptoms

Most clients with peptic ulcer disease have abdominal pain, which is usually confined to the epigastrium and does not radiate. It is most often described as having a "burning" quality. The client often complains of pain that disturbs sleep and also occurs one to several hours after meals. The pain may be relieved by eating food. Back pain suggests irritation of the pancreas by the ulcer. About 20% of clients may have bleeding as the first sign of the ulcer; hemorrhage, hematemesis, or melena may occur. Protracted vomiting secondary to scarring and resultant obstruction also is seen among those who have ignored earlier symptoms.

Diagnostic Findings

The diagnosis is suggested by the history and confirmed by results of an upper GI series or esopha-

;ogastroduodenoscopy (EGD). To differentiate be-ween benign and malignant ulcers, a gastric washing or biopsy for cytologic analysis may be performed. Typically, the hemoglobin and red blood cell values are low from chronic blood loss. Electrolytes are al-ered from vomiting.

MEDICAL AND SURGICAL MANAGEMENT

The effectiveness of dietary therapy in treating peptic ulcer disease is unknown. Foods known to in-crease acid production include milk and milk prod-ucts, alcohol, beverages containing caffeine and de-caffeinated coffee. Clients are provided with small frequent meals and are instructed to avoid eating foods that they find particularly irritating.

In the presence of *H. pylori*, eradication therapy is initiated. This includes the use of a combination of antibiotics, proton pump inhibitors, and bis-muth. Antacids are initially used to buffer stomach acid. They are not absorbed from the GI tract and therefore do not produce alkalosis, even when given in large doses. Cholinergic blocking agents, such as propantheline (Pro-Banthine), block the stimulating effects of acetylcholine; they also de-crease gastric motility. Anticholinergics are contra-indicated if partial obstruction is present because they further decrease the motility of an atonic stomach and add to the obstructive symptoms. Cimetidine (Tagamet), famotidine (Pepcid), nizati-dine (Axid), and ranitidine (Zantac) block hista-mine receptors. Sucralfate (Carafate) is a cytopro-tective agent that forms a seal over the ulcer, protecting it from irritation. Misoprostol (Cytotec), a synthetic prostaglandin, is used to sustain the mucosal layer especially among clients who require large doses or long-term treatment with aspirin or NSAIDs. Omeprazole (Prilosec) and lansoprazole (Prevacid) are gastric acid pump inhibitors, block-ing the final step in acid production at the surface of parietal cells.

Obstruction caused by edema and inflammation often subsides when gastric intubation is used con-currently with treatment for the ulcer. Treatment of hemorrhage includes complete rest, blood transfu-sions, and gastric lavage with saline solution. Iced saline solution is no longer used because of its poten-tial to cause hypothermia. Nothing is given by mouth, and IV fluids are administered until the bleeding has stopped. Endoscopic laser therapy or endoscopic injections of epinephrine into the ulcer bed may be used to control bleeding if more conserv-ative measures are unsuccessful.

Ulcers that persist despite medical interventions, repeatedly recur, cause severe hemorrhage, create un-relieved obstruction, cause perforation, or are predis-posed to malignant changes justify surgical interven-tions as described in Table 51–3.

If a total **gastrectomy** is performed, the client re-ceives vitamin B_{12} injections for life because without the stomach, the intrinsic factor necessary for absorp-tion of vitamin B_{12} is no longer produced. B_{12} therapy usually is not necessary for 1 or 2 years after surgery because the body uses very small amounts of this vit-amin and body reserves are usually sufficient for sev-eral years.

Clients with a gastrojejunostomy are at risk for de-veloping the **dumping syndrome** when they begin to take solid food. The syndrome, which produces weakness, dizziness, sweating, palpitations, abdomi-nal cramps, and diarrhea, is due to the rapid empty-ing (dumping) of large amounts of hypertonic *chyme* (a liquid mass of partly digested food) into the je-junum. The presence of this concentrated solution in the gut draws fluid from the circulating blood into the intestine, causing hypovolemia. The drop in blood pressure can produce syncope. As the syn-drome progresses, the sudden appearance of carbo-hydrates in the jejunum stimulates the pancreas to se-crete excessive amounts of insulin, which in turn causes hypoglycemia.

NURSING MANAGEMENT

Explore each symptom in depth. For example, if pain occurs, determine its type, onset in relation to eating food, location, and duration. Also obtain a di-etary history using relevant questions pertaining to foods that cause distress, the amount of food eaten at each meal, and whether eating food relieves pain. If necessary modify ingredients, temperature, or consis-tency of foods and present them in smaller portions on smaller plates so the client can continue eating. Give nutritional supplements, and if the client is re-ceiving tube feedings, reinstill gastric residual be-cause it contains partially digested nutrients. Note the client's bowel patterns and stool characteristics. Evaluate the client's emotional status and response to activity.

Monitor the nonsurgical client closely for med-ical complications. Assess vital signs and trends re-flecting fluid status. Assess gastric pH following guidelines in Nursing Guidelines 51–3. For a dis-cussion of appropriate nursing management of a surgical client refer to the nursing management sec-tion that accompanies the discussion of cancer of the stomach.

TABLE 51-3 **Surgical Procedures to Treat Peptic Ulcer Disease**

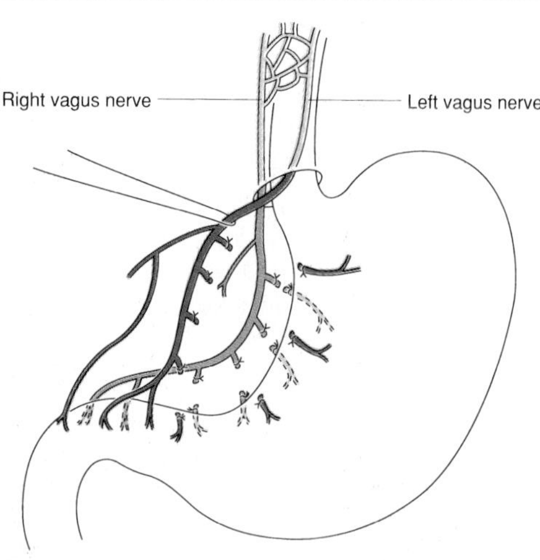

Name of Procedure	Description	Purpose
Vagotomy	A branch of the vagus nerve is cut.	To reduce gastric acid secretion
Pyloroplasty	The pylorus is repaired or reconstructed.	To expand the stomach outlet narrowed by scarring or improve gastric motility and emptying
Antrectomy	The antrum, the lower portion of the stomach including the pylorus, is removed.	To remove a somewhat benign ulcer in the lesser curvature of the stomach, which has not healed after 12 wk of medical treatment or has a history of recurring

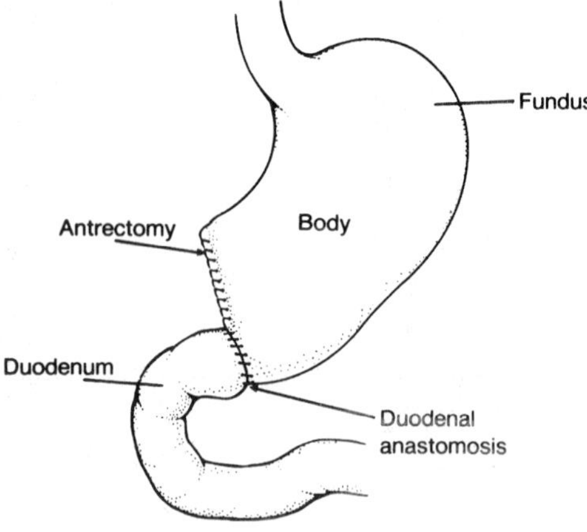

Name of Procedure	Description	Purpose
Gastroduodenostomy (Billroth I)	Part of the stomach (usually 2/3 to 3/4) is removed and the remaining portion of the stomach is connected to the duodenum. The procedure generally includes a vagotomy.	To remove an ulcerated area in the body of the stomach, which tends to have excess acid secretion and be prone to hemorrhage, perforation, and obstruction

(continued)

TABLE 51-3 *(Continued)*

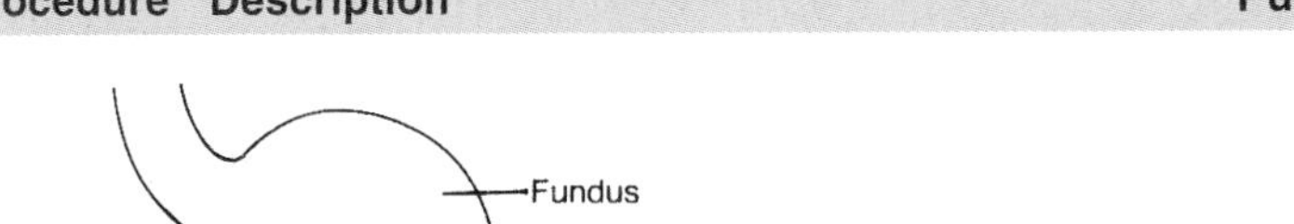

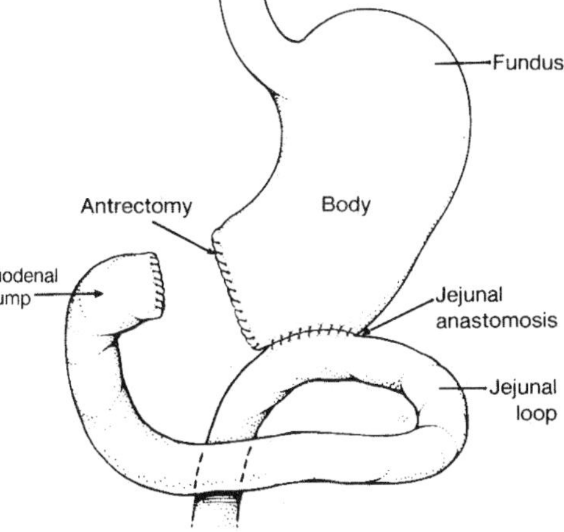

Name of Procedure	Description	Purpose
Gastrojejunostomy (Billroth II)	Same as for a Billroth I except the remaining portion is connected to the jejunum because there is extensive duodenal inflammation or perforation.	Same as for a Billroth I
Total *gastrectomy*	The entire stomach is removed and the esophagus is joined to the jejunum.	To remove an ulcer located high in the stomach near the gastroesophageal junction or to treat a gastric malignancy

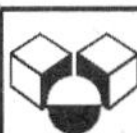

Nursing Guidelines 51-3

Assessing the pH of Aspirated Fluid

Purpose: To evaluate the effectiveness of antacid or histamine-2 antagonist therapy in peptic ulcer disease by aspirating stomach fluid and testing gastric pH
Desired pH range is 3 to 5.

- Obtain a pH test kit.
- Put on gloves.
- Verify that the distal tip of the client's nasogastric tube is within the stomach and has not migrated to the intestine.
- Use a separate syringe for withdrawing the test specimen because antacid residue or irrigating solution within the nasogastric tube will falsely raise the gastric pH.
- Connect the syringe to the tube.
- Instill a small amount of air to clear fluid from the gastric tube just before aspirating.
- Aspirate a small amount of fluid.
- Drop a sample of the gastric fluid onto a pH color indicator strip.
- Compare the color on the test strip with the color guide supplied in the test kit.
- Record the findings.

Nursing care of clients being treated medically for a gastric disorder includes, but is not limited to, the following:

Nursing Diagnosis and Collaborative Problems	Nursing Interventions
Risk for Fluid Volume Deficit related to vomiting, bleeding, diarrhea	Assist client to set a goal for minimum oral liquid intake during waking hours.
Goal: Fluid intake and output will be appropriate for the client's age and size.	Serve fresh liquids hourly.
	Provide a variety of choices to avoid monotony.
	If the client is receiving gastrostomy or nasogastric tube feedings, instill liberal amounts of water in addition to the feeding formula.
Activity Intolerance related to tissue hypoxia secondary to anemia	Minimize client activities that require exertion and result in fatigue.
Goal: Client will report increased, normal, or sufficient energy level for maintaining basic activities of daily living and self-care.	Schedule required nursing care to occur when the client is least fatigued.
	Delay completing an activity if the client develops signs of overexertion.

Anxiety related to observing blood loss, significance of diagnosis, and impending treatments **Goal:** Client will feel secure following support and explanations from nursing team.	Answer questions honestly and convey a positive outlook. Fully explain diagnostic test and treatment procedures. Never let the client feel ignored or abandoned; remain with the client or have a surrogate stay during periods of high anxiety. Always provide the client with a means of communication. Respond immediately to requests for assistance. Reassure the client that prompt treatment will be provided for new or ongoing problems, and keep the client informed of progress. Give prescribed medication to control anxiety. In cases of hemorrhage or hematemesis, make an effort to keep the client from seeing the blood loss. Remove bloody linen from the area as soon as possible.
Risk for Ineffective Individual Management of Therapeutic Regimen related to insufficient knowledge for safe self-care **Goal:** Client will describe and demonstrate knowledge and skills needed for safe self-care.	Provide information about the following topics: • Adherence to prescribed diet plan and medications • Medication schedule • Adverse effects and their management • Importance of well balanced diet, regular meal times, and identification of foods and beverages (eg, coffee, colas, alcohol) that cause discomfort • Drugs to be avoided or taken only as prescribed (eg, aspirin, NSAIDs, baking soda laxatives) • Importance of rest and reduction of stressful situations • Identification and appropriate response to complications • Scheduling of follow-up checkups with health care team as recommended

Cancer of the Stomach

Cancer of the stomach is a malignancy characterized by either an enlarged mass or ulcerating lesion that expands or penetrates several tissue layers.

ETIOLOGY AND PATHOPHYSIOLOGY

Malignancies of the stomach are common among Japanese, African Americans, and Latinos. Heredity and chronic inflammation of the stomach appear to be contributing factors. Although a single etiology has not been identified, achlorhydria, which may promote bacterial growth, and the chronic ingestion of toxins such as food preserved with nitrates or cooked over charcoal, are being linked to stomach cancer. When gram-negative microorganisms proliferate in the stomach, they produce a high level of nitrate reductase. This enzyme converts gastric nitrates to nitrites, which eventually become nitrosamines—known carcinogens. Cancer of the stomach often spreads to the lymph nodes and metastasizes to the spleen, liver, pancreas, or colon.

ASSESSMENT FINDINGS

Signs and Symptoms

Early symptoms are vague. As the tumor enlarges, symptoms include a prolonged feeling of fullness after eating, anorexia, weight loss, and anemia. The stool usually contains occult blood. Pain is a late symptom.

Diagnostic Findings

Diagnosis is made by a barium swallow and a biopsy of tissue obtained by gastroscopy. A gastric analysis may disclose absence of free hydrochloric acid. Computed tomography scanning or ultrasonography helps determine the depth of the cancer.

MEDICAL AND SURGICAL MANAGEMENT

A subtotal (partial) or total gastrectomy is the only curative approach to treating gastric cancer. The type and extent of surgery usually depend on tumor location, the symptoms, and amount of metastasis, if any. A subtotal gastrectomy preserves more normal digestion. Even though surgery may not achieve a complete cure, it may still be performed to control bleeding or relieve obstruction at the cardiac or pyloric junction. Chemotherapy with drugs such as 5-fluorouracil (5-FU) or doxorubicin (Adriamycin) and palliative radiation also may be used.

NURSING MANAGEMENT

The nurse's role in management of gastric cancer includes teaching the public, especially susceptible ethnic groups or clients with a family history of stomach cancer, how to change their dietary habits to reduce the predisposition for this disease. The nurse also may instruct high-risk groups, for instance those who have undergone vagotomy or who must take medications to reduce hydrochloric acid formation, on the early warning signs of cancer and the value of frequent health assessments. Nursing roles in managing clients undergoing surgery for gastric cancer are extensive.

NURSING PROCESS
The Client Undergoing Gastric Surgery

Assessment
Preoperative

In addition to performing the assessments for the client with a GI disorder, the nurse obtains a complete health, drug, tobacco, and allergy history. The nurse asks about how long the client has had symptoms, whether he or she can eat normally, whether weight has been lost and, if so, how much. Bowel sounds are assessed and the client is questioned about food intolerance and current dietary management. Bowel elimination patterns and stool characteristics are explored. In addition, the nurse assesses the client's understanding of diagnostic tests, the scheduled surgery, and preparations for surgery.

Nursing Diagnosis and Collaborative Problems	Nursing Interventions
Altered Nutrition: Less than Body Requirements related to anorexia, dyspepsia, vomiting, pain **Goal:** The client will obtain adequate nourishment to maintain weight.	Consult with physician and dietitian on modifying texture, temperature, and ingredients of client-preferred foods that are compatible with dietary needs. Evaluate client's ability to consume modified foods. Offer liquid nutritional supplements (Ensure, Enrich) if chewing or swallowing is impaired. Arrange to serve several small meals instead of a few large ones. Refer to agency policy or the information discussed in this chapter (see also Total Parenteral Nutrition in Chap. 22) if tube or gastrostomy feedings are necessary, Weigh the client daily. Report laboratory values such as a low blood cell count and hemoglobin, iron, serum protein, transferrin, and ferritin levels, which may indicate malnutrition.
Anxiety related to test results, diagnosis of serious illness, and surgery **Goal:** The client's anxiety will be restored to a mild level.	Call the client by name, making frequent eye contact and using touch appropriately. Acknowledge the client's feelings and show empathy if the client displays emotion. Encourage the presence and support of family member and other close caregivers. Give opportunities for family and client to ask questions and talk about tests or surgery. Explain the routine preparations for surgery; however, it may be best to explain some preparations, such as the insertion of a nasogastric tube, immediately before the procedure. Avoid rushing when preparing the client preoperatively; perform procedures with skill and dexterity. Incorporate your concern for the client's comfort and level of coping in preoperative activities. Respond promptly to the client's signal for assistance. Keep the client and family informed of progress and explain reasons for delays or modifications in previously described plans.
Knowledge Deficit related to preoperative preparations **Goal:** The client returns exercise demonstrations satisfactorily and acknowledges the purpose of equipment and procedures that may be used postoperatively.	Tell the client about common equipment that may be in place postoperatively such as an IV line, infusion pump, nasogastric suction, oxygen, urinary catheter, wound drain, cardiac monitor, and pulse oximeter. Prepare the client with reasons for taking frequent vital signs postoperatively. Explain that analgesics will be provided to reduce pain. Demonstrate and practice leg, deep breathing, and coughing exercises that the client will need to perform after surgery. Identify the approximate incisional area; explain the importance of adequate ventilation; and demonstrate how to splint the incision site. Keep the family informed of any information from the surgeon or staff during the intraoperative and postanesthesia period.

Postoperative Period

Refer to Standards for Postoperative Care in Chapter 24. When the client returns from surgery, assess vital signs and review the client's chart about the type of surgery performed and the client's progress during surgery and in the postanesthesia recovery unit. Inspect the surgical dressing for drainage and tubes or catheters for placement, patency, and type of drainage. Carefully observe nasogastric tube drainage for evidence of bleeding. Although the nasogastric tube may contain a small amount of dark blood when the client first returns from the operating room, the drainage should promptly return to the yellow-green of normal gastric secretions. Inspect the IV site and note the current rate and progress of fluid infusion. Document fluid intake and output as well as the client's level of consciousness and comfort. Closely monitor the client for the following complications:

- Change in the vital signs, especially low blood pressure, rapid pulse, and elevated temperature
- Extreme restlessness
- Difficulty breathing, increased respiratory rate, cyanosis
- Severe pain, especially after an analgesic has been given; pain in an area other than the operative site (eg, legs, head, or chest)
- Abdominal distention or rigidity
- Urinary output less than 35 mL/hr if catheterized, or failure to void within 8 hours of surgery
- Failure to pass flatus or stool more than 48 hours after surgery
- Profuse diaphoresis
- Excessive bloody drainage from the nasogastric tube, surgical drains, or surgical dressing
- Separation of the surgical wound edges
- Unusual color or odor of drainage

Postoperative nursing care of clients with stomach cancer includes, but is not limited to, the following:

Nursing Diagnosis and Collaborative Problems	Nursing Interventions
Altered Nutrition: Less than Body Requirements related to nausea, vomiting, distention after removal of nasogastric tube **Goal:** The client will retain food or fluids without discomfort from eating or drinking.	During the time the client cannot take oral nourishment, ensure uninterrupted infusion of IV solutions containing glucose, electrolytes, and vitamins. (For clients having GI tube or gastrostomy tube feedings, refer to discussions earlier in this chapter.) When eating is allowed, first offer sips of clear liquids and progress to full liquids, soft foods, and finally a normal diet if feasible.
Risk for Injury related to syncope secondary to dumping syndrome **Goal:** The client will be free of injury.	In clients with gastrojejunostomy, avoid syncope associated with the dumping syndrome and rebound hypoglycemia by providing the client with five or six small meals a day when food is allowed. Work with the dietitian to modify the diet to include reduced amounts of carbohydrate, especially simple sugars, with the remaining calories supplied by fat and protein sources. Withhold oral liquids at meals to avoid rapid emptying from the stomach. Provide them instead an hour after a meal. Encourage the client to lie down for about 30 minutes immediately after eating to help retain food longer in the stomach. Maintain bed rest if dizziness and weakness occur.
Risk for Impaired Tissue Perfusion related to inactivity **Goal:** Client will maintain adequate tissue perfusion as evidenced by strong peripheral pulses, absence of edema, and negative Homans' sign.	Position the client to promote circulation in the lower extremities. Apply elastic thromboembolism stockings. Supervise leg exercises every 2 hours while the client is awake. Help client ambulate as soon as possible. Provide adequate fluid intake to promote optimal vascular fluid volume.

Evaluation and Expected Outcomes

- Preoperatively, the client is adequately nourished to maintain weight and improve stamina for surgery. In addition, the client reports decreased anxiety and increased understanding of what to expect of the surgical process.
- Postoperatively, the client retains foods and fluids, does not sustain trauma, and has adequate peripheral circulation.

Client and Family Teaching

The type and extent of teaching depends on the surgery that is performed. If tube or gastrostomy feedings, tracheostomy care, and suction techniques will continue after discharge, involve the client and a family member in practicing these procedures while the client is still hospitalized. Identify where medical supplies can be purchased and offer a referral for home care from a local community agency. Other points to consider in the discharge teaching plan include:

Adhere to the diet (eg, foods to eat or avoid) recommended by the physician. Also adhere to the dietary, fluid, and positional modifications to avoid the dumping syndrome after a gastrojejunostomy.

- Take medications exactly as prescribed. Follow the directions on the label, paying particular attention to when the drug should be taken (eg, before, after, or with food or meals).
- Monitor weight weekly. Report any significant weight loss to the physician.
- Keep appointments for periodic medical follow-up.

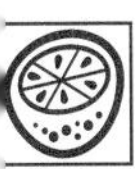

General Nutritional Considerations

Because fat delays gastric emptying, limit high-fat foods such as meat, high-fat dairy products, and rich desserts in clients with nausea.

Limit liquids with meals to minimize the feeling of fullness. Encourage a liberal intake of fluid between meals.

Hot foods may contribute to nausea.

Clients who avoid citrus fruits and juices because of reflux esophagitis may need a vitamin C supplement.

Intermittent cyclic and bolus tube feedings are physiologically preferable to continuous feeding for long-term use because they resemble a more normal pattern of intake, allowing hormone and enzyme levels to rise and fall rather than being constantly stimulated. Intermittent feedings may also decrease the risk of pneumonia.

Fat malabsorption, gastric stasis, and diarrhea are common after a vagotomy. Replacing some dietary fat long-chain triglycerides with medium-chain triglycerides (MCT) minimizes diarrhea and provides readily absorbed fat calories. Many commercial products, such as Osmolite and Isocal, contain MCT as the fat source. MCT oil can be used in place of vegetable oil in cooking, but it is unpalatable and expensive.

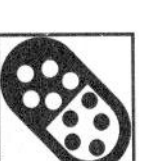

General Pharmacologic Considerations

Histamine-2 (H_2) antagonists decrease healing time and reduce the incidence of surgical intervention for the management of peptic ulcer. H_2 antagonists, such as ranitidine, are used for the short-term treatment of duodenal and gastric ulcers for managing gastroesophageal reflux disease.

Antacids may be given two to four times per day or as frequently as every 1 to 2 hours. Antacids are not administered within 1 hour of the H_2 antagonists. Antacids may cause diarrhea or constipation in some clients.

Sucralfate is administered 2 hours after an H_2 antagonist to ensure the absorption of the H_2 antagonist. Sucralfate is given for 4 to 6 weeks to ensure ulcer healing.

If the hospitalized client will self-administer a prescribed antacid, the nurse (1) demonstrates how to measure the drug in a medicine glass, (2) explains the importance of antacids in the treatment of dyspepsia, (3) explains the time of day the drug is to be taken (ie, every hour, every 2 hours on the even hour), (4) makes sure that the client has a clock or watch, (5) periodically checks the supply of the drug and measuring cups, and (6) checks to see if the client is taking the medication.

Although sodium bicarbonate (baking soda) is an antacid, it is readily absorbed from the GI tract and in large doses may produce alkalosis. Avoid sodium bicarbonate in clients for whom antacids have been prescribed to treat gastric disorders.

Consult the physician for changes in drug orders if a client cannot retain oral medications.

Never crush and administer an enteric-coated drug through any type of enteral feeding tube (nasogastric, nasoenteric, or gastrostomy).

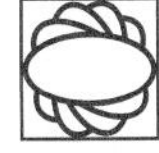

General Gerontologic Considerations

Severe and prolonged episodes of vomiting can be especially serious for older adults whose nutritional and fluid intake may be marginal; more profound electrolyte imbalances and severe dehydration can result.

Depression among older adults may be manifested by anorexia and weight loss.

Simple anorexia, which may have many causes, is not uncommon in older adults. To avoid malnutrition, older adults with anorexia are encouraged to eat four to six small, balanced meals per day.

Food preferences, economic status, and the inability of the older adult to chew because of tooth loss or ill-fitting dentures are considered when modifying a diet.

As individuals age, the gastric mucosa becomes thinner, predisposing them to superficial gastritis.

The presence of parietal cell antibodies among older adults can lead to pernicious anemia.

Older adults are more prone to developing gastritis, gastric bleeding, and gastric ulcers because they are regularly taking drugs, such as aspirin, to treat osteoarthritis.

Geriatric clients taking H_2 antagonists are prone to developing stress ulcers. In addition, confusion seems to develop more readily in older adults taking H_2 antagonists possibly because drug half-life increases when renal function is inadequate to excrete the drug metabolites.

With age, the salivary glands become less active and the numbers of taste buds are reduced, contributing to anorexia in the older adult.

The incidence of hiatal hernia increases with age. Hiatal hernia is more likely to develop in older women that in older men.

The older adult has a diminished gag reflex. This places the elderly client with esophageal diverticula at greater risk for aspiration.

SUMMARY OF KEY CONCEPTS

- Numerous upper GI disorders affect eating. Among them are anorexia, nausea and vomiting, cancer of the oral cavity; esophageal disorders including gastroesophageal reflux disease, hiatal hernia, esophageal varices, and cancer of the esophagus; and gastric disorders including gastritis, peptic ulcer disease, and cancer of the stomach.
- Cancer of the oral cavity is associated with a lesion or structural change about the lips, oral mucous membrane, tongue, or throat. The diagnosis is confirmed by a biopsy. Oral cancers are treated by surgical excision, radiation, and chemotherapy.
- Among alternative methods of oral nourishment are tube or gastrostomy feedings. Tube feedings are preferred when the client has normal intestinal absorption.
- When caring for a client receiving tube or gastrostomy feedings, the nurse instills the prescribed formula, irrigates the tubing with water, cleans and replaces equipment and formula to avoid bacterial contamination, and documents intake and output accurately. Care of the nose, stomal site, and oral care promote comfort and maintain the integrity of the skin and oral mucous membranes.
- Gastroesophageal reflux is a common disorder that can cause no symptoms at all or a number of associated symptoms and complications including pain and respiratory distress.
- Esophageal diverticula cause difficulty swallowing, belching, regurgitation, coughing, foul breath, and gurgling sounds in the chest. They are diagnosed by barium swallow and esophagoscopy and treated with dietary modifications or surgery.
- A hiatal hernia produces pressure or pain after eating, especially when lying down after the meal. The structural defect can be visualized with a barium swallow or esophagoscopy. Diet management, drugs, or surgery are treatments.
- Gastritis is generally characterized by epigastric discomfort. The diagnosis is usually made by linking the symptoms with some likely cause in the client's history. Treatment usually involves treating the cause, resting the stomach by restricting food, and temporarily decreasing gastric acidity with drugs.
- The chief symptom of an ulcer is epigastric pain or burning that is relieved by eating food. Diagnosis is made by barium swallow and esophagogastroduodenoscopy. Ulcers are generally treated by dietary management and drug therapy aimed at eradicating the *Helicobacter pylori* bacterial infection and controlling gastric acid. Severe hemorrhage, unrelieved obstruction, perforation, chronic recurrences, or malignant changes justify surgical interventions.
- Stomach cancer manifests few or vague early symptoms. As the disease progresses, the client may feel full after eating, experience anorexia and weight loss, and develop anemia from blood loss. Pain is a late symptom. The best response is obtained by surgically excising the tumor. Palliative treatment may include radiation and chemotherapy.
- Suggestions for relieving upper GI discomfort include eating small, frequent meals and avoiding alcohol, coffee, colas, tea, and spicy foods. Eliminating smoking also reduces gastric irritation. Aspirin should be avoided unless it is buffered or enteric coated. NSAIDs also irritate the stomach.
- Symptoms referred to as dumping syndrome occur when concentrated chyme surges into the small intestine, causing a shift in circulating blood volume and hypoglycemia from hyperinsulinism. The syndrome can be prevented by having the client eat small, frequent meals, keeping the content of food low in simple carbohydrates, eliminating beverages at meals, and lying down for 30 minutes after eating.
- Nursing management of clients undergoing gastric surgery includes ensuring adequate nutrition, reducing anxiety, and teaching about preoperative and postoperative care.

CRITICAL THINKING EXERCISES

1. An older adult client is admitted because of unexplained weight loss. What assessments are appropriate?
2. A 39-year-old traveling salesman skips breakfast and eats on an erratic schedule, usually at fast food establishments. When he does finish for the day, he orders a couple of cocktails before dinner. He smokes two packs of cigarettes a day. Lately he has been experiencing epigastric pain. What suggestions could you make to help relieve this client's discomfort?

Suggested Readings

Brozenec, S. A. (1996). Ulcer therapy update. *RN, 59*(9), 48–50, 52–54.

Consult stat. Reflux patients get heartburn relief from chewing gum. (1996). *RN, 59*(1), 61.

Farrington, E. (1996). Pediatric drug information. Cardiac toxicity with cisapride. *Pediatric Nursing, 22*(3), 256.

Gould, D. (1996). Hygienic practices...*Escherichia coli*. *Nursing Times, 92*(36), 76, 78, 80.

Hall, J. C. (1997). Learning about low-profile gastrostomy devices. *Nursing, 12*(2), 89–99.

National Institutes of Health. (1994). *NIH consensus statement. Helicobacter pylori in peptic ulcer disease* (12) 1–22, Washington, DC: Department of Health and Human Services.

Tolbert, C. G., & Pratt, J. C. (1996). Emergency! Bleeding gastric ulcer. *American Journal of Nursing, 96*(2), 48.

Chapter 52

Caring for Clients With Disorders of the Lower Gastrointestinal Tract

KEY TERMS

Abdominoperineal resection
Appendectomy
Appendicitis
Cantor tube
Colectomy
Crohn's disease
Diverticula
Diverticulitis
Diverticulosis
Fissure
Fistula
Fistulectomy
Fistulotomy
Harris tube
Hemorrhoidectomy
Hemorrhoids
Hernia
Hernioplasty
Herniorrhaphy
Inflammatory bowel disease
Irritable bowel syndrome
Intussusception
Miller-Abbott tube
Paralytic ileus
Peritonitis
Pilonidal sinus
Segmental resection
Short bowel syndrome
Skip lesions
Spastic colon
Tenesmus
Toxic megacolon
Ulcerative colitis
Ulcerative proctitis
Volvulus

LEARNING OBJECTIVES

On completion of this chapter, the reader will:

- List factors that contribute to constipation and diarrhea.
- Differentiate between Crohn's disease and ulcerative colitis.
- Describe the role of the nurse in relation to the use of tubes for intestinal decompression.
- Differentiate between diverticulosis and diverticulitis.
- Identify factors that contribute to forming an abdominal hernia.
- Describe the warning signs of colorectal cancer.
- List common problems that accompany anorectal disorders.

The lower gastrointestinal (GI) tract includes the small intestine from the duodenum to the anus (see Fig. 50–1 in Chap. 50). The material that moves down the intestinal tract is composed of food residues, microorganisms, digestive secretions, and mucus. The mixture of these substances are the components of feces. Disorders of the lower GI tract generally affect the absorption of nutrients, water, and electrolytes; the movement of feces toward the anus; and the elimination of dietary wastes.

Altered Bowel Elimination

Constipation

Constipation is a condition in which stool becomes dry, compact, and difficult to pass. People differ greatly in bowel habits. Some people normally have bowel movements every other day, whereas others have two or three movements a day. In differentiating normal from abnormal bowel elimination, the consistency of stools and the comfort with which they are passed are more reliable indicators than their frequency.

The consistency of the stool is greatly affected by the type and amount of food that is consumed. Diets that are high in fiber, such as those containing whole grains, fresh fruits, and uncooked vegetables, form a larger residual of cellulose, an insoluble, nondigestible product, in the bowel. Cellulose absorbs water; the combination of the two increases fecal volume, which speeds its passage through the lower GI tract, and softens the stool.

As fecal matter collects in the rectum, it presses on the internal anal sphincter, creating an urge to defecate, or eliminate stool. The signal to release stool is facilitated by peristalsis and distention of the colon. The gastrocolic reflex facilitates stool passage by accelerating peristalsis. This reflex is most active after eating, particularly after the first meal of the day.

ETIOLOGY AND PATHOPHYSIOLOGY

A diet low in fiber predisposes clients to constipation because the stools produced are smaller in volume and drier. Low-volume stools also are propelled more slowly through the lower GI tract. Whenever stool remains stationary in the bowel, moisture continues to be absorbed from the residue. Consequently, retention of stool, for any number of reasons, causes stool to become dry and hard. Constipation may result from:

- Insufficient dietary fiber and water
- Ignoring the urge or delaying defecation
- Emotional stress
- Use of drugs that tend to slow intestinal motility
- Inactivity
- Neurologic disorders that weaken an individual's ability to expel stool
- Intestinal disorders that tend to obstruct the passage of stool

Even the chronic use of laxatives or enemas may themselves produce constipation because they cause a loss of normal colonic motility and intestinal tone. They also dull the gastrocolic reflex.

ASSESSMENT FINDINGS

Signs and Symptoms

Bowel elimination is infrequent or irregular. Individuals who are constipated describe feeling bloated. The abdomen may be tympanic or distended and there may be hypoactive bowel sounds. Rectal fullness, pressure, and pain are experienced when the individual attempts to eliminate stool. What is passed is generally hard and dry. Rectal bleeding may result as the tissue stretches and tears while the person tries to pass the hard, dry stool. When a gloved and lubricated finger is inserted within the rectum, the stool may feel like small rocks, a condition referred to as *scyballa*.

Sometimes, when a constipated stool is retained for a long time, the client may begin passing liquid stool around an obstructive stool mass, a phenomenon sometimes misinterpreted as diarrhea. The liquid stool results from dry stool stimulating nerve endings in the lower colon and rectum, which increases peristalsis. The increased peristalsis sends watery feces from higher in the bowel around the retained stool.

Diagnostic Findings

A barium enema, proctosigmoidoscopy, or colonoscopy may be performed to identify the underlying cause of constipation.

MEDICAL AND SURGICAL MANAGEMENT

Constipation is best relieved by treating its cause. For more immediate relief, a laxative in oral or suppository form or an enema followed by prophylactic administration of a stool softener are prescribed. Dietary management is also promoted.

NURSING MANAGEMENT

In addition to the assessments performed on the client with a GI disorder, obtain a complete history as well as a drug history, including the frequency with which laxatives or enemas are used. In discussing bowel elimination with the client, determine the client's definition of constipation. Some clients are unaware that a daily bowel movement is not necessarily a rigid standard for proper bowel function. It also is important to obtain a description of the individual's bowel elimination pattern, such as its frequency, overall appearance and consistency of the stool, presence of blood, painful elimination, or effort necessary to pass stool. Monitor the client's bowel elimination. Assess the client's dietary habits, fluid intake, and activity level.

Examine the anal area, looking for fissures, redness, and hemorrhoids. Auscultate the abdomen for bowel sounds and palpate for distention and masses. Inspect the client's stool or gently insert a lubricated gloved finger within the anal canal to assess the characteristics of the unpassed stool.

The plan of care includes, but is not limited to, the following:

Nursing Diagnoses and Collaborative Problems	Nursing Interventions
Constipation **Goal:** A regular bowel elimination pattern will be established. Stools are soft and easily passed.	Urge the client to adopt dietary and exercise habits that foster normal elimination. Administer medically prescribed treatments and evaluate their effectiveness.

	Digitally remove impacted stool that the client cannot pass.
Pain related to rectal distention, stretching, and anal tears **Goal:** Rectal discomfort will be reduced or eliminated.	Apply a lubricant, such as K-Y jelly, in the rectum and around the anus using a gloved finger. Assist the client to soak the rectal area in a tub of warm water to relieve discomfort and to heal rectal fissures. Consult with the physician about applying an ointment with a topical anesthetic or a soothing medicated astringent.
Anxiety related to difficulty passing stool, treatment methods, abdominal discomfort **Goal:** Anxiety will be relieved.	Reassure the client dietary changes, greater fluid intake, and increased activity will promote bowel elimination. Provide privacy during elimination attempts and ensure that the client will not be interrupted. Assist client to use the toilet and bathroom rather than a bedpan. Help the client to a sitting position, if a bedpan is the only alternative. Explore techniques that relieve tension, such as looking through a magazine while using the toilet. Provide an air freshener if the client is self-conscious about lingering odors.

Client and Family Teaching

When constipation is related to dietary habits, decreased fluid intake, stress, lack of exercise, or other factors, suggest a high-fiber diet that includes plenty of raw fruits and vegetables, whole grain breads, and coarse brans and cereals (Box 52–1). To promote regularity, teach clients to drink eight or more full glasses of water and fruit juice daily because fructose is a natural laxative. Urge the client to schedule time to exercise each day because this promotes intestinal motility.

Advise the client to respond quickly to an urge to defecate and to allow sufficient time for bowel evacuation. Encourage the client to use the toilet at regular intervals, particularly after meals when the gastrocolic reflex is most active, or even in the absence of the urge to defecate. Provide privacy for bathroom times, and instruct the client to avoid excessive straining to have a bowel movement.

Discourage self-treatment with daily or frequent enemas or laxatives. Explain that chronic laxative use leads to a sluggish natural bowel function. Stress that laxatives containing a stimulant can be habit forming, requiring continued use and higher doses to maintain bowel function. Mention that stool softeners, such as fiber supplements containing psyllium or magnesium, are generally safer for long-term use. Reassure clients that daily evacuation is not necessary provided the stool is not hard and dry. The belief that a daily bowel movement is necessary can lead to a dependence on laxatives.

BOX 52-1 Dietary Modifications for Common Intestinal Problems

High-Fiber Diet to Manage Constipation

Adding fiber to the diet relieves constipation by adding bulk and moisture to the stool. The following foods increase dietary fiber:

- Bran and whole grains (100% bran, rolled oats, granola, wheat germ, brown rice, cornmeal)
- Legumes (dried peas, beans, lentils; split peas; black-eyed peas; pinto, kidney, navy beans; red or yellow lentils)
- Seeds and nuts (sesame, sunflower, poppy, crunchy peanut butter, popcorn)
- Fruits: raw (apples with skin, pears, oranges, melons, berries) and dried (prunes, dates, raisins)
- Vegetables: raw (sprouts, spinach, carrots, peppers, broccoli, cabbage) and steamed (peas, potatoes with skin)

Low-Residue Diet to Manage Diarrhea

Reintroducing food after a bout of diarrhea usually calls for a low-residue diet to reduce the volume of stool. The following foods may be used to manage diarrhea:

- Dairy products (all forms of milk, yogurt, pudding, cottage cheese) unless client is lactose intolerant
- Meat and meat substitutes (baked, steamed, roasted or pressure cooked poultry without skin; tuna or salmon; poached or boiled eggs)
- Fruits and vegetables (strained cooked, steamed without skins or seeds, applesauce, bananas)
- Grains (products made with refined flour such as white bread or soda crackers)

Diarrhea

Diarrhea is the frequent passage of liquid or semiliquid stool.

ETIOLOGY AND PATHOPHYSIOLOGY

Diarrhea may be due to many factors:

- Bacterial or viral infections affecting the intestine
- Lactose intolerance
- Food allergies or intolerances
- Uremia
- Intestinal disease such as diverticulitis, inflammatory bowel disease, ulcerative colitis, irritable bowel syndrome, malabsorption, or intestinal obstruction
- Rapid addition of fiber to the diet
- Eating highly spiced or seasoned food
- Overuse of laxatives
- Adverse effects of drugs, especially antibiotics or concentrated tube feeding formulas

Diarrhea results from increased peristalsis that rapidly moves the fecal matter through the GI tract. The swift velocity produces intestinal cramping and decreases the time for water to be absorbed from stool within the large intestine. Consequently, the stool is either very soft or liquid. Three major problems associated with severe or prolonged diarrhea include dehydration, electrolyte imbalances, and vitamin deficiencies. When diarrhea results from a disease that causes malabsorption, a nutritional deficiency may occur. The sudden onset of acute abdominal pain or a rise in temperature may indicate a perforation of the bowel.

ASSESSMENT FINDINGS

Signs and Symptoms

Stools are watery and frequent. In severe cases, blood and mucus pass with the stool. The client generally experiences urgency (**tenesmus**) and abdominal discomfort. Bowel sounds are hyperactive. Skin around the anus may become excoriated from contact with fecal matter.

Diagnostic Findings

Stool samples identify microorganisms or parasites that cause diarrhea. The stool also may test positive for the presence of blood. In chronic diarrhea, a proctosigmoidoscopy or colonoscopy demonstrates inflammation or alteration in the structural appearance of the mucosal layer of the large intestine.

MEDICAL AND SURGICAL MANAGEMENT

Mild diarrhea or diarrhea of short duration, such as that caused by a dietary change or acute illness, involves resting the bowel by limiting intake to clear liquids for one or two meals and gradually advancing to a regular diet. When diarrhea persists, when the stools are frequent and large, or when the person is very young, elderly, or debilitated, medical treatment may include one or more of the following:

- An antidiarrheal agent, such as diphenoxylate hydrochloride with atropine sulfate (Lomotil), loperamide hydrochloride (Imodium), or a combination product such as kaolin and pectin (Kaopectate)
- Fluid and electrolyte replacement by either the oral or the intravenous (IV) route
- Dietary adjustments, which may involve eliminating foods that cause diarrhea
- Total parenteral nutrition (TPN) if diarrhea is severe and prolonged and if the introduction of oral fluid and food results in another episode of diarrhea.

Chronic diarrhea depletes the bowel of helpful organisms and allows yeasts and fungi to thrive unchecked. To recolonize the bowel, capsules or granules containing *Lactobacillus acidophilus* (Bacid or Lactinex) are prescribed.

NURSING PROCESS
The Client With Diarrhea

Assessment

In addition to the assessments performed on the client with a GI disorder (see Chap. 50), obtain a complete health, dietary, allergy, and drug history. Be sure to include a history of newly prescribed drugs, such as antibiotics, and the pattern of laxative and enema use.

Ask the client about any recent incidence of constipation because diarrhea can occur if there is an impacted fecal mass. Observe the emotional status of the client because anxiety affects bowel motility.

To help determine a cause-and-effect relationship ask about the onset of diarrhea in relation to the possibility of eating tainted foods. Finding that others who ate the same food, have similar symptoms may support the possibility that the diarrhea is food related. Ask the client about recent foreign travel because some intestinal pathogens are transmitted by drinking unsanitary water or consuming uncooked food washed with contaminated water.

Depending on the severity of the diarrhea and the length of time it has been present, examine the anal area for redness or other tissue changes; use Standard Precautions when doing so. Auscultate the abdomen to identify characteristics of bowel sounds and palpate for distention and masses. Monitor the frequency and characteristics of the stools. The volume of liquid stools may be measured to assess fluid loss. Assess for signs of dehydration, electrolyte imbalance, and metabolic acidosis (see Chap. 21). Record daily weights and take vital signs to provide baseline data. Report the sudden onset of acute abdominal pain to the physician immediately. The plan of care includes, but is not limited to, the following:

Nursing Diagnoses and Collaborative Problems	Nursing Interventions
Diarrhea **Goal:** The client will develop a normal bowel elimination pattern.	Administer prescribed medications as directed to slow bowel motility. Avoid overmedicating the client who has excessive frequency by not exceeding the maximum dose allowed. Rest the bowel by restricting solid food for 8 hours or more. Avoid caffeinated beverages that stimulate GI motility when clear liquids are allowed. Provide buttermilk and active yogurt cultures containing *L. acidophilus* to restore a proper balance of intestinal bacteria being purged during diarrhea, but avoid their use if the client is lactose intolerant. Reintroduce low-residue foods gradually.
Pain (cramping) related to excessive peristalsis **Goal:** The client will experience relief from discomfort.	Discourage solid food temporarily. Help the client into a comfort position (eg, lying with the legs flexed toward the abdomen). Provide distracting activity (eg, watching television). Advise clients to avoid drinking carbonated beverages or using a straw because the resultant volume of swallowed air increases gas and cramping.
Risk for Fluid Volume Deficit related to frequent passage of watery stools, inadequate fluid intake **Goal:** Client's output will not exceed fluid intake.	Observe for signs of dehydration and electrolyte imbalances, especially hypokalemia and hyponatremia. When diarrhea is severe, provide water, clear liquids, and oral electrolyte solutions, such as Gatorade, when small amounts of fluids are allowed. Monitor IV fluid administration if dehydration develops. Report a urine output less than 240 mL in 4 hours.
Risk for Altered Nutrition: Less than Body Requirements related to anorexia or malabsorption secondary to rapid passage of stool through the gastrointestinal tract **Goal:** Client will maintain a stable weight.	Reintroduce small amounts of bland and low-residue foods (see Box 52-1). Restrict solid food again if food exacerbates the diarrhea. Notify physician if client cannot tolerate resumption of regular diet. Avoid milk products until client's tolerance of lactose is determined (temporary lactose intolerance may affect people who could previously tolerate milk). In cases of intolerance, ensure adequate calcium from nondairy food or mineral supplements. If appropriate, consult with physician about initiating total parenteral nutrition.
Impaired Skin Integrity related to mechanical and chemical trauma to the rectum **Goal:** Client's perianal tissue will be intact.	Provide premoistened, nonirritating, non–alcohol-based wipes rather than paper for the anal area. Or supply toilet tissue containing aloe. Wash the skin, rinse it well, and pat dry after each bowel movement. Apply a medicated ointment, such as one containing vitamins A and D or zinc oxide if skin appears reddened. Notify the physician if skin breakdown occurs.
Anxiety related to urgency, fear of incontinence, odors, other factors (specify) **Goal:** The client's anxiety will be restored to a tolerable level.	Acknowledge client's distress. Respond to signals for assistance as soon as possible. Provide bedside commode if client cannot walk to bathroom or keep a covered bedpan beneath the bed linens if this relieves client's insecurity. Empty the bedpan or commode as soon as possible and spray the room with air freshener. Avoid any nonverbal signals that cleaning the client or soiled equipment is disgusting. In instances of incontinence, protect the bed linen with disposable, absorbent pads placed under the client's buttocks.

Evaluation and Expected Outcomes

- The client's bowel elimination pattern is normal.
- Pain is absent and bowel sounds are normal.
- Intake and output are balanced.
- Preillness weight is attained.
- Skin excoriated by liquid feces is healed.
- Diarrhea-related anxiety has subsided.

Client and Family Teaching

Provide a list of foods and beverages to avoid. If medication is prescribed, explain the purpose and routine for its use and identify common side effects. Caution the client to avoid self-treatment of diarrhea and to consult the physician if the diarrhea does not respond to dietary restrictions and antidiarrheal medications. Advise the client to contact the physician also if the diarrhea is prolonged or accompanied by severe abdominal pain, if blood or mucus passes with stool, if fever develops or urine output decreases.

Irritable Bowel Syndrome

Irritable bowel syndrome (IBS), sometimes referred to as **spastic colon,** is not a disease. It is a cluster of symptoms that occur despite the absence of a disease process. IBS is described as a paroxysmal motility disorder primarily affecting the colon. Individuals with IBS experience alternating periods of constipation and diarrhea. One or the other elimination pattern predominates. Women are affected more often than men.

ETIOLOGY AND PATHOPHYSIOLOGY

Fluctuating intestinal motility tends to be the underlying symptom-producing factor. Because the autonomic nervous system affects motor function within the gastrointestinal tract, bowel motility is influenced by neuron stimulation and inhibition. When a parasympathetic neurotransmitter (eg, acetylcholine) is released, intestinal motility increases and diarrhea occurs. An opposite effect occurs when the smooth muscle of the gut responds to sympathetic neurotransmission. In some clients, IBS appears to intensify with stress.

ASSESSMENT FINDINGS

Signs and Symptoms

Most clients with IBS describe having chronic constipation with sporadic bouts of diarrhea. Some report the opposite pattern, although it is less common. Most experience various degrees of abdominal pain which may or may not be relieved by defecation. Many are bothered by belching and *flatulence* (intestinal gas). In general, symptoms do not awaken individuals from sleep. Some clients with IBS report feelings described as anxiety, insecurity, depression, or anger.

Weight generally remains stable, indicating that when diarrhea occurs, it is not accompanied by malabsorption of nutrients. When loose stools are inspected, though passed frequently, they are generally of low volume and may contain mucus. Blood is not generally found in the stool because the bowel is not locally inflamed.

Diagnostic Findings

Radiographic and endoscopic tests rule out other disorders with similar symptoms, such as peptic ulcer disease, colorectal cancer, diverticulosis, or inflammatory bowel disease.

MEDICAL AND SURGICAL MANAGEMENT

Dietary changes reduce flatulence and abdominal discomfort. By trial and error, the client eliminates common food sources that cause discomfort or intestinal gas such as beans, cabbage, and similar foods. At the same time, a high-fiber diet or a bulk-forming agent, such as products containing psyllium (eg, Metamucil), is prescribed to regulate bowel elimination. The fiber draws water into constipated stool and adds bulk to watery stool. An anticholinergic, such as dicyclomine (Bentyl), prescribed before meals, has an antispasmodic effect. Either a prescription or nonprescription antidiarrheal is used for temporary relief from diarrhea.

NURSING MANAGEMENT

Most clients with IBS are not hospitalized. Nurses become involved in care during diagnostic testing, follow-up visits, or hospitalization for a concurrent problem. During these encounters, gather a comprehensive data base of symptoms, help manage the problems associated with constipation and diarrhea, explain therapeutic treatment measures, evaluate the client's understanding of the regimen for self-care, and monitor the response to therapy. For more specific nursing interventions, refer to the preceding discussions of nursing management of clients with constipation and diarrhea.

Inflammatory Bowel Disease

Inflammatory bowel disease is a chronic disorder, characterized by exacerbations and remissions. **Ulcerative colitis** and **Crohn's disease** are collectively referred to as inflammatory bowel disease, or IBD. These two distinct disorders are grouped together because of their similar symptoms and treatments. The characteristics of these two diseases are summarized in Table 52–1. Because of similarity in presenting symptoms and results of diagnostic procedures, differential diagnosis may be difficult to make. Unlike IBS, IBD does not resolve without medical intervention.

Crohn's Disease

Crohn's disease is also called granulomatous colitis, ileitis, and regional enteritis. It is a chronic inflammatory condition that affects any portion of the GI tract, but predominantly the bowel in the terminal portion of the ileum. Its general onset is in young adulthood.

ETIOLOGY AND PATHOPHYSIOLOGY

The cause of Crohn's disease is unknown. Because there is an increased incidence among family members, a genetic predisposition is presumed. Other possible contributing factors include allergic and autoimmune responses triggered by diet or infectious microbial antigens. Recurrent attacks on the tissue are believed to be from an exaggerated immune response, which explains the chronic nature of the disease. Exacerbations seem to correlate with periods of stress accompanied by anxiety and depression. It is unclear whether the changes in emotional equilibrium contribute directly to the remanifestation of symptoms or if they are a secondary effect of coping with a chronic disease and concurrent stressors.

The inflammation in Crohn's disease extends transmurally through all the layers of the bowel, but the submucosal layer is most involved. Affected areas are characterized by hyperemia (increased blood supply), edema, and ulcerations. When examined endoscopically, inflamed areas alternate with healthy tissue. The inflamed areas occur randomly, a phenomenon described as **skip lesions**. The bowel is described as having a "cobblestone" appearance because of the deep ulcerations that form among the edematous tissue.

Fissures, which are small cracks in the tissue, fill with pus and abscesses form. Where adjacent loops of affected bowel or nearby tissue, such as the bladder or vagina, are in contact with one another, adhesions or connecting channels called **fistulas,** develop. Purulent drainage and stool pass through the fistula. Chronically inflamed areas may convert to a granuloma, a fibrotic mass, predisposing to intestinal obstruction.

ASSESSMENT FINDINGS

Signs and Symptoms

Usually, onset is insidious and the course of the disease variable. Generally most clients have abdominal pain, distention, and tenderness in the lower quadrants of the abdomen, especially on the right side. Pain may or may not be associated with eating. If eating causes abdominal cramping, defecation usually relieves the cramping. The client may have a history of chronic diarrhea and fatigue. Growth failure is a common early symptom in children and adolescents. Fever may be present. As Crohn's disease progresses, anorexia, weight loss, dehydration, and signs

TABLE 52-1 **Characteristics of Inflammatory Bowel Disease**

Characteristics	Crohn's Disease	Ulcerative Colitis
Onset of symptoms	Gradual	Abrupt
Location	Diffuse	Localized
Distribution	Can occur at any location in the GI tract, more commonly found in the ileum	Rectum to cecum
Type of lesion	Patchy, positioned between areas of normal tissue, and referred to as skip lesions	Continuous from rectum to cecum, without areas of healthy tissue
Extent of inflammation	May extend through all bowel layers; may be visible in the large intestine or invisible if located in the higher GI tract	Limited to mucosal lining
Blood in stool	Occult	Visible
Weight loss	Common	Less common
Perianal disease	Typical (fistula formation, abscesses)	Atypical
Extraintestinal symptoms (joint pain, skin lesions, inflammatory conditions of the eyes)	Common	Less common but can occur
Biopsy findings	Signs of chronic inflammation; granulomas	Signs of chronic inflammation; granulomas rare
Carcinogenesis	Rare	Common
Surgery	Does not relieve chronicity	Curative

of nutritional deficiencies occur. Some clients have a gradual increase in symptoms, whereas others have acute exacerbations alternating with remissions. The symptoms may go into remission spontaneously.

During the physical examination, palpation may reveal an abdominal mass. When the perineum and perianal areas are inspected, scars from previous fissures, skin tags, or evidence of fistula or perianal abscesses may be detected.

Diagnostic Findings

Stool cultures fail to reveal an etiologic microorganism or parasite, but occult blood and white blood cells are often found in the stool. Blood studies indicate anemia from chronic blood loss and nutritional deficiencies. The white blood cell count and erythrocyte sedimentation rate are elevated, confirming an inflammatory disorder. Serum albumin and electrolyte levels are low from malnutrition. Barium enema findings may show inflammation in the large intestine, but confirmation of the diagnosis requires endoscopic examination (colonoscopy or sigmoidoscopy) and biopsy to reveal the unique skip lesions and granuloma.

Clients with Crohn's disease are vulnerable to intestinal perforation during barium enema and endoscopy due to poor integrity of the bowel wall. They are monitored accordingly. Esophagogastroduodenoscopy with biopsy is indicated when inflammation is suspected in the upper GI tract. Upper GI series with small bowel follow-up allows for radiographic examination of the small intestine and identification of inflammation that cannot be evaluated by endoscopy.

MEDICAL MANAGEMENT

Treatment is supportive. The dietary approach varies, but a low-residue diet reduces irritation within the bowel. A high-calorie and high-protein diet helps replace nutritional losses from chronic diarrhea. Nutritional supplements may be needed, depending on the area of the bowel affected. When the small intestine is inflamed, some clients experience lactose intolerance, requiring avoidance of lactose-rich foods.

Some clients need an elemental diet formula, such as Tolerex, Vivonex, or Peptamen, in which proteins, fats, and carbohydrates are reduced to an easily absorbed form. Elemental diets effectively induce remission in Crohn's disease without medications. Unfortunately, clients are not allowed to eat or drink normally while on the elemental diet, making this treatment modality unacceptable for many. In addition, elemental formulas are not very palatable. Some may need to be administered through a nasogastric tube. Success with elemental diet therapy requires extensive education and client motivation. TPN may become necessary to provide intestinal rest. IV fluids, electrolytes, and whole blood are given to correct anemia and restore fluid and electrolyte balance.

Drug therapy involves supplementary vitamins, iron, antidiarrheal drugs, anti-inflammatory corticosteroids and 5-ASA medications, immune modulating agents, and antibiotics (Table 52–2). Vitamin and iron supplements are used for known deficiencies and malabsorption. Antidiarrheal agents, such as diphenoxylate (Lomotil) and loperamide (Imodium) are generally used sparingly and only when it is known that clients do not have an infection. Decreasing motility in cases of infection predisposes clients with IBD to **toxic megacolon**, a complication that is discussed in the section on ulcerative colitis.

Considered first-line treatment for IBD, 5-ASA drugs contain salicylate, which is bonded to a carrying agent that allows the drug to be absorbed in the intestine. These drugs work by decreasing the inflammatory response. The 5-ASA medications include sulfasalazine (Azulfidine), olsalazine (Dipentum) mesalamine (Asacol, Pentasa). Mesalamine is also available in enema or suppository form (Rowasa) and may be used for treating distal disease. Folic acid is generally recommended for clients taking sulfasalazine, which interferes with absorption of this nutrient. Corticosteroids (prednisone) are used during acute exacerbations of symptoms and when the symptoms cannot be controlled by 5-ASA drugs. Hydrocortisone is available in enema form (Cortenema) and is effective in controlling distal disease without a high risk for systemic side effects. Long-term corticosteroid use is undesirable due to potentially severe side effects, so the dose is generally tapered and discontinued when the symptoms are in remission. Failure to maintain remission necessitates the use of an immune-modulating agent such as mercaptopurine (6-MP) or azathioprine (Imuran). These agents often allow clients to discontinuance corticosteroids without exacerbating symptoms. Other immune modulators are cyclosporine (Sandimmune) and methotrexate (MTX). Antibiotics such as metronidazole (Flagyl) and ciprofloxacin (Cipro) are effective as an adjunct to treating Crohn's disease, especially related fistulas.

SURGICAL MANAGEMENT

Surgical treatment is reserved for complications such as intestinal obstruction, perforation, or fistula formation. Unlike surgical treatment for ulcerative colitis, removing the inflamed portion of the intestine does not alter disease progression or recurrence. Many clients who undergo surgery for Crohn's disease require additional surgery within a few years. Surgical removal of a large amount of intestine re-

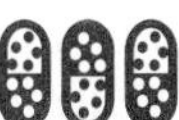

TABLE 52-2 **Drug Therapy for Disorders of the Lower Gastrointestinal Tract**

Drug Category/Drug Action	Side Effects	Nursing Considerations
Antidiarrheals		
bismuth subsalicylate (Pepto-Bismol)	Constipation, dark discoloration of oral mucous membranes and stools	Do not administer to clients who are allergic to aspirin or salicylates.
kaolin and pectin (Kaopectate)	Constipation, abdominal pain	Recognize that this drug may interfere with absorption of nutrients and other drugs.
diphenoxylate with atropine sulfate (Lomotil)	Sedation, dizziness, dry mouth, paralytic ileus, constipation	Monitor closely for proper bowel function. Advise client not to drive or operate dangerous machinery while taking this drug.
loperamide (Imodium)	Central nervous system (CNS) depression, abdominal pain, abdominal distention, nausea and vomiting, constipation	If necessary and prescribed, administer naloxone to counteract CNS depression from overdosage. Avoid prolonged use.
Laxatives, Cathartics and Bulk-Forming Agents		
bisacodyl (Dulcolax)	Abdominal cramping, nausea and vomiting, rectal irritation (from suppository form)	Advise client that prolonged use creates dependence on the product for regular defecation. Do not administer within 1 hour of milk or antacids.
magnesium preparations (milk of magnesia, magnesium citrate, magnesium oxide)	Abdominal cramping, diarrhea, nausea, vomiting	Monitor serum magnesium levels and avoid prolonged use, which may cause hypermagnesemia. Administer with caution in clients who have renal insufficiency. Explain that this drug may interfere with absorption of histamine-2 antagonists (cimetidine, Tagamet, ranitidine), phenytoin (Dilantin), steroids, and some antibiotics.
mineral oil	Leakage of oil from rectum, diarrhea, abdominal cramping	Recognize that mineral oil may cause lipid pneumonitis if aspirated. Do not administer to clients who are vomiting and therefore at risk for aspiration. Understand that prolonged use in high doses may result in poor absorption of fat-soluble vitamins (A, D, E, and K). Monitor serum levels of these vitamins.
polyethylene glycol (GoLYTELY, Colyte)	Nausea, vomiting, abdominal distention, abdominal cramping	Administer for bowel evacuation prior to GI test (ie, colonoscopy) Explain that large amounts must be administered (4–6 liters). Compliance may be difficult for some clients.
psyllium (Metamucil, Citrucel)	Nausea and vomiting, diarrhea, intestinal gas, abdominal cramping	Do not give if client has intestinal obstruction or fecal impaction. Some forms of psyllium require reconstitution with water and may gel within a short period.
Anti-inflammatory Drugs		
corticosteroids prednisone (Meticorten)	Cushingoid appearance, acne, water retention, weight gain, increased appetite, gastric irritation, ulcer formation, adrenal suppression, complications associated with prolonged use (osteoporosis, cataracts, growth retardation, decreased resistance to infection, decreased glucose tolerance, hypertension)	Monitor for side effects particularly with prolonged use. Administer with food to decrease gastric irritation. Encourage low-sodium diet to minimize water retention. Abrupt withdrawal may precipitate adrenal crisis. Monitor blood pressure accordingly. Because clients taking corticosteroids may not have a normal immune response to infection, monitor closely for signs of infection, prevent exposure through Standard Precautions, and encourage the client to consult the physician regularly.
5-ASA drugs sulfasalazine (Azulfidine), olsalazine (Dipentum), mesalamine (Pentasa, Asacol, Rowasa)	Headache, diarrhea, abdominal pain, cramping, rash, bone marrow suppression (sulfasalazine), photosensitivity (sulfasalazine)	Advise client to take drug(s) exactly as prescribed and to report signs of bone marrow abnormalities immediately (infection, fever, sore throat, rash, unusual bleeding or bruising).
Immune-Modulating Agents		
mercaptopurine (6-MP) azathioprine (Imuran)	Bone marrow suppression and increased vulnerability to infection, hair loss, arthralgia	Advise client to take drug(s) exactly as prescribed and to report signs of bone marrow abnormalities immediately (infection, fever, sore throat, rash, unusual bleeding or bruising).

sults in loss of absorptive surface, called **short bowel syndrome.** Massive bowel resection results in dependence on TPN, possibly for life. Removal of the colon requires a permanent ileostomy because there is a tendency for the disease to recur in any rectal pouch. Ileostomy is discussed in Chapter 53.

NURSING MANAGEMENT

In addition to the assessments performed on the client with a GI disorder, a thorough history is obtained, including a medical, drug, allergy, and diet history.

Determine the average number of stools passed each day and their appearance. Provide regular skin care to avoid breakdown (see previous nursing management section for diarrhea). Ask about weight loss and whether any foods increase the frequency of bowel movements or cause discomfort. Assess anxiety level and implement relief measures as needed.

Auscultate and lightly palpate the abdomen. Inspect the rectal area. Take vital signs and weigh the client. Measure and document intake and output. Advise the client to report whenever a bowel movement occurs so it can be inspected and a sample sent to the laboratory for occult blood and other analysis. The plan of care includes, but is not limited to, the following:

Nursing Diagnoses and Collaborative Problems	Nursing Interventions
Diarrhea related to malabsorption of food and water from the bowel **Goal:** Stools will be less frequent and more formed.	Determine the types of foods that alter bowel function and eliminate irritating food from the diet. If diarrhea is related to the quantity of food eaten, reduce portions and provide more frequent nourishment. Administer prescribed antidiarrheal drugs.
Risk for Altered Nutrition: Less than Body Requirements secondary to disease-related anorexia or malabsorption of nutrients **Goal:** Nutrition will be adequate and weight will remain stable or increase appropriately.	Weigh frequently to monitor for weight loss or failure to gain weight. Observe the amounts and types of food eaten. Assist the dietitian with calorie counts to allow complete evaluation of intake. Provide frequent small meals to reduce the gastrocolic reflex. Replace uneaten food with something more acceptable or arrange a consultation with a dietitian. Provide dietary supplements. Administer tube feedings and TPN as prescribed.
Risk for Fluid Volume Deficit related to loss of water in liquid stools, poor fluid intake **Goal:** Oral intake will approximate output; mucous membranes will be moist; urine output will be at least 500 mL/day.	Offer sips of fluid at frequent intervals. Provide a variety of easily tolerated beverages. Notify the physician if fluid output exceeds intake. Anticipate need for IV fluids.
Pain related to abdominal distention, rapid peristalsis **Goal:** Client will rate pain or discomfort at a lower level than initially experienced.	Administer prescribed antidiarrheals and antispasmodics. Encourage the client to assume a position of comfort. Encourage temporary fast or dietary changes to reduce discomfort. Identify activities that trigger acute episodes of cramping or pain. Suggest alternate activities when appropriate. Provide encouragement and support.
Activity Intolerance related to fatigue secondary to anemia and malnutrition **Goal:** Client will participate to a greater extent in performing self-care.	Eliminate unnecessary activities and divide those that are required into smaller tasks that can be performed between periods of rest. Ask client to identify times of peak strength and stamina and encourage client's input for scheduling routine activities. Communicate the information to the health care team. Postpone activities, when possible, if the client develops signs of exhaustion. Encourage progressive self-care as tolerance increases.
Ineffective Individual Coping related to changes in lifestyle secondary to chronic illness **Goal:** Client will ventilate feelings appropriately and seek positive alternatives to lifestyle changes.	Accept the client's method of coping with illness. Provide educational materials to help the client develop realistic expectations related to the disease and treatment. Encourage the client to express feelings when physical improvement occurs; suggest keeping a diary or journal or becoming involved in a support group of individuals with similar illnesses. Suggest imagery (to vent hostility against the disease) and creative pursuits (eg, painting, woodworking, or crafts) to redirect thoughts from chronic disease to positive activities.

Client and Family Teaching

Include the following topics in the plan for teaching the client and family about an IBD and Crohn's disease:

- Special dietary modifications and the importance of complying with them
- Name, purpose, dosage, and adverse effects of prescribed drugs
- Use of medications to control symptoms rather than cure the disease
- Importance of keeping all follow-up physician and laboratory appointment so potentially dangerous complications of disease and side effects of medications can be monitored
- Techniques for rectal hygiene and skin care
- Signs to report immediately to the physician such as more frequent bowel movements, extreme fatigue, severe abdominal pain, visible blood in the stool, adverse drug effects, or weight loss
- Recommendations for regular medical checkups, even when symptoms subside because clients with ulcerative colitis are prone to colon cancer

Clients who are discharged and need high levels of care, such as enteral feeding or TPN, require extensive teaching specific to their home care needs. Central venous catheter care and maintenance of TPN are a few examples of these special learning needs. Cover all technical procedures to be performed by the client or significant other thoroughly and allow time for the client or caregiver to perform them with nursing supervision before discharge. Make a referral to a home care agency to provide continuity of care and to ease the transition from acute care to home care.

Ulcerative Colitis

In ulcerative colitis, the chronic inflammation is generally limited to the mucosal and submucosal layers of the colon. The disease is most common in young and middle-aged adults, but it can occur at any age. Some clients experience prolonged remission, whereas others experience mild to severe (and potentially life-threatening) exacerbations.

ETIOLOGY AND PATHOPHYSIOLOGY

Although the exact cause of ulcerative colitis is unknown, some believe it is triggered by multiple factors, including infection, allergy, emotional stress, and autoimmunity. The connection between the disease and a malfunctioning of the immune system is supported by the fact that individuals with ulcerative colitis often have other coexisting immune-related disorders such as spondylitis of the spine, migratory arthritis, and uveitis.

Inflammation generally begins in the rectum and extends proximally in a continuous fashion. As a rule, no healthy tissue appears between inflamed areas, as in Crohn's disease. When inflammation remains confined to the most distal area of the large intestine, the client has **ulcerative proctitis**. When inflammation extends beyond the sigmoid colon, the client has *ulcerative colitis*. The lining of the colon tends to bleed easily. Ulceration may extend to the muscular layer of the bowel wall. Superficial abscesses form in depressions within the mucosa. Poor integrity of the bowel wall may lead to *toxic megacolon*, a complication in which the colon dilates and becomes atonic (lacks motility). The thin bowel wall is vulnerable to perforation under these conditions, leading to peritonitis, septicemia, and the need for emergency surgical repair.

ASSESSMENT FINDINGS

Signs and Symptoms

The onset of the disease is usually abrupt. The client experiences severe diarrhea and expels blood and mucus along with fecal matter. Diarrhea is accompanied by cramps. Eating precipitates cramping and diarrhea, resulting in anorexia and fatigue. The urge to defecate may come so suddenly and with such urgency that the client is incontinent (**encopresis**). For some clients this occurs during sleep. Despite intense tenesmus, the client may expel very little stool.

Diagnostic Findings

Barium enema reveals evidence of inflammation. Definitive diagnosis requires proctosigmoidoscopy or colonoscopy with biopsy. Endoscopic examination and biopsy of the lining of the colon reveals characteristic inflammatory lesions. These diagnostic studies are generally withheld in the presence of toxic megacolon, due to the high risk for perforation.

The stool is cultured for microorganisms or parasites that commonly cause diarrhea, but the results are negative. Stool analysis usually detects blood. Serum electrolyte and complete blood count values may be abnormal, reflecting the effects brought about by bleeding, inflammation, and severe diarrhea.

MEDICAL MANAGEMENT

Some clients are managed medically and helped into a remission. Medical treatment is primarily supportive. The diet is kept as normal as possible, but it is modified to increase caloric and nutritional content. Foods that are high in fiber irritate the intestine and are temporarily withheld during acute exacerbations. The client is instructed to temporarily refrain from eating foods associated with discomfort. Of course, if all foods cause discomfort, the symptoms are likely from the disease itself and not food. The client may be given TPN and intermittent lipid infusions to completely rest the bowel. The use of an elemental diet, as described with Crohn's disease, has not proved effective for ulcerative colitis.

Blood transfusions and iron are given to correct anemia. Parenteral fluids and electrolytes also may be needed. Because frequent bowel movements interfere with absorption of nutrients, supplementary vitamins are prescribed.

Medications used to treat Crohn's disease are also used to treat ulcerative colitis. See the previous section on Crohn's disease and Table 52–2 for a discussion of these drugs.

Corticosteroids, given orally, IV or rectally, are used if the disease does not respond to other measures. A dramatic relief of symptoms usually follows. To maintain a remission, the client may remain on therapy for weeks or months with as low a dose as possible. Although they are potentially dangerous, corticosteroids have helped many clients with this disease live longer and more comfortably and reduced mortality related to elective surgery.

SURGICAL MANAGEMENT

Surgery is necessary when the disease does not respond to medical treatment or when complications such as dysplastic tissue (a precancerous condition), perforation of the colon, or hemorrhage occur. Surgery is the definitive cure for ulcerative colitis. The current standard treatment is ileoanal pull through and anastomosis (see Chap. 53). This procedure is typically done in two stages, several weeks apart. In the first stage, the colon is removed and a rectal "pouch" is created from a section of the ileum. The rectal mucosa is removed to create a temporary ileostomy. In the second stage, the surgeon closes the ileostomy and connects the intestine to the rectum, allowing the client to defecate normally. When an emergency colectomy is performed (ie, for toxic megacolon or perforation), an anastomosis (rejoining of the bowel) may not be possible, necessitating creation of a permanent ileostomy.

NURSING MANAGEMENT

Compile a comprehensive data base and conduct frequent focused assessments to identify early changes in the symptoms, which may herald rapidly progressing complications. Until the disease is confirmed, prepare clients for diagnostic tests. Question radiographic and endoscopic protocols for harsh laxatives and cleansing enemas, when the client is experiencing severe diarrhea because bowel irritation and stimulation tend to aggravate the client's symptoms.

Once the diagnosis is confirmed, implement drug and fluid therapy. If antispasmodics and opiates are prescribed, administer them with great caution because they may trigger the development of toxic megacolon. Report any sudden onset of abdominal distention, severe pain, or fever in a client with acute ulcerative colitis. Observe the client receiving steroids for subtle changes because these drugs mask inflammatory symptoms accompanying complications. Gradually taper the dosage and frequency of steroids when they are no longer needed. Teach about the disease and measures for self-care as soon as the client is well enough to learn.

Refer to the section on the nursing management of a client with Crohn's disease for similar problems.

Acute Abdominal Inflammatory Disorders

Appendicitis and peritonitis are among conditions known as acute abdominal inflammatory disorders.

Appendicitis

Appendicitis is an inflammation of a narrow, blind protrusion called the vermiform appendix located at the tip of the cecum in the right lower quadrant (Fig. 52–1). Appendicitis can occur at any age but seems to be more common in adolescents and young adults. Appendicitis is difficult to diagnose at its onset because the initial symptoms resemble a host of other disorders such as gastroenteritis, an ovarian cyst, tubal pregnancy, or inflammation of the kidney or ureter.

ETIOLOGY AND PATHOPHYSIOLOGY

The inflammation begins when the opening of the appendix becomes narrowed or obstructed. The obstruction may be caused by a hard mass of feces, called a *fecalith*, a foreign body, local edema, or a tumor. The blockage interferes with the drainage of secretions from the appendix and they accumulate within the confined space. The appendix enlarges, distends, and the swelling compresses surrounding blood vessels. The locally damaged cells are then eas-

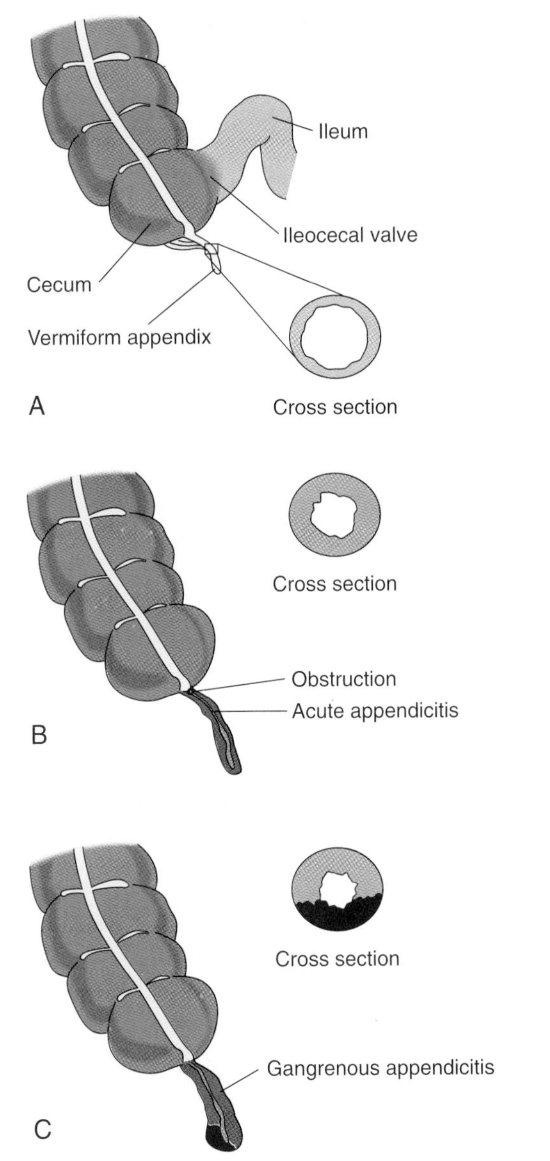

FIGURE 52-1. (*A*) Normal appendix. (*B*) Acute appendicitis resulting from obstruction (note the narrowing in the cross section). (C) Appendicitis and gangrene.

ily infected with bacteria from within the intestinal lumen. Unless the inflammation resolves, the appendix can become gangrenous or rupture, spilling bacteria throughout the peritoneal cavity.

ASSESSMENT FINDINGS

Signs and Symptoms

An attack of abdominal pain is the most frequent symptom of appendicitis. At first, the pain is generalized throughout the abdomen or around the umbilicus. Later, the pain localizes in the right lower quadrant of the abdomen at McBurney's point, an area midway between the umbilicus and the right iliac crest. Often the pain is worse when manual pressure near the region is suddenly released. This is called rebound tenderness. Slight or moderate fever, nausea, and vomiting may be present. The abdomen is tense and the client generally flexes the right hip to relieve the discomfort.

Diagnostic Findings

A white blood cell count reveals moderate leukocytosis. When a differential count of leukocytes is performed, it shows an ever-increasing number of immature neutrophils, indicating a progressive worsening of the inflammatory condition. A computed tomography (CT) scan or abdominal ultrasound of the abdomen shows enlargement at the cecum.

MEDICAL AND SURGICAL MANAGEMENT

Antibiotics are given and the client is restricted from eating or drinking while a decision is made about surgery. IV fluids are prescribed to meet the client's fluid needs. Analgesics may be withheld initially to avoid masking symptoms that may affect the diagnosis. If symptoms worsen, the surgeon performs an **appendectomy** to remove the appendix before it spontaneously ruptures. The appendix has no known function within the body. Its removal results in cure with no physiologic changes.

NURSING MANAGEMENT

Assess vital signs and client pain to detect early changes in the symptoms. Administer IV fluid therapy and observe the client's response to antibiotics if ordered. When analgesics are withheld, maintain an empathic attitude and facilitate comfort with positioning, imagery, and distraction.

When surgery is indicated, prepare the client quickly to avoid delay that may cause surgical complications. Soon after surgery, if no complications occur, ambulate the client and provide light nourishment. Convalescence may be rapid although postoperative progress depends on the client's age, general physical condition, and extent of complications. A healthy young adult can usually return to usual activities soon. However, advise these clients to avoid heavy lifting or unusual exertion for several months. For more specific nursing interventions when caring for a client undergoing surgery, see Chapter 24.

Peritonitis

In **peritonitis,** the peritoneum, a serous sac lining the abdominal cavity (Fig. 52–2) becomes inflamed.

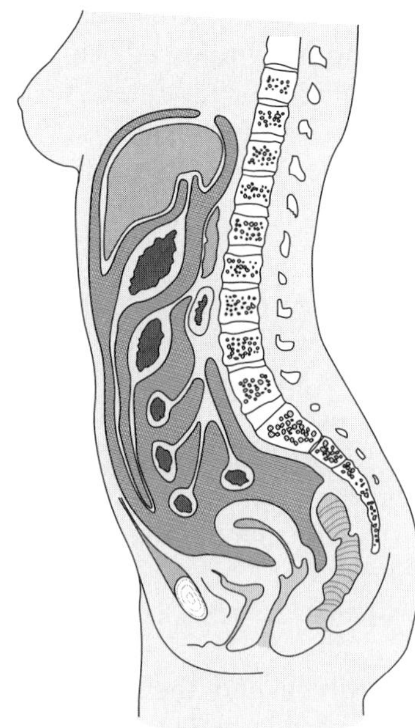

FIGURE 52-2. Abdominal organs enclosed within the peritoneum.

ETIOLOGY AND PATHOPHYSIOLOGY

Peritonitis may be caused by perforation of a peptic ulcer, the bowel, or the appendix; abdominal trauma, such as gunshot or knife wounds; ruptured ectopic pregnancy; or infection introduced during peritoneal dialysis, a procedure used to treat kidney failure.

Spillage of chemical contents and bacteria inflames the peritoneum, which leads to localized abscess formation or generalized inflammation. When generalized peritonitis occurs, vascular fluid shifts to the abdomen, lowering blood pressure, producing hypovolemic shock, or septic shock. If the condition is not treated promptly or adequately, death may follow.

ASSESSMENT FINDINGS

Signs and Symptoms

Symptoms include severe abdominal pain, distention, tenderness, nausea, and vomiting. Fever may be absent, initially, but the temperature rises as infection becomes established. The client avoids movement of the abdomen when breathing because movement increases pain. The knees may be drawn up toward the abdomen to lessen the pain. Lack of bowel motility typically accompanies peritonitis. The abdomen feels rigid and boardlike as it distends with gas and intestinal contents. Bowel sounds are typically absent. The pulse rate is elevated and respirations are rapid and shallow. If the peritonitis is unresolved, severe weakness, hypotension, and a drop in body temperature occur as the client nears death.

Diagnostic Findings

The results of a white blood cell count shows marked leukocytosis. Radiographs of the abdomen reveal the presence of free air and fluid within the peritoneum. A CT scan or ultrasonography identifies structural changes within abdominal organs.

MEDICAL AND SURGICAL MANAGEMENT

A nasogastric tube is used to relieve abdominal distention by suctioning the accumulated gas and stagnant upper GI fluids. Fluids and electrolytes are replaced IV to balance those relocated within the peritoneal cavity and lost through vomiting and drainage from gastric intubation. Large doses of antibiotics are prescribed to combat infection. Analgesics such as meperidine (Demerol) or IV morphine sulfate are ordered to relieve pain and promote rest. The perforation is surgically closed so that intestinal contents can no longer escape.

NURSING MANAGEMENT

Monitor the acutely ill client while completing preparations for diagnostic tests or surgery. Control pain with analgesics. Infuse IV fluids with secondary administrations of antibiotics. Pass a nasogastric tube and connect it to suction (see Chap. 51). Insert a urinary retention catheter. Assess the circulatory status by taking vital signs frequently and monitoring central venous and pulmonary artery pressures.

NURSING PROCESS
The Client Undergoing Surgery for Peritonitis

Assessment

Postoperatively, assess the client's vital signs, wound, wound drainage and drain, postanesthetic status, and need for pain medications and intestinal decompression. If recovery is prolonged, assess the need for nutritional measures such as TPN.

Diagnosis and Planning

Nursing management includes, but is not limited to, the following:

Nursing Diagnoses and Collaborative Problems	Nursing Interventions
Fear (of death) related to the severe symptoms and aggressive response of the health care team preoperatively **Goal:** Client will report that fear is reduced or has subsided entirely.	Relieve pain, which is usually the client's measurement of the seriousness of the condition. Control frantic activity that tends to alarm an already fearful client.

Remain with the client as much as possible, designate a surrogate to stay, or permit a supportive family member to remain with the client and be physically close enough to make skin contact.

Make frequent eye contact, call the client by name, and use touch appropriately.

If the client asks for a clergy person, arrange the referral. Briefly delay nursing actions, if possible, when the client is praying or meeting with spiritual counsel.

PC: Infection related to bacterial contamination of the abdominal cavity

Goal: Infection will be managed and minimized

Administer antibiotics as ordered.

Report increased abdominal distention, fever, changes in level of consciousness, and deviations in vital signs immediately.

Observe for delayed wound healing, redness, edema, drainage from incision.

Fluid Volume Deficit related to fluid losses and peritoneal shift

Goal: Client will maintain fluid balance with stable blood pressure (systolic pressure above 100 mm Hg) and urine output is at least 500 mL/day.

Maintain uninterrupted infusion of IV fluids at the prescribed rate.

Promptly restart any infusions that infiltrate.

Report urine output that falls below 50 mL/hr, blood in suctioned drainage, or systolic blood pressure under 100 mm Hg.

Pain related to generalized inflammation, surgical wound, abdominal distention

Goal: Pain will be brief, reduced, or eliminated within 30 minutes of an implemented nursing measure.

Initiate intestinal decompression as ordered.

Keep decompression tube free of kinks or obstructions.

Consult with the physician concerning the possibility of irrigating the tube to maintain its patency if drainage slows or stops and distention increases or the client begins to retch.

Replace improperly functioning suction equipment.

Replace obstructed decompression tube if obstruction cannot be removed by irrigation.

Assist the client gently with activity and position changes. Obtain assistance if necessary.

Avoid accidentally pressing on the abdomen.

Teach client how to splint incision for coughing and deep breathing.

Administer narcotic analgesics as ordered; monitor side effects of the medication, including depressed respiratory rate and decreased blood pressure.

Ineffective Breathing related to abdominal distention, pain

Goal: Client will have regular effortless respirations between 12 and 20/min.

Place the client in a Fowler's position to promote the collection of fluid below the diaphragm.

Maintain patency of the tube used for decompression.

Encourage slow but deep breathing on a regular basis.

Administer oxygen if arterial oxygen saturation, measured by pulse oximeter, falls below 90%.

Altered Oral Mucous Membrane related to mouth breathing secondary to intubation, reduced salivation

Goal: Lips and oral mucosa will return to moist and intact state.

Provide frequent mouth care and oral rinses.

Clean the mouth with moist swabs if the client is unable to use an oral rinse. If the client is allowed ice chips, provide them sparingly. Apply a moisturizing ointment or lip balm if the lips become dry.

Risk for Injury related to weakness, confusion, and disorientation

Goal: Client will remain free of injury.

Raise the side rails on the bed to prevent injury.

Check on the client frequently; respond to a call or signal for assistance promptly.

Relocate a confused or unstable client near the nursing station.

Place a bed monitor beneath the mattress that sounds an alarm if the client tries to ambulate without help.

Self-Care Deficit: Bathing/Hygiene related to postoperative weakness or pain

Goal: Client will participate in self-care independently or with assistance.

Provide hygiene during periods when the client's discomfort is reduced so that client can collaborate on what and how much assistance is needed.

Help with activities of daily living that are beyond the client's capabilities.

Risk for Impaired Tissue Integrity related to irritation from tape, separation of incision, displaced wound drainage tubing

Goal: Skin edges will approximate and heal without complication.

Support the incision when the client deep breathes and coughs.

Change the wound dressing when it becomes moist, soiled, or loose.

Pull tape securing the dressing toward the incision line rather than away from the wound to prevent disrupting healing.

Clean wound drainage from the skin with an antiseptic approved by the agency or physician.

Empty drainage containers frequently, especially before ambulating the client so that tubing is not displaced from within the wound.

Support the weight of the wound drainage container during ambulation by carrying it or pinning it to the client's gown or bathrobe below the insertion site.

Consult with the physician about removing every other suture one day and the remaining sutures on the next day to ensure that the wound has healed enough to remain closed.

Place devices, such as Steri-Strips across the suture removal site as temporary reinforcements.

Evaluation and Expected Outcomes

- Fear has diminished.
- Client is free of infection.
- Fluid loss has stopped and blood pressure is stable.
- Pain is controlled and decreasing.
- Breathing is spontaneous, deep; and effortless.
- Mucous membranes are moist and uncracked.
- Client is uninjured and tissues are healed.
- Client can participate in self-care.

Intestinal Disorders

Among intestinal disorders are blockages or obstructions. These are characterized by an interruption in the normal flow of intestinal contents.

Intestinal Obstruction

An intestinal obstruction can be nonmechanical or mechanical, partial or complete. In a *nonmechanical* obstruction peristalsis stops. This disorder is called an adynamic or **paralytic ileus.** A *mechanical* obstruction occurs when the intestinal lumen is blocked. An intestinal obstruction is extremely dangerous and may be fatal if not treated promptly.

ETIOLOGY AND PATHOPHYSIOLOGY

The intestine can become adynamic (lacking peristalsis) from an absence of normal nerve stimulation to intestinal muscle fibers, a common happening 12 to 36 hours after abdominal surgery. It can also occur from inflammatory conditions (ie, peritonitis), electrolyte disturbances (ie, hypokalemia), or adverse drug effects (ie, narcotics or cholinergic blockers). Even a vascular embolus or low blood flow during shock can interfere with the neuromuscular function of the bowel.

Mechanical obstructions result from a narrowing of the bowel lumen with or without a space-occupying mass, such as a tumor; *adhesions*, fibrous bands that constrict tissue; incarcerated or strangulated hernias; **volvulus,** a kinking of a portion of intestine; **intussusception,** a telescoping of one part of the intestine into an adjacent part; or impacted feces or barium (Fig. 52–3).

When the intestinal contents cannot move freely, the portion above the obstruction distends, whereas the portion below the obstruction is empty. If the obstruction is complete, no gases or feces are expelled rectally. Both forward and reverse peristalsis become forceful in an attempt to clear the obstruction. Stasis of the accumulating volume and the violent muscular peristaltic contractions potentiate the risk for intestinal rupture. Locally, the increased pressure pushes electrolyte-rich fluid from the intestine and capillaries into the peritoneal cavity. Failure of the mucosa to re-

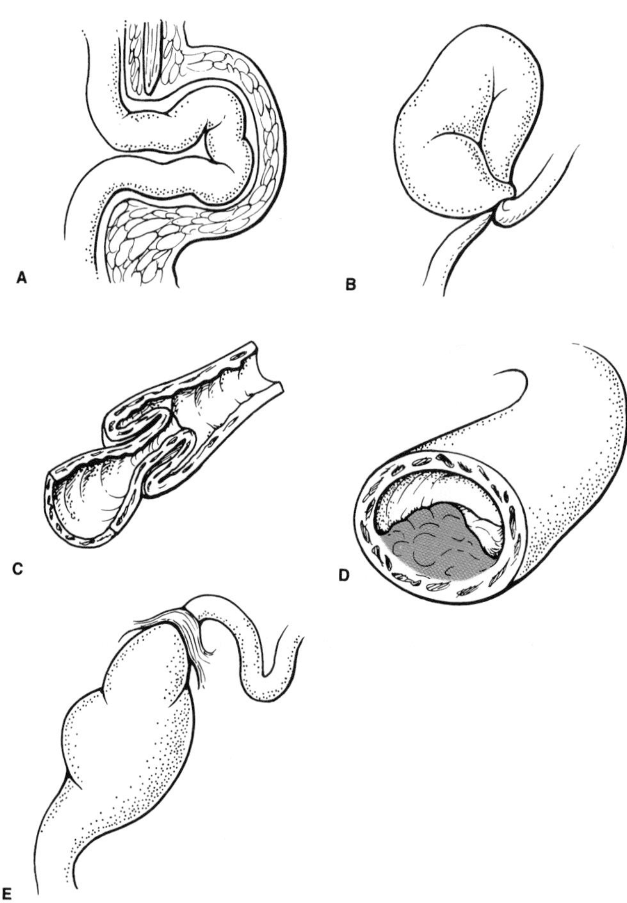

FIGURE 52-3. Major causes of intestinal obstructions. (*A*) Hernia. (*B*) Volvulus. (*C*) Intussusception. (*D*) Cancer. (*E*) Adhesions.

absorb the secretions contributes to water and electrolyte imbalances and shock. Increasing pressure on the bowel due to severe distention and edema impairs circulation and leads to necrosis and eventually gangrene of a portion of the bowel. Perforation of the gangrenous bowel, which results from pressure against weakened tissue, causes the intestinal contents to seep into the peritoneal cavity, resulting in peritonitis.

ASSESSMENT FINDINGS

Signs and Symptoms

Nausea and abdominal distention are common. When an obstruction occurs high in the GI tract, the client usually vomits whatever contents are in the stomach and small intestine. The emesis appears to contain bile or fecal material. If the obstruction is lower in the GI tract, vomiting may or may not occur. One or two bowel movements may occur soon after the intestine has been obstructed because the material already past the obstruction is being expelled. The client may experience severe intermittent cramps. Sudden, sustained pain, abdominal distention, and fever are symptoms of perforation.

In a nonmechanical obstruction, peristalsis is absent and therefore bowel sounds are not heard. In a mechanical obstruction, the bowel sounds are generally high pitched above the obstructed area. Pulse and respiratory rates are elevated. The blood pressure falls and the urine output decreases if shock develops.

Diagnostic Findings

A radiographic study of the abdomen shows air and fluid collecting within a segment of the intestine. A barium enema (used when the risk of perforation is low) pinpoints the location of the obstruction. Serum electrolytes may indicate low sodium, potassium, and chloride levels. Metabolic alkalosis is evidenced by arterial blood gas results. A complete blood count shows an increased white blood cell count in instances of infection. The hematocrit is elevated if dehydration develops.

MEDICAL AND SURGICAL MANAGEMENT

The client is supported medically while the cause and appropriate treatment of the obstruction are determined. The client receives nothing by mouth (NPO). IV fluids with electrolytes are administered to correct fluid and electrolyte imbalances and antibiotics are ordered to treat a potential infection.

To relieve intestinal distention, cramping, and vomiting and to reduce the potential for intestinal rupture with peritonitis, intestinal decompression is begun. Intestinal decompression is accomplished by suctioning large amounts of accumulated secretions and gas through a nasogastric tube or longer intestinal tube. Nasogastric tubes are used when there is partial obstruction or when the obstruction is located high in the small intestine. Box 52–2 presents information on decompression tubes. Decompression alone may be sufficient to relieve a nonmechanical obstruction or to relieve symptoms preoperatively in clients who are undergoing surgery for mechanical obstruction. In some cases, mechanical obstructions are treated during colonoscopy by removing obstructing polyps or destroying benign tumors with laser therapy or electrocautery. However, most mechanical obstructions require surgical treatment. Generally a section of the obstructed bowel is removed and then the proximal and distal sections are reconnected (bowel resection and anastomosis). A temporary or permanent ostomy (see Chap. 53) may be performed in some cases.

NURSING MANAGEMENT

In addition to the assessments performed on the client with a GI disorder, obtain complete medical, drug, and allergy histories. Assess fluid intake and output and take vital signs.

Document all symptoms and obtain detailed information about each. For example, if vomiting has occurred, gather information regarding its onset, amount, and color. If an intestinal tube has been inserted, monitor its progress (Nursing Guidelines 52–1).

The care of a client with an intestinal obstruction involves pain management, maintaining fluid balance to prevent deficits related to fluid shifts and losses from vomiting, and helping the client deal with fear related to severe, possibly life-threatening symptoms and an unstable condition.

Manage pain by maintaining the patency of the decompression tube and administering a prescribed narcotic analgesic as long as blood pressure and respiratory rate indicate it is safe to do so.

Maintain uninterrupted infusion of IV fluids. Shorten the siege of vomiting by maintaining intestinal decompression, even though intestinal fluid will be lost in the suctioning. Monitor urinary output hourly, and report output under 50 mL/hr, which may indicate that the client is going into shock.

Diverticular Disorders

Diverticula are sacs or pouches caused by herniation of the mucosa through a weakened portion of the muscular coat of the intestine or other structure (Fig. 52–4).

BOX 52-2 Intestinal Decompression Tubes and Their Uses

When intestinal intubation is needed, the physician may insert a Miller-Abbott, Cantor, or Harris tube, in much the same way as a nasogastric tube. These tubes range from 6 to 10 feet long. Then the nurse is responsible for monitoring their movement into the intestine.

Each type of tube is weighted at the end with a heavy substance, such as tungsten or mercury. Gravity helps to propel the weighted tip beyond the pylorus into the small intestine. Radiographic images are taken periodically to evaluate the tube's progress. Openings throughout the distal end provide channels through which to suction intestinal contents. The tubes are left in place until the intestinal lumen is patent and peristalsis resumes.

Miller-Abbott

The double-lumen **Miller-Abbott tube** is the most common type of intestinal tube. After it passes through the pylorus, mercury is instilled through one lumen to fill a reservoir at the tip of the tube. Label this lumen "mercury" to prevent accidental contact with mercury by staff caring for the client. Label the other lumen "suction." This is the lumen used to remove intestinal contents.

Cantor

The **Cantor tube** has just one lumen and a balloon-like bag on the end into which mercury is instilled with a needle before inserting the tube. Leakage does not occur because the needle does not make a hole large enough for the mercury to escape. The bag is elongated when the tube is inserted, so that it can be passed more easily and with less discomfort to the client.

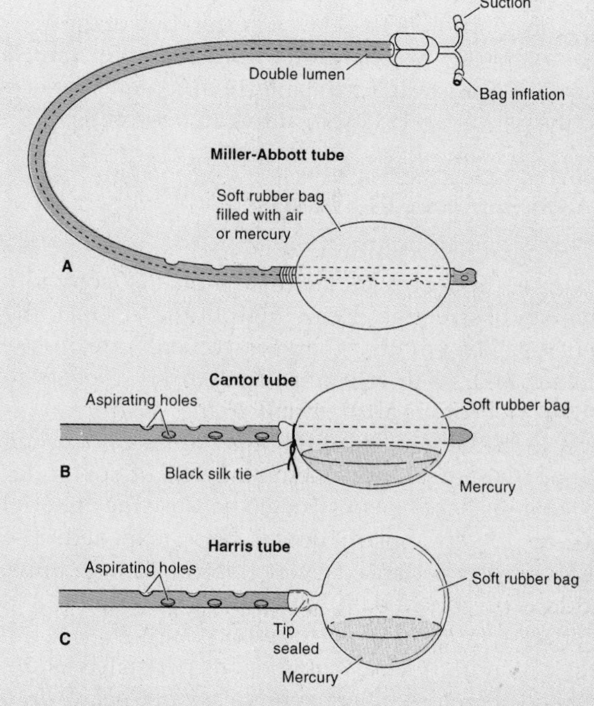

Tubes used for intestinal decompression. (*A*) Miller-Abbott. (*B*) Cantor. (*C*) Harris.

Harris

The single-lumen **Harris tube** is also weighted with mercury. A Y-tube is attached to the proximal end of the Harris tube. One end of the Y connects to suction and the other is clamped until it is used for irrigation. When irrigating this tube, place a clamp over the suction end of the Y-tube.

Diverticulosis and Diverticulitis

Asymptomatic diverticula are called **diverticulosis.** When the diverticula become inflamed, the term **diverticulitis** is used. Diverticula are common in the esophagus and the colon, especially in the sigmoid area in people over age 50.

ETIOLOGY AND PATHOPHYSIOLOGY

What causes diverticula is unknown. The incidence worldwide seems to be higher in countries, like the United States, where the diet is low in fiber. Most diverticula are thought to be due to weakness in the intestinal muscular layer associated with aging.

Diverticula become inflamed when fecal material becomes trapped within one or more blind pouches. The inflammation causes the tissue in the area to swell. If the localized swelling involves several diverticula in one area, the edema may be severe enough to cause an intestinal obstruction. Abscesses form when the inflamed tissue becomes infected with intestinal bacteria present in the bowel. The swollen, festering tissue has a potential for rupturing into the peritoneal cavity or forming a fistular connection with an adjacent organ such as the bladder.

ASSESSMENT FINDINGS

Signs and Symptoms

Constipation alternating with diarrhea, flatulence, pain and tenderness in the left lower quadrant, fever, and rectal bleeding may occur. A palpable mass may be felt in the lower abdomen. When the diverticula bleed, the stools appear maroon and are sometimes described as resembling "currant jelly."

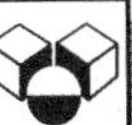

Nursing Guidelines 52-1

Managing Care of a Client With an Intestinal Tube

Preparations

- Auscultate and examine the abdomen for bowel sounds, distention, and tenderness.
- To provide a baseline for reference, measure abdominal girth, placing a measuring tape about the largest diameter of the abdomen.
- Mark the measuring location on the skin (with an indelible marker) to facilitate consistency when obtaining future comparison measurements.
- Assemble all the equipment the physician will need. If the Miller-Abbott tube is selected, label the tip of the adapter leading to the lumen through which mercury is instilled to avoid confusing which lumen to use for suction.

Tube Advancement

- After the physician inserts the tube, ambulate the client, if possible, to facilitate tube passage through the pylorus. When a radiographic image indicates that the tube has advanced beyond the stomach, position the client as follows:

—On the right side for 2 hours, then
—On the back in a Fowler's position for 2 hours, then
—On the left side for 2 hours.

- Observe the lines or numbers on the tube periodically to evaluate the tube's progressive movement and approximate anatomic location.
- Advance the tube several inches at specified intervals as directed to avoid tension as it descends into the intestine.
- Stabilize or tape the tube to the nose after a radiographic image verifies that the tube has reached the obstruction. Coil the excess length, securing it to the bedding or the client's hospital gown.
- Attach the proximal end to suction.
- Prepare for radiography to be performed daily to evaluate progress toward relieving the obstruction.

Removal

- Remove the tube once the obstruction is relieved or another treatment replaces intubation.
- Disconnect the tube from suction.
- If removing a Miller-Abbott tube, withdraw the mercury by aspirating it with a 10-mL syringe. Remove the mercury in the other types of tubes after the tube is withdrawn. For environmental reasons, do not discard the mercury; instead, place it in a biohazard container for proper disposal.
- Withdraw 6 to 10 inches of the tube between 10-minute pauses. When the tube is in the esophagus, as determined by 18 inches of length remaining within the client, flush the tube with a small amount of air to remove debris.
- Clamp the tube to prevent secretions from being deposited in the client's upper airway and instruct the client to hold the breath while the tube exits the esophagus.
- If removing a Cantor or Harris tube, grasp the bag of mercury with a forceps and withdraw it from the client's mouth when it reaches the oropharynx.
- Once the mercury is removed from the bag, remove the tube from the client's nose. Provide nasal and oral hygiene immediately afterward.

Diagnostic Findings

A barium enema shows an irregular mucosal wall. A colonoscopy helps visualize the areas of inflammation. A CT scan may be used as an alternative to a barium enema or colonoscopy because both require an aggressive bowel preparation that may be contraindicated when the large intestine is acutely inflamed. A complete blood count shows leukocytosis. A stool specimen may reveal occult blood.

MEDICAL AND SURGICAL MANAGEMENT

Diverticula noted during routine examination require no treatment if they do not cause symptoms. Avoiding foods that contain seeds of any kind is rec-

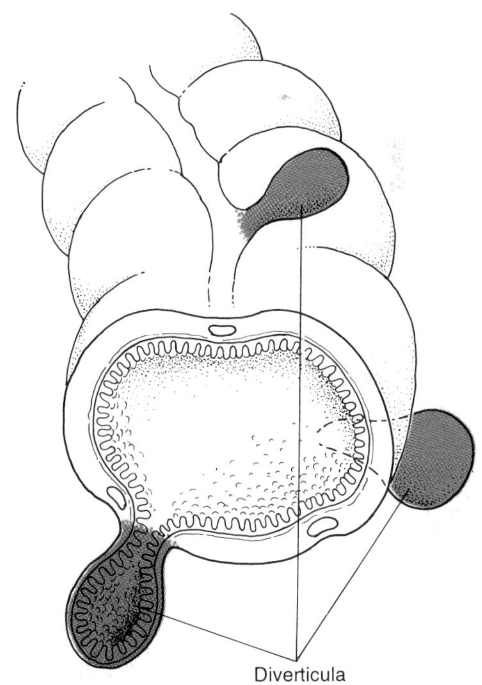

FIGURE 52-4. Intestinal diverticula, particularly common in the sigmoid colon of older adults, generally do not cause symptoms except for occasional rectal bleeding. However, they may become inflamed and infected from fecal matter that becomes lodged within the pouchlike herniations.

ommended. A high-fiber diet supplemented with bran or a prescription of a bulk-forming agent (Metamucil) helps to avoid constipation.

When symptoms occur, the diet is temporarily adjusted to low-residue foods. If the inflammation is severe and accompanied by pain and local tenderness, the client is maintained on IV fluids for several days with no oral intake. As the inflammation subsides under antibiotic therapy, oral fluids and food are reintroduced.

If the diverticulitis does not respond to medical treatment, or if complications such as perforation, intestinal obstruction, or severe bleeding occur, surgery becomes necessary. The portion of colon that contains the diverticula is removed, and the continuity of the bowel is re-established by joining the remaining portions of the colon. Depending on the location and extent of the disease and whether there is intestinal obstruction, a temporary colostomy may be necessary (see Chap. 53). The continuity of the bowel is restored and the colostomy is closed 3 to 6 weeks later.

NURSING MANAGEMENT

In addition to the assessments performed on the client with a GI disorder, obtain a history of symptoms, diet, drug use, and allergies. Take vital signs. Ask questions regarding pain, bowel elimination, and diet habits. Examine the abdomen for pain, tenderness, and masses.

Explain the underlying pathology and rationale for the treatment measures. Because dietary compliance reduces the potential for recurrent problems, consult the dietitian for dietary teaching. If surgery becomes necessary, prepare the client preoperatively and manage the postoperative care.

The nursing care of a client with a diverticular disorder includes, but is not limited to, the following:

Nursing Diagnoses and Collaborative Problems	Nursing Interventions
Diarrhea related to inflammatory process **Goal:** The client will pass stools regularly and easily; loose stools will cease.	Temporarily eliminate high-fiber foods because they irritate the lower bowel. Provide fluids, but restrict those containing caffeine. Reintroduce low residue food when the bowel quiets. Withhold oral nourishment and notify the physician if diarrhea intensifies.
Constipation related to delayed elimination secondary to low stool volume and dry feces, narrowing of the colon secondary to mucosal edema **Goal:** The client will pass stools regularly and easily; hard, dry stools will cease.	Provide a high-fiber diet, when the client can tolerate eating. Avoid refined and processed foods. Advise the client to drink at least eight 8-oz glasses of fluid daily, and honor the urge to defecate.
Pain related to inflammation and infection **Goal:** The client will be relieved of discomfort	Administer prescribed medications such as antidiarrheals, antispasmodics, and analgesics. Rest the bowel by restricting food or serving low-residue foods and implementing dietary changes. Show client how to assume a position of comfort and show concern for the client's pain. Provide distraction (TV, music) from pain.

Client and Family Teaching

A dietary consult or a list of foods to eat or avoid is necessary. Include the following points in the teaching plan:

- Follow the diet recommended by the physician. This will probably reduce pain and discomfort.
- Bran adds bulk to the diet. Unprocessed bran can be sprinkled over cereal or added to fruit juice.
- Avoid the use of laxatives or enemas except when recommended by the physician.
- Avoid constipation. Do not suppress the urge to defecate.
- Drink at least 8 to 10 large glasses of fluids each day.
- Take prescribed medications as directed, even if symptoms improve.
- Exercise regularly if the current lifestyle is somewhat inactive.
- If severe pain or blood in the stool occurs, see a physician immediately.

Abdominal Hernia

Although the term **hernia** refers to the protrusion of any organ from the cavity that normally confines it, it most commonly is used to describe the protrusion of the intestine through a defect in the abdominal wall. Certain areas within the abdominal wall are weaker than others and more vulnerable to the development of a hernia. These areas include the inguinal ring, the point on the abdominal wall where the inguinal canal egins; the femoral ring, at the abdominal opening of ne femoral canal; and the umbilicus.

If the protruding structures can be replaced in the odominal cavity, it is a *reducible hernia*. Placing the ient in a supine position and applying manual ressure over the area may reduce the hernia. An *irducible* or *incarcerated hernia* is one in which the inestine cannot be replaced in the abdominal cavity ecause of edema of the protruding segment and onstriction of the muscle opening through which has emerged. If the process continues withut treatment, the blood supply to the trapped segnent of bowel can be cut off, leading to gangrene. Vhen this results, it is referred to as a *strangulated ernia*.

ypes of Hernia

he most common types of abdominal hernia are *inuinal*, *umbilical*, *femoral*, and *incisional* (Fig. 52–5). nguinal hernias are the most common type. They re more prevalent in men than women. Umbilial and femoral hernias are more frequent among vomen.

INGUINAL HERNIA

The two types of inguinal hernia are direct and inlirect. A direct inguinal hernia extends through the nguinal ring and follows the spermatic cord in the nale client or its counterpart, the round ligament in a emale client. With an indirect inguinal hernia, the protrusion follows the posterior inguinal wall.

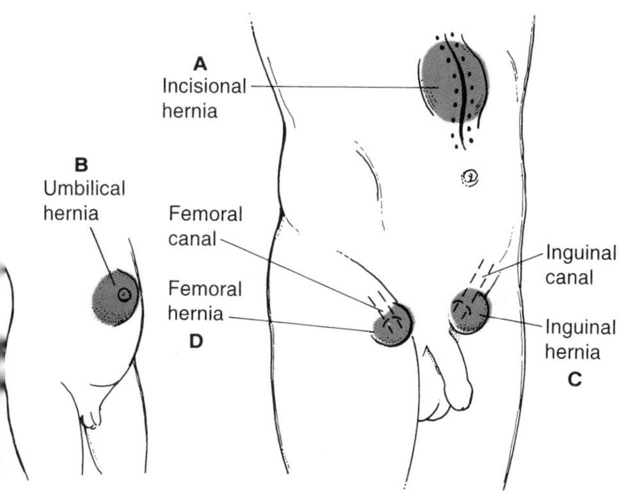

FIGURE 52-5. Types of hernia. (*A*) Incisional. (*B*) Umbilical. (C) Inguinal. (*D*) Femoral.

UMBILICAL HERNIA

An umbilical hernia usually occurs because the umbilical orifice fails to close shortly after birth. It is evidenced by a protrusion of the umbilicus. Obesity and prolonged abdominal distention also can result in an umbilical hernia.

FEMORAL HERNIA

A femoral hernia occurs where the femoral artery passes into the femoral canal, below the inguinal ligament. Femoral hernias have a high incidence of strangulation.

INCISIONAL HERNIA

An incisional hernia occurs through the scar of a surgical incision when healing has been impaired. Incisional hernias can be avoided by careful surgical technique, with particular emphasis on the prevention of wound infection. Obese or older clients and those who suffer from malnutrition are especially prone to the development of an incisional hernia.

ETIOLOGY AND PATHOPHYSIOLOGY

A hernia develops when intra-abdominal pressure increases such as while straining to lift something heavy, while having a bowel movement, or during forceful coughing or sneezing, and a segment of intestine moves into a weak area of abdominal muscle. In addition to the areas that are naturally predisposed to weakness, the abdominal wall may be thin or stretched due to an inadequate amount of collagen, a condition that may be present at birth or that develops as a result of aging, abdominal surgery, and obesity.

At first, the defect in the abdominal wall is small. As the hernia persists and the organs continue to protrude, the defect grows larger. Eventually the bowel becomes trapped within the weakened pouch. If the blood supply to the bowel is compromised, it becomes gangrenous.

ASSESSMENT FINDINGS

Signs and Symptoms

A hernia initially causes no symptoms other than a swelling on the abdomen. When instructed to cough or bear down, the protrusion is more obvious. Sometimes the swelling is painful, but the pain subsides when the hernia is reduced. Incarcerated hernias cause severe pain, and if not treated, they may become strangulated. If a strangulation occurs, the client suffers extreme abdominal pain, and the severe pressure on the loop of intestine protruding outside the abdominal cavity causes intestinal obstruction.

MEDICAL AND SURGICAL MANAGEMENT

Once a hernia forms, it tends to enlarge, leading to serious complications. Surgery is the only method of eliminating a hernia. Some clients, either because they are unwilling to have surgery or because they are not candidates for surgery, may wear a truss, an apparatus that presses over the hernia and prevents protrusion of the bowel. Or the client lies in a supine position while manual pressure is applied over the protruding area to reduce the hernia periodically. Some clients learn to do this themselves.

A **herniorrhaphy,** the surgical repair of a hernia, is the recommended treatment. When a herniorrhaphy is performed, the protruding intestine is repositioned within the abdominal cavity, and the defect in the abdominal wall is repaired. Herniorrhaphy is performed under local, spinal, or general anesthesia.

When a hernia is neglected for many years, the tissues in the area weaken, and postoperative healing may be impaired. Obese people, who have put off surgical repair for a prolonged period, are especially prone to recurrence of the hernia, despite surgical repair. For these cases, the surgeon may also perform a **hernioplasty** in which the weakened area is reinforced with wire, fascia, or mesh. The obese client is generally advised to lose weight before the surgery to lessen the possibility of recurrence.

Strangulation is an acute emergency. Unless surgery is performed promptly, blood flow to the intestine is impaired. If necrosis occurs, the gangrenous part of the intestine must be excised and portions of the intestine reconnected.

NURSING MANAGEMENT

If the client is managing herniation with a truss, and not undergoing surgery, the nursing process consists primarily of teaching. Teach the client ways to avoiding constipation, control a cough, and perform proper body mechanics. Inform the client of the signs indicating hernial incarceration and strangulation. Explain how to wear a truss and how to observe for and treat skin irritation from friction caused by continuous rubbing. Advise the client to keep the skin clean and dry or use cornstarch to absorb moisture. Tell the client that compression from a truss may produce localized edema from interference with lymphatic and venous blood flow.

When surgery is scheduled, prepare the client and manage the postoperative care (see Chap. 24). Assess clients undergoing surgery by obtaining a complete medical and drug history because malnutrition, diabetes, or concurrent use of corticosteroids or antimetabolite cancer drugs can affect wound healing. Obtain the client's allergy history, especially to seasonal inhalants (ie, ragweed pollen), and smoking history because sneezing and coughing can increase intra-abdominal pressure postoperatively and place the client at risk for weakening the surgical repair. Take vital signs and auscultate the lungs to identify infectious or respiratory risk factors. Document the client's weight and length of time the hernia has been present because these factors influence the potential for postoperative healing complications. Review the client's previous surgical experience. Assess the client's urinary and bowel patterns to determine if the client has any pre-existing problems affecting elimination. Postoperatively, inspect the scrotum of male clients because it is common for edema to occur after a surgical repair.

Client and Family Teaching

Hernia repairs are performed mainly on an outpatient basis; therefore, home care measures are given to the client and significant other who will provide care after discharge. Accompany verbal with written instructions about signs and symptoms of possible complications (ie, urinary retention, bleeding, infection) and to report these symptoms to the physician. Advise applying an ice pack to the inguinal area to prevent or relieve scrotal swelling. Other alternatives include elevating the scrotum on a pillow or applying a scrotal suspensory support. Include techniques for avoiding constipation and straining to have a bowel movement. Provide instructions to avoid strenuous exertion and heavy lifting until the physician determines that such activities can be safely undertaken. For clients who perform heavy physical labor, explore how they may modify the manner in which they perform their jobs, take an extended sick leave, or apply for a temporary leave of absence. Explain to those whose work is sedentary or light that they usually can return to full employment with few activity restrictions within a few weeks.

Cancer of the Colon and Rectum

Intestinal malignancies occur anywhere in the lower GI tract. Approximately 75% develop in the lower sigmoid colon and rectum. Colorectal cancer ranks second among causes of cancer deaths in the United States. The incidence of the disease increases with age. The American Cancer Society recommends routine flexible sigmoidoscopy for colorectal cancer screening in individuals over 50 years of age. This screening may be done for younger clients who have risk factors, such as a family history of colorectal cancer or ulcerative colitis.

ETIOLOGY AND PATHOPHYSIOLOGY

Many malignant colorectal tumors develop from benign adenomas present in the mucosal and submucosal intestinal layers. It is believed that genetic, environmental, and lifestyle factors spark the transformation from a benign state to a cancerous one. Catalysts seem to include chronic bowel inflammation, as in ulcerative colitis, and a lifetime pattern of eating low-fiber, high-fat foods.

Having a blood relative with this disease is a high-risk factor. Researchers have recently discovered a gene related to a familial type of colon cancer. Other genetic markers may yet be identified.

At some point the normal cells undergo mutation, which affects their proliferation and growth pattern. Some believe that an *oncogene*, a genetic messenger that stimulates tumor growth, is not adequately suppressed. Without growth inhibition, the neoplastic cells reproduce at a rapid rate and later go on to invade the muscle wall. Other research suggests that a gene mutation interferes with the ability of colon cells to copy their DNA molecule correctly.

While the malignant growth remains in situ (confined to its site of origin), it may change the shape of the stool—compressing it or making it appear pencil-like as it passes by the protruding mass. Untreated, the cancer extends to other organs by way of the mesentery lymph nodes or portal vein leading to the liver.

ASSESSMENT FINDINGS

Signs and Symptoms

The chief characteristic of cancer of the colon is a change in bowel habits, such as alternating constipation and diarrhea. Occult or frank blood may be present in the stool. Sometimes a client may feel dull, vague abdominal discomfort. Pain is a late sign of cancer. On physical assessment, the abdomen feels distended and a mass may be palpated in the abdomen or rectum.

Diagnostic Findings

Genetic screening may detect chromosomal markers for particular types of colon cancer. An elevated carcinoembryonic antigen (CEA) test result suggests a tumor. Unfortunately, a CEA test is not effective in identifying colorectal cancer in its earliest, most treatable stages. Unless the malignant growths are elevated from the mucosal wall, a barium enema may not provide conclusive evidence either. A tissue sample taken during proctosigmoidoscopy or colonoscopy usually detects malignant cells. A complete blood count may show a low erythrocyte count from chronic blood loss.

MEDICAL AND SURGICAL MANAGEMENT

When polyps are discovered during endoscopic examination, they are removed and examined. Even if the polyps are benign, the client continues to undergo periodic radiographic and endoscopic examinations to identify recurrent polyps or early malignant changes.

The primary treatment of colorectal cancer is surgical, but sometimes treatment involves a combination of surgery, radiation therapy, and chemotherapy. A colorectal tumor that is encapsulated may be removed without removing surrounding healthy tissue although this type of tumor may call for partial or complete surgical removal of the colon (**colectomy**). Occasionally, the tumor causes a partial or complete bowel obstruction. If the tumor is in the colon and upper third of the rectum, a **segmental resection** is performed. Using this procedure the surgeon removes the cancerous portion of colon and rejoins the remaining portions of the GI tract to restore normal intestinal continuity. Cancers in the lower third of the rectum are treated with an **abdominoperineal resection**—wide excision of the rectum and creation of a sigmoid colostomy. The surgical procedures used to treat cancers in the middle third of the rectum vary. A low resection with a temporary colostomy is usually attempted to preserve the anal sphincter.

If the cancer metastasizes, a colostomy may be performed to relieve an intestinal obstruction. In some cases the obstruction is relieved or bleeding is controlled with laser surgery.

NURSING MANAGEMENT

Advise and prepare clients for routine colorectal screening. Follow standard guidelines for collecting stool specimens and sending them to the laboratory for analysis (Box 52–3). Advise anyone who is asymptomatic, but whose stool tests are positive for blood, to undergo a proctosigmoidoscopy, the next step in cancer detection. Nursing management of the client with a colostomy is discussed in Chapter 53.

Anorectal Disorders

Hemorrhoids

Hemorrhoids are dilated veins outside or inside the anal sphincter (Fig. 52–6). Thrombosed hemorrhoids are veins that contain clots.

BOX 52-3 Testing Stool for Occult Blood

Seven Days Before the Test and Throughout the Testing Period

- Do not drink alcohol, or take aspirin, nonsteroidal anti-inflammatory drugs, vitamin C, or iron preparations.
- Check with the physician if anticoagulants, steroids, colchicine, which is used to treat gout, or cimetidine for peptic ulcer treatment has been prescribed.

Two Days Before the Test and Throughout the Testing Period

- Consume a high-fiber diet.
- Avoid red meat; chicken, turkey, and fish may be substituted.
- Avoid turnips, cauliflower, broccoli, cantaloupe, horseradish, and parsnips.

When Performing the Screening Test

- Collect stool within a toilet liner or bedpan.
- Use an applicator stick and remove a sample from the center of the stool.
- Apply a thin smear of stool onto the test area supplied with the screening kit.
- Take care to cover the entire space.
- Place two drops of developer solution onto the test area.
- Wait precisely 60 seconds.
- Observe for a blue color, indicating a positive reaction.*

*For more valid results, samples from several stools should be tested over a 3- to 6-day period.

ETIOLOGY AND PATHOPHYSIOLOGY

Chronic straining to have a bowel movement or frequent defecation with chronic diarrhea likely weakens the tissue supporting the veins. Pregnancy, prolonged labor, portal hypertension, or other intra-abdominal conditions that interfere with venous blood return aggravate the condition.

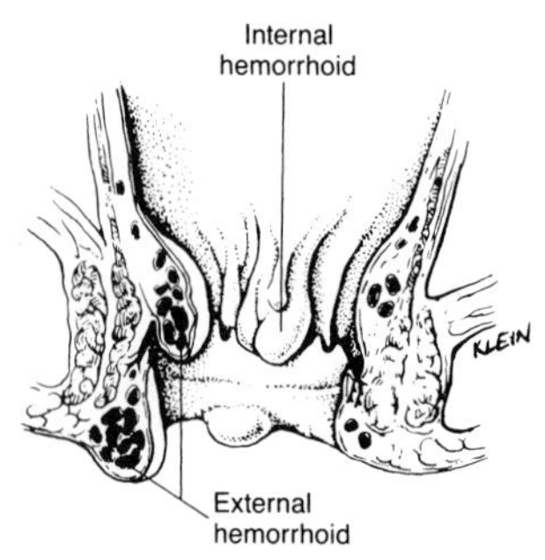

FIGURE 52-6. Internal and external hemorrhoids.

Probably, the veins near the anal sphincter are displaced downward from their natural location from a loss of supporting tissue. Without adequate connective tissue and smooth muscle support, the veins dilate and fill with blood. Dry stool passes by the engorged hemorrhoids and the mucosa is stretched and irritated giving rise to the local symptoms of burning, itching, and pain. Passing dry, hard stool causes the hemorrhoids to bleed.

ASSESSMENT FINDINGS

Signs and Symptoms

External hemorrhoids cause few symptoms, or they produce pain, itching, and soreness of the anal area. Internal hemorrhoids cause bleeding but are less likely to cause pain, unless they protrude through the anus. The amount of bleeding varies from an occasional drop or two of blood on toilet tissue or underwear to chronic loss of blood, leading to anemia. Thrombosed external hemorrhoids are painful but seldom cause bleeding.

External hemorrhoids appear as small, reddish blue lumps at the edge of the anus. Internal hemorrhoids usually protrude each time the client defecates but retract after defecation. As the masses grow larger, they remain outside the sphincter.

Diagnostic Findings

An anoscope, an instrument for examining the anal canal, or a proctosigmoidoscope allows visualization of internal hemorrhoids. A colonoscopy rules out colorectal cancer in which the symptoms are similar.

MEDICAL MANAGEMENT

Small external hemorrhoids may disappear without treatment, or the client may obtain relief through symptomatic treatment. The physician may recommend warm soaks, the application of an ointment that contains a local anesthetic for the relief of pain and itching, topical astringent pads to relieve swelling, a diet that corrects or prevents constipation, and a stool softener. In some cases the hemorrhoid is ligated (tied off) with a rubber band. Infrared photocoagulation, in which the protein and water in hemorrhoidal tissue is destroyed, is an alternative to traditional surgery.

SURGICAL MANAGEMENT

A **hemorrhoidectomy,** the removal of hemorrhoids, may be necessary in chronic and severe cases. The procedure is performed using conventional surgery or with laser surgery with the client receiving a local anesthetic or regional nerve block. An internal packing of lubricated gauze, external gauze dressing, or perineal pad is applied to absorb blood. A T-binder holds the absorbent material in place.

NURSING MANAGEMENT

Take a complete history, including drug and allergy histories. Because bleeding accompanies many colorectal disorders, ask the client to describe the bleeding as well as other related symptoms. Determine if there is a history of constipation or alternating diarrhea and constipation, and if any prescription or nonprescription drugs are used to treat the problem. Obtain a diet history, with particular attention to the type of foods (especially fiber) included in the diet. Put on gloves, drape the client, and inspect the anus. Take vital signs and determine whether the temperature is elevated. The nursing care of a client after anorectal surgery includes, but is not limited to, the following:

Nursing Diagnoses and Collaborative Problems	Nursing Interventions
Pain related to inflammation, swelling, impaired tissue integrity **Goal:** The client will report a reduction in pain within 30 minutes of nursing interventions.	Give prescribed analgesics to control pain. Medicate the client before performing a painful procedure (ie, removing wound packing). Advise client to lie prone or on the side to promote comfort. Apply a covered ice pack to the rectum. Provide a soft cushion for the client to sit on. The chair should not be so deep or low that the client must bear down when arising. Prevent pain with defecation by providing a liberal intake of fluids, a prescribed stool softener, and dietary fiber. Assist the client with a warm sitz bath especially after bowel elimination. Apply topical anesthetics or astringents, if prescribed.
Constipation or Risk for Constipation related to anticipated pain on defecation **Goal:** The client will develop or maintain regular and effortless bowel elimination.	Advise client to modify dietary habits, increase exercise, and drink adequate fluids. Administer a prescribed stool softener. Allow privacy and sufficient time for bowel elimination.
Risk for Infection related to contact between impaired tissue and bowel organisms. **Goal:** The client will be free of infection related to hemorrhoidectomy.	Keep the rectal area clean and dry. Wear gloves to change dressings using aseptic technique and to act as a barrier to bloody drainage. Advise client and health care team to wash hands before and after using the bathroom and after performing care.
Urinary Retention related to perianal tenderness **Goal:** The client will empty the bladder when it becomes full.	Assist client to the bathroom. Help male clients to stand at the toilet when the bladder becomes distended. Run water. The sound helps the client relax the urinary sphincter. Or have the client press over the bladder or bend from the waist to trigger relaxation of the urinary sphincter. If needed, consult the physician about inserting a straight catheter or administering a short-acting cholinergic drug, such as bethanechol (Duvoid, Urecholine).

Client and Family Teaching

Provide health teaching, as follows:

- Review the physician's home care instructions with the client.
- Demonstrate wound care to the client or responsible caregiver and provide an opportunity for returning the demonstration.
- To avoid constipation, provide dietary recommendations and offer a list of high-fiber foods.
- Emphasize the importance of an active lifestyle and increased fluid intake.
- Caution the client against the prolonged use of laxatives.
- To avoid transferring infectious microorganisms in the home, suggest using a liquid soap instead of bar soap. Remind everyone to use separate bath towels and washcloths.

Anorectal Abscess

An anorectal abscess is an infection with a collection of pus within an area between the internal and external sphincters.

ETIOLOGY AND PATHOPHYSIOLOGY

The original source of the infection may be microorganisms harbored within the intestine itself. This is a common finding among clients with Crohn's disease. However, anorectal infections also are transmitted from others through anal intercourse or from foreign bodies inserted into the rectum.

Generally, infectious microorganisms invade anal crypts, small tubular cavities within the anal skin and rectal mucosa. A purulent exudate collects and the pressure causes pain and swelling. The abscess may eventually develop into a fistulous tract.

ASSESSMENT FINDINGS

Signs and Symptoms

Clients with an anorectal abscess experience pain that is aggravated by walking and sitting or other activities that increase intra-abdominal pressure such as coughing, sneezing, and straining to have a bowel movement. A swollen mass is evident within the anus. Fever and abdominal pain develop if the abscess has extended into deeper tissues. Foul-smelling drainage may leak from the anus if the abscess spontaneously ruptures.

Diagnostic Findings

A culture of anal drainage reveals the infectious microorganism.

MEDICAL AND SURGICAL MANAGEMENT

Analgesics and sitz baths are prescribed to relieve symptoms. Antibiotic therapy is used to treat gonorrheal, staphylococcal, streptococcal, or other drug-sensitive bacteria. An incision and drainage to remove the infected material may be necessary. If a fistula has formed, deeper excision and removal of the fistulous tract are necessary.

NURSING MANAGEMENT

To limit the spread of infectious microorganisms, recommend scrupulous handwashing after a bowel movement, the use of separate hygiene articles, cleansing of the bath tub after each use, and the application of a condom if having anal intercourse. Refer to the nursing management of a client with hemorrhoids for additional nursing interventions.

Anal Fissure

An anal **fissure** (fissure in ano) is a linear tear in anal tissue. The fissure tends to ulcerate.

ETIOLOGY AND PATHOPHYSIOLOGY

Constipation is the leading cause of anal fissures. Other factors that may lead to producing a slitlike tear include eversion of the anus during vaginal delivery, and trauma to the anus, for example, during anal intercourse. When the anal canal is excessively stretched, the skin rips apart, exposing the underlying tissue.

ASSESSMENT FINDINGS

Signs and Symptoms

Severe pain and bleeding on defecation are common. If constipation was not an original problem, it becomes one; most clients with an anal fissure are reluctant to defecate because of the associated pain. The torn area may be visible when the anus is visually inspected, and the irregular surface of the fissure may be felt during a digital examination.

Diagnostic Findings

Anoscopy provides evidence of the altered integrity of the anal mucosa.

MEDICAL AND SURGICAL MANAGEMENT

Treatment includes applying anesthetic creams, ointments, or suppositories; taking sitz baths and analgesics; and preventing constipation. Surgical excision of the area may be necessary.

NURSING MANAGEMENT

Teach the client how to insert a suppository, how to take a sitz bath, and how to relieve constipation. Refer to the nursing management of a client with hemorrhoids for a discussion of postsurgical care of a client with an anorectal disorder.

Anal Fistula

An anal **fistula** (fistula in ano) is a tract that forms within the anal canal.

ETIOLOGY AND PATHOPHYSIOLOGY

When an anorectal abscess does not heal adequately, an inflamed tunnel develops connecting the area of the original abscess with perianal skin (Fig. 52–7). Purulent material drains from the opening.

ASSESSMENT FINDINGS

Signs and Symptoms

The client reports pain on defecation. The opening of the fistula appears red and pus leaks from the external opening of the fistula or can be expressed if the area is compressed. If the fistula is superficial, it feels cordlike on palpation.

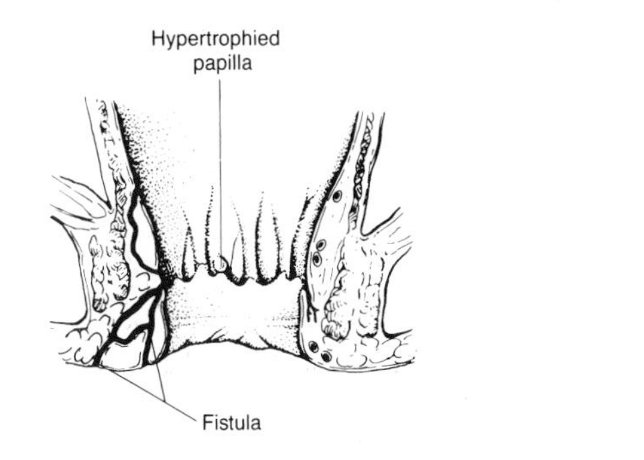

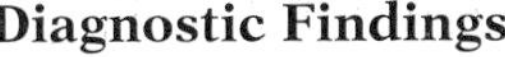

FIGURE 52-7. Anal fistula.

Diagnostic Findings

A proctosigmoidoscopy or colonoscopy may identify an IBD, such as Crohn's disease, which predisposes the client to an anorectal abscess or anal fistula.

SURGICAL MANAGEMENT

The entire fistula is opened (**fistulotomy**) with a guidewire to promote a continuous open pathway for drainage in two directions. In some cases it is necessary to remove the fistulous tract (**fistulectomy**). A stool softener and antibiotic may be prescribed.

NURSING MANAGEMENT

Teach the client to self-administer medications, to keep the anal region clean, and to avoid transferring microorganisms to other hygiene articles used in common with family members (ie, bar soap). For surgical nursing care, refer to the nursing management section that accompanies the discussion of clients with hemorrhoids.

Pilonidal Sinus

Pilonidal means "a nest of hair." The terms **pilonidal sinus** and *pilonidal cyst* are both used to describe the condition. A pilonidal sinus is actually an infection in hair follicles in the sacrococcygeal area above the anus (Fig. 52–8). However, other local infections, such as osteomyelitis and furuncles of the skin, have common presenting signs and symptoms and must be ruled out.

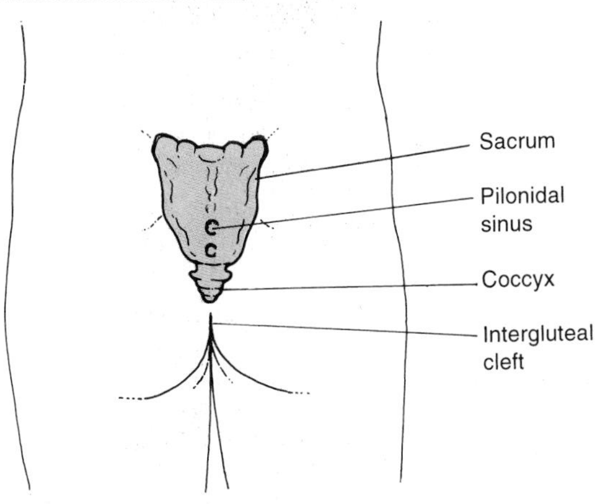

FIGURE 52-8. A pilonidal sinus may appear as a hairy dimple in the skin. It may not cause symptoms unless or until an infection occurs.

ETIOLOGY AND PATHOPHYSIOLOGY

The condition typically occurs after puberty. People who have a deep intergluteal cleft and those who have abundant hair in the perianal and lower back regions are predisposed to the condition. Inadequate personal hygiene, obesity, and trauma to the area also contribute to its development.

A sinus or cyst begins to form when the skin deep in the cleft softens due to being chronically moist. Stiff hairs then irritate and pierce the soft, macerated skin, becoming embedded in it. The irritation inflames the tissues. Infection readily follows because the break in the skin permits the entrance of microorganisms. Several channels may lead from the sinus to the skin.

ASSESSMENT FINDINGS

Signs and Symptoms

Pain and swelling at the base of the spine and purulent drainage occur. On inspection, the sinus opening may be located within the gluteal fold. Dilated pits of the hair follicles within the sinus are a unique characteristic.

SURGICAL MANAGEMENT

The abscess is drained and the tissue is incised. The sinus and all its connecting channels are laid open, and purulent material and hair are removed. Packing is inserted into the cavity and the wound heals by secondary intention. In some cases, the wound edges are approximated. However, healing by primary intention sometimes allows the purulent material to reform and collect, causing another abscess. Because the infection is localized, systemic antibiotics are not generally prescribed.

NURSING MANAGEMENT

Teach the client how to minimize discomfort and facilitate bowel elimination postoperatively. As appropriate, tell a family member how to remove the packing, clean the incised tissue, and redress the area.

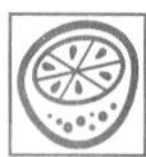

General Nutritional Considerations

A high-fiber diet is a vague term that does not quantify or qualify fiber content. Daily guidelines call for consuming between 6 and 11 servings of breads, cereals, and grains. This includes several servings of high-fiber bread (at least 2–5 g fiber/serving) and a serving of high-fiber cereal (at least 5 g fiber/serving).

Consume about one-half cup dried peas or beans (legumes) daily. They are a low-fat, high-fiber alternative to meat protein.

Take in between two and four servings of fruit daily. Most of the fiber is contained in the skin and seeds; fresh whole fruit is higher in fiber than canned fruit or fruit juice.

Eat between three and five servings of vegetables daily. The less peeling and scraping, the higher the fiber content. Because vegetables vary greatly in their fiber content, choose a variety.

Add coarse unprocessed wheat bran, a natural laxative, to the diet slowly. Start with 1 teaspoon daily and work up to 2 to 3 tablespoons daily to decrease the likelihood of flatus, distention, cramping, and diarrhea. Wheat bran can be mixed with juice or milk; added to muffins, quick bread, casseroles; and sprinkled over cereal, applesauce or other foods.

An excellent source of readily absorbed calcium for clients who are lactose intolerant is calcium-fortified orange juice. An 8-oz glass provides approximately the same amount of calcium as an 8-oz glass of milk, plus a significant amount of folic acid, potassium, and vitamin C.

Encourage client with diarrhea to consume potassium-rich foods as tolerated. These include bananas, canned apricots and peaches, apricot nectar, orange juice, grapefruit juice, tomato juice, fish, potatoes, and meat.

For clients with diverticulosis, a high-fiber diet excludes foods with husks and seeds (nuts, popcorn, cucumbers, strawberries, raspberries, tomatoes, corn, and breads containing sesame or poppy seeds) because they become trapped in the diverticula. In addition to lactose intolerance, some clients with Crohn's disease develop wheat or gluten intolerances during exacerbations of the disease, further complicating nutritional management.

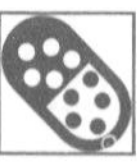

General Pharmacologic Considerations

Narcotics and sedatives decrease peristalsis and can result in constipation. Assess bowel function daily. A stool softener may be required to minimize the constipating effects of these drugs.

Habitual use of laxatives can decrease muscle tone in the large intestine resulting in constipation.

The misconception that a daily bowel movement is necessary may contribute to the overuse of laxatives.

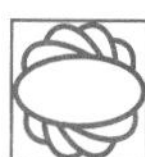

General Gerontologic Considerations

Constipation is a common problem in the older adult, and often is due to inadequate intake of dietary fiber, lack of exercise, and decreased fluid intake.

Older adults are encouraged to schedule regular health examinations, including screenings for colorectal cancer, because its incidence increases with age.

With age, peristaltic action of the GI tract decreases; therefore, the risk for constipation in the older adult increases.

Constipation can occur in an older adult who feels rushed when defecating or who is unable to get to the toilet in time.

An older adult with prolonged constipation, or one who goes from constipation to diarrhea, must be checked for a fecal impaction.

Older adults with appendicitis may not display the type of acute pain that younger individuals experience. Severe pain may be absent, minimal, or referred in the older adult, causing a delay in diagnosis and a greater incidence of complications.

SUMMARY OF KEY CONCEPTS

- Constipation can result from emotional stress, drugs that slow gastric motility, low fluid intake, low dietary fiber, laxative abuse, inactivity, and voluntary control of defecation.
- Diarrhea is associated with emotional stress, intestinal infections, malabsorptive and inflammatory disorders, food allergies, the rapid addition of fiber to the diet, misuse of laxatives, and side effects of drugs.
- Several differences distinguish Crohn's disease and ulcerative colitis. Crohn's disease may occur along any part of the GI tract, from mouth to anus, and inflammation may be transmural. Perianal complications are common and the risk for development of colorectal cancer is only slightly above that of the normal population. Ulcerative colitis involves only the colon, and inflammation is restricted to the mucosal layer. Perianal complications are rare and the risk for development of colorectal cancer is increased.
- When surgery is performed for the client with Crohn's disease, it only relieves complications, whereas it is considered curative for clients with ulcerative colitis.
- Appendicitis and peritonitis are two common acute inflammatory abdominal disorders. Appendicitis is a localized inflammation in a narrow, blind protrusion at the tip of the cecum. Peritonitis is a life-threatening complication that results when the peritoneal lining becomes inflamed.
- Intestinal obstructions may occur when the bowel is handled during abdominal surgery, secondarily to inflammatory conditions such as peritonitis, as a side effect of drugs (ie, narcotics or cholinergic blocking agents), from tumors, impacted feces or barium, adhesions, incarcerated hernia, volvulus, and intussusception.
- The Miller-Abbott, Cantor, and Harris tubes are used for intestinal decompression. The nurse is responsible for

preparing the client and assisting the physician with inserting, monitoring, and advancing the tube once it is in the stomach; assessing and maintaining its function; and removing it when the client's condition improves.

- Diverticulosis is a condition in which saclike pouches develop within the intestinal mucosa. Diverticulitis occurs when the diverticula become inflamed.
- Abdominal hernias commonly develop in the inguinal, femoral, umbilical, and incisional areas. They form during situations that increase intra-abdominal pressure, such as when lifting a heavy object, in places where the abdominal wall is weak.
- Warning signs of colorectal cancer include a change in bowel habits, passing blood in the stool, change in the shape of stool, and vague abdominal discomfort. Groups that are at risk for developing colorectal cancer include older adults, individuals who have a blood relative with the disease, those who have ulcerative colitis, and those who consume a high-fat, low-fiber diet.
- Five common anorectal disorders are hemorrhoids, anorectal abscess, anal fissure, anal fistula, and pilonidal sinus. Individuals with these problems commonly have rectal discomfort, a tendency toward constipation, and a potential for infection.

CRITICAL THINKING EXERCISES

1. The admitting department notifies the nursing unit to expect a client with ulcerative colitis. Based on the characteristics of the disease process, what assessments are essential to obtain at the time of admission?
2. As you assist an older adult with using a bedpan, you notice blood on the toilet tissue. What other data are appropriate to gather at this time?
3. What information is important to provide for a client who will shortly have a Miller-Abbott tube inserted?

Suggested Readings

Cox, J. (1995). Inflammatory bowel disease: Implications for the medical-surgical nurse. *MEDSURG Nursing, 4*(6), 427–437.

Lutz, B. H. (1996). Client challenge. Total parenteral nutrition in the older patient. *Home Healthcare Nurse, 14*(2), 123–125.

Hammerhofer-Jereb, K. (1996). Laparoscopic bowel resection? *RN, 59*(3), 22–25.

Marchiondo, K. (1994). When the Dx is diverticular disease. *RN, 57*(2), 42–47.

McConnell, E. A. (1996). Myths and facts about laparoscopic inguinal herniorrhaphy. *Nursing, 26*(9), 24j.

Ness, W. (1994). Silent problem. *Nursing Times, 90*(36), 67–68, 70.

Self-test. (1996). Understanding the gastrointestinal system...intestinal obstruction, pancreatitis, and hepatic encephalopathy. *Nursing, 26*(3), 28–29.

Warmkessel, J. H. (1997). Caring for a patient with colon cancer. *Nursing, 27*(4), 34–40.

Waterhouse, M. (1996). Why pain assessment must start with believing the patient. *Nursing Times, 92*(38), 42–43.

Additional Resources

National Foundation for Ileitis and Colitis
Crohn's and Colitis Foundation of America (CCFA)
386 Park Avenue South
17th floor
New York, NY 10016–8804
(800) 932–2423
http://www.ccfa.org/

Chapter 53

Caring for Clients With an Ileostomy or Colostomy

KEY TERMS

Abdominoperineal resection
Appliance
Colostomy
Continent ileostomy (Kock pouch)
Conventional ileostomy
Double-barrel colostomy
Enterostomal therapist
Ileoanal reservoir (anastomosis)
Ileostomy
Loop colostomy
Ostomate
Ostomy
Segmental resection
Single-barrel colostomy
Stoma

LEARNING OBJECTIVES

On completion of this chapter, the reader will:

- Identify and describe two types of intestinal ostomy procedures.
- Discuss the preoperative nursing preparation of a client undergoing ostomy surgery.
- List four complications associated with ostomy surgery.
- Describe the components used to apply and collect stool from an intestinal ostomy.
- Cite three reasons for changing an ostomy appliance.
- Describe how to change an ostomy appliance.
- Explain how stool is released from a continent ileostomy.
- Describe the two-part procedure that is performed when an ileoanal reservoir is created.
- List various types of colostomies.
- Explain three ways that clients with descending or sigmoid colostomies may regulate bowel elimination.

The term **ostomy** refers to an opening between an internal structure of the body and the skin. The most common intestinal ostomies are the **ileostomy**, an opening from the distal small intestine, and the **colostomy**, an opening from the colon (Table 53–1). Fecal material exits through a **stoma**, an opening on the exterior surface of the abdomen. Most ostomies are created in response to an inflammatory bowel disorder that fails to respond to medical treatment or complications such as rupture of a portion of intestine, irreversible obstruction, compromised blood supply to the intestine, or cancerous tumor.

Whether an ostomy is temporary or permanent, each client requires a plan of care adapted to the individual. The plan of care incorporates the client's preparation for surgery, recovery from surgery, and knowledge required for self-care.

Conventional Ileostomy

In the usual surgical procedure for a **conventional ileostomy**, the entire colon and rectum (total colectomy) are removed. The terminal end of the ileum is brought out through a separate area on the lower right quadrant of the abdomen slightly below the umbilicus, near the outer border of the rectus muscle (Fig. 53–1). The cut end is everted and sutured to the skin, a process referred to as creating a "matured" stoma.

When a conventional ileostomy is performed, stool and gas are continually released from the stoma. Fecal material discharged from an ileostomy is liquid or pastelike and contains digestive enzymes. The matured stoma promotes healing and provides a smooth peristomal area permitting the immediate postopera-

TABLE 53-1 **Types of Intestinal Ostomies**

Type	Stoma Location	Fecal Consistency	Fecal Control
Conventional ileostomy	Lower abdomen	Liquid	Never
Continent ileostomy	Lower abdomen	Liquid	By siphoning
Ascending colostomy	Middle right abdomen	Semiliquid	Never
Transverse colostomy	Center of the abdomen below the belt line	Semiliquid	Never
Descending colostomy	Middle left abdomen	Soft	Sometimes
Sigmoid colostomy	Lower left abdomen	Formed	Usually

tive application of an **appliance**, the collection device worn over a stoma. Clients with a conventional ileostomy wear an appliance at all times, and the appliance requires frequent emptying.

The Ostomy Appliance

Ostomy suppliers provide a variety of appliances to meet the individual needs of the **ostomate**. Basically all appliances consist of one-piece or two-piece devices that contain a pouch for collecting feces and a faceplate, or disk, that is attached to the abdomen with an opening through which the stoma protrudes (Fig. 53–2). The faceplate either adheres to the skin with a self-adhesive backing or requires other bonding substances such as an adhesive powder, paste, or wafer. Karaya gum is a common component in ostomy supplies. It becomes gelatinous when in contact with moisture and is used in place of an adhesive. This substance protects the skin as well as promote adhesion of the ostomy appliance. Karaya gum rings are used around the stoma. They are pulled or pushed into any shape and are ideal for correcting problems created by an ill-fitting appliance. Unlike rings made of rigid material, a karaya gum ring fits snugly around the stoma without injuring it.

A disposable, or temporary, appliance is preferred in the immediate postoperative phase because the size of the stoma continues to change, sometimes from one change of the appliance to the next. After the stoma heals and reaches its final size and shape, a permanent (reusable) appliance is fitted. Reusable equipment consists of a sturdier pouch with a custom-sized faceplate and "O" ring. The pouch is designed to fasten into position when pressed over the ring, much like snapping a lid on a plastic margarine tub. The pouch has a clamp at the bottom, which can be released when the pouch needs to be emptied. The pouch is fastened to a belt for more security. The belt supports the weight of the liquid fecal material and prevents the faceplate from being pulled away from the skin of the abdomen. Foam rubber, gauze, or flannel padding is placed under a belt if the belt cuts into the flesh. The client requires two sets of permanent appliances so that one can be cleaned periodically.

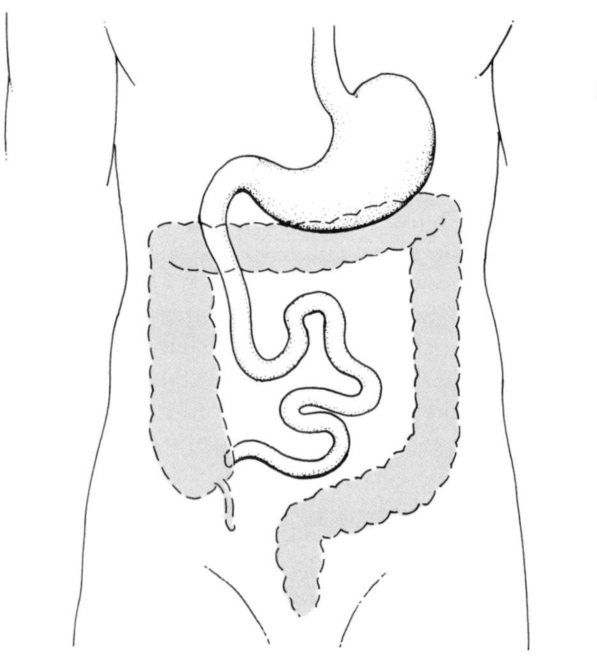

FIGURE 53-1. A conventional ileostomy.

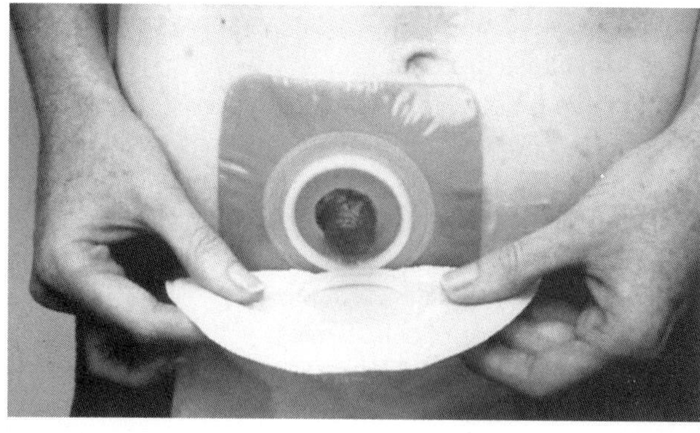

FIGURE 53-2. The ostomy appliance consists of an adhesive faceplate around the stoma and a collecting pouch. (Courtesy of Convatec, Princeton, NJ)

Preoperative Period

SURGICAL MANAGEMENT

Preoperatively, the physician explains the purpose for the surgical procedure along with its benefits and risks. The appearance and function of the stoma, where the stoma will be placed, and what is involved in its care are described. Potential risks from the total colectomy, such as bladder and sexual dysfunction due to possible parasympathetic nerve injury, are identified. Young male clients may wish to collect and store sperm for later use if children are desired.

If the client has been taking a corticosteroid before admission, the dose and frequency of administration are gradually reduced during the preoperative, intraoperative, and postoperative periods. Steroids interfere with healing but should not be discontinued abruptly. An antibiotic such as neomycin sulfate (Mycifradin) or kanamycin (Kantrex) is prescribed preoperatively to decrease the number of bacteria in the bowel and decrease the possibility of infection. Small meals of low-residue foods or liquids are recommended to reduce the fecal volume. The client's blood is typed and crossmatched so that blood transfusions may be given preoperatively to restore losses from gastrointestinal (GI) bleeding or to replace surgical blood loss. A bowel cleansing routine may be necessary to reduce the risk of infection by fecal contamination. This may be accomplished with laxatives, cleansing enemas, or administration of an intestinal lavage solution (ie, GoLYTELY, Colyte)

NURSING MANAGEMENT

Obtain complete medical, allergy, diet, and drug histories, especially of currently prescribed drugs. Evaluate the client's general physical and emotional status. Get a description of preoperative preparations the client may have been asked to perform, such as dietary modifications and antibiotic therapy. Perform a physical assessment with particular attention to inspecting the skin over the abdomen and auscultating bowel sounds. Document the client's vital signs and weight. Check the presurgical laboratory test results to determine if the blood cell counts and serum electrolytes are within normal ranges.

Closely monitor the client who has been treated with corticosteroids for signs and symptoms of adrenal insufficiency such as weakness, lethargy, hypotension, nausea, and vomiting as dosages are tapered (refer to the discussion of adrenal crisis in Chap. 56). Maintain nutritional and fluid support. Just before surgery, implement the medical orders for cleansing the bowel, inserting a nasogastric tube, and preparing the client for surgery.

Before surgery, the plan of nursing care includes, but is not limited to, the following:

Nursing Diagnoses and Collaborative Problems	Nursing Interventions
Risk for Infection related to malnutrition, suppressed inflammatory response secondary to corticosteroid therapy, surgically opening the intestine **Goal:** The client will remain free of infection.	Administer dietary support until food is restricted. Monitor temperature frequently, especially in clients receiving corticosteroids because they are at risk for infections and delayed wound healing. Observe for signs and symptoms of infection: wound drainage, pain, abdominal distention and increased pulse and respiratory rates. (The immunosuppressed client may not demonstrate a "typical" response to infection.) Wash hands before giving direct care. Protect client from visitors or health workers with infections. Screen potential roommates for infection.
Anxiety related to unfamiliarity with surgery and potential change in body image, bowel elimination, lifestyle **Goal:** The client will experience a reduction in anxiety.	Provide an overview of surgical preparations, explaining each procedure before it is performed to reduce the client's insecurity. Implement therapeutic communication techniques. Facilitate contact with the client's support system (family, clergy, close friends).
Risk for Ineffective Individual Coping related to potential change in body image **Goal:** The client will implement healthy coping techniques.	Arrange a visit with a member of a local ostomy organization, as appropriate and desired. This person can provide reassurance and practical information about living with an ostomy. Identify the following for the ostomy volunteer: type of visit (preoperative, postoperative, or both); the client's age, occupation, gender, physical handicaps (if any), and primary language (if other than English); and any information related to rehabilitation. Review printed materials from the ostomy association with the client. Answer questions that arise following the visit.

Client and Family Teaching

Health care teams hold several views about beginning ostomy instructions in the preoperative period. Some believe that this helps the client to accept the ostomy; others believe that this type of teaching creates premature stress and anxiety. Ostomy instruction, whether it is given preoperatively or postoperatively, is often provided by an **enterostomal therapist**. An enterostomal therapist is a nurse who has been certified to care for ostomates and manage their unique problems. The enterostomal therapist is an excellent resource for nurses providing direct care to ostomates. If the client expresses a readiness to learn or asks questions about ostomy care, provide information covering ostomy equipment and general principles of ostomy management. Arrange a preoperative visit with the enterostomal therapist.

Postoperative Period

SURGICAL MANAGEMENT

The rectum is packed with gauze during surgery to absorb drainage and promote gradual healing. The rectal pack is usually removed in 5 to 7 days. Afterward, irrigations may be ordered to promote healing. A nasogastric tube is used for GI decompression until normal bowel motility resumes. Fluid, electrolyte, and nutritional balances are maintained with intravenous (IV) fluids until oral nourishment is possible. Within several days, the nasogastric tube is removed and oral feedings begin. Antibiotic therapy continues into the postoperative period. Analgesics are prescribed for pain relief. Wound healing is monitored and complications that develop are managed.

Possible postoperative complications include intestinal obstruction, impaired blood supply to the stoma, stenosis of the stoma, and prolapse or excessive protrusion of the stoma. Intestinal obstruction is a serious complication. It may result from a twisted, strangulated, or incarcerated segment of the remaining intestine or a bolus of poorly chewed or inadequately digested food. When a collection of food causes obstruction, the physician may attempt to correct the problem by irrigating the stoma. If the bowel is twisted or strangulated, surgical intervention is necessary.

Prolapse or protrusion of the ileostomy is fairly common. If it is moderate (1 or 2 inches), no treatment is required. A severe prolapse of the stoma is a serious complication, however. If edema occurs, it may cause an obstruction and restrict stomal blood supply. Stomal necrosis results if the prolapse is not promptly and skillfully managed. Once the stoma prolapses, recurrence is likely.

NURSING PROCESS
The Client Recovering From Ostomy Surgery

Assessment

Review the medical record for information regarding the type of surgery and any problems encountered during surgery or immediately afterward. Perform routine postoperative assessments: Check vital signs and inspect the dressing and stoma (Table 53–2). Monitor the rate and progress of fluid and blood infusions. Check the function of the gastric suction. Measure intake and output. Inspect the collection appliance, special drains, packing, or tubes. Record all immediate postoperative findings to provide a data base. For a step-by-step discussion of how to replace an ostomy appliance, see Nursing Guidelines 53–1.

The postoperative nursing care plan, which includes standard pain (Chap. 20) and postsurgical interventions (Chap. 24), also includes, but is not limited to, the following:

Nursing Diagnoses and Collaborative Problems	Nursing Interventions
Risk for Altered Tissue Perfusion related to insufficient blood supply to stoma **Goal:** The client will have an adequate blood supply to the stoma.	Inspect the color of the stoma frequently. Report darkening of the stoma immediately. Measure the size of the stoma, using a gauge at each appliance change and be sure to allow an extra 1/8 inch in the appliance opening for clearance and potential swelling. Remove the appliance immediately if the client experiences discomfort; replace it with one with a larger opening.
Impaired Skin Integrity related to effect of fecal material and adhesives on the skin **Goal:** The client will maintain intact peristomal skin.	Frequently empty the ostomy appliance to avoid tension on the skin from the weight of drainage. Maintain skin integrity by gently removing the current ostomy appliance, providing fastidious skin and stomal care, and properly reapplying the appliance.
Bowel Incontinence related to absence of sphincter control, leakage from appliance **Goal:** Leaking and soiling with stool will be avoided.	Keep the appliance or collection device securely over the stoma at all times. Select an appliance that can be secured with a waist belt. Experiment with various adhesive products to find one that best prevents leakage.

Nursing Diagnosis	Interventions
	Use any of the following measures to prevent leaking: • Press the adhesive faceplate to the skin from the stomal edge outward to avoid forming wrinkles. • Ask the client to remain inactive for 5 minutes to allow time for the body heat to strengthen the adhesive bond. • Trap some air within the pouch so that the liquid feces drains to the bottom. • Make several pinhole-sized punctures at the upper edge of the pouch to allow gas to escape. • Requisition a sufficient supply of ostomy equipment to have on hand at all times. • Consult with an enterostomal therapist for difficult problems.
Risk for Infection related to fecal contamination of the surgical wound **Goal:** The client will be free of infection.	Apply dressing securely to protect incision from contact with fecal drainage. Change the ostomy pouch when it loosens. Clean away drainage that leaks near the incision.
Risk for Altered Sexuality Patterns related to anxiety concerning change in body image **Goal:** The client will plan modifications for maintaining sexual fulfillment.	Encourage men with sexual dysfunction to use methods, other than intercourse, to communicate their passion and sexually satisfy their partner. Reassure the client whose sexual function is unaffected by surgery that intercourse will not harm the healed ostomy.
Anxiety related to insecurity over results of surgery, change in bowel elimination, care of the stoma, soiling, and other changes **Goal:** The client will experience reduced anxiety.	Convey a calm and empathic attitude. Respect a reluctant client's initial refusal to look at the stoma, much less care for it. Confirm that stool is released unpredictably but that the volume is higher after consuming food; some soiling is inevitable soon after surgery until the intestine adapts to the altered anatomy; and volume will eventually decrease. Ensure that the appliance is secure. Change dressings and bedding promptly without showing any repulsion. Keep the room odor free by emptying the ostomy pouch frequently. Explain other methods for controlling odor, such as taking nonprescription chlorophyll compounds and putting charcoal into the ostomy pouch (ingested charcoal inhibits the absorption of oral drugs).
Body Image Disturbance related to perceived significance of surgical changes **Goal:** The client will accept changes in body image.	Allow the client time to grieve his or her loss. Help the client to gradually accept change. Do not coerce the client into looking at the surgical site; rather, describe the appearance of the stoma. Have the client participate in care in a minor way, such as cutting the opening in the faceplate. Gradually involve the client in more and more activities. Treat the altered bowel elimination as just a unique physical characteristic. Reassure the client that everyday clothing usually conceals the stoma and ostomy pouch completely.
Ineffective Individual Coping related to disturbed body image **Goal:** The client will cope effectively with body changes.	Ensure privacy when caring for the stoma. Do not disagree with or scold the client who expresses negative feelings; just listen patiently. Discuss with the client how the surgery may (in some cases) now permit activities that were impossible before. Point out signs of progress. Role-play scenarios that the client expects to be problematic. Meet with the client's partner separately so that he or she can express feelings and receive encouragement and support. Encourage contact with members of an ostomy support group.

Evaluation and Expected Outcomes

- Stoma appears red and shiny.
- Peristomal skin appears much like abdominal skin without redness or burning sensations.
- Stool is contained within ostomy pouch.
- Incision heals without infection.
- Client expects to resume sexual activity.
- Client openly discusses feelings and concerns with others (the nurse, family members, physician, visiting ostomates).
- Client observes ostomy care and participates, showing gradual acceptance of surgical alteration.
- In words and action, client develops a positive attitude toward resuming a normal life.

TABLE 53-2 **Characteristics of Healthy and Unhealthy Stomas**

Characteristics	Healthy Stoma	Unhealthy Stoma
Color	Bright pink or red	Dusky blue or black
Size	Comparable in diameter to the intestine from which it has been formed; may be somewhat large after surgery due to edema	Larger or smaller in comparison to size following resolution of postoperative edema
Opening	Patent, unobstructed	Tight or narrow
Surface	Moist, shiny with an overlying layer of mucus; may bleed slightly when being cleansed	Dull, dry; excessive bleeding
Length	Protrudes from or is just flush with the skin	Protrudes beyond 2 inches from the skin or retracts beneath it
Sensation	Painless	Peristomal burning
Function	Regular passage of feces	Sparse or absent elimination of feces

Client and Family Teaching

In logical steps and at a pace that allows for comprehension, teach the client and another family member about managing the ostomy, adopting dietary modifications, recognizing how drug therapy affects bowel elimination, and adjusting to various surgery-related changes, such as possible sexual dysfunction (Box 53–1). Additional aspects to include in the teaching plan include:

- Restricting oral intake only with medical supervision
- Eating slowly and chewing food well with the mouth closed to help lessen the development of gas
- Avoiding foods that cause discomfort, excessive gas, or loose stools
- Drinking extra fluids, especially in warm weather
- Dilating the stoma if the volume of stool decreases for some unexplained reason. To do this, cut the nail on the index or little finger, cover the finger with a finger cot, lubricate it thoroughly, then insert the finger gently into the stoma for a few minutes.
- Cleaning the pouch *thoroughly* to prevent odors
- Using an internal odor-absorbing substance or one that can be added to the pouch to control lingering or stubborn odors
- Using an old pouch or disposable pouch when medications or offending foods that cause disagreeable odors are excreted
- Slipping a plastic cover over the pouch to act as a second barrier against escaping odors
- Checking with a physician before self-administering any drug, especially a laxative or antidiarrheal

Continent Ileostomy (Kock Pouch)

A **continent ileostomy** or **Kock pouch** is the creation of an internal reservoir for the storage of GI effluent (discharged fecal material or liquid feces). The reservoir stores this effluent until the client removes it with a catheter. This eliminates the need for an external appliance.

SURGICAL MANAGEMENT

After removing the diseased portion of the ileum, the surgeon forms a reservoir with a portion of the terminal ileum and creates a nipple valve by telescoping (intussusception) the distal ileal segment into the reservoir. The surgeon then forms a permanent external stoma and anchors it to the abdominal wall (Fig. 53–3).

During the operation, the surgeon inserts a temporary catheter through the nipple valve and sutures the catheter in place so that its end protrudes from the external stoma. Then the surgeon packs the perineal area from which the lower intestine was removed with gauze. The packing remains in place for about 1 week.

NURSING MANAGEMENT

Reinforce the perineal packing, as needed, during the postoperative period. Check the abdominal dressing for drainage. Connect the stomal catheter, if ordered, to low, intermittent suction that empties the reservoir continuously, thereby preventing tension on healing suture lines. Check the ileal catheter frequently for signs of obstruction, that is, lack of fecal drainage or the client's complaint of feeling full in the area of the ileal pouch, or leakage of liquid stool around the catheter. Note the color and amount of drainage. Observe the size and color of the stoma. According to the written orders of the surgeon, administer either routine or as needed irrigations of the ileal catheter with small amounts of normal saline solution if the catheter appears to be obstructed. Keep the skin clean around the stoma. Change the gauze dressing over the stoma when it becomes wet with mucus

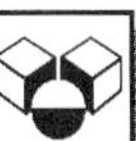

Nursing Guidelines 53-1

Changing an Ostomy Appliance

PURPOSE: To replace a full ostomy pouch with an empty one so that client remains clean and dry, infection and odor free, and surrounding skin is protected from breakdown resulting from leakage.

Assemble the needed equipment in one place: clean gloves, scissors, ostomy belt, a stoma gauge, faceplate, pouch, adhesive or protectant such as karaya paste, and cleaning materials such as gauze pads, water or adhesive solvent, and so forth.

- Wash hands and put on gloves.
- Empty the pouch when it is one-third full.
- Change the faceplate only when needed, that is, if it becomes loose, tight, or the client experiences discomfort. If the faceplate is changed too frequently, skin around the stoma may become raw and excoriated secondary to removal of protective layers of epithelium with the faceplate.
- If the ostomy appliance is being replaced routinely, schedule the change at a time when the gastrocolic reflex is less active. For many clients this time is early in the morning, before eating, or 2 or 3 hours after mealtime.
- Gently ease the faceplate from the skin. If the faceplate was applied with adhesive, roll the adhesive from the

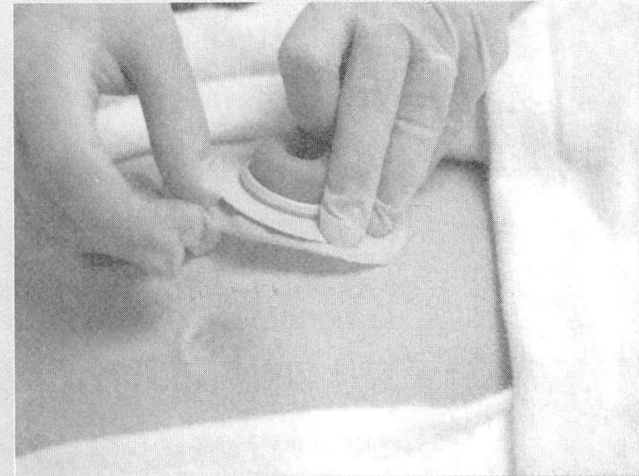

Removing faceplate. *(Courtesy of Ken Timby.)*

skin and appliance. If it does not roll off, use a small amount of solvent, which chemically loosens the adhesive bond. Because some solvents are irritating to the skin, apply solvent sparingly between the body and faceplate using a sprayer, medicine dropper, or a gauze pad. Avoid rubbing, which may further irritate the skin. Clean the area with soap and water and pat dry after a solvent has been used.
- Inform the client that the most common causes of discomfort are reactions to the adhesive or solvent used to remove it or irritation from leaking fecal drainage. In such cases, stinging, tingling, or itching may be experienced immediately after an appliance change, but these sensations should quickly subside. If a sensation is prolonged or intensified, the appliance should be removed regardless of whether it has been on for 1 hour or for several days. When using a new adhesive product, remember to patch test it first on nonirritated skin at the inner aspect of the client's forearm.
- After removing the faceplate and pouch, protect the peristomal area from drainage by placing a tissue cuff around the stoma or using a receptacle such as a small paper cup to collect the drainage. Use a soapy washcloth to clean the skin around the stoma and wipe the soap from the skin. Pat the area or allow it to air dry.
- Inspect the stoma and skin carefully. If excoriation is observed, use a temporary appliance or a hydrocolloid dressing, such as DuoDERM or Tegabsorb, to cover the excoriated skin to promote moist healing.
- Create an even surface for reapplying the pouch by filling irregular hollows in the peristomal skin with karaya paste before replacing the faceplate.

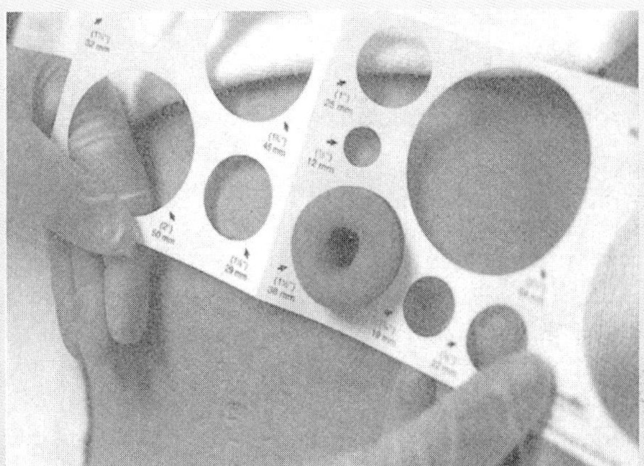

Measuring the stoma. *(Courtesy of Ken Timby.)*

- Measure the circumference of the stoma and cut a comparable hole in the faceplate, allowing 1/8-inch margin to account for potential swelling in a new stoma.
- Secure the pouch to the faceplate. Be sure to smooth out ridges or openings in the closure. Also be sure to seal the pouch.

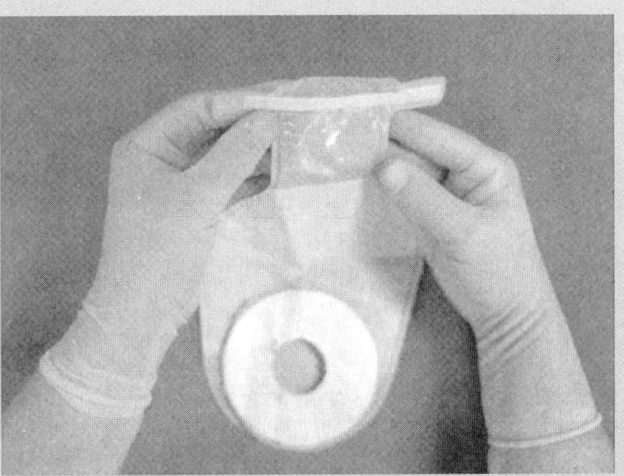

Sealing the pouch. *(Courtesy of Ken Timby.)*

- Peel the backing from the faceplate.
- Affix the faceplate to the skin.

BOX 53-1 Sexual Modifications for Ostomates

- Always practice good hygiene. Bathe and apply a fresh pouch before having sex.
- Disguise the pouch by enclosing it within a purse-string cloth cover.
- When anticipating sexual activity, avoid eating or drinking substances that activate the bowel or create a lot of gas.
- Fashion a cummerbund with a pocket or fold into which the pouch can be held.
- Remove the belt and temporarily secure the pouch to the skin with tape.
- If accidents happen, cultivate a sense of humor that may similarly relieve the anxiety of the sexual partner as well.
- Consult with members of a local ostomy group who also may provide support and counseling regarding sexual matters.

or serosanguineous drainage. As drainage decreases, change the dressing every 6 to 8 hours.

Monitor ileal output carefully during the entire postoperative period. As GI function resumes, the initial amount of ileal drainage usually is high. If excessive fluid and electrolyte loss continues, parenteral fluid and electrolyte replacement is necessary. When ileal drainage stabilizes, about 10 to 14 days after surgery, the physician removes the ileal catheter. The reservoir then holds the accumulating effluent until the nurse or client siphons it. Empty the reservoir initially, every 2 to 4 hours. As the capacity of the reservoir increases (usually in about 6 months), perform the procedure three or four times daily. For additional nursing management refer to the discussion that addresses similar problem experienced by a client with ileoanal reservoir.

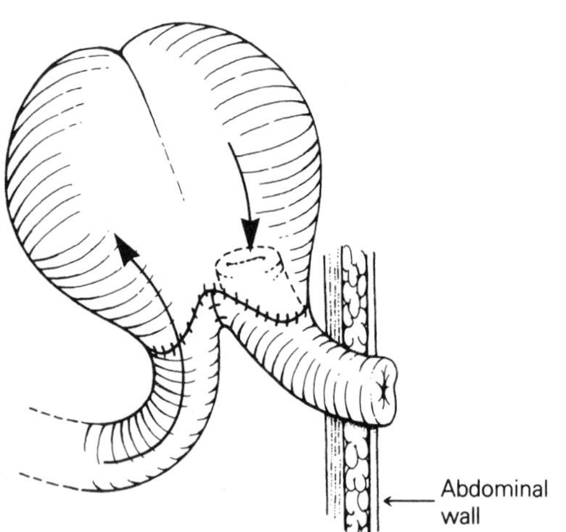

FIGURE 53-3. With a continent ileostomy, an internal reservoir is created by joining a loop of ileum and telescoping the distal segment to form a nipple valve. The distal segment is brought through the abdominal wall to create an external stoma. The arrows show the flow of GI effluent.

Client and Family Teaching

To assist the client in managing a continent ileostomy include the following information in the teaching plan. For tips on how to manage an obstructed catheter, see Box 53–2.

- To care for the stoma and catheter, assemble a clean catheter, lubricant, basin, tissues, irrigating syringe and solution, and gauze dressing.
- Sit on or beside the toilet or on the side of the bed.
- Warm the catheter to body temperature and lubricate the tip. Insert it about 2 inches into the stomal opening.
- Expect resistance when the catheter reaches the nipple valve (about 2 inches), which controls the retention of waste matter. Gently push the catheter a little further into the ileal pouch. At the same time, exhale or cough or bear down as if to pass stool until fecal material begins to drain.
- Direct the external end of the catheter into a basin or the toilet about 12 inches below the stoma.
- Allow 5 to 10 minutes for drainage to cease; then remove the catheter, clean it with soapy water, store it in a sealable plastic bag until needed again
- Wash the area around the stoma and pat the skin dry.
- Place an absorbent pad or dressing over the stoma

Ileoanal Reservoir

The **ileoanal reservoir** (also called an **ileoanal anastomosis**) (Fig. 53–4) is a procedure that maintains bowel continence. It is performed on selected clients who have chronic ulcerative colitis or whose disease does not affect the anorectal sphincter. Besides allow

BOX 53-2 Unblocking the Catheter in a Continent Ileostomy

If the catheter used to drain fecal matter or mucus from the internal reservoir becomes obstructed, suggest the following measures:

- Bear down as if to have a bowel movement.
- Rotate the catheter tip inside the stoma.
- Milk the catheter.
- If these are not successful, remove the catheter, rinse it, and try again.
- Notify the physician if these efforts do not result in any drainage.
- Never wait longer than 6 hours without obtaining drainage.

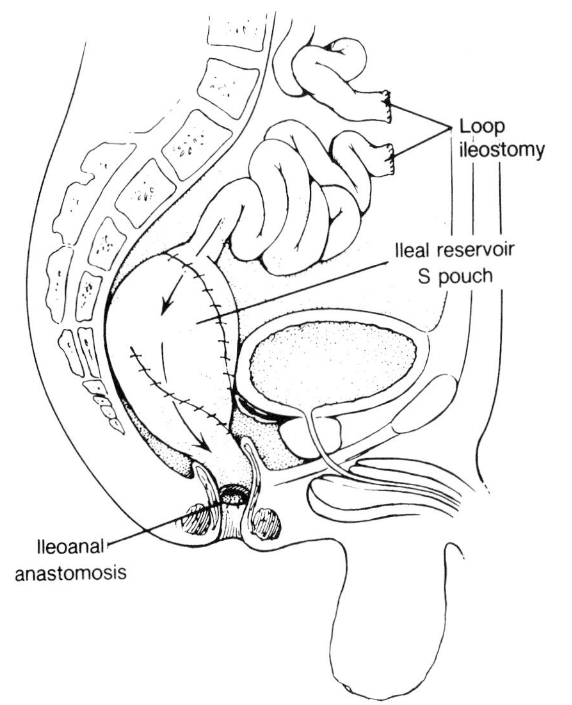

FIGURE 53-4. An ileoanal anastomosis joins a section of ileum to create an ileal reservoir. The distal end of the ileum is sutured above the anus. Intestinal effluent is temporarily discharged through the proximal stoma of a loop ileostomy until the second stage of surgery is performed.

ing the client to control bowel elimination, this procedure, as opposed to a conventional ileostomy with total colectomy, preserves nerve innervation to the male genitalia, and the client is unlikely to experience bladder dysfunction, impotence, or infertility.

SURGICAL MANAGEMENT

An ileoanal anastomosis is performed in two stages. In the first stage, the surgeon creates a temporary ileostomy, removes a large length of diseased colon down to the terminal section of the rectum above the anal sphincter, joins several distal loops of healthy ileum to form a pouch for holding stool, and connects the ileal reservoir to the anal cuff. After the first stage of surgery, clients experience an almost continuous mucous discharge from the anus and a frequent discharge of fecal material from the ileostomy. Initially, the client cannot control the frequent watery discharge.

The second stage is done 2 or 3 months later. At this time, the surgeon closes the temporary ileostomy and reunites the two sections of ileum. This establishes a normal flow of fecal material through the ileum to the reservoir. The fecal material, which is stored in the ileal reservoir, is then expelled from the anus. Control is achieved as edema subsides and the anal sphincter becomes stronger.

NURSING MANAGEMENT

The preoperative assessment of a client having either procedure is essentially the same as for the client with a conventional ileostomy. The postoperative assessment following the first stage of ileoanal reservoir surgery includes making the same observations and assessments as those for a conventional ileostomy. In addition, inspect the anal area for drainage, and check the drain or drainage tube in the presacral area if there is one. After the second stage, when the ileostomy is closed and the ileum connected to the anal reservoir, inspect the anal area and the operative sites for drainage.

Ordinarily, the postoperative plan of nursing care involves measures pertaining to general surgery and related client problems such as anxiety (see the Nursing Process: The Client Recovering From Ostomy Surgery). The nursing plan of care includes, but is not limited to, the following:

Nursing Diagnoses and Collaborative Problems	Nursing Interventions
Risk for Fluid Volume Deficit related to passage of liquid stools **Goal:** The client will maintain fluid balance.	Monitor administration of IV fluids. If infusions infiltrate, restart them as soon as possible so that the delay does not contribute to a fluid imbalance. Record intake and output; report a difference of more than 500 mL/day. Once oral intake can resume, provide between 2,000 and 3,000 mL/day of fluids containing sodium, potassium, and chloride to replace electrolytes in liquid stool.
Risk for Bowel Incontinence (second-stage ileoanal reservoir) related to poor sphincter control and high volume of liquid stool **Goal:** The client will be fecally continent.	Place and change disposable pads under the buttocks of the client with an ileoanal reservoir as needed. Encourage client to perform perineal exercises four to six times daily to reestablish anal sphincter control and enlarge the ileoanal reservoir. (Tell the client to tighten the anus as if trying to prevent a bowel movement. Hold the contraction for a count of 10 and relax.)
Impaired Skin Integrity related to effect of fecal material and adhesives on the skin, frequent bowel movements (ileoanal reservoir, second stage), other factors (specify) **Goal:** The client will acquire or maintain intact peristomal skin.	Place an absorbent pad beneath the client. Clean the anus with warm, soapy water to remove mucus or stool. (Clients with a first-stage ileoanal reservoir can use a squirt bottle to clean the perianal area or toilet tissue with aloe to avoid skin irritation.)

Pat the skin dry.

Cover the stoma with a gauze pad or temporary ostomy bag.

Use an adhesive or karaya seal appliance with a drainable pouch for clients who have liquid or semiliquid stool.

To prevent irritation, apply a protective cream or ointment around the skin that comes into contact with the stoma.

Provide sitz baths to gently clean the perianal area.

Client and Family Teaching

Include the following in the teaching plan:

- Continue performing perineal strengthening exercises daily.
- Apply protective ointments or creams as recommended by the physician.
- Inspect the anal area daily by using a hand-held mirror. Contact the physician if the anal area becomes sore or skin changes (eg, ulceration, bleeding) are apparent.
- Use a thin sanitary shield or disposable, lined underwear to absorb fecal drainage until anal sphincter control is achieved.

Colostomy

A colostomy is an opening in the large bowel created by bringing a section of the large intestine out to the abdomen and fashioning a stoma. The presence of a cancerous lesion, an ulcerative inflammatory process, multiple polyposis, or traumatic injury to the bowel are indications for a colostomy.

Types

A temporary or permanent colostomy may be created in the ascending, transverse, descending, or sigmoid areas of the colon (Fig. 53–5). The consistency of the fecal material ranges from semiliquid to formed depending on the intestinal area from which the colostomy is formed (see Table 53–1). A sigmoid colostomy, and sometimes a descending colostomy, may be controlled with regular irrigations, thus eliminating the need to constantly wear an appliance.

The stoma may be found anywhere from the lower right, center, to mid or lower left positions on the abdomen. Words like single-barrel, double-barrel, or loop are used to describe the appearance of the colostomy.

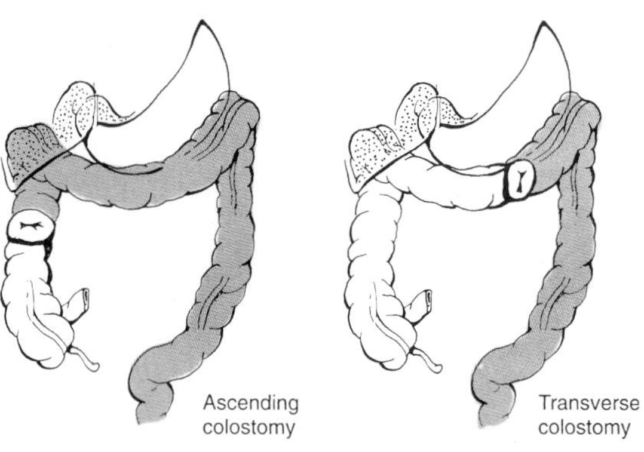

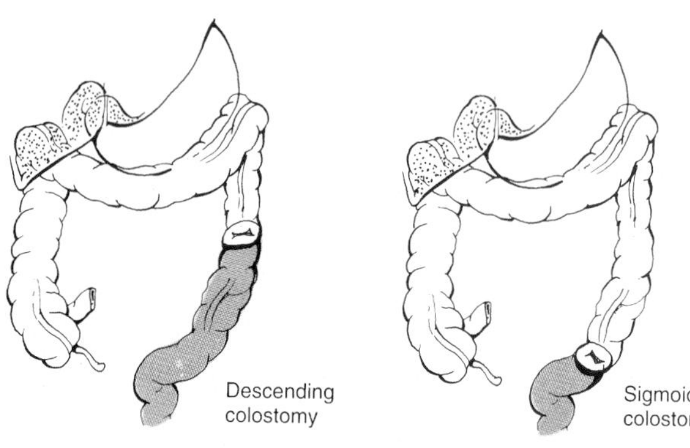

FIGURE 53-5. Various kinds of colostomies.

SURGICAL MANAGEMENT

Single-Barrel Colostomy

The term **single-barrel colostomy** indicates that the ostomy has a single stoma through which fecal matter passes. The colon is cut above the diseased area and the healthy end is brought through the abdominal wall to form the matured stoma. The diseased portion of the bowel is removed with the remaining distal end closed for later reconnection (**segmental resection**). For tumors in the lower third of the sigmoid, that portion, the rectum, and anus may be surgically removed through a perineal incision in a procedure referred to as an **abdominoperineal resection**. After performing an abdominoperineal resection, the surgeon leaves a temporary drain or pack in the perineal area. It is removed in about 1 week and irrigations of the perineal wound may be ordered.

Double-Barrel Colostomy

A **double-barrel colostomy**, which is most often performed in the transverse section of the large intestine, contains both a proximal and distal stoma. Each stoma is everted and sutured in place. Fecal material is expelled from the proximal stoma. The distal stoma leads from the lower portion of the cut bowel to the anus. Because fecal drainage has been diverted, the distal portion of the bowel does not pass feces, but mucus may be expelled from the anus and from the distal stoma. When a double-barrel colostomy has been performed, the physician is asked to identify the distal and proximal stomas. A diagram is provided within the medical record and the nurse may duplicate it on the nursing care plan. This information is essential when assessing bowel function and if an irrigation is required. Irrigation (Clinical Procedure 53–1) may be ordered for both the proximal and distal portions of the bowel or for only the proximal portion.

A double-barrel colostomy often is temporary and usually performed to rest a portion of the bowel to treat a disorder such as acute diverticulitis. The interval before re-establishing the continuity of the bowel may be 16 months or longer. When the diseased portion of the bowel is removed or healed, the bowel is reconnected and functions normally. In the mean time, the stoma may need irrigation (Box 53–3).

Loop Colostomy

A **loop colostomy** indicates that a loop of bowel has been lifted through the abdomen; it is supported

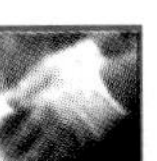

Clinical Procedure 53-1
Performing a Standard Colostomy Irrigation

PURPOSE

- Regulation of bowel elimination
- Preparation of the bowel for diagnostic or surgical procedures

EQUIPMENT

- Receptacle for the irrigant
- Tubing
- Soft catheter (with or without a cone tip)
- Irrigation sleeve or sheath for fecal return
- Irrigant (ie, water or saline solution)
- Water-soluble lubricant
- Clean gloves

Nursing Action	Rationale
ASSESSMENT	
Check the medical orders.	Collaborates nursing activities with medical treatment
Check the client's identification.	Prevents errors
Explain the procedure to the client.	Allows for assessment of the client's learning needs and provides an opportunity for teaching Also allows the client to understand that he or she will learn this activity as a part of self-care, and will be used to establish bowel control
PLANNING	
Plan the initial irrigation for the fourth or fifth day after surgery. The most widely advocated method for irrigation is the standard method, which consists of a daily scheduled irrigation with 500 to 1,500 mL water.	Allows time for healing to begin and bowel function to resume
Obtain and assemble the necessary equipment and prepare the irrigant.	Prevents unnecessary delays in the plan of care
Explain the procedure, its purpose and intended effect to the client. Then provide for the client's privacy.	Decreases client anxiety
IMPLEMENTATION	
Ask the client to sit on a toilet seat or a chair in front of the toilet with the irrigation sheath directed into the toilet bowl.	Decreases the risk of spillage of fecal material
Wash your hands and put on gloves.	Reduces the transmission of microorganisms (from the nurse to the client and from the client to the nurse)
Purge air from the tubing by allowing the irrigation solution to flow to the tip of the catheter. Clamp the tubing to prevent further flow of the irrigation solution.	Prevents introduction of air into the intestine, which can increase cramping

continued

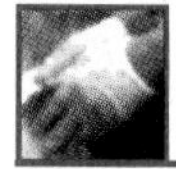

Clinical Procedure 53-1
Continued

Lubricate the distal end of the catheter with water-soluble lubricant.	Eases introduction of the catheter into the stoma
Hang the container of irrigant so that the bottom of the solution bag is about 12 inches above the client's stoma. Then, slowly and gently insert the tip of the catheter into the stoma and advance it 2 to 3 inches into the stoma.	Facilitates introduction of the catheter into the stoma

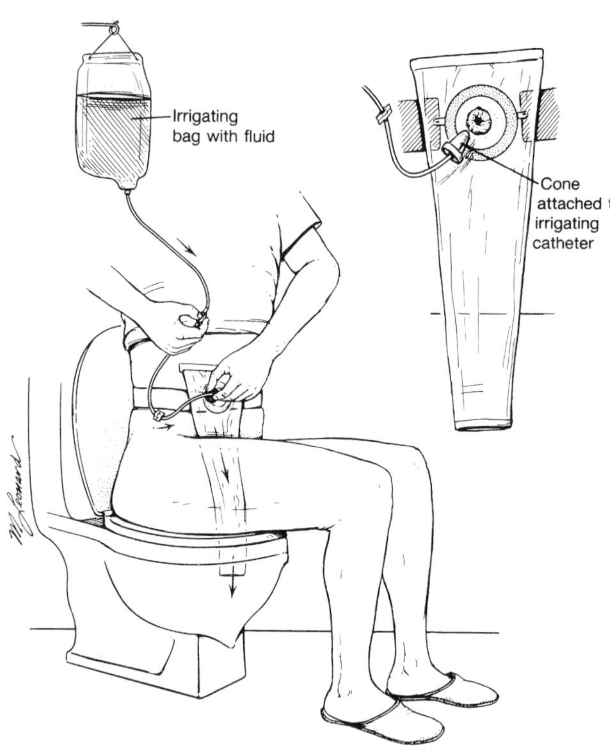

If resistance is felt, remove the irrigation tip, release the clamp on the tubing and gently reinsert the catheter while the solution is flowing.	Relieves obstruction from hard stool or tissue
Allow the irrigant to flow slowly and gradually into the stoma.	Prevents cramping from rapid instillation
If cramping occurs clamp the tubing and instruct the client to take a few deep breaths. Continue irrigating once the cramp subsides.	Allows time for the cramp to pass
If water escapes from the stoma as fluid is being introduced, clamp the tubing until it ceases. If a catheter tip is used instead of a cone, introduce the catheter further into the stoma—but never more than 6 inches.	Prevents leakage of irrigant
When the prescribed amount of solution has been instilled, remove the catheter and allow the client to remain on the toilet or close off the end of the irrigation sleeve and allow the client to walk about. Complete drainage may take up to 30 minutes but varies with the person.	Allows for drainage from the stoma. Mild activity stimulates evacuation
If irrigant fails to return properly, gently massage the lower abdomen, or have the client take several deep breaths and relax or reposition the body (gently twisting at the waist from side to side or standing up or sitting straighter). If these measures do not work, notify the physician.	Encourages the return of fluid that may be trapped behind hard stool.

continued

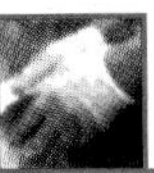

Clinical Procedure 53-1
Continued

Observe the expelled effluent. Watery, slightly colored return without stool suggests a clean bowel; return that is full of stool suggests that additional irrigation is needed.	Allows for evaluation of the effectiveness of the irrigation. Helps to determine the need for further irrigation.
Repeat the procedure, if indicated, using no more than 2 liters of water at a time.	Permits proper elimination. Using less than 2 liters of water avoids water intoxication resulting from absorption through the bowel wall.
Remove the irrigation sheath. If it is disposable, discard it. If it is reusable, wash and store it according to the manufacturer's directions.	Allows the equipment to be reused, as appropriate.
Document the time the irrigation was performed, the amount of irrigant used, the results of the procedure, and the client's response.	Provides a record of nursing activity and the client's tolerance.

in place with a glass rod or plastic butterfly device. About 24 to 72 hours after surgery, the anterior wall of the loop is opened at the client's bedside or in a treatment room either by incising the bowel or using a cautery machine to form the stoma. The posterior wall of the bowel is left intact, which results in a proximal and distal opening to the bowel.

By delaying the opening of the intestinal loop, the initial healing of the incision occurs without danger of contamination. Opening the bowel does not cause any discomfort because the bowel lacks pain receptors. When a loop colostomy is opened, the bed and client's clothing are well protected. Prepare the client for the pungent odor of cauterized tissue, which subsides shortly, and the initial gush of fecal material. Use a temporary ostomy pouch to receive the initial flow of liquid feces.

BOX 53-3 Alternatives to Standard Irrigation

If the client has a double-barrel colostomy, irrigate the proximal stoma in the same manner as a single-barrel colostomy. However, to irrigate the distal stoma, try the following:

- Have the client sit on a toilet or a bedpan because the irrigation fluid and a small amount of mucus will leave by way of the anus. During the immediate postoperative period, necrotic tissue also may be expelled.
- Use a bulb syringe, short catheter, container of solution, plastic sheath or apron, and an emesis basin as another technique for irrigation. This method calls for several instillations of 250 to 500 mL solution at a time sometimes twice a day. Some clients have found this method effective for controlling spillage for 24 hours or more. It may be used as an alternate choice when the standard method cannot be used.

NURSING MANAGEMENT

The nursing management during the preoperative period is similar to that for clients having an ileostomy. However, because a colostomy may be performed for cancer of the colon or rectum, the client may be more anxious about the procedure.

After the client returns from surgery, nursing assessments include taking vital signs, checking dressings, and monitoring nasogastric tubes and IV infusions. The nurse reviews the client's chart for the type of colostomy and the location of the stoma(s). If an abdominoperineal resection was performed, the drain or packing in the perineal area is checked and the characteristics of the drainage are noted.

Vital signs are monitored every 4 hours or as ordered. The temperature is taken by other than the rectal route. Report a sudden elevation in temperature, over 38.3°C (101°F), or an increase in pain and abdominal tenderness or distention to the physician immediately. Check the surgical dressing frequently in the early postoperative period, and observe the characteristics of the stoma. Monitor urine output and the volume of suctioned gastric secretions. Report a marked decrease in urine output or a urine output of less than 500 mL/day is reported to the physician immediately.

Postoperatively, nasogastric decompression is carried out and the client's fluid and electrolyte status are monitored (see Chap. 51). An indwelling catheter may be used to relieve abdominal pressure as well as prevent urine retention during the first few days after surgery.

In addition to standard postsurgical measures for maintaining the airway, relieving pain and anxiety, the care of a client after colostomy surgery includes but is not limited to the following. Strategies for maintaining skin integrity as well as dealing with altered sexuality (see Box 53–1) and altered body image were discussed previously.

Nursing Diagnoses and Collaborative Problems	Nursing Interventions
Risk for Bowel Incontinence related to unpredictable bowel elimination pattern **Goal:** The client will not experience accidental soiling.	Be sure the ostomy appliance remains intact. Eliminate unpredictable bowel elimination from a descending or sigmoid colostomy by irrigating the colostomy or inserting a suppository well within the stoma on a regular basis to eliminate fecal elimination for 1 to 3 days.
Risk for Diarrhea or Constipation related to changes in bowel motility **Goal:** The client will maintain expected consistency of feces according to location of the colostomy.	*Diarrhea* Urge the client to identify (by trial and error) irritating or poorly tolerated foods. Recommend eliminating the offending foods or reducing the amount to be eaten. Report increased stool volume, watery stool consistency, nausea, vomiting, or abdominal pain to the physician; even ostomates can have gastroenteritis. *Constipation* Gently dilate the stoma with a lubricated gloved finger to help expel stool. Increase fluid intake, particularly if the client has a fever or illness or perspires a lot. Advise regular meals; dieting or fasting may decrease stool volume and slow elimination. Provide foods containing fiber to increase stool moisture. Offer foods that promote elimination, such as coffee or stewed prunes. Help the client implement stress management techniques if slow motility is stress-related. Consult with the physician about prescribing a suppository, laxative, or irrigation if the constipation is unrelieved by these measures.
Risk for Infection related to potential for wound contamination with fecal organisms **Goal:** The client will remain free from infection.	Maintain optimum nutrition. Keep the incision free of fecal contamination with techniques used for a client with an ileostomy. Administer prescribed antibiotics as ordered to maintain adequate blood levels of the drug.
Social Isolation related to odor, accident (leakage, soiling of clothes) **Goal:** The client will continue to interact socially with others.	Make frequent contact with the client, especially during time when no other nursing activity is scheduled. This will set an example of how other people will accept the client after surgery. Teach the client how to control odors as discussed in the care of the client with an ileostomy.
Ineffective Individual Coping related to perceived lifestyle changes **Goal:** The client will cope effectively with lifestyle changes	Explore ways that the client has coped effectively in the past and encourage the use of those methods. Suggest new coping techniques that others have found useful, such as keeping a journal or diary, investing energy in a worthwhile project, or learning as much as possible about the disease and its treatment from experts.

Client and Family Teaching

Teach the client how to care for the colostomy. Assist the client with a demonstration of the irrigating procedure, if possible, and outline nonirrigation methods for keeping the ostomy patent and establishing a regular pattern of bowel elimination (Box 53–4). The time between the use of these methods and eventual regularity is unique to each client. Explain that natural methods are the least predictable for regulating the bowel, but many clients learn to recognize subtle clues that the bowel will be moving. They then have sufficient time to reach a bathroom and eliminate in private.

Also demonstrate skin and stoma care and appliance application and removal. Divide the material that must be learned into small units. Demonstrate one aspect of care, have the client return the demonstration, and add additional material when the client feels self-confident. Reinforce verbal information and demonstrated skills with printed material that may be available from ostomy associations or the enterostomal therapist. Arrange a dietary consultation to discuss nutrition and food modifications. Try to include the following points in the teaching plan:

BOX 53-4 Regulating Bowel Elimination Without Irrigating

Some ostomates learn to regulate bowel elimination without irrigating frequently. The following tips may be encouraging to new ostomates, who may be able to establish regular elimination patterns.

- Insert a suppository, such as glycerin or bisacodyl (Dulcolax), into the stoma. The suppository should be recommended by the physician. Up to 7 days or more of daily use may be needed before a regular elimination pattern is established. Initially movements may occur three or four times daily, but each day movements should decrease until only one or two movements occur daily.

Other methods to stimulate bowel elimination and a regular schedule include:

- Drinking prune or fruit juice
- Eating fiber-rich foods and dried fruits and performing mild exercise
- Using a stool softener, mineral oil, or milk of magnesia if recommended by the physician

- Changes in the size and color of the stoma vary with activity and emotional status. Anger or extreme annoyance may cause the stoma to turn red or purple. Small beads of blood may ooze from the surface. Fright may cause the stoma to blanch. These are normal reactions and are insignificant as long as the tissues revert to their normal state when the cause is alleviated.
- A regular diet can be eaten, but gas-forming foods can be avoided to control intestinal gas.
- In most cases, increasing the amount of fiber in the diet and drinking extra water corrects constipation.
- Diarrhea may be related to diet. Eliminating food items that result in diarrhea may help to control the problem. If diarrhea persists for more than 2 days, however, contact the physician.
- Eating slowly with the mouth closed and chewing food well will decrease the amount of gas that results chiefly from swallowing air rather than from digestion.
- With the exception of tightly fitted clothing, no adjustment needs to be made in the type of clothing worn. Clients who require a firm support (eg, those who wear girdles, have back problems, or wear braces) may find a stoma shield helpful in preventing irritation or undue pressure on the stoma.
- Check body weight weekly. Contact the physician if there is a sudden weight loss or gain.
- Perform irrigations at about the same time each day. The best time to irrigate is after a meal because food in the digestive tract stimulates peristalsis and defecation.
- The physician may recommend that the schedule for irrigations gradually progress to every other day, every third day, or even twice a week. If constipation occurs, contact the physician regarding a change in the irrigation schedule.
- Travel or activities outside the home need not be restricted. Kits that contain all the materials needed for irrigation and changes of the colostomy appliance are available. The necessary items also may be assembled individually and placed in a waterproof container.

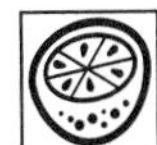

General Nutritional Considerations

A low-fiber diet may be prescribed for 6 to 8 weeks after ostomy surgery to prevent irritation and slow transit time. Thereafter, small amounts of foods containing fiber are added individually to the diet so that the client's tolerance can be evaluated. Foods not tolerated initially may be reintroduced weeks or months later.

One to 2 quarts of fluid are needed to replace liquid lost from decreased water reabsorption from the bowel. Reassure the client that extra fluids do not contribute to watery stools, but rather are excreted as urine. Fluid restriction should not be undertaken as a means of controlling liquid feces. Likewise, extra sodium may be needed.

Foods that may produce odorous gas include beans, corn, chocolate, coconut, green pepper, legumes, onions, vegetables of the cabbage family, beets, simple sugars, pork, oat bran, dark rye and pumpernickel breads, carbonated beverages, beer and other alcoholic beverages, and fried foods.

Because they may be linked to stomal obstruction in clients with ileostomy, the following items can be avoided: fibrous vegetables (ie, celery and cabbage), bamboo shoots, nuts, and foods with kernels.

Supplements of the fat-soluble vitamins (A, D, E, K) and parenteral injections of vitamin B_{12} are used to prevent deficiencies in clients who have had most or all of the ileum removed. Decreased bile salt absorption causes diarrhea and steatorrhea; a low-fat diet supplemented with medium-chain triglycerides may be used to minimize symptoms and maintain adequate caloric intake.

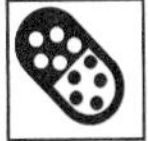

General Pharmacologic Considerations

Some medications, especially vitamins, antibiotics, and antituberculosis drugs, cause particularly strong odors that cling to the appliance. A list of drugs capable of imparting an odor to an ostomy appliance can be obtained from an ostomy association or ostomy appliance manufacturers.

Enteric-coated products and some modified-release forms of drugs, such as slow-release beads and layered tablets, should be avoided by clients with an ileostomy because they may pass through without being absorbed. When changing the ileostomy appliance, check the contents of the appliance for undissolved—and therefore unabsorbed—capsules. This means the client has not received the desired effect of the medication, and the physician should be contacted.

Some preparations such as Slow-K (potassium chloride) leave a "ghost" of the wax matrix coating, but that does not indicate the drug has been unabsorbed. Clients with an ileostomy may need monthly vitamin B_{12} injections because the terminal ileum may be compromised to such an extent as to interfere with its dietary absorption.

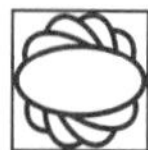

General Gerontologic Considerations

When teaching an older adult about ostomy care, present the material in brief sessions. Supplement the instructions with illustrations and written directions.

Teach a family member or another responsible person how to perform ostomy care in case the client is temporarily unable to assume responsibility for this task. Always provide the telephone number of an individual to contact (ie, the enterostomal therapist) if problems occur after discharge.

Difficulty in changing the appliance, skin care, irrigation of the colostomy stoma, and care of the permanent appliance may be encountered by the older adult ostomate because of chronic disorders such as poor vision and arthritis. Consult with an enterostomal therapist regarding which equipment may best meet the client's individual needs. If it is believed that the older adult client will be permanently unable to assume care for an ostomy, arrangements for daily care will have to be made. Depending on the situation, a family member, visiting nurse, or a home health care nurse will have to assume this responsibility. In some instances, transfer to a skilled nursing facility or nursing home may be necessary.

Older ostomates are particularly vulnerable to emotional distress, including loss of self-esteem and increased anxiety. Actively listen as the older adult expresses concerns and fears over adjusting to and caring for the ostomy and being rejected by family and friends.

Never assume that an older adult is not concerned about the effects of the ostomy on sexuality. Provide an opportunity for the older adult to discuss sexual concerns.

SUMMARY OF KEY CONCEPTS

- The two general types of intestinal ostomy procedures are an ileostomy, in which the ileum is opened onto the skin of the abdomen, and a colostomy, in which a section of the large intestine is opened onto the skin of the abdomen.
- Before an ostomy is created, the procedure and routine for care are explained. An antibiotic is given to sterilize the bowel and a bowel cleansing routine is carried out. Steroids, if they are currently prescribed, are gradually discontinued and the client's nutritional status is improved. Blood transfusions may be given. Teaching about ostomy care begins. A nasogastric tube is inserted just before surgery or during the surgical procedure while the client is under anesthetized.
- Complications that may occur following ileostomy surgery include intestinal obstruction, loss of blood supply to the stoma, stenosis of the stoma, and prolapse or retraction of the stoma.
- Nursing management of the client undergoing gastric surgery includes maintaining adequate nutrition, minimizing anxiety, preventing injury, maintaining adequate tissue perfusion, and patient teaching.
- A basic appliance used to collect stool from an intestinal ostomy consists of an adherent faceplate or disk, for protecting the skin and holding the appliance in place over the stoma, and a pouch for collecting the feces.
- An ostomy appliance is changed when it becomes loose, tight, or uncomfortable. It is emptied when it is one-third full or the client feels it is necessary.
- The main steps in changing an ostomy appliance include easing it from the skin, cleaning the stoma and peristomal skin, measuring and cutting the correct opening for the faceplate, attaching the pouch to the faceplate, and positioning the faceplate over the stoma.
- Stool is removed from a continent ileostomy by inserting a catheter through a nipple valve made of ileal tissue and siphoning the liquid stool.
- An ileoanal reservoir is a two-part procedure in which the surgeon removes the diseased portion of the colon then forms a pouch with a portion of the terminal ileum and connects it to the anus. Stool is temporary released through an ileostomy. Later the ileostomy portion is reconnected to the ileoanal pouch and stool is released through the anus.
- A colostomy may be created in the ascending, transverse, descending, or sigmoid areas of the large intestine. Depending on whether the fecal diversion is temporary or permanent, a single-barrel, double-barrel, or loop colostomy may be constructed out of the healthy bowel.
- Many individuals who have a colostomy, especially in the descending or sigmoid areas, may be able to regulate bowel elimination by regular colostomy irrigations, evacuating the bowel with the use of a suppository, or using dietary modifications to influence bowel elimination.

CRITICAL THINKING EXERCISES

1. In what ways is the care of a 20-year-old client with an ileostomy different from that of a 60-year-old client with a colostomy?

2. A client with an ileostomy is disturbed by the need to empty liquid stool from his appliance so frequently. He intends to reduce his intake of fluids. What information is important to give this client?
3. What recommendations are appropriate for the client with a colostomy who has been experiencing an unusual amount of intestinal gas?

Suggested Readings

Bradley, M., & Pupiales, M. (1997). Essential clements of ostomy care. *American Journal of Nursing, 97*(7), 38–45.

Bryant, G. (1992). When the bowel is blocked. *RN, 55*(1), 58.

Epps, C. K. (1996). The delicate business of ostomy care. *RN, 59*(11), 32–37, 53.

MacArthur, A. (1996). Sexuality and the stoma: Helping patients to cope. *Nursing Times, 92*(39), 34–35.

Pontieri-Lewis, V. (1996). Focus on wound care. Utilizing a team approach to wound management. *MEDSURG Nursing,* 5(6), 427–429.

Additional Resources

Wound Ostomy and Continence Nurses Society (formerly International Association for Enterostomal Therapy)
2755 Bristol Street
Suite 110
Costa Mesa, CA 92626
(714) 476–0268
http://www.social.com/health/nhic/data/hr1700/hr1725.html

Ostomy International
http://www.ostomyinternational.org/webforum/ioawtocf.htm

United Ostomy Association, Inc.
4500 East 9th Avenue
Denver, CO 80222
(303) 530–2506
http://www.unitedwaydenver.org/iris/mj0q5mi1.htm

Chapter 54

Caring for Clients With Disorders of the Liver, Gallbladder, and Pancreas

KEY TERMS

Alpha-fetoprotein
Ascites
Biliary colic
Caput medusae
Cholecystitis
Choledocholithiasis
Cholelithiasis
Cirrhosis
Cullen's sign
Encephalopathy
Esophageal gastric tamponade
Esophageal varices
Fetor hepaticus
Hepatic lobectomy
Hepatitis
Hepatorenal syndrome
Injection sclerotherapy
Laparoscopic cholecystectomy
Lithotripsy
Open cholecystectomy
Pancreatectomy (partial, total)
Pancreatitis
Peritoneal venous shunt
Portal hypertension
Radical pancreaticoduodenectomy (Whipple procedure)
Steatorrhea
T-tube
Turner's sign
Variceal banding

LEARNING OBJECTIVES

On completion of this chapter, the reader will:

- List common findings manifested by clients with cirrhosis.
- Discuss four complications that often accompany cirrhosis.
- Identify the modes of transmission of viral hepatitis.
- Describe nursing measures following a liver biopsy.
- Discuss the nursing management of clients with a medically or surgically treated liver disorder.
- Identify a factor that contributes to cholecystitis.
- List five signs or symptoms of cholecystitis.
- Identify four methods for medically managing cholecystitis.
- Name two techniques for removing the gallbladder.
- Discuss the nursing management of clients with a T-tube.
- Discuss the nursing management of clients undergoing medical or surgical treatment of a gallbladder disorder.
- Describe the treatment of acute and chronic pancreatitis.
- Discuss the nursing management of clients with pancreatitis.
- Describe the treatment of pancreatic carcinoma.
- Discuss the nursing management of clients undergoing pancreatic surgery.

The liver, gallbladder, and pancreas play important roles in digestion. Poor function of these accessory organs impairs the digestive process and the overall nutritional status of the client. In addition, these organs are responsible for other physiologic activities (see Chap. 50).

Anatomy of the Liver

The liver has two major lobes—right and left—and two small lobes—the caudate and quadrate lobes—located on the undersurface (Fig. 54–1). It is supported by intra-abdominal pressure and various attachments called *ligaments*, or *mesenteries*, which connect the liver to the adjacent intestines, abdominal wall, and diaphragm. Unless it is abnormally enlarged, the liver is usually not palpable.

The liver has various functions (Box 54–1) and a rich blood supply. It receives arterial blood from the *hepatic artery*, an indirect branch of the aorta. The *portal vein* transports blood from the intestinal tract to the liver. After it has traversed vascular pathways in-

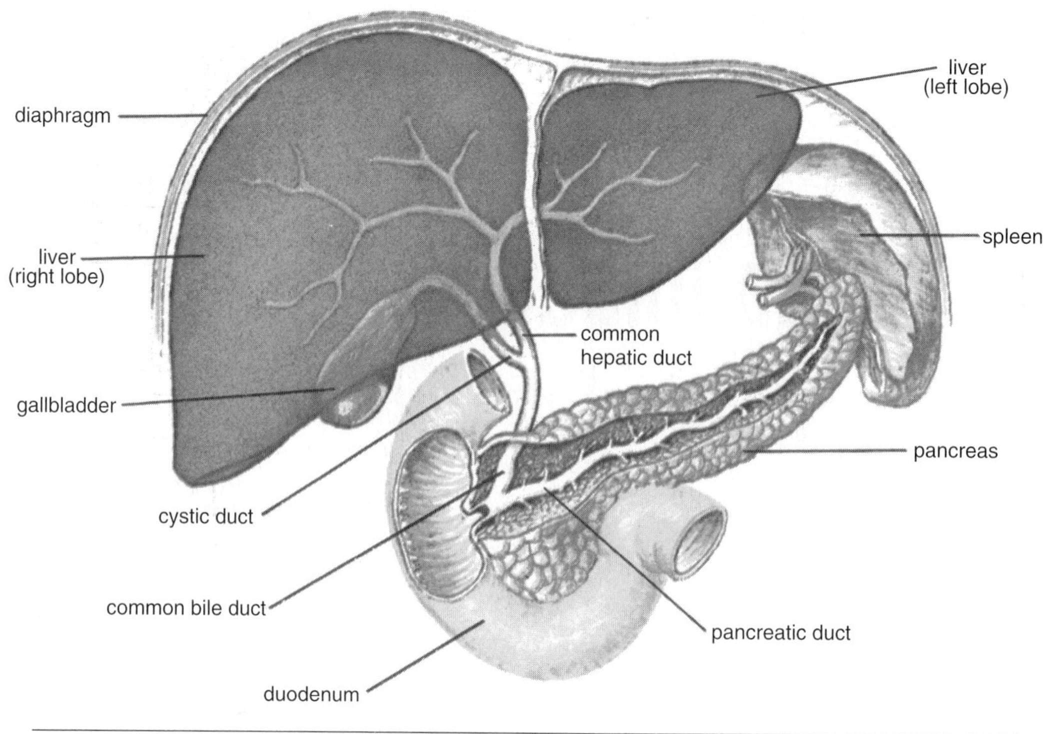

FIGURE 54-1. The liver.

side the liver, the blood is collected by the hepatic veins and transported to the inferior vena cava and then back to the heart (Fig. 54–2).

Microscopically, the internal structure of the liver includes smaller branches of the hepatic artery, the hepatic and portal veins, the lymphatics, and the bile ducts. The cellular constituents of the liver are the *hepatic parenchymal cells*, which perform most of the liver's metabolic functions, and the *Kupffer cells*, which engage in the immunologic, detoxifying, and blood-filtering actions of the liver.

BOX 54-1 Functions of the Liver

- Forms and excretes bile
- Uses, transforms, and distributes vitamins, proteins, fats, and carbohydrates
- Stores energy-yielding glycogen
- Synthesizes factors needed for blood coagulation (eg, prothrombin and fibrinogen)
- Detoxifies endogenous and exogenous chemicals (including drugs), bacteria, and foreign elements that may be harmful
- Forms immunizing substances, including gamma globulin

Jaundice (Icterus)

Jaundice, also called *icterus*, is a greenish yellow discoloration of tissue. It is a sign of disease but not itself a unique disease. Jaundice is caused by an abnormally high concentration of the pigment *bilirubin* in the blood. Total bilirubin concentration normally ranges between 0.2 and 1.0 mg/dL blood. If serum bilirubin levels reach 3 mg/dL or higher, jaundice is visible, notably on the skin, mucous membranes of the mouth, and especially the sclera. Jaundice occurs in a multitude of diseases that directly or indirectly affect the liver. It is probably the most common sign of a liver disorder.

To understand the scope and significance of jaundice, it is important to know how bile is formed and excreted. When red blood cells are old or injured, they are picked up by the spleen and bone marrow, where they are broken down by mononuclear phagocytes. Hemoglobin released from these red blood cells is then reduced to the compound known as *unconjugated, free* or *indirect, bilirubin*. This type of bilirubin is then carried by the blood to the liver, where further chemical processes transform it into *conjugated*, or *direct, bilirubin*. The conjugated bilirubin formed by the liver enters the bile ducts, reaches the intestine, and is transformed into urobilinogen. Some of the urobilinogen is changed into urobilin, the brown pigment of stool, some is excreted in the urine, and some is carried back to the liver by the bloodstream for re-excretion in the bile.

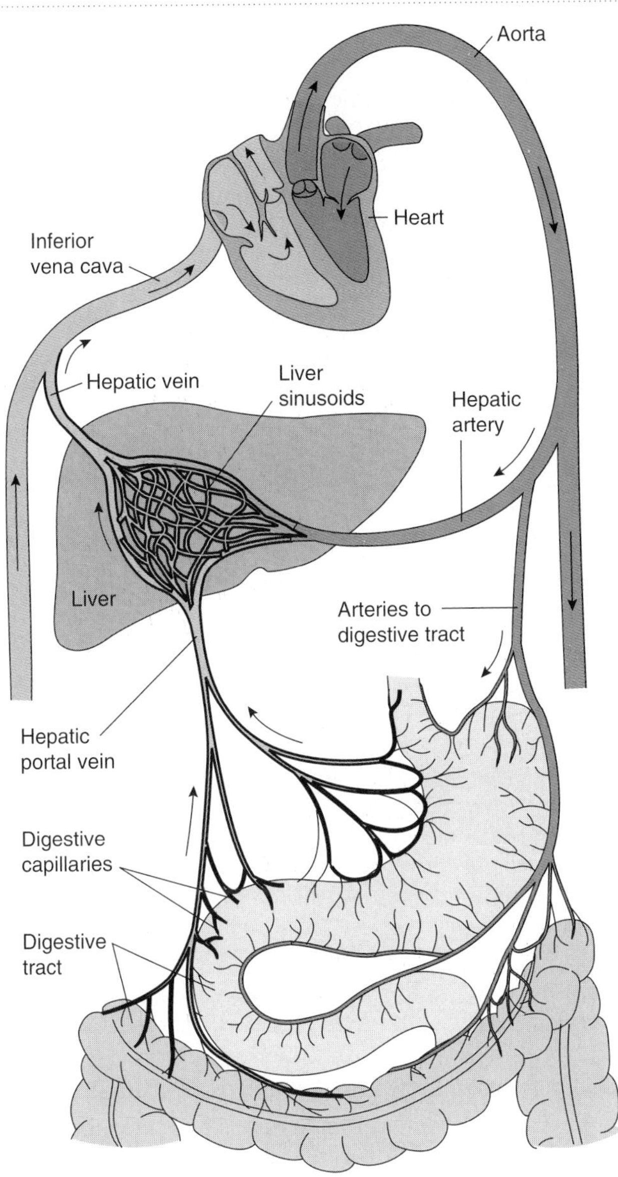

FIGURE 54-2. Hepatic blood supply and circulation.

There are three forms of jaundice: (1) *hemolytic jaundice*, caused by an excess of destroyed red blood cells (see Chap. 38); (2) *hepatocellular jaundice*, caused by liver disease; and (3) *obstructive jaundice*, caused by a block in the passage of bile between the liver and intestinal tract. Because unconjugated and conjugated bilirubin are distinct and can be differentiated chemically, they are important in the differential diagnosis of diseases that produce jaundice.

Cirrhosis

Cirrhosis is a degenerative disorder of the liver from generalized cellular damage. There are several types of cirrhosis: Laennec's, postnecrotic, biliary and cardiac.

ETIOLOGY AND PATHOPHYSIOLOGY

Once the liver cells become irreversibly damaged, they are replaced with nonfunctional fibrous connective scar tissue. This leads to considerable anatomic distortion, including partial or complete occlusion of blood channels within the liver. The liver becomes increasingly unable to carry out its many functions. Consequently, there are disturbances in digestion and metabolism, defects in blood coagulation, fluid and electrolyte imbalance, and an impaired ability to metabolize hormones and detoxify chemicals. Portal hypertension, esophageal varices, ascites and hepatic encephalopathy are complications of advanced cirrhosis and are discussed later.

Laennec's (portal, alcoholic, nutritional, or toxic) *cirrhosis*, the most common type, is associated with chronic alcohol intake, usually coincidental with poor nutrition. It also can follow chronic poisoning with certain chemicals, such as carbon tetrachloride, a cleaning agent, or ingestion of hepatotoxic drugs.

Postnecrotic cirrhosis results from destruction of liver cells secondary to an infection, such as hepatitis, or metabolic liver disease.

Biliary (primary, secondary) *cirrhosis* may be the result of chronic obstruction or inflammation of the bile ducts or unknown etiology.

Cardiac cirrhosis is associated with right-sided congestive heart failure and constrictive pericarditis (see Chap. 35).

ASSESSMENT FINDINGS

Signs and Symptoms

The client's history often correlates with factors that predispose to cirrhosis such as chronic alcohol use, hepatitis, and exposure to toxins. Clients with cirrhosis typically experience chronic fatigue, anorexia, dyspepsia, nausea, vomiting, and altered bowel elimination (diarrhea or constipation), all of which are accompanied by weight loss. Abdominal discomfort and shortness of breath are common complaints and are due to organ compression from the enlarged liver. Many indicate that they have nosebleeds, bleeding from the gums, or bruise easily. The skin may itch (*pruritus*) from an accumulation of bile salts.

When examining a client with cirrhosis, the size of the liver, and sometimes the spleen, is increased causing the abdomen to appear distended. The skin, sclera, or oral mucous membrane appear jaundiced. Edema may be present in the legs and feet. Veins over the abdomen may be dilated. Because the dysfunctional liver cannot fully metabolize estrogen, men may present with *gynecomastia* (enlarged breasts) and testicular atrophy. *Palmar erythema* (bright pink palms) and cutaneous *spider angiomata* (tiny, spider-like blood vessels visible on the surface of the skin) are also related to an inability to inactivate estrogen.

Diagnostic Findings

A liver biopsy, which reveals hepatic fibrosis, is the most conclusive diagnostic evidence. A liver biopsy is obtained by percutaneous method on the nursing unit, using mild sedation (see Clinical Procedure 54–1), or through a surgical incision. Prolonged prothrombin time and low platelet count resulting from liver disease place the client at high risk for hemorrhage. Other tests used to examine the liver include computed tomographic (CT) scan, magnetic resonance imaging (MRI), and radioisotope liver scan, all of which may demonstrate the liver's enlarged size, nodular configuration, and distorted blood flow. Blood values appear in Box 54–2.

MEDICAL AND SURGICAL MANAGEMENT

No specific cure for hepatic cirrhosis exists. The principal aim of therapy is to prevent further deterio-

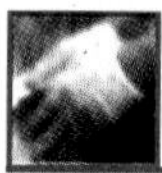

Clinical Procedure 54-1
Assisting With a Percutaneous Liver Biopsy

PURPOSE

- To provide a sample of liver tissue for the differential diagnosis of liver disease and/or evaluating the extent of liver damage

EQUIPMENT

- Soft tissue biopsy needle or kit of the physician's choice
- Sterile drape
- Antimicrobial skin preparation solution, such as povidone-iodine (Betadine)
- Sterile gloves sized appropriately for the surgeon
- Sterile dressing and tape
- Small pillow or towel roll
- Containers with solutions appropriate for the specimen being obtained (eg, formalin, gluteraldehyde)
- Clean gloves
- Monitoring devices specified by institutional policy

Nursing Action	Rationale
ASSESSMENT	
Check the medical orders.	Coordinates nursing activities with medical treatment
Assess the client's understanding of the procedure.	Assesses the client's learning needs and provides an opportunity to reinforce what the client has learned
Obtain baseline vital signs and check the client's identification.	Allows identification of complications during and after the procedure and prevents errors
PLANNING	
Ensure that the surgeon has the most current laboratory results prior to performing the procedure.	Allows for evaluation of additional risks from the procedure, such as bleeding. If coagulation problems remain uncorrected, for example, the surgeon may wish to postpone the procedure.
Obtain and assemble the necessary equipment.	Prevents unnecessary delays in care
Provide for the client's privacy.	Decreases client anxiety
Make sure the client has signed an informed consent form.	Ensures that the client and physician have discussed the procedure, including risks and benefits and possible alternatives
IMPLEMENTATION	
Wash your hands and put on gloves.	Reduces the transmission of microorganisms (from the nurse to the client and from the client to the nurse).
Assemble equipment to be used by the physician, maintaining sterility as packages are opened.	Prevents errors, maintains sterility of the equipment, and prevents infection
Administer sedative medications, as ordered.	Promotes client comfort, decreases anxiety

continued

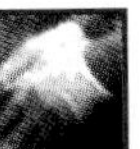

Clinical Procedure 54-1
Continued

Nursing Action	Rationale
Tell the client to lie supine with the right arm behind the head. 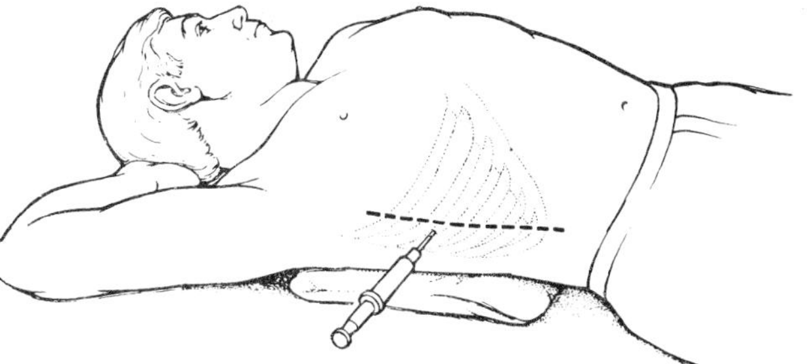	Positions the client properly for the procedure
Provide reassurance to the client as the site is cleaned and covered with a sterile barrier drape. Remind the client to keep the hands away from the sterile area.	Reduces anxiety and prevents contamination of the site by unexpected patient movement
After the physician instructs the client to take a deep breath and hold it while the needle is introduced and withdrawn, remind the client that this process takes only a few seconds.	The physician's instructions facilitate entry of the biopsy needle into the liver while minimizing the risk of injury to other organs; the nurse's instructions provide reassurance and minimize anxiety.
Monitor vital signs throughout the procedure.	Evaluates client tolerance of the procedure and signals arising complications (eg, bleeding, perforation of other abdominal organs)
Place a pressure dressing over the biopsy site and instruct the client to lie on the right side for a specified period of time. If ordered, place a small pillow or towel roll under the right side to apply additional pressure	Decreases the risk of bleeding
Continue monitoring vital signs at regular intervals according to institutional policy.	Allows detection of complications from the procedure or from sedatives
Monitor the biopsy site at regular intervals for bleeding, swelling, and hematoma.	Allows detection of bleeding from the biopsy site
Assess breath sounds immediately after the procedure and at regular intervals. Immediately report diminished or absent breath sounds in any of the lung fields.	Allows detection of pneumothorax, a complication that can occur when the lung is inadvertently punctured by the biopsy instrument
Assess the abdomen and check temperature at regular intervals. Immediately report fever, abdominal distention, rigidity, or pain.	Detects perforation of abdominal organs and subsequent peritonitis
Carefully label the tissue specimen containers and ensure their transport to the appropriate laboratory.	Prevents errors
Document the time of the procedure, client tolerance, vital signs, and disposition of specimens.	Provides a record of nursing activity and the client's response

ration by abolishing underlying causes and to preserve whatever liver function remains.

Various approaches are used for relieving the symptoms associated with the disorder. The physician may order a diet high in carbohydrates, proteins, and vitamins. Because absorption of the fat-soluble vitamins (A, D, E, and K) is impaired, special attention is given to supplementation of these vitamins. Protein intake is restricted in clients with advanced liver disease because it increases the amount of ammonia in the intestine, precipitating hepatic encephalopathy. Malnutrition is treated with enteral or parenteral feedings. Vitamin K is used to correct coagulopathy. Vitamin B complex, vitamin C, and iron

BOX 54-2 Common Blood Test Findings in Cirrhosis

Blood studies of clients with cirrhosis are likely to show:

- Increased unconjugated and conjugated bilirubin
- Increased liver enzymes ALT, AST, ALP
- Low red blood cell count—cells appear large
- Decreased leukocytes and thrombocytes
- Low fibrinogen level
- Prolonged prothrombin time
- Low serum albumin level
- Increased globulin level
- Hypokalemia

ALP, alkaline phosphatase; ALT, alanine transaminase; AST, aspartate transaminase.

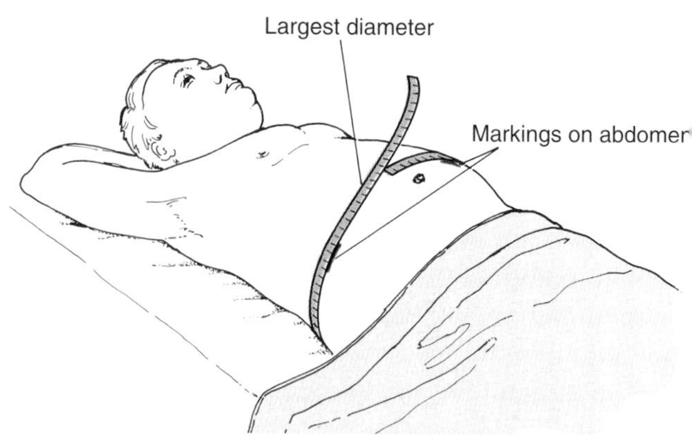

FIGURE 54-3. To measure abdominal girth, place a tape measure about the largest diameter of the abdomen. Make guide marks on the skin so that future measurements are obtained from the same site.

may also be prescribed. Intravenous (IV) albumin may be given in severe hypoproteinemia, and blood transfusions may be necessary for anemia. Sodium intake is carefully regulated and is often restricted because of the potential for water retention, which can lead to edema, circulatory congestion, and heart failure. Fluid intake may also be restricted.

BOX 54-3 Liver Transplants and Organ Donation

The United Network for Organ Sharing (UNOS) is the nonprofit policy-making organization that administers the Organ Procurement and Transplantation Network. After a transplant team evaluates a potential transplant recipient, the person's name is added to the national UNOS waiting list. Each time a donor organ becomes available, a list of potential recipients is generated, based on factors that include genetic similarity, organ size, medical urgency, and time on the waiting list.

Although most liver transplantations are performed using organs from cadaver donors, "living related donor" programs have been established at some centers. In these programs, which particularly benefit children, a portion of the liver from a living donor is used. After transplantation surgery, the organ recipient requires lifelong drug therapy (ie, cyclosporine, tacrolimus) to suppress the immune system and prevent rejection of the transplanted organ.

Because few organs are available in comparison to the many needed, potential recipients may succumb to liver failure while waiting for a donor organ. The cost of liver transplantation is extremely high, and many clients with liver disease are poor candidates for this type of surgery because of their fragile medical condition. As a result, the decision to transplant an organ is made only after careful scrutiny by the client, the client's family, and the transplant team.

Liver transplantation is an option for treating liver failure as well as chronic liver disease (Box 54–3).

NURSING MANAGEMENT

If the client has active alcoholism on admission, monitor vital signs closely. A rise in blood pressure, pulse, and temperature correlates with alcohol withdrawal. Alcohol withdrawal must be recognized and treated appropriately along with the client's other presenting symptoms (see Chap. 16).

Weigh the client daily and keep an accurate record of intake and output. If the abdomen appears enlarged, measure it according to a set routine (Fig. 54–3). Because of the anorexia that accompanies severe cirrhosis, the client may tolerate frequent, small, semisolid or liquid meals rather than three full meals a day. Carefully evaluate the client's response to drug therapy because the liver is unable to metabolize many substances. Report any change in mental status or signs of gastrointestinal (GI) bleeding immediately because they indicate secondary complications. When discharge teaching is begun, include abstinence from alcohol and all nonprescription drugs unless approved by the physician.

NURSING PROCESS
The Client With a Liver Disorder

Assessment

Obtain complete diet, drug, and allergy histories and a history of symptoms from the client or family. Depending on the circumstances, in-depth questioning may be necessary to obtain information that may help establish or confirm a diagnosis. Contributing factors such as exposure to toxic chemicals, a history of hepatitis, or long-term alcohol abuse may be revealed.

In addition to evaluating the client's physical and mental condition, perform a physical examination. Pay special attention to the client's ventilation, abdominal size, weight, the presence or absence of jaundice, and other symptoms of liver disease. Maintain and analyze food intake and fluid records. Review laboratory and diagnostic studies and the physician's progress notes daily to assess the client's response (or lack of response) to therapy.

Diagnosis and Planning

Additional nursing measures include, but are not limited to, the following:

Nursing Diagnoses and Collaborative Problems	Nursing Interventions
Ineffective Breathing related to ascites, liver enlargement **Goal:** The client will breathe without effort.	Assist the client to a Fowler's or orthopneic position. Elevate the head. Assess respiratory tolerance to activity and modify activity if necessary. Provide supplemental oxygen if the client becomes short of breath. Observe for increased respiratory distress when the client is asleep.
Pain related to pressure on abdominal organs and tissue damage **Goal:** The client will report relief from discomfort.	Acknowledge the client's discomfort, convey empathy and caring, and collaborate on methods for relieving the pain. Position the client frequently to relieve pressure. Administer prescribed analgesics as prescribed. Use distraction techniques; encourage the client to listen to music or engage in an activity that does not require much energy such as a word puzzle or hand-held computer game.
Altered Nutrition: Less than Body Requirements related to anorexia, use of alcohol as a source of food, chronic gastritis, other factors (specify) **Goal:** The client will obtain the nourishment needed to meet metabolic needs.	Provide small, frequent meals so that client eats without feeling overwhelmed by volumes of food. Consult the dietitian if the client's anorexia continues for ways to provide preferred foods that complement the prescribed diet. Provide high-carbohydrate snacks or supplements to meals. Reduce dietary fat because bile needed for fat digestion may be insufficient. Restrict protein if encephalopathy develops. Implement total parenteral nutrition (TPN), if necessary.
Diarrhea related to blood in the GI tract and fats in the stool secondary to impaired bile production **Goal:** The client will experience regular bowel elimination with formed stool.	Work with the dietitian and physician on dietary modifications. Aim for a nutritious, low-residue diet that does not irritate the bowel. Maintain an adequate fluid intake. Administer prescribed antispasmodics or antidiarrheals to slow hyperperistalsis.
Fluid Volume Excess related to peripheral edema, ascites, sodium retention or **Fluid Volume Deficit** related to bleeding, diarrhea **Goal:** The client will maintain fluid balance, with stable blood pressure, adequate urine output, and decreased ascites and peripheral edema.	*Fluid volume excess:* Administer prescribed diuretics and a salt-restricted diet to reduce edema and ascites (excess fluid lies trapped within the interstitial spaces as peripheral edema and in the peritoneal cavity as ascites). If albumin is administered IV, monitor lung sounds and urine output. Report signs of vascular overload. *Fluid volume deficit:* Provide oral liquids within the fluid restrictions. Regulate and maintain IV fluid infusions at the prescribed rate. Control losses from diarrhea.
Impaired Skin Integrity related to pruritus, bleeding tendencies, edema **Goal:** The client will have intact skin with no signs of pressure ulcers.	If pruritus exists, avoid drying types of soaps for bathing. Relieve itching with moisturizing lotions, sponge baths with tepid water, cornstarch or oatmeal baths, or antipruritic ointments. Request bed linen and clothing laundered in hypoallergenic cleaning agents. If the client scratches, cut fingernails short; suggest wearing light cotton gloves, especially while sleeping. Apply a cool pack to the skin to temporarily block the itching sensation. Give intramuscular injections and IV fluids with small-gauge needles (when possible); apply firm, prolonged pressure to the injection or discontinued infusion site to prevent hematoma.

	Use a transparent dressing or paper tape rather than adhesive tape tears that may injure the skin with removal. Change the client's position every 2 hours or more if needed. To minimize damage from muscle wasting and weight loss, provide skin care for bony prominences with each position change.
Activity Intolerance related to ascites, anemia, fatigue, other factors (specify) **Goal:** The client will be able to participate in gradually increased levels of activity.	Adjust activity within the tolerance of the client. Consult with the client on when energy levels seem to be highest and perform more strenuous activities at that time. Determine which activities are essential and carry them out between rest periods. Depending on the client's capabilities, assist partially or completely with activities of daily living.
Risk for Infection related to decreased antibody production **Goal:** The client will not acquire an infection. Temperature will be normal; venipuncture sites will not appear red or tender; breath sounds will be clear; and there will be no unusual drainage.	Protect clients with liver disease from others with contagious diseases. Perform conscientious handwashing before providing direct care. Keep the environment clean. Change dressings over IV sites according to agency policy and follow principles of asepsis. Wear a mask and gloves when changing a central venous catheter dressing when this site is used to administer TPN. Use filtered tubing when instilling TPN and replace the tubing according to the agency's infection control policies
Risk for Injury related to mental changes (eg, confusion and disorientation), impairment of clotting factors secondary to liver dysfunction **Goal:** The client will not fall or have other injuries.	Relocate the confused or disoriented client to a room near the nursing station for closer observation. Apply a bed monitor that sounds an alarm if the client tries to get out of bed without assistance. Encourage family members to take shifts staying with the client, especially if the client tries to pull out IV lines or tubes.
Altered Thought Processes related to increased serum ammonia levels and liver failure **Goal:** The client will become reoriented and will be treated with respect and dignity if comatose.	Reorient the confused client verbally. If the client is comatose, continue to talk assuming that the client can hear but cannot respond. Guard against saying anything that would be distressing. Continue to provide explanations before performing any procedure.
Anxiety related to symptoms (eg, hematemesis and tarry stools), diagnosis, other factors **Goal:** The client will be relaxed and express confidence in the skill of caregivers.	Tell the client about the plan for treatment and the routine for care. Make explanations brief and avoid the use of medical jargon. Repeat explanations because anxiety interferes with attention and concentration. Encourage contact between the client and those who are supportive. Respond as quickly as possible to the client's signal for assistance. Demonstrate manual skill when carrying out procedures or operating equipment. If the client's condition changes suddenly, remain calm, but implement emergency measures as quickly as possible. Coordinate assistance from other health professionals when other than nursing skills are needed.

Evaluation and Expected Outcomes

The client:

- Breathes effortlessly.
- Reports freedom from pain.
- Is well-nourished.
- Experiences bowel regularity without diarrhea.
- Exhibits fluid balance and stable blood pressure; edema and ascites decrease.
- Shows no evidence of pressure ulcer formation.
- Exhibits increased tolerance for activity.
- Remains free of infection and injury.
- Becomes reoriented and ammonia levels drop.
- Demonstrates confidence in the health care team.

Client and Family Teaching

Provide educational information specific to the client's liver disorder. Refer the client to the American Liver Foundation (or similar organization) for education and information about available support groups. Additional discharge teaching depends on the type and cause of the liver disorder and the physician's prescribed or recommended home care.

The following topics are appropriate for a teaching plan:

- Following the diet recommended by the physician; consult a dietitian if a special diet (ie, a low-sodium diet to prevent edema and ascites) is required
- Avoiding situations that could further damage the liver, for example drinking alcohol, taking tranquilizers, or inhaling toxic chemicals such as benzene or vinyl chloride
- Taking frequent rest periods, especially if fatigue occurs during activity
- Avoiding exposure to people with known infections
- Continuing skin care
- Avoiding nonprescription drugs (especially aspirin and products that contain aspirin because they contribute to bleeding problems) unless approved by the physician
- Being prepared for rejection as a blood donor because of liver disease
- Contacting the physician immediately about: vomiting of blood tarry stools, extreme fatigue, yellow skin, light-colored stools

Complications of Cirrhosis: Portal Hypertension

ETIOLOGY AND PATHOPHYSIOLOGY

In the scarred cirrhotic liver, intrahepatic veins may be compressed. Consequently, blood backs up into the *portal system*, the venous pathway through the liver. The portal system consists of the gastric veins from the stomach, the mesenteric vein from the intestines, the splenic vein from the spleen and pancreas, and portal vein, which all drain into and through the liver and out the hepatic veins into the inferior vena cava. This congestion and increase of fluid pressure is called **portal hypertension.** As the normal pathway for blood is obstructed, the collateral veins become distended and engorged with blood (Fig. 54–4). These collateral vessels develop primarily in the esophagus (**esophageal varices**), the rectum (hemorrhoids), and on the surface of the abdomen (**caput medusae**).

Signs and Symptoms

Ascites, the accumulation of fluid in the peritoneal cavity, results from portal hypertension and other factors associated with liver disease. Ascites, visible abdominal veins, and hemorrhoids are indicators of portal hypertension.

MEDICAL AND SURGICAL MANAGEMENT

Methods for treating portal hypertension aim to reduce fluid accumulation and venous pressure. Sodium is restricted and a diuretic, usually an aldosterone antagonist, such as spironolactone (Aldactone), is prescribed (Table 54–1). Administration of a beta-blocker, such as propranolol (Inderal), reduces blood pressure and lowers pressure within the portal system.

Portal hypertension is relieved surgically by bypassing the circulation around the liver and reconnecting the portal vein to an adjacent systemic vein. This lowers the pressure within the portal circulation and decreases the pressure within the collateral vessels.

Complications of Cirrhosis: Esophageal Varices

Dilated, bulging esophageal veins are referred to as *esophageal varices*. A single dilated bulging esophageal vein is referred to as a varix.

ETIOLOGY AND PATHOPHYSIOLOGY

Esophageal varices, which are overfilled due to portal hypertension, are especially vulnerable to bleeding because they lie superficially in the mucosa, contain little elastic tissue to protect them when pressure rises, and are easily traumatized by rough food or chemical irritation.

Signs and Symptoms

Bleeding, which may be slight but chronic, or occur massively and rapidly is a cardinal sign. Massive bleeding from esophageal varices is a life-threatening emergency requiring immediate intervention. Once bleeding begins, it is aggravated by clotting disorders common to liver damage.

Diagnostic Findings

Esophageal varices are confirmed by barium swallow or esophagoscopy.

MEDICAL AND SURGICAL MANAGEMENT

Measures for treating portal hypertension reduce the potential for bleeding varices. In addition, bleeding may be prevented with a soft diet and elimination of alcohol, aspirin, and other substances that are locally irritating. Antitussives and stool softeners are prescribed, when the client is symptomatic, to reduce coughing or straining, which tends to increase vascular pressure.

Esophageal varices are also treated with **injection sclerotherapy** or **variceal banding.** In injection sclerotherapy, the physician passes an endoscope orally and locates the varix, passes a thin needle through the endoscope into the varix, and injects a sclerosing agent (such as sodium tetradecyl or sodium morrhuate) directly into the varix. The sclerosing agent solidifies the

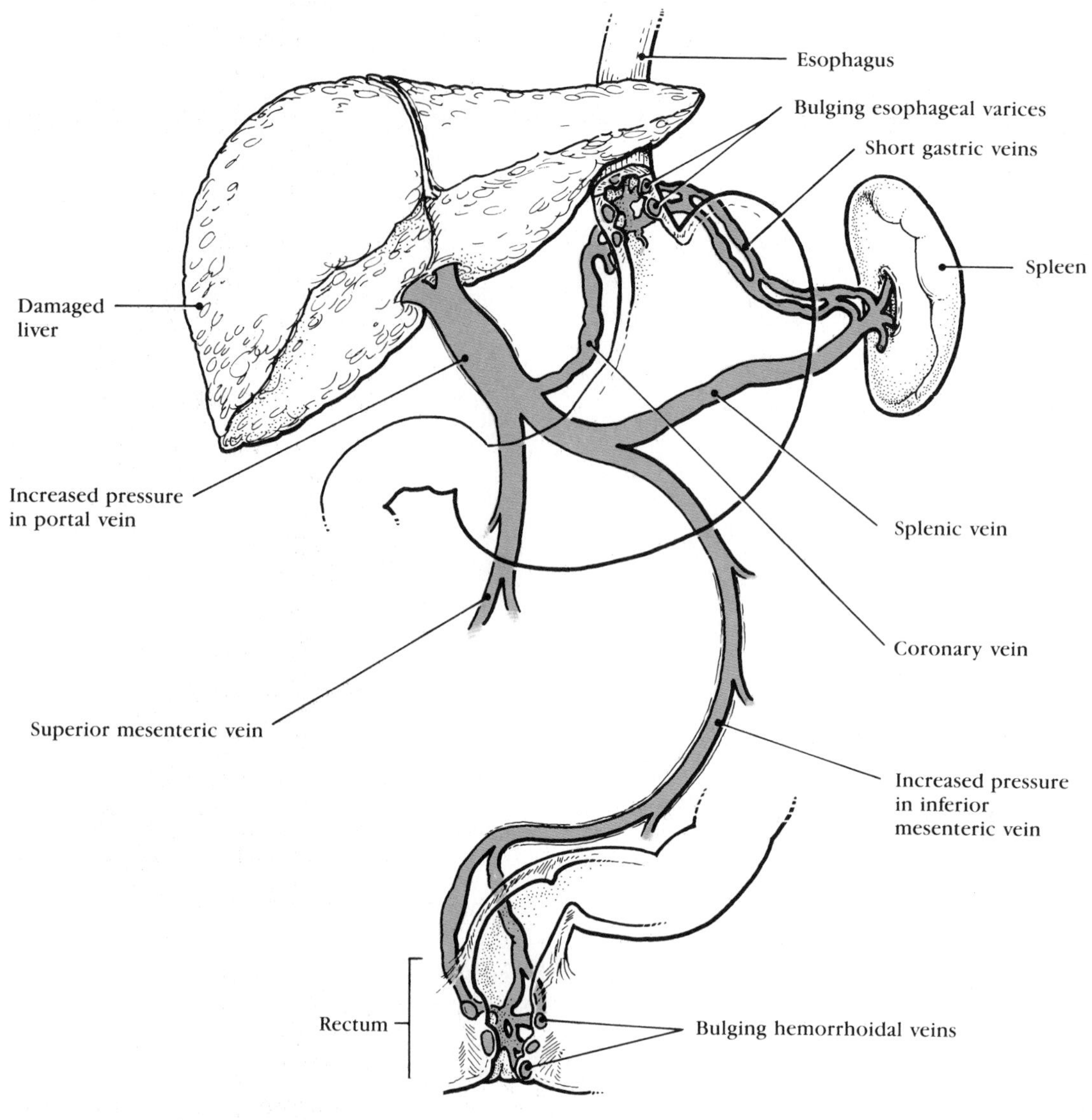

FIGURE 54-4. In portal hypertension, collateral vessels become dilated.

varix and stops circulation to it. In variceal banding, another endoscopic procedure, the physician uses a device that holds small rubber bands at the end of the endoscope. After locating the varix, the physician places a rubber band over it. The band restricts blood flow to the varix, and the varix sloughs off after a few days. Persistent portal hypertension allows for the reformation of varices, making it necessary to repeat sclerotherapy or banding procedures regularly.

If severe bleeding occurs, blood transfusions are administered. Bleeding is controlled by instilling tepid saline solution through a nasogastric tube or by **esophageal gastric tamponade** (compression). Tamponade is accomplished by exerting pressure internally on the hemorrhaging veins with a multilumen balloon tube, such as the Sengstaken-Blakemore tube or Minnesota tube (Fig. 54–5). Clots are removed by suction and irrigation to reduce protein by-products from digested blood (see Hepatic Encephalopathy). During the bleeding episode, vasopressin (Pitressin) may be administered IV. This drug causes vasoconstriction and reduces blood flow within the portal system.

Complications of Cirrhosis: Ascites

Ascites is a collection of fluid in the peritoneal cavity.

ETIOLOGY AND PATHOPHYSIOLOGY

Undoubtedly portal hypertension is a major underlying factor in the development of ascites. It leads to a cascade of events, referred to as the **hepatorenal**

TABLE 54-1 **Selected Medications Used for Liver, Gallbladder, and Pancreatic Disorders** 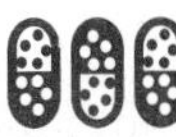

Drug Category/Drug Action	Side Effects	Nursing Considerations
For Liver Disorders		
Procoagulant vitamin K (AquaMEPHYTON, Mephyton, Konakion) Promotes blood coagulation in bleeding conditions resulting from liver disease	Dizziness, transient hypotension, rapid and weak pulse, diaphoresis, flushing, skin rash, anaphylaxis	Instruct the client not to take additional vitamin supplements unless specifically directed to do so by the physician. Assess adequacy of therapy by measuring prothrombin time.
Aminoglycoside antibiotic kanamycin (Kantrex) Decreases intestinal bacteria, thereby decreasing serum ammonia level	Diarrhea, cramping, ototoxicity, nephrotoxicity	Administer orally to decrease intestinal bacteria and serum ammonia levels. Note that discoloration does not indicate the loss of potency. Assess adequacy of therapy by measuring serum ammonia levels.
Laxative and ammonia reduction agent lactulose (Cephulac, Chronulac, Constilac, Duphalac, Heptalac, Portalac) Degrades intestinal bacteria	Diarrhea, cramping, abdominal distention, flatulence, nausea, vomiting, belching, hypernatremia	Because acidic stools will excoriate the perianal area, perform careful cleansing after bowel movements to maintain skin integrity. Monitor serum sodium level for hypernatremia. Assess adequacy of therapy by measuring serum ammonia levels.
Bile acid sequestrant cholestyramine (Questran) Reduces pruritus by binding bile salts for excretion in feces	Headache, anxiety, vertigo, dizziness, insomnia, fatigue, tinnitus, constipation, hematuria, dysuria, skin rash, muscle and joint pain	Give all other drugs at least 1 hour before or 4 hours after cholestyramine because drug interferes with absorption of fat-soluble vitamins (A, D, E, and K), as well as many other drugs. Mix powder with liquid. Taking the medication in its dry form causes esophageal irritation and severe constipation.
Potassium-sparing diuretic spironolactone (Aldactone, Spirotone) Promotes excretion of sodium and water, particularly in cases of acities	Headache, drowsiness, lethargy, confusion, ataxia, diarrhea, gastric bleeding, cramping, vomiting, urticaria, skin eruptions, hyperkalemia, dehydration, hirsutism, agranulocytosis	To enhance absorption, give with meals. Protect drug from light. Monitor serum electrolytes, intake and output, weight. Administer in the morning to prevent nocturia. Avoid potassium supplements and salt substitutes.
Immune agents interferon alfa-2b, recombinant (Intron A) Promotes viral-fighting capacities	Dizziness, confusion, paresthesia, lethargy, depression, insomnia, anxiety, fatigue, amnesia, malaise, hypotension, chest pain, anorexia, nausea, diarrhea, abdominal pain, dyspepsia, constipation, stomatitis, gingivitis, transient impotence, gynecomastia, leukopenia, anemia, thrombocytopenia, dyspnea, cough, rash, pruritis, alopecia, dermatitis, flulike symptoms (fever, fatigue, chills, headache, muscle aches), back pain, diaphoresis	Administer intramuscularly or subcutaneously for chronic hepatitis. Administer at bedtime to minimize daytime drowsiness. Monitor for flulike symptoms. Monitor blood studies for hematologic side effects. Explain to the client the increased risk for infection when taking this drug. Advise avoiding contact with those who have an acute illness and those who have recently received oral polio vaccine. The client should not receive vaccines prepared with live virus, unless specifically instructed to do so by the physician.
Immunosuppressives cyclosporine (Sandimmune) Prevent rejection of transplanted organ	Tremor, headache, seizures, confusion, paresthesia, hypertension, gum hyperplasia, nausea, vomiting, diarrhea, nephrotoxicity, hepatotoxicity, anemia, leukopenia, thrombocytopenia, hemolytic anemia, acne, flushing, infection, hirsutism, anaphylaxis, gynecomastia	Administer from a glass container or dropper to minimize adherence of the drug to container walls. Monitor cyclosporine blood levels to ensure that the client's level is within therapeutic range. Monitor renal function, blood urea nitrogen (BUN) and creatinine levels. Monitor liver enzyme levels for hepatotoxicity. Because the client is at increased risk for infection when taking this drug, advise against contact with those who have an acute illness and those who have recently received oral polio vaccine. The client should not receive vaccines prepared with live virus, unless specifically instructed to do so by the physician.

(*continued*)

TABLE 54-1 *(Continued)*

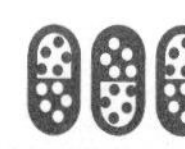

Drug Category/Drug Action	Side Effects	Nursing Considerations
tacrolimus (Prograf, FK-506) Prevent rejection of transplanted organ	Headache, tremor, insomnia, paresthesia, hypertension, peripheral edema, diarrhea, nausea, constipation, abnormal liver function test, anorexia, abdominal pain, abnormal renal function, elevated creatinine or BUN levels, oliguria, hyperkalemia, hypokalemia, hyperglycemia, hypomagnesemia, anemia, leukocytosis, thrombocytopenia, pleural effusion, dyspnea, atelectasis, pruritus, rash, back pain, ascites, anaphylaxis	Monitor for neurotoxicity and nephrotoxicity, especially in clients who receive high doses, or who have renal dysfunction. Monitor serum magnesium and electrolyte levels and blood glucose levels. Monitor liver enzymes. Inform client of an increased risk for infection when taking this drug. The client should avoid contact with those who have an acute illness and those who have recently received oral polio vaccine. The client should not receive vaccines prepared with live virus, unless specifically instructed to do so by the physician.
For Gallbladder Disease		
Gallstone-dissolving agents chenodiol—also called chenodeoxycholic acid (Cheodiol, Chenix) Suppresses hepatic synthesis of cholesterol and cholic acid	Diarrhea, cramping, heartburn, constipation, nausea, anorexia, epigastric distress, elevated liver enzymes, possible hepatotoxicity	Administer orally to dissolve gallstones; may require long-term therapy for effectiveness. Monitor the client's liver enzyme levels. Avoid administering during pregnancy.
urosdiol (Actigall) Suppresses hepatic synthesis of cholesterol and inhibits intestinal absorption of cholesterol	Headache, fatigue, anxiety, depression, sleep disorders, rhinitis, nausea, vomiting, dyspepsia, metallic taste, abdominal pain, biliary pain, diarrhea, constipation, flatulence, cough, pruritis, rash, dry skin, urticaria, alopecia, myalgia, back pain	Administer orally to dissolve cholesterol-related gallstones; may require long-term therapy for effectiveness and may be helpful in promoting bile flow in liver disease. Monitor the client's liver enzyme levels.
For Pancreatic Disorders		
Pancreatic enzymes pancreatin (Creon, Boglan, Panazyme, Donnazyme, Entozyme) pancrelipase (Pancrease, Cotazym, Creon 10 and Creon 20, Protilase, Ultrase, Viokase, Zymase) Promote digestion and fat, protein, and carbohydrate absorption	Nausea, diarrhea, allergic reactions, perianal irritation	Administer with meals and with snacks. Monitor stool consistency. Open capsules and sprinkle onto a small quantity of soft food. Do not combine with foods that have a low pH. Do not crush or chew tablets. Expect dosage to vary with degree of malabsorption, amount of fat in diet, size of the meal and enzyme activity of individual preparations.

syndrome. These events ultimately alter fluid distribution and interfere with fluid excretion.

When pressure increases within the portal system, serum proteins are forced into the peritoneal cavity. The proteins draw plasma by osmosis from the circulating blood. The kidneys respond to the decrease in blood volume and drop in renal blood pressure by initiating the renin–angiotensin–aldosterone system (see Chap. 34). In response, the body conserves sodium ions, which further contributes to fluid retention. Antidiuretic hormone (ADH) also may be suppressed by low renal blood volume. ADH causes water to be reabsorbed rather than eliminated as urine. These combined factors promote the accumulation of fluid within the abdomen.

ASSESSMENT FINDINGS

Signs and Symptoms

The cardinal sign of ascites is accumulation of fluid within the abdomen. Ascites is visible as extensive and massive abdominal swelling.

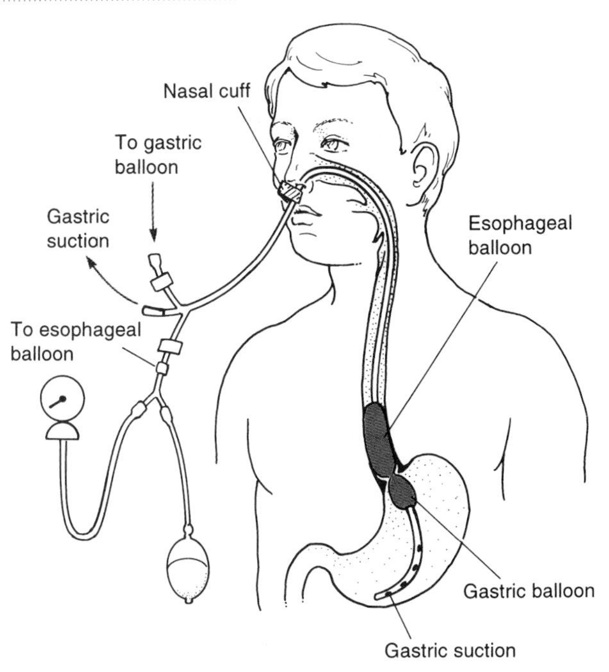

FIGURE 54-5. The Sengstaken-Blakemore tube has three separate openings; one lumen inflates the gastric balloon, another inflates the esophageal balloon, and the third one is used to aspirate blood from the stomach.

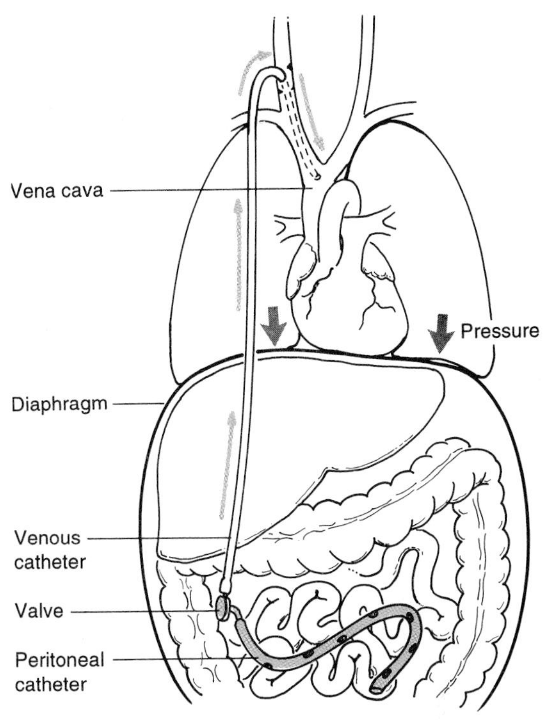

FIGURE 54-6. A peritoneal venous shunt for recirculating ascitic fluid. Changes in pressure during ventilation open and close the intraperitoneal valve, which moves fluid from the peritoneum into venous circulation.

MEDICAL AND SURGICAL MANAGEMENT

Abdominal paracentesis may be performed to remove ascitic fluid. The removal of abdominal fluid is achieved rapidly by carefully introducing a needle through the abdominal wall and allowing the fluid to drain. This usually eases severe discomfort resulting from distention and relieves breathing difficulty secondary to a high volume of abdominal fluid pressing on the diaphragm and lungs.

Up to 6 to 8 liters of fluid may be removed over 60 to 90 minutes. Albumin is simultaneously infused IV to pull fluid back into the vascular space. Blood pressure and urine output are monitored to evaluate the effects of the fluid shifts. Diuretic therapy is prescribed if the circulatory volume becomes excessive.

Additional treatment includes maintenance diuretic therapy and a sodium-restricted diet. The potassium-sparing diuretic spironolactone (Aldactone) may be chosen because this drug specifically antagonizes the hormone aldosterone. Reversing the effects of aldosterone causes excretion of sodium and water, retention of potassium, and reduction of ascitic fluid.

If ascites repeatedly develops despite conservative treatment, the physician surgically inserts an internal catheter to redirect the ascitic fluid back into the vascular space. A continuous **peritoneal venous shunt** (LeVeen shunt) diverts fluid from the peritoneal cavity to the jugular vein (Fig. 54–6).

Complications of Cirrhosis: Hepatic Encephalopathy

Hepatic **encephalopathy** is a central nervous system (CNS) manifestation of liver failure that often leads to coma and death.

ETIOLOGY AND PATHOPHYSIOLOGY

This neurologic complication seems related to an increased serum ammonia level, but not singularly. Ammonia forms in the intestine by bacterial action on ingested proteins. The liver normally detoxifies the ammonia by converting it to urea, which is then excreted by the kidneys. A failing liver, as in advanced cirrhosis, can no longer break down ammonia and the ammonia, therefore, accumulates in the blood. Ammonia can cross the blood–brain barrier and enter brain cells where it interferes with brain metabolism, cell membrane pump mechanisms, and neurotransmission.

ASSESSMENT FINDINGS

Signs and Symptoms

Indications of the CNS effects include disorientation, confusion, personality changes, memory loss, a flapping tremor called *asterixis*, a positive Babinski reflex, the odor of sulfur to the breath referred to as **fetor hepaticus,** and lethargy to deep coma. Symptoms usually worsen after the client eats a meal high in protein or has active GI bleeding because both dietary protein and digested blood cells increase ammonia volume in the intestine.

Diagnostic Findings

Besides an elevated serum ammonia level, electroencephalography (EEG) may show abnormal waveforms.

MEDICAL AND SURGICAL MANAGEMENT

Treatment of hepatic encephalopathy includes eliminating dietary protein, removing residual protein, such as blood if the client had a recent GI hemorrhage, and depleting intestinal microorganisms with drugs, laxatives, and enema therapy. Antibiotics, such as neomycin (Mycifradin) or kanamycin (Kantrex), which are poorly absorbed from the GI tract, are prescribed also to destroy intestinal microorganisms and thereby decrease ammonia production. Serum ammonia concentration is also decreased by administering lactulose (Cephulac). In the colon, lactulose splits into lactic acid and acetic acid, attracts the ammonia from the blood, and forms a compound that can be eliminated in the feces. Levodopa (L-dopa), a precursor of dopamine, restores normal neurotransmission within the brain. Supportive measures include administering IV fluids containing electrolytes and multivitamins or total parenteral nutrition (TPN). The prognosis for clients with hepatic encephalopathy is grim. Only a few survive without liver transplant.

Hepatitis

Hepatitis is an inflammation of the liver. The disease may be acute or chronic.

ETIOLOGY AND PATHOPHYSIOLOGY

The liver may become inflamed shortly after being exposed to hepatotoxic chemicals or drugs, after lengthy alcohol abuse, or by invasion with an infectious microorganism. The most common cause of hepatitis is a viral infection, which is the focus here. The viruses that infect the liver are identified by letters (A, B, C, D, and E) (Table 54–2). They are distinguished by their mode of transmission and incubation period.

Once the virus invades the hepatocytes (liver cells), it alters the cells' structure. This sets up an immune reaction in which the infected cells become inflamed and dysfunctional. During the active disease process, the uptake, conjugation, and excretion of bilirubin is affected. Most people recover from the acute infection, but a few suffer from *chronic active hepatitis* during which liver damage continues. In *chronic persistent hepatitis,* liver damage does not worsen, but it does not improve either, and the liver remains enlarged. Some clients go on to develop cirrhosis; a few deteriorate rapidly with liver failure and die unless a liver transplant is performed. Invasion of the transplanted liver by the virus is common.

ASSESSMENT FINDINGS

Signs and Symptoms

In some instances, the signs and symptoms of the various forms of hepatitis are indistinguishable. The signs and symptoms for the three phases of hepatitis are:

- *Preicteric phase*: nausea; vomiting; anorexia; fever; malaise; arthralgia; headache; right upper quadrant discomfort; enlargement of the spleen, liver, and lymph nodes; weight loss; rash; and urticaria
- *Icteric phase*: jaundice, pruritus, clay-colored or light stools, dark urine, fatigue, anorexia, and right upper quadrant discomfort. Symptoms of the preicteric phase may continue.
- *Posticteric phase*: liver enlargement may still be seen, and malaise and fatigue may continue even though other symptoms of the disease subside.

Not all clients with hepatitis experience all the symptoms listed above, and the severity of any one symptom may vary. Even though the symptoms are categorized, all clients with hepatitis do not necessarily develop jaundice.

Diagnostic Findings

The blood can be serologically analyzed to detect specific viral antibodies; however, it may take some time. The white blood cell count is elevated as is the serum bilirubin level. Liver enzymes (alanine transaminase [ALT] and aspartate transaminase [AST]) levels rise during the incubation period and begin to fall once the symptoms appear. In chronic cases, a liver biopsy confirms the disease and its severity.

MEDICAL AND SURGICAL MANAGEMENT

Treatment is symptomatic and includes bed rest, a balanced diet given as small, interval feedings, and IV administration of fluids if the client is extremely ill or has a low oral fluid intake. Multivitamin therapy is initiated if the client eats poorly. In some cases, antiemetics are given to relieve vomiting, but usually drug therapy is avoided until the liver recovers. Re-

TABLE 54-2 **Viral Agents Causing Hepatitis**

Virus	Mode of Transmission	Incubation Period	Related Facts
Hepatitis A (HAV)	Oral route from the feces and saliva of infected persons, water, food, and equipment contaminated with the virus	3–5 wk	Formerly called *infectious hepatitis* The virus is found in the blood of infected people, but it is not spread in this way Sporadic outbreaks may occur in college dormitories, camps, prisons, or in communal living with an infected person
Hepatitis B (HBV)	Infected blood or plasma; needles syringes, surgical or dental equipment contaminated with infected blood; also sexually transmitted through vaginal secretions and semen of carriers or those actively infected	2–5 mo	Formerly called *serum hepatitis* Considered a factor in developing liver cancer Some infected people become carriers
Hepatitis C (HCV)	Infected blood, blood products, and probably sexual contact	2–20 wk	Formerly called *non-A* and *non-B hepatitis* (NANB) May be caused by other undiscovered viruses besides HCV Causes mild symptoms May lead to chronic hepatitis Up to half may become carriers
Hepatitis D (HDV)	Same as HBV	Same as HBV	Also called *delta hepatitis* Cannot infect alone; occurs as a dual infection with HBV Clinically is quite severe
Hepatitis E (HEV)	Same as HAV	Longer than HAV, but less than HCV	Found more in underdeveloped countries with substandard sanitation and water quality

combinant interferon alfa-2b (Intron A) may be given to individuals with chronic hepatitis B, C, and D to force the virus into remission. For patients with chronic disease that does not respond to medical treatment, a liver transplant may be performed.

NURSING MANAGEMENT

Use preventive techniques to control the spread of the hepatitis virus , and teach the family and general public how to reduce the risk of infection (Nursing Guidelines 54–1). Focus nursing management in the early stages of hepatitis on maintaining physical rest, supporting the client's nutritional intake, and preventing complications. Before discharge, teach self-care measures to promote health and avoid transmitting the infection to others (see Nursing Process: The Client With a Liver Disorder). If the client develops chronic active or persistent hepatitis and requires a liver transplant, see Nursing Process: The Client Undergoing Surgery for a Liver Disorder for additional nursing management.

Tumors of the Liver

A tumor of the liver is an abnormal mass of cells in the liver. Liver tumors may be benign or malignant. If malignant, the tumor may be a primary lesion (classified as a *hepatoma*) or a metastasis from some other site.

ETIOLOGY AND PATHOPHYSIOLOGY

Primary malignancies are rare but appear to have a higher incidence in people with previous hepatitis B virus infection or cirrhosis, especially those with the postnecrotic form. The most common malignant tumor of the liver is a metastatic lesion from the breast, lung, or GI tract. Causes of benign tumors of the liver are tuberculosis and fungal and parasitic infections. Oral contraceptives and anabolic steroids also have been implicated in the development of benign hepatic lesions.

Tumor cells grow at an accelerated rate. They function in a disorganized manner and eventually impair the physiologic activities of the liver. The tumor may obstruct bile flow, leading to jaundice, liver failure, portal hypertension, and ascites.

ASSESSMENT FINDINGS

Signs and Symptoms

Symptoms of a liver tumor may be vague and can be confused with those of cirrhosis. Jaundice is common. Once the tumor is sufficiently large, the client may report pain in the right upper quadrant. Weight loss and debilitation are common. Bleeding tendencies are noted. Eventually the abdomen becomes distended from liver enlargement and related ascites.

Diagnostic Findings

Alpha-fetoprotein (AFP), a serum protein normally produced during fetal development, is a marker indicating a primary malignant liver tumor. The total bilirubin and serum enzyme (ALT, AST, ALP) levels are elevated. A liver scan, ultrasonography, MRI, or CT scan identify the tumor and its location. A biopsy identifies the specific type of tumor cells.

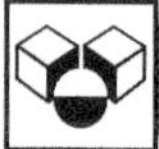

Nursing Guidelines 54-1

Techniques for Preventing Viral Hepatitis

Preventing Hepatitis A*

- Receive hepatitis A (HAV) vaccine, especially when considered at high-risk (health care workers, day-care workers, foreign travel).
- Obtain immune globulin (IG) injection if exposed (in household or sexual contacts with infected individuals) to hepatitis without previous immunization.
- Observe Standard Precautions. Wear gloves if hands come into contact with body fluids, wear gown and face shield if body fluids may be splashed.
- Require child care staff to wear gloves during diaper changes and to perform adequate hand washing.
- Perform conscientious handwashing, even after removing gloves.
- Screen food handlers.
- Avoid eating from public salad bars and buffets that do not have sneeze guards or other hygienic device and practices to prevent food contamination.
- Use liquid soap dispensers and hand dryers in public restrooms rather than bar soap and cloth towels.
- Avoid placing fingers and hand-held objects in mouth.
- Do not share cigarettes, eating utensils, or beverage containers.
- Avoid eating raw seafood or seafood harvested from possibly polluted water.
- Use a pocket mask when giving pulmonary resuscitation.
- Drink bottled water in underdeveloped countries. Avoid ice unless it was made from bottled water.

Preventing Hepatitis B†

- Receive hepatitis B vaccine HBV vaccine, especially if in a high-risk category (dialysis, blood dyscrasias, IV drug abuser, homosexual, health care worker, school teacher).
- Adhere to American Academy of Pediatrics guidelines for immunization.
- Obtain hepatitis B immune globulin (HBIG) if exposed to hepatitis B and not previously vaccinated within 24 hours but no later than 7 days after blood contact.
- Observe Standard Precautions (wear gloves if hands may come into contact with body fluids, wear gown and face shield if body fluids may be splashed).
- Do not recap needles.
- Dispose of needles and other sharp objects in a puncture-resistant container.
- Use a condom when engaging in sexual intercourse.
- Do not share razors, fingernail tools, toothbrushes, or any personal care item that may come into contact with blood or body fluids.
- If contemplating surgery, investigate the possibility of donating and storing your own blood for later use.
- Wear a mouth shield when giving mouth-to-mouth resuscitation.

**Prevention of hepatitis A also prevents hepatitis E; no vaccine or postexposure treatment is available for hepatitis E.*

†Prevention of hepatitis B also prevents hepatitis C and D; no vaccine or postexposure treatment is available for hepatitis C or D.

MEDICAL AND SURGICAL MANAGEMENT

If the tumor is confined to a single lobe of the liver a **hepatic lobectomy** may be attempted for the removal of primary malignant or benign tumors. Metastatic tumors usually are considered inoperable because they often are scattered throughout the liver. The frequency of metastasis and poor survival rate generally discourages liver transplantation as a therapeutic option. For malignant tumors, short-term improvement may be achieved using IV chemotherapy or infusions directly into the hepatic artery or within the peritoneum. Doxorubicin hydrochloride (Adriamycin) and 5-fluorouracil (5-FU) are common choices for drug therapy. Unfortunately, results from chemotherapy tend to be transient.

NURSING MANAGEMENT

In the terminal stages of the disease, keep the client as comfortable as possible by administering analgesics, supporting ventilation compromised by ascites, and reducing the discomfort from pruritus. When the liver fails and coma develops, institute safety measures and continue performing total care. While the client is alert, provide support—for the client and the family—as both begin grieving their potential losses. As appropriate, make referrals for hospice care. Additional nursing management depends on the client's symptoms and treatment (see Nursing Process: The Client With a Liver Disorder and Nursing Process: The Client Undergoing Surgery for a Liver Disorder).

NURSING PROCESS
The Client Undergoing Surgery for a Liver Disorder

Assessment

Determine if the client will be undergoing a lobectomy or a liver transplant (see Chap. 24 for a discussion of general nursing management throughout surgery). Postoperative assessments include vital signs and checking the function of drains and tubes. Continually observe the client for potential complications (ie, hemorrhage, shock, infection, rejection if a transplant has been done, electrolyte imbalances, and hepatic coma). In addition, observe the client with cirrhosis for signs of alcohol withdrawal. Perform standard postsurgical assessments to evaluate the client's breathing pattern, airway patency, pain, and infection.

Diagnosis and Planning

Additional nursing management includes, but is not limited to, the following:

Nursing Diagnoses and Collaborative Problems	Nursing Interventions
Hyperthermia related to infection, rejection **Goal:** The client's body temperature will remain at 101°F or below.	Report temperature elevation immediately because the physician may order blood or wound cultures or increase the dosage of immunosuppressant drugs if rejection is suspected following a liver transplant. Cover the client only with a sheet if the temperature is elevated and chilling has ceased. Apply cool cloths to the forehead. Sponge the skin to promote heat loss through evaporation. Place the client on a hypothermia pad if the physician approves its use. Administer prescribed antipyretics when the fever rises above the range the physician thinks acceptable (usually exceeding 101°F or 38.3°C). Encourage a liberal fluid intake.
Risk for Altered Nutrition: Less than Body Requirements related to nausea, vomiting, sluggish peristalsis **Goal:** The client's weight will be stable; oral nourishment will be taken and well tolerated.	Initially administer nutrition IV until bowel sounds resume and the client passes flatus or stool. After removing the nasogastric tube, give the client small sips of clear liquids to avoid causing nausea and vomiting. Progress the diet to full liquids and then a soft diet according to the client's tolerance. If the client cannot eat for an extended period, explore the need for TPN.
Self-Care Deficits related to pain and weakness **Goal:** The client's basic needs will be met and he or she will be able to participate in activities of daily living.	Carry out or assist with basic needs until the client can begin participating more fully in self-care and other activities of daily living.

Evaluation and Expected Outcomes

- The client's body temperature remains stable below 101°F.
- The client tolerates food and nourishment meets metabolic needs; weight stabilizes.
- The client exhibits greater capacity for self-care; pain and weakness decrease.

Client and Family Teaching

Postoperative teaching depends on the diagnosis, the type and extent of surgery, and the physician's orders. It may be necessary to reinforce the physician's recommendations and explanations of future treatment modalities. If the client has a malignant tumor, further treatment and prognosis are explained by the physician and reinforced by the nurse. Include the following points in the teaching plan:

- Follow the diet recommended by the physician.
- Take planned rest periods during the day and avoid heavy lifting.
- Take medications exactly as prescribed. Follow the directions on the label, particularly with regard to taking the drug before, after, or with food or meals.
- Record weight weekly or as recommended by the physician. Report any significant weight gain or loss to the physician.
- Contact the physician if any of the following occur: significant weight gain or increase in the size of the abdomen, fever, nausea, vomiting, vomiting of blood (bright red, coffee ground), tarry stools, difficulty in concentrating, jaundice, swelling of the ankles.
- Make and keep appointments for periodic follow-up office visits.

Disorders of the Gallbladder

Cholelithiasis and Cholecystitis

Cholelithiasis is a term used to denote stones that form in the gallbladder. Gallstone formation represents the most common abnormality of the *biliary system*, which refers to the gallbladder and ducts that carry bile (Fig. 54–7). If the stones are located within

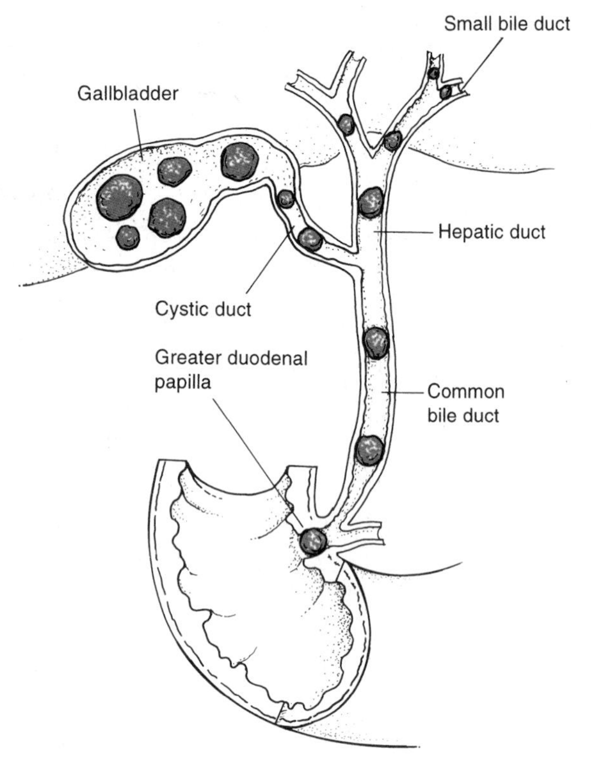

FIGURE 54-7. Gallstones may form in many locations within the biliary tree.

the common bile duct, the condition is referred to as **choledocholithiasis.** The formation of stones often leads to **cholecystitis,** an inflammation of the gallbladder. The inflammation may be chronic or acute.

ETIOLOGY AND PATHOPHYSIOLOGY

Cholelithiasis and cholecystitis are intimately related, and the two conditions almost always coexist. Their incidence increases progressively with aging. Gallstones occur more frequently in women than in men, particularly those who are middle-aged or have a history of multiple pregnancies, diabetes, and obesity. The cause of cholelithiasis remains unestablished, but bile stasis and infection are suspected. The formation of pigmented stones is associated with hemolytic anemias that increase the amount of free bilirubin; cholesterol-type stones are linked to a high-fat diet or predisposition to hypercholesterolemia.

Symptoms tend to occur when one or more gallstones partially or totally impairs the passage of bile, causing the gallbladder to distend with stored bile. The bile stasis causes inflammation and swelling. Each time the person eats fatty foods, *cholecystokinin*, a hormone secreted by the small intestine, stimulates the gallbladder to send bile for its digestion. The gallbladder responds by contracting forcefully. Discomfort occurs from a combination of the inflammation and contractile spasms. Digestion problems result from the reduction or absence of bile. If the swelling and distended volume are unrelieved, the gallbladder can become necrotic or rupture causing subsequent peritonitis.

ASSESSMENT FINDINGS

Signs and Symptoms

Initially clients experience belching, nausea, and right upper abdominal discomfort, with pain or cramps after a meal containing fried, greasy, spicy, or fatty foods. Symptoms become acute when a stone blocks the flow of bile from the gallbladder. With acute cholecystitis, clients usually are very sick with fever, vomiting, tenderness over the liver, and severe pain called **biliary colic.** The pain may radiate to the back and shoulders. The gallbladder may be so swollen that it becomes palpable. Slight jaundice may be noted. The urine appears dark brown and the stools may be light colored.

Diagnostic Findings

Various tests are performed to rule out other disorders that mimic similar symptoms. Eventually, the stones and structural changes in the gallbladder are imaged by means of cholecystography (gallbladder imaging), ultrasonography, CT scan, or radionuclide imaging. Percutaneous transhepatic cholangiography distinguishes jaundice caused by liver disease from that of jaundice due to gallbladder disease. Endoscopic retrograde cholangiopancreatotomy (ERCP) locates stones that have collected within the common bile duct. Clients with jaundice have an elevated bilirubin level and leukocytosis findings correlate with inflammation. In addition, serum liver enzymes also may be elevated. The prothrombin time may be prolonged due to interference with absorption of vitamin K.

MEDICAL MANAGEMENT

When the gallbladder is acutely inflamed, the client takes nothing by mouth (NPO). Instead, a nasogastric tube is inserted and antibiotics and parenteral fluids are prescribed until the inflammation subsides. Treatment of mild or chronic cholecystitis involves a low-fat diet. To relieve pain and discomfort, analgesics, anticholinergics, and even nitroglycerin are prescribed. Fat-soluble vitamins may be ordered to compensate for their reduced absorption. A bile-binding resin, such as cholestyramine (Questran), is prescribed to relieve pruritus.

Clients who are a surgical risk and whose gallstones appear radiolucent on diagnostic studies receive oral bile acids, either chenodeoxycholic acid henodiol, Chenix) or ursodeoxycholic acid (urso-iol, Actigall), in an attempt to dissolve the gall-ones. These drugs, which may take between 6 and 2 months to be effective, are only moderately suc-essful. The success rate is greatest when the stones re small, but there is a high rate of recurrence within years.

Dissolving the stones by direct contact may be at-mpted by instilling a solvent, methyl terbutyl ether, ito the gallbladder or common bile duct through a ercutaneously placed catheter. If successful, the ones clear in hours or a few days. The rate for recur-nce at this time is unknown.

Lithotripsy, a nonsurgical procedure using shock aves generated by a machine called a lithotriptor, ay break up some types of gallstones. The shock aves are directed at the gallbladder while the anes-etized client lies in a special kind of water tank. Af-r the shock waves fragment the gallstones, they are moved by endoscopy or direct contact dissolution.

Stones within the common bile duct can be re-oved by performing a *sphincterotomy* (opening of the sphincter of Oddi where the common bile duct joins the duodenum) using an endoscope. The stone is snared or retrieved using a basket-like attachment on the endoscope.

SURGICAL MANAGEMENT

Laparoscopic cholecystectomy is the preferred surgical procedure for gallbladder removal. It is the treatment of choice for about 80% of clients with gall-bladder disease. The procedure requires general anesthesia, but the surgery is performed with an en-doscope inserted within one of three or four small puncture sites in the abdomen (Fig. 54–8). After in-flating the abdomen with carbon dioxide to displace abdominal structures and provide a better view, the surgeon drains the gallbladder, dissects the vessels and ducts, and then grasps and removes the gallblad-der. Next the surgeon staples the puncture sites closed and covers the incisions with a light dressing. Most clients return home in the evening or the morn-ing after the procedure. Although a nasogastric tube

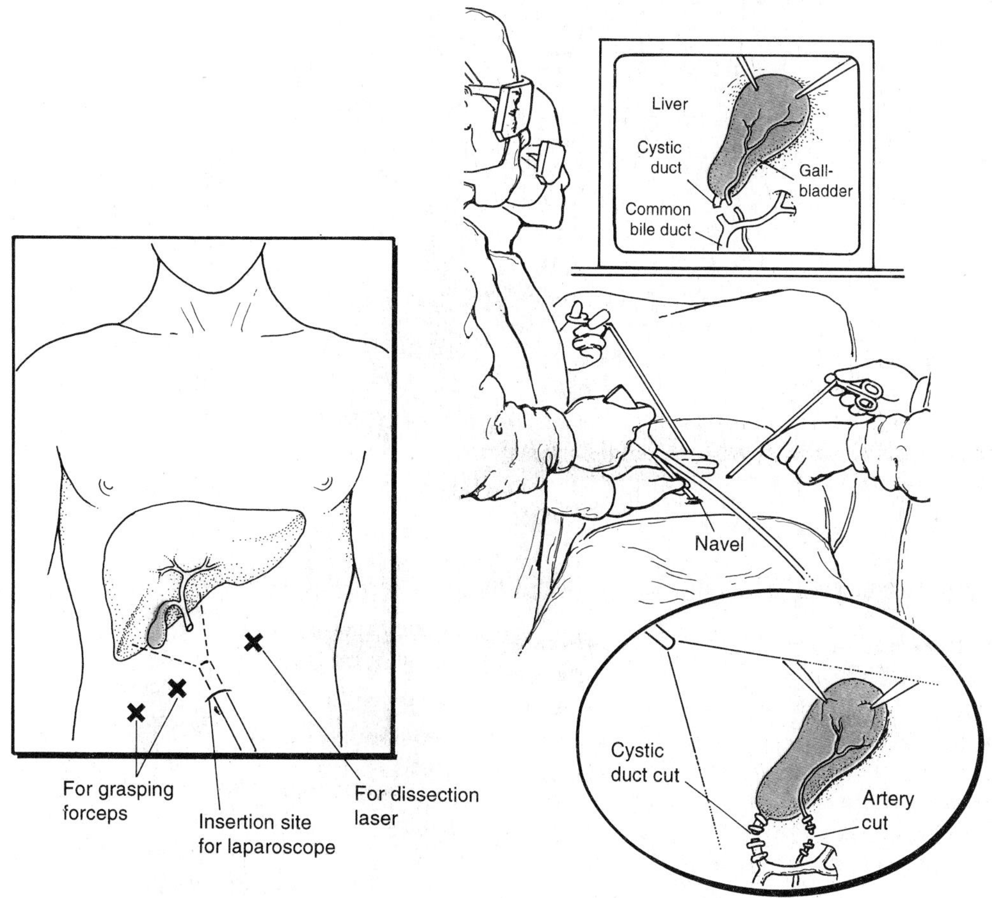

FIGURE 54-8. In laparoscopic cholecystectomy, the abdominal organs are viewed on a TV monitor while the gallbladder is removed.

may have been inserted during surgery, it is removed before the client is awake and alert. Mild analgesics are administered to relieve minor discomfort. The client may eat food once the effects of the anesthetic subside. A prolonged recovery period is usually unnecessary. Most clients resume normal activities within a week.

For some clients laparoscopic removal is not possible. When the gallbladder is extremely distended and fragile due to inflammation and infection or contains unusually large or multiple stones, it may be dangerous to remove it through a small abdominal opening. In these cases, the surgeon performs an **open cholecystectomy**. This procedure involves a *laparotomy* (abdominal incision). A Penrose drain, a wide, flat rubber tube, or a vacuum drain, a plastic tube connected to a bulb or other collecting device, is inserted within the wound to remove serosanguineous fluid. Postoperatively, clients experience a lengthy period of gastric decompression, acute postoperative pain, and about a week of hospitalization followed by a 6-week recovery period after discharge.

During cholecystectomy, a *choledochotomy*, surgical opening and exploration of the common bile duct, may be performed. A **T-tube** (a tube used to drain bile) is generally inserted while the surgical wound heals (Fig. 54–9). The T-tube is brought through the abdomen near the incision and connected to gravity drainage. Bile salts such as dehydrocholic acid (Decholin) may be prescribed to promote drainage.

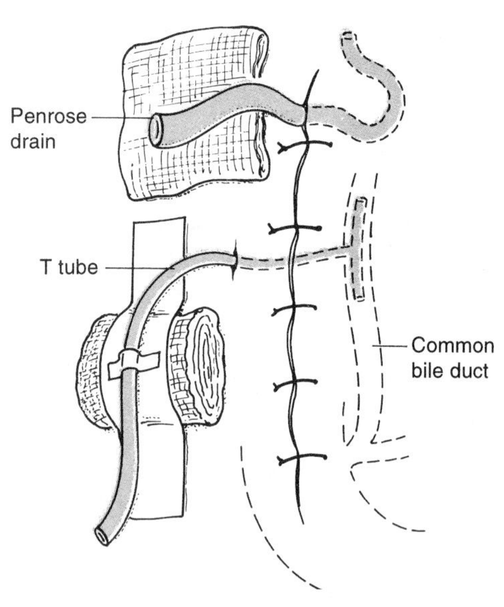

FIGURE 54-9. After an open cholecystectomy, a wound drain removes exudate from the area formerly occupied by the gallbladder, and a T-tube diverts bile, which is still being formed by the liver.

NURSING MANAGEMENT

During an attack of biliary colic, ensure that th client rests, monitor the client's ability to digest bland liquid diet, and administer prescribed ant spasmodics or analgesics. If gastric decompression required, insert a nasogastric tube and connect it t suction (see Chap. 51). If lithotripsy or another proce dure is initiated to remove the stones, observe th client closely after the procedure for increased pai shock, or signs of internal bleeding.

The general plan of care for a client with a mec ically treated gallbladder disorder includes, but is nc limited to, the following:

Nursing Diagnoses and Collaborative Problems	Nursing Interventions
Pain related to inflammation, gallstones, or tissue trauma from nonsurgical treatment	When certain types of foods (usually fatty foods) cause pain, omit them from the diet
Goal: The client will experience a reduction or elimination of pain.	Provide frequent, small meal
	As prescribed, administer a narcotic analgesic, such as meperidine (Demerol), and smooth muscle relaxants to re lieve severe pain that cannot controlled by other measures
	Question any order for morphin sulfate. This drug causes spasms in the common bile duct and the sphincter of Odc resulting in increased pain.
Anxiety related to concern over significance of symptoms, unfamiliarity with diagnosis	Relieve insecurity and dispel fantasized fears by providing the client with information about his or her condition.
Goal: The client will report reduced anxiety because of increased knowledge about self-care and health maintenance	Explain gallbladder function, reasons for the pain, and the tionale of treatment measure
	Reinforce or clarify explanations of planned procedures, such as lithotripsy. Provide time for asking and answerir questions.
	Be sure to inform the client even if the gallbladder is removed, the liver still produc bile, which is transported to intestine.

Same-Day Surgery

When outpatient or laparoscopic surgery is sche uled, be sure the client receives thorough presurgic instruction and laboratory testing and understan the consent form. On the day of surgery, comple preoperative skin preparation, insert an IV line, ar administer sedation. After the client recovers frc

NURSING CARE PLAN 54-1

Managing the Care of a Client With an Open Cholecystectomy

Potential Problems and Nursing Diagnoses	Nursing Management	Outcome Criteria
Pain related to tissue trauma	Administer analgesics. Support incision during coughing and deep breathing. Reposition the client gently. Maintain the patency of the nasogastric tube and T-tube, if present. Empty the drainage from a vacuum drain, if present, before ambulation and support the collection device during ambulation.	Pain is controlled.
PC: Pneumonia **Risk for Ineffective Airway Clearance** related to inadequate coughing and deep-breathing secondary to incisional pain	Medicate the client when appropriate. Place in Fowler's position. Instruct client to take a slow deep inspiration and expiration. If breaths are shallow, use an incentive spirometer. • With the mouthpiece in place, have the client inhale slowly through the mouth to the 500 to 1,000-mL mark. • Instruct to hold the breath for 2 to 5 seconds. • Remove the mouthpiece during expiration. • Repeat 5 to 10 times every 2 hours according to tolerance. If lung sounds are moist, splint the incision and instruct the client to voluntarily cough several times in succession near the end of exhalation until feeling the need to inhale again.	Clear breath sounds are heard throughout the lungs; no fever.
PC: Thrombophlebitis **Risk for Impaired Tissue Integrity** related to venous stasis secondary to inactivity	Coach the client to pump each calf, plantar flexing and dorsiflexing the foot and to follow with rotating the ankles as if making a circle with each great toe. Next, advise client to flex and extend each leg at the knee; repeat 5 to 10 times every 2 hours. Remove and reapply elastic stockings once per shift. Ambulate three times daily.	Homans' sign is negative.
PC: Dehydration/Electrolyte Imbalance **Risk for Fluid Volume Deficit** related to fluid losses	Maintain IV infusions at prescribed rate. Measure intake and output. Provide oral fluids when nasogastric tube is removed.	Urine output is $\geq$ 500 mL/day; serum electrolytes are within normal ranges.
Risk for Impaired Skin Integrity related to contact with wound or T-tube drainage	Remove dressing when moist. Clean skin with betadine and allow to air dry. Apply several gauze fluffs about the Penrose drain and cover with an ABD pad. Apply a sterile pouch about the drain if volume is profuse. Secure dressing with hypoallergenic tape or Montgomery straps. Keep drainage collector for T tube below incision and maintain connection to gravity drainage.	Skin around drain remains nonirritated.

continued

NURSING CARE PLAN 54-1
Continued

	Consult with enterostomal therapist or physician on using a skin protectant such as zinc oxide ointment around the T-tube if drainage leaks around tube.	
Risk for Infection related to compromised skin at incision site	Perform handwashing before changing dressing. Follow aseptic principles when changing dressing. Instruct client not to touch incision or drainage tube sites. Change dressing as soon as it becomes moist.	Skin edges approximate; no unusual redness, tenderness, or drainage. Wound heals when drains are removed.
Risk for Ineffective Management of Therapeutic Regimen related to insufficient knowledge for self-care	Explain or refer low-fat or calorie-controlled diet instruction to dietitian, include that alcohol should be avoided for several months to avoid irritating the pancreas. If drug prescriptions are given, instruct on drug action, schedule for administration, side effects. Demonstrate and have client or a family member return demonstration of wound care, how to change the dressing, and care of the T-tube and drainage collector. Advise notifying the physician if the incision or drain wound appears red, tender, swollen, purulent drainage is observed, or the output from the T-tube increases (this may indicate obstruction below the T-tube). Refer to a home health care agency if client is not able to manage wound care. Explain that stools may be loose and frequent for awhile due to a continuous trickle of bile into the digestive system because the gallbladder no longer stores it. Inform client to report if stools become clay colored or urine turns dark brown, or if jaundice occurs. Recommend to avoid lifting anything over 5 lb for at least a month to prevent developing an incisional hernia. Review the date, time, and place of the postsurgical follow-up appointment.	Repeats discharge instructions accu rately; given list of written instructions; demonstrates wound care satisfactorily; appointment card for physician follow-up is provided.

anesthesia and before discharge, provide intensive instruction to the client and the accompanying caregiver regarding self-care. Give written instructions for reference. In accord with agency policy, perform follow-up measures, such as telephoning the client on the day after surgery to inquire about recovery progress.

Cholecystectomy

Ask the client to describe symptoms experienced before admission such as the type and location of pain or discomfort. Find out whether and which specific foods cause pain or discomfort and othe problems, such as nausea, vomiting, or abdomina cramping. Inspect the skin and sclera for jaundic and palpate the abdomen for tenderness. Perforn routine presurgical and postsurgical assessment when the client returns from surgery (Nursing Car Plan 54–1). If a T-tube is in place after an open chole cystectomy, maintain tube patency by keeping th collector *below* the level of the incision. This prevent bile from flowing back into the duct. Never clamp T-tube without a physician's order. As healing oc curs, the physician may direct that the T-tube b clamped temporarily before a meal and reopened later after eating.

Measure bile drainage every 8 hours. If more than 500 mL of bile drains within 24 hours or if drainage is significantly reduced, notify the physician. Take care is taken to prevent tension on the tubing, which may dislodge its internal placement. A return of normal color to stool and urine indicates that bile is being deposited normally within the GI tract.

Client and Family Teaching

Among the many aspects of care for clients with gallbladder disease are diet and drug therapy. As the client desires, schedule a consultation with a dietitian. Provide a complete list of foods to be avoided, and show the client how to read the labels of all food products to determine their fat content.

When applicable, explain the purpose of drug therapy, the schedule to follow for its administration, and point out potential side effects. Inform the client that the medication must be continued, even if symptoms disappear, and that frequent monitoring of the effect of drug therapy is necessary. Reinforce the importance of contacting the physician immediately if severe pain, jaundice, or a fever occurs or if the color of the stools or urine changes.

Disorders of the Pancreas

Pancreatitis

Pancreatitis, an inflammation of the pancreas, may be acute and fatal or chronic with a long history of relapse and recurrent attacks.

Acute Pancreatitis

ETIOLOGY AND PATHOPHYSIOLOGY

Acute pancreatitis tends to develop in people with a history of biliary tract disease, trauma to the abdomen, hyperparathyroidism, or high alcohol intake. Alcohol causes edema of the duodenum and decreases the tone of the sphincter of Oddi, creating a condition in which duodenal contents can move into the pancreatic duct. However, for unknown reasons, acute pancreatitis can develop in clients without any predisposing factors.

Inflammation is generally initiated by a reflux of bile and duodenal contents into the pancreatic duct, which activates the exocrine enzymes that the pancreas produces. Swelling of the opening to the pancreatic duct impairs or even obstructs the release of enzymes that digest proteins (proteases), carbohydrates (amylase), and fats (lipase) as well as bicarbonate, which neutralizes chyme as it enters the small intestine. As the enzymes build up within the gland, they begin to digest the tissue of the pancreas itself, a process referred to as *autodigestion*. Eventually, endocrine functions are also impaired as the gland is destroyed. Hyperglycemia results from an imbalance of glucagon, insulin, and somatostatin.

Necrosis and hemorrhage of the gland, peritonitis, severe fluid and electrolyte imbalance, shock, pleural effusion, adult respiratory distress syndrome, and blood coagulation problems ensue. When fatty tissue around the pancreas is digested by lipase, calcium binds with the released fatty acids. In rare cases, this reduces the level of circulating calcium to a dangerous degree, resulting in tetany and convulsions.

ASSESSMENT FINDINGS

Signs and Symptoms

The most common complaint of clients with pancreatitis is severe mid-upper abdominal pain, radiating to both sides and straight through to the back. Nausea, vomiting, and flatulence usually are present. The client may describe the stools as being frothy and foul smelling, a sign of **steatorrhea,** a greater than normal amount of fat in the stool, from poor fat digestion. The symptoms—aggravated after the client eats fatty foods or drinks alcohol—are relieved when the client sits up and leans forward or curls into a fetal position.

Physical inspection may disclose jaundice. Bowel sounds are diminished or absent with accompanying distention, and the abdomen is tender to palpation. A bluish gray discoloration to the skin about the umbilicus (**Cullen's sign**) or on the flanks (**Turner's sign**) indicates that blood is being released from the injured pancreas. The client may be hypotensive, feverish, and tachycardic. Breathing is shallow from severe pain. *Chvostek's sign* (facial twitching when the skin over the facial nerve is tapped) and *Trousseau's sign* (spasms of the fingers when a blood pressure cuff is inflated) indicate low calcium levels.

Diagnostic Findings

Elevated serum and urine amylase, lipase, and liver enzyme level accompany significant pancreatitis. If the common bile duct is obstructed, the bilirubin level is above normal. Blood glucose levels and the white blood cell counts can be elevated. Serum electrolyte levels (calcium, potassium, and magnesium) are low. Pancreatic edema and necrosis appear on CT scan with vascular enhancement. Various endoscopic examinations may be performed to assist the differential diagnosis.

MEDICAL MANAGEMENT

Medical treatment concentrates on relieving pain, reducing pancreatic secretion, restoring fluid and electrolyte losses, and preventing or treating systemic complications such as respiratory distress syndrome, acute (renal) tubular necrosis, and bleeding abnormalities.

The client usually receives nothing by mouth, and a nasogastric tube is inserted and connected to suction. This relieves nausea, distention, and vomiting, and reduces stimulation of the pancreas by gastric contents that otherwise may enter the duodenum. Along with general fluid therapy for hydration purposes, albumin may be given IV to pull fluid trapped in the peritoneum back into the circulation. Atropine or other anticholinergic drugs are given to reduce the activity of the vagus nerve, which stimulates the pancreas. IV antibiotic therapy is prescribed to prevent localized abscesses from forming or treat systemic sepsis. If *pseudocysts* (fibrous capsules filled with fluid, blood, enzymes, and tissue debris) develop, they may be located by CT scan and drained by percutaneous needle aspiration. Improvement, if it is forthcoming, usually occurs in about a week. A clear liquid diet is initially prescribed with a slow progression to a low-fat diet. Alcohol, caffeine, and pepper, which are digestive stimulants, are withheld.

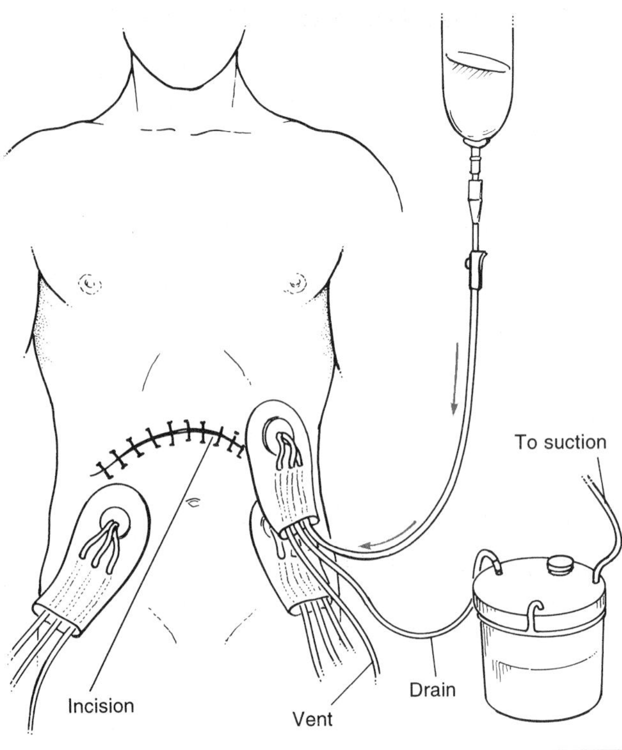

FIGURE 54-10. The peritoneum is continuously irrigated and drained to remove necrotic debris caused by acute pancreatitis

SURGICAL MANAGEMENT

In severe cases, the abdomen is opened to debride necrotic tissue. Every 2 to 3 days, the process is repeated in an attempt to prevent the spread of infection. Multiple sump drains, inserted into the cavity to remove debris, are attached to continuous irrigation (Fig. 54–10). If acute cholecystitis or obstruction of the common duct is thought to be a coincidental or inciting factor, drainage and simple stone removal may be necessary.

NURSING MANAGEMENT

Nursing management involves monitoring the client for life-threatening changes, alcohol withdrawal if substance abuse is part of the client history, and performing the prescribed treatment measures. The nurse is responsible for inserting a nasogastric tube, maintaining its patency, and infusing IV fluids. If gastric decompression is prolonged, the client may be nourished with jejunal feedings of a low-fat formula or TPN. Blood glucose levels must be monitored closely. Clients with acute pancreatitis require frequent administrations of analgesics.

Most clients with acute pancreatitis are severely ill. Continuously monitor intake and output, especially urine volume. If the physician inserts a pulmonary artery or central venous catheter, monitor pressure measurements. Track the client's heart rhythm by continuous cardiac monitoring because electrolyte imbalances can produce arrhythmias. Continue performing other assessments consisting of vital signs, lung sounds, and serum electrolyte values. Observe for bleeding tendencies also. If severe respiratory problems develop, anticipate intubating the client and initiating mechanical ventilation. Report any sudden change in the clients's general condition or symptoms (ie, pain or abdominal distention) to the physician immediately.

When surgery is performed, infuse irrigation solution and ensure that suction is functioning effectively. Provide skin care if pancreatic drainage leaks from the sump drain sites.

Chronic Pancreatitis

Chronic pancreatitis is a prolonged and progressive inflammation of the pancreas.

ETIOLOGY AND PATHOPHYSIOLOGY

Intermittent attacks of pancreatic inflammation may recur from time to time after an initial episode. This is often the case in alcoholic clients who do not remain abstinent or in those who repeatedly reform gallstones that lodge in the common bile duct. However, for some individuals, there is no particular identifiable cause.

With chronicity, the gland undergoes fibrotic scarring due to the recurring inflammation. The pancreas hardens and partial to complete loss of exocrine and endocrine functions occurs as pancreatic tissue is destroyed.

ASSESSMENT FINDINGS

Signs and Symptoms

In chronic pancreatitis, persistent pain, weight loss, and digestive disturbances including flatulence and diarrhea occur. If pseudocysts form, they contribute to the severity of the symptoms by putting pressure on adjacent organs or by rupturing. If secondary diabetes develops, the client may experience an increase in appetite, thirst, and urination. A firm mass may be palpated in the upper left quadrant. The urine may be dark and the stools light colored and foul smelling. Fatty streaks appear in the stool. With the loss of plasma proteins from the blood, peripheral edema and ascites develop.

Diagnostic Findings

Abnormal laboratory findings are the same for chronic pancreatitis as for acute disease. CT scans, MRI, ultrasonography, and endoscopic retrograde studies of the pancreas show similar diagnostic results as those performed on individuals with acute pancreatitis. A glucose tolerance test shows an impaired ability to metabolize carbohydrates because of malfunctioning endocrine cells within the islets of Langerhans.

MEDICAL AND SURGICAL MANAGEMENT

Treatment depends on the cause and whether the pancreatic duct is obstructed. If the duct is not obstructed, treatment consists of abstinence from alcohol, a clear liquid to bland, fat-free diet, and correction of associated biliary tract disease or hyperparathyroidism. The client who adheres to treatment may have good results.

Drug therapy with meperidine (Demerol) is ordered in deference to morphine sulfate. Narcotics are prescribed cautiously. Insulin and digestive enzyme deficiencies are treated by diet, insulin, and pancreatic enzyme replacement therapy using pancreatic enzymes, such as pancreatin (Creon, Bioglan, Panazyme, Donnazyme, Entozyme) or pancrelipase (Pancrease, Cotazyme, Creon 10 and Creon 20, Protilase, Ultrase, Viokase, Zymase), which help to digest and absorb fats, proteins, and carbohydrates (Box 54–4).

When surgery is part of treatment, part or all of the pancreas (**partial** or **total pancreatectomy**) may be removed. If there is scarring, with stricture and stenosis of portions of the pancreatic duct, various surgical measures can be performed to attempt reconstitution of the duct. A *pancreatojejunostomy* (joining of the pancreatic duct to the jejunum) can relieve ductal obstruction.

NURSING MANAGEMENT

Administer prescribed analgesics. Keep in mind that the client may exhibit tolerance or may develop tolerance due to a cross-addiction to alcohol. Monitor the client for signs of alcohol withdrawal that may occur within the first 24 hours of admission. Also implement measures to manage nutrition and blood glucose level and administer insulin accordingly. Institute therapeutic skin care to prevent breakdown from frequent, loose stools. If surgery is planned, manage preoperative and postoperative care. Begin diabetic and diet teaching before discharge. As appropriate, provide referrals to a community substance abuse rehabilitation program.

BOX 54-4 Providing Pancreatic Enzyme Replacement Therapy

- Consult with the physician before administering the enzyme if the client has an allergy to pork or beef.
- If an antacid or histamine antagonist is also prescribed, check with the pharmacist as to the possibility of an interaction* and the best manner in which to schedule their administration.
- Give the enzyme replacement immediately before or with each meal and snack.
- Sprinkle the powdered or granular form over small portions of cold or cool food or mix with milk or water.
- Take care not to inhale the enzyme particles.
- Do not crush enteric-coated enzyme tablets.
- Caution the client to avoid chewing enzyme capsules or enteric-coated tablets.
- Monitor for the normal appearance and characteristics of stool to evaluate the effectiveness of enzyme replacement therapy.

*See General Pharmacologic Considerations at the end of the chapter.

NURSING PROCESS
The Client With Pancreatitis

Assessment

Initial assessment includes a history of symptoms experienced before admission as well as a complete medical history. Ask about the frequency and amount of alcohol ingestion and determine when the last drink was consumed as a method of evaluating if or how soon withdrawal symptoms may occur. For reliability, include family members in compiling assessment data, if possible, especially if the client's condition is serious. During the interview, obtain a description of pain with respect to location, type, severity, and circumstances that aggravate or relieve it. Gently palpate the abdomen especially the epigastric area for pain, tenderness, distention, or rigidity.

Include an immediate evaluation of vital signs because shock often is an outstanding symptom of acute pancreatitis. Compile a description of the client's general appearance and inspect the skin for Cullen's and Turner's signs. Weigh the client for later comparisons. As ordered, collect stool for inspection or laboratory testing. Blood glucose records may be initiated. If the client is hyperglycemic, urine may also be tested for ketones.

Diagnosis and Planning

Additional nursing management includes, but is not limited to, the following:

Nursing Diagnoses and Collaborative Problems	Nursing Interventions
Ineffective Breathing related to pain and inflammation and ascites **Goals:** The client will breathe efficiently at regular intervals and lungs will be clear.	Elevate the head of the bed and provide rest at the first sign of dyspnea. Monitor arterial oxygenation with pulse oximetry and report episodes of desaturation to the physician. Observe the client's color and effort necessary to breathe. Relieve breathing-related pain by administration of prescribed analgesics, being careful to report inadequate pain relief. The client may need a higher dosage due to drug tolerance. Promote comfort by having the client sit upright or assume a side-lying position with the knees flexed. Inform the physician of a sudden increase of pain accompanied by a rigid abdomen, signs that the pancreas has ruptured. Monitor the client's response to dietary modifications designed to ease breathing such as small but frequent bland, low-fat meals. Also administer histamine antagonists or anticholinergic drugs as prescribed.
Risk for Fluid Volume Deficit related to vomiting, gastric decompression, diarrhea, fluid shifts **Goal:** The client will be sufficiently hydrated.	If the client is not NPO, encourage oral liquids within prescribed dietary limitations. Try to match intake with output. If a fluid deficit occurs, notify the physician and implement prescribed fluid therapy.
Risk for Altered Nutrition: Less than Body Requirements related to nausea, vomiting, pain, malabsorption **Goal:** Nausea and vomiting will be controlled; weight will stabilize or increase; and client will follow prescribed diet.	Keep the client NPO during an acute episode, but maintain caloric intake with prescribed glucose solutions to which vitamins, electrolytes, and insulin may be added. Because extended IV therapy does not provide optimum nutrition, collaborate with the physician on instituting jejunal tube feedings or TPN to avoid weight loss and catabolism of body tissue. After removing the nasogastric feeding tube, give clear liquids, progressing to a soft bland, low-fat diet with recommended diabetic modifications. Once pancreatic enzyme therapy begins, monitor for constipation (constipation indicates that the enzyme dosage is too high).
Diarrhea related to impaired fat and protein digestion **Goal:** Bowel elimination will be normal.	Administer prescribed medications and replace fluids and electrolytes. Ensure a low-fat diet.
Risk for Impaired Skin Integrity related to diarrhea, skin contact with pancreatic drainage **Goal:** Skin will remain intact or heal in response to nursing measures.	Clean rectal area after each bowel movement. Use lubricated wipes rather than paper toilet tissue and avoid scented wipes, which may contain skin irritants. Apply zinc oxide or other medicated barrier ointments to the perianal tissue or cover excoriated skin with a hydrocolloid dressing (DuoDERM). Apply an ostomy device over a karaya disk around abdominal sump drainage tubes.
Risk for Impaired Physical Mobility related to prolonged inactivity	Encourage the client to move about as actively as possible and to participate in performing activities of daily living.

Goal: Muscle size and tone will be preserved; joints will remain flexible.	Ambulate as soon as possible at distances the client can tolerate. Supplement passive range of motion if the client fails to fully move all joints independently. When feasible, provide sandbags or weights for arm exercises to restore strength.
Risk for Injury related to alcohol withdrawal **Goal:** Vital signs will remain stable with no evidence of seizures.	Monitor for CNS stimulation, an indication that the depressant effects of alcohol are wearing off. Look for hand tremors and emotional irritability. Report a heart rate over 100, diastolic blood pressure over 100 mm Hg, or temperature over 100°F (36.6°C). Minimize environmental stimuli. Be prepared to administer prescribed sedatives. Pad the side rails if seizures are possible and keep an oral suction machine at the bedside. If a seizure occurs, protect but do not restrain the client. Afterward, clear the airway and administer oxygen briefly.

Evaluation and Expected Outcomes

- Client breathes deeply at a rate of 12 to 20 breaths per minute, maintains adequate pulmonary ventilation with reduced pain and inflammation.
- Fluid intake and output are balanced.
- Nourishment is sufficient to prevent weight loss and malnutrition.
- Client attains normal bowel elimination patterns.
- Skin remains intact.
- Client is active and mobile.
- No injuries are sustained.

Client and Family Teaching

Most clients with pancreatitis require a prolonged recovery period. Reinforce the treatments prescribed or recommended by the physician. The following instructions are common:

- Follow the written instructions for a bland, low-fat, calorie-controlled diet.
- Eat four or more small meals daily.
- Take prescribed medications, including enzyme replacements, as directed.

If alcohol abuse is known to cause acute or chronic pancreatitis, strongly encourage the client to avoid *all* alcoholic beverages. Discuss a self-referral to Alcoholics Anonymous or a medical treatment center. Urge the family to attend Al-Anon meetings. (If insulin administration is necessary because of diabetes mellitus, see Chap. 57.)

Carcinoma of the Pancreas

Carcinoma of the pancreas may occur in the head, body, or tail of the gland. Some tumors are primary lesions, whereas many are metastases from other locations. Because tumors of the head of the pancreas tend to cause obstructive jaundice, they are usually diagnosed earlier. Nevertheless, most are discovered late in the disease and invariably have a lethal prognosis.

ETIOLOGY AND PATHOPHYSIOLOGY

Besides pancreatitis, factors that correlate with pancreatic cancer include diabetes mellitus, a high-fat diet, and chronic exposure to carcinogenic substances (ie, petrochemicals). Although data are inconclusive, a relationship may exist between cigarette smoking and high coffee consumption (especially decaffeinated coffee) and development of pancreatic carcinoma.

When sufficient malignant cells accumulate, they block the pancreatic duct, producing symptoms similar to chronic pancreatitis. There is some question as to whether the pancreatitis is a precursor or consequence of tumor development. Tumors in the body or tail of the pancreas can press on the portal vein and lead to the formation of varices and bleeding. Once a tumor develops, it tends to grow rapidly. It may spread to adjacent structures, such as the liver or spleen, by the time symptoms are serious enough for the client to seek medical assistance.

ASSESSMENT FINDINGS

Signs and Symptoms

Symptoms may not appear until the disease is far advanced. The most common symptoms are left upper abdominal pain that may be referred to the back, jaundice, anorexia, and weight loss. The client may describe light-colored stools but dark urine, typical symptoms of obstructive jaundice. Pruritus may accompany jaundice. A mass may be palpated in the left upper quadrant. The mass may be a tumor or an enlarged gallbladder, which tends to expand due to obstruction in the passage of bile. Ascites may be present in the late stages of the disease. Some clients develop thrombophlebitis from pancreatic tumor products that increase the blood's coagulability.

Diagnostic Findings

Abdominal ultrasonography or CT scan demonstrates pancreatic enlargement but does not indicate the underlying cause. A biopsy obtained by ERCP or percutaneous needle aspiration provides evidence of malignant cells.

Elevated serum amylase, alkaline phosphatase, and bilirubin levels support the evidence that the pancreas is diseased, but they do not confirm carcinoma. The level of carcinoembryonic antigen (CEA) is elevated, but the elevation it is not as specific a tumor marker as CA 19–9.

MEDICAL AND SURGICAL MANAGEMENT

The prognosis for cure is poor. In some cases, resection of a tumor at the head of the pancreas is possible by **radical pancreaticoduodenectomy (Whipple procedure).** This involves removing the head of the pancreas, resecting the duodenum and stomach, and redirecting the flow of secretions from the stomach, gallbladder, and pancreas into the jejunum. The tumor may be irradiated during surgery or radioactive seeds may be implanted. Because metastasis to the spleen is so common, some surgeons may also perform a splenectomy. Rather than do an extensive resection, others are inclined to do a total pancreatectomy. This radical surgery then creates a malabsorption syndrome and historically brittle diabetes that must be treated in the postoperative phase. Some of the complications associated with this surgery also include bleeding tendencies caused by a vitamin K deficiency and liver and kidney failure.

A *cholecystojejunostomy*, a rerouting of pancreatic and biliary drainage, may be done to relieve obstructive jaundice. This is considered a palliative measure only. For inoperable tumors, radiation therapy or chemotherapy with 5-fluorouracil (5-FU) or mitomycin (Mutamycin) may be tried. This form of treatment does not cure the disease. Despite treatment with surgery, chemotherapy, or radiation therapy, most clients die within 3 to 12 months after the onset of symptoms.

NURSING MANAGEMENT

Nursing management for those treated medically is the same as for any client with a terminal malignant disorder. On initial assessment, evaluate the client's general physical condition and obtain a history of all symptoms present before admission. Assess onset of symptoms, weight loss, bleeding tendencies, and the type of pain or abdominal discomfort. Physical assessment includes inspection for jaundice, a visual examination of the stools and urine, and palpation of the abdomen for tenderness and distention. Obtain blood or urine samples for analysis and detection of glucose. Record vital signs and weight, and assess nutritional status.

Preoperative Care

Candidates with severe anorexia and weight loss are poor risks for immediate surgery. These clients may receive IV fluids, TPN, or a special diet preoperatively to improve nutritional status and correct any fluid or electrolyte imbalances. Almost all surgical clients will have a nasogastric tube inserted.

Nursing management for clients undergoing palliative surgery is essentially the same as for those having general abdominal surgery. However, expect the color of the skin, stools, and urine to return to near normal color once the biliary obstruction is relieved. Clients undergoing the Whipple procedure or one of its variations require more intensive nursing management.

Postoperative Care

Observe this client postoperatively for complications such as shock, pancreatic abscess formation, and hemorrhage. Postoperative nursing management measures for pain control, anxiety, impaired skin integrity are discussed in Chapter 24. Immediate postoperative assessments include vital signs and a review of the chart for the type and extent of surgery. Check the surgical dressing. Check all drains and tubes for patency. Note the amount and color of drainage throughout the entire postoperative course. Closely observe for signs of bleeding, such as easy bruising, blood in the urine or stool, or bleeding from the incision, drains, or tubes. Also monitor for signs of infection (elevated temperature, increased pain, abdominal distention, abdominal tenderness, and purulent drainage from the incisional site).

Auscultate lung sounds and monitor level of consciousness. Assess pain using a pain rating scale from 1 to 10 and monitor blood glucose levels several times each day. Note the color of the urine and stools compared with the trends in the bilirubin levels. Check bowel sounds at least once per shift. Follow principles of asepsis when providing direct care. Change or reinforce dressings when they become moist. Empty drainage collection devices before they become full, taking care to avoid contaminating the drainage port. Follow agency policy for changing IV sites, tubing, and infusing solutions. Reassign staff with potentially infectious symptoms to assignments that do not require direct client care or advise them to take sick leave. Discourage family or friends who may be ill from visiting until they are well.

Additional nursing management measures include, but are not limited to, the following:

Nursing Diagnoses and Collaborative Problems	Nursing Interventions
Risk for Impaired Tissue Perfusion related to predisposition for clot formation	Apply antiembolism stockings and then remove them for 20 minutes each shift before reapplying them.

Goal: The client will have adequate venous circulation to prevent blood clots; no Homans' sign; and no tissue swelling or chest pain.	To promote venous circulation, assist the client with as much movement and activity as the client can tolerate. Have the inactive client perform leg exercises every 2 hours. Avoid gatching the knees of the bed or allowing the client to sit for long periods in a chair without elevating or moving the legs. Keep the client well hydrated. Report a positive Homans' sign and any sudden chest pain, a sign of pulmonary embolism.
Ineffective Airway Clearance related to ineffective coughing secondary to pain from large upper abdominal surgical incision, prolonged period of anesthesia, and mechanical ventilation (if the Whipple procedure was performed) **Goal:** The client will maintain clear lungs and a clear airway, deep breathe independently, and cough effectively.	Suction the client's endotracheal tube because mucous production increases due to the artificial airway and effective coughing is impossible because the tube separates the glottis. Once the client is disconnected from the ventilator, encourage coughing and deep breathing hourly.
Risk for Altered Nutrition: Less than Body Requirements related to digestive and metabolic changes **Goal:** The client will have stable weight, normal blood glucose levels, no evidence of fat in the stools, healed wounds, and adequate dietary and caloric intake.	Provide temporary nourishment with IV fluids, TPN, or tube feedings. Once oral nourishment is allowed, monitor the client's response and arrange small frequent meals that are better tolerated than large meals. Follow medical orders for testing blood glucose levels and administering insulin to promote carbohydrate metabolism. Administer pancreatic enzymes with each meal and snack.
Impaired Skin Integrity related to inactivity, pruritus, damage to skin cells from radiation, other factors (specify) **Goal:** The client will experience skin integrity and skin will remain intact over bony prominences.	Change the client's position every 2 hours. Massage bony prominences that blanch with pressure relief to increase circulation. Consult with the physician on using a special bed or pressure-relieving mattress. Make sure that sheets are smooth and that the client does not lie on drainage tubes. Support nutritional measures as soon as bowel sounds are active. Relieve itching and prevent scratching. Bathe the client with tepid water and do not rub the skin after radiation therapy. Avoid using soap, lotion, or creams on the irradiated skin unless approved by the physician. Advise wearing loose clothing and avoiding exposure of irradiated skin to direct sunlight. Secure surgical dressing with a roller bandage or Montgomery straps rather than tape.
Anticipatory Grieving related to future losses **Goal:** The client will develop coping mechanisms to effectively deal with emotionally traumatic information and a terminal condition. The client will receive and accept support from family members, close friends, and the health care team.	Facilitate a response to the prognosis the client received. Do not inhibit crying or other methods the client uses to deal with the reality of the situation at hand. Allow as much contact as possible and open communication with those whom the client finds supportive and assist the client to complete unfinished business. Offer a referral to a hospice organization or support services such as the "I Can Cope" program sponsored by the American Cancer Society.

Client and Family Teaching

Include the following in a teaching plan:

- Schedules and techniques for administering prescribed medications
- How to check the blood or urine for glucose and ketones
- Recommended diet
- Importance of drinking fluids and eating an adequate diet
- Care of the skin (particularly the skin around the incision)
- Symptoms to report to the physician: jaundice, dark urine, bleeding tendencies, vomiting, tarry stools, increased pain, swelling of the extremities, abdominal enlargement, decreased urine output, weight loss, calf pain
- Future schedule for follow-up visits, radiation therapy, or chemotherapy

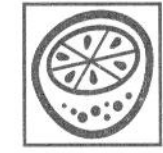

General Nutritional Considerations

A high-protein diet of 1.5 to 2.0 g/kg is used to promote liver cell regeneration in clients with hepatitis. To spare protein, 3000 to 4000 calories are recommended. Fat is allowed as tolerated. Small, frequent meals help maximize intake.

For clients with cirrhosis, there is often a small margin of error regarding protein intake. Too much protein may precipitate hepatic encephalopathy; too little protein intake results in body protein catabolism, with the same effect as eating too much protein. As little as 0.74 g/kg of protein (normal RDA for protein is 0.8 g/kg) may achieve positive nitrogen balance without promoting CNS symptoms. Tolerance and intake are monitored closely; protein allowance is determined on a meal-to-meal basis for critical clients.

Some studies suggest that specially formulated mixtures of amino aids may help prevent encephalopathy by correcting the abnormal amino acid profile seen in clients with cirrhosis. Although clients with chronic encephalopathy may benefit from these supplements that are high in branched-chain amino acids, controlled studies have failed to confirm that they are beneficial to clients with acute encephalopathy.

Coffee, both regular and decaffeinated, causes a significant increase in plasma cholecystokinin, the hormone that stimulates gallbladder contraction. Clients with symptomatic gallstones should avoid coffee. All other diet modifications are based on individual tolerance, including fat intake. Although some clients with gallbladder disease are bothered by eating fat, some studies indicate that fat intolerance is no more common among clients with gallbladder disease than among the general population.

If motility and absorption are not impaired, malnourished clients may be given nasojejunal feedings of an elemental formula during an acute attack of pancreatitis; their extremely low fat content causes only minimal pancreatic stimulation. TPN is used cautiously; some clients with pancreatitis cannot tolerate a high-glucose concentration even with insulin coverage. IV lipids are used sparingly when pancreatitis is related to hyperlipidemia.

General Pharmacologic Considerations

Many drugs are potentially hepatotoxic. Liver impairment may occur in some persons with normal, short-term doses, prolonged use, or high doses. Examples of drugs capable of causing hepatotoxicity are the penicillins, acetaminophen (Tylenol), methotrexate, and allopurinol (Zyloprim).

Oral bile acids given to dissolve gallstones can be hepatotoxic; frequent monitoring of liver function is necessary.

Barbiturates, narcotics, and any drug metabolized or detoxified by the liver are *contraindicated* or *used with caution* in clients with liver disease.

The effectiveness of a conventional pancreatic enzyme such as pancrelipase (Ilozyme) is increased when the gastric pH is 4 or above; but enteric-coated preparations such as pancreatin (Panteric) require a pH of under 4 to 5 to avoid being broken down in the stomach.

Clients with carcinoma of the head of the pancreas usually require vitamin K before surgery to correct a prothrombin deficiency.

Chenodiol (Chenix) and urosdiol (Actigal) dissolve gallstones until they are able to pass out of the bile ducts, but they do not prevent stones from recurring. Gallstones do recur in up to 50% of the clients treated with a gallstone dissolving agent. It is important that the client keep all follow-up appointments with the physician.

Tacrolimus (Prograf) is used for the prevention of organ rejection in clients who have a liver transplant. The drug should be given orally if possible. Intravenous (IV) administration is used only if the client is unable to take the drug orally because there is an increased risk of anaphylactic shock when the drug is given IV.

A vaccination to prevent hepatitis B (Recombivax B) is available for administration to prevent the disease. The vaccination is administered intramuscularly in the deltoid muscle in three doses. The second dose is given 1 month after the first dose, and the last dose is given 6 months later.

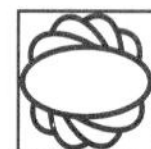

General Gerontologic Considerations

Although hepatitis A commonly is found in younger people, older adults may develop hepatitis through contact with younger people who have the disease such as grandchildren, waiters, or supermarket or nursing home employees.

Older adults may recover more slowly from surgery on the gallbladder. They also are more prone to develop postoperative complications, such as pneumonia and thrombophlebitis, because of an inability to move about in bed, adequately perform deep breathing exercises, and ambulate shortly after surgery.

Disease of the gallbladder is common in older adults. The incidence of gallstones is greater in older women than in men. Approximately 33% of the abdominal surgeries performed in adults over age 70 are for disorders of the gallbladder and biliary tree.

With age the liver loses weight, becomes more fibrous, and takes on a brownish color. However, function is not significantly affected unless disease is present.

While recurrent severe pain is the predominant symptom of chronic hepatitis in young to middle-aged adults, older adults report the pain with chronic hepatitis as mild or absent.

Hepatitis B vaccination is not routinely given to older adults. In general, older adults should receive the vaccine only if they are traveling to areas where they may be exposed to the disease. Immunogenecity is somewhat reduced in the elderly.

SUMMARY OF KEY CONCEPTS

- Jaundice, a sign that accompanies many diseases, results from destruction of red blood cells, liver disorders, or biliary obstruction.
- Cirrhosis is a disease in which the liver becomes fibrotic and dysfunctional. Laennec's cirrhosis, the most common

form of the disease, is associated with malnutrition, chronic alcoholism, and exposure to hepatotoxic drugs and chemicals.

- Individuals with cirrhosis have an enlarged liver, jaundice, prominent abdominal veins, spider-like veins on the face and chest, digestive disturbances, and a tendency to bleed easily. Men may develop gynecomastia and testicular atrophy.
- Once cirrhosis occurs, clients are prone to developing portal hypertension, esophageal varices, ascites, and hepatic encephalopathy.
- Hepatitis, an inflammation of the liver, can be caused by several viruses that are spread by the oral route from feces or through blood or body fluids.
- Hepatitis A and E are prevented by vaccination, conscientious handwashing, Standard Precautions, and appropriate sanitation measures. Hepatitis B is prevented with a series of vaccinations. Following Standard Precautions and avoiding transfusions with donated blood reduces the risk of acquiring hepatitis B, C, and D.
- Liver tumors are associated with previous liver infections, cirrhosis, oral contraceptives, or anabolic steroids and may occur as metastatic lesions from the breast, lung, or GI tract.
- In caring for the client after liver biopsy, the nurse places the client in a right, side-lying position, compresses the liver by placing a pillow or rolled towel beneath the right rib margin, and keeps the client inactive to prevent excessive bleeding.
- Gallbladder inflammation may be due to bile stasis that leads to gallstone formation and infection.
- Clients with cholecystitis experience digestive problems, particularly after eating fatty foods, and tenderness or right upper abdominal pain radiating to the back and shoulders. Bile duct obstruction is characterized by jaundice, dark urine, and light-colored stools.
- Cholecystitis may be managed by a low-fat diet, bile acid therapy to dissolve stones, lithotripsy to disintegrate stones, or endoscopy with a basket-like attachment that snares stones in the comon bile duct.
- Permanent relief of cholecystitis can be achieved surgically by endoscopic removal or an open cholecystectomy.
- When a T-tube is placed within the bile duct, the nurse reports drainage over 500 mL/day, maintains the tube's patency, promotes dependent drainage, prevents tension on the tubing, and never clamps the tube without specific directions from the surgeon.
- The nursing management of a client undergoing cholecystectomy includes pain control, infection prevention and promotion of airway clearance, prevention of thrombophlebitis, prevention of dehydration and electrolyte imbalance, promotion of skin integrity, and client teaching.
- Pancreatitis results from autodigestion of the gland.
- Acute pancreatitis is life-threatening; chronic pancreatitis may recur after an initial episode.
- The client with pancreatitis is supported with diet modifications and symptomatic treatment. Eventually, the client may resume a bland, calorie-controlled, low-fat diet, but alcohol is a lifelong restriction. Pancreatic enzymes and insulin also may be prescribed. Surgically, stones may be removed from the common bile duct to relieve the inflammation, the pancreas may be totally or partially removed, or a new route for pancreatic drainage may be created surgically.
- Carcinoma of the pancreas is deadly because many clients remain asymptomatic during the early stage thus delaying diagnosis, and the tumor has a tendency for rapid metastasis to adjacent organs.
- Radical treatment of pancreatic cancer usually involves removing the head of the pancreas, resecting the duodenum and stomach, and redirecting the flow of secretions from the stomach, gallbladder, and pancreas into the jejunum. Surgery may be accompanied by radiation and chemotherapy.
- Nursing management of the client undergoing pancreatic surgery includes promoting skin integrity, effective airway clearance, adequate nutrition, and adequate coping mechanisms.

CRITICAL THINKING EXERCISES

1. A client has jaundice. What assessment questions help determine the cause of the jaundice?
2. How would you reassure someone who is interested in becoming a nurse, yet has reservations because of potentially acquiring a blood-borne disease, such as hepatitis B?
3. Describe the differences between a laparoscopic cholecystectomy and an open cholecystectomy.

Suggested Readings

Ambrose, M. S., & Dreher, H. M. (1996). Pancreatitis: Managing a flare-up. *Nursing, 26*(4), 33–40.

Chappell, S. M. (1997). Anxiety in liver transplant patients. *MED-SURG Nursing, 6(2), 98–103.*

Finlay, T. (1996). Making sense of the care of patients with pancreatitis. *Nursing Times, 92*(32), 38–39.

Granley, P. P. (1995). Living related liver transplantation (LRLT) in children: Focus on issues. *Pediatric Nursing, 21*(6), 523–525.

Kirton, C. A. (1996). Physical assessment. Assessing for ascites. *Nursing, 26*(4), 53.

Meissner, J. E. (1996). Caring for patients with liver cancer. *Nursing, 26*(1), 52–53.

Murphy, M., & Rossi, M. (1995). Managing ascites via the Tenckhoff catheter. *MEDSURG Nursing, 4*(6), 468–471.

Roberts, A. (1996). Systems of life. The pancreas. *Nursing Times, 92*(28), 42–44.

What's new in drugs. Tacrine users now need fewer liver checks. (1995). *RN, 58*(12), 78.

Additional Resources

American Liver Foundation
14256 Pompton Avenue
Cedar Grove, NJ 07009
(800) Go Liver
http://sadieo.ucsf.edu/alf/alffinal/homepagealf.html

United Network for Organ Sharing
Patient and Public Information
(888) TXINF01
http://www.unos.org/

American Digestive Health Foundation
7910 Woodmont Avenue
7th Floor
Bethesda, MD 20814
(301) 654–2055
http://www.gastro.org/

National Cancer Institute
Office of Cancer Communications
31 Center Drive
MSC 2580
Bethesda, MD 20892–2580
(800) 4-CANCER

13

Caring for Clients With Endocrine Problems

Chapter 55

Introduction to the Endocrine System

KEY TERMS

Adenohypophysis
Adrenal cortex
Adrenal glands
Adrenal medulla
Adrenocorticotropic hormone
Antidiuretic hormone
Calcitonin
Corticosteroids
Estrogen
Feedback loop
Follicle-stimulating hormone
Glucagon
Glycogenolysis
Hormones
Hypophysis
Hypothalamus
Insulin
Islets of Langerhans
Luteinizing hormone
Melatonin
Neurohypophysis
Ovaries
Oxytocin
Pancreas
Parathormone
Parathyroid glands
Pineal gland
Pituitary gland
Progesterone
Prolactin
Radionuclide
Radioimmunoassay
Nuclear scan
Somatotropin
Testes
Testosterone
Tetraiodothyronine
Thymosin
Thymus gland
Thyroid gland
Thyroid-stimulating hormone
Triiodothyronine

LEARNING OBJECTIVES

On completion of this chapter, the reader will:

- Identify the chief function of endocrine glands.
- Describe the general function of hormones.
- Explain the relationship between the hypothalamus and the pituitary gland.
- Discuss how levels of hormones are regulated.
- List endocrine glands and the hormones they secrete.
- Outline information included when taking the health history of a client with an endocrine disorder.
- Describe physical assessment findings suggestive of an endocrine disorder.
- List examples of laboratory and diagnostic tests that identify endocrine disorders.
- Discuss the nursing management of clients undergoing diagnostic tests to detect endocrine dysfunction.

The endocrine glands (Fig. 55–1) secrete hormones directly into the bloodstream. This characteristic distinguishes them from exocrine glands, which release secretions into a duct.

Hormones are chemicals that accelerate or slow physiologic processes. They circulate in the blood un til they reach receptors in target cells or other endocrine glands (Fig. 55–2). Hormones play a vital role in regulating homeostatic processes such as:

- Metabolism
- Growth
- Fluid balance
- Electrolyte balance
- Reproductive processes
- Sleep and awake cycles

Table 55–1 presents an overview of the hormones involved in the endocrine system.

Anatomy and Physiology

Pituitary Gland

Many endocrine glands respond to stimulation from the pituitary gland. The **pituitary gland** (or **hypophysis**) is connected by a stalk to the hypothalamus in the brain (Fig. 55–3). The pituitary is divided into three lobes: the anterior lobe (**adenohypophysis**), the intermediate lobe (pars intermedia), and the posterior lobe (**neurohypophysis**). The pituitary gland is called the master gland because it regulates the function of other

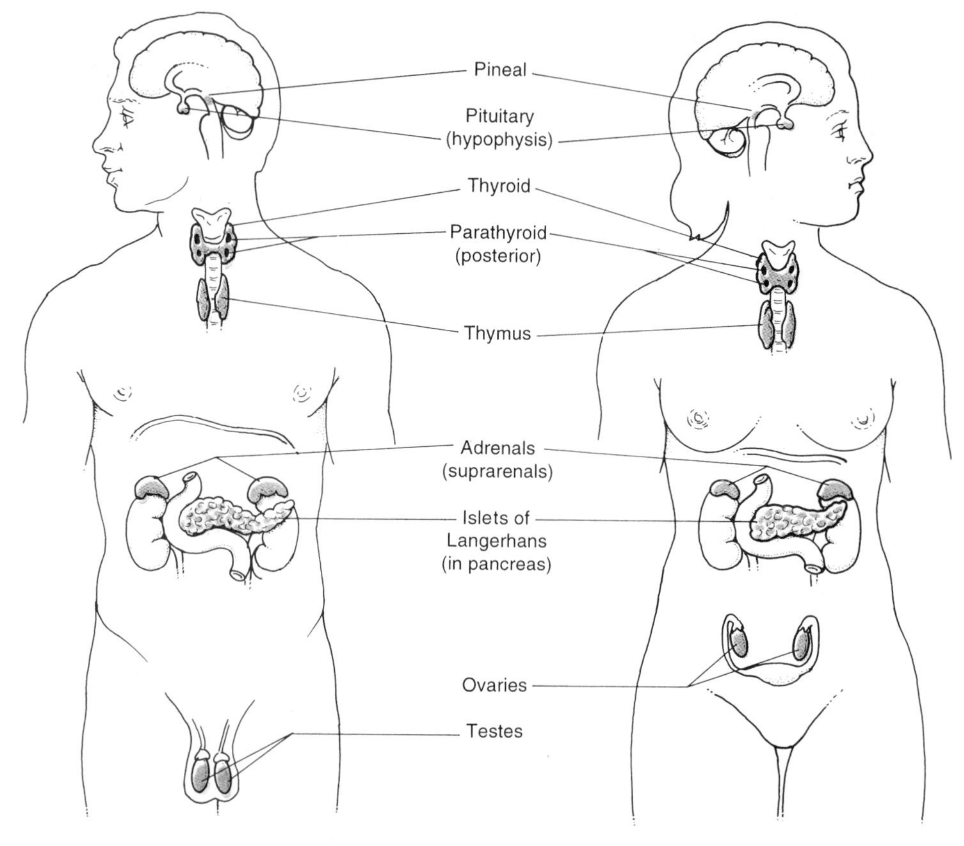

FIGURE 55-1. The glands of the endocrine system.

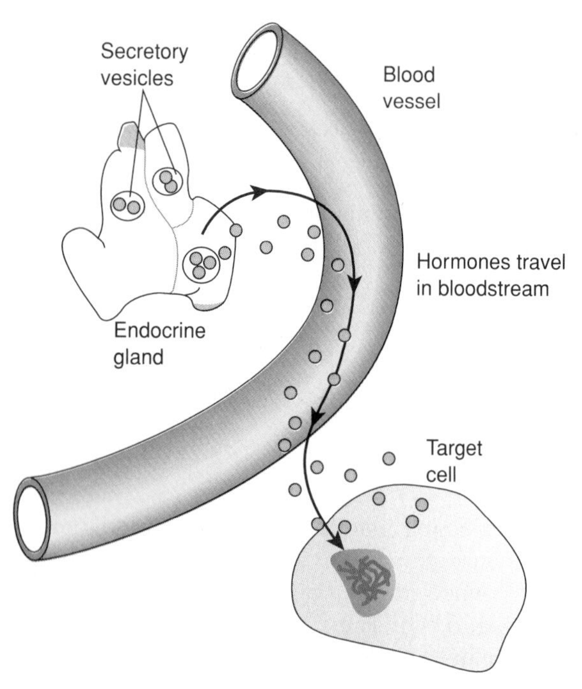

FIGURE 55-2. Transmission of hormones.

endocrine glands. The term is somewhat misleading because the hypothalamus influences the pituitary gland.

HYPOTHALAMUS

The **hypothalamus,** a portion of the brain between the cerebrum and the brain stem, stimulates and inhibits the pituitary gland. It sends nerve impulses to the posterior lobe of the pituitary gland and releasing factors to the anterior lobe. When stimulated, each respective lobe secretes a variety of hormones (Fig. 55–4).

HORMONE REGULATION

Hormone levels are controlled by a feedback loop. A **feedback loop** is a mechanism through which hormone production is turned off and on (Fig. 55–5). Feedback can be either negative or positive. Most hormones are secreted in response to negative feedback; when levels decrease, the releasing gland is stimulated. In positive feedback the opposite occurs, keeping concentrations of hormones within a stable

TABLE 55-1 **Endocrine Hormones**

Gland	Hormone Released	Hormone Function	Hormone Regulator
Posterior pituitary	**Antidiuretic hormone (ADH)**	Increases water absorption from kidney; raises blood pressure	Hypothalamic secretions, blood osmolarity
	Oxytocin	Stimulates contraction of pregnant uterus and release of breast milk after childbirth	Hypothalamic secretions, uterine stretch, suckling
Anterior pituitary	**Somatotropin** (growth hormone)	Stimulates bone and muscle growth; promotes protein synthesis and fat mobilization	Hypothalamic secretions
	Prolactin	Promotes production and secretion of milk after childbirth	Hypothalamic hormones
	Thyroid-stimulating hormone (TSH)	Stimulates production and secretion of thyroid hormones	Blood thyroxine levels; hypothalamic secretions
	Adrenocorticotropic hormone (ACTH)	Stimulates adrenal cortex to secrete cortisol and other steroids	Corticotropin-releasing hormone (CRH) from the hypothalamus; blood cortisol levels
	Luteinizing hormone (LH) in females and interstitial cell-stimulating hormone (ICSH) in males	Initiates ovulation and the secretion of sex hormones in both genders	Hypothalamic secretions, estrogen and testosterone levels
	Follicle-stimulating hormone (FSH)	Stimulates development of ovum in ovaries and sperm in testes	Hypothalamic secretions, progesterone
Thyroid	Tetraiodothyronine (thyroxine or T_4 and triiodothyronine or T_3)	Increases oxygen consumption and heat production; stimulates, increases, and maintains metabolic processes	TSH regulated by thyrotropin-releasing hormone (TRH) from the hypothalamus
	Calcitonin	Inhibits calcium release from bone thus lowering blood calcium levels	Blood calcium concentrations
Parathyroids	Parathyroid hormone (PTH)	Increases blood calcium by stimulating calcium release from bone; decreases blood phosphate level	Calcium concentrations in blood
Thymus	Several thymosin and thymopoietin hormones; thymic humoral factor; thymostimulin; factor thymic serum	Stimulates T-cell development in thymus and maintenance in other lymph tissue; involved in some B cells developing into antibody-producing plasma cells	Not known
Pineal gland	Melatonin	Involved in circadian rhythms; antigonadotropic effect; exposure to light decreases release	Exposure to light–dark cycles
Adrenal medulla	Epinephrine (adrenaline)	Constricts blood vessels in skin, kidneys, and gut, which increases blood supply to heart, brain, and skeletal muscles, leads to increased heart rate and blood pressure; stimulates smooth muscle contraction; raises blood glucose levels	Sympathetic nervous system
	Norepinephrine	Constricts blood vessels; increases heart rate and contraction of cardiac muscles; increases metabolic rate	Sympathetic nervous system
Adrenal cortex	Corticosteroids Glucocorticoids Mineral corticoids Androgens	Regulates blood glucose by affecting carbohydrate metabolism; affects growth; decreases effects of stress and anti-inflammatory agents	ACTH; stress and serum electrolyte concentrations

(continued)

TABLE 55-1 *(Continued)*

Gland	Hormone Released	Hormone Function	Hormone Regulator
	Mineralocorticoids (mainly aldosterone)	Regulates sodium, water, and potassium excretion by the kidney	Renin and angiotensin
	Gonadocorticoids (mainly androgens—male sex hormones)	Contribute to secondary sex characteristics (particularly after menopause)	ACTH
Pancreas (islets of Langerhans)	Insulin	Lowers blood sugar; increases glycogen storage in liver; stimulates protein synthesis	Blood glucose concentrations
	Glucagon	Stimulates glycogen breakdown in liver; increases blood sugar (glucose) concentration	Blood glucose and amino acid concentration
Ovary follicle	Estrogens	Develop and maintain female sex organs and characteristics; initiates building of uterine lining	FSH and LH
Ovary (corpus luteum)	Progesterone and extrogens	Influences breast development and menstrual cycles; promotes growth and differentiation of uterine lining; maintains pregnancy	FSH
Testes	Androgens (mainly testosterone)	Develop and maintain male sex organs and characteristics; aid sperm production	FSH and ICSH

Note: Words in bold type are key terms
Adapted from Campbell, N. A. (1996). *Biology* (4th ed.). Redwood City, CA: Benjamin/Cummings.

range at all times. Most endocrine disorders result from overproduction or underproduction of specific hormones.

Thyroid Gland

The **thyroid gland** is located in the lower neck anterior to the trachea (Fig. 55–6). It is divided into two lateral lobes joined by a band of tissue called the isthmus. The thyroid concentrates iodine from food and uses it to synthesize **tetraiodothyronine** (thyroxine or T_4) and **triiodothyronine** (T_3). These two hormones regulate the body's metabolic rate. Another hormone, **calcitonin,** inhibits the release of calcium from bone into the extracellular fluid. A rise in the serum calcium level stimulates the release of calcitonin from the thyroid gland.

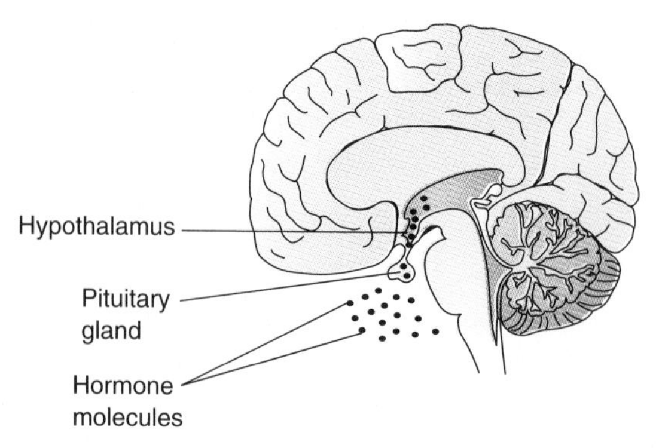

FIGURE 55-3. The hypothalamus regulates pituitary activity.

Parathyroid Glands

The **parathyroid glands** are four small bean-shaped bodies embedded in the lateral lobes of the thyroid (Fig. 55–7). The upper parathyroids are found posteriorly at the junction of the upper and middle third of the thyroid. The lower parathyroids typically lie among the branches of the inferior thyroid artery. They secrete **parathormone,** which regulates the metabolism of calcium and phosphorus.

Thymus Gland

The **thymus gland** is located in the upper part of the chest above or near the heart. The thymus gland secretes **thymosin,** which aids in developing T lymphocytes, a type of white blood cell that is involved in immunity (see Chap. 41). This gland is large during childhood but usually shrinks by adulthood. Functional disorders of the gland are rare.

Pineal Gland

The **pineal gland** is attached to the thalamus in the brain. It secretes melatonin. **Melatonin** aids in regu-

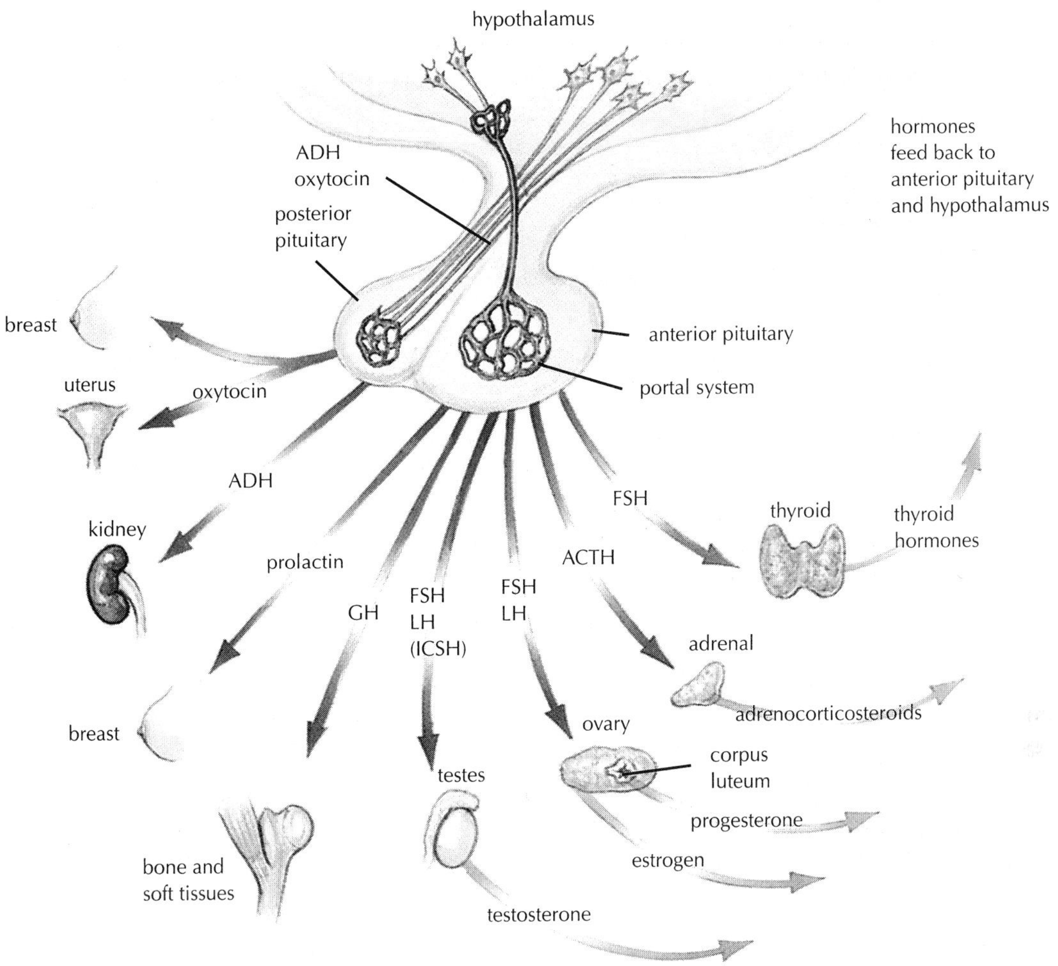

FIGURE 55-4. Pituitary hormones.

ating sleep cycles and mood (see Chap. 14). Melatonin is believed to play a role in hypothalamic-pituitary interaction.

Adrenal Glands

The **adrenal glands** are located above the kidneys (Fig. 55–8). The outer portion is called the cortex and

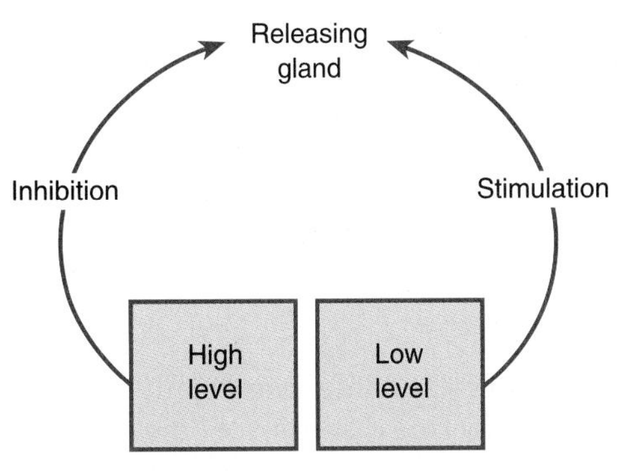

FIGURE 55-5. A feedback loop regulates hormone levels.

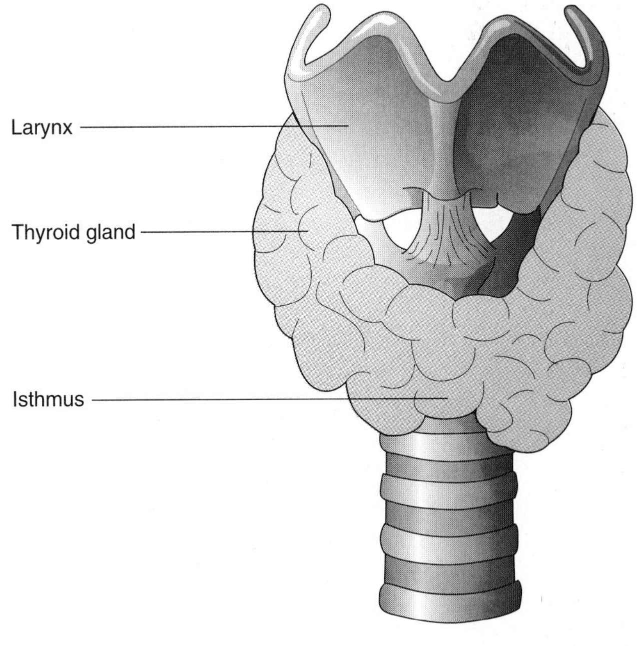

FIGURE 55-6. The thyroid gland is divided into two lateral lobes joined by a band of tissue called the isthmus.

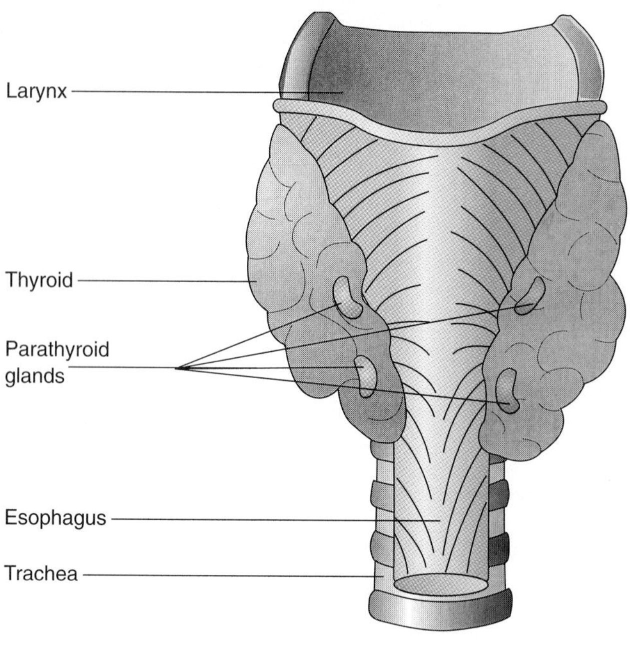

FIGURE 55-7. The parathyroid glands.

the inner portion is the medulla. The **adrenal cortex** manufactures and secretes glucocorticoids, mineralocorticoids, and small amounts of sex hormones. Collectively, these hormones are called **corticosteroids.** Glucocorticoids and mineralocorticoids are essential to life and influence many organs and structures of the body. Glucocorticoids affect body metabolism, suppress inflammation, and help the body to withstand stress. Mineralocorticoids, primarily aldosterone, maintain water and electrolyte (sodium, potassium, chlorides) balances.

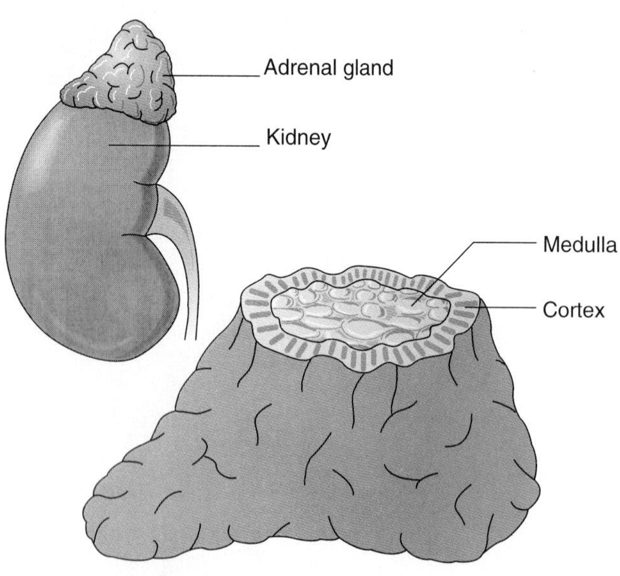

FIGURE 55-8. Each adrenal gland lies on top of a kidney. The cortex and medulla secrete hormones.

The **adrenal medulla** secretes epinephrine and norepinephrine. These two hormones are released in response to stress or threat to life. They facilitate what has been referred to as the fight or flight response (see Chap. 11). Many organs respond to the release of epinephrine and norepinephrine. Responses include an increase in blood pressure and pulse rate, dilatation of the pupils, constriction of blood vessels, bronchodilation, and a decrease in peristalsis.

Pancreas

The **pancreas** lies below the stomach with the head of the gland close to the duodenum (Fig. 55–9). The pancreas is both an exocrine and an endocrine gland. The exocrine portion secretes digestive enzymes that are carried by the common bile duct to the small intestine. The hormone-secreting cells of the pancreas, called the **islets of Langerhans,** release **insulin,** a hormone necessary for the metabolism of glucose, and glucagon. **Glucagon** increases blood sugar levels by stimulating **glycogenolysis,** the breakdown of glycogen into glucose, in the liver. Together glucagon and insulin maintain a relatively constant level of blood sugar.

Ovaries and Testes

The sex glands, the **ovaries** of the female and the **testes** of the male, are important in the development of secondary sex characteristics, the manufacture of hormones, and the development of the ovum (female) and sperm (male).

The hormone produced by the testes is **testosterone,** which is involved with the development and maintenance of male secondary sex characteristics such as facial hair and a deep voice. The hormones produced by the ovaries are the **estrogens** and **progesterone.** The functions and roles of these hormones are discussed in Chapters 58 and 60.

Assessment

Health History

The health history becomes important in the diagnosis of many endocrine disorders. Some endocrine disorders are inherited or have a tendency to occur in

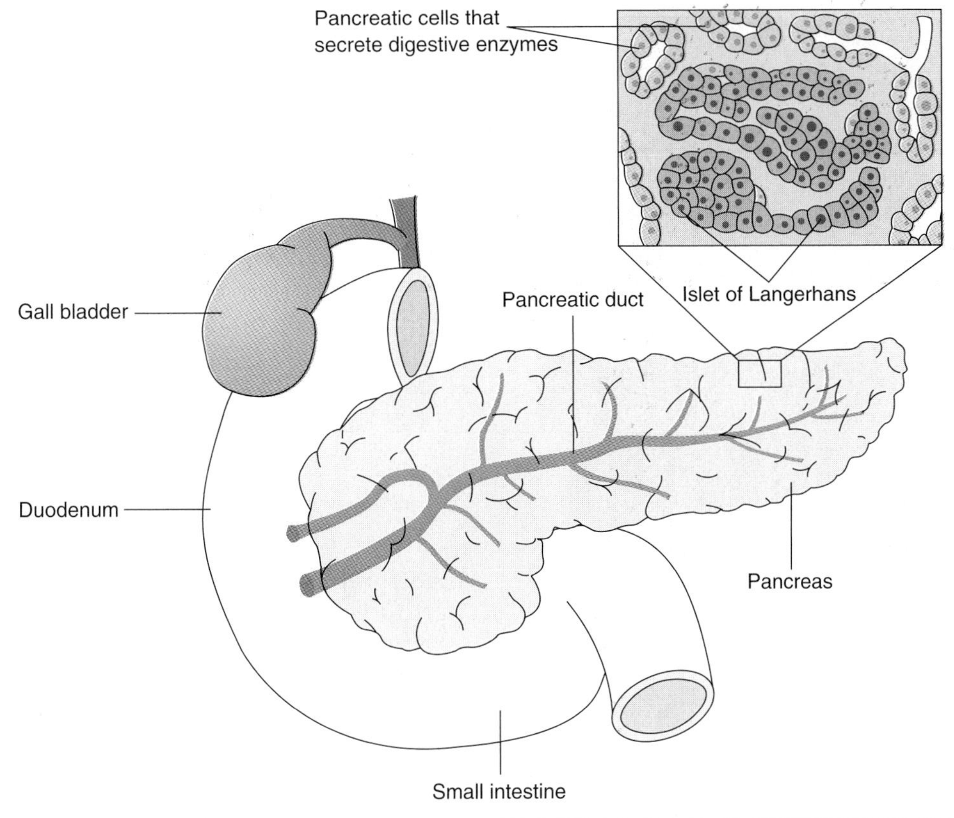

FIGURE 55-9. The pancreas secretes hormones from the isles (singular, islet) of Langerhans. Digestive enzymes are released from the common bile duct.

milies; therefore, a complete family history is essenal. Obtain diet and drug histories also. Document an lergy to iodine, a component of contrast dyes, or afood, and inform the physician. Also report hether the client has had a test that used iodine (eg, travenous pyelography, gallbladder series) within e past 3 months. This information is essential before thyroid test is carried out. Identify the current mptoms. Sometimes the symptoms of endocrine isorders are vague or resemble other physical or ental disorders. Examples are fatigue, personality anges, inability to sleep, and frequent urination. At ther times symptoms are dramatic, such as a change mental acuity or sudden weight loss.

hysical Examination

btain the client's height, weight, and vital signs and ote the general physical appearance. Examine body ructures to detect evidence of hyper- or hyposecreon of hormones (see Chaps. 56 and 57 for assessment ndings unique to specific endocrine glands). Inspect the skin for excessive oiliness, dryness, excessive or absent areas of pigmentation, excessive hair growth or loss of hair, and skin breaks that heal poorly. Examine the shape and color of the nails and determine whether they are thin, thick, or brittle. Examine the eyes for **exophthalmos,** abnormal bulging or protrusion of the eyes (Fig. 55–10), and periorbital swelling. Observe the client's facial expression and general features. Visually inspect the neck for thyroid enlargement. Gently palpate the thyroid gland (Fig. 55–11). Repeated or forceful palpation of the thyroid can result in a sudden release of a large amount of thyroid hormones, which can have serious implications. Note the pulse rate and rhythm. Examine the extremities for edema and changes in pigmentation. Auscultate the lungs for abnormal sounds. Examine outstretched hands for the presence of tremors. Determine if there is any loss of motor function or a decrease in sensitivity to pain or touch in the extremities.

Assess the client's mental and emotional status. Determine the client's ability to process information and respond to questions. Evaluate the client's demeanor, such as dull, apathetic, or extremely nervous.

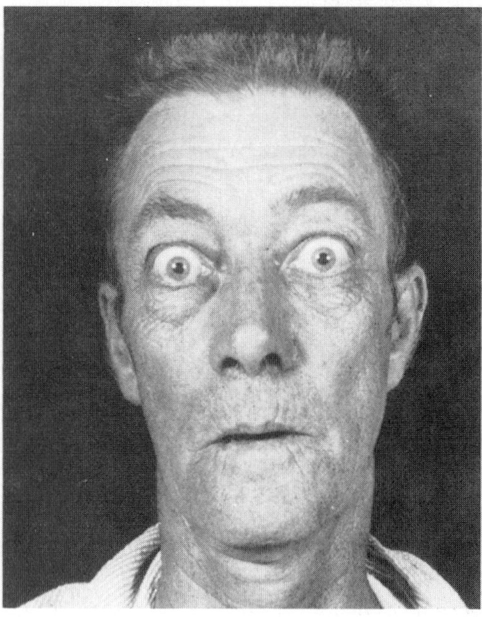

FIGURE 55-10. Exophthalmos in a person with hyperthyroidism.

Diagnostic Tests

The type and extent of laboratory and diagnostic testing depends on the tentative medical diagnosis. Because the physical symptoms may be vague, multiple and varied laboratory tests may be necessary to ultimately determine the etiology of the client's symptoms. A complete blood count and chemistry profile are performed to determine the client's general status and to rule out disorders.

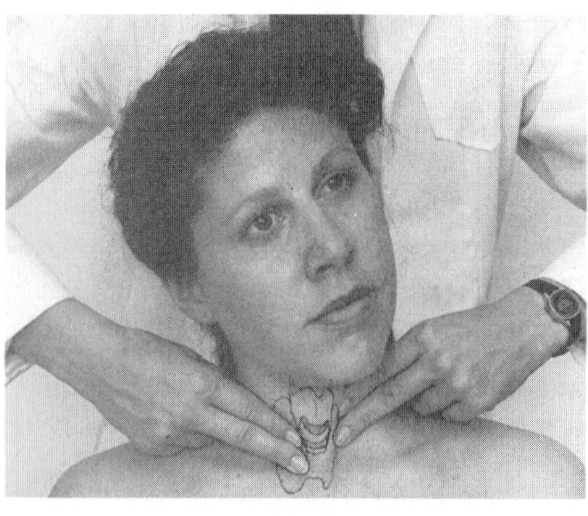

FIGURE 55-11. With the head slightly tilted to the side and the fingers laterally displacing the thyroid, the thyroid is palpated as the person swallows. The examination is repeated on the opposite side.

Hormone Levels

Measuring hormone levels helps evaluate the fur tioning of some endocrine glands. These tests inclu blood cortisol levels (morning and evening) to dete mine adrenal hyper- or hypofunction, antidiure hormone (ADH) levels in blood to determine t presence or absence of ADH, blood testosterone le els to detect increased or decreased total testostero levels, and total thyroxine (blood) to identify diseas associated with increased or decreased thyroid hc mone levels.

Radiography, Computed Tomography Scan, Magnetic Resonance Imaging

Radiographs of the chest or abdomen are taken to d tect tumors as well as to determine organ size ar placement. A computed tomography (CT) scan magnetic resonance imaging (MRI) is performed detect a suspected pituitary tumor or to identify cal fications or tumors of the parathyroid glands.

Radionuclide Studies

A **radionuclide** is an atom with an unstable nucle that emits electromagnetic radiation as alpha, beta, gamma particles. A radioactive iodine uptake te (RAI, ^{131}I uptake) or thyroid-stimulating hormo test are radionuclide studies performed to determi thyroid function.

A **radioimmunoassay** determines the concentratic of a substance in blood plasma. Venous blood sampl are required for radioimmunoassay tests. A radioa tively labeled substance (hormone, protein, antibodi antigens) is combined in the laboratory with a blo sample to determine the quantity of the substance be identified. For example, a T_3 determination by r dioimmunoassay evaluates thyroid function.

A **nuclear scan** uses a radioactive substance that taken orally or injected intravenously. The dose of t radioactive substance is larger than the dose used f radionuclide studies. Certain endocrine organs a visualized or their activity determined by means special equipment. Examples of scans include thyro scan, adrenergic tumor scan, and parathyroid scan.

Nursing Management

Prepare the client for laboratory and diagnostic tes ing. Explain the general purpose of the test, type test, and how it will be performed. Encourage t ent and family to ask questions and discuss the results with the physician.

Consult the institution's procedure manual and physician's orders for the required preparation each diagnostic procedure. Some tests, such as a scan, require no special preparation other than a general explanation. Fasting is required for some tests; others require temporary elimination of certain foods from the diet. Explain to the client his or her participation in the test. For example, the client may required to save all voided urine for a period of time or return for additional testing.

If a client is anxious about the use of radioactive materials for tests, offer assurance that these substances are safe and ordinarily pose no danger to the client or others.

General Nutritional Considerations

me health foods, especially sea salt and kelp, are high in iodine. A diet history includes the use of any type of health food or health food supplements.

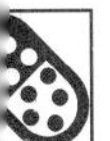

General Pharmacologic Considerations

a client has recently taken a drug that contains iodine or has had radiographic contrast studies that used iodine, thyroid test results may be inaccurate. Other drugs (eg, salicylates and corticosteroids) also affect the results of thyroid tests. All drugs presently taken or taken within the past 3 months are entered on the laboratory request slip.

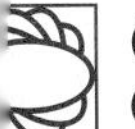

General Gerontologic Considerations

der adult clients may forget the instructions for a diagnostic test. Printed directions can be given to outpatients and, when possible, reviewed with a family member. This is especially important if test preparations or participation in the test are complicated.

hen obtaining a drug history before a diagnostic examination in an older adult, it may be necessary to consult a family member or the caregiver to confirm drugs currently being taken or those taken within the last several months.

SUMMARY OF KEY CONCEPTS

The chief characteristic of endocrine glands is that they are ductless; they secrete hormones directly into the bloodstream.

- Hormones are chemicals that speed up or slow down physiologic processes.
- The hypothalamus, a portion of the brain between the cerebrum and the brain stem, stimulates and inhibits the pituitary gland.
- Hormone levels are controlled via a feedback loop. When hormone levels decrease, the releasing gland is stimulated. In positive feedback the opposite occurs.
- The hormones of the anterior pituitary gland are:, growth hormone (GH), adrenocorticotropic hormone (ACTH), thyroid-stimulating hormone (TSH), follicle-stimulating hormone (FSH) and interstitial cell-stimulating hormone (ICSH), luteinizing hormone (LH), and prolactin. The hormones of the posterior pituitary are antidiuretic hormone (ADH) and oxytocin. The thyroid secretes tetraiodothyronine (thyroxine, or T_4), triiodothyronine (T_3), and calcitonin. Parathormone is the hormone produced by the parathyroid gland. The adrenal cortex manufactures and secretes a group of hormones known collectively as corticosteroids; the adrenal medulla secretes epinephrine and norepinephrine. Insulin and glucagon are hormones released by the pancreas. The hormone produced by the testicles is testosterone. The hormones produced by the ovaries are the estrogens and progesterone.
- In a health history the nurse obtains information about the client's past illnesses, family diseases, allergy history—especially to iodine, a list of medications the client takes, and a description of the client's symptoms.
- A head-to-toe examination is performed during which normal and abnormal data are noted. Of particular significance is the presence of exophthalmos, dry or oily skin, increased skin pigmentation, hand tremors, anxiousness, or apathy.
- The nursing management of clients undergoing diagnostic tests for endocrine disorders includes explaining the purpose for each test and how it is conducted, preparing the client for each test, collecting specimens, and instructing the client about care after the test.

CRITICAL THINKING EXERCISES

1. Explain why the pituitary gland is considered the master gland and give some examples that support the terminology.
2. Discuss the meaning of a feedback loop and explain its purpose.

Suggested Readings

Bullock, B. L. (1996). *Pathophysiology: Adaptations and alterations in function* (4th ed.). Philadelphia: Lippincott-Raven.

Fuller, J., & Schaller-Ayers, J. (1994). *Health assessment: A nursing approach* (2nd ed.). Philadelphia: J. B. Lippincott.

Memmler, R. L., Cohen, B. J., & Wood, D. L. (1996). *Structure and function of the human body* (6th ed.). Philadelphia: Lippincott-Raven.

Fischbach, F. T. (1996). *A manual of laboratory diagnostic tests* (5th ed.). Philadelphia: Lippincott-Raven.

Roberts, A. (1995). The adrenal glands. *Nursing Times, 91*(45), 34–36.

Chapter 56

Caring for Clients With Disorders of the Endocrine System

KEY TERMS

Acromegaly
Addisonian crisis
Adrenal insufficiency
Adrenalectomy
Carpopedal spasm
Chvostek's sign
Cushingoid syndrome
Diabetes insipidus
Goiter
Hyperparathyroidism
Hyperplasia
Hyperthyroidism
Hypoparathyroidism
Hypophysectomy
Hypothyroidism
Myxedema
Pheochromocytoma
Simmonds' disease
Syndrome of inappropriate antidiuretic hormone secretion
Tetany
Thyroiditis
Thyrotoxic crisis
Trousseau's sign

LEARNING OBJECTIVES

On completion of this chapter the reader will:

- Describe the physiologic effects of hypo- and hypersecretion of the pituitary, thyroid, parathyroid and adrenal glands.
- Identify the symptoms of hyperthyroidism.
- Identify symptoms of adrenal crisis.
- Describe the symptoms of pheochromocytoma.
- Identify the symptoms of Cushing's disease.

A disorder of any one of the endocrine glands can profoundly affect other endocrine glands as well as many major body systems. When caring for clients with endocrine disorders, the nurse must consider not only the management of the endocrine disorder itself but also the effects of the disorder on other organs and systems.

Disorders of the Pituitary Gland

Pituitary disorders are usually the result of excessive or deficient production and secretion of a specific hormone. When oversecretion of growth hormone (GH) occurs prior to puberty, before the ends of the long bones are fully united (epiphyseal union), gigantism results. Oversecretion of GH during adulthood results in **acromegaly.** Conversely, an absence of pituitary hormonal activity causes panhypopituitarism, or **Simmonds' disease.**

Acromegaly (Hyperpituitarism)

Acromegaly is a condition in which an oversecretion of GH occurs after the epiphyses of the long bones have sealed.

ETIOLOGY AND PATHOPHYSIOLOGY

Acromegaly is the result of **hyperplasia** (increase in the number of cells) or a tumor of the anterior pituitary.

The most common tumor of the pituitary is an adenoma, which is benign. As with other cranial tumors, a benign pituitary tumor becomes a space-occupying lesion and can exert an effect on other cerebral structures (see Chap. 45).

ASSESSMENT FINDINGS

Signs and Symptoms

A client with acromegaly has coarse features, a huge lower jaw, thick lips, a thickened tongue, a bulging forehead, a bulbous nose, and large hands and feet (Fig. 56–1). When the overgrowth is due to a tumor, headaches caused by pressure on the sella turcica are common. Partial blindness may result from pressure on the optic nerve. The heart, liver, and spleen may be enlarged. Despite enlarged tissues, muscle weakness is common, and hypertrophied joints may become painful and stiff. Osteoporosis of the spine and joint pain develop. Many men become impotent, and women may have amenorrhea (absence of menstruation), increased facial hair, and deepened voices (Fig. 56–2).

Diagnostic Findings

Skull radiography, magnetic resonance imaging (MRI), and computed tomography (CT) reveal pituitary enlargement. Bone radiographs show a thickening of the long bones and bones of the skull. Radioimmunoassay shows increased plasma levels of GH. The results of a glucose tolerance test show the same or increased levels of GH in a client with acromegaly and decreased GH levels in a normal person.

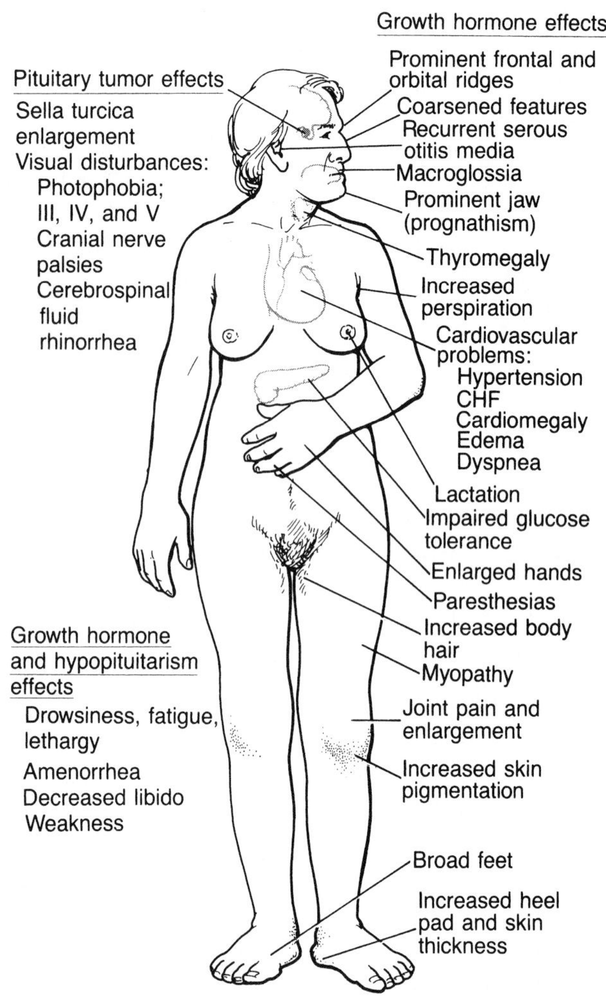

FIGURE 56-2. Clinical manifestations of acromegaly.

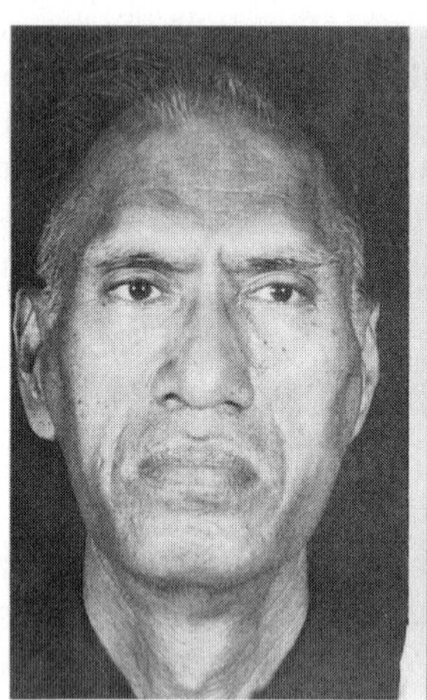
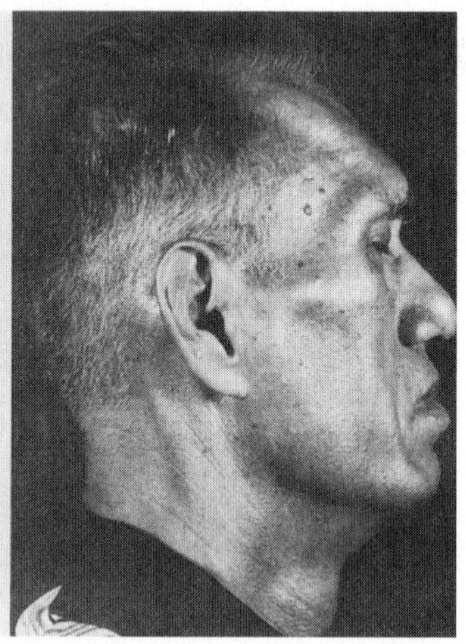

FIGURE 56-1. A 64-year-old man with acromegaly. Note the prominent, "lantern-like" jaw, the large zygomatic arches and supraorbital ridges, and the sloping "beetle brow." The bony overgrowth often results in a comparative hollowing of the temporal region. The nose and ears are enlarged, and the latter may be calcified. The skin folds are exaggerated, the skin is tough and oily, and there is enlargement of the sebaceous glands and pores.

MEDICAL AND SURGICAL MANAGEMENT

Acromegaly is treated by surgical removal of the pituitary gland (**hypophysectomy**) or by radiation therapy with consequent destruction of the pituitary. Even if the disease is arrested successfully, physical changes are irreversible. If the tumor is removed or destroyed by radiation therapy, replacement therapy with thyroid hormone, corticosteroids, and sex hormones is necessary.

Medical treatment includes bromocriptine mesylate (Parlodel), an antiparkinsonism drug that inhibits release of GH in clients with acromegaly. Parlodel is used alone or in conjunction with pituitary irradiation or surgery to reduce the serum GH level.

NURSING MANAGEMENT

Nursing priorities include correction of a fluid volume excess or deficit, relief of pain, and improved nutrition. Carefully measure fluid intake and output. Weigh the client daily and observe for signs of fluid volume excess or deficit. Notify the physician of a sudden or steady weight loss or gain.

Severe psychological stress may occur because of the prominent physical changes, impotence, and decreased libido. Discuss physical changes, body image, and sexual dysfunction to assist the client to cope with changes. If the client expresses concern over sexual dysfunction, bring it to the physician's attention. Referral to a sex therapist could be indicated.

Skeletal changes can cause mild to severe musculoskeletal pain. Evaluate the pain, noting the type and location. Give analgesics as ordered and note whether the client reports relief from pain.

Simmonds' Disease (Panhypopituitarism)

Simmond's disease is a rare disorder caused by destruction of the pituitary gland followed by an absence of pituitary hormonal activity.

ETIOLOGY AND PATHOPHYSIOLOGY

Events such as postpartum emboli, surgery, tumor, and tuberculosis can destroy pituitary function. The hormones of the anterior pituitary are generally affected: GH (bones and muscles), adrenocorticotropic hormone (ACTH; adrenals), thyroid-stimulating hormone (TSH; thyroid), follicle-stimulating hormone (FSH; ovaries), luteinizing hormone (LH), interstitial cell-stimulating hormone (ICSH; testes), and prolactin (breasts).

ASSESSMENT FINDINGS

Signs and Symptoms

The gonads and genitalia atrophy. Because of an impairment of pituitary stimulus, the thyroid and adrenals fail to secrete adequate amounts of hormones. Signs and symptoms of hypothyroidism, hypoglycemia, and adrenal insufficiency (Addison's disease—see later discussion) are apparent. The client ages prematurely and becomes extremely cachectic.

Diagnostic Findings

The results of laboratory tests show decreased hormone levels (eg, thyroid, corticosteroid, male and female hormones).

MEDICAL MANAGEMENT

Treatment includes administration of substitute hormones for the glands that depend on the pituitary for stimulation. If untreated, the disease is fatal. GH replacement is necessary only for children. Deficiency of TSH requires replacement with levothyroxine (Synthroid) or liothyronine (Cytomel), for the client's lifetime. Males receive testosterone and females receive estrogen, as well as FSH and LH for both sexes.

NURSING MANAGEMENT

Administer all hormone replacements as prescribed. It is important to teach the client to adhere to the medication schedule and not omit a dose. Monitor blood hormone levels.

Assess the client's mental status, emotional state, energy level, and appetite. Be alert to altered nutrition. Four to six small meals are often better tolerated than three regular meals.

Diabetes Insipidus

Diabetes insipidus is an endocrine disorder that develops when there is insufficient antidiuretic hormone (ADH) from the posterior pituitary gland.

ETIOLOGY AND PATHOPHYSIOLOGY

Diabetes insipidus can be caused by head trauma that damages the pituitary and by primary or metastatic brain tumors. There are some congenital incidences in which symptoms occur shortly after birth. It can also occur after hypophysectomy, surgical removal of the pituitary gland.

Antidiuretic hormone, secreted by the posterior pituitary, regulates the reabsorption of water in the kidney tubules. Lack of ADH secretion results in the production of large volumes of dilute urine.

ASSESSMENT FINDINGS

Signs and Symptoms

Urine output for a 24-hour period may be as high as 20 liters. The urine is dilute, with a specific gravity of 1.002 or less. The excretion of urine cannot be controlled by limiting the intake of fluids. Thirst is excessive and constant. The need for drinking and voiding frequently limits activities. Weakness, dehydration, and weight loss develop.

Diagnostic Findings

If a fluid deprivation test is performed, fluids are withheld for 8 to 12 hours, and urine specific gravity and osmolarity are determined at the beginning and end of the test. Failure to concentrate urine during the time of fluid deprivation is characteristic of this disorder. Urinalysis reveals virtually colorless urine of low specific gravity. Measurement of the 24-hour urine output reveals an abnormally large urine output.

MEDICAL MANAGEMENT

Desmopressin (DDAVP) nasal solution and lypressin (Diapid) nasal spray are synthetic drugs with ADH activity that reduce the urine output to 2 to 3 L/24 hours (see Nursing Guidelines 56–1). If the client is unable to take oral fluids to meet an excessive fluid volume loss, intravenous (IV) fluids are necessary.

NURSING MANAGEMENT

Nursing measures to correct fluid volume deficit include closely monitoring the rate of IV infusions to ensure that the prescribed amount is given over the required period and measuring fluid intake and output. If the client is acutely ill, extremely dehydrated, fails to take oral fluids, or medical treatment is being initiated, measure urine output at 30-minute intervals. Weigh the client daily to identify weight gain or loss and observe for signs of fluid excess or deficit. Notify the physician of sudden or steady weight gain or loss. Assure the patient that symptoms can be controlled with treatment.

Syndrome of Inappropriate Antidiuretic Hormone Secretion

The **syndrome of inappropriate antidiuretic hormone secretion** (SIADH) is characterized by renal reabsorption of water rather than its normal excretion.

ETIOLOGY AND PATHOPHYSIOLOGY

Causes of SIADH include lung tumors, central nervous system disorders, brain tumors, cerebrovascular accident, head trauma, and drugs such as vasopressin, general anesthetic agents, oral hypoglycemics, and tricyclic antidepressants. The continued release of ADH results in increased fluid volume and hyponatremia (decreased serum sodium level).

ASSESSMENT FINDINGS

Signs and Symptoms

Water retention, headache, muscle cramps, and anorexia develop. As the condition becomes more severe, nausea, vomiting, muscle twitching, and changes in the level of consciousness occur.

Diagnostic Findings

Diagnosis is based on symptoms and a history of a disorder associated with SIADH. Serum sodium levels and serum osmolarity are decreased. Urine sodium and osmolarity are high.

MEDICAL MANAGEMENT

When possible, treatment is aimed at eliminating the underlying cause. Osmotic diuretics, such as mannitol (Osmitrol), and loop diuretics, including furosemide (Lasix), help to correct water retention. Severe hyponatremia is treated with IV administration of a 3% hypertonic sodium chloride solution.

NURSING MANAGEMENT

Closely monitor fluid intake and output and vital signs. The level of consciousness is carefully assessed, and changes are immediately reported to the physician. Assess the client closely for signs of fluid overload (confusion, dyspnea, pulmonary congestion, hypertension), and hyponatremia (weakness, muscle cramps, anorexia, nausea, diarrhea, irritability, headache, and weight gain without edema).

Client and Family Teaching

Give the client and family extensive information about the medication schedule and the adverse effects of drug therapy, especially if several medications are prescribed. Emphasize the importance of adhering to the medication schedule and not omitting a dose.

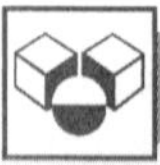

Nursing Guidelines 56-1

Teaching the Client Self-Administration of Nasal Spray

- Hold bottle upright.
- Place nozzle in nostril while in sitting position.
- Spray prescribed number of times in each nostril.
- Do not inhale medication.
- Report nasal irritation to the physician.

Disorders of the Thyroid Gland

Thyroid disorders are difficult to detect because the symptoms are vague until the disease advances to a severe level. Treatment is often long-term, and the client requires periodic follow-up to monitor response to the treatment. Thyroid disorders include hyperthyroidism, thyrotoxic crisis, hypothyroidism, thyroid tumors, and endemic and multinodular goiters.

Hyperthyroidism

Hyperthyroidism is also called Graves' disease, Basedow's disease, thyrotoxicosis, or exophthalmic goiter.

ETIOLOGY AND PATHOPHYSIOLOGY

There is no one etiologic factor for hyperthyroidism. It has been suggested that it may be an autoimmune or inherited disorder. Hypersecretion of thyroid hormones can be produced by thyroid tumors, pituitary tumors, and hypothalamic malignancies. It also may be the result of stress or infection. The metabolic rate increases because of oversecretion of thyroid hormones thyroxine (T_4) and triiodothyronine (T_3). Both T_4 and T_3 increase the body's metabolic rate. The disorder is more common in women than in men.

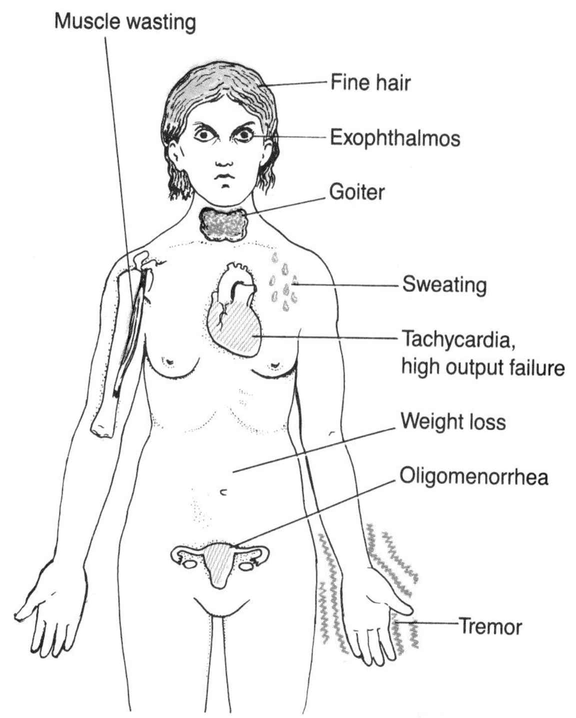

FIGURE 56-3. Clinical manifestations of hyperthyroidism.

ASSESSMENT FINDINGS

Signs and Symptoms

Symptoms vary from mild to severe. Clients with well developed hyperthyroidism are characteristically restless despite feeling fatigued and weak, highly excitable, and constantly agitated. Fine tremors of the hands occur, resulting in unusual clumsiness (Fig. 56–3). Individuals cannot tolerate heat, and experience an increased appetite with weight loss. Diarrhea also occurs. Visual changes, such as blurred or double vision, can develop. Exophthalmos, seen in clients with severe hyperthyroidism, is due to enlargement of muscle and fatty tissue that surrounds the rear and sides of the eyeball (Fig. 56–4). Swelling of the neck caused by the enlarged thyroid gland often is visible. The signs and symptoms of hyperthyroidism and hypothyroidism are compared in Table 56–1.

Diagnostic Findings

The protein-bound iodine, free T_3, thyroglobulin, and serum T_3 and T_4 levels are elevated. The TSH level is decreased. Thyroid ultrasonography shows an enlarged thyroid gland. A thyroid scan indicates an increased uptake of radioactive iodine (^{131}I and ^{123}I). The results of a radioactive iodine (RAI) uptake study show an increased uptake of iodine.

MEDICAL AND SURGICAL MANAGEMENT

Antithyroid drugs, such as propylthiouracil (PTU, Propyl-Thyracil) and methimazole (Tapazole), are given to block the production of thyroid hormone. Potassium iodide (Lugol's solution) is prescribed in combination with an antithyroid drug. Antithyroid medications should be avoided during pregnancy because they can induce hypothyroidism, or cretinism, in the fetus. These and other drugs used to treat thyroid disorders are listed in Table 56–2.

^{131}I is used to destroy hyperplastic thyroid tissue by radiation. The thyroid is quick to remove iodine,

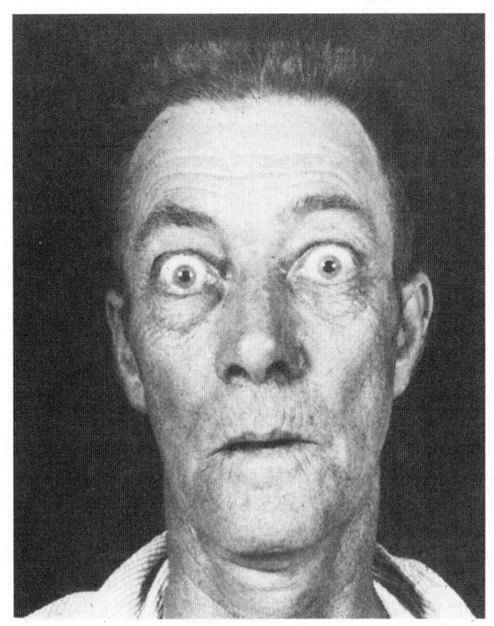

FIGURE 56-4. Thyroid enlargement with exophthalmos.

TABLE 56-1 **Symptoms of Thyroid Dysfunction**

Body System or Function	Hyperthyroidism	Hypothyroidism
Metabolism	Increased, with symptoms of increased appetite, intolerance to heat, elevated body temperature, weight loss despite increased appetite	Decreased, with symptoms of anorexia, intolerance to cold, low body temperature, weight gain despite anorexia
Cardiovascular system	Tachycardia, moderate hypertension	Bradycardia, moderate hypotension
Central nervous system	Nervousness, anxiety, insomnia, tremors	Lethargy, sleepiness
Skin and skin structures	Flushed, warm, moist	Pale, cool, dry; face appears puffy, hair coarse; nails thick and hard
Ovarian function	Irregular or scant menses	Heavy menses, may be unable to conceive, loss of fetus also possible
Testicular function		Low sperm count

including radioactive iodine, from the bloodstream. Antithyroid drugs may be given for 6 months or more before the administration of ^{131}I. If no remission of symptoms occurs, a second and perhaps a third dose of ^{131}I are given. About 6 to 8 weeks after the initial dose of ^{131}I, most clients notice some remission of symptoms. The extended time lag before symptoms are relieved is a disadvantage of this treatment method. A more common and unfortunate result of treatment is hypothyroidism because it is difficult to accurately determine the precise amount of thyroid tissue that will be destroyed by radiation. This complication may not occur until long after the administration of ^{131}I, and clients must remain under medical supervision for many years.

Subtotal thyroidectomy (partial removal of the thyroid gland) is an effective treatment for hyperthyroidism. Total thyroidectomy (removal of thyroid gland) may be performed if a neoplastic tumor is present. Clients commonly receive antithyroid drug therapy for several weeks preoperatively to prevent a dramatic release of thyroid hormones into the bloodstream during surgery.

NURSING MANAGEMENT

Monitor heart rate and blood pressure at regular intervals. Record the client's sleep pattern and daily weights. Inform the client that the effects of antithyroid therapy usually do not become evident until the excess thyroid hormone stored in the thyroid gland has been secreted into the bloodstream. This process may take several weeks or more. If radioactive iodine is used to destroy thyroid tissue, tell the client that it does not seriously affect other tissues. Possible transient effects after the use of ^{131}I and ^{123}I are nausea, vomiting, malaise, fever, and gland tenderness.

Thyrotoxic Crisis

Thyrotoxic crisis is an abrupt form of hyperthyroidism that is a life-threatening event.

ETIOLOGY AND PATHOPHYSIOLOGY

Thyrotoxic crisis is thought to be triggered by extreme stress, infection, diabetic ketoacidosis, trauma, toxemia of pregnancy, or manipulation of a hyperactive thyroid gland during surgery or physical examination. Although this condition is rare, it may occur in people with undiagnosed or inadequately treated hyperthyroidism.

The oversecretion of T_3 and T_4 is followed by a release of epinephrine. Metabolism is markedly increased. The adrenal glands produce excess corticosteroids in response to the stress created by this hypermetabolic state.

ASSESSMENT FINDINGS

Signs and Symptoms

The temperature may be as high as 41°C (106°F), the pulse rate is rapid, and cardiac arrhythmias are common. There may be persistent vomiting, extreme restlessness with delirium, chest pain, and dyspnea.

Diagnostic Findings

The diagnosis is based on the symptoms and a recent medical history that indicates symptoms of severe hyperthyroidism. Laboratory tests, such as serum T_3 and T_4 determinations, may be used to confirm the diagnosis. In thyrotoxic crisis, serum thyroid determinations are markedly elevated.

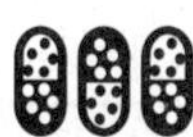

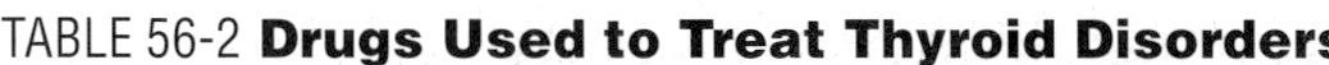

TABLE 56-2 **Drugs Used to Treat Thyroid Disorders**

Drug Category/Drug Action	Side Effects	Nursing Considerations
Antithyroid Agents		
methimazole (Tapazole) Inhibits synthesis of thyroid hormones. propylthiouracil (PTU) Inhibits synthesis of thyroid hormones.	Paresthesias, nausea, agranulocytosis, bleeding, skin rash, diarrhea, vomiting	Avoid use during pregnancy. Monitor blood tests for bone marrow depression. Give in three equal doses at 8-hour intervals Client teaching: notify physician if fever, sore throat, unusual bleeding or bruising, malaise occur.
Iodides		
strong iodine solution (Lugol's solution) Inhibits synthesis and release of T_3 and T_4.	Iodism: metallic taste, burning mouth, sore teeth and gums, stomach upset, diarrhea, skin rash	Monitor for symptoms of acute iodine toxicity: vomiting, abdominal pain, diarrhea, circulatory collapse. Dilute with fruit juice or water, drink with straw to avoid staining teeth.
Radioactive Iodine		
sodium iodine ^{131}I and ^{123}I Used in diagnostic scans; destroys thyroid tissue in hyperthyroidism and thyroid malignancies.	Allergy to iodine, nausea, vomiting	Precautions with body fluids 24 hours following diagnostic test. Monitor for signs of hypothyroidism.
Beta-Adrenergic Blockers		
propranolol (Inderal) Reduces symptoms of hyperthyroidism—tachycardia, tremors, nervousness.	Nausea, vomiting, diarrhea, constipation, bradycardia, congestive heart failure, arrhythmias, hypoglycemia	Monitor cardiac function. Give with meals. Instruct client not to discontinue abruptly. Assess blood sugar regularly for diabetic clients.
Thyroid Hormone Replacement Drugs		
thyroid desiccated (Armour Thyroid, S-P-T, Thyrar, Thyroid Strong) thyroid hormones T_3 and T_4 in their natural state levothyroxine (L-thyroxine, Synthroid) liothyronine (T_3, Cytomel, Triostat) liotrix (Thyrolar) Increases metabolic rate of body tissues.	Hyperthyroidism: tachycardia, tremors, headache, nervousness, insomnia, diarrhea, weight loss, heat intolerance	Monitor response closely. Monitor thyroid function tests. Usually required for lifetime. Given as single daily dose before breakfast. Thyroid preparations interact with digitalis, estrogen, beta blockers, hypoglycemics, and anticoagulants.

MEDICAL MANAGEMENT

Immediate treatment is necessary. Antithyroid drugs such as propylthiouracil or methimazole are used to block the synthesis of thyroid hormones. A corticosteroid may be given IV to replace depletion that results from overstimulation of the adrenals during the hypermetabolic state. IV sodium iodide prevents the release of thyroid hormones by the thyroid gland. Propranolol (Inderal), a beta blocker, reduces the effect of thyroid hormones on the cardiovascular system. Supportive therapy includes IV fluids, antipyretic measures, and oxygen therapy.

NURSING MANAGEMENT

The client with thyrotoxic crisis is acutely ill. Monitor vital signs, especially the temperature, at frequent intervals. Failure to respond to an antipyretic drug requires other measures, such as a cooling blanket or the application of ice. A cool room may also be used to reduce body temperature. All therapeutic treatment measures are given as ordered because the situation must be corrected as soon as possible.

Hypothyroidism

Hypothyroidism occurs when the thyroid gland fails to secrete an adequate amount of thyroid hormones.

ETIOLOGY AND PATHOPHYSIOLOGY

This condition may originate within the thyroid (primary hypothyroidism) or within the pituitary, in which case insufficient TSH is secreted. Regardless of the condition's cause, the result of inadequate thyroid hormone secretion is a slowing of all metabolic processes (see Table 56–1). Severe hypothyroidism is called **myxedema.** Advanced, untreated myxedema can progress to myxedema coma. Signs of this life-threatening event are hypothermia, hypotension, and hypoventilation. A hypothyroid client experiencing infection, trauma, excessive chills, or taking drugs such as narcotics, sedatives, or tranquilizers, can lapse into a myxedema coma.

ASSESSMENT FINDINGS

Signs and Symptoms

The signs and symptoms are opposite in many respects to those of hyperthyroidism. The metabolic rate and physical and mental activity are slowed. The client is lethargic, lacks energy, dozes frequently during the day, is forgetful, and has chronic headaches. The face takes on a masklike unemotional expression, yet the client often is irritable. The tongue may be enlarged and the lips swollen, and there may be edema of the eyelids. The temperature and pulse rate are decreased, and there is an intolerance to cold. The weight increases despite a low caloric intake. The skin is dry, and hair characteristically is coarse and sparse and tends to fall out. Menstrual disorders are common. Constipation may be severe. The voice is low pitched and hoarse, and speech is slow. Hearing may be impaired. There may be numbness or tingling in the arms or legs that is unrelieved by position change.

Hypothyroidism may lead to enlargement of the heart caused by pericardial effusion and an increased tendency toward atherosclerosis and heart strain. Anemia also may be present. Early recognition of hypothyroidism is difficult because many of the symptoms are nonspecific and may not be sufficiently dramatic to bring the client to the physician. This condition can go untreated for years.

Diagnostic Findings

In primary hypothyroidism, levels of TSH are increased because of the negative feedback to the pituitary gland (see Chap. 55). The RAI uptake may be decreased. The T_3 and T_4 levels show no response in primary untreated hypothyroidism but may show a response if hypothyroidism is due to failure of the pituitary to secrete TSH.

MEDICAL MANAGEMENT

Hypothyroidism is treated with thyroid replacement therapy (see Table 56–2). Thyroid hormone in the form of desiccated thyroid extract, or with one of the synthetic products, such as levothyroxine sodium (Synthroid) or liothyronine sodium (Cytomel), are oral thyroid preparations. A low dose of thyroid hormone is given initially and then increased or decreased as needed.

NURSING MANAGEMENT

The client is observed for the adverse effects of thyroid replacement therapy. Dyspnea, rapid pulse rate, palpitations, precordial pain, hyperactivity, insomnia, dizziness, and gastrointestinal disorders—in other words, signs of *hyper*thyroidism—may be seen if the dose of thyroid hormone is too high. Once replacement therapy has begun, a dramatic change may be seen in a few weeks.

NURSING PROCESS
The Client With Hypothyroidism

Assessment

Obtain medical, drug, and allergy histories, and a thorough description of symptoms. Check vital signs and weight. Look for symptoms of thyroid disease such as lethargy, fatigue, anorexia, weight gain, hair loss, brittle nails, and cold intolerance.

Diagnosis and Planning

The nurse's focus when managing the care of a client with hypothyroidism includes, but is not limited to, the following:

Nursing Diagnoses and Collaborative Problems	Nursing Interventions
Activity Intolerance related to fatigue and depressed cognitive processes **Goal:** Client will demonstrate increased ability to tolerate activities.	Assess client's tolerance to activities. Allow adequate time for rest between activities. Assist with hygiene and other self-care activities as needed.

Constipation related to decreased bowel function **Goal:** Client will reestablish normal bowel function.	Assess client's bowel function. Provide high-fiber foods. Encourage adequate fluid intake. Encourage increased physical activity such as short walks within client's tolerance.
Altered Body Temperature related to hyposecretion of thyroid hormones **Goal:** Client's body temperature will be maintained.	Assess body temperature and report deviations from client's usual values. Provide extra warmth with blankets or clothing. Protect from exposure to cold or drafts.
Knowledge Deficit related to need for lifelong thyroid replacement therapy **Goal:** Client will verbalize need for hormone replacement, describe effects of over- or underdosage.	Teach reasons for hormone replacement therapy. Explain therapeutic effects of therapy, that symptoms will gradually resolve. Teach signs of over- and underdosage of medication. Assist client to develop a schedule for taking medication each day. Explain the need for continued follow-up to monitor hormone status.
PC: Myxedema and Myxedema Coma **Goal:** Myxedema or myxedema coma will be managed and minimized.	Assess client for decreases in pulse, respirations, and temperature. Assess client for changes in level of consciousness, difficulty waking client, or increasing confusion. Carefully administer analgesics; avoid administering sedatives or hypnotics.

Evaluation and Expected Outcomes

- The client reports feeling rested and meets self-care needs.
- The client has regular stoolswithout discomfort.
- The client reports feeling comfortable, not cold, in a normal temperature setting.
- The client describes the medication regimen, possible side effects, and precautions.

Client and Family Teaching

The symptoms associated with hyperthyroidism and hypothyroidism often affect the client's learning and retention ability. Carefully explain the treatment regimen, including the dose of the medications and possible adverse effects that may occur during therapy. If a special diet has been recommended, obtain a dietary consultation and review sample diets with the client. Develop a teaching plan to include the following:

- Weigh self weekly; keep a record of symptoms and weight in case the dose of the medication needs to be adjusted.
- Avoid stressful situations.
- Maintain good nutrition.
- Notify the physician if symptoms worsen or adverse drug effects occur.

Thyroid Tumors

Tumors of the thyroid can cause hyperthyroidism. They are more commonly benign, but all nodules must be evaluated.

ETIOLOGY AND PATHOPHYSIOLOGY

A follicular adenoma is the most common benign thyroid lesion. A lump is more likely to be benign for adult women with symptoms of hyperthyroidism or hypothyroidism. Papillary carcinoma is the most common malignant lesion, which generally occurs in individuals who received radiation treatments to the head and neck region in the past. It tends to spread only to nearby lymph nodes and rarely spreads to other parts of the body. The cure rate of thyroid cancer depends on the type of tumor present.

ASSESSMENT FINDINGS

Signs and Symptoms

Symptoms are vague, and the client may be unaware of the lesion. Often a routine physical examination reveals a nodular thyroid. As the tumor enlarges, the client often notices a swelling in the neck. Benign tumors cause symptoms of hyperthyroidism in some clients. Malignant tumors can cause voice changes, hoarseness, and difficulty swallowing.

Diagnostic Findings

The diagnosis is confirmed by biopsy of the lesion. Thyroid cancer is suspected when the gland is firm and palpable and when the results of RAI show poor concentration in the suspicious area.

MEDICAL AND SURGICAL MANAGEMENT

If there are no symptoms of hyperthyroidism with a benign nodule, treatment usually is not needed. The nodule is examined yearly. If the enlargement results in such symptoms as difficulty swallowing and a noticeable swelling in the neck, surgical removal of the lesion is considered. Although treatment of malignant lesions varies, a thyroidectomy (total or subtotal) is typically performed. A modified or radical neck dissection is indicated if there is metastasis. After a thyroidectomy, replacement therapy (consisting of thyroid hormones) is given to supply thyroid hormones and to suppress pituitary TSH so that it no longer stimulates growth of residual thyroid tissue. ^{131}I is administered to destroy remaining thyroid tissue as well as to treat lymph node metastasis, if present.

NURSING MANAGEMENT

If the thyroid tumor is malignant, the physician explains the planned treatment and expected outcome. Provide emotional support, especially if the tumor has metastasized and radical surgery is necessary.

When RAI is used after surgery, the client is isolated and placed on radiation precautions (see Chap. 19). Handle body fluids carefully to prevent spread of contamination.

Endemic and Multinodular Goiters

The word **goiter** refers to an enlargement of the thyroid gland.

ETIOLOGY AND PATHOPHYSIOLOGY

A goiter is caused by a deficiency of iodine in the diet, by the inability of the thyroid to use iodine, or by relative iodine deficiency caused by increasing body demands for thyroid hormones.

Nontoxic goiter (also called simple or colloid goiter) is an enlargement of the thyroid, usually without symptoms of thyroid dysfunction. Nodular goiters contain one or more areas of hyperplasia. This type of goiter appears to develop for essentially the same reasons as an endemic goiter.

ASSESSMENT FINDINGS

Signs and Symptoms

The thyroid gland enlarges and there is a sense of fullness in the neck area. Continued gland enlargement eventually results in difficulty swallowing and breathing as the thyroid presses on the trachea and esophagus. When the gland has enlarged, it is visible as a swelling in the neck. Nodular goiters also produce enlargement, but the gland has an irregular surface on palpation (Fig. 56–5).

Diagnostic Findings

A thyroid scan shows an enlarged gland and a decreased uptake of ^{131}I. Tests of thyroid function are performed, but results may or may not be abnormal and, thus, inconclusive.

MEDICAL MANAGEMENT

Treatment depends on the cause. If the diet is deficient in iodine, foods high in iodine, such as seafood or iodized salt, are recommended. Potassium iodide to supplement iodine intake may be given. In some instances, a thyroidectomy is recommended, especially when the gland is grossly enlarged.

NURSING MANAGEMENT

If the client has respiratory distress because of the enlarged thyroid, closely observe the respiratory status. Elevate the head of the bed to relieve respiratory symptoms. Provide a diet high in iodine and use

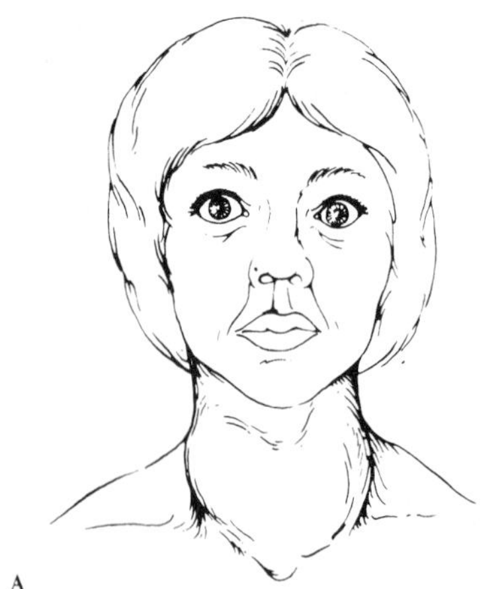

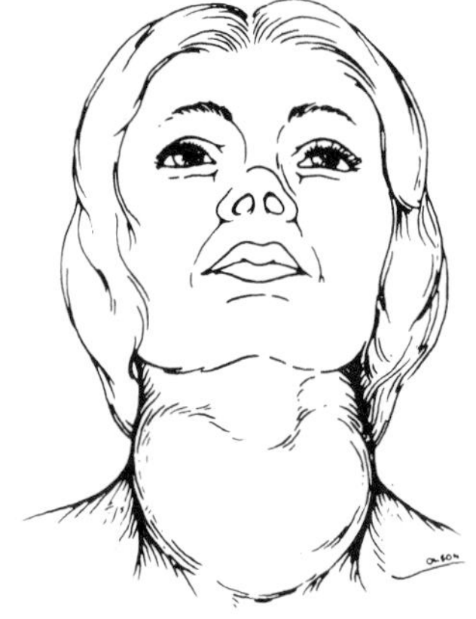

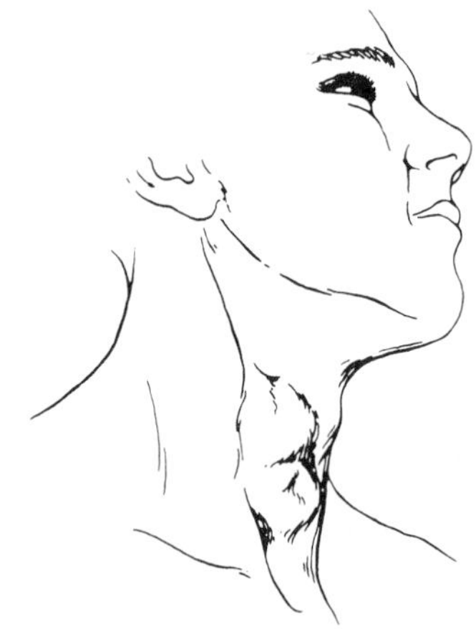

FIGURE 56-5. Thyroid abnormalities. (*A*) Diffuse toxic goiter (Graves' disease) with exophthalmos. (*B*) Diffuse nontoxic goiter. (C) Nodular goiter. (Judge, R.D., Zuidema, G.D., & Fitzgerald, F.T. [Eds.]. [1982] *Clinical diagnosis* [4th ed.] Boston: Little, Brown).

iodized salt. The natural iodine content is highest in seafoods and in variable amounts in bread, milk, eggs, meat, and spinach. A soft diet may be necessary if the client has difficulty swallowing.

Thyroiditis

Thyroiditis, or inflammation of the thyroid gland, can be acute, subacute, or chronic.

ETIOLOGY AND PATHOPHYSIOLOGY

Acute thyroiditis, more common in children, appears to be the result of a bacterial infection of the gland. Subacute thyroiditis can follow an upper respiratory viral infection and is relatively rare. More common is Hashimoto's thyroiditis, a chronic form of thyroiditis. It is believed to be an autoimmune disorder.

ASSESSMENT FINDINGS

Signs and Symptoms

Signs and symptoms of acute thyroiditis include high fever, malaise, and tenderness and swelling of the thyroid gland. Subacute thyroiditis produces symptoms of a swollen and painful gland, chills, fever, and malaise approximately 2 weeks after a viral infection. Hashimoto's thyroiditis is manifested by enlargement of the thyroid and, in some cases, symptoms of hypothyroidism.

Diagnostic Findings

In acute thyroiditis, laboratory test results show an elevated white blood cell count and normal thyroid function. In subacute thyroiditis, the results of some thyroid tests, such as T_3 and T_4, reveal elevated levels. RAI shows a decrease in iodine uptake. In Hashimoto's thyroiditis, there are high titers of antithyroid antibodies, and RAI shows an increase in iodine uptake.

MEDICAL AND SURGICAL MANAGEMENT

Acute thyroiditis requires administration of appropriate antibiotics. The treatment of subacute thyroiditis is symptomatic and includes analgesics for pain and discomfort. Corticosteroid medication also may be prescribed to reduce inflammation. The treatment of Hashimoto's thyroiditis includes thyroid hormone replacement therapy. Surgery is required if the gland becomes excessively large.

NURSING MANAGEMENT

Management depends on the type of thyroiditis and the severity of symptoms. Give antipyretics for fever. Elevate the head of the bed if the client has difficulty breathing. Offer a soft diet if the gland is markedly enlarged and the client has difficulty swallowing.

The Client Having Thyroid Surgery

NURSING PROCESS
Care of the Client Before Thyroid Surgery

Preoperative Period

Assessment

Obtain complete medical, drug, and allergy histories. To decrease bleeding during surgery, a short course of treatment with an antithyroid drug preparation may be ordered at least 2 weeks before scheduled thyroidectomy. If preoperative medications are prescribed, it is important to determine whether the client has completed the course of therapy.

Perform a physical assessment while avoiding palpation of the thyroid gland because manipulation of the gland may release additional amounts of thyroid hormones (see Chap. 55).

Assess the client's understanding of what to expect before and after the surgical procedure. Show the client how to support his or her head when rising from bed to avoid straining the neck incision (Fig. 56–6). Inform the client that a dressing will be applied to the front of the neck.

Diagnosis and Planning

The preoperative nursing management includes, but is not limited to, the following:

Nursing Diagnoses and Collaborative Problems	Nursing Interventions
Anxiety related to pending surgery **Goal:** The client's anxiety will be mild.	Allow the client time to talk and ask questions about surgery and what further treatments may be necessary if a malignant tumor is found.
Knowledge Deficit related to postoperative preventive self-care **Goal:** The client demonstrates head support technique, deep breathing and leg exercises.	In addition to the usual preoperative preparations, show the client how to support the head when rising to a sitting position (see Fig. 56-6). Instruct the client how to perform deep breathing and leg exercises.

Evaluation and Expected Outcomes

- The client reports a decrease in anxiety and verbalizes feelings about the surgery.

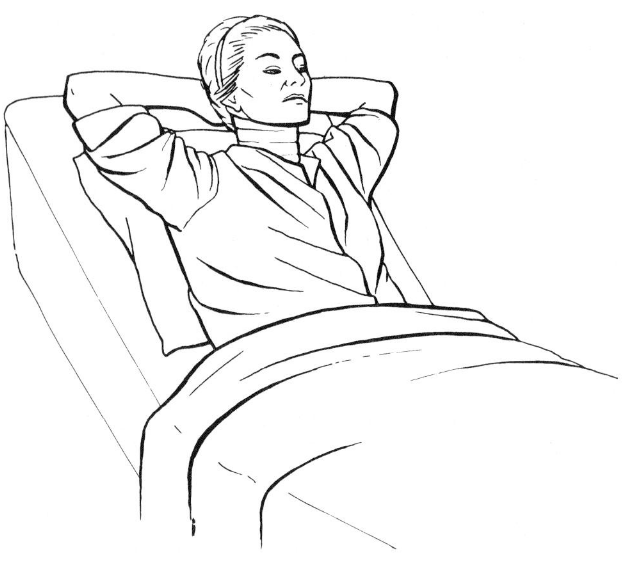

FIGURE 56-6. After a thyroidectomy, the client uses the hands to support the head while rising to a sitting position. This type of support helps avoid strain to the neck muscles and surgical incision.

- The client is able to describe the postoperative course of treatment.

Postoperative Period

Complications associated with thyroid surgery include hemorrhage, airway obstruction, paralysis of the recurrent laryngeal nerve (responsible for speech), hypoparathyroidism, and hypothyroidism. The latter complication may not be apparent for several days or weeks after surgery. Rarely, thyrotoxic crisis occurs as a result of excessive manipulation of the gland during surgery. It may be seen within the first 12 hours after surgery.

NURSING PROCESS
Care of the Client After Thyroid Surgery

Assessment

Immediately on return from surgery, take vital signs, assess the client for a patent airway, and inspect the dressing for bleeding or drainage. Ask the client to say a few words to check the voice for tone, pitch, and hoarseness. Minor voice changes are normal after thyroid surgery.

An infrequent postoperative complication is **tetany** (muscle hypertonia with spasm and tremor), which is caused by a low concentration of calcium resulting from the accidental removal of the parathyroid glands during thyroidectomy. The client may complain of muscle cramps and numbness and tingling of the arms and legs.

Diagnosis and Planning

The nursing plan of care includes, but is not limited to, the following:

Nursing Diagnoses and Collaborative Problems	Nursing Interventions
PC: Tetany **Goal:** Tetany will be managed and minimized.	Assess for Chvostek's and Trousseau's signs (Fig. 56–7 and Fig. 56–8). Note crowing respirations and dyspnea, caused by laryngeal spasm. If these symptoms are present, notify the physician immediately. The treatment is IV calcium.
PC: Thyrotoxic Crisis **Goal:** Thyrotoxic crisis will be managed and minimized.	Assess for hyperthermia, tachycardia, chest pain, cardiac arrhythmias, and altered level of consciousness. If these symptoms are present, notify the physician immediately. Place a suction machine at the client's bedside. Obtain an emergency tracheostomy tray in case respiratory obstruction develops. Have IV calcium available.
Risk for Ineffective Airway Clearance related to compression of the trachea from edema of the glottis or bleeding **Goal:** The client's airway will remain patent.	Observe the client for signs of respiratory obstruction. Notify the physician immediately if apparent because this serious problem must be treated within minutes by the insertion of an endotracheal tube or by tracheostomy. Encourage the client to breathe deeply every 2 hours the first postoperative day, but postpone coughing unless medically ordered, to avoid strain on the incision and precipitation of bleeding. The postoperative orders are checked to determine the surgeon's preference in this matter. Auscultate the lungs every 4– 8 hours.
PC: Hemorrhage/Bleeding **Goal:** The client's wound will remain free from infection.	Monitor vital signs every 1 to 4 hours. Inspect the surgical dressing at frequent intervals for bleeding and drainage. Attend to the client's complaints of a sense of fullness in or around the surgical incision. Check for oozing around the back of the neck; blood may not be evident on the front of the dressing.

	During the first 24 postoperative hours, pass a hand behind the client's neck to see whether it feels damp. When the client is turned, check the dressing and bed linen for blood.
Risk for Aspiration related to aryngeal and tracheal reflex depression **Goal:** The client will swallow ood and fluids safely without aspiration.	Ensure that the client is sitting upright and is fully alert. Instruct the client to take fluids in small amounts when oral fluids are allowed.
Pain related to tissue trauma **Goal:** The client reports pain relief and improved comfort evel.	Give analgesics for pain, which usually is minimal. Keep the client in a supine position with the head slightly elevated. Place pillows under the head, neck, and shoulders to support these structures, to prevent excessive pulling on and possible separation of the incision. Support the head when the client's position is changed to reduce pain or discomfort.
Risk for Impaired Communication related to laryngeal nerve injury, vocal cord paralysis, or respiratory obstruction **Goal:** The client will regain normal speech.	Ask the client to speak a few words every 2 to 4 hours, but keep talking to a minimum during the first 2 postoperative days. Report severe hoarseness or other voice changes to the physician. Provide bedside humidification to relieve hoarseness.

Evaluation and Expected Outcomes

- No complications develop.
- The client maintains normal ventilation, free from obstruction.
- The client is comfortable or pain-free.
- The client's speech returns to normal.

Client and Family Teaching

Before discharge, instruct the client in the care of the surgical wound and to avoid excessive strain on the wound until it is healed. Because the incision is made in a neck crease, the healed scar is barely visible. If a client appears concerned about scarring, suggest that the client wear clothing that covers the neck until the scar is almost invisible.

Discuss the symptoms of hypothyroidism, hyperthyroidism, and hypoparathyroidism with instructions to immediately notify the physician if they occur. If medication is prescribed, review the dosage and adverse effects of each drug with the client and family. Develop a teaching plan to include:

- Techniques for wound care
- The need to follow the prescribed medical regimen: Take thyroid replacement medication in the morning to avoid insomnia and central nervous system stimulation and at the same time each day.
- Side effects that require notification of the physician, such as chest pain, tachycardia, and dyspnea

Disorders of the Parathyroid Glands

When the parathyroid gland dysfunctions, hyperparathyroidism or hypoparathyroidism develops. Calcium and phosphorous levels are affected.

Hyperparathyroidism

Hyperparathyroidism can be a primary or secondary condition.

ETIOLOGY AND PATHOPHYSIOLOGY

The most common cause of primary hyperparathyroidism is an adenoma of one of the parathyroid glands. In primary hyperparathyroidism, excessive secretion of parathyroid hormone (parathormone) results in increased urinary excretion of phosphorus and loss of calcium from the bones. The bones become demineralized as the calcium leaves and enters the bloodstream. Renal stones may develop as calcium becomes concentrated in the urine.

In secondary hyperparathyroidism, the parathyroid glands secrete an excessive amount of parathormone in response to hypocalcemia (low serum calcium level), which may be caused by vitamin D deficiency, chronic renal failure, large doses of thiazide diuretics, and excessive use of laxatives and calcium supplements.

ASSESSMENT FINDINGS

Signs and Symptoms

Excessive calcium in the blood depresses the responsiveness of the peripheral nerves, accounting for fatigue and muscle weakness. The muscles become hypotonic (loss of or decrease in muscle tone). Cardiac arrhythmias may develop. Because the bones have lost calcium, there is skeletal tenderness and pain on bearing weight; the bones may become so demineralized that they break with little or no trauma (pathologic fractures). Other possible effects include nausea, vomiting, and constipation.

Large amounts of calcium and phosphorus passing through the kidneys predisposes to the formation of stones in the genitourinary tract, pyelonephritis, and uremia.

Diagnostic Findings

The diagnosis is made on the basis of elevated serum calcium and decreased serum phosphorus levels in the absence of other causes of hypercalcemia. The results of a 24-hour urine test show increased urine calcium levels. Skeletal radiographs show a loss of calcium from bones. An MRI or a CT scan identifies a parathyroid adenoma if present. Parathormone levels are elevated in hyperparathyroidism.

MEDICAL AND SURGICAL MANAGEMENT

Secondary hyperparathyroidism is managed by correcting the cause (eg, vitamin D therapy for a vitamin D deficiency, correction of renal failure, calcium-restricted diet). Sodium and phosphorous replacements are often ordered. Hormone replacement with synthetic calcitonin (Calcimar) is avoided because it is associated with allergic reactions and drug resistance. The latter is due to antibodies that neutralize the hormone.

The only treatment for primary hyperparathyroidism is surgical removal of hypertrophied gland tissue or of an individual tumor of one of the parathyroid glands. Before surgery, the physician determines the number of glands to be removed, based on the cause of hyperparathyroidism and laboratory and diagnostic test results. One or more of the parathyroids are left in place because they are necessary for calcium and phosphorus metabolism.

NURSING MANAGEMENT

Closely measure the client's intake and output. Observe for signs of urinary calculi from hypercalcemia, flank pain, and decreasing urine output. Encourage a large volume of fluid to keep the urine dilute. Assess the client's ability to perform self-care and provide a safe environment to prevent falls and other injury. Provide rest periods and monitor fatigue level.

The primary nursing responsibility is teaching the client about the effects of the disease, the planned medical management, and the importance of following the prescribed treatment. If the client undergoes surgery, the nursing management is similar to that for thyroid surgery. In addition, the client is observed for symptoms of hypoparathyroidism.

Hypoparathyroidism

Hypoparathyroidism is a deficiency of parathormone that results in hypocalcemia.

ETIOLOGY AND PATHOPHYSIOLOGY

Parathormone regulates calcium balance by increasing absorption of calcium from the gastrointestinal tract and bone resorption of calcium. Hypocalcemia affects neuromuscular functions. It causes hyperexcitability, resulting in spastic muscle contractions and paresthesias (abnormal sensations).

The most common causes of hypoparathyroidism are trauma to the glands and inadvertent removal of all or nearly all these structures during thyroidectomy or parathyroidectomy. The idiopathic form of this disorder is rare but may be autoimmune in origin or caused by the congenital absence of the parathyroids.

ASSESSMENT FINDINGS

Signs and Symptoms

The main symptom of acute, sudden hypoparathyroidism is tetany. The client may report numbness and tingling in the fingers or toes or around the lips. A voluntary movement may be followed by an involuntary jerking spasm. Muscle cramping may be present. Tonic (continuous contraction) flexion of an arm or a finger may occur. If the facial nerve (immediately in front of the ear) is tapped, the client's mouth twitches and the jaw tightens (positive **Chvostek's sign;** see Fig. 56–7). A positive **Trousseau's sign** may be elicited

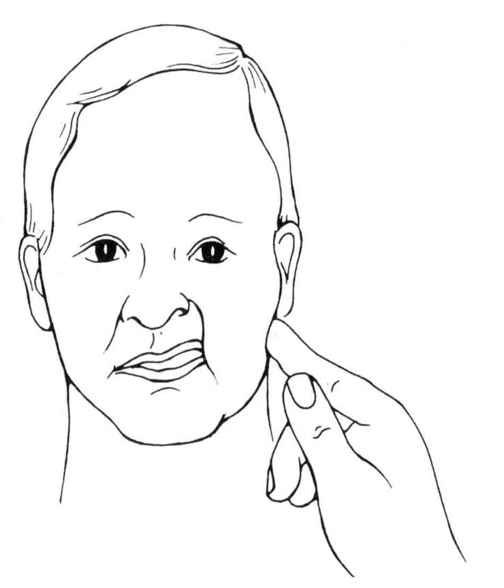

FIGURE 56-7. Tapping of the facial nerve approximately 2 cm anterior to the earlobe elicits the Chvostek's sign in patients with hypocalcemia or hypomagnesemia.

by placing a blood pressure cuff on the upper arm, inflating it between the systolic and diastolic blood pressures, and waiting 3 minutes. The client is observed for spasm of the hand (**carpopedal spasm**), which is evidenced by the hand flexing inward (see Fig. 56–8).

Laryngeal spasm can occur in the larynx, causing dyspnea, with long, crowing respirations as air tries to get past the constriction. Cyanosis may be present, and the client is in danger of asphyxia and cardiac arrhythmias. Nausea, vomiting, abdominal pain, and seizures can develop.

In chronic hypoparathyroidism, neuromuscular irritability, constipation or diarrhea, numbness and tingling of the arms and legs, loss of tooth enamel, and muscle pain are experienced. Positive Chvostek's and Trousseau's signs may or may not be elicited, depending on the degree of hypocalcemia.

Diagnostic Findings

The serum calcium level is decreased, the serum phosphorus level is increased, and the urine levels of both are decreased. In chronic hypoparathyroidism, radiographs show increased bone density.

MEDICAL MANAGEMENT

Tetany and severe hypoparathyroidism are treated immediately by the administration of an IV calcium salt, such as calcium gluconate. Endotracheal intubation and mechanical ventilation may be necessary if acute respiratory distress occurs. Bronchodilators also are used. Parathyroid replacement therapy is not the usual treatment because of its associated incidence of allergic reactions. If used, drug resistance develops in approximately 2 weeks.

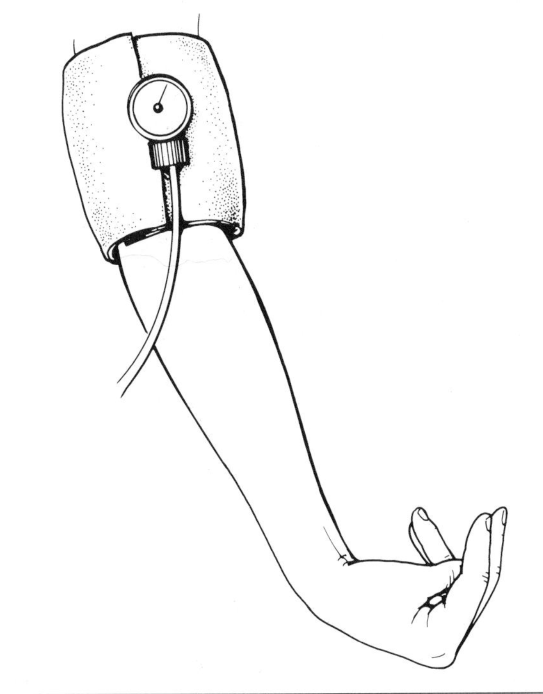

FIGURE 56-8. Trousseau's sign is evidenced by carpopedal spasms.

Long-term treatment after trauma to or inadvertent removal of the parathyroids includes administration of oral calcium, vitamin D, or vitamin D_2 (calciferol), which increases the serum calcium level. The dose is related to the degree of hypocalcemia, which is determined by frequent monitoring of serum and urine calcium levels. A diet high in calcium and low in phosphorus usually is recommended.

NURSING MANAGEMENT

Be alert for signs of tetany. Assess for Chvostek's and Trousseau's signs. Monitor the client with chronic hypoparathyroidism for increasing severity of symptoms.

Be prepared to administer IV calcium salt. Observe the client when administering IV calcium for adverse effects, such as flushing, cardiac arrhythmia (usually a bradycardia), tingling in the arms and legs, and a metallic taste. Local tissue necrosis may occur if the IV fluid escapes into surrounding tissues. Monitor serum calcium levels to determine the effectiveness of therapy.

If the client has chronic hypoparathyroidism, obtain complete medical, drug, and allergy histories. Examine the client for symptoms of the disorder, primarily for the effect of hypocalcemia on the nervous system. Assess the arms and legs for evidence of muscle spasm. Auscultate the lungs because the client may have dyspnea or other respiratory difficulty. When taking vital signs, pay particular attention to heart rate and rhythm.

Keep an emergency tracheostomy tray, mechanical ventilation equipment, artificial airway, and endotracheal intubation equipment at the bedside if the client has severe hypocalcemia. An IV line may be inserted for the emergency administration of calcium. Observe the client at frequent intervals for respiratory distress, and notify the physician immediately if this problem occurs.

Until hypocalcemia is corrected, assist the client with activities of daily living. Movement, noise, and other environmental disturbances can trigger muscle contractions or convulsions. Keep stress to a minimum until serum calcium levels approach normal and symptoms are relieved.

Client and Family Teaching

Clients who require lifetime treatment of the disorder need careful review of the prescribed treatment. Because normal calcium levels depend on drug and diet therapy, stress the importance of these two aspects of treatment. Consultation with a dietitian may be necessary to provide a list of foods to include or avoid in the prescribed diet.

Give the client a list of the symptoms of hypercalcemia and hypocalcemia, either of which can occur if the dose of the prescribed drug is too high or too low or if the drug is omitted. Emphasize the need to contact the physician immediately if one or more symptoms occur. Remind the client that the physician may need to periodically adjust the dose of the drug, and therefore, it is important to recognize the symptoms associated with hypercalcemia and hypocalcemia.

Develop a teaching plan to include one or more of the following:

- Drugs must be taken at the doses and intervals prescribed.
- Drug doses must not be increased, decreased, or omitted unless advised by the physician. Increasing the dose can cause symptoms of hypercalcemia; decreasing or omitting the dose can cause the original symptoms to return.
- If the prescribed dose cannot be taken because of nausea, vomiting, or severe diarrhea, contact the physician.
- Adherence to the recommended diet is necessary. Food labels must be read carefully so that foods that are and are not part of the diet can be included or avoided, respectively.

Disorders of the Adrenal Glands

Adrenal dysfunction includes pathology of the outer portion of the adrenal gland, the cortex, which synthesizes and secretes the hormones known as steroids: mineralocorticoids, glucocorticoids, and androgens or estrogens. Disorders of the adrenal glands also involve the medulla, the inner portion, which secretes catecholamines norepinephrine (noradrenalin) and epinephrine (adrenalin). Proper secretion of these hormones is essential to life.

Adrenal Insufficiency (Addison's Disease)

Adrenal insufficiency is classified as either primary or secondary.

ETIOLOGY AND PATHOPHYSIOLOGY

Primary adrenal insufficiency (Addison's disease) results from destruction of the adrenal cortex by diseases such as tuberculosis. The disease also could be an autoimmune disorder where adrenal tissue is destroyed by antibodies formed by the individual's immune system. In many instances, the cause is unknown.

The consequences of decreased adrenal cortical function include a decreased amount of available glucose and hypoglycemia. The glomerular filtration rate of the kidneys slows dramatically, causing decreased urea nitrogen excretion.

Secondary adrenal insufficiency is the result of surgical removal of both adrenal glands (bilateral adrenalectomy), hemorrhagic infarction of the glands, hypopituitarism (caused by pituitary failure or surgical removal of the pituitary), or suppression of adrenal function by the administration of corticosteroids. Clients with secondary adrenal insufficiency after bilateral adrenalectomy or surgical removal of the pituitary gland do not experience true adrenal insufficiency because corticosteroids are administered to replace the hormones no longer secreted by the adrenals.

ASSESSMENT FINDINGS

Signs and Symptoms

The symptoms of primary and secondary adrenal insufficiency are similar. A decrease in or absence of adrenocortical hormones leads to the symptoms of adrenal insufficiency (Box 56–1).

Clients with primary adrenal insufficiency usually experience symptoms over a period of time. Clients with secondary adrenal insufficiency develop symptoms suddenly or over a period of several days to weeks.

BOX 56-1 Signs and Symptoms of Adrenal Insufficiency

- Increased urinary excretion of sodium and retention of potassium followed by dehydration and a reduction of blood plasma volume
- Weakness, fatigue, dizziness, hypotension, postural hypotension, hypothermia
- Vascular collapse because of poor myocardial tone, decreased cardiac output, weak and irregular pulse
- Weight loss, anemia, anorexia, gastrointestinal symptoms
- Nervousness, periods of depression
- Hypoglycemia caused by a deficiency of the hormones that facilitate the conversion of protein into glucose; episodes of hypoglycemia may occur 5 to 6 hours after eating; the period before breakfast is an especially dangerous time
- Abnormally dark pigmentation, especially of exposed areas of the skin and mucous membranes, and a decrease in hair growth (primary adrenal insufficiency)

Diagnostic Findings

A synthetic dose of ACTH, cosyntropin (Cortrosyn), is administered intramuscularly as a screening test for adrenal function. In primary adrenal insufficiency, an absent or a low cortisol response indicates adrenal insufficiency. In secondary insufficiency, there is a less significant decrease in serum cortisol levels.

The serum cortisol level is decreased. Serum sodium and fasting blood glucose levels are low, and serum potassium, calcium, and blood urea nitrogen levels are increased. The white blood cell count is often elevated. A glucose tolerance test shows evidence of hypoglycemia. In Addison's disease, the glucose level in the bloodstream does not rise as high as normal and returns to its fasting level more quickly than it would under normal conditions. The fasting blood glucose level may be low. Radiographs of the adrenals show calcification. An abdominal CT scan reveals atrophy of the adrenal glands.

MEDICAL MANAGEMENT

Clients with primary adrenal insufficiency require daily corticosteroid replacement therapy for the rest of their lives. Fludrocortisone (Florinef), a synthetic corticosteroid preparation that possesses glucocorticoid and mineralocorticoid properties, is frequently selected for replacement therapy. An additional glucocorticoid can be necessary, depending on the client's response to therapy.

Treatment for secondary adrenal insufficiency caused by bilateral adrenalectomy or pituitary failure is the same as treatment for primary adrenal insufficiency. Treatment of secondary adrenal insufficiency resulting from discontinuation of corticosteroid therapy or hemorrhagic infarction of the gland is variable and depends on the ability of the adrenals to return to normal function.

NURSING MANAGEMENT

If the client is not given or does not take the medication, acute adrenal crisis can develop (see the next section). This also applies to clients on long-term corticosteroid therapy for the treatment of disorders such as allergies, rheumatoid arthritis, and collagen diseases who abruptly discontinue taking their prescribed steroid. If the drug is to be discontinued, the dose *must be tapered* over time.

Nursing management of the client with primary adrenal insufficiency is essentially the same as that of the client with secondary adrenal insufficiency because the major problem in both types is a lack of adrenal cortical hormones. The client with secondary adrenal insufficiency because of surgery (bilateral adrenalectomy, surgical removal of the pituitary) has a controlled deficiency that is corrected with hormone replacement therapy.

Take vital signs at frequent intervals. Hypoglycemia may be seen in clients with primary adrenal insufficiency. These clients must *never* receive insulin by error because insulin would lower the blood glucose to a critically low level that could result in brain damage, coma, or death.

NURSING PROCESS
The Client with Addison's Disease

Assessment

Obtain a complete health history that includes presence or absence of weight loss, salt craving, nausea and vomiting, abdominal cramps, diarrhea, muscle weakness, and decreased stress tolerance.

Diagnosis and Planning

The nursing plan of care includes, but is not limited to, the following:

Nursing Diagnoses and Collaborative Problems	Nursing Interventions
Risk for Fluid Volume Deficit related to inadequate fluid intake, fluid loss secondary to inadequate adrenal hormone secretion **Goal:** The client's fluid intake will be 1500 to 3000 mL/day.	Keep careful records of fluid intake and urine output. Weigh the client daily. Notify the physician if dehydration, signs of hyponatremia, or progressive weight loss occurs. Encourage the client to drink fluids and eat the prescribed diet to maintain fluid and electrolyte balance. If serum sodium levels are decreased, instruct the client to add salt to food. If excessive perspiration occurs, increase fluid and salt intake.
PC: Hypoglycemia **Goal:** Episodes of hypoglycemia will be managed and minimized.	If a meal is delayed because of diagnostic tests or for other reasons, keep the fasting period to a minimum. Observe for symptoms of hypoglycemia: hunger, headache, sweating, weakness, trembling, emotional instability, visual disturbances, and, finally, disorientation, coma. If these symptoms are noted, contact the physician immediately. Instruct the client to remain in bed. Offer five or six small meals per day rather than three regular meals to control hypo-

	glycemic episodes. If the client is eating three meals per day, give between-meal snacks of milk and crackers.
Fatigue related to fluid, electrolyte, and glucose imbalances **Goal:** The client will demonstrate increased energy by independently meeting self-care needs.	Assist with bathing and grooming as needed. Provide rest periods between activities. Control environmental stimuli to promote rest.
Risk for Injury related to hypotension, muscle weakness **Goal:** The client will remain free from injury due to falls.	If dizziness occurs on sitting, tell the client to lie down again. Take the blood pressure if symptoms such as weakness and faintness occur. Keep the side rails raised. Instruct the client to ask for assistance in getting out of bed. Emphasize the importance of getting out of bed slowly.

Evaluation and Expected Outcomes

- The client's fluid intake approximates output; electrolytes remain within normal limits.
- The client has sufficient energy for ADLs.
- No injuries occur.

Client and Family Teaching

Explain to client and family about adrenal insufficiency and the importance of lifetime corticosteroid replacement. Develop a teaching plan to include:

- *Lifetime corticosteroid replacement therapy is necessary. A dose must never be omitted, increased, or decreased.* If the prescribed drug is not taken, adrenal insufficiency, which is serious and life-threatening, will occur.
- The body has limited ability to handle stress of any kind. Seek medical attention for dosage readjustment whenever there is stress. Examples of stress include an infection, a motor vehicle accident (even if not noticeably hurt), a family crisis, and a heavy work load.
- Avoid exposure to infections and excessive fatigue.
- If an infection (eg, sore throat, upper respiratory tract infection) or other type of illness occurs, contact the physician immediately because an increase in the medication dose may be necessary.
- Vomiting, diarrhea, or any other condition that prevents the medication from being taken orally or interferes with proper absorption of the drug requires immediate medical attention because parenteral administration will be necessary. (The physician instructs the client on the procedures to follow if the medication cannot be taken orally.)
- Wear identification, such as a Medic Alert tag or bracelet, stating that the wearer has adrenal insufficiency. If an accident or other problem occurs, medical personnel must be made aware of the need for corticosteroids.
- Follow the diet recommended by the physician.

Acute Adrenal Crisis (Addisonian Crisis)

Clients with either primary or secondary adrenal insufficiency have the potential to develop an **Addisonian crisis**, a life-threatening emergency.

ETIOLOGY AND PATHOPHYSIOLOGY

Acute adrenal crisis occurs when there is a sudden failure of the adrenal glands. Because the hormones of the adrenal cortex are prominent in effecting the body's adaptive reactions to stress, clients with Addison's disease may develop acute adrenal crisis when faced with extreme stress. Even uncomplicated surgery requires more physiologic adaptive ability than a client with Addison's disease usually possesses. Salt deprivation, infection, trauma, exposure to cold, overexertion, or any abnormal stress can cause adrenal crisis. Acute adrenal crisis can occur when corticosteroid therapy is suddenly stopped. If untreated, coma and death result.

ASSESSMENT FINDINGS

Signs and Symptoms

Adrenal crisis may occur suddenly or gradually. It may begin with anorexia, nausea, vomiting, diarrhea, abdominal pain, profound weakness, headache, intensification of hypotension, restlessness, or fever. Unless the corticosteroid dose is increased to meet the demand, the client progresses to acute adrenal crisis. The blood pressure becomes markedly decreased, and shock develops.

Diagnostic Findings

A diagnosis is based on symptoms and history. Case finding can show an omission of daily corticosteroid therapy. (See Diagnostic Findings for adrenal insufficiency.)

MEDICAL MANAGEMENT

Adrenal crisis is an emergency; death may occur from hypotension and vasomotor collapse. Corticosteroids are given IV in solutions of normal saline and glucose. Antibiotics are administered because of an extremely low resistance to infection.

NURSING MANAGEMENT

Two important nursing tasks are the recognition of signs and symptoms of adrenal crisis and the accurate administration of corticosteroid drugs.

A client with a diagnosis of adrenal insufficiency is a candidate for acute adrenal crisis; therefore, constantly observe for this problem. Administer the correct dose of corticosteroid therapy at the correct time. *Doses must never be omitted or abruptly discontinued because this can result in adrenal crisis.*

Once the condition is recognized, take vital signs frequently with special attention to the heart rate and rhythm. Observe the client for signs of hyponatremia and hyperkalemia. Keep the client warm and as quiet as possible until treatment is instituted and the condition is stabilized.

Pheochromocytoma

Pheochromocytoma is a tumor of the adrenal medulla that causes increased hyperfunction of the adrenal gland.

ETIOLOGY AND PATHOPHYSIOLOGY

A pheochromocytoma is generally a benign tumor that causes the adrenal gland to produce an excessive secretion of the catecholamines epinephrine and norepinephrine. Episodes can be triggered by exercise, emotional distress, trauma such as surgery, manipulation of the tumor, and postural changes. Excessive secretion of epinephrine leads to hypertension and increases the potential for cerebrovascular accident, palpitations, and tachycardia.

ASSESSMENT FINDINGS

Signs and Symptoms

Symptoms include elevated blood pressure (intermittent or, more frequently, persistent), tremors, nervousness, sweating, headache, nausea, vomiting, hyperglycemia, polyuria, and vertigo.

Diagnostic Findings

The level of vanillylmandelic acid in a 24-hour urine specimen is markedly increased. Urinary catecholamine determination on the same or a different specimen may be elevated. CT, MRI, ultrasonography, aortography, and retrograde pyelography will reveal the tumor. A drop in blood pressure after phentolamine (Regitine) injection supports the presence of a pheochromocytoma.

MEDICAL AND SURGICAL MANAGEMENT

Treatment involves surgical removal of the tumor by means of unilateral adrenalectomy (removal of one adrenal gland). Phentolamine (Regitine) is given preoperatively and intraoperatively to control hypertensive episodes. Alpha-adrenergic blockers, such as phenoxybenzamine (Dibenzyline), are used to control hypertension preoperatively or when surgery is contraindicated or to treat a malignant pheochromocytoma. Medical treatment includes metyrosine (Demser), an enzyme inhibitor that reduces synthesis of catecholamines to decrease hypertensive attacks.

NURSING MANAGEMENT

Monitor the blood pressure closely when drug therapy is initiated and when the dose is changed. Notify the physician of a sudden decrease in the blood pressure. If the client undergoes adrenalectomy, assess for signs and symptoms of acute adrenal insufficiency (see earlier discussion).

Cushing's Syndrome (Adrenocortical Hyperfunction)

Cushing's syndrome is the opposite of Addison's disease.

ETIOLOGY AND PATHOPHYSIOLOGY

An overproduction of adrenocortical hormones results from (1) overproduction of ACTH by the pituitary gland, with resultant hyperplasia of the adrenal cortex and excessive production and secretion of glucocorticoids, mineralocorticoids, and androgens; (2) benign or malignant tumors of the adrenal cortex; or (3) prolonged administration of high doses of corticosteroid preparations. A complication of this disorder is peptic ulcers. Hyperadrenalism affects most body systems.

ASSESSMENT FINDINGS

Signs and Symptoms

Physical examination reveals muscle wasting and weakness resulting from extensive protein depletion. Carbohydrate tolerance is lowered, and signs and symptoms of diabetes mellitus develop (see Chap. 57). There is a redistribution of fat, leading to facial fullness and the characteristic moon face and buffalo hump. The skin is thin, and the face is ruddy. There is a susceptibility to infection because of a depressed production of white blood cells. Symptoms of infection may be masked.

Because the blood vessels are fragile, the client bruises easily, and striae often form over extensive skin areas. Wounds are slow to heal, and the bones become so demineralized that the client may have backache, kyphosis, and collapse of the vertebra. Sodium and water are retained, and peripheral edema and hypertension develop. Mood changes and depression may be seen; a psychosis occasionally develops. In women, Cushing's syndrome may produce masculinization with hirsutism and amenorrhea. The term **cushingoid syndrome** describes the physical changes that occur with this disorder (Figs. 56–9 and 56–10).

Diagnostic Findings

Diagnosis is tentatively based on the physical changes. Urine levels of 17-hydroxycorticosteroids (17-OHCS) and 17-ketosteroids (17-KS) are almost always increased. Plasma and urine cortisol levels are increased. An overnight dexamethasone suppression test is used as an initial screening. The client takes 1 mg oral dexamethasone; the next morning plasma cortisol levels are obtained. If these results are above normal (5 mg/dL), 0.5 mg dexamethasone is given every 6 hours, and 24-hour urine collections are tested for 2 consecutive days. Normal readings show decreased 17-OHCS and 17-KS levels.

Laboratory blood test results show increased serum sodium, decreased serum potassium, and increased blood glucose levels. Abdominal radiographs, CT scan, or MRI may show adrenal enlargement, and an IV pyelogram (IVP) may show changes in the renal shadow caused by an abnormally large adrenal gland.

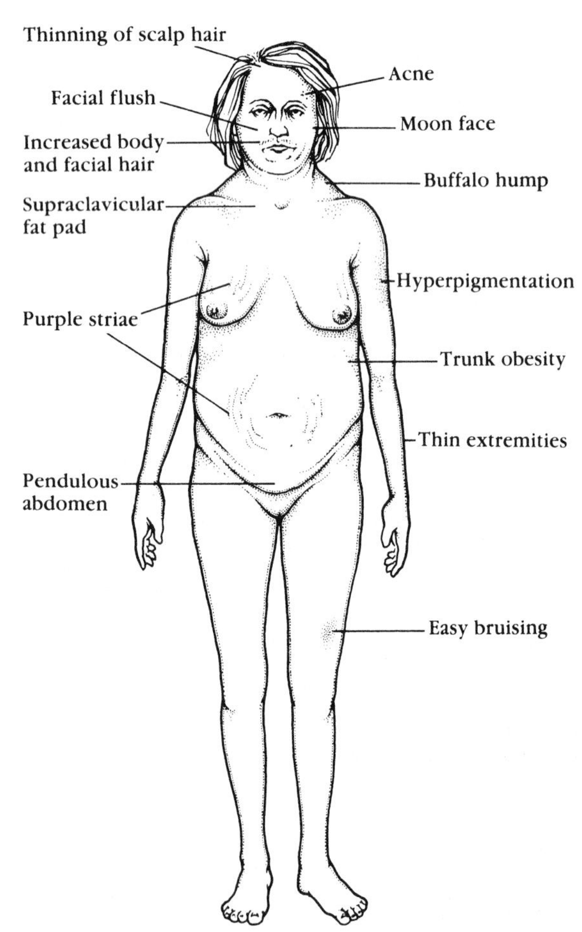

FIGURE 56-9. The symptoms of Cushing's disease. (Beyers, M., & Dudas, S. [Eds.]. [1984]. *The clinical practice of medical surgical nursing* [p. 71]. Boston: Little, Brown.)

MEDICAL AND SURGICAL MANAGEMENT

Treatment depends on whether the disease is caused by a tumor or by adrenal hyperplasia and is directed toward removing the cause of the disorder and lowering plasma cortisol levels. Radiation therapy to or removal of the pituitary may be used if there is adrenal hyperplasia. Bilateral adrenalectomy may be preferred if both adrenals are involved.

Drug therapy includes diuretics for edema as well as an antihypertensive agent. A diet low in sodium and carbohydrates controls edema and elevated blood glucose level. Antibiotics are used to treat infection.

If cushingoid syndrome is the result of exogenous administration of a corticosteroid preparation, the drug is slowly withdrawn by tapering the dose over a period of days or weeks. In some instances, as in the treatment of a disorder such as leukemia, or to prevent rejection of transplanted organs, the syndrome is allowed to persist.

NURSING MANAGEMENT

Management depends on the severity of symptoms as well as the proposed method of treatment.

NURSING PROCESS
The Client with Cushing's Syndrome

Assessment

Obtain thorough medical, drug, and allergy histories. Assess for symptoms of an adrenal disorder: altered skin pigmentation and integrity, decreased energy level, mental changes, sexual dysfunction, and changes in appetite, weight, and bowel patterns.

Monitor vital signs every 4 hours, and test the blood or urine (or both) for glucose three or four times per day. Inform the physician if the urine tests positive for glucose or the blood glucose level is elevated.

Observe the color of each stool and test for occult blood. Report the occurrence of epigastric pain or discomfort, a change in the color of the stool, or a stool testing positive for blood.

Diagnosis and Planning

The plan of care includes, but is not limited to, the following:

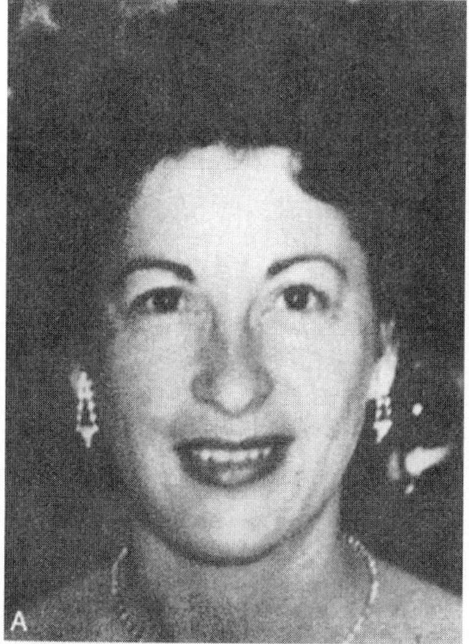

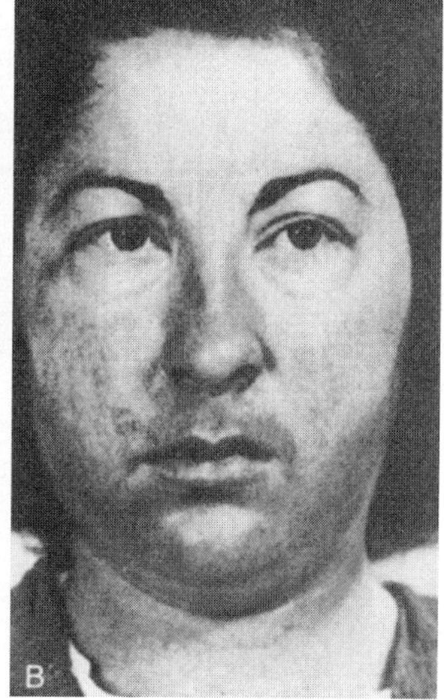

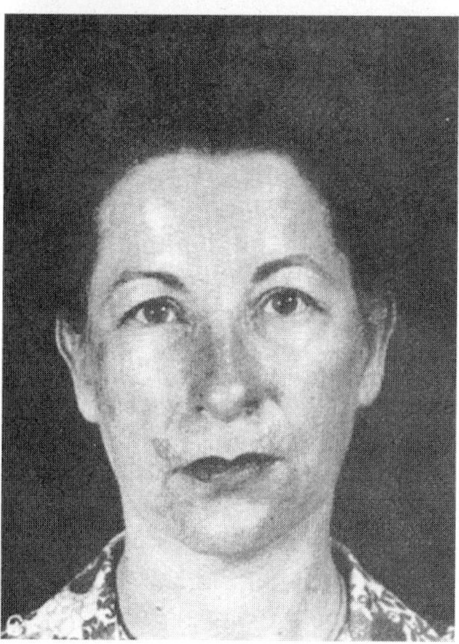

FIGURE 56-10. Progressive facial changes in a woman with Cushing disease. (*A*) Before onset of the illness. (*B*) Preoperative. (*C*) One year after surgery.

Nursing Diagnoses and Collaborative Problems	Nursing Interventions
Fluid Volume Excess related to sodium and water retention **Goal:** The client's fluid volume will be normal as evidenced by equivalent fluid intake and output volumes.	Examine extremities for an increase or decrease in edema. Measure intake and output weekly or as ordered. Administer diuretics. Provide a sodium-restricted diet.
Risk for Impaired Skin Integrity related to thinning of skin and edema **Goal:** The client's skin will remain intact.	Inspect the skin over bony prominences daily for signs of breakdown. Encourage the client to change positions frequently. Prevent skin abrasions and the development of pressure ulcers. Exercise care when performing tasks that may damage the skin, such as removing the tape when discontinuing an IV infusion.
Fatigue related to muscle wasting and protein depletion **Goal:** The client will demonstrate energy to complete activities of daily living.	Provide frequent rest periods between activities. When muscle wasting or pain secondary to osteoporosis is severe, give the client complete care and assistance with all activities.
Risk for Infection related to immunosuppression **Goal:** The client will be free from infection.	Observe the client for signs and symptoms that indicate an infection: a skin injury that does not heal, rise in temperature, sore throat, or cough. Immediately notify the physician. Make every effort to prevent the client from being exposed to infectious microorganisms.

	Limit or avoid the client's exposure to people with a known infection.
Risk for Injury related to demineralization of bones **Goal:** The client will be safe from injury such as bone fracture.	Protect the client from falls and other types of injury. Use side rails and instruct the client to seek assistance to get out of bed. Advise the ambulatory client to wear shoes rather than slippers to prevent falls.
Risk for Emotional Disturbance related to mood changes and depression **Goal:** The client's mood will stabilize with absence of depressive symptoms.	Assess the client's mental status at frequent intervals. If behavior changes or signs of depression arise, discuss changes with the physician. Explain that mood swings are part of the disorder and will resolve with treatment.
Body Image Disturbance related to changes in appearance **Goal:** The client will express a positive self-image.	Provide the client opportunities to express feelings over physical changes. Explain that if the cause of the disorder can be eliminated, some of the physical changes gradually improve, but that other physical changes, such as striae and kyphosis, are permanent. Offer suggestions, such as wearing loose clothing, if the client expresses concern over physical changes.

Evaluation and Expected Outcomes

- Fluid volume is normal; no evidence of edema or weight gain.
- The client meets self-care needs without fatigue.
- Temperature and white blood cell count are within normal limits.
- The client's skin is free from breakdown, with minimal petechiae.
- The client is free from injury, such as pathologic fractures.
- The client demonstrates normal range of moods.
- Client copes effectively with physical changes.

Client and Family Teaching

If a cushingoid appearance is caused by corticosteroid therapy and the dose is to be tapered over time, give the client and family a detailed explanation of the tapering schedule. Review the directions printed on the prescription container with the client. *Emphasize the importance of strict adherence to the tapering schedule.* Suggest using a calendar to enter the dosage for each day of the tapering schedule. Write the entire tapering schedule on a card and instruct the client to cross off each day.

Depending on many factors, such as age and severity of the disorder, clients with Cushing's syndrome may or may not be scheduled for adrenalectomy or removal or irradiation of the pituitary. Until such time as further treatment is scheduled, emphasize the importance of continued medical supervision. Develop a teaching plan to include:

- Avoid trauma to the skin.
- Contact the physician if sores or cuts do not heal or they become infected, if easy bruising occurs, or if stools are dark or black.
- Follow the recommended diet; read food labels carefully.
- Avoid exposure to infection.
- Avoid nonprescription drugs unless approved by the physician.
- Weigh self weekly and report marked weight gain or edema to the physician.

Hyperaldosteronism

The secretion of aldosterone, a mineralcorticoid, is regulated by serum levels of potassium and sodium, the renin–angiotensin mechanism, and ACTH. The hypersecretion of aldosterone creates extreme electrolyte imbalances.

ETIOLOGY AND PATHOPHYSIOLOGY

Primary hyperaldosteronism is caused by a benign aldosterone-secreting adenoma of one of the adrenals or by an adrenal malignant tumor, or its cause may be unknown. Secondary hyperaldosteronism can be caused by disorders or conditions such as pregnancy, congestive heart failure, narrowing of the renal artery, and cirrhosis.

Excessive secretion of aldosterone results in increased reabsorption of sodium and water and excretion of potassium by the kidneys. Figure 56–11 presents an overview of the renin–angiotensin–aldosterone cycle.

ASSESSMENT FINDINGS

Signs and Symptoms

Headache, muscle weakness, increased urine output, fatigue, hypertension, and cardiac arrhythmias are seen.

Diagnostic Findings

Serum potassium levels are decreased and serum sodium levels are increased in the absence of other causes, such as diuretic therapy or diarrhea. The serum bicarbonate level, serum aldosterone level, and plasma renin levels are increased. CT or MRI may rule out or locate an adrenal tumor. Adrenal venography may identify small tumors that cannot be seen by CT scanning.

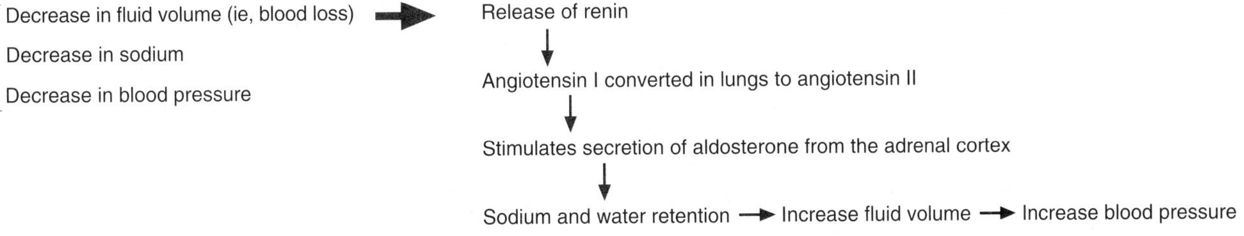

FIGURE 56-11. The renin–angiotensin–aldosterone cycle.

MEDICAL AND SURGICAL MANAGEMENT

If hyperaldosteronism is caused by an adrenal tumor, unilateral adrenalectomy may be performed. Medical management may include administration of spironolactone, a potassium-sparing diuretic, and an antihypertensive agent to control blood pressure. A sodium-restricted diet may be necessary.

NURSING MANAGEMENT

Monitor vital signs every 4 hours, or as ordered. Report marked elevations to the physician. Measure fluid intake and output. Weigh the client every 2 to 7 days. Examine the extremities daily for edema. Observe the client for signs of hypokalemia and hypernatremia (see Chap. 21).

Adrenalectomy

Adrenalectomy is performed to remove tumors of the adrenal gland(s). In some instances, removal of the ovaries and testes, and removal of both adrenal glands, which also secrete male and female hormones, is considered to control cancerous tumors of the breast and prostate, which depend on hormones for growth.

The adrenals are surgically approached by means of an abdominal incision or a flank incision under and following the position of the 12th rib. The abdominal incision usually is long because adequate exposure is needed for the adrenals, which lie posteriorly. The flank incision is the same surgical approach used for kidney surgery.

Nursing Management

PREOPERATIVE PERIOD

Major goals include a reduction in anxiety and an understanding of the preparations for surgery and the events that may occur during the postoperative period.

If the client has a pheochromocytoma, monitor the blood pressure at frequent intervals before surgery. When bilateral adrenalectomy is to be performed, IV administration of a solution containing a corticosteroid preparation may be started the morning of surgery. Some surgeons prefer to initiate corticosteroid administration during surgery, at the time of removal of the adrenals. Additional preparations are the same as for the client having general surgery (see Chap. 24).

Keep the client with a pheochromocytoma on bed rest, and reduce anxiety-provoking events to a minimum. The client who requires surgery to halt progression of a metastatic disease may be anxious as well as depressed, and needs time to talk about the surgery and anticipated results.

POSTOPERATIVE PERIOD

When the client returns from surgery, review the surgical record because the nursing postoperative observations and management depend on whether one or both adrenal glands were removed.

In addition to the complications that are associated with general anesthesia, observe the client for such problems as hemorrhage, atelectasis, and pneumothorax because the adrenals are located close to the diaphragm and the inferior vena cava. Monitor vital signs at frequent intervals, and closely observe the client for signs of adrenal insufficiency, which may occur in the following situations:

- When the prescribed dose of a corticosteroid preparation is inadequate to meet the client's individual needs (bilateral adrenalectomy)
- When the remaining adrenal gland does not produce a sufficient amount of hormone to meet the client's needs (unilateral adrenalectomy)
- When the prescribed dose of a corticosteroid preparation is not given.

If symptoms of adrenal insufficiency occur, notify the physician immediately.

Prescribed corticosteroid must never be omitted; corticosteroid replacement is essential to life.

NURSING PROCESS
The Client Undergoing An Adrenalectomy

Assessment

Check vital signs as soon as the client returns to the unit to establish a data base. Closely observe the client for potential acute adrenal crisis (see earlier discussion).

Monitor blood studies for electrolyte imbalances. Assess the client closely for any signs of infection and continue to monitor pulse, blood pressure, temperature, breath sounds, and urinary output postoperatively.

Diagnosis and Planning

The nursing plan of care includes, but is not limited to, the following:

Nursing Diagnoses and Collaborative Problems	Nursing Interventions
Pain related to tissue trauma **Goal:** The client's pain will be minimized.	Give an analgesic for pain before the pain increases. Assess and note the client's response to the analgesic. Offer comfort measures such as massage, skin care, and emotional support.
Ineffective Airway Clearance related to inadequate coughing secondary to incisional pain **Goal:** The client's airway will be clear as evidenced by normal breath sounds and respiratory rate and effort.	Support the incision firmly when turning or changing the client's position, and apply firm support over the incision when the client deep breathes and coughs. Change the client's position every 2 hours. Encourage deep breathing and coughing every 2 hours. Assist the client who has undergone bilateral adrenalectomy with turning on either side. Auscultate the lungs daily, and report abnormal findings and inability to cough and deep breathe to the physician.
Risk for Infection related to decreased cortisol secretion or immunosuppression secondary to steroid therapy replacement **Goal:** The client's wound is clean and dry, with no signs of infection.	Notify the physician if there is a change in vital signs or purulent drainage on the dressing or if pain is not controlled with analgesics. Inspect the wound at the time of each dressing change. Notify the physician if excessive redness, swelling of the suture line, or purulent drainage is noted. Observe strict aseptic technique for all procedures.
Risk for Injury related to postural hypotension, weakness secondary to adrenal insufficiency **Goal:** The client will be free from injury.	Assist with ambulatory activities and observe for weakness and dizziness. Notify the physician of continued episodes.

Evaluation and Expected Outcomes

- The client reports relief from pain and general increase in comfort level.
- Lungs are clear to auscultation; coughs and breathes effectively.
- No evidence of infection.
- Remains injury-free.

Client and Family Teaching

Give the client who has undergone bilateral adrenalectomy detailed instructions for postdischarge management (Box 56–2).

Disorders of the Ovaries and Testes

Disorders associated with the female and male reproductive systems are covered in Chapters 58 and 60 respectively.

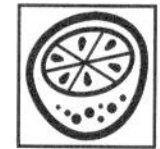

General Nutritional Considerations

Clients with hyperthyroidism may need 4500 to 5000 calories or more to maintain normal weight. A liberal protein intake of 100 g or more, combined with a liberal carbohydrate intake, is recommended. Clients experiencing steady weight loss despite eating large amounts of food are often frustrated and discouraged. Encourage frequent meals and the intake of nutritionally dense foods (ie, fortified milkshakes, foods fortified with skim milk powder, eggs, cheese, butter, or milk).

Until normal metabolism is restored, clients with myxedema experience weight gain even if calorie intake is low. After hormone replacement therapy begins, the client may stil

BOX 56-2 Discharge Instructions for the Client After an Adrenalectomy

Teach the client about the:

- Function of the adrenal glands and importance of adhering to the prescribed treatment regimen
- Care of the surgical wound until healed
- Medication schedule
- Need for obtaining adequate rest, eating a well balanced diet, complying with ongoing medical supervision, avoiding infections and stressful situations, carrying identification indicating surgical removal of the adrenal glands, seeking immediate medical help if unable to take the prescribed corticosteroid drug or if symptoms of adrenal insufficiency and adrenal crisis develop

need to follow a low-calorie diet to attain or maintain normal weight. A high fiber intake helps alleviate constipation and promotes satiety. Additional diet modifications, such as low fat, low cholesterol, and low sodium are necessary if the client has cardiovascular complications.

Clients with hyperparathyroidism should drink at least 3 to 4 liters of fluid daily to dilute the urine and prevent the formation of renal stones. It is especially important that the client drink fluids before going to bed and periodically throughout the night to avoid concentrated urine.

In addition to calcium and vitamin D supplements, clients with hypoparathyroidism may be prescribed a high-calcium, low-phosphorus diet, even though the diet is difficult to achieve because milk and milk products (the richest sources of calcium) are also high in phosphorus.

Clients with Addison's disease who are treated with cortisone may require a high sodium intake of at least 4 to 6 g/day. A high sodium intake is contraindicated for clients receiving fludrocortisone (Florinef) because it is a sodium-retaining hormone. Potassium requirements are determined on an individual basis. Frequent meals, including a large bedtime snack, that are high in protein and moderate in carbohydrate are recommended to avoid hypoglycemia. Concentrated sugars are restricted.

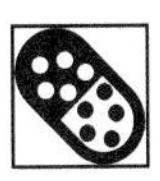

General Pharmacologic Considerations

Substances that contain iodine, such as some cough medicines and dyes administered for radiographs of the gallbladder, IV pyelograms, and bronchograms, can interfere with the results of some thyroid tests.

The most serious adverse effect of the antithyroid drugs is agranulocytosis. Agranulocytosis occurs most often in the first 2 months of therapy and necessitates discontinuing the drug. The patient must be instructed to report sore throat, fever, chills, headache, malaise, weakness, or unusual bleeding or bruising.

Antithyroid drugs are administered at 8-hour intervals around the clock, unless directed otherwise by the physician.

During the initial therapy with a thyroid preparation, the most common adverse reactions are signs of hyperthyroidism (which would indicate an overdosage of the drug). Adverse reactions other than symptoms of hyperthyroidism are rare.

The dosage of a thyroid preparation may need to be decreased or increased over a period of time until the optimal dose is attained. A full therapeutic response of thyroid hormone replacement therapy may not be evident until the patient has concluded several weeks of therapy, but early effects may be observed within 48 hours of the initial dose.

Florinef is a mineralocorticoid with some glucocorticoid activity. It is commonly prescribed after a bilateral adrenalectomy and for the management of adrenocortical insufficiency. The more common adverse reactions to Florinef include frontal and occipital headache, arthralgia, edema, and hypertension. Dosage increases may be necessary during stressful periods to prevent drug-induced adrenal insufficiency.

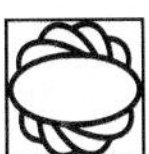

General Gerontologic Considerations

Changes in hormone levels may occur with age. While levels of thyroxine (T_4) tend to remain constant, levels of triiodothyronine (T_3) may decrease with age. Parathyroid hormone levels tend to increase with age. There is an increased incidence of nodules and small goiters on the thyroid gland of the older adult.

The symptoms of thyroid disease in older adults are often atypical or minor and easily attributed to other problems. For example, the older adult may not experience restlessness or hyperactivity and may not appear nervous. Symptoms seen most often in older adults include anorexia, weight loss, palpitations, angina, and atrial fibrillation. The most reliable thyroid function test to diagnose hyperthyroidism in an older adult is a serum thyroxine (T_4) level.

Hypothyroidism is difficult to identify in an older adult because the symptoms closely resemble normal aging—for example, anorexia, constipation, weight loss, muscular weakness and pain, joint stiffness, apathy, and depression.

Dosages of thyroid replacement drugs are lower in the older adult, and drug therapy is initiated slowly with increases given cautiously. The older adult receiving thyroid replacement therapy is at increased risk for adverse reactions associated with cardiac function.

SUMMARY OF KEY CONCEPTS

- When there is oversecretion of GH in a young person, before the ends of the long bones are fully united (epiphyseal union), gigantism results. Oversecretion of GH during adulthood results in acromegaly.
- Simmonds' disease is a rare disorder that results from the destruction of the pituitary gland. All pituitary hormonal function ceases.
- Diabetes insipidus is a lack of ADH secretion in response to a decreased vascular volume and increased osmolarity, resulting in a lack of conservation of fluid by the kidneys and decreased concentration of urine.
- SIADH occurs because of an excessive release of ADH, resulting in increased water retention and hyponatremia (decreased serum sodium level).
- In hyperthyroidism, the metabolic rate increases because of an oversecretion of thyroid hormones. Symptoms include heat intolerance, weight loss, restlessness, excitability, agitation, fine hand tremors, tachycardia, nervousness, insomnia, diarrhea, exophthalmos, and swelling of the neck.
- Thyrotoxic crisis (thyroid storm) is a severe form of hyperthyroidism caused by oversecretion of T_3 and T_4 followed by a markedly increased metabolic rate.
- Hypothyroidism occurs when the thyroid gland fails to secrete an adequate amount of thyroid hormones. The rates of all metabolic processes slow. Severe hypothyroidism is called myxedema. Hypothyroidism may originate within the thyroid or within the pituitary, in which case insufficient TSH is secreted.

- Treatment of benign thyroid tumors may not be necessary if no symptoms of hyperthyroidism are present. Malignant tumors may be treated by thyroidectomy. Radioactive iodine may be administered to destroy remaining thyroid tissue as well as to treat lymph node metastasis, if present.
- A goiter may be caused by a deficiency of iodine in the diet, by the inability of the thyroid to use iodine, or by relative iodine deficiency caused by increasing body demands for thyroid hormones.
- In primary hyperparathyroidism, excessive secretion of parathyroid hormone (parathormone) results in increased urinary excretion of phosphorus and loss of calcium from the bones. In secondary hyperparathyroidism, the parathyroid glands secrete an excessive amount of parathormone in response to hypocalcemia.
- The most common causes of hypoparathyroidism are trauma to the glands and inadvertent removal of all or nearly all these structures during thyroidectomy or parathyroidectomy.
- Addison's disease results from destruction of the adrenal cortex. Certain diseases also can affect the adrenal cortex, or this may be an autoimmune disorder. Secondary adrenal insufficiency may be caused by surgical removal of both adrenal glands (bilateral adrenalectomy), hemorrhagic infarction of the adrenals, hypopituitarism (caused by pituitary failure or surgical removal of the pituitary), or suppression of adrenal function by the administration of corticosteroid drugs.
- Adrenal crisis can begin gradually with anorexia, nausea, vomiting, diarrhea, abdominal pain, profound weakness, headache, intensification of hypotension, restlessness, and fever. Unless the dosage of the corticosteroid is increased to meet the demand, the client progresses to acute adrenal crisis. The blood pressure becomes markedly decreased, and adrenal shock is present. If untreated, coma and death can occur.
- A pheochromocytoma is a tumor, usually of the adrenal medulla, that causes excessive secretion of the catecholamines epinephrine and norepinephrine. Symptoms include hypertension, tremors, nervousness, sweating, headache, nausea, vomiting, hyperglycemia, polyuria, and vertigo.
- Symptoms of Cushing's syndrome include muscle wasting and weakness, decreased carbohydrate tolerance, moon face, buffalo hump, thin skin, ruddy face, susceptibility to infection, easy bruising, striae, impaired wound healing, demineralization of the bones, edema, hypertension, and mood changes. In women, masculinization, hirsutism, and amenorrhea may be seen.
- Excessive secretion of aldosterone results in increased reabsorption of sodium and water and excretion of potassium by the kidneys.
- Unilateral adrenalectomy usually does not require hormone replacement because the remaining adrenal gland probably can supply a sufficient amount of adrenal hormones. Bilateral adrenalectomy requires glucocorticoid and mineralocorticoid replacement therapy.

CRITICAL THINKING EXERCISES

1. When caring for a client receiving fludrocortisone (Florinef) orally after bilateral adrenalectomy, the nurse in charge asks the nursing staff for suggestions on how to be sure the client receives these medications on time and as ordered. What suggestions could you give?
2. A client had a thyroidectomy this morning. It is now 8 PM, and she is complaining of difficulty swallowing clear liquids and a fullness in her throat. Her blood pressure is normal, but her pulse rate is elevated. You do not see drainage on the surface of her dressing. What actions would you take at this time?

Suggested Readings

Clayton, L. H., & Dilley, K. B. (1998). Cushing's syndrome. *American Journal of Nursing, 98*(7), 40–41.

Corsetti, A., & Buhl, B. (1994). Managing thyroid storm. *American Journal of Nursing, 94*(11), 39.

Healy, P. F. (1995). Self-test. Caring for patients with endocrine disorders. *Nursing, 25*(9), 22.

Jankowski, C. B. (1996). Irradiating the thyroid: How to protect yourself and others. *American Journal of Nursing, 96*(10), 50–54.

McConnell, E. A. (1996). Myth & facts...about thyroid disease. *Nursing, 26*(4), 17.

McKennis, A., & Waddington, C. (1997). Nursing interventions for potential complications after thyroidectomy. *ORL Head and Neck Nursing, 15*(1),27–35.

Moore, S., & Haughey, B. H. (1997). Surgical treatment for thyroid cancer. *AORN Journal, 65*(4),710–716.

O'Donnell, M. (1997). Emergency! Addisonian crisis. *American Journal of Nursing, 97*(3), 41.

Wallymahmed, M. (1997). Practice. Growth hormone deficiency in adults. *Nursing Times, 93*(23), 50–51.

What's new in drugs. Octreotide enters the market against acromegaly. (1996). *RN, 59*(1), 69, 71.

Additional Resources

American Thyroid Association, Inc.
Montefiore Medical Center
11 East 210th Street
Bronx, NY 10467
(717) 882–6047

Endocrine Nurses' Society
P.O. Box 229
West Linn, OR 97068
(503) 494–3714

National Adrenal Diseases Foundation
505 Northern Boulevard
Great Neck, NY 11021
(516) 487–4992

Pituitary Tumor Network Association
38 South Wendy Drive
Newbury Park, CA 91320
(805) 499–9973

Chapter 57

Caring for Clients With Diabetes Mellitus

KEY TERMS

Diabetes mellitus
Diabetic coma
Diabetic ketoacidosis
Fasting blood glucose
Glycosuria
Glycosylated hemoglobin
Hyperglycemia
Hyperinsulinism
Hyperosmolar hyperglycemic nonketotic syndrome
Hypoglycemia
Ketones
Ketonemia
Kussmaul respirations
Oral glucose tolerance test
Polydipsia
Polyphagia
Polyuria
Postprandial glucose
Renal threshold

LEARNING OBJECTIVES

On completion of this chapter, the reader will:

- Define and distinguish the two types of diabetes mellitus.
- Identify the three classic symptoms of diabetes mellitus.
- Explain the source of ketones.
- Name three laboratory methods used to diagnose diabetes mellitus.
- Describe the methods used to treat diabetes mellitus.
- Explain the cause of diabetic ketoacidosis.
- List three main goals in the treatment of diabetic ketoacidosis.
- Identify two physiologic signs of hyperosmolar hyperglycemic nonketotic syndrome.
- Describe the treatment of hyperosmolar hyperglycemia nonketotic syndrome.
- Explain the cause and treatment of hypoglycemia.
- List common complications of diabetes mellitus.
- Differentiate between the symptoms of hypoglycemia and hyperglycemia.
- Discuss the nursing management of the client with diabetes mellitus.

Diabetes Mellitus

Diabetes mellitus is a metabolic disorder of the pancreas in which glucose intolerance results from varying degrees of insulin insufficiency. Although no age group is exempt, diabetes is most frequently seen in people between ages 40 and 60.

The two major groups of diabetes mellitus are:

- Type I—insulin-dependent diabetes mellitus (IDDM), characterized by cessation of insulin production by the pancreas. Type I diabetes occurs in juveniles.
- Type II—adult-onset non–insulin-dependent diabetes mellitus (NIDDM), characterized by a deficiency in the secretion of insulin or a decrease in the sensitivity of the tissues to insulin (insulin resistance).

ETIOLOGY AND PATHOPHYSIOLOGY

The exact cause of diabetes mellitus is unknown, but certain risk factors play a role in the development of type II. Persons at risk for developing diabetes mellitus include those with a family history of diabetes, obesity, mothers giving birth to large infants, and persons with premature manifestation of arteriosclerosis. It appears that the development of diabetes mellitus could involve a combination of factors rather than a single factor.

Research supports the theory that the cause of type I is genetic, immunologic, or viral. Diabetes mellitus tends to run in families although a specific diabetic gene has not been isolated. Autoimmune dysfunction can cause total destruction of the islets of Langerhans in the pancreas, giving rise to type I diabetes mellitus.

Insulin is secreted into the bloodstream by the beta cells of the islets of Langerhans. Diabetic individuals have less insulin available than their metabolic processes require. Because insulin is required to move the glucose from the bloodstream to the liver and cells for use, the glucose remains within the bloodstream.

Excess glucose in the blood is called **hyperglycemia.** Some glucose in the blood is excreted by the kidneys. Glucose is usually found in the urine (**glycosuria**) when the level rises over 180 mg/dL in the blood. This is called the **renal threshold** for glucose.

To eliminate glucose, water also is excreted. Therefore, one of the symptoms of untreated diabetes is **polyuria** (excessive urine production). The client experiences urinary frequency and large amounts of urine are passed each time. Because so much water is lost in the urine, **polydipsia** (excessive thirst) occurs, but the fluid intake is often not enough to compensate for water loss, leading to dehydration.

While the needed glucose is being wasted, the body's requirement for fuel continues. The diabetic person feels hungry and eats more (**polyphagia**). Hunger and weakness increase and weight is lost. To meet the rising need for energy, which now cannot be obtained from glucose, fats and proteins are metabolized. Normally when fat is metabolized, ketones are formed in the liver and transported to muscle and other tissue, where they serve as a source of energy. **Ketones** are chemical intermediate products in the metabolism of fat, such as beta-hydroxybutyric acid, acetoacetic acid, and acetone (note two of them are acids). All three are toxic if they accumulate in the body, a condition called ketoacidosis.

If ketones are produced faster than they can be oxidized in tissues, they accumulate in tissues and body fluids. Ketones are buffered by the bicarbonate buffer system. Thus, **ketonemia** (an increase in ketones in the blood) causes a decrease of alkali (base) reserve. **Kussmaul respirations** (fast, deep, labored breathing) are common in ketoacidosis. Acetone, which is volatile, can be detected on the breath by its characteristic odor. If treatment is not initiated, the outcome is circulatory collapse, renal shutdown, and death. This complex is known as **diabetic coma** (though severe ketoacidosis can be present without the client's being comatose).

Anything that causes glycogen depletion in the liver, thereby increasing the need for oxidation of fat (eg, insulin deprivation, infection, surgery, anesthesia, vomiting), can result in an excess of ketones. Infection and surgery invite ketosis and diabetic coma because they increase the demand for insulin that the diabetic's pancreas cannot produce. In addition, clients with diabetes mellitus are at greater risk for vascular disorders such as cerebrovascular accidents, myocardial infarction, renal failure, blindness, and neuropathy.

ASSESSMENT FINDINGS

Signs and Symptoms

The three classic symptoms of diabetes mellitus a polyuria, polydipsia, and polyphagia. Addition symptoms include weight loss, weakness, thirst, fa tigue, and dehydration. These signs and symptom have an abrupt onset in individuals with type I dia betes. Those with type II diabetes have a gradual or set of symptoms.

Diagnostic Findings

Although diabetes mellitus is a highly comple disease, a diagnostic test for its detection is extremel simple. Normally, urine contains no detectable glu cose or ketones; in this disease, both may be presen Because glucose is not adequately used by the body, is excreted in urine. If fats are metabolized faster tha the body can use the ketone bodies, they also appea in the urine. The relative ease of these urinary test helps to facilitate early detection of diabetes (Nursin Guidelines 57–1).

Because glucose in the urine is not always an indi cation of diabetes mellitus, and not all diabetics ex crete glucose the urine, other tests are necessary to es tablish the diagnosis. These tests include a fastin blood glucose, a postprandial glucose, and an ora glucose tolerance test (Box 57–1). Another method o testing for blood glucose is with a glucometer (Fig 57–1). This instrument measures glucose from a fin ger stick blood sample (Clinical Procedure 57–1) Close monitoring of blood glucose levels can delay the onset of complications associated with diabetes. Man physicians are now recommending self-monitorin of blood glucose levels with a glucometer for individ uals taking insulin, individuals with unstable dia-

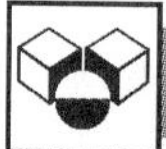

Nursing Guidelines 57-1

Performing Urine Glucose Testing

Method: Test-tape™ and Diastix™

- Client empties the bladder to eliminate glucose and ketones that have been stored in the bladder for hours; save this specimen in case the client cannot void later.
- Encourage the client to drink water; ask the client to void in 30 minutes.
- For the client with an indwelling catheter, clamp the catheter for 30 minutes and take the specimen directly from the catheter, not the drainage bag.
- Test the second voided specimen to detect current concentration of glucose and ketones.
- Dip the testing strip into the urine and wait for the recommended time.
- Observe the color change and document the results.

BOX 57-1 Diagnostic Tests for Diabetes Mellitus

Test	Implementation	Diagnostic Result
Fasting blood glucose	Blood specimen obtained after 8 hours of fasting.	In the nondiabetic the glucose level will be between 70 and 110 mg/dL. In the diabetic, glucose is > 120 mg/dL.
Postprandial glucose	Blood sample taken 2 hours after a high-carbohydrate meal.	In the nondiabetic the glucose level will be between 70 and 110 mg/dL. In diabetes mellitus (DM), the result is > 120 mg/dL.
Oral glucose tolerance test	Diet high in carbohydrates is eaten for 3 days. Client then fasts for 8 hours. A baseline blood sample is drawn and a urine specimen is collected. An oral glucose solution is given and time of ingestion recorded. Blood is drawn at 30 minutes and 1, 2, and 3 hours after the ingestion of glucose solution. Urine is collected simultaneously. Drinking water is encouraged to promote urine excretion.	In the nondiabetic the glucose returns to normal in 2 to 3 hours and urine is negative for glucose. In the diabetic, blood glucose level returns to normal slowly; urine is positive for glucose.
Glycosylated hemoglobin	Single blood sample	The amount of glucose stored by the hemoglobin is elevated above 7.0% in the newly diagnosed client with DM, in one who is noncompliant, or in one who is inadquately treated.

betes, or individuals with frequent hypoglycemic episodes. Self-monitoring with a glucometer is helpful for individuals taking an oral hypoglycemic agent to determine the effects of diet, exercise, and medications.

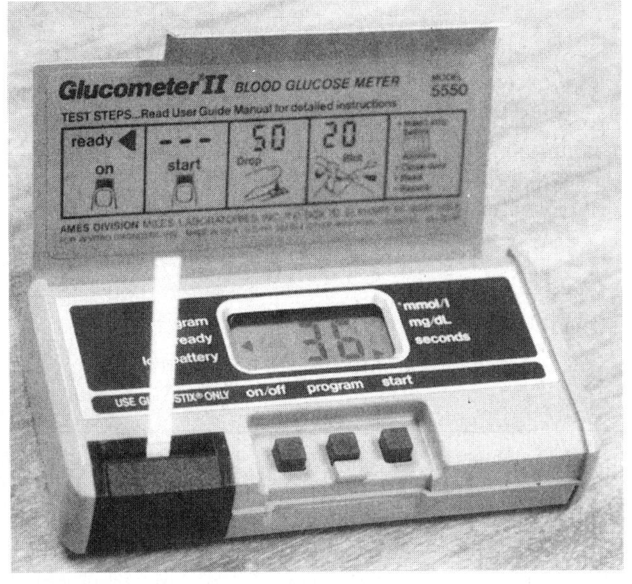

FIGURE 57-1. The Glucometer II is an example of a glucose self-testing device that can be used by the client or members of the health care team.

MEDICAL MANAGEMENT

Treatment depends on many factors, such as the type of diabetes and the ability of the pancreas to manufacture insulin, and involves combinations of the following:

- Diet
- Exercise
- Insulin
- Oral hypoglycemic agent
- Weight control

Diet

Diet is part of treatment for every individual with diabetes. Formulation of a diabetic diet depends on the individual's sex, age, height and weight, activity level, occupation, state of health, former dietary habits, and cultural background. When dietary allowances (calories, percentages of carbohydrates, fats, and proteins) are prescribed, the client is given a formal diet to follow and a list of substitutions and exchanges to vary the diet.

Some individuals can control their diabetes by diet alone. These individuals have a mild form of diabetes, with some insulin being produced by the pancreas. The overweight diabetic client is placed on a weight reduction diet because diabetes is exacerbated by excess weight.

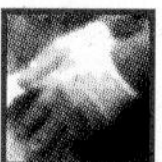

Clinical Procedure 57-1
Using a Glucometer to Monitor Blood Glucose

PURPOSE	EQUIPMENT
• To monitor blood glucose levels and effectiveness of treatment	• Glucometer and test strips • Lancet, lancet holder • Gloves • Paper tissue

Nursing Action	Rationale
ASSESSMENT	
Check the client's medical record to review trends in blood sugar measurements and if insulin coverage is ordered.	Establishes baseline and informs nurse of treatment plan
Check that glucometer has been calibrated at least once in the last 24 hours. Check the date on the test strips and compare code number of test strip with programmed code number in glucometer.	Ensures validity of test results

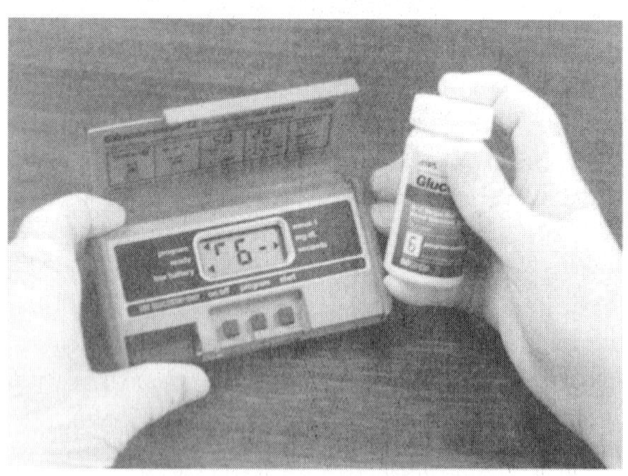

Comparing code number on test strip bottle to glucometer code number. (Courtesy of Ken Timby.)

Nursing Action	Rationale
Inspect the client's fingers and thumb for a nontraumatized area; the earlobe is an acceptable alternative.	Avoids secondary trauma
PLANNING	
Collect equipment.	Promotes efficient time management
IMPLEMENTATION	
Have the client wash his or her hands with soap and warm water and towel dry.	Reduces microorganisms and dilates capillaries
Place lancet in lancet holder.	Lancet holder delivers sharp, measured thrust.
Wash your hands and don gloves.	Provides a barrier against contact with blood.
Apply the lancet to a nontraumatized area, avoiding the central pad of the fingertip and release the spring.	Avoids puncturing an area where there are nerve endings

continued

Exercise

Exercise helps metabolize carbohydrates, thus decreasing insulin requirements. It improves circulation, which is compromised in the diabetic client. Exercise also lowers cholesterol and triglyceride levels and improves muscle tone. An exercise program for the diabetic client specifies the type of exercise and the length of time the exercise is performed. The program is tailored to the client's age, sex, occupation, abilities, and preferences. Most important, the client should exercise consistently each day. Sporadic periods of exercise are discouraged because wide fluctuations in blood glu-

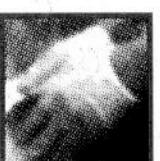

Clinical Procedure 57-1
Continued

Nursing Action	Rationale
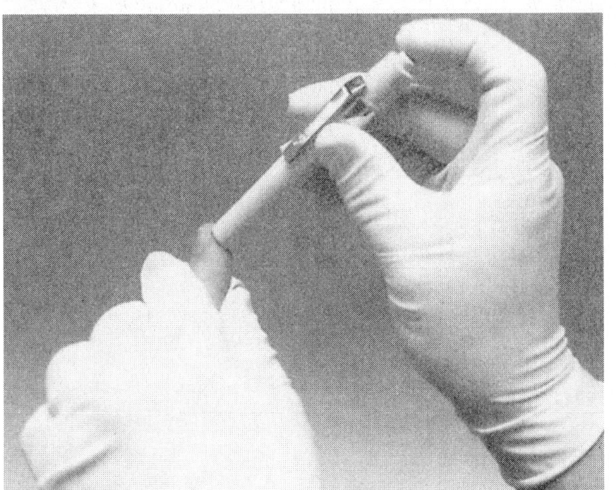 *Puncture made with lancet holder. (Courtesy of Ken Timby.)*	
Hold the finger or thumb so that a large hanging drop of blood forms.	Uses gravity to aid in collecting blood
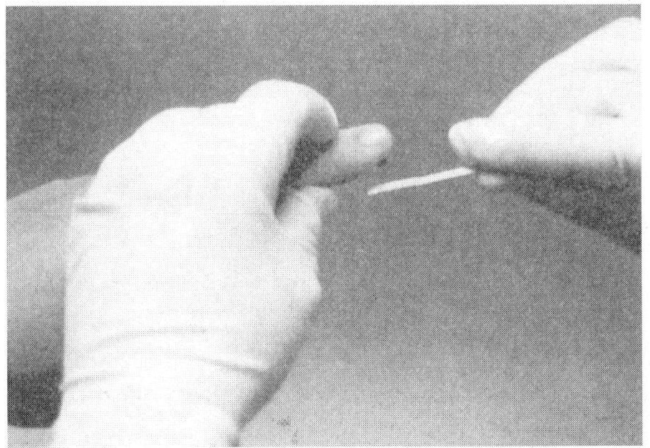 *One large drop of blood is necessary for test. (Courtesy of Ken Timby.)*	
Touch the drop of blood to the test strip, making sure the test area is completely covered.	Ensures accurate test results
Press the start button on the glucometer.	Activates timer
Offer the client a Band-Aid.	Absorbs blood and controls bleeding
Blot and reblot blood for 1 to 2 seconds when machine beeps.	Removes excess blood

continued

cose levels can occur. It is necessary to regulate food and insulin requirements during times of increased activities.

Insulin

Insulin is available as purified extracts from beef and pork pancreas. It is biologically similar to human insulin. There are two methods for deriving human insulin: genetic engineering using strains of *Escherichia coli*, a microorganism found in the gastrointestinal tract, and chemical modification of pork insulin. Human insulin appears to cause fewer allergic reactions than insulin obtained from animal sources.

Insulin is inactivated by gastrointestinal juices and, therefore, must be injected. Table 57–1 includes commonly used insulin preparations. The prepara-

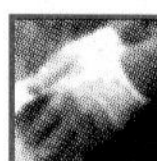

Clinical Procedure 57-1
Continued

Nursing Action	Rationale
Insert the test strip into the window of the glucometer and shut the door immediately after blotting and before the timer reaches zero.	Ensures accurate test results; prevents light from altering test results

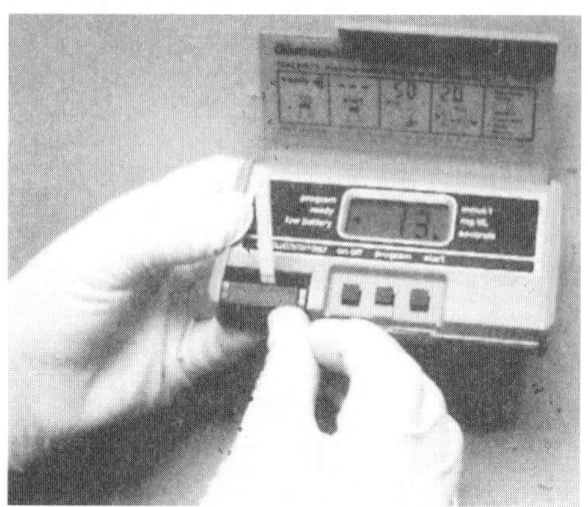

Inserting the test strip. (Courtesy of Ken Timby.

Nursing Action	Rationale
Observe the number displayed on the screen at the end of the test.	Indicates the current level of blood glucose
Remove the test strip and compare the color change with the color code on the test strip container.	Provides a method for checking the accuracy of the displayed glucose measurement
Press the sharp tip of the lancet into its plastic protector and dispose of the lancet in a puncture-resistant container.	Prevents needle stick injury

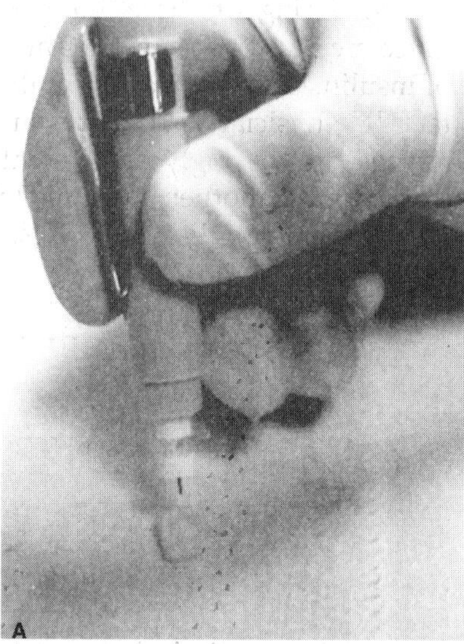

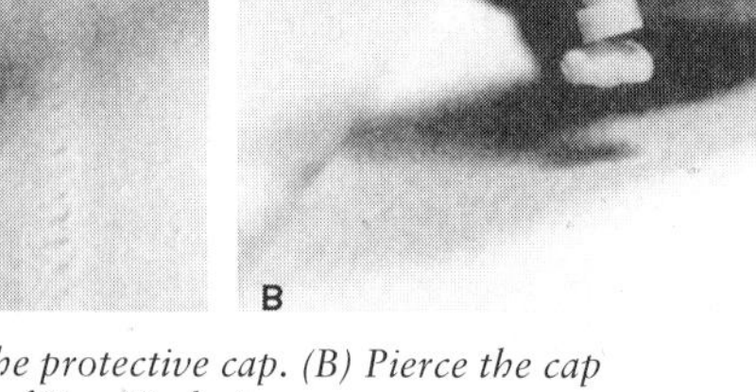

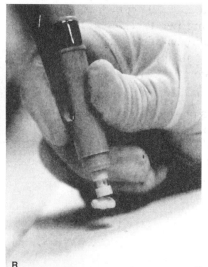

(A) Position used lancet above the protective cap. (B) Pierce the cap with the sharp point. (Courtesy of Ken Timby.)

Nursing Action	Rationale
Clean light window with a dry, lint-free cloth.	Keeps light window free of debris that may impair light detection
Remove gloves and wash hands.	Reduces the number of microorganisms
Record the glucose measurement in the client's record and report blood sugar level to nurse in charge.	Documents and communicates essential data needed for making treatment decisions

TABLE 57-1 **Insulin Preparations**

Insulin	Onset (hours)	Peak (hours)	Duration (hours)
Very rapid acting			
insulin lispro (Humalog)	15 minutes	1–2	3–4
Short acting			
regular insulin (Humulin R)	30 minutes–1 hour	1–3	6–8
Intermediate acting			
isophane insulin suspension (NPH, Humulin N)	1–1.5	4–12	24
insulin zinc suspension (Lente)	1–2.5	7–15	24
70/30 insulin	1–3	2–16	24
Long acting			
protamine zinc insulin suspension (PZI)	4–8	14–24	36
extended insulin zinc suspension (Ultralente)	4–8	10–30	>36

tions are divided into four categories: very rapid acting, rapid acting, intermediate acting, and long acting.

Administration of Insulin

Insulin is prescribed in units. U100 means that 1 mL contains 100 units of insulin. The physician specifies both the dosage and the type of insulin to be used. When combining two types of insulin, one of which is regular insulin, withdraw the regular insulin into the syringe *first* (Nursing Guidelines 57–2).

Insulin is administered in several ways:

- A disposable needle and syringe (Fig. 57–2)
- A cartridge that is prefilled with a specific type of insulin; the number of desired units is selected by turning a dial and locking the ring.
- An access port; the client inserts a subcutaneous access port into the skin, changing sites every 3 days. Each dose of insulin is injected into the port, eliminating multiple punctures over a 3-day period.
- An insulin pump for those who need better blood glucose control, is battery powered, and requires insertion of a special needle into subcutaneous tissue, changed every 1–3 days.

Oral Hypoglycemic Agents

Oral hypoglycemic agents act by stimulating the beta cells of the pancreas to secrete more insulin. Individuals with little or no pancreatic insulin-secreting activity cannot use these agents.

Oral hypoglycemic agents are indicated for the individuals with one of more of the following:

- Type II adult-onset diabetes
- Fasting blood glucose less than 200 mg/dL
- Insulin requirement of less than 40 units/day
- Absence of ketoacidosis
- Absence of renal or hepatic disease

The timing of the administration of oral hypoglycemic agents is as important as the administration of insulin. Give these drugs at the time ordered. Contact the physician if a client is unable to take the prescribed oral hypoglycemic agent because of nausea, vomiting, or another problem. Table 57–2 lists examples of oral hypoglycemic drugs.

NURSING MANAGEMENT

Obtain a complete medical, drug, and allergy history, including a list of all symptoms and their duration. Inquire when the client was diagnosed with diabetes and the presence of a family history of diabetes. If the client is a diagnosed diabetic, record the prescribed treatment regimen. Check if any complications associated with diabetes have occurred and the treatment instituted for each.

Weigh the client and perform a complete head-to-toe physical examination because diabetes affects many systems. Look for any changes that could be the result of diabetes, including:

- Changes in the skin over insulin injection sites, if used, skin breaks that appear to be healing poorly; presence of ulcerations or evidence of infection

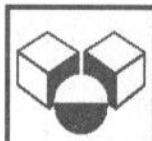

Nursing Guidelines 57-2

Combining Insulins

- Cleanse rubber stoppers of both vials of insulin.
- Instill an amount of air into the longer-acting insulin that is equal to the volume of insulin that will be withdrawn. Take care not to insert the needle into the insulin.

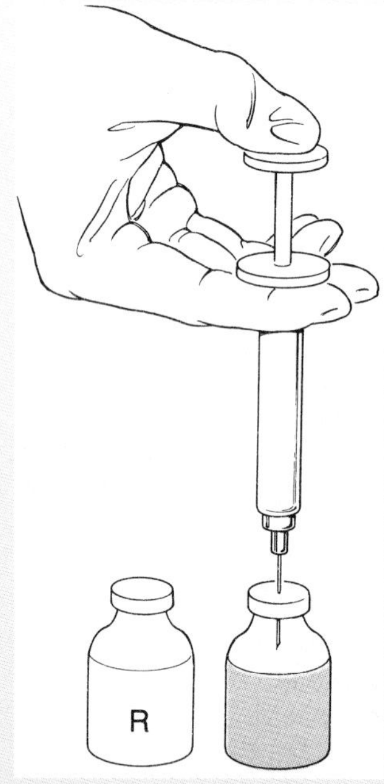

Instilling air into vial with additive insulin.

- Inject amount of air into short-acting insulin vial that is equal to amount of insulin to be withdrawn; invert vial and withdraw the prescribed amount of short-acting insulin.

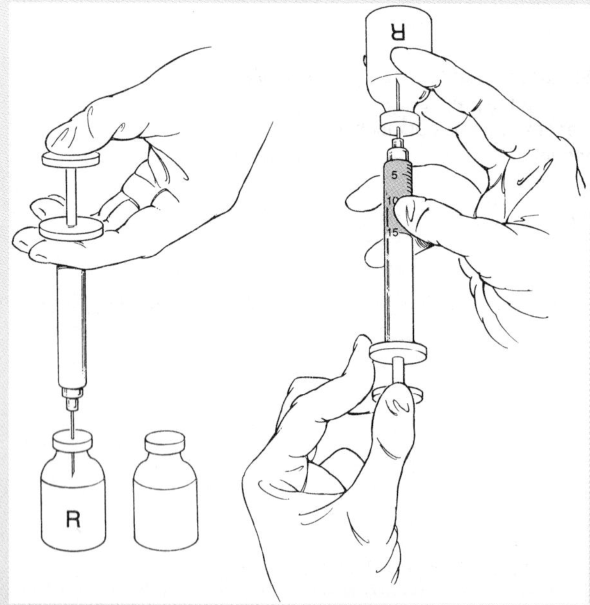

Instilling air then withdrawing from additive-free vial.

- Withdraw prescribed amount of insulin from longer-acting insulin.

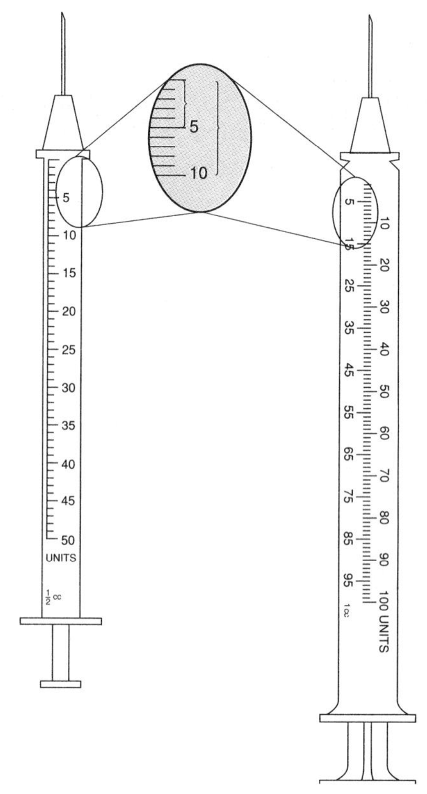

FIGURE 57-2. A Lo-Dose (50 U) insulin syringe (*left*) and a 100U insulin syringe (*right*).

- Vital signs, peripheral pulses, temperature of the extremities, inspection of the extremities for edema or changes in color
- Decreased visual acuity and visual changes such as blurred or double vision
- Muscle atrophy, weakness, or loss of sensation

Complications of Diabetes Mellitus

Some individuals, despite careful control of their disease, develop one or more serious complications over time. Some of these complications can be controlled when detected in the early stages.

Diabetic Ketoacidosis

Diabetic ketoacidosis (DKA), a type of metabolic acidosis, is an outcome of an acute insulin deficiency (Fig. 57–3).

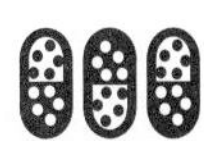

TABLE 57-2 **Oral Hypoglycemic Drugs**

Drug Category/Drug Action	Side Effects	Nursing Considerations
First-Generation Sulfonylureas		
acetohexamide (Dymelor) Stimulates insulin release in NIDDM, type II.	Anorexia, nausea, vomiting, hypoglycemia	Give before breakfast and before evening meal. Monitor serum and urine glucose levels. Avoid during pregnancy. Intermediate acting (12–24 hours)
chlorpropamide (Diabinese) As above	As above	As above Long acting (72 hours)
tolazamide (Tolinase) As above	As above	As above Intermediate acting (10–14 hours)
tolbutamide (Orinase) As above	As above	As above Short acting (6–12 hours)
Second-Generation Sulfonylureas		
gilmepride (Amaryl) Stimulates insulin release, more potent than first-generation sulfonylureas.	Increased risk of cardiovascular mortality, anorexia, nausea, vomiting, heartburn, diarrhea, hypoglycemia, allergic skin reactions	Give before breakfast. Monitor urine and serum glucose levels. Avoid during pregnancy. Client must avoid alcohol. Teach client: diet, exercise, signs and symptoms of hypoglycemia and hyperglycemia, avoidance of infection, do not discontinue medication.
glipzide (Glucotrol) As above	As above	As above Onset of action 1–1.5 hours Duration 10–16 hours.
glyburide (DiaBeta, Glynase Pres Tab, Micronase) As above	As above	As above Onset of action 2–4 hours Duration 24 hours
Alpha-Glucosidase Inhibitors		
acarbose (Precose) Delays digestion of carbohydrates, effects are additive to sulfonylureas in NIDDM, type II.	Abdominal pain, flatulence, diarrhea, hypoglycemia	Give t.i.d with first bite of each meal. Monitor urine and serum glucose levels. Inform client of gastrointestinal side effects.
miglitol (Glyset) As above	As above	As above
Biguanide Compound		
metformin (Glucophage) Increases production of insulin in NIDDM, type II.	Anorexia, nausea, heartburn, diarrhea, lactic acidosis, hypoglycemia, allergic skin reactions	Monitor urine and serum glucose levels. Avoid during pregnancy. Client to avoid use of alcohol. Instruct client not to discontinue medication.
Insulin-Enhancing Agent		
troglitazone (Rezulin) Increases effects of circulating insulin.	Causes few side effects, does not cause hypoglycemia	Give once daily in morning.

ETIOLOGY AND PATHOPHYSIOLOGY

Diabetic ketoacidosis can develop despite the client's compliance to the prescribed treatment regimen. These clients are often severe diabetics whose disease is hard to control (brittle diabetes). On occasion, a client admitted to the hospital in DKA is an undiagnosed diabetic. Other causes of this serious event are infection and noncompliance with the treatment regimen. (See the discussion of ketoacidosis under Pathophysiology of Diabetes Mellitus.)

ASSESSMENT FINDINGS

Signs and Symptoms

Early symptoms can be vague and become more definite and serious as increasing amounts of ketones

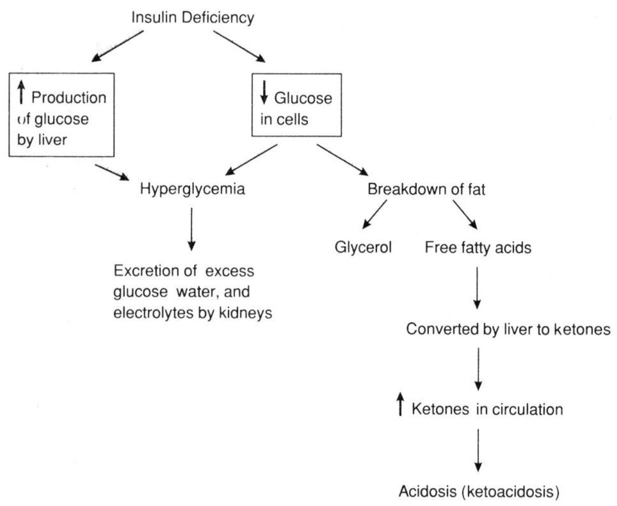

FIGURE 57-3. Development of ketoacidosis.

accumulate in the bloodstream. Weakness, thirst, anorexia, vomiting, drowsiness, and abdominal pain develop. The cheeks are flushed, and the skin and mouth are dry. The breath has an odor of acetone. Kussmaul respirations are often evident. The pulse is rapid and weak. The blood pressure is low. If the condition is severe, the client can become comatose. If the client is unconscious, restlessness is seen. If DKA is untreated, death will result.

Diagnostic Findings

Blood glucose levels are elevated. Urine contains glucose and ketones. The blood pH ranges from 6.8 to 7.3. The serum bicarbonate level is decreased.

MEDICAL MANAGEMENT

Treatment depends on the severity of DKA. The main goals of treatment are: (1) to reduce the elevated blood glucose, (2) to correct fluid and electrolyte imbalances, and (3) to clear the urine and blood of ketones. To accomplish these goals, insulin is given, usually intravenously (IV). Insulin reduces the production of ketones by making glucose available for oxidation by the tissues and by restoring the liver's supply of glycogen. Regular insulin added to an IV solution is given for its rapid effect. The amount of insulin and the rate of infusion depend on the blood glucose levels. Periodic monitoring of serum electrolytes and blood glucose levels is necessary. The urine is tested for glucose and ketones.

NURSING MANAGEMENT

If the client is comatose, keep the airway patent, and suction the oral cavity as necessary. Monitor IV infusions closely. Take vital signs at frequent intervals. Keep the physician informed of the client's response, or lack of response, to therapy. See the Nursing Management of the Client With Diabetes Mellitus for additional nursing care.

Hyperosmolar Hyperglycemic Nonketotic Syndrome

In contrast to DKA, this disorder does not involve ketosis and acidosis. Severe fluid and electrolyte imbalances occur.

ETIOLOGY AND PATHOPHYSIOLOGY

Hyperosmolar hyperglycemic nonketotic syndrome (HHNKS) often occurs as a result of a serious illness. Because of persistent hyperglycemia, fluid moves from the intracellular compartment to the extracellular compartment. Diuresis occurs with a subsequent loss of sodium and potassium. HHNKS is more common is older diabetic clients. It is also seen in the nondiabetic individual with severe burns, renal dialysis, or total parenteral nutrition.

ASSESSMENT FINDINGS

Signs and Symptoms

Hypotension, mental changes, extreme thirst, dehydration, tachycardia, and fever develop. Neurologic signs include paralysis, lethargy, coma, and seizures. Symptoms of hypokalemia and hyponatremia are usually present. Physical examination reveals dry mucous membranes and poor skin turgor.

Diagnostic Findings

Blood glucose levels are exceedingly high and serum potassium and sodium levels are low. The serum osmolarity level is increased.

MEDICAL MANAGEMENT

Treatment includes the administration of insulin and correction of fluid and electrolyte imbalances. A central venous pressure manometer is used to monitor fluid balance.

NURSING MANAGEMENT

The client is assessed for signs of electrolyte imbalances and dehydration. Closely monitor the client's response to treatment; hydration status with intake, output, and skin turgor; and electrolyte studies. Additional management depends on symptoms. See Nursing Management of the Client With Diabetes Mellitus.

Hypoglycemia

Hypoglycemia is always a potential adverse reaction to insulin and oral hypoglycemic agents.

ETIOLOGY AND PATHOPHYSIOLOGY

When there is too much insulin (**hyperinsulinism**) in the bloodstream relative to the amount of available glucose, **hypoglycemia** occurs. The blood glucose level falls below 60 mg/dL. If the condition is untreated, permanent brain damage could result or death can occur.

ASSESSMENT FINDINGS

Signs and Symptoms

The pattern of symptoms varies somewhat from person to person, depending on the degree of hypoglycemia, the individual reaction, and the type of insulin taken. Initial symptoms include weakness, headache, nausea, drowsiness, nervousness, hunger, tremors, malaise, and excessive perspiration. Some clients have characteristic personality or behavior changes. Confusion, aphasia, delirium, and vertigo can occur. If hypoglycemia is not corrected, symptoms can progress to difficulty with coordination. The client may complain of double vision. If left untreated, unconsciousness and seizures can develop.

Although symptoms vary, a pattern is exhibited whenever the client has had too much insulin and too little food. The sequence can be extremely rapid, with unconsciousness or seizures occurring before other symptoms are recognized.

When a diabetic person is found unconscious, DKA or hypoglycemia needs to be ruled out. These conditions are direct opposites: in ketoacidosis, the blood glucose level is high; in hypoglycemia, it is low. The nurse and client must be familiar with the symptoms of hyperinsulinism (hypoglycemia) and hypoinsulinism (hyperglycemia) so that these can be recognized in their early stages (Table 57–3).

Diagnostic Findings

Diagnosis is based on symptoms, client history, and blood glucose levels. The history is important in differentiating between DKA and hypoglycemia. If the client had insulin and has not eaten, it is most likely that hypoglycemia is present. If the client has eaten and has not taken or received insulin, it is most likely DKA is present. Recognition of hypoglycemia must be immediate; therefore, a bedside glucometer test, as well as sharp assessment skills, are important.

MEDICAL MANAGEMENT

The medical treatment for a hypoglycemic reaction is administration of a simple carbohydrate, such as 50% glucose IV. Glucagon is given to increase alertness and to stimulate the liver to release glycogen. Clients who are conscious can drink orange juice with added sugar or eat candy.

NURSING MANAGEMENT

If the client is conscious and able to swallow, give orange juice, candy, warm tea or coffee with sugar, a cola beverage, honey, or an oral dextrose solution. Administer dextrose IV if the client is unconscious. Whenever a client with diabetes mellitus is on a hospital unit, keep quick-acting carbohydrates available.

TABLE 57-3 **Characteristic of Hyperglycemia and Hypoglycemia**

Characteristic	Hyperglycemia	Hypoglycemia
Predisposing factors	Insufficient or omitted insulin Concurrent infection Dietary indiscretion Gastrointestinal upset	Excessive insulin Unusual exercise Too little food
Onset	Slow; hours to days	Sudden; minutes
Mental status	Drowsy	Disoriented; eventually becomes comatose
Skin	Flushed, dry, hot	Pale, moist, cool
Blood pressure	Low	Normal
Pulse	Rapid, weak	Normal or slow, bounding
Respiration	Air hunger	Normal to rapid, shallow
Hunger	Absent	Often present
Thirst	Present	Absent
Vomiting	Present	May be absent
Urine glucose	Present in large amounts	Absent in second voided specimen
Response to treatment	Slow	Rapid

(Adapted from Lilly Research Laboratories, Diabetes mellitus.)

In a severe reaction, the client needs repeated feedings before the symptoms abate.

Stay with the client until the pronounced symptoms are corrected. The regulation of glucose metabolism is difficult for about 24 hours. Observe the client at frequent intervals for further episodes of hypoglycemia.

The nurse can prevent hypoglycemia by:

- Ensuring that the meal is served within 15 to 30 minutes after very rapid-acting or rapid-acting insulin is administered
- Informing the physician immediately if nausea, vomiting, or diarrhea occur, or if the client refuses to eat
- Ensuring that the client eats the prescribed diet and between-meal snacks
- Administering the correct type and dose of insulin at the prescribed times

Additional nursing management of hypoglycemia depends on the symptoms presented. See Nursing Management of the Client With Diabetes Mellitus.

Vascular Disturbances and Neuropathies

Diabetic clients are especially at risk for developing circulatory problems and peripheral neuropathies.

ETIOLOGY AND PATHOPHYSIOLOGY

Neuropathy is the result of poor glucose control and decreased circulation to nerve tissue. The incidence of arteriosclerosis in diabetic persons is higher than that in nondiabetic individuals. It is believed that circulating insulin plays a role in arteriosclerosis. Many vascular changes seen in diabetic clients are not seen in nondiabetic clients. A consistent finding in diabetic clients is thickening of the walls of some capillaries, arterioles, and venules. Diabetic individuals also have a higher incidence of coronary artery disease and increased cholesterol levels.

Any part of the body can be affected by vascular disturbances and diabetic neuropathy. The retina of the eye (diabetic retinopathy), the kidneys (nephropathy), and the legs are particularly affected. The lower extremities are vulnerable to changes brought about by decreased blood supply to the tissues.

In diabetic clients, the retinal capillaries tend to develop multiple tiny aneurysms, accompanied by small points of hemorrhage and by exudates. The scarring from repeated hemorrhages eventually cause blindness. The incidence of cataracts is also higher in diabetic individuals.

ASSESSMENT FINDINGS

Signs and Symptoms

A wide variety of manifestations of the vascular disorders occur. Chest pain, kidney failure, numbness in the extremities, impotence, and visual changes are examples of indications of changes in the blood or nerve supply to a body organ or part.

Peripheral vascular changes are one of the more common complications associated with diabetes. Because of a decreased blood supply, the extremities are often pale and cool. Leg cramps can occur. Gangrene can develop if the blood supply to the extremities is markedly diminished. Uncontrolled infection leads to skin ulcers.

Diagnostic Findings

Fluorescein angiography identifies the degree of retinopathy. Angiography and Doppler ultrasonic flow studies indicate peripheral vascular disease. Renal function studies, such as renal angiography and intravenous pyelography, detect renal involvement. Additional studies depend on the type of complication.

MEDICAL AND SURGICAL MANAGEMENT

Uncontrolled gangrene of the extremities can result in amputation. The lower extremities are most often involved. Retinal hemorrhages are treated with laser therapy, which seals off the retinal blood vessel. Renal failure requires dialysis or renal transplantation.

Surgery is an enormous stress on the body. The diabetic client's glucose levels are likely to increase with a concomitant increased demand for insulin. The health care team closely monitors the client's blood glucose levels during the surgery and for several days postoperatively.

NURSING MANAGEMENT

Nursing management is geared toward the type of vascular disturbance and the signs and symptoms experienced by the client.

NURSING PROCESS
The Client With Diabetes Mellitus

Assessment

Obtain a complete health history to determine the type of diabetes, the hypoglycemic medication, type and dosage, current symptoms including polyphagia, polydipsia, and polyuria, sores that are not healing, visual changes, and changes in mental status.

Diagnosis and Planning

The nursing plan of care of the client with diabetes includes, but is not limited to, the following:

Nursing Diagnoses and Collaborative Problems	Nursing Interventions
PC: Hyperglycemia **Goal:** The client's blood glucose levels will be maintained within normal limits.	Monitor blood glucose levels and urine for glucose and ketones. Assess client for signs and symptoms of hyperglycemia. Give insulin on schedule at set time before meals.
PC: Hypoglycemia **Goal:** The client's incidence of hypoglycemia will be managed and minimized.	Recognize the signs and symptoms of hypoglycemia. Give concentrated sugar if hypoglycemia occurs.
Risk for Fluid Volume Deficit related to polyuria and dehydration **Goal:** The client will maintain proper fluid balance.	Monitor intake and output. Assess for signs of dehydration. Encourage oral fluid intake.
Alteration in Nutrition related to imbalance of insulin, food and physical activity **Goal:** Client will achieve and maintain nutritional balance.	Encourage client to eat prescribed meals and snacks, record same. Administer insulin as prescribed with alterations as necessary for delayed eating or diagnostic procedures. Ensure the correct timing of insulin injections and meals. Precise timing is most important with very rapid-acting and rapid-acting insulins. Reinforce the importance of compliance with the prescribed diet and insulin regime.
Knowledge Deficit related to diabetes self-management and information **Goal:** The client will verbalize and demonstrate knowledge of diabetes and self-management of illness.	Assess client's ability and willingness to learn about diabetes and self-management. Teach client about insulin and how to self-administer using proper technique. Allow client opportunities to practice administering insulin. Teach client how to monitor blood glucose, using a glucometer. Arrange for the dietitian to teach client about proper diet and exercise.
Risk for Injury related to neuropathy, retinopathy, and vascular insufficiency **Goal:** The client will be free from injury.	Examine skin daily for sores that do not heal. Assess client for changes in sensation, pain, or muscle weakness. Assess client for visual changes, blurring, or diminished sight. Assess peripheral circulation paying special attention to lower extremities. Reinforce need for daily foot care (Nursing Guidelines 57-3). Teach client and family to watch for signs of complications and seek medical help for same.
Anxiety related to diagnosis of diabetes and complications of diabetes **Goal:** The client will verbalize a decrease in anxiety regarding diagnosis of diabetes and possible complications.	Allow client time to talk about feelings regarding disease, administering insulin, possible complications. Provide verbal, written, and audiovisual information about disease and self-care. Provide information regarding support groups available to client. Develop and implement a teaching plan geared to client's level of understanding.
Risk for Impaired Skin Integrity related to susceptibility to infection and poor wound healing secondary to vascular disturbances **Goal:** The client's skin will remain intact with no evidence of breakdown or infection.	Assess client's skin daily for signs of breakdown, poor healing, change in color or temperature, pruritus, or infection. Keep skin dry to avoid irritation. Pay special attention to creases and folds of skin to prevent fungal infection. Rotate insulin injection sites (Fig. 57-4) to prevent insulin lipoatrophy (atrophy of subcutaneous fat) and lipohypertrophy, or swelling. Give each injection one-half to 1 inch away from the previous injection. Examine client's feet daily for blisters, cuts, or bruises; check between toes, and keep feet clean and dry.

Evaluation and Expected Outcomes

- Blood glucose levels are normal.
- The client is well-hydrated.
- The client eats the prescribed diet and verbalizes understanding of restrictions and allowances.
- The client demonstrates knowledge and skills to manage disease.
- No evidence of trauma.
- The client is comfortable with managing the disease.
- The client's skin remains intact.

Client and Family Teaching

Some hospitals use a diabetic teaching team comprised of nurses and dietitians who are responsible

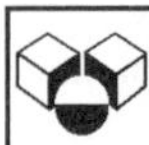

Nursing Guidelines 57-3

Teaching Clients Foot Care

Instruct diabetic clients and their families to:

- Inspect the feet daily for blisters, corns, calluses, long or ingrown nails, or any reddened areas; use a mirror if necessary to visualize all aspects of the foot.
- Wash the feet daily in warm (not hot) water.
- Dry the feet thoroughly, being careful to dry between the toes.
- Keep toenails short and cut straight across.
- Apply a moisturizer to feet daily.
- Do not use razor, abrasive, or commercial products to remove corns or calluses.
- Use lamb's wool between toes that overlap.
- Wear well fitting shoes that fit comfortably when first worn; do not wear rubber, plastic, or vinyl shoes that cause the feet to perspire. Consult physician about wearing sneakers.
- Never go barefoot.
- Visit a podiatrist regularly for foot care.
- Wash, dry, and cover any injuries with sterile gauze and call health care provider immediately for evaluation.
- Notify the physician about a blister, abrasion, or foot injury.

for teaching the diabetic client. When a diabetic teaching team is available, reinforce the material presented during teaching sessions with the client. If a diabetic teaching team is not available, help develop and institute a teaching plan using individualized or group sessions for teaching.

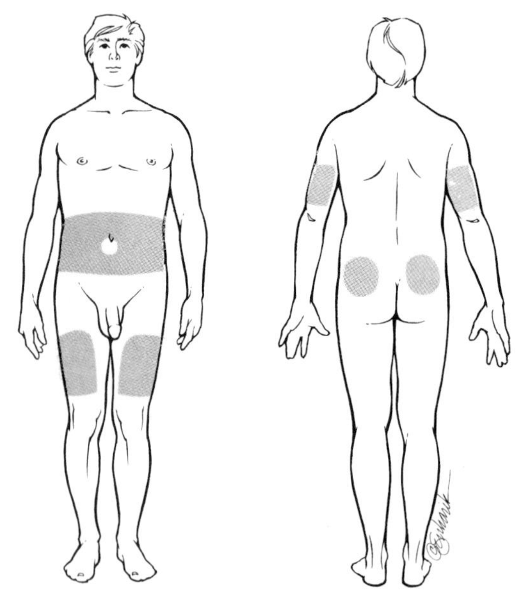

FIGURE 57-4. Sites for insulin injection.

The extent of the teaching program depends on whether the client has been diabetic for a period of time or is a new diabetic; even those who have had the disorder for years may have inaccurate ideas about their disorder and treatment regimen.

Before teaching begins, confer with the physician regarding:

- Type of diet to be followed
- Medication regimen (insulin or hypoglycemic agent)
- Materials to be used for insulin administration, such as needle and syringe, an insulin injection device, such as Novolin PenFill, an insulin pump, or an injection port
- Monitoring of blood glucose levels, self-testing devices (glucometer), and the suggested brand to be used
- Materials to be used for urine testing, frequency of urine testing
- Additional information to be presented, such as skin care, signs of DKA, HHNKS, and hypoglycemia

Whenever possible, include the family in a diabetic teaching program because one or more family members may assume some or all of the responsibility for the treatment regimen.

To allow the client and family member time to understand material, plan a teaching program that presents material in small steps. Begin teaching by explaining diabetes, what it is, why treatments are necessary, and the various methods of treatment. Use audiovisual materials to enhance learning. Emphasize that the treatment of diabetes is highly individualized; the treatment of one person cannot be compared with that of another.

If the client requires insulin, use a chart to explain how to rotate insulin injection sites. The American Diabetes Association in its 1998 *Clinical Practice Recommendations* now advocates rotating insulin injections within only one anatomic region to ensure consistent rates of absorption (Rausch, 1998). Abdominal injections are absorbed fastest and have the least variability in the rate of absorption. If the physician has recommended the use of a glucometer to monitor blood glucose levels, allow time for the client to use the glucometer and monitor his or her own blood glucose levels.

Develop a teaching plan to include the following general areas that apply to all individuals with diabetes:

- Signs and symptoms of hyperglycemia and hypoglycemia
- The importance of weight reduction, if necessary

- Methods of terminating hypoglycemia: orange juice, Prolycen (a commercial product containing glucose), 2 or 3 teaspoons of honey, hard candy, and glucose tablet
- Problems that require contacting the physician include skin infection, pain in the extremities, visual problems, change in color or temperature of the skin of the extremities, frequent episodes of hypoglycemia, prolonged nausea and vomiting, and illness (especially a severe illness).
- Follow the exercise regimen suggested by the physician. During exercise, carry some food or other physician-approved form of glucose if symptoms of hypoglycemia occur. This is especially important for individuals taking insulin or those subject to episodes of hypoglycemia while taking an oral hypoglycemic agent.
- Seek physician approval for using foods containing artificial sweeteners.
- When using foods containing an artificial sweetener, the fats, proteins, and carbohydrates in these foods still have to be counted within the prescribed diet.
- Read food labels because sugar, fat, and protein contents must be counted in the diet.
- Products labeled as "low calorie" and "dietetic" are not synonymous with "no sugar." These products may contain sugar.
- Drink adequate amounts of water, especially in warm weather, when exercising, and when perspiring.
- Take special care of the feet.
- Arrange yearly appointments with an ophthalmologist for a comprehensive eye examination.
- If ill, consult the physician regarding dosage adjustments for insulin or oral hypoglycemic agent.

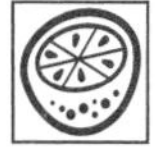

General Nutritional Considerations

Nutrition therapy is the cornerstone of treatment for all diabetics, regardless of the client's weight, blood glucose levels, or use of medication. There is no longer one diabetic diet that is appropriate for all individuals; meal plans are individualized according to the assessment data and treatment goals. Traditional assumptions that sugar causes a diabetic's blood glucose levels to rise too high and too quickly no longer hold true. Today, consistency in the total amount of carbohydrate consumed is considered a more important factor influencing blood glucose level than is the type of carbohydrate eaten.

Because most Type I diabetics are of normal weight, calorie allowances are calculated for weight maintenance. Weight loss is the focus of nutrition intervention for Type II diabetics. Clinical symptoms may immediately improve by a low calorie diet, and even a mild to moderate weight loss (eg, 10 to 20 pounds) can lower blood glucose levels and improve insulin action. Because gradual weight loss is easier to maintain than rapid loss, and because weight fluctuations can be detrimental to long-range goals, a 1/2 to 1 pound loss per week is recommended.

The most recent diet recommendations issued by the American Diabetes Association in 1994 state that saturated fat intake should provide less than 10% of total calories to reduce the risk of cardiovascular disease, and that polyunsaturated fat provide up to 10% of total calories. The percentage of total fat in the diet is determined by assessment data; 30% calories from total fat may be appropriate for normal-weight clients with normal lipid levels, whereas lower fat diets may promote weight loss in obese clients. Unless the client has nephropathy, protein recommendations for diabetics are the same as for the general public, approximately 10–20% of total calories. The remainder of calories in the diet are provided by carbohydrates; consistency in the total amount of carbohydrates consumed daily is emphasized.

The nutrition recommendations for diabetes are merely guidelines; the actual content of the diet depends on the client's assessment data and ability and willingness to change eating habits. The diet should be designed so that a minimal amount of adjustment is needed. Goals can best be met by providing information in stages, beginning with basic information and progressing to in-depth details, if the client is so motivated. Some clients never progress beyond basic information, which is acceptable as long as goals are met.

The use of exchange lists simplifies meal planning, eliminates the need for daily calculations, and offers variety. Clients are given a meal pattern that specifies how many servings from each food exchange are allowed at each meal and snack. Factors that influence which and how many exchanges are allowed at what times include the total calorie allowance, the type of medication used, and the client's preferences and lifestyle.

Elderly diabetics who are not treated with medication may simply be told to avoid "sugar."

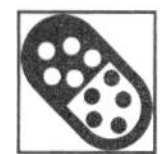

General Pharmacologic Considerations

The three important properties of insulin are onset, when the insulin first begins to act in the body; peak, the time when insulin is exerting maximum action; and, duration, the length of time the insulin remains in effect.

Oral hypoglycemic agents are usually used to treat those who can be controlled on 40 or fewer units of insulin per day.

The measurement of insulin must be accurate because clients may be sensitive to minute dose changes. The client is observed for signs of hypoglycemia at the expected onset and again at the peak of action.

Hospital policy may dictate the actions to be taken when a client taking insulin or an oral hypoglycemic agent experiences hypoglycemia. Most hospitals approve of the administration of oral glucose, fruit juice, Karo syrup and water, ginger ale, and others if the client can safely swallow. The unconscious or semiconscious client requires IV administration of 50% dextrose or glucagon.

The client receiving a hypoglycemic agent is observed for signs of hypoglycemia. The time when the reaction might occur is not predictable and could be from 30 to 60 minutes to several hours after the drug is ingested.

Make certain that the patient understands that insulin and the oral hypoglycemic drugs are used to control hyperglycemia, but do not cure diabetes.

The sulfonylureas may interact with other drugs such as the diuretics, antihypertensives, and thyroid preparations and, depending on the specific drug, may increase or decrease the effects of the sulfonylurea.

The oral hypoglycemic drugs may be used in conjunction with insulin therapy in some insulin-dependent diabetics; this reduces the insulin requirement and decreases the incidence of hypoglycemic reactions.

Use of alcohol with the oral hypoglycemic drugs may result in abdominal cramps, nausea, flushing, headache, and hypoglycemia.

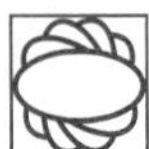

General Gerontologic Considerations

Diabetes mellitus is especially prevalent among the elderly. Many older diabetics can learn to care for themselves if they are given sufficient time, instruction, and help in overcoming disabilities of age.

Although it is useful for a family member to learn how to care for the older adult with diabetes, be certain to actively include the client unless it is evident that the client cannot safely assume responsibility for his or her own treatment.

Some older clients experience difficulty in administering their insulin because of problems such as decreased visual acuity or arthritis. The nurse must evaluate the client's ability to self-administer insulin before a teaching program is developed.

A variety of aids, such as a magnifier that fits over the syringe, are available for clients who experience difficulty in preparing insulin for injection.

The eating and sleeping habits of the elderly are often different from those of young or middle-aged persons and are taken into consideration when planning meals and selecting the proper type and dosage of insulin or oral hypoglycemic agent.

Good foot care is especially important in the older adult because other diseases common in the elderly, such as peripheral vascular disease and osteoarthritis, increase the risk of complications related to the feet. A podiatrist should be consulted at regular intervals.

Cognitive problems as seen in older adults with depression, dementia, or Alzheimer's disease can interfere with the management of diabetes.

Because older adults generally take several drugs, the nurse should review all drugs (both prescription and nonprescription) for any that may interact with the oral hypoglycemic drugs.

SUMMARY OF KEY CONCEPTS

- Diabetes mellitus is a metabolic disorder of the pancreas in which glucose intolerance results from varying degrees of insulin insufficiency. Insulin is secreted into the bloodstream by the beta cells of the islets of Langerhans in the pancreas. Diabetic persons produce less insulin than their metabolic processes require.
- The two major groups of diabetes mellitus are type I, insulin-dependent diabetes mellitus, and type II, non–insulin-dependent diabetes mellitus.
- The three classic symptoms of diabetes mellitus are polyuria, polydipsia, and polyphagia.
- Ketones are chemical intermediate products in the metabolism of fat. If ketones are produced faster than they can be oxidized in the tissues, they accumulate in tissues and body fluids.
- Four laboratory methods of diagnosing diabetes mellitus are the fasting blood glucose test, an oral glucose tolerance test, a glycosylated hemoglobin test, and a postprandial blood glucose test.
- Diabetic ketoacidosis is an acute insulin deficiency followed by a decrease in glucose in body cells and an increased production of glucose by the liver. An increase in production of glucose and the inability of the cells to use glucose for energy results in hyperglycemia. The need for an energy source results in a breakdown of fat into glycerol and free fatty acids, which are converted by the liver to ketones. This increase in ketones in the circulation leads to DKA.
- The main goals of treatment of DKA are: (1) to reduce the elevated blood glucose, (2) to correct fluid and electrolyte imbalances, and (3) to clear the urine and blood of ketone bodies.
- Hyperosmolar hyperglycemic nonketotic syndrome is manifested by hyperglycemia and hyperosmolarity and often occurs as a result of an event, such as an acute illness. Because of persistent hyperglycemia, fluid moves from the intracellular compartment to the extracellular compartment. Diuresis occurs, and there is a loss of sodium and potassium. Ketosis and acidosis do not occur as in DKA.
- Treatment of HHNKS includes the administration of insulin and correction of fluid and electrolyte imbalances.
- When there is too much insulin (hyperinsulinism) in the bloodstream in relation to the amount of available glucose, hypoglycemia occurs. The treatment for hypoglycemic reaction is the administration of a quick-acting carbohydrate.
- The complications of diabetes mellitus include diabetic ketoacidosis, HHNKS, hypoglycemia, and vascular disturbances and neuropathies.
- The treatment of diabetes mellitus involves diet, exercise, insulin or an oral hypoglycemic agent, and weight control.
- The nursing management of the client with diabetes mellitus includes maintaining normal blood glucose levels, minimizing the incidences of hypoglycemia, maintaining fluid and nutrition balance, teaching self-management, reducing the risk for injury, minimizing anxiety, and maintaining skin integrity.

CRITICAL THINKING EXERCISES

1. A client with diabetes mellitus has not followed the diet prescribed by his physician. What information would you include in a teaching plan for this client, and what approach would you take to reinforce the importance of diet in the management of diabetes?
2. Explain the differences between the signs and symptoms of hyperglycemia and hypoglycemia.
3. Describe the techniques for mixing two types of insulin.

Suggested Readings

Anderson, S. (1994). Care tips for managing patients with diabetes. *American Journal of Nursing, 94*(9), 36–38.

Drass, J. A. (1996). Caring for patients with non-insulin dependent diabetes mellitus. *Nursing, 26*(9), 48–49.

Drass, J. A. (1996). Caring for patients with insulin-dependent diabetes mellitus. *Nursing, 26*(8), 46.

Drass, J. A., & Peterson, A. (1996). Type II diabetes: Exploring treatment options. *American Journal of Nursing, 96*(11), 45–50.

Lupo, M. M. (1997). Focus on wound care: An overview of foot disease associated with diabetes mellitus. *MEDSURG Nursing, 6*(4), 225–229.

Rausch, M. (1998). Update on insulin administration. *American Journal of Nursing, 98*(7), 55.

Reising, D. L. (1995). Acute hyperglycemia: Putting a lid on the crisis. *Nursing, 25*(2), 33–40.

Wilson, B. A. (1994). What nurses don't know about managing NIDDM. *MEDSURG Nursing, 3*(2), 152–154.

Additional Resources

American Diabetes Association
1600 Duke Street
Alexandria, VA 22314
(800) DIABETES
http://www.diabetes.org

Lilly Education Center
Managing Your Diabetes
www.lilly.com/diabetes

The National Institute of Diabetes and Digestive Kidney Diseases
National Institutes of Health
http://www.niddk.nih.gov/

14

Sexual Structures and Reproductive Function

Chapter 58

Caring for Female Clients With Disorders of Pelvic Reproductive Structures

KEY TERMS

Amenorrhea
Carcinoma in situ
Cervicitis
Conization
Cystocele
Dilatation and curettage
Dysmenorrhea
Dyspareunia
Endometrial ablation
Endometriosis
Fertilization
Fibroid tumor
Fistula
Gynecologic examination
Hormone replacement therapy
Hysterectomy
Implantation
Libido
Menarche
Menopause
Menorrhagia
Menstrual diary
Menstruation
Metrorrhagia
Oligomenorrhea
Oophorectomy
Ova
Ovulation
Papanicolaou smear
Pelvic inflammatory disease
Premenstrual syndrome
Puberty
Rectocele
Salpingo-oophorectomy
Toxic shock syndrome
Vaginitis

LEARNING OBJECTIVES

On completion of this chapter, the reader will:

- Name three reproductive processes that are associated with sexual maturation.
- Explain the processes of ovulation, fertilization, and implantation, and menstruation.
- Name at least four conditions that deviate from normal patterns of menstruation.
- Describe how to keep a menstrual diary and discuss its purpose.
- Discuss therapeutic techniques for managing menstrual disorders.
- Discuss the nurse's role in caring for clients with menstrual disorders.
- List several physiologic consequences of menopause and the benefits of hormone replacement therapy.
- Name four infectious and inflammatory conditions that commonly occur in women and one cause for each.
- Describe the signs and symptoms that differentiate three types of vaginal infections.
- Discuss methods that may help prevent vaginal infections or their recurrence.
- Describe the technique for inserting vaginal medications.
- Name at least four aspects of nursing care for clients with pelvic inflammatory disease.
- Give at least two suggestions that can help women avoid toxic shock syndrome.
- List four structural abnormalities that can affect the female reproductive system and describe how they affect fertility or sexuality.
- Discuss methods the nurse can use to help a client decide on an appropriate treatment for endometriosis.
- List three problems experienced by women who develop vaginal fistulas and discuss how the nurse can help the client manage them.
- Give examples of information that is appropriate when teaching a client to use a pessary.
- Explain the term cancer *in situ* and how it applies to the prognosis of women with gynecologic malignancies.
- Identify which types of reproductive cancers are more common than others and methods for promoting an early diagnosis.

- Discuss the nursing diagnoses and potential complications that occur among clients who undergo a hysterectomy and the nursing interventions that are important to include in their care.
- Give two reasons that explain the high lethality associated with ovarian cancer.
- Name three possible causes of vaginal cancer.
- Discuss the nursing management of a client who has a radical vulvectomy for vulvar cancer.
- Give examples of discharge instructions that are appropriate to teach clients who have had a radical vulvectomy.

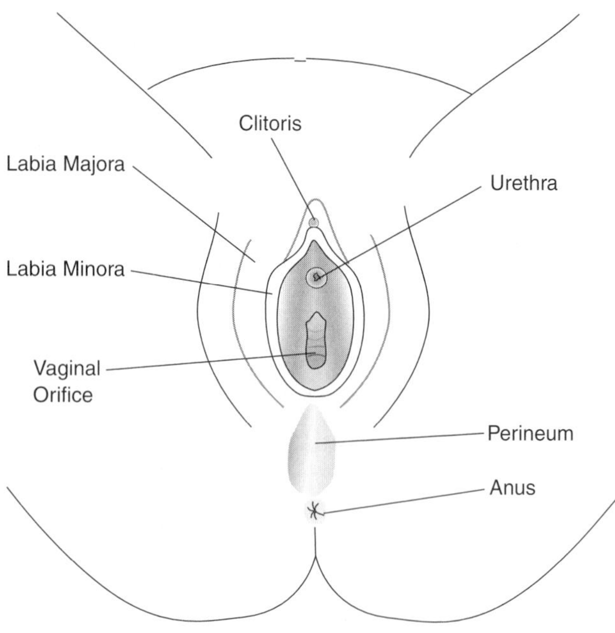

FIGURE 58-1. Female external genitalia.

Diseases or disorders of pelvic reproductive structures can have a profound effect on a female's health and sexuality. Some common problems for which adult women seek health care include disturbances in menstruation, infectious and inflammatory disorders, structural abnormalities, and benign and malignant tumors of the reproductive system.

Anatomy and Physiology

External and Internal Structures

The female reproductive system consists of external and internal structures. The external structures include the breasts (see Chap. 59) and female genitalia (Fig. 58–1). The genitalia are comprised of the vaginal orifice (opening), the *labia majora*, the *labia minora*, and the *clitoris*.

The internal structures of the female reproductive system (Fig. 58–2) consist of two *ovaries*, two *fallopian tubes*, the *uterus*, and the *vagina*. The two ovaries (female gonads) lie behind and slightly below the ends of the fallopian tubes. Each ovary contains thousands of **ova** (sing., *ovum*), all of which are present at birth. The ovaries secrete two hormones: *estrogen*, which is responsible for secondary sexual characteristics such as breast development and the preparation of the uterus for conception, and *progesterone* (discussed later).

After **puberty,** which is the onset of sexual maturation, and up to **menopause,** the termination of female fertility, three processes occur: ovulation, pregnancy, and menstruation.

Ovulation

The role of the internal reproductive structures is to release and transport ova and to support the implantation and nourishment of a fertilized ovum. The cyclical release of an ovum is known as **ovulation** and occurs under the influence of pituitary hormones.

Ovulation is initiated monthly by the anterior pituitary hormone known as follicle-stimulating hormone (FSH). It triggers the maturation of a follicle within one of the ovaries and an increased production of ovarian estrogen. A second pituitary hormone, luteinizing hormone (LH), causes the mature follicle to rupture, thereby releasing an ovum from the ovary (Fig. 58–3). After the ovum is released, movement of the cilia at the end of the fallopian tube combined with muscular contractions of the tube itself draw the ovum toward the uterus.

Meanwhile the *endometrium*, the inner lining of the uterus, becomes thick and vascular from the secretion of estrogen. The ruptured follicle is transformed into the *corpus luteum*, a small body filled with yellow fluid. The corpus luteum secretes *progesterone*, a hormone that sustains the lining of the uterus should fertilization occur.

Pregnancy

Pregnancy occurs as a result of fertilization and implantation. **Fertilization,** the union of an ovum and a *spermatozoon* (pl., *spermatozoa*), normally occurs in the fallopian tube. At the moment a sperm penetrates the ovum the number of chromosomes is complete, making it possible for an embryo to develop. The fertilized ovum, or *zygote*, then proceeds down the uterus

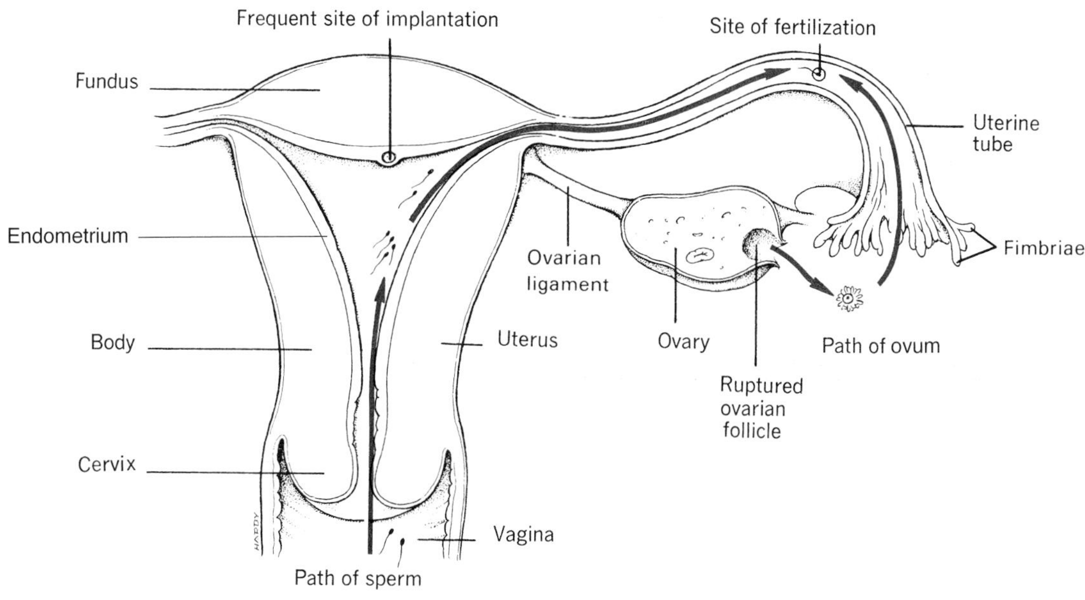

FIGURE 58-2. Schematic drawing of female reproductive organs, showing path of ovum from ovary into fallopian tube, path of spermatozoa, and the usual site of fertilization and implantation.

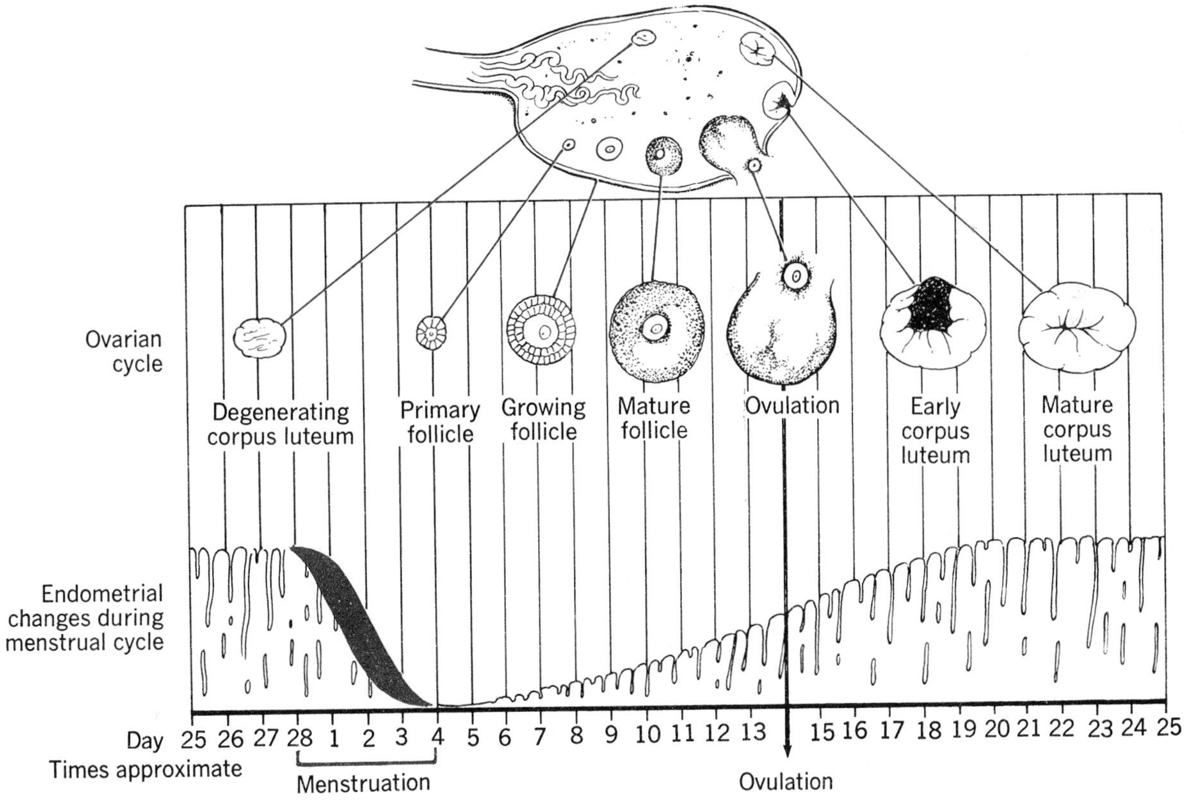

FIGURE 58-3. Normal menstrual cycle.

and attaches itself within the endometrium, a process referred to as **implantation.** Once fertilization and implantation occur, the pituitary production of FSH is inhibited so that ovulation is temporarily halted.

Menstruation

If the ovum is not fertilized, the production of progesterone by the corpus luteum begins to decrease until it changes from a yellow to a white spot on the ovary (*corpus albicans*). Without the high level of progesterone, the endometrium degenerates and is shed, a process referred to as **menstruation.** Menstruation begins about 2 weeks after ovulation. Menstrual flow usually lasts 4 to 5 days, with a normal loss of 30 to 60 mL of blood. Women who have a heavy *menses*, or menstrual flow, lose more blood. After menstruation, the endometrium becomes thicker and more vascular again in preparation for a possible pregnancy. Because of these hormone-dependent changes, the microscopic characteristics of the uterus are in a cyclical state of transition. Thus, it is important that each gynecologic specimen sent to the laboratory is marked with the date of the beginning of the client's last menstrual period (LMP).

Assessment

History

To ensure a thorough baseline history, obtain the following information:

- General health and family history
- Age of **menarche,** the first menstruation
- Date of client's LMP, description of the menstrual pattern and flow, other symptoms associated with menstruation
- Risks for sexually transmitted diseases (see Chapter 61)
- Pregnancy history: number of pregnancies, number of live births, number of stillborn births, type of fetal abnormalities
- Abortion history
- Contraceptive practices
- Age of menopause, symptoms associated with menopause, and use of estrogen replacement therapy (ERT)
- Date of last gynecologic and breast examination, including mammograms and Papanicolaou smears
- Prior treatments or surgery for a gynecologic disorder
- Drug, allergy, substance abuse, and smoking history
- Symptoms of present disorder, such as painful intercourse or characteristics of vaginal discharge, and length of time present

Gynecologic Examination (Pelvic Examination)

A physician, clinical nurse specialist, physician's assistant, or nurse practitioner performs the **gynecologic examination,** an inspection and palpation of pelvic reproductive structures. Inspection of the external genitalia and adjacent structures occurs first, followed by the inspection of the vaginal wall and cervix using a bivalve speculum. Next, one or two fingers of a lubricated, gloved hand are placed into the vagina. By vaginal-abdominal palpation, the structures beyond the vaginal orifice are examined and the position, size, and contour of the uterus, ovaries, and other pelvic structures are assessed. At the end of the examination, a gloved finger is inserted into the rectum to palpate the posterior surface of the uterus.

In preparation for the test, the nurse obtains examination gloves, lubricant, several sizes of bivalve speculums, a light source, and materials for obtaining a Papanicolaou smear (see next discussion). The nurse is sensitive to the fact that many women dislike having gynecologic examinations because they anticipate discomfort, are embarrassed, and have anxiety over possible diagnoses. See Nursing Guidelines 58–1.

Diagnostic Tests

CYTOLOGIC TEST FOR CANCER (PAPANICOLAOU SMEAR)

A **Papanicolaou smear** (Pap smear) is an important cancer screening tool. It involves obtaining a sample of *exfoliated* cells (dead cells that are shed). The specimens, which are best obtained 2 weeks after the first day of the LMP, are removed by scraping and brushing tissue during the pelvic exam. The test is used mainly to detect early cancer of the cervix and secondarily to determine estrogen activity as it relates to menopause or endocrine abnormalities. See Box 58–1 for classification system.

The American Cancer Society recommends that all women at the age of 18 (or earlier if sexually active) have an initial Pap smear. Pap smears are then repeated yearly for 3 years, then every 3 years if the results for the three prior tests are normal. The nurse advises the client to avoid intercourse for 2 days and douching for 1 day before the test. When assisting with the exam, the nurse obtains the required materials, prepares the client, and labels and preserves the specimens (Clinical Procedure 58–1).

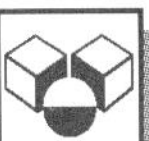

Nursing Guidelines 58-1

Assisting the Client Undergoing a Pelvic Examination

- Have the client void before the examination.
- Ask the client open-ended questions to promote verbalizing anxiety.
- Provide information on what to expect during the examination and when results from tissue samples will be available.
- Answer questions and use the opportunity to educate the client on health maintenance and health promotion activities.
- Have a blanket available.
- Assist the client to assume a lithotomy position immediately before the examination.
- Put pleasing posters on the walls or ceiling to help distract the client.
- Guide the client to breathe deeply during examination.

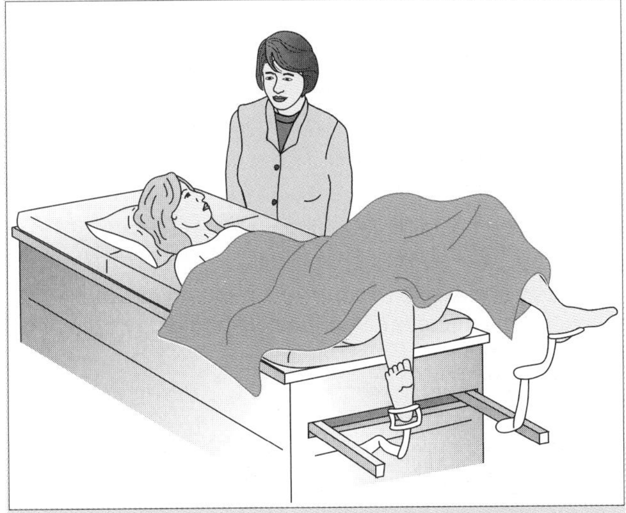

Client in lithotomy position, ready for pelvic examination.

CERVICAL BIOPSY

A cervical biopsy is performed when a Pap smear is positive or questionable. Tissue is obtained by punching out multiple small samples or by **conization,** removing a larger cone-shaped section of cervical tissue. Conization is an invasive surgical procedure that is performed on an outpatient basis; it is also used to treat early stage cervical cancer.

If the client is premenopausal, schedule the biopsy for 1 week after the end of a menstrual period when the cervix is least vascular. Tell the client that cramps and slight spotting may occur afterwards. Recommend a mild analgesic for discomfort. Advise the client to report severe pain or heavy bleeding.

BOX 58-1 Papanicolaou Classification System

Papanicolaou findings are described using the following numerical system:

Class 1	Absence of atypical or abnormal cells
Class 2	Atypical cells but no evidence of malignancy
Class 3	Suggestive of but not conclusive for malignancy
Class 4	Strongly suggestive of malignancy
Class 5	Conclusive for malignancy

ENDOMETRIAL SMEARS AND BIOPSY

Diagnosing cancer of the endometrium, the inner lining of the uterus, is accomplished by aspirating endometrial tissue specimens or performing an endometrial biopsy. Of the two, the endometrial biopsy is more accurate. A smear is obtained by inserting a flexible cannula through the cervix and into the uterine cavity. The cannula is attached to a syringe that is used to aspirate secretions. This procedure usually is performed without anesthesia.

To obtain a biopsy specimen, a dilating instrument called a uterine sound is inserted through the cervical opening. A tissue sample is then obtained with a scraping instrument called a curette or by aspiration. This procedure can be performed in the physician's office without anesthesia.

DILATATION AND CURETTAGE

Dilatation and curettage (D and C) is a surgical procedure in which the cervix is stretched open and the endometrium scraped (curettage). Dilatation and curettage is done to diagnose or treat a variety of gynecologic problems such as abnormal uterine bleeding and to remove fetal and placental tissue. Samples of endometrial scrapings are obtained when the client is under general or light intravenous (IV) anesthesia. A vaginal and cervical pack is usually left in place and a sterile perineal pad applied before the client leaves the operating room. See Nursing Guidelines 58–2 for examples of discharge instructions.

ENDOSCOPIC EXAMINATIONS

Endoscopic examinations are diagnostic procedures that use a lighted instrument inserted into the body for the purpose of visualizing structures not otherwise accessible. They are less invasive and more economical than using surgical techniques.

Culdoscopy, performed under local or general anesthesia, allows visualization of the uterus, broad

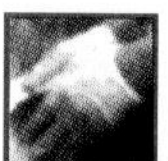

Clinical Procedure 58-1
Assisting with the Collection of a Papanicolaou Smear

PURPOSE

- To collect and appropriately preserve cells from the vagina, cervix, and endocervix (inside the cervix)

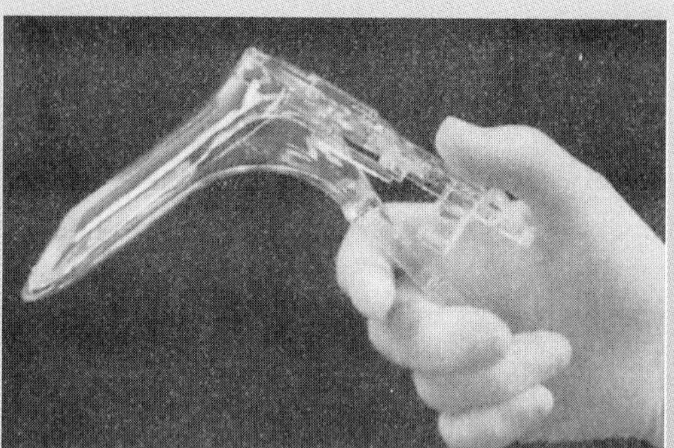

Vaginal speculum. (Courtesy of Ken Timby.)

EQUIPMENT

- Vaginal speculum
- Clean gloves
- Examination light
- Long, soft applicators and spatula

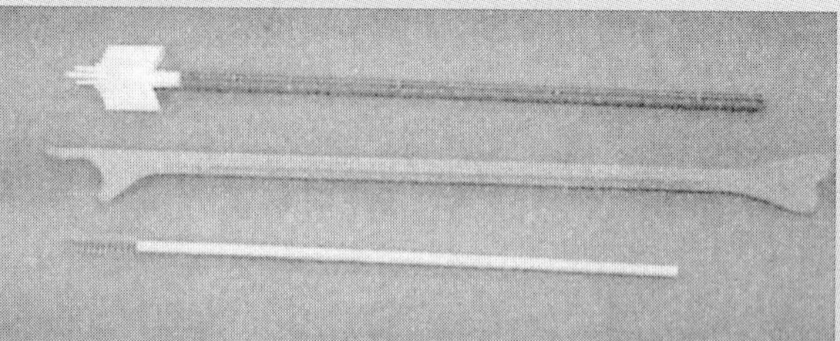

Applicators and spatula for obtaining cervical and vaginal specimens. (Courtesy of Ken Timby.)

- Three glass slides
- Chemical fixative
- Container for the slides

Nursing Action	Rationale
ASSESSMENT	
Determine the identity of the client on whom the examination will be performed.	Prevents errors
Find out if the client has ever had a pelvic examination before.	Provides a basis for teaching
Ask if the client is currently menstruating or had intercourse within the last 24 to 48 hours.	Interferes with microscopic examination of collected specimens; the examiner may wish to delay obtaining the specimens
Inquire if the client has douched in the last 24 hours.	Suggests a need to reschedule the Pap smear because an adequate sample of cells and secretions may not be available
Ask the client's age, the date of the last menstrual cycle, the number of pregnancies and live births, and a description of symptoms such as bleeding or drainage, or pain characteristics.	Provides data with which to compare cellular specimens with hormonal activity and to provide clues as to possible pathology and the need for additional tests
Determine if and what type of birth control is being used if the client is premenopausal.	Correlates the influence of prescribed hormones on cellular specimens
For oral contraceptives, identify the name of the drug and dosage.	
Ask menopausal clients if they are taking estrogen replacements, the brand name, and dosage.	Correlates the influence of prescribed hormones on cellular specimens
Observe for impaired strength or joint limitation.	Suggests the need to modify the examination position
PLANNING	
Explain the procedure and give the client an opportunity to ask questions.	Tends to reduce anxiety
Provide an examination gown and direct the client to empty her bladder.	Facilitates palpation of the uterus and ovaries
Mark one slide with an "E" for endocervical, another with "C" for cervical, and the last with a "V" for vaginal.	Identifies the location from which the specimens are taken
Arrange to be with the client during the examination especially if the examiner is a man.	Relieves anxiety and reduces the potential for claims of sexual impropriety

continued

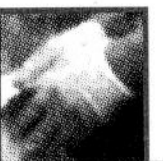

Clinical Procedure 58-1
Continued

Nursing Action	Rationale
IMPLEMENTATION	
Place the client in a lithotomy position or use an alternate position, such as Sims' or dorsal recumbent positions if the client is disabled.	Provides access to the vagina
Cover the client with a cotton or paper drape.	Maintains modesty
Introduce the examiner to the client if the two are strangers.	Tends to reduce anxiety by extending common courtesies
Fold back the drape just before the examination begins.	Exposes the genitalia
Direct the examination light from behind the examiner's shoulder toward the vaginal opening.	Illuminates the area facilitating inspection
Wet the speculum with warm water.	Provides comfort during insertion; lubricant interferes with cellular examination
Prepare the client to expect the momentary insertion of the speculum and explain that a loud click may be heard as it is locked in place.	Tends to reduce anxiety and aids in relaxation
Hand the examiner a soft-tipped applicator, the spatula, and another applicator in that order.	Facilitates collection of cells for the Pap smear
Hold the slide marked "E" so the examiner can roll the specimen across the slide; follow a similar pattern as the second and third samples are collected from the cervix and vagina.	Deposits intact cells according to their source

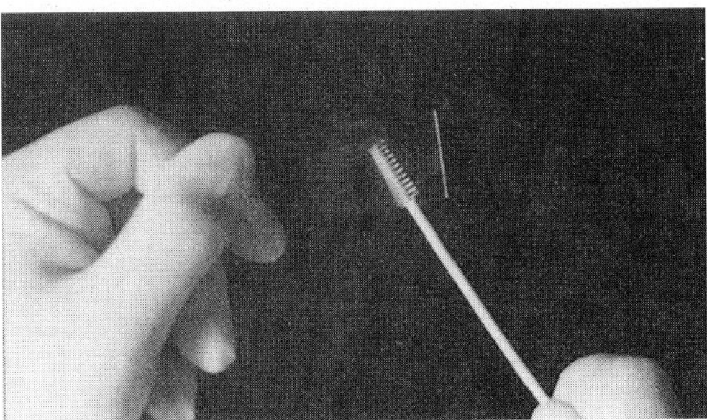

Transferring secretions to a glass slide. (Courtesy of Ken Timby.)

Nursing Action	Rationale
Position a lined receptacle so the examiner can dispose of each collection device and the speculum after they are used.	Controls the spread of microorganisms
Place each slide in a chemical fixative solution or spray it with a similar chemical.	Preserves the integrity of the specimens

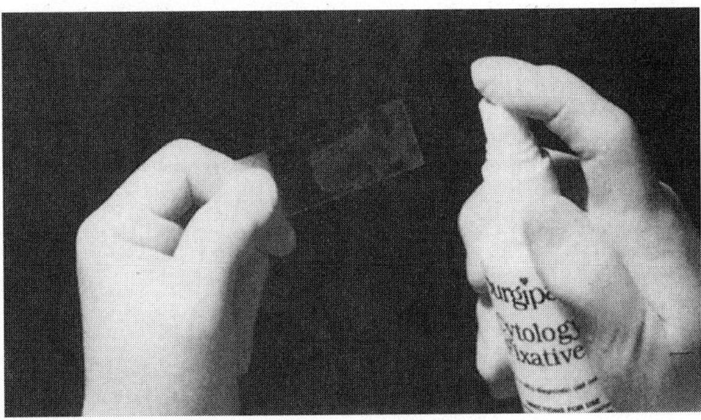

Preserving specimen. (Courtesy of Ken Timby.)

continued

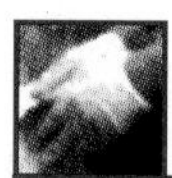

Clinical Procedure 58-1
Continued

Nursing Action	Rationale
Lower both feet simultaneously from the stirrups and assist the client to sit up.	Reduces strain on abdominal and back muscles
Assist the client from the room after she has dressed.	Maintains client safety
Label the specimens with the client's name, date, and any other required data, such as the date of the last menstrual period.	Ensures that the specimens are identified correctly
Remove gloves and wash hands.	Reduces the number of microorganisms on the hands
Arrange for the specimens to be transported to the laboratory.	Facilitates efficiency in obtaining test results

ligaments, and fallopian tubes by inserting an endoscope through an incision made in the posterior vaginal wall. Ectopic pregnancy and pelvic masses can be visualized. Afterwards, observe the client for signs of internal bleeding and symptoms of shock.

Laparoscopy is an examination of the interior of the abdomen using a special endoscope called a laparoscope. It is inserted through a small incision located one-half inch below the umbilicus. Two or three liters of carbon dioxide or nitrous oxide gas are introduced into the peritoneal cavity to separate the intestines from the pelvic organs and facilitate visualization. Laparoscopy is used to detect an ectopic pregnancy, perform a tubal ligation, obtain ovarian tissue for biopsy, and detect pelvic abnormalities. The nurse can tell the client undergoing laparoscopy that she will experience discomfort in the shoulder as a result of the instillation of gas. The incisional sites should be checked for bleeding afterwards and discomfort relieved with a prescribed analgesic.

A *colposcopy* is a procedure used to visualize the cervix and vagina. A speculum is inserted into the vagina, and the surface areas are examined with a light and magnifying lens (colposcope). A cervical biopsy and Pap smear can be taken at this time.

Nursing Guidelines 58-2

Client Education After Dilatation and Curettage

Following a D and C, clients are instructed to:

- Expect slight cramping and a dark, bloody discharge that may last a few days to several weeks.
- Report bright red bleeding, foul vaginal drainage, a fever, or pain that is intolerable despite mild analgesia.
- Change soiled perineal pads frequently and avoid tampons.
- Shower rather than take tub baths for 3 or 4 days.
- Refrain from strenuous exercises and heavy household cleaning for 4 to 5 days after which full activity may be resumed.
- Wipe from front to back following bowel elimination to avoid introducing microorganisms into the vaginal canal or urethra.
- Delay intercourse and douching for 1 to 2 weeks or until the physician indicates that they may be resumed.

HYSTEROSALPINGOGRAM

A *hysterosalpingogram* is a radiographic examination that visualizes the uterus and fallopian tubes. It is used to detect deviations such as adhesions and to determine fallopian tube patency, other tubal abnormalities, or congenital malformations of these structures. A cannula is inserted into the cervix and contrast media injected. Fluoroscopic or radiographic films are then taken. Bowel preparation is usually necessary to clear the intestine of gas and fecal material that interferes with proper visualization of the uterus and fallopian tubes.

ABDOMINAL ULTRASONOGRAPHY (SONOGRAM)

Ultrasonography aids in visualizing soft tissue by recording the reflection of sound waves. An abdominal ultrasound detects pelvic abnormalities such as tumors and the size and location of fetal and placental tissue. Instruct the client to drink at least a quart of water 45 minutes to an hour before the test and not to void until after the test is completed. A full bladder facilitates the transmission of the ultrasound waves and elevates the bowel away from the other pelvic organs. Solid food may be restricted for 6 to 8 hours to avoid obscuring the image with gas and intestinal contents.

LABORATORY TESTS

Various laboratory tests, such as a complete blood cell count, hemoglobin, and serum electrolytes, are ordered to obtain a baseline of the client's health status. Culture and sensitivity tests are ordered if an infection is suspected. Ovarian hormone activity is evaluated by tests such as total urine estrogen and urine pregnanediol.

Disorders of Menstruation

Premenstrual Syndrome

Premenstrual syndrome (PMS), also known as *late luteal dysphoric disorder,* is a group of physical and emotional symptoms that occur in some women 7 to 10 days before menstruation. Its cause is unknown; however, it has been proposed that PMS is due to an estrogen excess or progesterone deficit or both, hypothalamic-pituitary dysregulation, or the effect of reproductive hormones on brain chemicals such as endorphins, melatonin and serotonin. Women experience a combination of symptoms including weight gain; headache; nervousness; irritability; personality changes; depression; abdominal bloating; pain or tenderness of the breasts; breast enlargement; craving for sweets; swelling of the ankles, feet, and hands; anxiety; or increased physical activity. Diagnosis is based on data from a **menstrual diary** (Fig. 58–4) in which the client has kept daily recordings of her symptoms for at least 2 months. The classic finding is that the client is symptom free during the period between the onset of menstruation and ovulation.

Treatment of PMS depends on the severity and type of symptoms experienced. Hormonal drug ther-

Diagnostic Diary A: Evaluation of PMS Symptoms

NAME ______________________

YEAR ______________________

Grading of Symptoms:
0—*No Symptoms* 2—*Moderate Symptoms*
1—*Mild Symptoms* 3—*Severe Symptoms (i.e., Disabling)*

DAY OF CYCLE	1	2	3	4	5	6	7	8	9	10	11	12	13	14	15	16	17	18	19	20	21	22	23	24	25	26	27	28	29	30	31
DATE																															
MENSES																															

PSYCHOLOGICAL SYMPTOMS

Depression																															
Anxiety																															
Irritability																															
Lethargy																															
Insomnia																															
Forgetfulness																															
Confusion																															

PHYSICAL SYMPTOMS

Swelling																															
Breast Tenderness																															
Abdominal bloating																															
Palpitations																															
Weight gain																															
Constipation																															
Headache																															
Rhinitis																															

PAIN SYMPTOMS (Usually NOT associated with PMS)

Menstrual cramps																															
Painful intercourse																															
Pelvic pain																															
Backache																															

Morning weight (lb)																															

FIGURE 58-4. Example of a diary kept by the patient for tracking premenstrual symptoms. (Chihal HJ. Premenstrual Syndrome: A Clinic Manual, 2nd ed. Dallas, Essential Medical Information Systems, 1990, pp 80–81.)

apy is aimed at manipulating the cyclic fluctuation in estrogen and progesterone. This is accomplished with oral contraceptives, progesterone therapy, synthetic androgens, or gonadatropin-releasing hormone (GnRH) analogues such as histrelin (Supprelin) and nafarelin (Synarel) for 6 months. In some instances, short-term therapy with tranquilizers or antidepressants are indicated. Nonnarcotic analgesics, such as mefenamic acid (Ponstel), ibuprofen (Motrin), and naproxen (Anaprox) are given for discomfort.

Encourage clients to make healthy lifestyle changes such as exercising, eating nutritiously, and managing stress more effectively to augment the medical treatment. Explain how to maintain an accurate menstrual diary. Help the client identify dietary sources of sodium so that she can restrict salt consumption during the second half of her menstrual cycle. Explain drug therapy using oral contraceptives and stress the importance of taking nonsteroidal anti-inflammatory drugs (NSAIDs) with food or after meals to avoid gastric distress. Tell the client who takes a GnRH analogues that because estrogen levels are pharmacologically suppressed, she may experience vaginal dryness that can make intercourse uncomfortable and a loss of bone density similar to osteoporosis (see nursing management of menopause for additional interventions).

Dysmenorrhea

Dysmenorrhea is painful menstruation and may be primary or secondary. *Primary dysmenorrhea* usually is idiopathic, and no abnormality is found. *Secondary dysmenorrhea* is a result of other disorders such as endometriosis, displacement of the uterus, or fibroid uterine tumors. Symptoms are lower abdominal pain and cramping, which may become more severe with fatigue, cold, and tension. Dysmenorrhea is treated with mild nonnarcotic analgesics and by treating the underlying cause if one is identified.

For symptomatic relief of pain and discomfort, suggest local applications of heat, such as a warm shower, heating pad, or water bottle. Demonstrate how to assume a knee–chest position (Fig. 58-5) to relieve discomfort caused by *retroversion* (backward tilt) of the uterus. Encourage the client to obtain adequate rest, nutrition, and relief from stress to facilitate coping with periodic discomfort.

Amenorrhea and Oligomenorrhea

Amenorrhea is the absence of menstrual flow. *Primary amenorrhea* is the term used when a female of reproductive age has never menstruated. If menstruation stops after menstrual cycles have occurred, it is called *secondary amenorrhea*. Secondary amenorrhea occurs normally during pregnancy, after menopause, sometimes throughout lactation, and when the ovaries or uterus are surgically removed. **Oligomenorrhea** is infrequent menses. It is perfectly normal for adolescent girls to experience oligomenorrhea for a year or more before they establish regular menses.

Oligomenorrhea and amenorrhea usually are caused by endocrine imbalances resulting from pituitary disorders or hypothyroidism, the stress response, or severely lean body mass. Female athletes, women with anorexia nervosa, or women with debilitating diseases can have such low levels of estrogen that menstruation ceases. Treatment focuses on correction of the underlying cause. Clients with eating disorders (see Chap. 15) require referral to appropriate psychiatric specialists.

Menorrhagia

Menorrhagia is excessive bleeding at the time of normal menstruation. It may be quantified as menstrual flow that lasts more than 7 days, that requires the use of an additional two pads per day, or that extends 3 or more days longer than usual. It can be caused by endocrine, coagulation, or systemic disorders.

Drug Therapy

Symptomatic relief is accomplished with NSAIDs, progestins, and oral contraceptives with combinations of estrogen and progestin. NSAIDs reduce *prostaglandins*, biologic chemicals that exist in endometrial tissue where they exert a stimulating effect on the uterus. *Progestins*, natural and synthetic forms of progesterone, transform the proliferative endometrium into a secretory endometrium that simulates a pregnant state. When combination oral contraceptives are administered, they produce a "pill period," which is characterized by light menstrual bleeding.

Surgical Therapy

A D and C is performed for symptomatic relief; however, effectiveness sometimes lasts only 1 to 2 months. **Endometrial ablation** (detachment of the lining of the uterus) by photodynamic therapy or uterine balloon therapy is a potential nonsurgical alternative. When *photodynamic therapy* is used, a photosensitive substance is applied to endometrial tissue after which a laser probe is inserted through the cervix. The absorption of laser light by the tissue causes the endometrium to slough, in contrast to being removed with a surgical curette. *Uterine balloon therapy* produces the same effect by introducing a heated balloon into the uterus for 8 minutes. Both of these procedures are gaining popularity because they are cost effective. The post-treatment course is similar to that following a D and C. Refer to Nursing Guidelines 58–2 for client education.

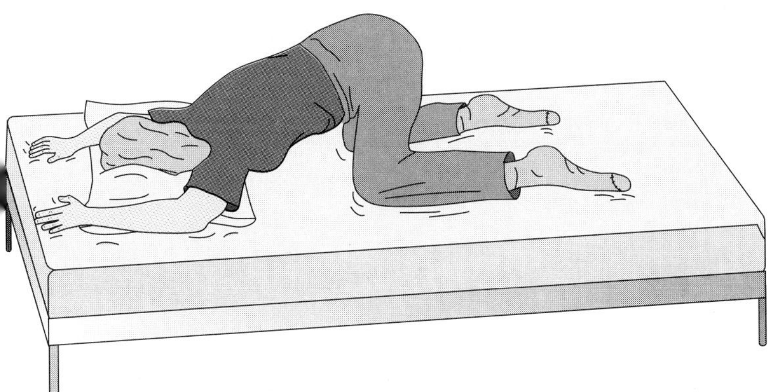

FIGURE 58-5. Knee–chest position.

Metrorrhagia

Metrorrhagia is vaginal bleeding at a time other than a menstrual period. The amount of blood is not important; the fact that it occurs unexpectedly *is* significant. Irregular bleeding is often due to an erratic stimulation of or response to pituitary or ovarian hormones, especially in adolescent and perimenopausal females. Some women spot for a day or two midway between menstrual periods. This functional bleeding is attributed to ovulation and is not considered abnormal. However, other causes for atypical bleeding include uterine malignancies, cervical irritation, or breakthrough bleeding that occurs with ERT or low-dose oral contraceptives. Intermenstrual or postcoital (after intercourse) bleeding needs to be evaluated promptly. Treatment depends on the underlying cause.

Advise the client with unexplained bleeding to see a physician. For metrorrhagia or any menstrual disorder, the role of the nurse is the same: gather appropriate information; assist with gynecologic examinations; offer suggestions for relieving discomfort; instruct clients about their drug therapy; prepare clients for surgical interventions; care for them during recovery; and provide specific health-teaching instructions.

Menopause

Menopause (change of life) is the cessation of the menstrual cycle. The *climacteric* or *perimenopausal period* refers to the time during which ovarian activity gradually ceases; the *postmenopausal period* begins 1 year after menstruation ceases. Menopause normally occurs between the ages of 45 and 55. Surgical menopause, which results when the ovaries are removed, occurs at any age.

Menopause is a natural physiologic process. The changes in hormone levels that accompany menopause cause a variety of reproductive and systemic effects. Some women have symptoms so mild and transitory that they go noticed; other women experience severe symptoms. Some women seek health care to reduce the risk for osteoporosis and cardiovascular disease that occur when estrogen production decreases.

ETIOLOGY AND PHYSIOLOGY

Menopause occurs when ovarian function diminishes. Levels of estrogen and progesterone are reduced, ovulation gradually ceases, menstruation becomes irregular until it stops, and natural reproductive capacity ends. As the levels of estrogen and progesterone drop, the hypothalamus attempts to raise them by releasing GnRH which stimulates the anterior pituitary gland to release FSH and LH. The surge of hypothalamic-pituitary stimulation is thought to be responsible for altered temperature, sleep, and mood-regulating mechanisms. Estrogen deficiency causes thinning of the vaginal walls, breast and uterine atrophy, and loss of bone density. The risks for heart disease and stroke increase with estrogen reduction. Depression, should it occur, is felt to be related more to an individual's perception of the social or psychological implications of menopause rather than biologic factors.

ASSESSMENT FINDINGS

Signs and Symptoms

Changing menstrual patterns including irregular periods and scanty or sometimes unusually copious menstrual flow signal the onset of menopause. Vasomotor disturbances such as hot flashes and sweats, sleep disturbance, irritability or depression, vaginal dryness, diminished **libido** (interest or desire for sex), or **dyspareunia** (discomfort during intercourse) are not uncommon and are often the symptoms for which women seek treatment.

Diagnostic Findings

A cytologic examination of vaginal and cervical smears (Pap smear) shows a decrease in estrogen production.

MEDICAL MANAGEMENT

The decision to administer **hormone replacement therapy** (HRT), or estrogen combined with progestin, is made for each client on an individual basis. If HRT is indicated, it is prescribed in the lowest appropriate dose. It is believed that estrogen in small doses can help prevent osteoporosis and reduce the atherosclerotic process. The slight risk of endometrial or breast cancer is outweighed by the seriousness of future myocardial infarction, stroke, hip fracture, and kyphosis.

It may be necessary to treat some of the symptoms associated with menopause. Vaginal itching and drying is prevented or reduced by drugs such as an estrogen or cortisone cream or ointment. Low-dose androgens are added to the hormone replacement regimen to restore an interest in sexual activity. Antidepressants or minor tranquilizers are prescribed for women experiencing emotional problems.

NURSING MANAGEMENT

The nurse collects a data base that includes a menstrual, reproductive, and sexual history and prepares and supports the client during physical and diagnostic examinations. Health teaching addresses topics such as normal developmental changes during middle adulthood (see Chap. 7), coping strategies, health promotion techniques, methods to achieve symptomatic relief, and treatment-related information.

Client Teaching

Because normal and abnormal structural changes are easily confused, the nurse recommends regular gynecologic and breast examinations during and after menopause. The nurse also gives the following suggestions:

- Use bland skin creams or lotions to reduce skin dryness.
- Develop a planned exercise program to prevent weight gain and loss of calcium from the bones.
- Increase calcium intake by eating calcium-rich foods or take a supplement.
- Take HRT by the oral, transdermal, or vaginal route, as prescribed.
- Discuss breakthrough bleeding or menses that may occur with HRT with the physician. The dose or a different combination of hormones may eliminate this effect.
- Cultivate new interests and hobbies or resume those that have been abandoned because of other responsibilities.

Infectious and Inflammatory Disorders of the Female Reproductive System

Vaginitis

Vaginitis is a condition in which the vagina is inflamed.

ETIOLOGY AND PATHOPHYSIOLOGY

Vaginal inflammation is caused by chemical or mechanical irritants such as feminine hygiene products, allergic reactions, age-related tissue changes (atrophic vaginitis with menopause), and the most common etiology, infections. The pathogenic microorganisms frequently associated with vaginitis are the bacteria *Gardnerella vaginalis*, the protozoan *Trichomonas vaginalis*, and the yeast (fungus) *Candida albicans* (also see Chap. 61).

Although the vagina is self-protected by mucus-secreting cells and an acidic environment (pH of 3.5–4.5), the tissue may still become disrupted. Some situations predispose to vaginitis because they alter one or the other protective mechanism. For example, antibiotics or frequent douching eliminate the bacilli that promote an acidic vaginal environment. Decreased estrogen at menopause reduces the thick, moist consistency of vaginal tissue. Pregnant women, those with unregulated diabetics, and those who take oral contraceptives containing estrogen have an excess of glycogen in vaginal mucus, which supports the growth of microorganisms.

ASSESSMENT FINDINGS

Signs and Symptoms

An abnormal vaginal discharge is the primary symptom of vaginal infection, and the characteristics of the discharge are often indicative of the infecting organism (Table 58–1). The discharge is often accompanied by itching, burning, redness and swelling of surrounding tissues.

Diagnostic Findings

Diagnosis is confirmed by visual and microscopic examination of secretions.

MEDICAL MANAGEMENT

Infectious vaginitis is remedied by using drugs to which the microorganism is particularly sensitive. They include antifungal, antiprotozoal, and antibiotic

TABLE 58-1. **Characteristics of Vaginal Infections**

Microorganism	Color of Discharge	Consistency	Odor	Other Symptoms
Candida albicans	Curdy white	Thick	Strong	Burning with urination
Trichomonas vaginalis	Yellow-white	Foamy	Foul	Severe itching
Gardnerella vaginalis	Gray-white	Watery	Fishy	More discharge after intercourse

agents (Table 58–2). In some cases, the sexual partner is also infected and the vaginitis recurs if both are not treated simultaneously.

Atrophic vaginitis is relieved with estrogen replacement administered as a topical cream. If the client has diabetes mellitus, regulating blood sugar is an important aspect of treatment.

NURSING MANAGEMENT

The nurse informs the client not to douche before the physical examination because washing away the secretions removes the characteristics of the vaginal discharge and interferes with obtaining an adequate diagnostic smear.

Client Teaching

After diagnosis, the nurse may insert the first dose of vaginal medication while teaching the client how to repeat the technique (Clinical Procedure 58–2). Nonprescription drugs for the treatment of yeast infections are available. The nurse informs clients that although these drugs are usually effective, the initial diagnosis of vaginitis is best made by a physician. The nurse emphasizes the importance of completing the course of therapy.

The nurse also informs the client that routine douching when asymptomatic should be avoided, but to combat vaginitis, the client may douche once or twice a day for 1 week with a solution of 1 tablespoon of white vinegar to 1 pint of water (Reeder,

TABLE 58-2. **Drug Therapy for Vaginitis**

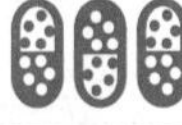

Drug Category/Example	Side Effects	Nursing Considerations/Client Education
Antiprotozoal		
metronidazole (Flagyl) Antiprotozoal-trichomonicidal mechanism of action unknown. Used in the treatment of trichomoniasis and *Gardnerella vaginalis.*	Headache, dizziness, ataxia, unpleasant metallic taste, anorexia, nausea, vomiting, diarrhea, darkening of the urine	Contraindicated in first trimester of pregnancy. Sexual partner may need to be treated. Instruct client to complete therapy. Take with food if gastrointestinal upset occurs. Avoid alcoholic beverages and alcohol-containing products—a severe reaction may occur. Expect that darkening of the urine may occur.
Antifungal		
clotrimazole (Gyne-Lotrimin), meconazole (Monistat), terconazole (Terazol), tioconazole (Vagistat). Disrupts fungal cell membrane causing cell death. Used in the treatment of candidiasis.	Cramping, nausea, vomiting, slight urinary frequency, erythema, stinging	Obtain culture before initiating therapy. Administer cream or vaginal tablets high into the vaginal canal, instruct client to remain recumbent for 10–15 min or administer at bedtime. Treatment continues through menses if necessary. Instruct partner to use a condom to prevent reinfection. Partner may have to be treated. Use a sanitary pad to prevent staining underwear.
Antibiotic		
sulfisoxazole (Gantrisin) Prevents cell replication by competing with the enzyme involved in the synthesis of intracellular proteins. Used in the treatment of vaginitis, chlamydia trachomatis infections.	Headache, nausea, vomiting abdominal pain, agranulocytosis photosensitivity, hematuria	Discontinue immediately if hypersensitivity reaction occurs. Administer or inform client to take medication on an empty stomach with a full glass of water. Complete drug therapy as ordered. Inform client of potential side effects. Tell client to report blood in urine, rash, fever, difficulty breathing, drowsiness, nausea, vomiting or diarrhea.

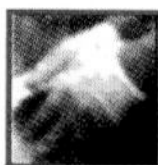

Clinical Procedure 58-2
Inserting Vaginal Medication

PURPOSE

- To implement medical treatment of vaginitis
- To demonstrate medication administration to a client

EQUIPMENT

- Bath blanket for draping
- Clean gloves
- Lubricant
- Vaginal applicator
- Medication
- Paper tissues
- Sanitary pad

Nursing Action	Rationale
ASSESSMENT	
Check the medical orders.	Collaborates nursing activities with medical treatment
Read and compare the label on the medication at least three times.	Prevents errors
Inspect the applicator for signs of rough or chipped surfaces.	Prevents injury
PLANNING	
Give the client an opportunity to void.	Promotes client comfort
Cover the client's pelvis and legs with a bath blanket.	Demonstrates respect for privacy
Help the client to assume a dorsal recumbent position.	Facilitates medication administration

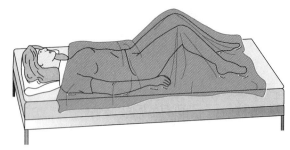

Client in dorsal recumbent position.

Nursing Action	Rationale
IMPLEMENTATION	
Wash your hands and don clean gloves.	Reduces the potential for transferring and acquiring infection
Load the applicator with medication; some are solid tablets, others are vaginal suppositories, or creams.	Facilitates depositing the medication deep within the vagina

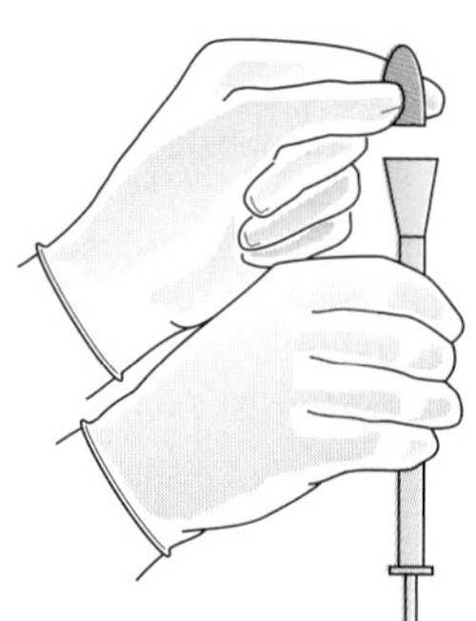

Loading medication into applicator.

continued

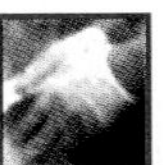

Clinical Procedure 58-2
Continued

Nursing Action	Rationale
Lubricate the tip with K-Y gel.	Reduces friction and eases comfort during insertion
Ask the client to let her knees fall outward.	Relaxes the perineum and facilitates visualization
Separate the labia and insert the applicator within the vagina 2 to 4 inches or the depth recommended by the drug company in the package insert.	Locates the medication well within the vagina

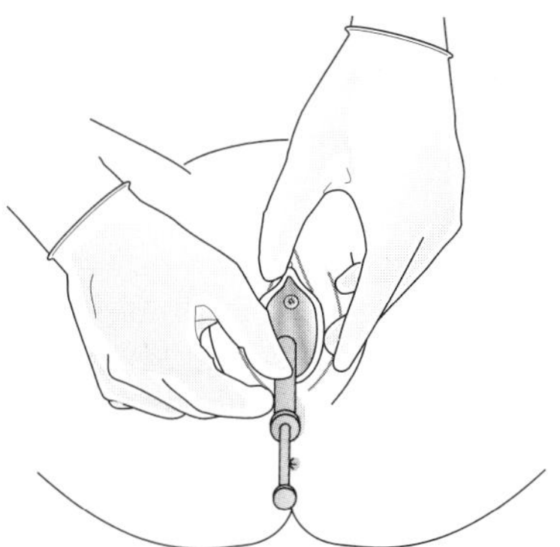

Inserting applicator.

Nursing Action	Rationale
Depress the plunger of the applicator	Deposits the medication into the client's vagina
Remove the applicator and place it on a clean tissue.	Supports principles of asepsis
Wipe the lubricant from the vulva and labia.	Demonstrates concern for the client's comfort
Apply a clean sanitary pad.	Absorbs vaginal discharge and excess medication
Suggest that the client remain recumbent for at least 10 to 30 minutes.	Prevents premature loss of the medication
Wash the applicator with soap and water if it is reusable; otherwise discard it in a lined container.	Removes debris and microorganisms from equipment
Remove gloves and wash hands.	Reduces transient microorganisms from the hands
Explain to the client that the best time for instilling vaginal medication is before retiring for sleep.	Facilitates retention of the medication

Martin, & Koniak, 1992). Taking acidophilus (lactobacillus) in capsule form or eating yogurt containing active cultures of lactobacillus can replenish normal vaginal microorganisms. Sitz baths are recommended to relieve itching, burning, and swelling of the vulva and perineum. Skin protectants containing zinc oxide promote healing. Additional suggestions for preventing a recurrence of vaginal infections are offered during health teaching (see Nursing Guidelines 58–3).

Cervicitis

Cervicitis is an inflammation of the cervix.

ETIOLOGY AND PATHOPHYSIOLOGY

Cervical inflammation is caused by infectious microorganisms, decreased estrogen levels during menopause, trauma during gynecologic procedures, or as a consequence of inserting tampons or vaginal medication applicators. Streptococcal, staphylococcal, gonorrheal, and chlamydial (see Chap. 61) infections are the most common etiology. The potential is greater during pregnancy and after childbirth when the microorganisms are able to enter cervical tissue through small lacerations. The infection can travel upward through uterine and tubal structures leading to pelvic inflammatory disease (PID) (see later discussion). Inflammation and subsequent formation of scar tissue increase the potential for ectopic preg-

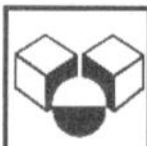

Nursing Guidelines 58-3

Preventing Vaginal Infections

Teach the client to do the following:

- Bathe daily with particular attention to perineal hygiene.
- Wipe from front to back after voiding and bowel movements.
- Avoid feminine hygiene products and douching more than once per week.
- Wear cotton undergarments and change them daily.
- Refrain from wearing layers of clothing, such as underwear plus pantyhose plus slacks, that increase warmth and interfere with air circulation about the genital area.
- Change from a wet swimsuit as soon as possible.
- Wash hands and devices that are inserted into the vagina, such as medication applicators, douche tips, and diaphragms, and store them in clean containers.
- Change sanitary pads before they become saturated; substitute a sanitary pad for a tampon at night.
- Use a condom or avoid intercourse if either client or her sex partner has genitourinary symptoms.

nancy or difficulty conceiving. Chronic cervicitis decreases the amount and quality of cervical mucus and alters the pH, both of which are underlying causes of infertility.

ASSESSMENT FINDINGS

Signs and Symptoms

Early cervicitis may fail to produce any symptoms. However, the client eventually spots or bleeds intermenstrually or develops a vaginal discharge. Dyspareunia (painful intercourse) or slight bleeding after sexual intercourse may occur. Severe cervicitis sometimes causes a sensation of weight in the pelvis.

Diagnostic Findings

Diagnosis is made by visual examination of the cervix. Microscopic examination of cervical smears identifies the causative microorganism.

MEDICAL MANAGEMENT

Douches and local or systemic antibiotics are the treatment of choice for acute cervicitis. Chronic cervicitis is treated with electrocautery. Frank bleeding requires cervical or vaginal packing or electric coagulation of the bleeding vessel. Healing often takes 6 to 8 weeks. Severe chronic cervicitis is treated by conization (removal of the diseased portion of the cervical mucosa). This outpatient procedure uses an instrument that simultaneously cuts tissue and coagulates the bleeding area. Dilatation is done if there is cervical stenosis. Successful treatment eliminates the inflammation, relieves the symptoms, and aids fertility.

NURSING MANAGEMENT

The nurse schedules treatment procedures 5 to 8 days after the end of the menstrual period to reduce the potential for bleeding. The nurse positions the client as for a gynecologic examination and explains that a momentary cramping sensation may be felt during the electrocautery procedure.

Client Teaching

After electrocautery, the nurse instructs the client to:

- Rest more than usual for 1 to 2 days.
- Avoid straining or heavy lifting.
- Rest in bed and report if slight bleeding does occur; frank bleeding requires a return visit to the physician.
- Expect a grayish green, malodorous discharge about 3 weeks after cautery.
- Anticipate slight bleeding about the 11th day.
- Return for a follow-up visit to the physician in 2 to 4 weeks.
- Abstain from sexual relations until tissues are healed.
- Plan for healing that may take 6 to 8 weeks.

Pelvic Inflammatory Disease

Pelvic inflammatory disease (PID) is an infection of the pelvic organs except the uterus. These include the ovaries (oophoritis), fallopian tubes (salpingitis), pelvic vascular system, and pelvic supporting structures.

ETIOLOGY AND PATHOPHYSIOLOGY

Microorganisms enter pelvic structures through the cervix from the vagina (Fig. 58–6). The cause is usually bacterial with gonococci and *Chlamydia trachomatis* being the most common pathogens. The infection travels up the uterus to the fallopian tubes (salpingitis) and ovaries (oophoritis) and can result in pelvic abscess or peritonitis as pus from the infected tubes leaks into the abdomen.

ASSESSMENT FINDINGS

Signs and Symptoms

Signs and symptoms include an infectious malodorous discharge, backache, severe or aching abdominal and pelvic pain, a bearing-down feeling, fever, dyspareunia, nausea and vomiting, menorrha-

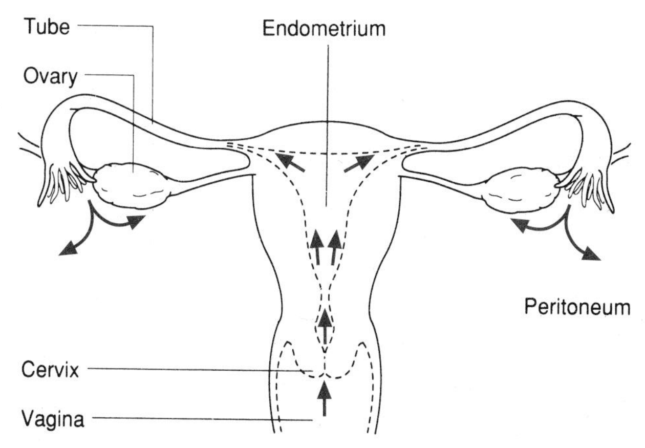

FIGURE 58-6. Pelvic inflammatory disease involves the ascending spread of microorganisms.

gia, and dysmenorrhea. Some women experience milder symptoms such as pain during a pelvic examination. Severe infection may cause urinary symptoms.

Diagnostic Findings

Diagnosis is based on symptoms as well as a gynecologic examination. A culture and sensitivity test of the vaginal discharge is obtained to identify the causative microorganism. Ultrasonography, magnetic resonance imaging (MRI), or computed tomography (CT) may disclose a pelvic abscess.

MEDICAL MANAGEMENT

Hospitalization with complete bed rest is often necessary. Parenteral or oral antibiotics are administered as soon as culture and sensitivity tests are obtained. IV fluids are ordered if the client is dehydrated and antipyretics are used if the temperature is elevated. A ruptured pelvic abscess requires emergency surgery.

NURSING PROCESS
The Client With Pelvic Inflammatory Disease

Assessment

A complete medical, drug, and allergy history is obtained, and the client is asked to describe all symptoms. A vaginal smear may be necessary. If the client is an outpatient, she is asked to not douche for 48 hours before being examined. If the client is admitted to the hospital and a vaginal smear is to be taken, she is asked if she has douched within the last 48 hours.

Diagnosis and Planning

The nurse's focus when managing the care of a client hospitalized with PID includes, but is not limited to the following:

Nursing Diagnoses and Collaborative Problems	Nursing Interventions
Potential Complication: Sepsis related to systemic spread of pathogenic microorganisms	Monitor vital signs and results of white blood cell counts.
	Maintain intravenous site and administer parental fluids and antibiotic therapy as scheduled.
Goal: The nurse will manage and minimize sepsis.	Keep the client in a semi-sitting position to facilitate pelvic drainage and minimize upward extension of infection.
Risk for Infection Transmission related to direct or indirect contact with infectious microorganisms	Provide the client with a private room with a toilet and sink.
Goal: No nosocomial infections will occur among other clients or staff that can be traced to the client with the primary infection.	Follow contact isolation precautions. Wrap and dispose of soiled perineal pads in a lined biohazard container. Bag soiled linen according to infection control policies of the institution.
	Leave a disposable stethoscope and paper thermometers in the room for assessments. Wash hands after removing gloves.
	Clean the cover on the blood pressure cuff with a disinfectant when the client is discharged.
	Instruct housekeeping personnel to damp mop the client's room after cleaning other clients' rooms and change the mop head when finished.
Pain related to inflamed tissue and pelvic congestion	Administer prescribed analgesic. Provide diversional activities to distract client from pain.
Goal: The client's comfort will be maintained within a level of tolerance.	Position for comfort and limit unnecessary activity.
Risk for Impaired Skin Integrity related to excoriating potential of vaginal drainage	Wash the perineum well with soap and water every 4 hours. Pat or blot the skin dry.
Goal: The vulvar and perineal tissue will be intact.	Change perineal pads frequently.

Evaluation and Expected Outcomes

- Vital signs and white blood cell count are normal.
- Infection control measures are effective.
- Pain or discomfort is relieved or eliminated.
- Genital tissue is free of redness and excoriation.

Client Teaching

After discharge from the hospital, the nurse tells the client to temporarily abstain from sexual intercourse to prevent extending the infection and infecting the partner. Additionally, the nurse explains that preventing subsequent episodes of PID can be accomplished by seeking medical attention when symptoms of infection, such as a feeling of pressure in the pelvic area, burning on urination, or vaginal drainage first appear. Early treatment prevents the infection from moving up the reproductive tract and resulting in complications such as peritonitis, abscess formation, and obstruction of the fallopian tubes. When early treatment of acute PID is delayed or inadequate, the infection may become chronic.

Toxic Shock Syndrome

Toxic shock syndrome (TSS), a type of septic shock (see Chap. 22), is a life-threatening systemic reaction to the toxin produced by several kinds of bacteria. Some causative microorganisms include *Staphylococcus aureus*, *Streptococcus pyogenes*, and *Clostridium sordellii*. TSS also occurs in men and in nonmenstruating women with soft tissue and postoperative infections.

ETIOLOGY AND PATHOPHYSIOLOGY

Toxic shock syndrome is associated with the use of super-absorbent tampons that are not changed frequently and internal contraceptive devices that remain in place longer than necessary.

The syndrome occurs when virulent bacteria reproduce suddenly and abundantly within the body and remain unchecked by normal physiologic defense mechanisms. The bacteria produce chemicals that cause blood vessels to dilate, which keeps the major portion of the blood volume in the periphery, reduces cardiac output, and causes severe hypotension (shock). The toxin also seems to inhibit the ability of affected cells to use oxygen (Porth, 1994).

ASSESSMENT FINDINGS

Signs and Symptoms

A sudden onset of high fever, chills, tenderness or pain in the muscles, nausea, vomiting, diarrhea, hypotension, hyperemia (increased redness and congestion) of vaginal mucous membranes, disorientation, and headache occurs. The skin is warm despite the fact that the client is in shock. A rash that first appears on the palms of the hands or the body a few hours after the infection later results in a shedding of the superficial layer of the skin (desquamation). The pulse is rapid and thready.

Diagnostic Findings

The infecting microorganism is found in cultures of specimens from the vagina, blood, urine, or other sites. The blood urea nitrogen (BUN), serum creatinine, and serum bilirubin levels are increased. The serum enzymes aspartate transaminase and alanine transaminase are elevated. The platelet count may be decreased.

MEDICAL MANAGEMENT

Circulation is supported with IV fluids while combating the infection with IV antibiotic therapy. Some drugs that are used include oxacillin (Prostaphlin), nafcillin (Nafcil), and methicillin (Staphcillin). Potent adrenergic drugs such as dopamine (Intropin) or dobutamine (Dobutrex) are given to counteract peripheral vasodilation and maintain renal perfusion. Oxygen is given to promote aerobic metabolism at the cellular level.

NURSING MANAGEMENT

Assess vital signs at frequent intervals. Administer the first dose of antibiotics immediately and as ordered thereafter. Apply pressure to venipuncture sites or injection sites to control bleeding and oozing if the platelet count is low. Carefully measure intake and output. Any sudden decrease in the urinary output or a urinary output of less than 500 mL/day is reported to the physician.

Client Teaching

Before discharge, teach the client preventive measures such as using perineal pads rather than tampons or changing tampons frequently if they are used. Tell clients who use a diaphragm, vaginal sponge, or cervical cap for birth control to remove the device within 24 hours after being used. Emphasize handwashing and keeping vaginal devices clean.

Structural Abnormalities

Endometriosis

Endometriosis is a condition in which tissue that histologically and functionally resembles that of the endometrium is found outside of the uterus. The atypical locations for endometrial tissue include the ovaries, the pelvic cavity, and occasionally the abdominal cavity.

ETIOLOGY AND PATHOPHYSIOLOGY

The cause of endometriosis is not clearly understood. It may be due to remnants of embryonic tissue that remain in the abdominal cavity. Another possible cause is retrograde menstruation, in which the fallopian tubes expel fragments of endometrial tissue that eventually become implanted outside the uterus.

The ectopic tissue responds to stimulation by estrogen and, perhaps, to progesterone. The tissue bleeds when the endometrium of the uterus is shed, but unfortunately, there is no outlet for the extrauterine bleeding. The trapped blood causes pain and ultimately adhesions in the peritoneal cavity. If the fallopian tubes are affected, they may become occluded and result in sterility. If endometrial tissue is enclosed in an ovary, a chocolate cyst (named because of its collection of dark blood) develops. Occasionally this cyst ruptures, spilling old blood and endometrial cells into the pelvic or abdominal cavity. The condition is naturally relieved when endometrial tissue atrophies after menopause or regresses during pregnancy.

ASSESSMENT FINDINGS

Signs and Symptoms

Severe dysmenorrhea and copious menstrual bleeding are typical symptoms. Dyspareunia and pain on defecation may be experienced. Rupture of a chocolate cyst results in severe abdominal pain that can mimic other abdominal pathologies such as appendicitis or bowel obstruction.

Diagnostic Findings

A pelvic examination reveals fixed, tender areas in the lower pelvis. Restricted mobility of the uterus due to adhesions may be noted. A laparoscopy confirms the diagnosis.

MEDICAL AND SURGICAL MANAGEMENT

Endometriosis is cured by natural or surgical menopause. However, many women are managed medically as long as possible to maintain the potential for having children later.

Estrogen–progestin contraceptives are administered to keep the client in a nonbleeding phase of her menstrual cycle for about 9 months. The goal is to control the ectopic tissue so that the client is symptom free for several years. The progestin norethindrone (Norlutin) and the synthetic androgen danazol (Danocrine) are effective in causing atrophy of endometrial tissue.

Without destroying the possibility for childbearing, surgery is performed to remove the cysts, as much of the ectopic tissue as possible, and lyse adhesions caused by bleeding. Laparoscopy is used to remove small areas of endometrial tissue as well as relieve adhesions. However, endometriosis that is widespread throughout the pelvic organs may necessitate a *panhysterectomy*, removal of the uterus, both fallopian tubes, and ovaries.

NURSING MANAGEMENT

Obtain a complete reproductive history. Have the client describe all symptoms, including the length of time symptoms have been present, type and location of pain, number of days of menses, amount of menstrual flow, and regularity or irregularity of the menstrual cycle.

Offer information on methods for relieving menstrual pain (see discussion of dysmenorrhea) and assist the client through the decision-making process as it applies to family planning and medical or surgical treatment of endometriosis before natural menopause. Some techniques for resolving decisional conflict include the following:

- Reinforce or clarify explanations of treatment options and the consequences of each option.
- Emphasize that the condition does not require an immediate decision and avoid giving advice or influencing the client's opinions.
- Suggest that the client include her significant other in discussion of options.
- Offer the option of seeking a second medical opinion.
- Suggest listing the pros and cons of each option to help determine which choice is most compatible with her values and goals.

Refer to the information on nursing management of clients undergoing a hysterectomy (later in this chapter) for those who choose that treatment option.

Client Teaching

The nurse emphasizes the importance of adhering to the prescribed medication schedule, if that is the client's choice, and the importance of regular gynecologic evaluations. The nurse instructs the client to seek care if pain increases, the menstrual flow is extremely heavy, or pregnancy occurs.

Vaginal Fistulas

A **fistula** is an unnatural opening between two structures. The opening may be between a ureter and the vagina (*ureterovaginal fistula*), between the bladder and the vagina (*vesicovaginal fistula*) (Fig. 58–7), or between the rectum and the vagina (*rectovaginal fistula*).

ETIOLOGY AND PATHOPHYSIOLOGY

Vaginal fistulas are caused by cancer, radiation treatment, surgical or obstetric injury, congenital anomaly, or a complication of ulcerative colitis. They result in the continuous drainage of urine or feces from the vagina. The vaginal wall and the external genitalia become excoriated and often infected. The client may not void through the urethra because urine does not accumulate in the bladder.

ASSESSMENT FINDINGS

Signs and Symptoms

The client reports that urine or stool leaks from the vagina.

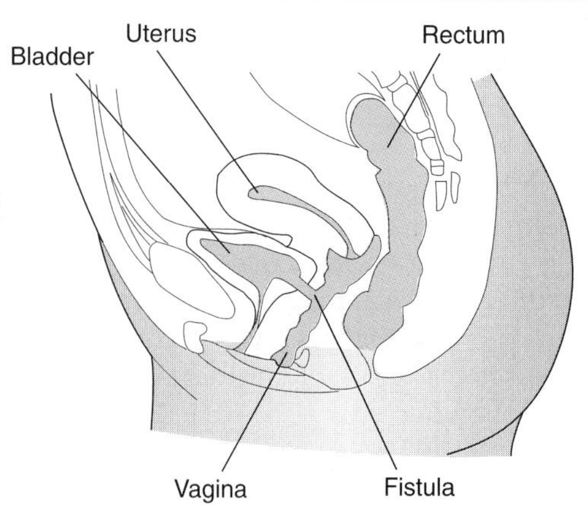

FIGURE 58-7. Vesicovaginal fistula with an opening between the bladder and the vagina.

Diagnostic Findings

Diagnosis is made by physical examination of the vaginal wall. A sterile probe is inserted if the fistula is easily seen or a dye (usually ethylene blue) is used to detect the exact location of the fistula. When a vesicovaginal fistula is suspected, the colored dye is injected into the bladder through a urethral catheter. A ureterovaginal fistula requires IV administration of the dye. An IV pyelogram (IVP) detects the flow of radiopaque dye through the lower genitourinary tract. A rectovaginal fistula is located by looking for fecal drainage on the posterior vaginal wall.

MEDICAL AND SURGICAL MANAGEMENT

Surgery is performed after inflammation and edema have disappeared. This may require months of treatment. Sometimes the tissues are in such poor condition that surgical repair is not possible. In the meantime, or if the fistula cannot be repaired, symptomatic treatment to reduce the risk for infection and manage skin excoriation is provided.

NURSING MANAGEMENT

The nurse's focus when managing the care of a client with a vaginal fistula includes implementing and teaching measures for maintaining skin integrity, helping the client maintain self-esteem, and offering suggestions for promoting sexuality if the client experiences sexual repercussions as a consequence of the condition.

The nursing care plan may include the following as well as others.

Nursing Diagnoses and Collaborative Problems	Nursing Interventions
Risk for Low Self-Esteem related to leaking of urine and stool, body and environmental odors **Goal:** The client's self-esteem will be maintained or restored as evidenced by a positive self-image and self-confidence.	Recommend wearing disposable, absorbent incontinence briefs or perineal pads with protective panties, changing and laundering clothing or bed linens as soon as possible. Let the client know that commercial deodorizers are available for use in the home. Recognize positive attributes when they are demonstrated. Affirm that the client is capable of managing odor and elimination problems. Provide genuine feedback on self-care and hygiene measures.
Risk for Impaired Skin Integrity related to continuous skin contact with urine or stool **Goal:** The client's skin will remain intact and integrity will be restored.	Advise daily bathing and frequent perineal hygiene with premoistened disposable wipes. Apply a skin protectant, such as collodion, over intact skin, or a skin barrier, such as zinc oxide or karaya paste to excoriated skin. Teach the client how to take sitz baths and administer cleansing douches. Explain that mixing a perfumed scent with a fecal or urine odor may intensify the odor as well as irritate the area. Inform the client that powders may cake and cause irritation or a superficial skin infection. A thin dusting of plain cornstarch may be used but must be thoroughly washed off when the area becomes soiled with feces or urine.
Altered Sexuality Patterns related to embarrassment over vaginal drainage **Goal:** The client will engage in satisfying sexual activity.	Recommend scheduling sexual intercourse to allow for hygienic preparation (eg, bathing, perineal care). Point out that attractive lingerie, soft music, and scented candles may overcome emotional barriers to sex. Suggest reclining on an absorbent, disposable pad. Propose substituting the shower, private swimming pool, or a hot tub as a place for intercourse. Encourage using alternate means of reaching orgasm other than vaginal intercourse such as manual or mechanical stimulation.

Surgical treatment ultimately may become necessary.

Preoperative and Postoperative Nursing Care

The nurse administers neomycin (Mycifradin), kanamycin (Kantrex), or another prescribed antibiotic to clean the bowel of microorganisms before repair of a rectovaginal fistula. A light, low-residue diet is provided to keep stool soft. The nurse gives an enema and a cleansing vaginal irrigation the morning of surgery, and inserts an indwelling catheter to keep the bladder empty.

After surgery, serosanguineous vaginal drainage on the perineal pad is normal. The absence of urine or feces from the vagina indicates healing of the repaired fistula. The nurse prevents pelvic pressure and stress on the suture line by monitoring catheter drainage closely. The pressure of a full bladder due to an obstructed catheter may break down the surgical repair and cause the fistula to reappear. Prevent and relieve pressure on perineal structures. Warm perineal irrigations and heat-lamp treatments are effective in promoting healing and lessening discomfort. Douches are used during the postoperative period to remove drainage, keep the suture area clean, and lessen chances of infection. About the third or fourth postoperative day, a rectal suppository or a stool softener may be ordered to prevent straining when having a bowel movement.

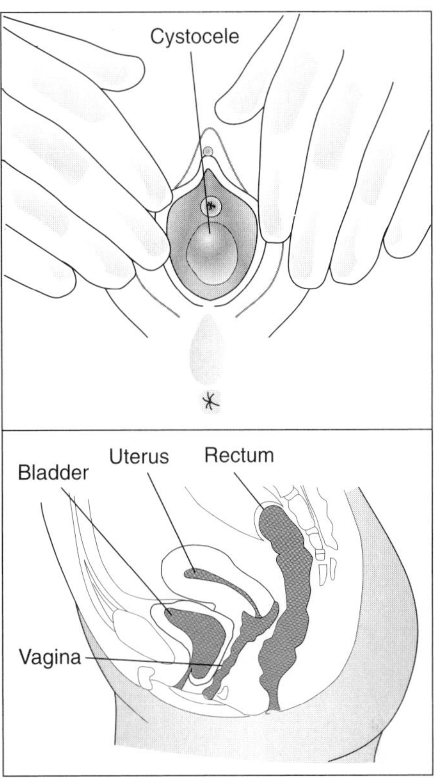

FIGURE 58-8. Cystocele. Relaxation of the anterior vaginal wall permits downward bulge of bladder on straining.

Pelvic Organ Prolapse

The term *prolapse* indicates a structural protrusion. Women experience any number of problems of this nature within the vagina. They include cystocele, rectocele, enterocele, and uterine prolapse.

A **cystocele** (Fig. 58–8) is the bulging of the bladder into the vagina. Herniation of the rectum into the vagina is called a **rectocele** (Fig. 58–9). An *enterocele* is a protrusion of the intestinal wall into the vagina. A *uterovaginal prolapse* is the downward displacement of the cervix anywhere from low in the vagina to outside the vagina.

ETIOLOGY AND PATHOPHYSIOLOGY

Pelvic organ prolapse is a consequence of congenital or acquired weaknesses in the muscles and fascia that are needed to support pelvic structures. Common causes include unrepaired postpartum tears; stretching during pregnancy and childbirth or with tumorous masses, ascites, and obesity; and postmenopausal atrophy. As the pelvic floor relaxes, the uterus, rectum, intestine, and bladder, alone or in combination, herniate downward. Structural displacement of the bladder and bowel leads to alterations in urinary and bowel elimination. Uterine tissue that protrudes below the vaginal

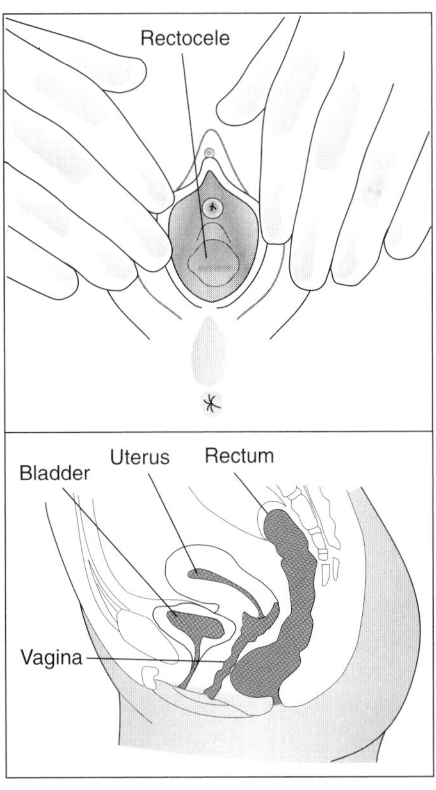

FIGURE 58-9. Rectocele. Relaxation of the posterior vaginal wall permits bulging of the rectum into the vagina on straining.

orifice is subject to irritation from clothing or rubbing against the thighs while walking; ulceration and infection frequently follow. Clients with severe uterovaginal prolapse are at greater risk for cervical cancer.

The functional consequences of pelvic organ prolapse can be disruptive. The client often experiences difficulty standing for long periods of time, walking with ease, lifting, and other activities that are hard to avoid.

ASSESSMENT FINDINGS

Signs and Symptoms

Clients with a cystocele may experience *stress incontinence*—a little urine seeps every time the woman coughs, sneezes, laughs, bears down, or strains. Cystitis (inflammation of the bladder), discussed in Chapter 64, results from the stagnation of urine in the bladder. Constipation is often a problem for those with a rectocele. In some instances, the client has to put her finger into the vagina and apply pressure to the posterior vaginal wall to reduce the herniation before being able to evacuate stool. Symptoms of a uterovaginal prolapse include backache, pelvic pain, fatigue, and a feeling that "something is dropping out," especially when lifting a heavy object, coughing, or standing for prolonged periods.

Diagnostic Findings

Diagnosis is confirmed during a pelvic examination and visual inspection of the vagina. Urinary tests are performed to reproduce stress incontinence or to determine the volume at which a client senses an urgent need to void. A Pap smear determines the client's estrogen status.

MEDICAL AND SURGICAL MANAGEMENT

A pessary, which is a firm doughnut-shaped or ring device, may be inserted in the upper vagina to reposition and give support to the uterus when surgery cannot be done or the client declines surgery. Kegel's exercises, also known as pelvic floor strengthening exercises (see Chap. 63), are recommended when there is stress incontinence.

Surgical repairs are done transvaginally. The surgical repair of a cystocele is called *anterior colporrhaphy*. Repair of a rectocele is called *posterior colporrhaphy*. Repair of the tears (usually old obstetric tears) of the perineal floor is called *perineorrhaphy*. A vaginal hysterectomy (see later discussion) is done to remove a completely prolapsed uterus.

NURSING MANAGEMENT

The nurse obtains a comprehensive medical history including the chief complaint and symptoms, inserts a catheter for diagnostic testing; assists with the pelvic examination and collection of specimens, and provides appropriate health teaching based on the physician's plan for treatment.

Client Teaching

The client is shown how to remove, clean, and reinsert a pessary. The following information is included:

- Remove the pessary and then thoroughly wash it with warm soapy water, followed by rinsing and drying.
- Inspect the pessary to be sure that all secretions have been removed.
- Apply a sterile lubricant to the pessary before it is reinserted. Discomfort may indicate that it has been inserted incorrectly, the pessary has moved, or that it is causing irritation. Contact the physician if these problems occur.
- See the physician immediately if a white or yellow discharge from the vagina develops. It may indicate an infection.
- Assume the knee–chest position for a few minutes once or twice a day to keep the pelvic organs and the pessary in good position.
- Avoid heavy lifting and straining when having a bowel movement.

Those not wishing to manage their own pessary are told to see their physician at least every 2 months or sooner if vaginal discharge or changes in voiding develop.

After an anterior colporrhaphy, some women have temporary difficulty voiding or emptying the bladder completely. For this reason, clients are discharged with a retention catheter in place or are taught to perform clean intermittent catheterization (see Chap. 62) for 7 to 10 days until they are able to void sufficiently to empty the bladder. The client is taught Kegel's exercises after surgical repairs.

Uterine Displacement

In some women, the uterus, which is normally flexed about 45 degrees anteriorly with the cervix positioned posteriorly, is displaced. *Anteflexion* describes a uterus that is bent forward on itself. In *retroflexion*, the uterus tilts backward (the opposite of anteflexion). *Retroversion*, the most common displacement, refers to the posterior tilt of the uterus while the cervix tilts anteriorly.

ETIOLOGY AND PATHOPHYSIOLOGY

Displacement usually is congenital; sometimes backward displacement is due to childbearing or scar tissue that forms in clients who have endometriosis or PID. Positional displacement may not cause any noticeable problems, or it may be the underlying reason for discomfort during menstruation and intercourse. Some cases of infertility are due to retrodisplacement of the uterus.

ASSESSMENT FINDINGS

Signs and Symptoms

Clients with a malpositioned uterus describe having backache, dysmenorrhea, or dyspareunia. Sometimes the client seeks a medical examination to investigate the reason pregnancy has not occurred.

Diagnostic Findings

A bimanual pelvic examination locates the abnormal position of the uterus.

MEDICAL AND SURGICAL MANAGEMENT

If the displacement causes severe discomfort, or if the sterility can be corrected, abdominal surgery is performed to relocate and suture the uterus to a more natural position. Age or complicating diseases sometimes make surgery too great a risk. Under such circumstances, the displacement is reduced by inserting a pessary, which repositions the uterus, and having the client assume the knee–chest position several times a day.

NURSING MANAGEMENT

The nurse performs an initial interview, collects pertinent data, and assists with the gynecologic examination. If surgery is performed, the nurse assesses the client for complications, manages wound drains, maintains patency of the indwelling catheter, inspects vaginal packing, and notes the condition of dressings. Deep breathing, pain management, and early ambulation are included in the postoperative management.

Client Teaching

If a pessary is used to correct the prolapse, show the client how to remove, clean, and reinsert it. Explain how to assume a knee–chest position and describe activity level and hygiene measures. Schedule medical follow-up or inform the client to do so.

Tumors of the Female Reproductive System

Uterine Leiomyoma

A *leiomyoma*, sometimes shortened to *myoma*, is a benign uterine growth principally consisting of smooth muscle and fibrous connective tissue. Myomas, which are the most common tumor in the female pelvis, are often referred to as **fibroid tumors.**

ETIOLOGY AND PATHOPHYSIOLOGY

The development of fibroids is believed to be stimulated by estrogen. Tumors may be small or large, single or multiple. Growth usually is slow except during pregnancy. They shrink during and after menopause. Fibroids can occur in various locations in the uterus (Fig. 58–10): *subserous* (below the serous membrane), *intramural* (within the wall), and *submucous* (below the mucous membrane). The latter are most frequently associated with excessive menstrual bleeding.

ASSESSMENT FINDINGS

Signs and Symptoms

When symptoms exist, menorrhagia is most common. There can be a feeling of pressure in the pelvic region, dysmenorrhea, anemia (from loss of blood), and malaise.

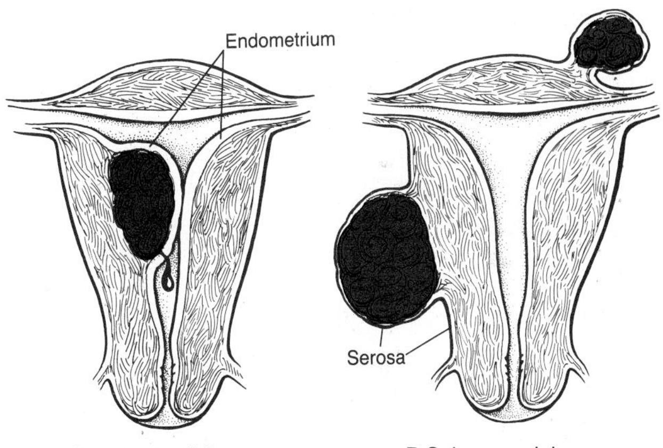

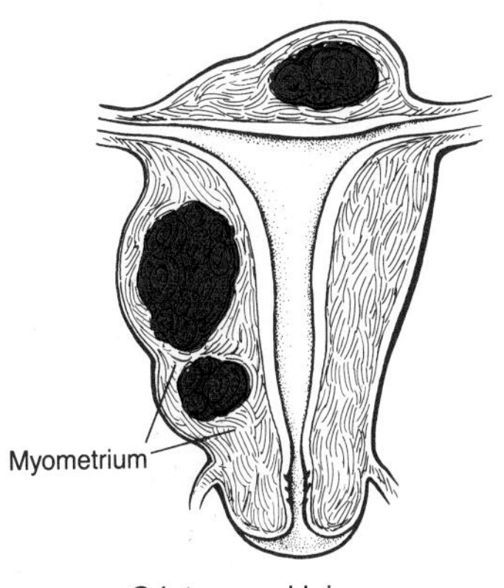

FIGURE 58-10. Sites of leiomyoma.

Diagnostic Findings

Benign uterine tumors may be detected during a pelvic examination. A Pap smear is done to rule out a malignancy. A sonogram reveals uterine and fibroid size. Microscopic examination of the excised tumor confirms the diagnosis.

MEDICAL AND SURGICAL MANAGEMENT

Treatment of benign uterine tumors is governed by a number of factors. A symptomatic tumor in a woman who wishes to have children is watched closely. The client receives a gynecologic examination every 3 to 6 months. A Pap smear is repeated every 6 to 12 months.

When the client has abnormal bleeding, a D and C is performed to determine the cause of bleeding or to control the bleeding. Although a D and C does not remove the tumor, it may make more extensive surgery unnecessary. A *myomectomy* (surgical removal of the tumor only) through an abdominal incision or with a laparoscope inserted through the cervical canal, preserves the uterus if the tumor is benign or a woman of childbearing years wishes to become pregnant in the future. A hysterectomy is performed when symptoms are severe and incapacitating, if the client is past childbearing years, or a future pregnancy is not wanted.

NURSING MANAGEMENT

The nurse assists with the gynecologic examination, reinforces medical explanations, and provides preoperative instructions. During the postoperative time frame, the nurse assists in the safe recovery of the client (see Nursing Care Plan 58–1 that accompanies the discussion of cervical and endometrial cancer).

Cervical and Endometrial Cancer

Cervical cancer, which affects the lowest portion of the uterus, is the second most frequently occurring malignancy of the female reproductive system (breast cancer is first). Cancer of the endometrium affects the lining of the uterus usually in the area of the fundus or corpus and is more common in postmenopausal women.

ETIOLOGY AND PATHOPHYSIOLOGY

Cancer of the cervix has its peak incidence among women between the ages of 35 and 50 and is associated with risk factors that include:

- Being born to mothers treated with diethylstilbestrol (DES) while pregnant
- Becoming sexually active at an early age
- Having multiple sexual partners, or having intercourse with a high-risk man (one who has had multiple partners or penile condyloma [warts])
- Acquiring genital infections caused by the human papilloma virus (HPV)
- Having chronic cervicitis secondary to uterine prolapse
- Having a history of cigarette smoking
- Having had pelvic radiation

The risk of endometrial cancer increases after the age of 50 especially among those women taking estrogens without the addition of progesterone for 5 or more years during and after menopause. Other risk factors include early menarche, late menopause, never having been pregnant (nulliparity), and obesity.

Cervical and endometrial cancers probably begin as premalignant lesions that later undergo malignant changes. The localized malignancy is referred to as **carcinoma in situ** (CIS). Untreated, it will subsequently invade other areas of the uterus and adjacent tissue.

ASSESSMENT FINDINGS

Signs and Symptoms

Bleeding is the earliest and most common symptom of both endometrial and cervical cancer. In early cervical cancer spotting occurs first, especially after slight trauma such as douching or intercourse. The bleeding from endometrial cancer can be mistaken for menorrhagia in premenopausal women. Late symptoms for both include pain, symptoms of pressure on the bladder or bowel, and the generalized wasting associated with advanced cancer.

Diagnostic Findings

All vaginal bleeding is investigated, first by a gynecologic examination, then by diagnostic tests. Cervical cancer is detected with Pap smears and biopsies of suspicious tissue. Cells obtained by endocervical aspiration or endometrial biopsy during a hysteroscopy identify abnormal cells higher in the uterus. Radiography, MRI, or CT scanning are used to determine if there is metastasis; barium studies or an IVP are ordered to determine bowel or bladder metastasis. Both types of cancer are classified according to stages (Table 58–3).

MEDICAL AND SURGICAL MANAGEMENT

Treatment of cervical and endometrial cancer depends on the stage of the tumor. Prognosis depends

TABLE 58-3. **Stages of Uterine Cancers**

Type	Stage	Description
Cervical	0	Cancer in situ
	I	Limited to the cervix
	II	Extends beyond the cervix to the upper two-thirds of the vagina
	III	Involves the lower third of the vagina and is fixed to the pelvic wall
	IV	Involves the rectum, bladder, or extends beyond the true pelvis
Endometrial	0	Cancer in situ
	I	Confined to the corpus
	II	Involves the corpus and cervix
	III	Extends outside the uterus, but not the true pelvis
	IV	Involves the rectum, bladder, or extends outside the true pelvis

Adapted from Federation Internationale de Gynecologic et Obstetrique.

on how early the cancer is diagnosed. Methods for treating cervical and endometrial cancer include one of various **hysterectomy** (removal of uterus) procedures (Box 58–2), external or internal radiation therapy, and chemotherapy (see Chap. 19).

The uterus is removed using an abdominal or vaginal approach—the choice generally depends on the pathology and the condition of the client. An abdominal approach is always used for a radical hysterectomy. The vaginal approach has fewer complications, reduced recovery time, and a lower cost. Laparoscopically assisted vaginal hysterectomy, a combination of surgical and endoscopic techniques, is being used to perform vaginal hysterectomies that otherwise would have been performed abdominally.

NURSING MANAGEMENT

A major role of the nurse is educating all women to have regular gynecologic examinations and Pap smears. Theoretically, all uterine cancers begin *in situ.* Therefore, regular cytologic (cell) examinations increase the potential for an early diagnosis before invasion occurs.

Specific nursing management depends on the selected treatment. In the interim between diagnosis and treatment, the nurse offers emotional support and information about the various options for treatment. See Chapter 19 for discussion of radiation therapy or chemotherapy and nursing management techniques.

Preoperative and Postoperative Nursing Care

Preoperative preparations vary depending on the surgeon's preference and the planned surgical approach (abdominal or vaginal). A douche is given prior to a vaginal hysterectomy, and an enema is given before either surgery. The nurse inserts an indwelling catheter preoperatively and administers an antibiotic, usually one of the cephalosporins, peri-, intra-, or postoperatively to prevent infection. For general postoperative care, refer to perioperative standards of care found in Chapter 24; for postoperative care specific to an abdominal hysterectomy, refer to Nursing Care Plan 58–1.

Client Teaching

Depending on the client's treatment, the teaching plan includes some or all of the following:

- Take any prescribed medications as ordered. Seek care if adverse drug effects occur.
- Avoid heavy lifting, sexual intercourse, vigorous physical exercise, and douching until permitted by the physician.
- Ambulate at intervals and avoid sitting in one position for a prolonged period of time.
- Clean the incision as directed.
- Seek medical care if any of the following signs and symptoms occur: fever; redness, swelling, pain, or drainage of the incision; vaginal discharge that has a foul odor; vaginal bleeding; pain in the chest, abdomen, or legs.
- Avoid constipation and straining to have a bowel movement. Drink plenty of fluids. If constipation occurs, contact the physician.

BOX 58-2 **Types of Hysterectomies**

Total hysterectomy	Removal of the entire uterus and cervix
Subtotal hysterectomy	Removal of the uterus only, with a stump of the cervix left intact
Panhysterectomy	Removal of the uterus, fallopian tubes, and ovaries
Radical hysterectomy	Removal of the uterus, cervix, ovaries, and fallopian tubes; part of the upper vagina and some pelvic lymph nodes also may be removed at this time
Pelvic exenteration	Removal of all reproductive organs, rectum, colon, bladder, distal ureters, iliac blood vessels, and pelvic lymph nodes and peritoneum

NURSING CARE PLAN 58-1
Postoperative Management of the Client With a Total Abdominal Hysterectomy

Potential Problems and Nursing Diagnoses	Nursing Management	Outcome Criteria
Pain related to surgery, inactivity	Assess type of pain, intensity; location, onset, and duration; administer analgesics as ordered; change position q 2 hr; encourage active exercises; maintain correct body alignment; use pillows to support back and legs as needed	Client reports decreased discomfort; pain adequately controlled with analgesics
Potential Complication: Thrombophlebitis	Remove and reapply antiembolic stockings q 8 hr; encourage active leg exercises q 2–4 hr; assess lower extremities for color, warmth, pain, redness, blanching, or other changes in sensation q 4 hr; do not use pillows behind the knees or raise the foot gatch while client is in a supine position; ambulate as ordered	Negative Homans' sign
Potential Complication: Urinary Retention	Measure intake and output; palpate lower abdomen for distention q 4 hr; if client is voiding in small amounts, measure urine each voiding (to detect retention with overflow); report any decrease in urine output to physician; encourage a liberal fluid intake; ambulate as ordered	Voiding in sufficient quantity
Potential Complication: Abdominal Distention; Paralytic Ileus	Encourage ambulation; auscultate abdomen q 4 hr for bowel sounds; palpate abdomen q 4 hr for signs of rigidity; insert rectal tube if ordered; report signs of abdominal distention or rigidity or sudden absence of bowel sounds to physician immediately	Bowel sounds normal; abdomen soft; passes flatus
Potential Complication: Vaginal Bleeding or Hemorrhage	Record number of perineal pads used; record color, amount, type of vaginal drainage; report excessive bleeding or passage of clots to physician immediately; monitor vital signs q 4 hr	Normal postoperative vaginal drainage; vital signs within normal range
Risk for Disturbance in Body Image related to misconceptions of physical and sexual consequences of surgical procedure	Give the client an opportunity to verbalize perceptions and fears Clarify that a hysterectomy does not physically compromise libido, ability to achieve orgasm, cause premature aging, depression, or masculinization	The client has a realistic understanding of the physical outcomes of surgery
Knowledge Deficit related to onset of menopause secondary to removal of ovaries in premenopausal women	Discuss the physiologic effects of menopause with the client Explain the action, frequency for administration, side effects, and benefits of taking hormone replacement therapy Inform the client to continue to have regular Pap smears if the cervix remains	The client accurately paraphrases health teaching related to surgical menopause

Ovarian Cysts and Benign Ovarian Tumors

A *cyst* is a membranous sac filled with fluid, cells, or both. Ovarian cysts, which are benign, are filled with fluid. Benign ovarian tumors are noncancerous growths of solid tissue.

ETIOLOGY AND PATHOPHYSIOLOGY

The exact etiologic mechanism for the variety of ovarian cysts and tumors is essentially unknown, but endocrine dysfunction has been implicated in some types. Follicular cysts are thought to develop when a ripening ovum fails to be released. Another type forms when the corpus luteum fails to regress after ovulation and continues to produce progesterone. Chocolate cysts are secondary to endometriosis. Ovarian cysts and benign tumors tend to affect menstruation and fertility depending on the specific type. Some benign tumors have a potential to become malignant (Porth, 1994).

ASSESSMENT FINDINGS

Signs and Symptoms

Pressure in the lower abdomen, backache, menstrual irregularities, and pain may be experienced. The pain can be mistaken for the pain of appendicitis, ureteral stone, or other abdominal disorders. Clients with tumors associated with or influenced by hypothalamic, pituitary, or adrenal hormones can develop hirsutism (growth of facial hair), atrophy of the breasts, and sterility.

Diagnostic Findings

Tumors and cysts may be detected during a pelvic examination. Ultrasonography and laparoscopy are used to determine tumor size. Surgery is the only means for confirming a diagnosis of a benign tumor or cyst.

MEDICAL AND SURGICAL MANAGEMENT

Some ovarian cysts and benign tumors require no treatment or are treated with oral contraceptives to provide symptomatic relief. If the cyst ruptures, surgery, which can entail complete **oophorectomy** (removal of the ovary), removal of the tissue (oophorocystectomy) only, or a **salpingo-oophorectomy** (removal of the ovary and fallopian tube), is required.

NURSING MANAGEMENT

The nurse explains measures for relieving menstrual discomfort and provides referrals to support groups that are devoted to infertile women. The preoperative preparation and postoperative management are the same as for any client having abdominal surgery and a general anesthetic (see Chap. 24). Following surgery some women develop abdominal distention, which is relieved by ambulating, inserting a rectal tube, or applying an abdominal binder.

Client Teaching

Inform the client who has had surgery but not a hysterectomy to continue having regular gynecologic examinations and Pap smears because she is still at risk for uterine cancer.

Cancer of the Ovary

Although other types of female reproductive system cancers occur with greater incidence, ovarian tumors are the leading cause of death from gynecologic malignancies (National Institutes of Health, 1994). Its lethality is largely because tumors of the ovary present with nonspecific symptoms and therefore are frequently far advanced and inoperable by the time they are diagnosed.

ETIOLOGY AND PATHOPHYSIOLOGY

It is believed that some ovarian tumors have a hereditary link, whereas others arise from ovarian cysts. Recent research has shown that the more times a woman ovulates during her lifetime, the greater the risk for ovarian cancer. Certain individuals in the population tend to develop ovarian cancer more often than others. They include nulliparous women, those with a family history of ovarian cancer, and those who have been diagnosed with other types of cancer such as endometrial, colon, or breast cancer.

Malignant tumors of the ovary are classified according to the type of cell from which they originate. Most are epithelial, followed by germ cell (an ovum) tumors. Other types are very rare.

ASSESSMENT FINDINGS

Signs and Symptoms

In the beginning, clients experience vague lower abdominal discomfort. As the tumor grows larger, urinary frequency and urgency may develop because of pressure on the bladder. Later, ascites, weight loss, severe pain, and gastrointestinal symptoms occur.

Diagnostic Findings

A mass may be felt during a pelvic examination. Many physicians feel that ovarian enlargement found on pelvic examination requires surgical exploration. Laboratory studies measuring tumor marker antigens, such as alpha-fetoprotein, carcinoembryonic antigen (CEA) and CA 125, are ordered. Transvaginal and transabdominal ultrasound and Doppler imaging of ovarian vessels are used in an effort to detect early stage ovarian cancer. An abdominal CT scan, proctoscopy, barium study, chest radiograph, and IVP are done to detect metastasis to other areas. A positive diagnosis is made by microscopic examination.

MEDICAL AND SURGICAL MANAGEMENT

Preventive measures are recommended to at-risk populations. They include having at least two full-term pregnancies followed by breast-feeding and using oral contraceptives for more than 5 years. In addition, prophylactic bilateral oophorectomy is recommended for women at risk for hereditary ovarian cancer syndrome after they reach the age of 35 or after childbearing is completed. Following diagnosis of a malignant tumor, the diseased ovary is removed. A total hysterectomy may or may not be performed. If both ovaries are removed, HRT may be prescribed.

Surgical treatment, which reduces the tumor load, is followed by chemotherapy. The current antineoplastic drug regimen of choice is a combination of cisplatin (Platinol) and paclitaxel (Taxol), although combinations of other drugs such as cyclophosphamide (Cytoxan) and carboplatin (Paraplatin) may be used as alternatives (National Institutes of Health, 1994). The use of radiation therapy rather than chemotherapy is controversial at this time.

NURSING MANAGEMENT

Only a small percentage of clients with malignant tumors of the ovary survive 5 or more years despite intensive treatment. The emotional impact of the diagnosis requires support and understanding on the part of the nurse and other members of the health team. Many of these clients are young, the treatment is difficult, and the prognosis is poor. Preoperative and postoperative nursing care is similar to that of others who undergo abdominal surgery (See preoperative and postoperative care in the nursing management discussion of the client with cervical and endometrial cancer). See Nursing Care Plan 58–1 for nursing diagnoses and interventions for the client undergoing a total abdominal hysterectomy.

Cancer of the Vagina

Cancer of the vagina is rare and usually is seen in women older than 40.

ETIOLOGY AND PATHOPHYSIOLOGY

The incidence of vaginal cancer is higher among women infected with the *human papilloma virus* (HPV), a sexually transmitted microorganism (see Chap. 61), and among those who use a pessary, but neglect removing and cleaning the device. Studies have shown a relationship between taking of diethylstilbestrol (DES) during early pregnancy and the development of vaginal carcinoma in the (young) female offspring. DES is no longer used to treat problems associated with pregnancy.

The upper posterior third of the vagina is the most common site of vaginal cancer. Metastatic lesions may occur in the cervix or adjacent areas such as the vulva, uterus, or rectum.

ASSESSMENT FINDINGS

Signs and Symptoms

Abnormal vaginal bleeding usually is the predominant symptom. Dyspareunia also may occur.

Diagnostic Findings

Visual examination of the vaginal canal discloses the lesion. A biopsy then confirms the diagnosis.

MEDICAL AND SURGICAL MANAGEMENT

Cancer of the vagina is treated according to the extent of the tumor. Most clients undergo laser photovaporization treatments although a partial or total vaginectomy is a possibility. Radiation therapy also is used. Complications, such as fistulas and bleeding, arise from the tumor itself and from radiation therapy. These complications are difficult to correct and control.

NURSING MANAGEMENT

The poor prognosis and complications associated with vaginal cancer and its treatment present a nursing challenge. Keep the client as comfortable as possible and change bedding and clothing frequently. Urine or fecal drainage from the fistulas make odors difficult to control, but a room deodorizer and frequent gown and linen changes help.

Client Teaching

The nurse encourages all women who took DES during a pregnancy to tell their daughters and advise them to have complete gynecologic examinations at regular intervals. Following treatment, clients may profit from techniques to reduce the discomfort during sexual intercourse that is caused by narrowing of the vagina. Some suggestions include:

- Using K-Y gel or prolonged foreplay to lubricate the vagina.
- Having one's sex partner dilate the vagina with fingers before penetration with the penis.
- Taking a slower pace during sexual activities.

Cancer of the Vulva

Cancer of the vulva, the external female genitalia, is a relatively rare malignancy. It usually occurs in women older than 60, but there has been a recent rise in cases among younger women. Vulvar cancer is highly curable when diagnosed in an early stage.

ETIOLOGY AND PATHOPHYSIOLOGY

Infections with carcinogenic agents like HPV and type-2 herpes simplex virus (HSV-2) increase the risk for vulvar cancer (see Chap. 61). These infections are treatable, but not curable, which explains the lifelong threat for genital cancer.

Atypical cells, which appear as white or pigmented raised patches, most commonly involve the labia majora. The cancer also occurs in the labia minora, clitoris, and Bartholin glands. Due to the widespread presence of the viruses in the vulvar epithelium and their potential for carcinogenesis, multiple cancerous sites may coexist or occur again after treatment. Although the cancer is slow growing, it can and does spread to the vagina, urethra, and anus via regional lymph nodes.

ASSESSMENT FINDINGS

Signs and Symptoms

Pruritus and genital burning are the most frequent early symptoms. Later, a bloody discharge, enlarged lymph nodes, ulceration and swelling of the vulva, and a visible mass develop. Eventually, severe pain is experienced. As the cancer ulcerates, a bloody, and sometimes purulent, discharge from the vulva occurs.

Diagnostic Findings

The lesions are first noted during inspection of the genitalia. Application of acetic acid tends to accentuate the abnormal tissue. Diagnosis is confirmed by biopsy.

MEDICAL AND SURGICAL MANAGEMENT

Vulvectomy (removal of the vulva) with or without the removal of lymph nodes (*radical vulvectomy*) is the standard for treatment. However, laser photovaporization is being used as an alternative to preserve the cosmetic appearance of the genitalia, especially if the lesions do not exceed a depth of 3 mm. The efficacy of preoperative chemotherapy plus radiation before surgery for advanced disease is being investigated.

When cancer of the vulva is inoperable, wet dressings and perineal irrigations with a deodorizing solution help to control the odor and the infection that usually occur in the ulcerating neoplasm. Narcotic analgesics usually are necessary in the terminal stage of the disease.

NURSING MANAGEMENT

The nurse offers emotional support while the client awaits the results of the biopsy. If surgery is the selected method of treatment, the nurse provides appropriate preoperative and postoperative care.

Preoperative and Postoperative Nursing Care

The client is instructed to begin the initial preoperative skin preparation by washing the lower abdomen, genitalia, perineum, and upper thighs with antibacterial soap for several days before surgery. On the day of surgery, the nurse inserts a Foley catheter and provides standard teaching for deep breathing and leg exercises. Antibiotic therapy may begin before the operative procedure.

The nurse plans measures to prevent postoperative complications, manage pain, relieve edema in the lower extremities, prevent wound infection, and preserve and restore skin integrity. The nurse will also intervene therapeutically to assist the client in maintaining an acceptable body image, preparing for the resumption of sexual function, and performing self-care activities after discharge.

Refer to perioperative standards of care in Chapter 24. Additionally, the nurse's responsibilities include, but are not limited to the following:

Nursing Diagnoses and Collaborative Problems	Nursing Interventions
Pain related to tissue trauma and swelling	Administer prescribed analgesics liberally.
Goal: The client's pain will be relieved to a tolerable level.	Apply an air mattress or eggcrate mattress to the bed for comfort. Place the client in a semirecumbent position to relieve pressure on the sutures. Modify the client's position at least every 2 hours. Use as many pillows as necessary to promote comfort.
	When in a lateral position, bend and support the upper leg on pillows to prevent tension on the operative area.
Potential Complication: Thrombophlebitis related to venous stasis	Assess for and report calf pain on dorsiflexion or calf tenderness. Remove and reapply antithrombotic stockings or pneumatic leg compression device at regular intervals each day. Ensure that client is performing leg exercises while in bed and ambulating as tolerated.
Goal: The nurse will manage and minimize risk for the development of thrombophlebitis.	
	Administer prescribed anticoagulants; monitor laboratory tests for therapeutic levels.

Impaired Peripheral Tissue Perfusion related to compromised lymphatic and venous circulation secondary to excision of lymph nodes and ligation of blood vessels	Elevate the lower extremities whenever possible. Dangle the client the evening of surgery and assist to ambulate on a daily basis.
Goal: Dependent edema will be absent by the time of discharge.	
Risk for infection related to compromised skin integrity in close proximity to the rectum	Perform conscientious handwashing before caring for the wound.
Goal: There will be no wound infection as evidenced by temperature within normal ranges, no wound tenderness or purulent drainage, and normal white blood cell count.	Inspect and change perineal dressing following principles of asepsis. Cleanse the anus with moistened antiseptic wipes following bowel elimination. Empty surgical drains and catheter drainage bag aseptically. Observe and record the appearance and amount of drainage.
Impaired Skin Integrity related to unresolved tissue healing	Irrigate the wound with sterile saline, hydrogen perioxide, or a medically prescribed antiseptic solution at least three times daily. Dry the wound with a heat lamp or hair dryer.
Goal: The wound will become approximated.	Give warm sitz baths after sutures have been removed. Cover intact skin with a transparent or air and water occlusive dressing to protect it from moist drainage. Support surgical drain during periods of ambulation. Explore the need to refer the client for home health nursing if family or significant member is unavailable for postdischarge wound care.
Risk for Disturbance in Body Image related to emotional distress secondary to amputated genitalia	Ensure privacy when assessing the wound or carrying out treatment measures. Keep the client clean, odor free, and well groomed to promote feeling attractive.
Goal: The client will maintain a positive self-image as evidenced by interacting with others and resuming previous lifestyle activities.	Listen when the client expresses emotions regarding her changed appearance. Encourage significant others to be genuinely attentive and to express acceptance through hand holding, sitting close, or other actions that express continued regard for the client.
Risk for Sexual Dysfunction related to anatomic changes in external genitalia	Act as a liason for information between the client and her surgeon as to the physical consequences of surgery.
Goal: The client will find satisfactory techniques for experiencing sexual intimacy.	Role play or encourage discussions regarding sexual issues between the client and significant other. Explore the idea of using a vaginal dilator, liberal lubrication, and a side-lying position for intercourse once healing is complete. Suggest that the client seek a referral from her physician to a sexual counselor if sexual issues are unresolved.

Client Teaching

Before being discharged, the nurse can instruct the client on the following measures for self-care:

- Wound healing will take as long as 6 months.
- Elevate the legs and wear antiembolic stockings to reduce dependent edema in the lower extremities.
- Eat a high-protein diet with sources of vitamin C to promote healing.
- Try to stand and straddle the toilet when attempting to void after the catheter is removed in 7 to 10 days so that urine is directed into the toilet rather than running down the leg or perineum.
- Cleanse the periurethral area with water or normal saline in a plastic drink container with a spout after urination.
- Continue to take the prescribed stool softener after discharge.
- Take a sitz bath using a portable basin after each bowel movement.
- Report any unusual odor, fever, fresh bleeding, separation of the wound margin, inability to void or constipation, and perineal pain.

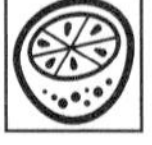

General Nutritional Considerations

Although some studies suggest that megadoses of vitamin B_6 relieve PMS symptoms, large doses (ie, 500 mg) can cause sensory neuropathy, which disappears after supplement use stops. Until the relationship between nutrients and PMS is more clearly defined, self-medicating with megadoses of vitamins and minerals should be discouraged.

Soy is rich in naturally occurring compounds called phytoestrogens (plant estrogens), which are similar to the body's own estrogen. Some studies suggest that increasing the intake of soy products may help alleviate menopausal symptoms such as hot flashes and vaginal dryness. Interestingly, women from Asian countries, where soy intake is high, report a low incidence of menopausal symptoms.

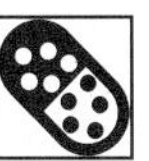

General Pharmacologic Considerations

Estrogen therapy can cause nausea and vomiting, pigmentation of the nipple and areola, and uterine bleeding. Stress incontinence may occur. Sodium may be retained, leading to excessive storage of intercellar fluid and edema. Diuretics and a low-sodium diet help relieve this situation. Large doses of estrogen sometimes cause the mobilization of calcium into the bloodstream, damaging the kidney when it excretes the excess calcium.

Because synthetic estrogen hormones cause thromboembolic phenomena, the client is instructed to contact the physician if tenderness, pain, swelling, or redness occur in the legs. If vaginal bleeding occurs during hormonal therapy, the client should contact the physician because the dose may need to be adjusted.

When androgen therapy is prescribed, clients may have increased bone pain after the first few injections. As therapy continues, pain frequently lessens, some recalcification of bone occurs, and the client has an increased appetite and gains weight. Androgen therapy may cause fluid retention, increased libido, and distressing symptoms of virilization, such as deeper voice and increased facial and body hair.

To prevent loss of bone mass in post menopausal women unable to tolerate ERT, the drug alendronate (Fosamax) may be prescribed. Alendronate acts to prevent bone reabsorption. Do not give the drug with milk or milk products because calcium inhibits absorption of the drug. The drug is best absorbed when given in 8 ounces of water on arising in the morning. The patient is instructed to avoid lying down and to remain upright for at least 30 minutes after the drug is taken to prevent dyspepsia and esophageal irritation.

When antibiotics are taken for a long time or if repeated courses of antibiotic therapy are necessary, an overgrowth of yeastlike fungi that usually exists in small numbers in the vagina can occur, resulting in vaginitis.

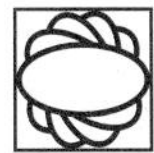

General Gerontologic Considerations

Older women may develop perineal pruritus. An effort is made to discover the cause of the pruritus; it may require asking questions about diet, type of clothing worn, presence of a vaginal discharge, and so on. The client also may be tested for glucose in the blood and urine, and a pelvic examination may be performed to rule out other abnormalities, such as cervicitis, cystocele, rectocele, or cancer of the vulva, cervix, or uterus.

When an older client has a uterine prolapse, surgery may not be considered because of complicating chronic disorders. A pessary may be used to return the uterus to its normal position in the pelvis.

The female genitalia changes during the aging process. The vulva atrophies, causing a loss of vascularity and elasticity. This can result in irritation or excoriation of the tissue. Pubic hair thins and the labia majora and minora became smaller.

Vaginal flora changes with age causing the environment to become more alkaline and predisposing the older woman to vaginitis.

Hot flashes, which occur in approximately 75% of all perimenopausal women, are accompanied by increased perspiration, vasodilation, and a 10% to 20% increase in pulse rate. Estrogen, progesterone, combinations of the two, or clonidine may be used to alleviate symptoms.

SUMMARY OF KEY CONCEPTS

- Three reproductive processes associated with sexual maturation are ovulation, pregnancy, and menstruation.
- Common conditions that occur in relation to or alter menstrual patterns are premenstrual syndrome, dysmenorrhea, amenorrhea, oligomenorrhea, menorrhagia, metrorrhagia, and menopause.
- Menstrual disorders generally result in one or more of the following problems: absent, scant, or excessive bleeding; discomfort that ranges from mild to severe; and emotional consequences that may require psychological adaptation.
- A menstrual diary in which a woman correlates her symptoms in relation to the days preceding and following menstruation may help in the diagnosis of menstrual disorders, especially premenstrual syndrome.
- Menstrual disorders are managed medically with drugs, such as hormone therapy, analgesics, oral contraceptives, antidepressants, antianxiety drugs, or surgically with more invasive procedures such as a dilatation and curettage or endometrial ablation.
- The nurse's role in managing menstrual disorders is to gather appropriate information, assist with gynecologic examinations, offer suggestions for relieving discomfort, instruct clients about their drug therapy, prepare clients for surgical interventions, care for them during recovery, and provide specific health teaching instructions.
- Menopause, a universal experience for all women, can be accompanied by vasomotor disturbances such as hot flashes and sweating, vaginal thinning and dryness, and atrophy of reproductive organs.
- When estrogen production decreases, women have an increased risk for developing osteoporosis and coronary artery disease. The risk is diminished and physiologic symptoms reduced with hormone replacement therapy.
- Women are subject to infectious and inflammatory conditions such as vaginitis, cervicitis, pelvic inflammatory disease, and toxic shock syndrome. Most of these conditions are due to an invasion of pathogenic microorganisms; another etiology is local trauma.
- Vaginitis may be caused by a yeast infection that results in a thick discharge with white flecks that has an unpleasant odor, a protozoan infection that causes a frothy yellowish discharge with disgusting odor, and a bacterial infection characterized by a gray discharge that smells fishy.

- Clients with vaginal infections are taught preventive techniques such as wiping correctly following bowel elimination, keeping the vaginal area clean and dry, avoiding routine douching, and avoiding intercourse if a sex partner is symptomatic.
- Clients with vaginal infections are taught to insert antimicrobial medications by assuming a dorsal recumbent position, loading the applicator, inserting it 2 to 4 inches, and remaining in a reclined position overnight if possible.
- When caring for a client with pelvic inflammatory disease, the nurse implements interventions that aid in monitoring and managing sepsis, reducing the risk for transmitting the infectious agent to others, reducing pain, and preventing or restoring skin integrity.
- To prevent the occurrence of toxic shock syndrome, women are advised to use perineal pads during menstruation, avoid using super-absorbent tampons, change tampons frequently, and remove internal contraceptive devices after their use.
- Some women develop structural abnormalities such as endometriosis, vaginal fistulas, pelvic organ prolapse, or uterine displacement. Endometriosis and uterine displacement may reduce the potential for conception. Vaginal fistulas may impair expressing affection via sexual intercourse. Pelvic organ prolapse can affect bladder control and bowel elimination or increase the risk for cervical irritation in the case of a uterovaginal prolapse.
- Clients who are faced with a decision on how to treat endometriosis may be assisted by reinforcing the physician's explanations, clarifying misinformation, suggesting a second medical opinion, encouraging consultation with the client's significant other, helping the client identify pros and cons of each option, and advocating for the client's final choice.
- Clients with vaginal fistulas are at risk for low self-esteem, impaired skin integrity, and altered sexuality patterns. The nurse helps manage these problems by implementing measures that disguise the drainage and its odor, cleaning and protecting the skin, and suggesting ways to modify sexual intercourse.
- Clients who must use a pessary are taught to remove it periodically, clean and dry it before reinsertion, and assume a knee–chest position once or twice a day to maintain its location.
- Cancer in situ is a term that refers to a localized noninvasive malignancy. Several gynecologic cancers, such as cervical malignancies, have a long period of time during which they remain in situ. Consequently, this increases the potential for early diagnosis and more favorable prognosis.
- The most common types of cancer affecting the pelvic reproductive organs are cervical and endometrial cancer. Many gynecologic malignancies are easily diagnosed by having regular gynecologic examinations, Pap smears and biopsies that may be performed in the physician's office.
- When caring for a client who undergoes a hysterectomy, the nurse focuses on care that prevents, reduces, or eliminates problems such as blood loss, pain, wound infection, impaired venous circulation, urinary retention, abdominal distention, and change in body image. Complications such as hemorrhage, thrombophlebitis, and anuria are managed, if they occur.
- Ovarian cancer has a more lethal outcome because its onset is accompanied by vague symptoms and it tends to be diagnosed after it has invaded adjacent or distant tissue.
- Vaginal cancer is triggered by cellular changes secondary to a localized viral infection, chronic irritation from internal vaginal devices, or spread from some other primary site.
- Vulvar cancer, the rarest of all gynecologic malignancies, tends to have the most physically traumatic outcome from surgical treatment because it involves amputation of the external genitalia. Postoperative nursing care focuses on caring for the wound, preventing wound infection, and helping the client cope with the change in body image and sexual expression.

CRITICAL THINKING EXERCISES

1. What information could be shared with a person who discredits the validity of premenstrual syndrome as a physiologic disorder?
2. Discuss information that is appropriate to document in a menstrual diary and how to record the information for analysis.
3. Identify possible reasons why an adult woman becomes amenorrheic or experiences oligomenorrhea.
4. Discuss the measures that are appropriate to recommend to reduce the incidence of gynecologic cancers.
5. Describe the physiologic, psychological, and social consequences of menopause.
6. To gain empathy for the sexual adjustment a couple may experience after a woman undergoes a radical vulvectomy, explore how you or some other woman might react if a male sex partner lost his external genitalia. Men may choose to respond to this question by describing their response to a female sex partner whose genitalia are surgically excised.

Suggested Readings

Bates, B., Binkley, L. S., & Hoekleman, R. A. (1995). *A guide to physical examination and history taking* (6th ed.). Philadelphia: J. B. Lippincott.

Bullock, B. L. (1996). *Pathophysiology, adaptations and alterations in function* (4th ed.). Philadelphia: Lippincott-Raven.

Crandall, S. G. (1997). Menopause made easier. *RN, 60*(7), 46–50.

Garner, C. (1997). Endometriosis: What you need to know. *RN, 60* (1), 27–31.

Lamb, M. A. (1990). Psychosexual issues: The woman with gynecologic cancer. *Seminars in Oncology Nursing, 6*(3), 237–243.

Lieb, S. M. (1996). Benefits of hormone replacement therapy for menopause and osteoporosis. *Surgical Services Management,* 2(10), 16–18.

National Institutes of Health. (1994, April 5–7). *Ovarian cancer: Screening, treatment, and followup.* (NIH Consensus Statement 12, 3). Bethesda, MD: Author.

Novak, J. C., & Broom, B. L. (1995). *Maternal and child health nursing* (8th ed.). St. Louis: Mosby–Year Book.

Porth, C. M. (1994). *Pathophysiology, concepts of altered health states* (4th ed.). Philadelphia: J . B. Lippincott.

Reeder, S. J., Martin, L. L., & Koniak, D. (1992). *Maternity nursing: Family, newborn, and women's health care* (17th ed.). Philadelphia: J. B. Lippincott.

Rudy, D. R., & Bush, I. M. (1992). Hysterectomy and sexual dysfunction: You can help. *Patient Care, 26*(15), 67–76.

Scura, K. W., & Wipple, B. (1997). How to provide better care for the postmenopausal woman. *American Journal of Nursing, 97*(4), 36–43.

Shurpin, K. M. (1997). Clinical snapshot: Ovarian cancer. *American Journal of Nursing, 97*(4), 34–35.

Thompson, S. D., & Szukiewicz-Nugent, J. M. (1996). When ovarian cancer strikes. *Nursing, 26*(10), 33–38.

Additional Resources

RESOLVE (Nationwide Infertility Support Group)
(617) 623–0744

Organization of Parenting Through Surrogacy (OPTS)
P.O. Box 213
Wheeling, IL 60090
(847) 394–4116
Fax (847) 394–4165

National Adoption Clearinghouse
11426 Rockville Pike
Suite 410
Rockville, MD 20852
(301) 231–6512

Endometriosis Association
8585 North 76th Place
Milwaukee, WI 53223
(800) 992–3636

Cancer Information Service
Building 31
Room 10A16
9000 Rockville Pike
Bethesda, MD 20892
(800) 4-CANCER

Hysterectomy Educational Resources Services (HERS)
(610) 667–7757

Chapter 59

Caring for Clients With Breast Disorders

KEY TERMS

Breast abscess
Breast cancer
Breast reconstruction
Breast self-examination
Clinical breast examination
Fibroadenoma
Fibrocystic breast disease
Lumpectomy
Lymphedema
Mammography
Mastitis
Mastopexy
Mammoplasty
Modified radical mastectomy
Partial (or segmental) mastectomy
Reduction mammoplasty
Simple (or total) mastectomy
Subcutaneous mastectomy

LEARNING OBJECTIVES

On completion of this chapter, the reader will:

- List four signs and symptoms that are common among breast disorders.
- Name and describe three techniques for obtaining a breast biopsy.
- Name two infectious and inflammatory breast disorders and explain how they are acquired.
- Discuss health teaching that may help prevent or eliminate infectious and inflammatory breast disorders.
- Identify two benign breast disorders and describe their similarities and differences.
- Explain how and when to perform breast self-examination.
- Give the current recommendations for mammography.
- Name groups that are at high risk for developing breast cancer.
- List common signs and symptoms of breast cancer.
- Name three methods for treating breast cancer.
- Name and describe six surgical techniques used to remove a malignant breast tumor.
- Give two criteria that are used when selecting a mastectomy procedure.
- Name a serious complication of breast cancer treatment.
- Discuss the nursing management of clients who undergo surgical treatment for breast cancer.
- List four sites to which breast cancer commonly metastasizes.
- Name and describe three cosmetic breast procedures that mastectomy clients may elect to have done.
- Name and describe three cosmetic breast procedures that women with nondiseased breasts may elect to have done.

The breasts are glands that produce milk after pregnancy. Although the most dramatic changes occur in the breast during preparation for lactation, the mammary glands are part of the female reproductive system and they respond to the hormonal cycle associated with ovulation and menstruation, pregnancy, and lactation.

Anatomy and Physiology

The breasts contain the mammary glands, a network of ducts that carry milk to the nipple (Fig. 59–1). The breasts manufacture milk from elements in the blood, a process not yet fully understood. The area has an abundant supply of blood vessels and

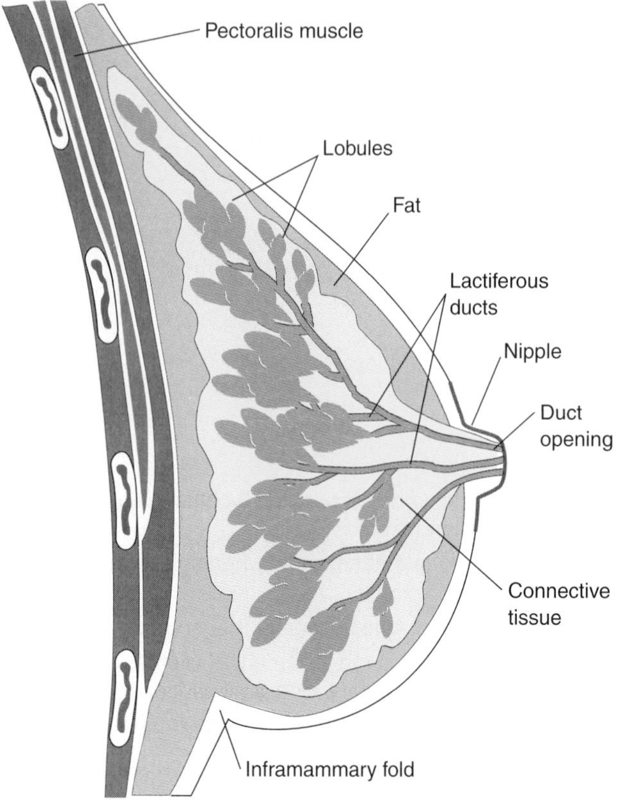

FIGURE 59-1. Breast structures.

lymphatics. The axillary lymph nodes and the internal mammary lymph nodes drain the breasts.

Estrogen secreted by the ovaries brings about the growth and development of the mammary duct systems. Progesterone, secreted by the corpus luteum of the ovary, stimulates lactation as does the hormone prolactin.

Assessment

Breast Examination

Clinical breast examination is performed when the client has a gynecologic examination. The examiner notes breast size and symmetry and any unusual changes in the skin of the breasts and nipples. The breasts and the axilla are then palpated for masses, lymph nodes, tenderness, and other abnormalities.

Disorders of the breast may be manifested by one or more signs or symptoms in Box 59–1 among adult women of all age groups. Therefore, regular **breast self-examination** (BSE), described and illustrated in Nursing Guidelines 59–1, is an important way for women to discover early breast changes.

BOX 59-1 Signs and Symptoms Common to Breast Disorders

- Pain, tenderness, fullness of the breast
- Breast mass(es)
- Nipple discharge
- Change in breast appearance

Mammography

Mammography (mammogram) is a radiographic technique used to detect cysts or tumors of the breast, some of which may be too small to palpate. Mammography is used as a screening test for breast cancer (Fig. 59–2). The American Cancer Society recommends that women begin receiving annual mammograms at age 40 (Box 59–2). The need for mammograms before the age of 40 depends on factors such as a family history of breast cancer, a past history of benign breast disease, incisional or excisional breast biopsies, or other conditions that interfere with accurate BSEs.

NURSING MANAGEMENT

Explain the radiographic procedure and instruct the client to omit using a deodorant with aluminum hydroxide or body talc to avoid artifacts on the x-ray film. If the client forgets or was not provided with this information, have her wash the axillae just before the test. Determine how often the client performs BSEs and have her demonstrate or describe the technique; teach women who are unfamiliar with BSE techniques how to do them. Ensure privacy throughout the examination. Advise clients to have their mammograms at the same health agency or arrange for records to be transferred so that previous mammograms can be compared.

Breast Biopsy

A breast biopsy is performed to determine if a breast lesion is malignant. A specimen of tissue from the breast may be obtained in one of three ways: incisional biopsy, excisional biopsy, or aspiration biopsy.

Incisional biopsy is performed in the operating room, where one or more sections of tissue are removed. The specimen is frozen quickly and examined microscopically by a pathologist while the client remains anesthetized. If the tissue is negative (ie, benign), the remainder of the benign tissue is removed (if it had not been completely removed for biopsy), the incision closed, and the client sent to the recovery room. If the removed specimen is found to be malignant, the surgeon may then perform the surgical pro-

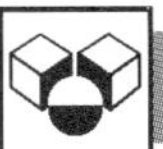

Nursing Guidelines 59-1

Teaching Breast Self-Examination

- Examine your breasts 3 days after the end of menstruation or monthly on a date of your choice if you no longer menstruate.
- Begin the examination in the shower when the breasts are wet and soapy and again after the shower when laying down with a folded towel under the shoulder on the side being examined.
- Use light, medium, and firm pressure applied with the pads of three fingers when checking each breast.
- Move your fingers in circles, spokes of a wheel, or rows, but follow the same technique with each BSE.

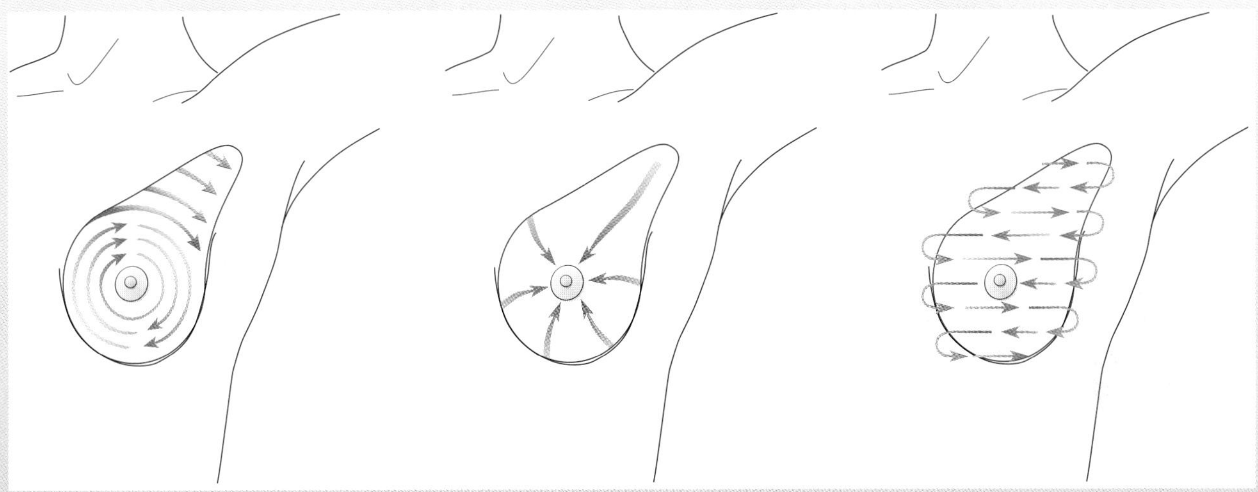

- Feel every part of each breast including the nipple area and the armpit to the collar bone.
- Raise your arms over your head and look at the breasts in a mirror.
- Look for changes in breast shape, size, and contour; puckering (dimpling) of the skin; or areas that appear red.
- Squeeze each nipple and look for liquid drainage.

cedure that offers the best chance of cure. The decision to operate immediately when there is a malignancy is thoroughly discussed with the client prior to surgery.

Some surgeons prefer an *excisional biopsy*, which is the removal of the entire lesion. The excised specimen is examined later and more comprehensively by a pathologist. Clients may be discharged from the hospital before the results of the biopsy are obtained, or they may remain hospitalized. If the lesion is malignant, the biopsy results and the proposed treatment are discussed with the client.

Aspirational biopsy, a procedure usually performed on an outpatient basis, uses a needle and syringe to obtain a sample of the suspicious tissue. A local anes-

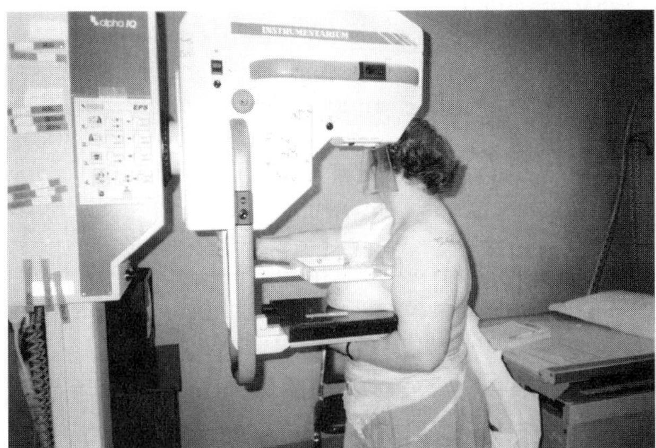

FIGURE 59-2. A client undergoing mammography.

BOX 59-2 Guidelines for Mammography

The American Cancer Society's Breast Cancer Advisory Committee (1997) recommends that all women have a mammogram:

- Initially at age 40
- Every 1 to 2 years thereafter through age 49
- Yearly at age 50

thetic is first injected around the area, and a sample of tissue is removed. The tissue sample is examined by a pathologist.

NURSING MANAGEMENT

Allow the client time to ask questions and listen to concerns before the breast biopsy is performed. The client may have concern not only over the procedure but also over the results of the biopsy and a possible diagnosis of cancer.

An aspiration biopsy usually causes minimal discomfort after the procedure, but there may be redness and soreness in the area. Instruct the client to notify the physician if drainage or bleeding from the biopsy site is more than slight or if increased redness, pain, or fever occurs. Incisional and excisional biopsies require sutures, but pain is usually minimal and can be relieved with a mild analgesic.

Provide instructions regarding wound care, use of a mild analgesic, wearing a supportive bra, and timing of a follow-up appointment. Review the signs and symptoms that suggest wound infection.

Infectious and Inflammatory Breast Disorders

Mastitis

Mastitis, an inflammation of breast tissue, most commonly occurs in women who are breast-feeding. It may occur in one or both breasts.

ETIOLOGY AND PATHOPHYSIOLOGY

Breast inflammation is caused or contributed to by one or more plugged lactiferous ducts or an infectious agent that enters through cracked or fissured nipples. Ducts become plugged as a consequence of infrequent nursing, failure to alternate breasts at each feeding, or a poorly nursing infant.

Lactating breasts have an elaborate blood supply and ductal system that easily supports microbial growth. If an infection develops, the most common causative microorganism is *Staphylococcus aureus,* which often is resistant to antibiotic therapy. The infectious process occurs as a result of inadequate maternal handwashing, or from an infant infected by microorganisms on the hands of nursery personnel, or from organisms on the mother's skin.

ASSESSMENT FINDINGS

Signs and Symptoms

Breast tenderness, pain, and redness are accompanied by fever and malaise. The breast later becomes swollen, firm, and hard. A crack in the nipple or areola develops and the axillary lymph nodes enlarge. On rare occasions a breast abscess develops.

Diagnostic Findings

A culture and sensitivity test on expressed breast milk identifies the infectious agent.

MEDICAL MANAGEMENT

Appropriate antibiotic therapy based on culture and sensitivity tests is given for 10 days. For organisms that are penicillin resistant, oxacillin (Prostaphlin), cephalosporins such as cefazolin (Kefzol), or vancomycin (Vancocin) are given. Analgesics are prescribed for pain.

NURSING MANAGEMENT

The nurse assists with taking the health history (which includes identifying allergies to antibiotics), prepares the client for a physical examination, and collects the specimen of breast milk using standard precautions and aseptic principles.

Client Teaching

Client teaching includes information for self-administering antibiotic medications, reinforces principles of medical asepsis, and identifies techniques to promote comfort and temporary alternatives to breast-feeding.

Teach the client to:

- Take antibiotic medication for the full time that it is prescribed.
- Report the occurrence of side effects of the medication such as rash, gastrointestinal upset, and opportunisitc infections in the mouth or vagina.
- Perform scrupulous handwashing before touching the breast.
- Bathe or shower regularly.
- Wear a supportive brassiere.
- Avoid wearing breast shields that trap breast milk and moisture around the nipple.
- Apply warm soaks to the breast or let warm water from a shower flow over the breast.
- Express milk with a breast pump until the infection is resolved sufficiently to resume breast-feeding.

Breast Abscess

A **breast abscess** is a localized collection of pus within breast tissue.

ETIOLOGY AND PATHOPHYSIOLOGY

When an abscess occurs in the breast, it is most frequently a complication of postpartum mastitis. Purulent exudate accumulates in a confined, local area of breast tissue.

ASSESSMENT FINDINGS

Signs and Symptoms

The client experiences the signs and symptoms of mastitis, but in the case of an abscess, pus may drain from the nipple.

Diagnostic Findings

The diagnosis is based on physical examination of the breast. A culture and sensitivity of nipple drainage identifies the infecting microorganism and indicates to which antibiotics it is sensitive.

MEDICAL AND SURGICAL MANAGEMENT

The client usually is hospitalized and placed on contact isolation precautions because the soiled dressings are highly infectious. The client is started on intravenous antibiotic therapy. The abscess may be incised, drained, and packed.

NURSING MANAGEMENT

Remove and reapply dressings following aseptic principles. Use a binder to hold the dressing in place so that the frequent removal of tape does not irritate the skin. Apply zinc oxide to the surrounding skin to avoid maceration from irritating drainage or wound compresses. Support the arm and shoulder with pillows to reduce swelling. Instruct the client not to shave axillary hair on the side with the abscess until healing is complete.

The mother who is temporarily separated from her newborn will need emotional support. If she decides to terminate breast-feeding, apply a tight fitting brassiere.

Benign Breast Lesions

Fibrocystic Breast Disease

Fibrocystic breast disease, also called *mammary dysplasia* (abnormal development of breast tissue) or *chronic cystic mastitis*, is a benign breast condition that affects women primarily between the ages of 30 and 50.

ETIOLOGY AND PATHOPHYSIOLOGY

Fibrocystic disease occurs as a result of hormonal changes that occur during the menstrual cycle. The condition may also be aggravated by caffeine and nicotine.

When the disorder develops, single or multiple breast cysts appear in one or both breasts. The cysts increase in size and become increasingly tender in proportion to the secretion of estrogen. Cyst formation tends to continue throughout the reproductive years. Some disappear, though others may remain permanently. The condition resolves with menopause.

Although a correlation between fibrocystic disease and breast cancer was reported years ago, studies indicate that there is no cause and effect relationship between the two conditions. However, women with fibrocystic disease may mistake a cancerous mass for a fibrocystic mass and delay medical diagnosis, perform BSE less vigorously due to breast tenderness, or fail to palpate a malignant mass disguised by scar tissue from a previous incisional biopsy.

ASSESSMENT FINDINGS

Signs and Symptoms

Fibrocystic disease of the breast may cause no symptoms, but many women report having tender or painful breasts and feeling one, but more often, multiple lumps within breast tissue. The symptoms are most noticeable from midway onward in the menstrual cycle. They abate at the time of menstruation.

Diagnostic Findings

A preliminary diagnosis is made by examination of the breasts. The characteristic breast mass of fibrocystic disease is soft to firm, movable, and unlikely to cause nipple retraction. Fluid from the cysts is aspirated for cytologic examination, or an incisional biopsy is performed. If the results are questionable, mammography and ultrasonography are performed to distinguish a cystic lesion from a solid malignant tumor.

MEDICAL AND SURGICAL MANAGEMENT

Mild discomfort is relieved with an analgesic such as aspirin or ibuprofen (Advil). For severe symptoms, oral contraceptives or danazol (Danocrine), a synthetic androgen, and bromocriptine (Parlodel), a semisynthetic ergot derivative that mimics prolactin inhibitory factor, are prescribed (Table 59–1). Occasionally, one or more cysts are removed surgically.

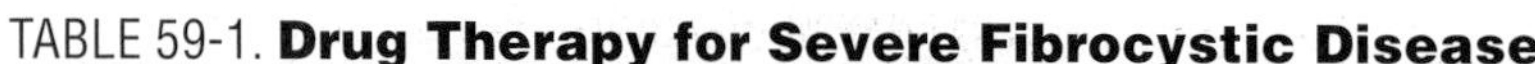

TABLE 59-1. **Drug Therapy for Severe Fibrocystic Disease**

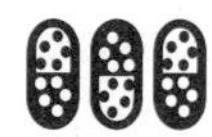

Drug/Mechanism of Action	Side Effects	Nursing Considerations
Hormone:		
Synthetic androgen		
danazol (Danocrine) Decreases estrogen and progesterone levels by suppressing FSH and LH.	Acne, deepened voice, weight gain, flushing, vaginitis, enlarged clitoris, nervousness, emotional lability, fluid retention, headache, fatigue, liver dysfunction	Arrange for periodic history and physical because long-term use increases chances of side effects and medical supervision is required. Cancer should be ruled out before treatment is initiated. Begin during menstrual period to ensure that client is not pregnant and instruct client to use a nonhormonal form of birth control. Inform client of possible side effects, that masculinizing can occur, and to report occurrence of any unusual developments.
Progestins		
medroxyprogesterone (Provera, Amen) Hinders estrogen's effect on breast tissue.	Breakthrough bleeding, spotting, amenorrhea, rash, acne, weight gain, edema, depression, thrombophlebitis, migraine, loss of vision, photosensitivity	Arrange for periodic history and physical as noted above. Have client mark drug administration days on the calendar. Inform client of possible side effects including signs and symptoms of thrombophlebitis and embolism. Instruct client to use a reliable method of birth control and sunscreen and to report any visual disturbances.
Estrogen and progesterone combinations		
estradiol and norethindrone (Ortho-Novum 10/11) Oral contraceptives suppress ovarian secretion of estrogen and oppose estrogen's effect on breast tissue.	Headache, dizziness, thromboembolism, nausea, breakthrough bleeding, depression, anxiety	Continued medical supervision is required; arrange for physical exam, Pap smears and breast exams at least yearly. Discuss side effects with client and instruct on signs and symptoms of thrombophlebitis and embolism. Instruct client not to smoke and to report the occurrence of any side effects.
Ergot Derivative		
bromocriptine (Parlodel) Binds with prolactin-secreting cells of the anterior pituitary; inhibits the release of prolactin.	Nausea, vomiting, diarrhea, constipation, headache, drowsiness, nasal congestion, hypotension	Take initial dose at bedtime; take with meals thereafter. Change positions slowly. Use a reliable contraceptive. Report any side effects.

Widespread disease that causes severe discomfort is treated with partial mastectomy. Care is taken to preserve the areola to provide a cosmetic appearance to the breast after surgery.

NURSING MANAGEMENT

The nurse obtains a health history and asks focused questions about the characteristics and timing of symptoms in relation to the menstrual cycle. During diagnostic examinations, the nurse prepares and supports the client, labels tissue or fluid specimens, and arranges for laboratory analysis.

Client Teaching

The nurse teaches the client with fibrocystic disease to:

- Perform BSE monthly using the same technique and become familiar with the feel and location of cystic masses.
- Schedule a breast examination with a physician every 6 months or anytime a new or unusual lump develops.
- Follow the American Cancer Society's Breast Advisory Committee's Guidelines for mammography (see Box 59–2).
- Wear a well fitting, supportive bra day and night.
- Take mild analgesics or prescription medications according to label directions.
- Apply cold compresses to the breasts when symptomatic.
- Avoid smoking, coffee, chocolate, and cola drinks.
- Restrict activities that may cause trauma to the breasts such as playing soccer or other sports where the breasts are unprotected.

Fibroadenoma

A **fibroadenoma** is a solid, benign breast mass that is composed of connective and glandular tissue. This type of breast lesion generally occurs in women during late adolescence or young adult years, but occasionally is found in older women as well.

ETIOLOGY AND PATHOPHYSIOLOGY

The cause of fibroadenomas is unknown. However, there may be a hormonal influence because the mass is growth stimulated during pregnancy and shrinks after menopause.

The benign tumor is classically a single nodule that grows slowly in nonpregnant women until it becomes a fixed, stable size. It usually does not enlarge and regress with each menstrual cycle like those in fibrocystic disease, and it, too, is *not* considered precancerous.

ASSESSMENT FINDINGS

Signs and Symptoms

A fibroadenoma presents as a painless, nontender lump in the breast. The lesion is usually encapsulated, mobile, and firm when palpated. If the size of the mass is large, the breasts may appear asymmetrical.

Diagnostic Findings

Ultrasound can reveal physical characteristics unique to a fibroadenoma versus malignant mass with a higher degree of accuracy than mammography (Greenfield et al., 1997). In the case of very young women—an atypical age for breast cancer—an excisional biopsy is only performed when and if the mass changes or becomes larger. If the mass is detected in a woman with a higher risk for developing breast cancer, such as one with a family history or one in a higher age group, a biopsy is performed to validate that the tissue is indeed benign.

MEDICAL AND SURGICAL MANAGEMENT

Based on the diagnostic findings, the client and her physician decide to either continue to observe the mass or excise it. Surgery involves removal of the benign tumor, but not a mastectomy. The client is discharged a few hours after recovery from anesthesia.

NURSING MANAGEMENT

The client receives emotional support while the diagnosis is tentative because finding a mass in the breast conjures up fears that it may be malignant.

Client Teaching

The nurse teaches the client to:

- Continue monthly BSE and follow recommendations for mammography.
- Consult a physician if the characteristics of the mass change or if a pregnancy occurs.

If surgery is performed, instructions include to:

- Keep the wound clean and covered until the incision heals.
- Wear a firm, supportive brassiere to reduce incisional discomfort.
- Follow label directions for taking a mild nonnarcotic analgesic to relieve minor pain that may last 1 to 3 days.
- Contact the surgeon to schedule a postoperative evaluation or call immediately if there is exceptional incisional pain or if swelling, wound drainage, or a fever develops.

Malignant Breast Disorders

Cancer of the Breast

One woman in eight develops **breast cancer,** a mass of abnormal cells. Although breast cancer does occur in men, the ratio is approximately 1:150 cases in women. Deaths among women from breast cancer are second only to cancer of the lung. When the disease is discovered and treated early, the 5-year survival rate for small lesions is about 80% or better. A breast cancer preventive study, funded by the National Cancer Institute—the lead agency in the United States for cancer research—has determined that taking the drug tamoxifen (Nolvadex) can prevent breast cancer in women who are at high risk (1998).

ETIOLOGY AND PATHOPHYSIOLOGY

Certain factors appear to increase the chance of developing breast cancer. Being female, over age 30, and having a family history of breast cancer are the most common risk factors. Relatives of women with breast cancer who carry a defective gene (BRCA1 and BRCA2) are very likely to develop breast cancer. Additional factors include exposure to ionizing radiation in childhood and adolescence, previous breast cancer, a history of colon or endometrial cancer, chronic alcohol consumption, early menarche, late menopause, obesity, and women who have had no children or who have had children after age 30.

Each normal breast contains 15 to 20 lobes connected by ducts to smaller lobules (see Fig. 59–1). The most common type of malignancy is ductal cancer, followed by lobular cancer, and inflammatory breast cancer, which is quite uncommon. Some malignant breast tumors are hormone dependent, wherein tumor growth is enhanced by the presence of estrogen or progesterone. Regardless of the type or its etiology, untreated cancer spreads elsewhere through the axillary lymph nodes.

ASSESSMENT FINDINGS

Signs and Symptoms

The primary sign of breast cancer is a painless mass in the breast, most often in the upper outer quadrant (Fig. 59–3). The tumor may have been developing *in situ* for as long as 2 years before becoming palpable. Other signs of breast cancer include a bloody discharge from the nipple, a dimpling of the skin over the lesion, retraction of the nipple, and a difference in size between one breast and the other. The lesion may be fixed or movable, and axillary lymph nodes may be enlarged. Many of these signs depend on several factors, such as the type and location of tumor and the length of time the tumor has been present.

Diagnostic Findings

Mammography detects breast lesions. The radiologist can often differentiate between a benign and malignant tumor on radiograph. Diagnosis is confirmed by biopsy and microscopic cell examination.

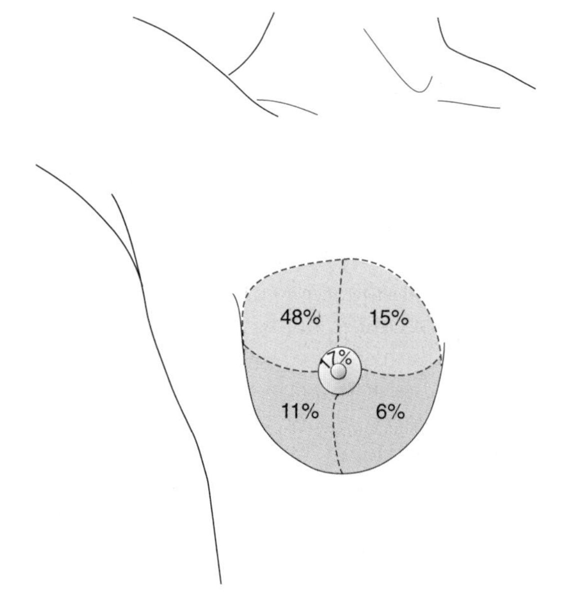

FIGURE 59-3. Locations of primary malignant breast tumors.

MEDICAL AND SURGICAL MANAGEMENT

Treatment depends on the stage of the breast tumor (Fig. 59–4). It includes surgery, which may be combined with chemotherapy, including hormone therapy, and radiation therapy. Clinical trials using immunotherapy are currently in progress.

Surgery

Surgery is performed immediately after obtaining the results of the biopsy or shortly thereafter. The type of surgery that is recommended depends on the stage of the tumor and the client's informed decision about treatment options (Table 59–2). The current trend is to perform the least mutilating procedure necessary to obtain a favorable prognosis. When compared to more extensive types of mastectomy procedures, breast conserving surgery such as lumpectomy, partial mastectomy, and segmental mastectomy have demonstrated equivalent outcomes in terms of survival rate for treatment of early stage breast cancer (National Institutes of Health, 1990).

In complex surgical procedures such as modified radical or radical mastectomy, drains may be inserted to remove serous fluid that collects under the skin. Removing fluid promotes healing and reduces the potential for infection. Also, a skin graft may be required to close the wound if a radical mastectomy is performed. Pressure dressings are applied to both the donor and recipient graft sites.

Lymphedema, soft tissue swelling from an accumulation of lymphatic fluid, occurs in some women after breast cancer surgery. The condition is a consequence of removing or irradiating the axillary lymph nodes. It is evidenced by temporary or permanent enlargement of the arm and hand on the side of the cancerous breast. Impaired lymphatic circulation predisposes to disfigurement, reduced range of motion, heaviness of the limb, skin changes, infection, and in severe cases, tissue necrosis that may require amputation of the limb.

The prognosis for women whose tumors are hormone stimulated is enhanced by removing the ovaries. The additional surgery inhibits the growth of the primary tumor or metastatic tissue derived from the primary tumor elsewhere in the body.

Depending on circumstances, chemotherapy and chemotherapy plus radiation therapy are common surgical adjuncts. The choice depends on factors

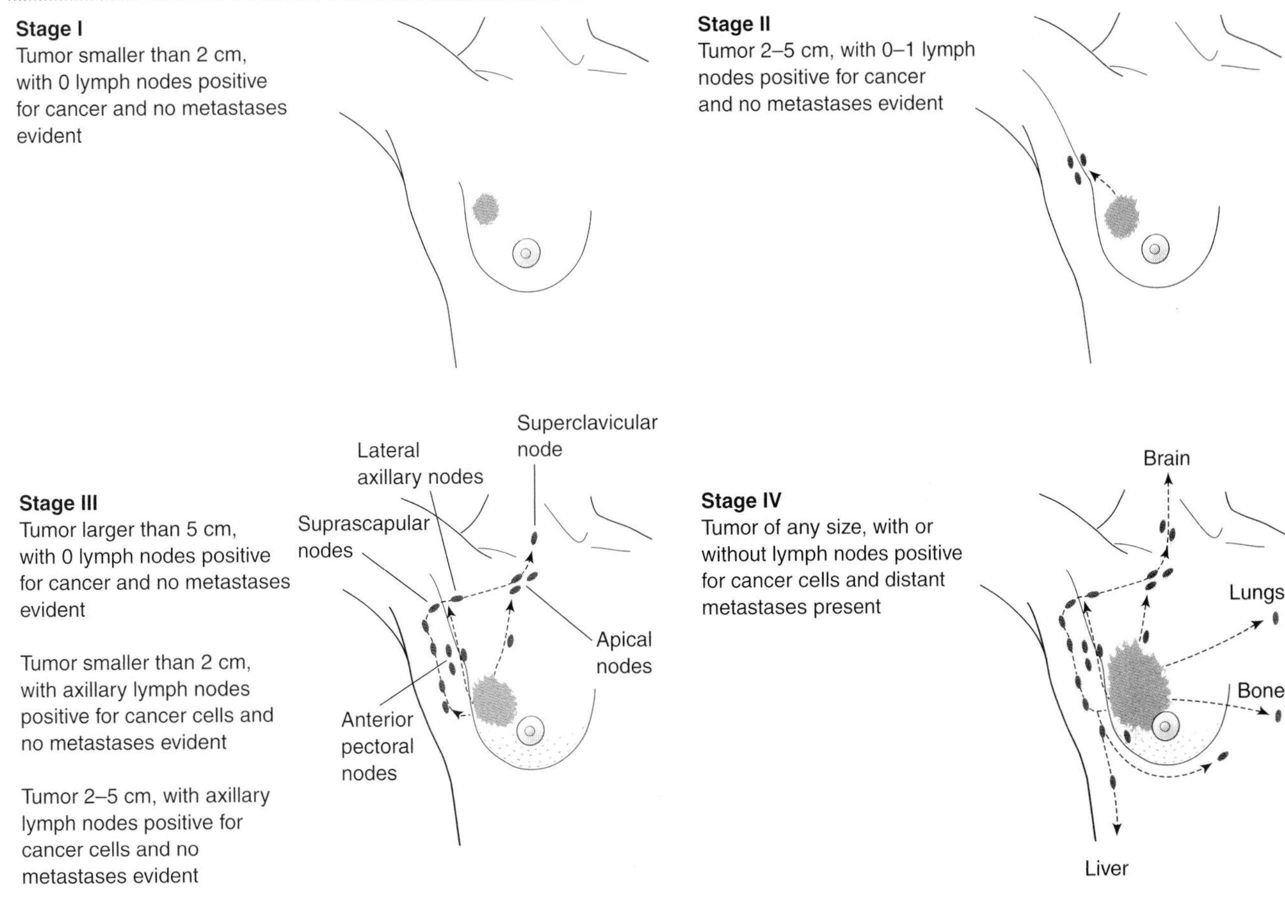

Stage I
Tumor smaller than 2 cm, with 0 lymph nodes positive for cancer and no metastases evident
Stage II
Tumor 2–5 cm, with 0–1 lymph nodes positive for cancer and no metastases evident
Stage III
Tumor larger than 5 cm, with 0 lymph nodes positive for cancer and no metastases evident
Tumor smaller than 2 cm, with axillary lymph nodes positive for cancer cells and no metastases evident
Tumor 2–5 cm, with axillary lymph nodes positive for cancer cells and no metastases evident
Superclavicular node
Lateral axillary nodes
Suprascapular nodes
Apical nodes
Anterior pectoral nodes
Stage IV
Tumor of any size, with or without lymph nodes positive for cancer cells and distant metastases present
Brain
Lungs
Bone
Liver

FIGURE 59-4. Breast cancer stages.

such as the the type of cancer and stage of the tumor, presence or absence of metastasis, and the age of the client. Bone marrow transplantation may be used if the breast cancer resists other forms of treatment.

Chemotherapy

One or more of the following drugs are given:

- An antiestrogen drug, such as tamoxifen (Nolvadex), for postmenopausal women whose tumor is hormone dependent.
- An antiprogestin drug mifepristone (RU486) blocks progesterone-dependent breast cancers as determined by progesterone receptor assay on excised tissue.
- Androgen therapy for advanced breast cancer in postmenopausal women using testolactone (Teslac).
- Single or combined antineoplastic agents, such as cyclophosphamide (Cytoxan), doxorubicin (Adriamycin), fluorouracil (5-FU), methotrexate, and prednisone. Antineoplastic drugs also are combined with drugs mentioned earlier that influence hormonal physiology.

Radiation Therapy

Radiation therapy can be given before or after surgery. If the surgeon finds that the axillary nodes contain cancer cells, a series of radiation treatments may be ordered prophylactically.

NURSING MANAGEMENT

The nurse encourages anyone who detects breast changes to see a physician immediately. The nurse prepares the client for surgery and assists with her or his safe recovery. Men who undergo a mastectomy do not face the extreme physical changes, but they still require emotional support because of the diagnosis. For breast-conserving procedures, nursing care focuses on wound management and discharge instructions.

TABLE 59-2. **Surgical Procedures for Breast Cancer**

Procedure	Description	Illustration
Lumpectomy	Only the tumor is removed; some axillary lymph nodes may be excised at the same time for microscopic examination.	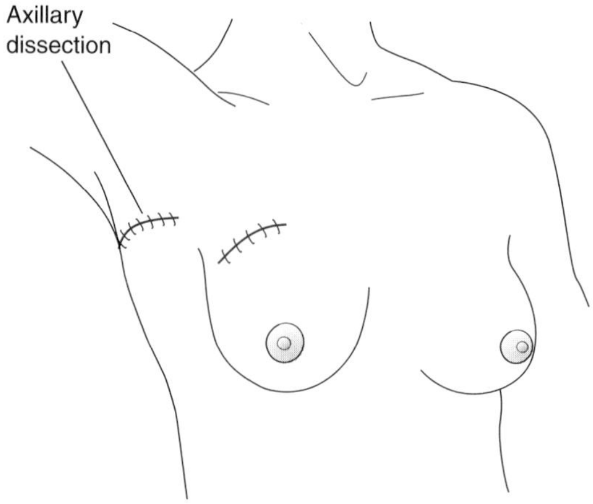 Axillary dissection
Partial or segmental mastectomy	The tumor and some breast tissue and some lymph nodes are removed.	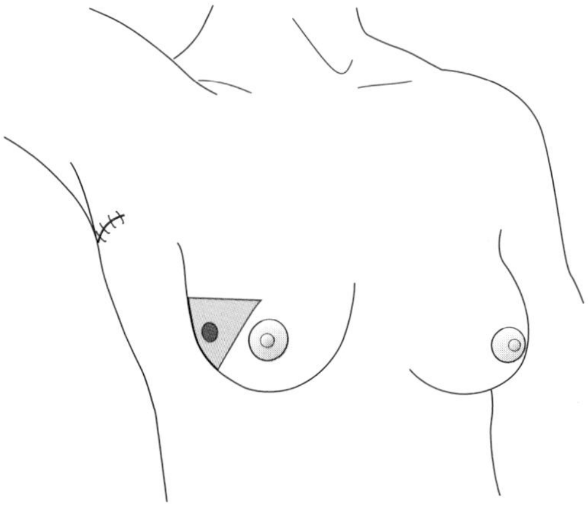
Simple or total mastectomy	All breast tissue is removed. No lymph node dissection is performed.	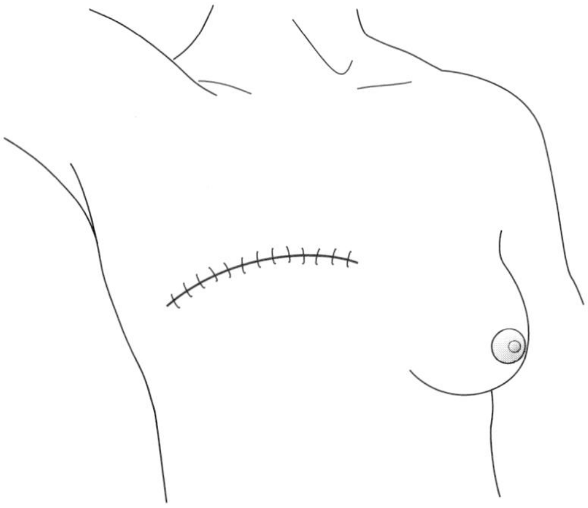

(continued)

TABLE 59-2. *(Continued)*

Procedure	Description	Illustration
Subcutaneous mastectomy	All breast tissue is removed, but the skin and nipple are left intact.	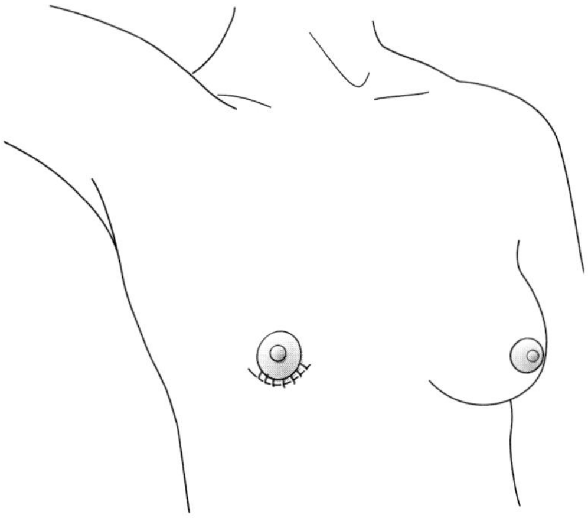
Modified radical mastectomy	The breast, some lymph nodes, the lining over the chest muscles and the pectoralis minor muscle are removed.	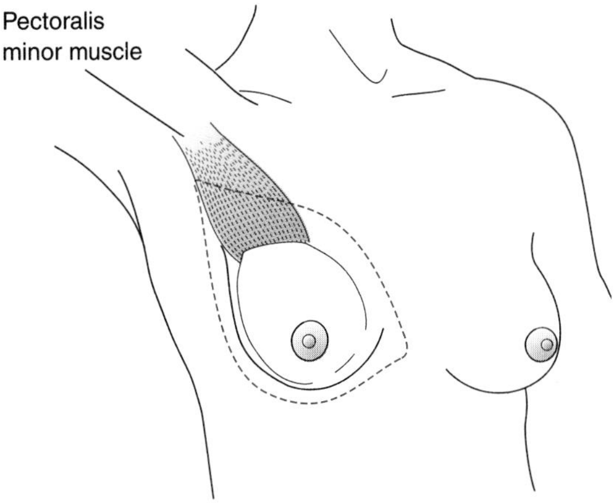 Pectoralis minor muscle
Radical mastectomy	The breast, axillary lymph nodes, and pectoralis major and minor muscles are removed. In some instances, sternal lymph nodes also are removed.	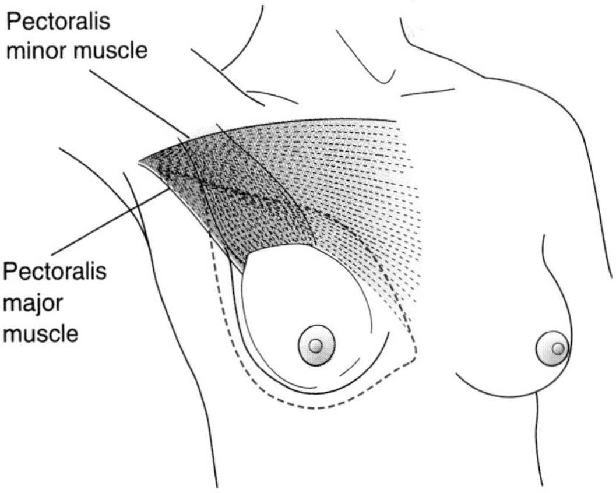 Pectoralis minor muscle Pectoralis major muscle

NURSING PROCESS
The Client Undergoing a Modified Radical or Radical Mastectomy

Assessment

A complete medical, drug, allergy, and family history is obtained. Vital signs are taken, and the client is weighed.

The client's records are reviewed for information about the location of the breast lesion, the diagnostic tests performed before admission (if any), and the information the physician has given the client about the type and extent of surgery.

Diagnosis and Planning

See Chapter 24 for the perioperative standards of care. In addition to standard care, the nursing management of a client undergoing a modified radical or radical mastectomy includes, but is not limited to the following:

Nursing Diagnoses and Collaborative Problems	Nursing Interventions
Preoperatively **Anxiety** and **Fear** related to undergoing an unfamiliar experience and the potential consequences of the disease and its treatment **Goal:** The client will indicate an increase in emotional comfort.	Provide an opportunity for the client to express feelings and discuss concerns. Answer any and all questions or consult with other health team members in matters that involve their expertise. Collaborate with the physician on arranging for a visit from a *Reach to Recovery* or *I Can Cope* volunteer sponsored by the American Cancer Society. Do not stifle crying; stay with the client when emotions are overwhelming. Encourage the client's significant other or whomever the client turns to for support to remain with the client as much and as long as possible. Keep the client informed of the routine that will be followed in preparation for surgery and care afterwards.
Knowledge Deficit related to surgical routines **Goal:** The client will be able to paraphrase the preoperative and postoperative routine.	Explain that the arm on the surgical side may be elevated and movement away from the body (abduction) may be temporarily restricted.
Postoperatively **Potential Complication: Hemorrhage and Shock** **Goal:** Hemorrhage and shock will be managed and minimized.	Monitor vital signs according to agency routines. *Do not take the blood pressures on the arm on the side of the mastectomy.* Check the color and amount of blood loss from the wound and drain, if one is present. Feel underneath the client's side or back for obscured evidence of bleeding. Administer intravenous fluids or blood transfusions at the rate prescribed.
Risk for Ineffective Breathing and **Ineffective Airway Clearance** related to pain, weak cough, and presence of bulky dressing **Goal:** The client will be well oxygenated as evidenced by an oxygen saturation of 90% or above and clear lung sounds.	Instruct the client to deep breathe and cough every 2 hours during waking hours or use an incentive spirometer. Splint the incision to reduce discomfort. Administer oxygen as prescribed. Instruct the client to self-administer analgesia prior to deep breathing and coughing if a patient-controlled analgesia (PCA) pump is being used.
Pain related to tissue trauma **Goal:** The client's discomfort will be controlled within a tolerable level.	Administer pain medication liberally according to prescribed dose and frequency. Avoid arm injections on the same side as the surgery. Monitor response to analgesia 30 minutes after administration or more frequently if PCA is in use. Pin the tubing of the drain or the drain collection chamber to the client's gown to avoid pulling at the insertion site. Implement nursing techniques such as changing positions, relaxation, distraction, and guided imagery (see Chap. 20) to supplement or complement analgesia. Collaborate with the physician if pain control is inadequate.
Impaired Skin Integrity and Risk for Infection secondary to surgical wound **Goal:** The incision will heal as evidenced by intact skin. The client will be free of infection as evidenced by absence of wound drainage, temperature and white blood cell count within normal range.	Limit movement, especially abduction, of the arm on the side of surgery until the wound edges are intact. Inspect the wound for pockets of swelling, for drainage, odor, redness or separation of the suture line. Check the color and amount of blood loss from the wound and drain. Feel underneath the client's side or back for obscured evidence of bleeding.

	Empty and re-establish negative suction in tissue drains at least once per shift. Administer antibiotic therapy as prescribed. Monitor the trend in temperature and white blood cell counts. Allow the client to shower after the sutures and drains are removed.
Risk for Impaired Peripheral Tissue Perfusion (lymphedema) related to compromised flow of lymphatic fluid **Goal:** Tissue swelling will be controlled as evidenced by loose skin over the arm and hand.	*Do not take blood pressures, give injections, administer intravenous infusions, or have blood drawn from the arm on the side of the mastectomy.* Support and elevate the arm on the side of the mastectomy with pillows so it is kept higher than the heart. Place the arm in a sling when the client ambulates initially; eventually the arm can be positioned at the client's side. Show the client how to squeeze and release a soft rubber ball or a rolled pair of cotton socks several times a day to promote venous and lymphatic circulation. Remove and reapply an elastic roller bandage from the fingers to the axilla twice a day, or insert the affected arm into a pneumatic sleeve, an air-filled device that mechanically pumps the arm for a half hour or the prescribed amount of time twice a day. Assess the hand for swelling, dusky color, delayed nail blanching, coldness, and tingling. Report abnormal findings.
Impaired Physical Mobility related to alteration in pectoral chest muscles **Goal:** The client will achieve full range of arm motion.	Start active exercises of the affected arm on the first or second postoperative day or later if the physician indicates a need to postpone them (skin grafts may need additional time to heal). Begin with flexing and extending the fingers, wrist, and elbow. Later, encourage the client to use the affected arm to perform oral hygiene, hair combing, and face washing. Show the client how to face and "finger-walk" up a wall in the room. Mark the client's progress with masking tape so that the height can be exceeded with subsequent efforts. Loop a rope or cord around a shower rod and raise and lower each arm in pulley fashion. Tie a string or rope to a door knob and have the client turn the rope in a circular fashion.
Risk for Injury related to change in center of gravity secondary to extensive removal of chest tissue **Goal:** The client will not fall.	Assist the client during periods of ambulation. Walk on the client's unaffected side. Instruct the client to keep the shoulders level and the muscles relaxed when walking.
Grieving related to loss of breast **Goal:** The client will express grief and deal with losses.	Avoid trying to diminish the significance of the loss. Acknowledge the client's grief and reinforce that feeling angry or sad is normal and expected. Stay with the client and ensure privacy during emotional periods. Avoid administering prescribed sedatives or tranquilizers as a substitute for spending time with the client. Encourage sharing with those who can be empathic like another breast cancer survivor.
Risk for Disturbance in Body Image, Ineffective Individual Coping, Altered Sexual Patterns related to feeling a loss of physical attractiveness and sexual desirability **Goal:** The client will accept body changes, use positive coping strategies, and experience satisfactory sexual activity.	Suggest that the client pad a bra with one or two cotton socks until a prosthesis is fitted in 6 to 8 weeks. Inform the client that cosmetic breast reconstruction is an option to discuss with the surgeon. Advocate that the client and sexual partner openly express to each other how they are affected emotionally by the surgery. Discuss methods of dealing with the absence of the breast during sexual activities such as no or low lighting during intercourse, or wearing the upper portion of lingerie.

Evaluation and Expected Outcomes

Preoperative

- Anxiety is reduced.
- Demonstrates understanding of preoperative preparations
- Demonstrates understanding of postoperative management, including coughing, deep breathing, and leg exercises.
- Demonstrates understanding of the type of surgery and potential postsurgical treatment modalities.
- Openly discusses and asks questions about surgery.

Postoperative

- Bleeding is controlled; shock does not occur.
- Gas exchange is adequate.
- Pain is controlled.
- Incision heals without complications.
- Circulation is maintained in operative arm; arms are comparable size.
- Uses arm and hand of operative side.
- Performs postmastectomy exercises.
- No injuries occur.
- Adjusts to loss of breast.
- Openly discusses care of the incision; asks questions about home care.

Client Teaching

Most clients are not hospitalized long after mastectomy. Therefore, it is important to provide early discharge instructions and possibly make arrangements for home care. Before discharge:

- Explain wound and drain care or to arrange for home health nursing.
- Assess availability of family assistance at home.
- Look for and report any signs of infection or impaired wound healing such as drainage or significant pale or dusky appearance to the skin around the incision.
- Stress continuation of arm exercises.
- Arrange for follow-up examinations by the surgeon.
- Instruct the client on the self-administration of prescribed drug therapy.
- Tell the client to expect that there will be some residual numbness or tingling on the chest wall and the inner side of the arm from the axilla to the elbow, which may take as long as a year to resolve.
- Suggest applying cream or lotion to the arm if the skin tends to be dry.
- Explain that when selecting a prosthesis, those that are filled with fluid assume natural contours like the other breast, feel like normal breast tissue, and even radiate body warmth.
- Advise against lifting or carrying objects that weigh over 15 lb and vigorous repetitive movements with the affected arm.
- Discourage sleeping on the affected arm or wearing constrictive clothing that impairs circulation.
- Reinforce that blood pressures, injections, drawing blood, or starting intravenous infusions are contraindicated in the arm on the side of the mastectomy.
- Recommend wearing gloves while doing yard or housework to prevent injuries that may heal slowly or become infected.
- Advise using an electric razor for shaving axillary hair.
- Instruct to continue to perform monthly BSE on the intact breast and have the intact breast clinically examined each year by a physician along with a mammogram.

Metastatic Breast Cancer

Despite treatment even in the early stages of breast cancer, some women develop metastatic disease.

PATHOPHYSIOLOGY

Lymph nodes are most commonly involved in metastasis, with bone and pulmonary involvement following in order of frequency. The brain and liver may also become involved.

ASSESSMENT FINDINGS

Signs and Symptoms

Metastases often cause pain in the new site. When bone becomes involved, *pathologic fractures* (a fracture after slight or no trauma) are possible.

Diagnostic Findings

Radiographs of the lungs, spine, or other areas of the body are used to detect metastases. Magnetic resonance imaging or computed tomography scanning may also be performed. These studies are done before or after treating the primary tumor.

MEDICAL MANAGEMENT

Treatment is aimed at providing the greatest period of *palliation* (relieving symptoms without curing the disease) for the client. It varies with the physician and specific type of metastasis. Large doses of estrogen or testosterone sometimes alleviate the pain, weight loss, and malaise of metastatic cancer. Intramuscular androgen (testosterone) therapy is used especially when metastases are to bone. All forms of treatment carry the possibility of unpleasant effects and complications. For palliative purposes, radiation therapy may be used to treat regional or distant metastases (especially to bone), or local tumor recurrence of the chest wall.

NURSING MANAGEMENT

For nursing care of the client undergoing chemotherapy or radiation and caring for the terminally ill client with cancer see Chapters 19 and 25.

Cosmetic Breast Procedures

Some women undergo various cosmetic breast procedures, collectively referred to as **mammoplasty,** for a number of reasons, but primarily to improve their appearance.

Breast Reconstruction

Breast reconstruction is a surgical procedure in which the area of a mastectomy is refashioned to simulate the contour of a breast and optionally create the nipple and areola. The procedure is accomplished by using either an artificial implant filled with saline or autogenous (self) tissue. Reconstruction can begin at the time of a mastectomy if sufficient skin is spared, or it can be performed later.

ARTIFICIAL IMPLANTS

Before an implant can produce an optimum cosmetic appearance, the skin and tissue on the chest wall is expanded to provide a large enough space to fill and approximate the size of the remaining breast. Tissue expansion is achieved by stretching the chest wall over several months with an inflatable or saline-filled pocket (Fig. 59–5).

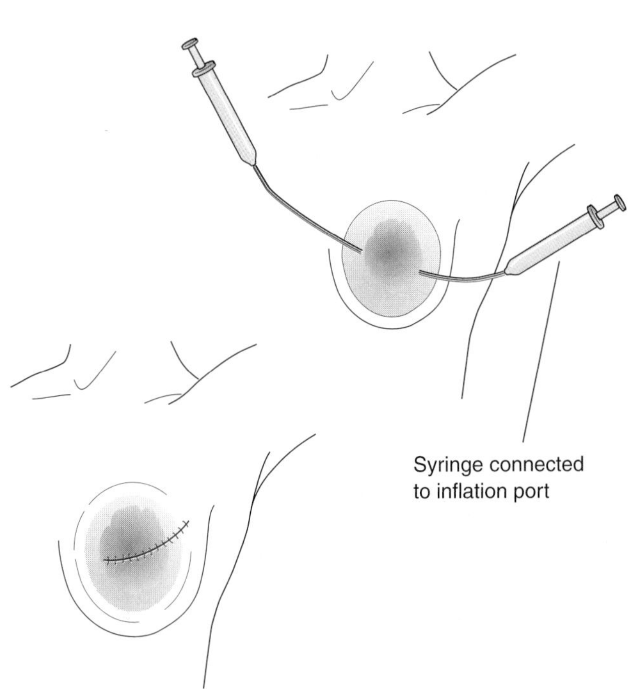

FIGURE 59-5. Tissue expander and breast implant.

Although there has been no definitive proof of a correlation between silicone implants and connective tissue and autoimmune diseases (Gabriel et al., 1994; Sancbez-Guerrero, Colditz, & Karlson, 1995), silicone implants are no longer used except in clinical studies. Saline implants are now used for breast enhancement procedures.

AUTOGENOUS TISSUE

Reconstructing the breast with autogenous tissue provides a more natural look and feel to the breast. The tissue is harvested similarly to a "tummy tuck" (abdominoplasty) from the rectus abdominis muscle along with its adjoining skin and fat (Fig. 59–6). Other donor sites such as a portion of the latissimus dorsi or gluteal muscles may be used. Removing donor tissue tends to leave a physical deformity some of which may be more obvious than others.

If a woman desires a nipple, it is reconstructed from tissue from the opposite nipple, the ear, or toe. Tissue for the areola is selected from a site with a sim-

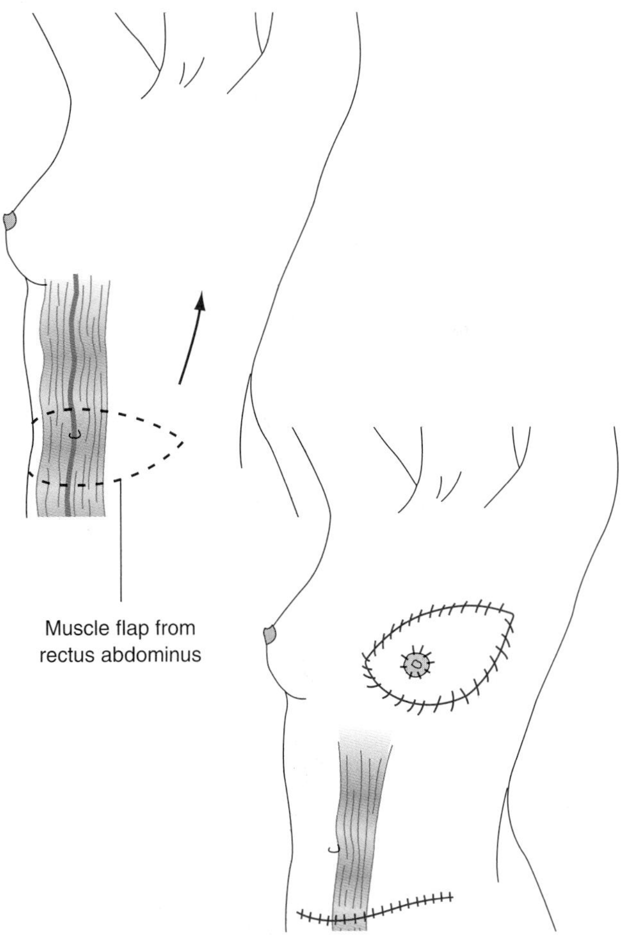

FIGURE 59-6. Autogenous breast reconstruction.

ilar color match like the inner thigh or vaginal labia. It may also be created by pigmented tattoo.

OPPOSITE BREAST REDUCTION

The size of a reconstructed breast is limited by the amount of tissue that remains; thus, there may be potential asymmetry. Opposite breast reduction is a surgical procedure that is performed to reduce the volume of a healthy breast so it more closely resembles the size of a reconstructed breast. The procedure, although done for different reasons, is the same as a reduction mammoplasty.

Reduction Mammoplasty

A **reduction mammoplasty** is an overnight surgical procedure in which glandular breast tissue, fat, and skin are removed bilaterally to decrease the size of large pendulous breasts. Most candidates for a reduction mammoplasty wear a size D cup or larger brassiere, experience discomfort in the shoulders or back, skin irritation beneath the breasts, difficulty in finding suitable clothing, self-consciousness, or low self-esteem.

To reduce the size of the breasts, an incision is made around the nipple through which tissue is removed. The loose skin is tightened to reposition the areola and nipple. The client is discharged with a bulky chest dressing and sometimes a small wound drain.

Breast Lift

Ptosis, or drooping, of the breast(s) is corrected with a breast lift or more technically, **mastopexy.** The sagging skin and low nipple placement that occur as a consequence of weight loss and aging are corrected similarly to reduction mammoplasty although the incision and scar line are smaller and the recovery time is shorter. In some cases the size or contour of the breast is enhanced with breast augmentation techniques.

Breast Augmentation

Women who wish to enlarge their breasts may choose *breast augmentation*, which is similar to reconstructing the breast using an artificial implant.

Nursing Management

Maintain the client in a semi-Fowler's position following cosmetic breast surgery to promote drainage from the operative site. Give analgesics for pain and inspect the operative site for changes in color and temperature. Maintain dressings and support bras to minimize stretching of the tissues and suture line.

Client Teaching

Provide clients undergoing cosmetic breast surgery with information that applies to the type of surgery being performed. General guidelines include:

- Have a mammogram to verify that there are no malignancies before having any cosmetic surgery.
- Continue to perform BSE and have clinical breast examinations (inspection and palpation) by the physician.
- Expect reduced sensation in the nipple, a certain amount of scarring, and temporary discomfort when moving the arms and shoulders following cosmetic breast surgery.
- Wear a soft bra for 3 to 6 weeks postoperatively except when bathing or taking a shower.
- Avoid activities, such as vigorous sports, which may result in injury to the the breasts until healing is complete.

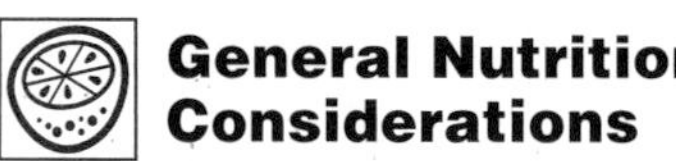

General Nutritional Considerations

Although once suspected as a risk factor, studies have failed to prove that a high-fat diet increases the risk of breast cancer. Studies on the protective role of fruits and vegetables, soy, and fiber are also inconclusive. The strongest link between diet and breast cancer is with alcohol: drinking more than one alcoholic drink per day may increase the risk of breast cancer by 40%. It is possible that the greatest effect of nutrition on breast cancer occurs during puberty or adolescence, when breasts are still forming.

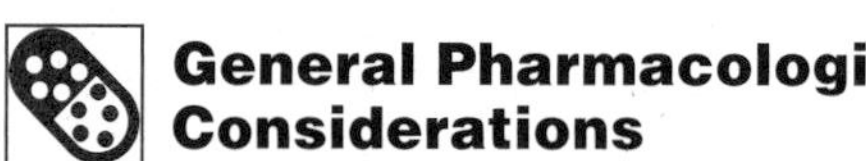

General Pharmacologic Considerations

Metastases of breast cancer to soft tissue and bone may respond to antineoplastic drugs. These drugs may cause bone marrow depression, granulocytopenia, anemia, nausea and vomiting, hypotension, dermatitis, malaise, diarrhea, and stomatitis.

Pain management is an important issue in managing patients with breast cancer metastasis. The opioid analgesics morphine and fentanyl are the drugs most often used for relief of cancer pain. Morphine can be given orally, rectally, subcutaneously, intravenously, and intramuscularly, and via epidural catheter. Fentanyl (Duragesic) is given transdermally for pain. Patients taking these drugs must be monitored for adverse reactions that include excessive sedation, confusion, weakness, hypotension, constipation, dry mouth, nausea, vomiting, and anorexia.

When administering danzol (Danocrine) for fibrocystic breast disease, amenorrhea may occur, especially with higher doses. Treatment with danazol for fibrocystic disease usually continues for 4 to 6 months and may be continued up to 9 months, if necessary, to eliminate cystic lesions. Inform the patient to notify the health care provider if regular menses do not resume within 90 days after discontinuing the drug.

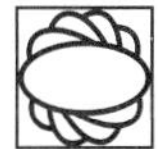

General Gerontologic Considerations

Many breast disorders that are hormonally influenced regress after menopause.

The risk for breast cancer increases with age. Older adult women need to continue performing monthly BSE and have yearly clinical breast examinations and mammograms.

With age the breast tissue atrophies causing sagging and hanging of the breast. Fibrotic changes may cause some retraction of the nipple in women.

In the older client, surgery for breast cancer may be limited to a lumpectomy or simple mastectomy.

Occasionally breast tumors that have been present for years become more evident with age, making detection easier.

SUMMARY OF KEY CONCEPTS

- Clients with breast disorders may exhibit one or more of the following signs and symptoms: breast pain, tenderness, or fullness; a cystic or solid breast mass; nipple discharge; and a change in the normal appearance of the breast.
- Three techniques for analyzing cells of a breast lesion include incisional, excisional, and aspirational biopsy. These diagnostic procedures involve removing some or all of the suspicious tissue or a portion of tissue fluid.
- Mastitis and breast abscess are two infectious and inflammatory breast conditions that are common among breast-feeding mothers. They are acquired as a consequence of an obstruction in the ducts that deliver milk from the nipple or colonization by pathogenic microorganisms.
- Breast-feeding mothers may prevent or eliminate infectious and inflammatory disorders by nursing their infants regularly, offering the opposite breast at each feeding, and ensuring that their hands and breasts are clean.
- Fibrocystic breast disease and fibroadenoma are two benign breast conditions that usually occur in premenopausal woman. They each are discovered by palpating one or more lumps within the breast. Clients with fibrocystic disease experience more discomfort just prior to menstruation. Those with a fibroadenoma are often asymptomatic; their breast mass does not enlarge or regress during the menstrual cycle.
- Breast self-examination is performed monthly by inspecting the breasts and nipples visually and palpating the entire breast tissue that extends into the axilla and the axillary lymph nodes.
- The current recommendations for mammography are that all women at age 40 should have an initial mammogram; thereafter through the age of 49, women should have mammography repeated every 1 to 2 years; at the age of 50 all women should have yearly mammograms.
- Groups that are at higher risk for developing breast cancer include women with close blood relatives with breast cancer, aging women, women who are obese, had an early menarche, late menopause, and women who have had no children or who have had children after age 30. Additional risk factors include those exposed to ionizing radiation as children or adolescents, women already diagnosed with cancer of the breast or elsewhere, and those who consume a high-fat, high-calorie diet.
- Signs and symptoms of breast cancer are a painless mass in the breast, bloody discharge from the nipple, a dimpling of the skin over the lesion, retraction of the breast nipple, and a difference in size between the breasts.
- Breast cancer is treated by surgery, chemotherapy, and radiation therapy, or any combination of these three.
- Surgical approaches for removing a malignant breast tumor include: lumpectomy, partial mastectomy, total mastectomy, subcutaneous mastectomy, modified radical mastectomy, and radical mastectomy.
- The current tendency is to perform the least mutilating surgical procedure necessary to obtain a favorable prognosis.
- Lymphedema occurs in some women after breast cancer treatment. It causes disfigurement and increases the lifetime potential for infection and poor healing.
- The nursing management of clients with breast cancer includes relieving their anxiety and fear and providing preoperative preparation and postoperative care. Postoperatively, the nurse monitors for surgical complications, promotes adequate breathing, reduces pain, promotes venous and lymphatic circulation, cares for the surgical wound, initiates hand and arm exercises, prevents falls, supports the client during the normal grief process, helps the client cope with body changes and sexual consequences, and teaches the client how to manage self-care after discharge.
- Breast cancer commonly spreads from the axillary lymphatics to the bones, lungs, brain, and liver.
- Following a modified radical or radical mastectomy some women elect to have a breast reconstructed either with an artificial implant or with autogenous tissue. In some cases the opposite breast is reconstructed to achieve bilateral symmetry.
- Women who feel a need to change the size, shape, or contour of normal breasts may have a reduction mammoplasty, breast lift, or breast augmentation.

CRITICAL THINKING EXERCISES

1. How might the signs and symptom differ among women with fibrocystic breast disease, a fibroadenoma, and malignant breast tumor.
2. What advice is appropriate for preventing breast cancer?

3. Discuss the options that are available for cosmetic breast reconstruction.

Suggested Readings

Gabriel, S. E., O'Fallon, W. M., Kurland, L. T., et al. (1994). Risk of connective tissue diseases and other disorders after breast implantation. *New England Journal of Medicine, 330,* 1697–1702.

Greenfield, L. J., Mulholland, M. W., Oldham, K. T., et al. (1997). *Surgery, scientific principles and practice* (2nd ed.). Philadelphia: Lippincott-Raven.

Harwood, K. (1996). Straight talk about breast cancer. *Nursing, 26*(10), 39–44.

Jeffries, E. (1997). Home health care for patients receiving one-day mastectomy. *Home Healthcare Nurse, 15*(1), 30–37.

National Institutes of Health. (1990, June 18–21). *Early stage breast cancer. Consensus statement.* (Vol. 8, No. 6). Bethesda, MD: Author.

Norwood, S. L. (1990). Fibrocystic breast disease: An update and review. *Journal of Obstetric, Gynecologic, and Neonatal Nursing, 19*(2), 116–121.

Sanchez-Guerrero, J., Colditz, G. A., & Karlson, E. W. (1995). Silicone breast implants and the risk of connective tissue diseases and symptoms. *New England Journal of Medicine, 332,* 1666–1670.

Wolfe, S. (1997). The great mammogram debate. *RN, 60*(8), 40–44.

Additional Resources

OBGYN Net
http//www.obgyn.net
American Cancer Society
http://www.cancer.org/
National Cancer Institute Information Service
(800) 4-CANCER
Y-ME National Breast Cancer Organization
(800) 221–2141
Breast Implants
c/o Food and Drug Administration
HFE-88
Rockville, MD 20857
Implant Hotline
(800) 532–444

Chapter 60

Caring for Clients With Disorders of the Male Reproductive System

KEY TERMS

Benign prostatic hyperplasia
Cryptorchidism
Digital rectal examination
Ejaculation
Epididymitis
Impotence
Orchiectomy
Orchitis
Orchiopexy
Prostatectomy
Prostatic specific antigen
Retrograde ejaculation
Semen
Spermatogenesis
Testicular self-examination
Transillumination
Tumor markers
Vasectomy

LEARNING OBJECTIVES

On completion of this chapter, the reader will:

- List the external and internal structures of the male reproductive system.
- Identify at least three possible consequences of disorders that affect the male reproductive system.
- Give four examples of structural disorders that affect the male reproductive system.
- Explain the technique and purpose for performing testicular self-examinations.
- List three infectious or inflammatory conditions and identify how they are acquired.
- Discuss two erectile disorders and explain their effects on fertility and sexuality.
- Identify two methods for treating impotence.
- Describe the nursing plan of care for a client who receives a penile implant.
- Explain how prostatic hyperplasia compromises urinary elimination and the symptoms it produces.
- Discuss the nursing management of a client undergoing a prostatectomy.
- Compare and contrast three male reproductive cancers as to age of onset, incidence, and treatment outcomes.
- List the home care instructions following a vasectomy.

The physiologic functions of the male reproductive structures include generation of gender-specific sexual characteristics, and the manufacture and transportation of sperm and seminal fluid. The lower urinary tract and reproductive system structures are so closely associated that disorders frequently affect both systems. Congenital or acquired structural abnormalities, infectious and inflammatory conditions, erection disorders, benign prostatic enlargement, and cancer are all threats to male reproductive health.

Anatomy and Physiology

External and Internal Structures

The external male genitalia consists of the *penis* and *scrotum*. The *testes* (sing., testis) lie within the scrotum and are responsible for spermatogenesis, sperm production, and secretion of testosterone. *Testosterone* is the male sex hormone that pertains to the development and maintenance of secondary male sex characteristics. The structures that extend from the testes, the *epididymides* (sing., epididymis), *vas deferens* (or ductus deferens), *seminal vesicles*, *prostate gland*, and *bulbourethral* (Cowper's) *glands* (Fig. 60–1), form a complex secretory and ductal system. Their functions are to nurture and enhance the motility of sperm and ensure their survival once they are released from the body. The *prostate gland* is an accessory sex organ that surrounds the urethra at the neck of the bladder. It secretes fluid that neutralizes acidic vaginal secretions.

Spermatogenesis and Ejaculation

Under the influence of follicle-stimulating hormone (FSH) and testosterone, sperm are manufactured and sustained in the *seminiferous tubules* of the testes until they are motile—a process that takes approximately 64 days. They then pass into the epididymides and vas deferens where they complete their maturation. The seminal vesicles that empty into the vas deferens produce *seminal fluid*, which adds volume to the sperm and nourishes them after ejaculation.

Ejaculation is the discharge of **semen,** the fluid that contains the sperm, from the body. The process of ejaculation occurs as a result of rhythmic contraction of the muscles of the vas deferens and the penis during orgasm and sexual climax. The normal volume of ejaculate is 2.5 to 6 mL, which contains an average of 400 million spermatozoa (Bullock, 1996). A count of less than 20 to 50 million spermatozoa per mL results in infertility.

Assessment

History

A general health and family history is obtained (see Chap. 4) as is a detailed sexual history. A sexual history includes questions that elicit information on:

- Risks for sexually transmitted diseases
- Contraceptive practices
- Ability to achieve or sustain an erection

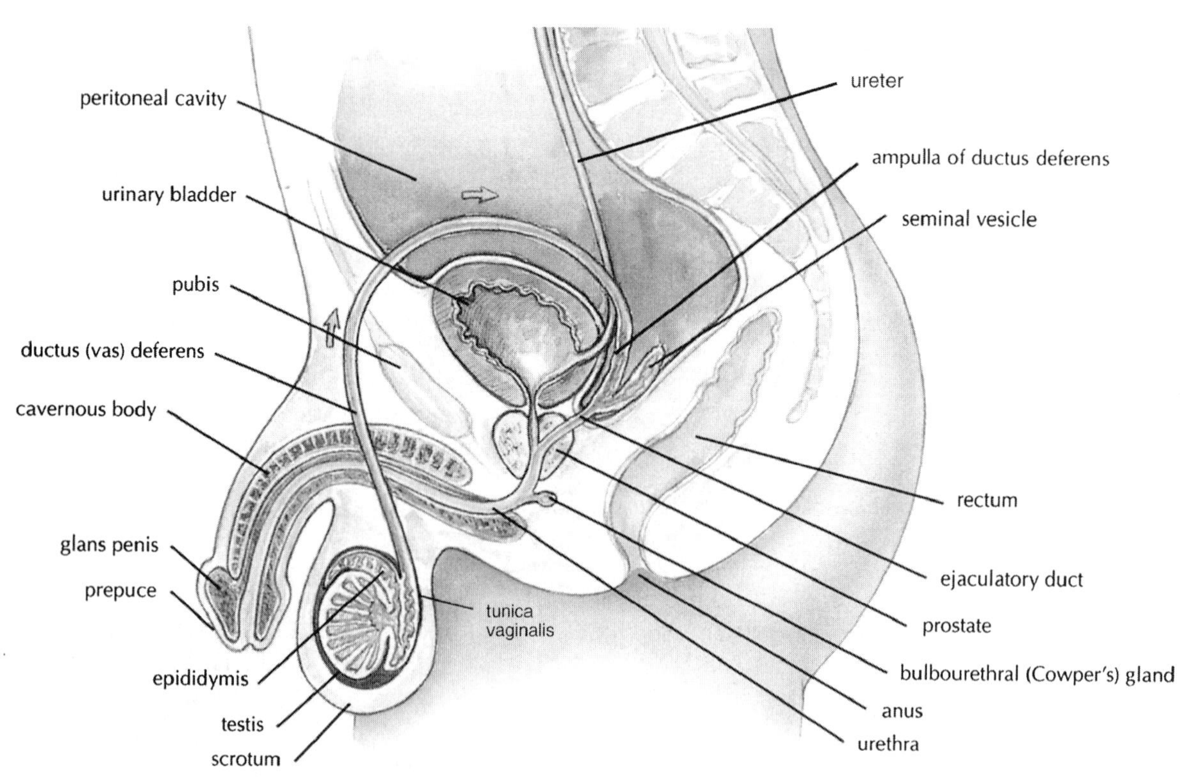

FIGURE 60-1. Anatomy of male reproductive system. Arrows show path of sperm.

- Pain during sexual intercourse
- Premature ejaculation or other concerns of a sexual nature
- Inability of a sex partner to conceive
- Prior treatment (including drug therapy, diagnostic tests, or surgery) that relate to the genitourinary system.

Physical Examination

The external genitalia are inspected, looking for abnormalities such as skin lesions and urethral discharge. The testes are palpated for tumors and the scrotum examined. **Transillumination,** shining a light through the scrotum, provides clues about the density of scrotal tissue. A **digital rectal examination** (DRE) is performed to assess the prostate for size as well as evidence of tumor. Yearly DREs are recommended for men over 40 or 50 years of age.

Diagnostic Tests

Several diagnostic tests are commonly performed to evaluate the male genitourinary tract. See Nursing Guidelines 60–1 for appropriate nursing care.

TRANSRECTAL ULTRASONOGRAPHY

Transrectal ultrasonography (sonogram) is a test in which a lubricated probe is inserted into the rectum to obtain a view of the prostate gland from various angles. The test is indicated in cases where the prostate gland is enlarged or the prostate specific antigen (see later discussion) is elevated.

CYSTOSCOPY

In a *cystoscopy*, an illuminated optical instrument called a cystoscope is inserted into the meatus to inspect the bladder, prostate, and urethra. This aids in evaluating the degree of encroachment by the prostate on the urethra.

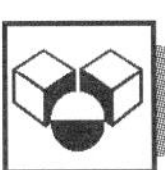

Nursing Guidelines 60-1

Nursing Management of the Client Undergoing Genitourinary Diagnostic Testing

Test	Preprocedure Care	Postprocedure Care
All tests	Explain procedure, answer questions in a calm and reassuring manner. Use techniques of therapeutic communication to provide an opportunity for client to express concerns. Talk with client and inform him of each step as test proceeds.	Assist client to resume a comfortable position and clean up gels or lubricants. Answer questions about when test results will be available and when normal activity can resume. Provide client with written posttest instructions, if applicable.
Ultrasound of the prostate	Assure client that test is not painful; administer or have client self-administer an enema; encourage client to focus on breathing slowly to reduce anxiety.	Assist client in removing excess lubricant. Explain that client may resume normal activities.
Prostatic biopsy	Inform client that a local anesthetic may be used to minimize discomfort; administer or have client self-administer an enema if a rectal approach is used.	Provide information about site care. Instruct client that sitz baths and a mild analgesic will reduce discomfort. Tell client that a prophylactic antibiotic will be given and stress that medication be taken as ordered.
Testicular biopsy	Inform client that a local anesthetic will be administered.	In the case of an incisional rather than a needle biopsy, instruct the client to refrain from tub baths until the sutures are removed.
Cystoscopy	Inform client that he will experience bladder fullness and a strong desire to void. Inform client that an anesthetic lubricant will be instilled into the urethra to minimize discomfort and facilitate passage of cystoscope.	Instruct client to monitor voiding pattern and to report any bleeding or difficulty urinating. Inform client that prophylactic antibiotics will be given and stress that medication be taken as ordered.

TISSUE BIOPSY

A needle biopsy of prostatic tissue is obtained for analysis by the perineal or rectal approach. A testicular biopsy is obtained for evaluation of spermatozoa production or to diagnose a testicular malignancy.

CULTURES

Cultures are obtained from urethral secretions, skin lesions, or urine. Prostatic fluid can be expressed during a DRE and also sent for culture.

FERTILITY TESTS

Fertility studies include a semen analysis to determine the sperm count, sperm motility, and the presence of abnormal sperm. Other laboratory tests may include measuring the level of plasma luteinizing hormone (LH), which is necessary for the release of testosterone from the testes. A decrease in the blood level of LH may be responsible for decreased testosterone production and infertility.

TUMOR MARKERS

Tumor markers are substances synthesized by tumors that are released into the circulation in excessive amounts. The **prostatic specific antigen** (PSA) assay is a blood test that detects prostate cancer. Although an elevated PSA does not always indicate a malignancy, it is now possible to differentiate free PSA in total PSA. High percentages of free PSA are more often associated with benign disease, whereas low percentages of free PSA indicate malignancy. Regular PSA tests assist in the early diagnosis and staging of prostatic cancer, and in evaluating the effectiveness of the cancer treatment. Other blood tests that suggest the presence of cancer are elevated levels of alpha-fetoprotein (AFP), beta-human chorionic gonadotropin (bHCG), and total urine estrogens. Alkaline and acid phosphatase blood tests determine if prostatic cancer has spread to the bone.

Structural Abnormalities

Structural abnormalities of the male genitalia may be congenital or acquired. These various abnormalities, including cryptorchidism, torsion of the spermatic cord, disorders of the foreskin, and benign scrotal swelling, often require surgical repair. Nursing management after these surgeries is similar.

Cryptorchidism

Cryptorchidism is a condition in which one or both testes fail to descend into the scrotum. The undescended testis(es) may lie in the inguinal canal, in the abdominal cavity, or, rarely, in the perineum or femoral canal. The scrotum is essentially empty, but otherwise the client is asymptomatic. During childhood or at puberty, undescended testes occasionally find their way into the scrotum without treatment. At least one testis must be within the scrotum to ensure production of sperm.

The cause of undescended testes is unknown. However, the longer the testis(es) remains undescended during childhood, the greater the potential that fertility will be compromised. If the condition is not corrected by age 2, the seminiferous tubules atrophy and fibrose. Some male clients are treated with a short trial of androgen hormone therapy when the condition is diagnosed. If a response is not noted within a brief period of time (3–6 weeks), surgery to secure the testis within the scrotum, called **orchiopexy**, is performed (Kelley, 1997). A second consequence of undescended testes is a 20% to 40% greater risk for testicular cancer (see later discussion).

NURSING MANAGEMENT

All men, especially those who have had cryptorchidism, are taught to perform **testicular self-examination** (Fig. 60–2) to detect the presence of an abnormal mass within the scrotum. Instruct clients to examine the testicles monthly, preferably when warm, such as in the shower.

After surgery, inspect the dressing. Check for the presence of a rubber band secured to the upper thigh. The rubber band provides traction on the relocated testes. Ensure that the traction remains taut.

Torsion of the Spermatic Cord

Torsion means to twist. In this case, it is the spermatic cord that twists, kinking the artery and compromising blood flow to the testicle (Fig. 60–3). The condition occurs in prepubescent boys and in men whose spermatic cords are congenitally unsupported in the *tunica vaginalis,* the membrane surrounding the testes. A sudden, sharp testicular pain is reported and local swelling is seen. The pain may be so severe that nausea, vomiting, chills, and fever occur. Torsion may follow severe exercise, but it also may occur during sleep or after a simple maneuver such as crossing the legs. Physical examination reveals an extremely tender testis. Elevation of the

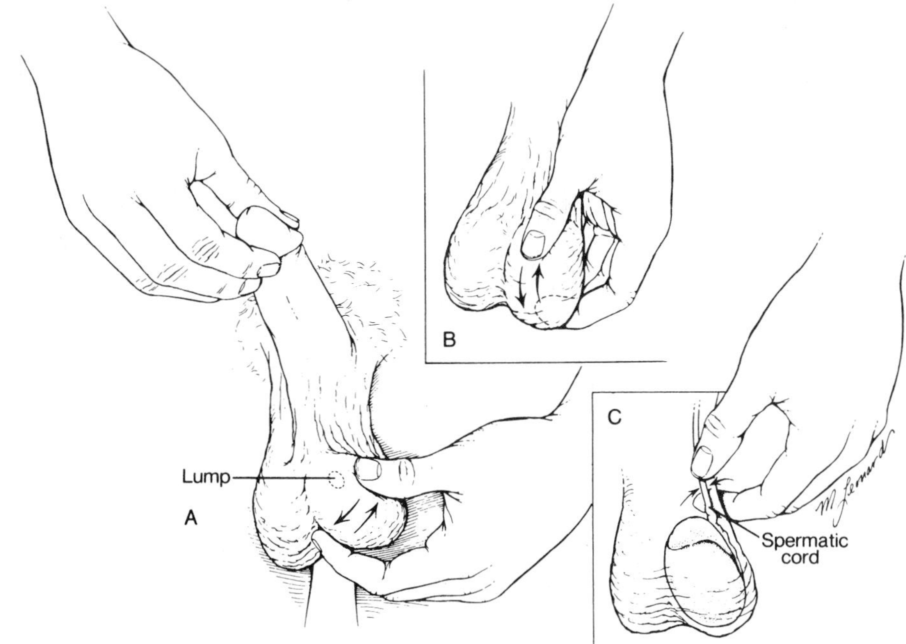

FIGURE 60-2. Testicular self-examination should be performed monthly. The testicles should be examined when warm, such as when bathing or showering. Roll each testicle between the thumb and index finger of one hand, both vertically and horizontally, while supporting the penis.

scrotum intensifies the pain by increasing the degree of twist.

Immediate surgery is necessary to prevent atrophy of the spermatic cord and preserve fertility. The torsion is reduced, excess tunica vaginalis is excised, and the testis is anchored with sutures in the scrotum. A prophylactic procedure may be performed on the opposite side.

NURSING MANAGEMENT

Preoperatively, administer prescribed analgesia to relieve pain. Following surgery, apply a scrotal support, especially when the client is out of bed. Inspect the dressing for signs of drainage. Give antibiotics if medically ordered. Report any sudden onset of pain to the physician.

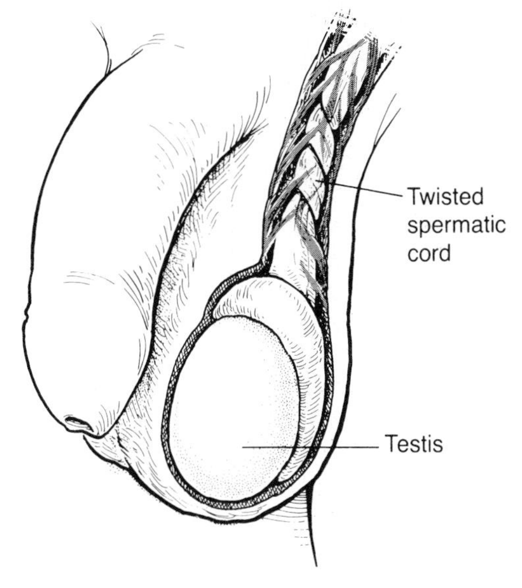

FIGURE 60-3. Torsion of the spermatic cord

Phimosis and Paraphimosis

Phimosis and paraphimosis are conditions that occur among uncircumcised male clients when the opening of the foreskin is constricted. *Phimosis* refers to an inability to retract the foreskin (prepuce); *paraphimosis* is a strangulation of the glans penis due to an inability to replace the retracted foreskin. These phimotic conditions are often caused by a congenitally small foreskin; however, chronic inflammation at the glans penis and prepuce secondary to poor hygiene or infection are also etiologic factors. Clients with phimosis report pain with erection and intercourse and difficulty cleaning under the foreskin. Clients with paraphimosis experience painful swelling of the glans. If the condition continues, severe edema and urinary retention may occur. Circumcision is recommended to permanently relieve these conditions; if surgery is not indicated, the client is instructed to wash under the foreskin daily and seek care if unable to retract the tissue.

Hydrocele, Spermatocele, and Varicocele

The suffix, *cele*, indicates a swelling. *Hydrocele*, *spermatocele*, and *varicocele* all present as a swelling of the scrotum (Fig. 60–4), but in each case, the conditions are

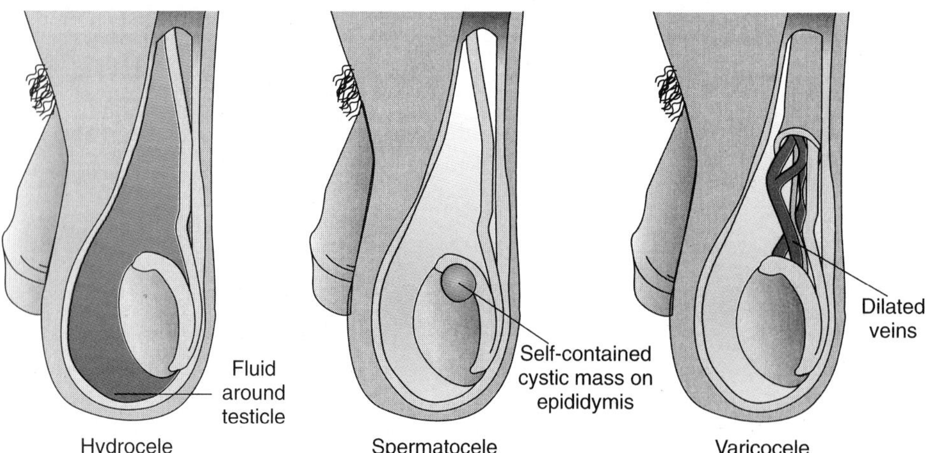

FIGURE 60-4. Causes of scrotal swelling

somewhat different. Often, hydrocele and spermatocele are not clinically significant and do not require treatment; however, varicoceles are thought to be an underlying cause of male infertility and may be surgically repaired (Table 60–1).

Infectious and Inflammatory Conditions

Prostatitis

Prostatitis is an inflammation of the prostate gland and is most often caused by microorganisms that reach the prostate by way of the urethra. *Escherichia coli* and microbes that cause sexually transmitted diseases (see Chap. 61) are often responsible, but in some instances no evidence of bacterial infection is found. Occasionally, a psychosexual problem may be the suspected cause of the client's symptoms. In any case, inflammation causes glandular swelling and tenderness. Because the prostate surrounds the urethra, a combination of genitourinary problems develops. Clients experience perineal pain or discomfort, unusual sensation preceding or following ejaculation, low back pain, fever, chills, dysuria, and urethral discharge. Treatment consists of up to 30 days of antibiotic therapy, mild analgesics, and sitz baths.

NURSING MANAGEMENT

The nurse stresses that sexual partners need to be treated also. The nurse tells the client to avoid caffeine, prolonged sitting, and constipation, and to reg-

TABLE 60-1 **Comparison of Hydrocele, Spermatocele, and Varicocele**

Condition and Etiology	Description	Signs and Symptoms	Diagnostic Aids	Medical and Surgical Management
Hydrocele				
Congenital defect; injury; infection; lymph obstruction; tumor; side effect of radiation; or unknown cause	Accumulation of as much as 100 mL of lymphatic fluid between the testis and tunica vaginalis	Swollen testicle; heaviness in scrotum or lower back; may be asymptomatic; pain if testicular blood flow is impaired	Palpation; transillumination	No treatment if asymptomatic; aspiration of fluid as a temporary measure; surgical excision of fluid-filled sac; treatment of primary condition (ie, infection)
Spermatocele				
Unknown cause	Epididymal, sperm-containing cyst	Small, freely movable mass; usually asymptomatic, may be painful if large	Palpation; transillumination	No treatment unless cyst is large and causes pain
Varicocele				
Incompetent valves in the spermatic veins	Venous dilation with damage to elastic fibers and hypertrophy of vein walls	Feeling of heaviness in scrotum; may be asymptomatic or have pain and swelling	Palpation; auscultation of venous rush; ultrasound; blood flow studies	No treatment, surgical ligation, or sclerosing

ularly drain the prostate gland through masturbation or intercourse. The client is instructed to comply with antibiotic therapy and use a mild analgesic for pain.

Epididymitis and Orchitis

An inflammation of the epididymis (**epididymitis**) (Fig. 60–5) and testis (**orchitis**) (Fig. 60–6) occurs alone or simultaneously (*epididymo-orchitis*). Common causes are an extension of the infectious agent causing prostatitis or an infection elsewhere in the body. Noninfectious epididymitis may occur as a result of long-term indwelling catheter use or as a result of genitourinary procedures such as cystoscopy or prostatectomy. Orchitis without epididymal involvement is associated with a viral mumps infection that occurs after puberty and may result in testicular atrophy and sterility. Bilateral epididymitis frequently leads to permanent *azoospermia* (absence of sperm), especially when the infection recurs frequently or when it becomes chronic.

The chief complaint is pain and swelling in the inguinal area and scrotum. Fever and chills occur with bacterial infections, and the urine contains pus and bacteria. Inspection reveals a markedly swollen testis and epididymis and scrotal skin that is red and tense. It is important to differentiate epididymitis from testicular torsion because torsion is a surgical emergency. Treatment consists of bed rest, scrotal elevation, analgesics, anti-inflammatory agents, and comfort measures such as local cold applications. Antibiotic therapy is initiated to eliminate the infectious agent. An *epididymyectomy* (excision of the epididymis) is performed on clients who have recurrent, chronic or intractable infections, but this results in sterility if it is performed bilaterally.

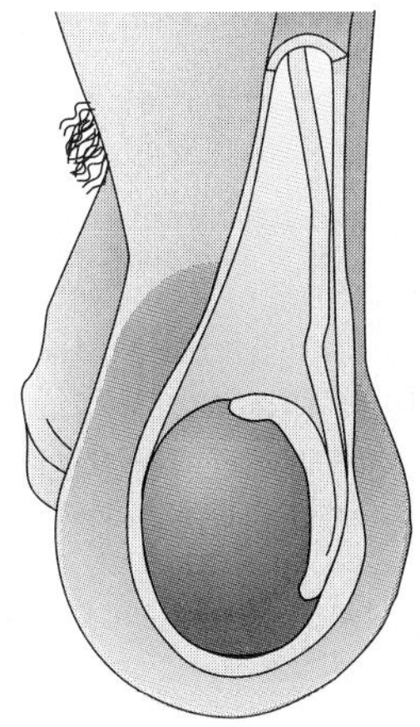

FIGURE 60-6. Acute orchitis.

NURSING MANAGEMENT

Elevate the scrotum with a folded towel, a four-tail bandage, or adhesive taped across the upper thighs (Fig. 60–7) to relieve pain by lessening the weight of the testes. Place an ice bag under the tender scrotum, not on top of it or leaning against it. Avoid keeping the cold bag constantly next to the skin because it may damage tissue. Use a routine such as on 60 minutes, off 30 minutes. As with any infection, encourage copious fluid intake.

Home care includes instructions to continue taking prescribed antibiotics, to take sitz baths, apply local heat after scrotal swelling subsides, and to avoid lifting and sexual intercourse until symptoms are relieved.

Nurses also advocate for infant and childhood immunizations against infectious diseases, such as mumps, to reduce potential adult complications such as orchitis.

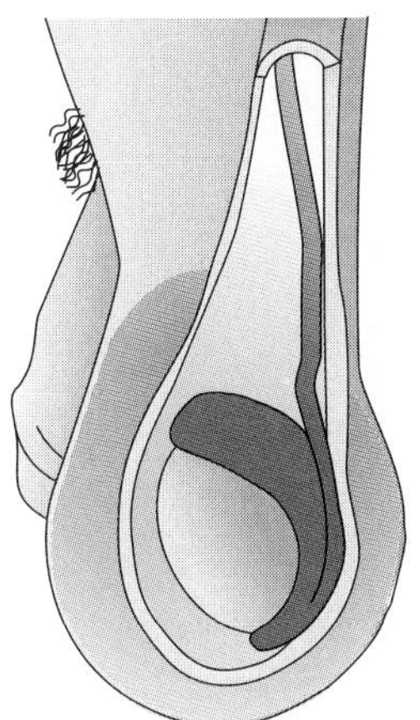

FIGURE 60-5. Acute epididymitis.

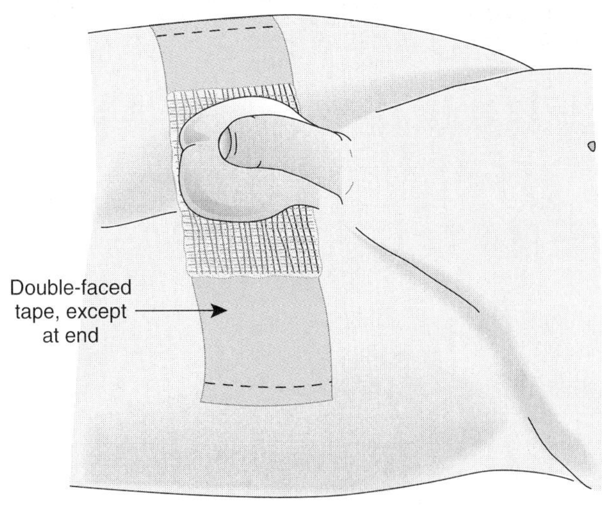

FIGURE 60-7. Technique for scrotal elevation.

Erection Disorders

Priapism

Priapism is a condition in which the penis becomes engorged and remains persistently erect in the absence of any sexual stimulation.

The underlying etiology is generally a vascular problem, a medical condition that causes blood to thicken, or a side effect of medications, including those prescribed to treat impotence. The engorged penis produces significant discomfort, interferes with arterial blood flow, and, in some cases, urinary elimination. If the erection lasts for longer than 6 hours, the tissue may be sufficiently damaged to result in impotence.

Treatment options include administering vasoconstrictive medications such as terbutaline (Brethine) or phenylephrine (Neo-Synephrine) or draining the trapped blood with a needle placed in the side of the penis. If these interventions fail, emergency surgery is performed to temporarily shunt blood out of the corpus cavernosum. Respect for the client's feelings and understandable embarrassment is extended throughout interactions.

Impotence

Impotence is the inability to achieve or maintain an erection sufficiently rigid for sexual activity. There must be multiple or persistent incidences of failed erection for the disorder to be considered pathologic. It is often a consequence of inadequate blood flow to the penis or rapid emptying of blood once it accumulates. Aging, testosterone insufficiency, side effects of drug therapy, atherosclerosis, hypertension, and complications of diabetes mellitus are common causes. Impotence also may be related to anxiety or depression. A *nocturnal penile tumescence test* is used to determine if the client is experiencing spontaneous erections during sleep. The test involves applying paper bands about the shaft of the penis at bedtime and observing if the bands are broken in the morning. Absence of nocturnal erections supports a physical rather than emotional cause for impotence.

Several approaches exist to help restore sexual function. Substituting other drugs for those that cause impotence or treating the contributing cause may restore *potency* (erectile ability). Some elect to facilitate penile engorgement by attaching a vacuum device to the penis or self-injecting drugs such as papaverine (Pavatine), phentolamine (Regitine), or alprostadil (Caverject) into the corpus cavernosa to achieve an erection. The drug sildenafil (Viagra) facilitates penile erection by producing smooth muscle relaxation in the corpus cavernosa, facilitating an inflow of blood. Sildenafil is taken orally about 1 hour before sexual activity. It has no erectile effect in the absence of sexual stimulation. Vascular surgery is an option for some clients, but many clients choose a surgically implanted penile prosthesis (Fig. 60–8). One type contains a saline reservoir that is pumped to fill the implant when sexual activity is desired and the other type maintains the penis in a semierect state at all times.

If the client prefers to self-inject a vasodilator, the nurse provides instruction on technique, suggested frequency of injections, and side effects. If the client

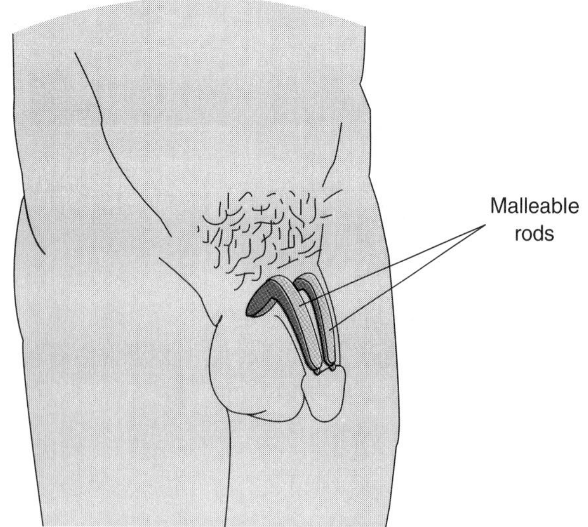

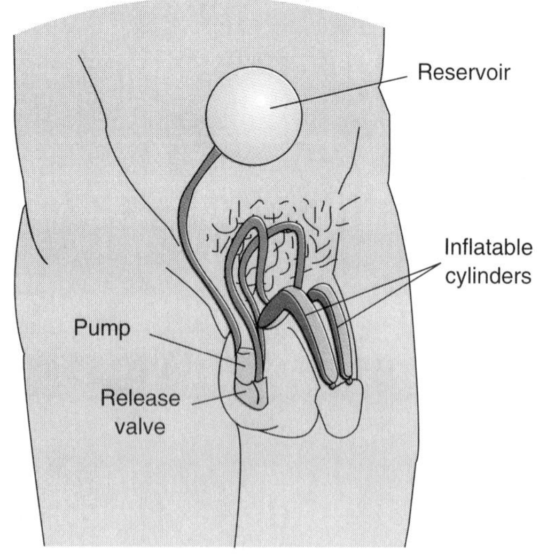

FIGURE 60-8. Examples of penile implants.

undergoes a penile implant, the nurse assesses for surgical complications, implements measures to ensure a safe recovery, and provides instructions to promote self-care (Nursing Care Plan 60–1).

Benign Prostatic Hyperplasia

When there is an increase in the number of cells in a structure, the condition is referred to as *hyperplasia*. If the cells are nonmalignant, it is called *benign hyperplasia*. Thus, **benign prostatic hyperplasia** (BPH) indicates that the prostate gland contains more than the usual number of normal cells. When the gland enlarges, the condition is known as *benign prostatic hypertrophy*.

ETIOLOGY AND PATHOPHYSIOLOGY

Benign prostatic hyperplasia occurs as men age. The outward expansion of the gland is not of any clinical importance. Inward encroachment, however, diminishes the diameter of the prostatic section of the urethra and interferes with emptying the bladder (Fig. 60–9).

NURSING CARE PLAN 60-1

Postoperative Management of the Client With a Penile Implant

Nursing Diagnosis and Collaborative Problems	Nursing Interventions	Outcome Criteria
Pain related to tissue injury and swelling	Offer analgesia as prescribed. Elevate genitalia with a rolled towel. Apply ice pack to incision and replace as needed. Suspend linen over lower pelvis with a bed cradle.	Pain is reduced or eliminated.
Risk for Bleeding related to inadequate hemostasis	Assess for frank bleeding or enlarging hematoma. Ensure that implant is semirigid to provide local pressure.	Blood loss is minimal and genitalia are within size expected postoperatively.
Risk for Urinary Retention related to urethral compression	Monitor urinary output. Report an inability to void or void a sufficient quantity.	Voids without difficulty and empties bladder.
Risk for Impaired Skin Integrity related to dermal deterioration secondary to tight prostheses	Look for pale, thin skin near the glans penis. Report signs of inadequate capillary perfusion and skin erosion.	Skin in the operative area is supple and intact.
Risk for Self-Esteem Disturbance related to fear of ridicule	Explain purpose for inspection. Provide privacy and draping during assessments. Avoid unprofessional comments about the client's reasons for or outcome of surgery. Provide opportunities for client to privately share his feelings about his changed appearance. Describe techniques for concealing the semierect appearance of the penis, such as wearing untucked shirts and pleated trousers or pants with an elastic waist.	Client has positive self-esteem and values the outcome of the procedure.
Risk for Ineffective Management of Therapeutic Regimen related to lack of knowledge concerning postoperative course after discharge	Identify the period for sexual abstinence (3–6 weeks). Instruct on how to inflate and deflate inflatable prosthesis. Advise to avoid contact sports. Explain that heavy lifting must be avoided for at least 3 weeks.	Heals without complications.

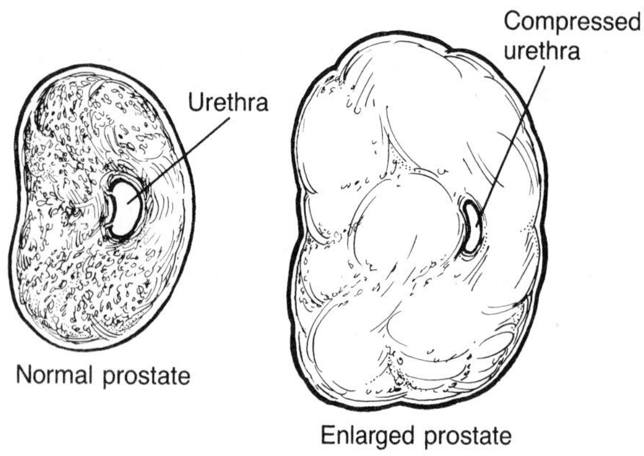

FIGURE 60-9. Comparison of normal prostate and enlarged prostate.

ASSESSMENT FINDINGS

Signs and Symptoms

The symptoms of BPH appear gradually. At first the client notices that it takes more effort to void. Eventually, there is a narrowing of the urinary stream and decreased force. The bladder empties incompletely. As residual urine accumulates, there is an urge to void more often and nocturia occurs. Because residual urine is a good culture medium for bacteria, symptoms of cystitis (inflammation of the bladder) may develop (see Chap. 64).

Diagnostic Findings

A DRE reveals an enlarged and elastic gland. Cystoscopy exposes the extent of the infringement on the urethra and the effects on the bladder. Intravenous and retrograde pyelograms and blood chemistry tests give information about possible damage to the upper urinary tract due to urinary retention. Measurement of a significant quantity of residual urine adds to the data that confirm the diagnosis. The PSA test may be slightly elevated. Transrectal ultrasonography indicates prostatic size and helps rule out the possibility that a malignancy is causing the enlargement.

MEDICAL AND SURGICAL MANAGEMENT

In the early stages of BPH the progression of prostatic enlargement is monitored with periodic digital examinations. Drug therapy is the second line of treatment (Table 60–2). Terazosin (Hytrin), an alpha-adrenergic blocker, helps relax the muscles in the prostate and relieve urinary symptoms. Finasteride (Proscar), an androgen hormone inhibitor, can be used to decrease symptoms and also appears to arrest the progression of prostate enlargement in some clients.

Other forms of treatment are used when glandular enlargement results in pronounced symptoms. The aim of all surgical procedures for BPH is to enlarge the bladder outlet (Table 60–3). Surgeries preformed through the urethra include *transcystoscopic urethroplasty*, *transurethral prostatectomy* (TURP), *transurethral incision of the prostate* (TUIP), and *transurethral laser incision of the prostate* (TULIP). Operations such as *suprapubic, retroperitoneal, or perineal prostatectomy* are preformed through an external incision (Fig. 60–10). In almost all cases, a continuous bladder irrigation is ordered after TURP to remove blood clots and residual tissue.

After a TURP, clients experience retrograde ejaculation, a condition in which the semen is deposited in the bladder rather than discharging through the urethra at the time of orgasm, rendering the client sterile. Following a TURP and open prostatectomies, men may have temporary or permanent urinary incontinence depending on the procedure used and the sur-

TABLE 60-2 **Drug Therapy for Benign Prostatic Hyperplasia**

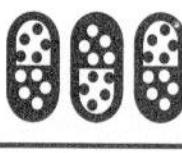

Drug Category/Example	Side Effects	Nursing Considerations
Hormonal Agents		
finasteride (Proscar) Inhibits the conversion of testosterone into a potent androgen (DHT) on which the prostate depends; causes the gland to shrink.	Loss of libido, impotence, decreased ejaculate, adversely affects fetal development	Monitor urinary output. Avoid handling the drug if pregnant. Instruct to use a condom to prevent fetal exposure. Explain that sexual changes are reversible after drug is discontinued. Inform the client that it may take 6 months or longer to achieve full benefit.
Alpha-Adrenergic Blockers		
terazosin (Hytrin) Reduces the tone of smooth muscle in the bladder neck and prostatic urethra.	Hypotension, dizziness, nausea, urinary frequency, incontinence, edema, fatigue, headaches	Monitor urinary elimination patterns and postural blood pressure changes. Administer drug at bedtime to reduce orthostatic hypotension. Warn to change position slowly. Weigh regularly for evidence of fluid imbalance.

TABLE 60-3 **Invasive Procedures for Prostatic Enlargement**

Procedure	Description
Transurethral Approaches	
Transcystoscopic urethroplasty	The balloon tip of a catheter is inflated for 10 to 20 minutes to stretch the prostatic urethra.
Urethral stent or coils	A flexible tube is permanently placed in the urethra to dilate the lumen.
Thermotherapy	A heated instrument inserted within a urethral catheter destroys prostatic tissue, but preserves the urethra.
Transurethral resection of the prostate (TURP)	Part of the prostate is removed with a cutting instrument inserted through an endoscope.
Transurethral incision of the prostate (TUIP)	No tissue is removed; the bladder outlet is enlarged by making an incision in the prostate, which relieves pressure on the urethra.
Transurethral laser incision of the prostate (TULIP)	A laser is used to incise and destroy prostate tissue.
Open Surgical Approaches	
Suprapubic prostatectomy	The prostate gland is removed by making a midline abdominal incision into the bladder. A suprapubic catheter, also known as a cystostomy tube, and a Foley catheter are inserted.
Retropubic prostatectomy	The prostate gland is removed through an abdominal incision, but the bladder is not entered.
Perineal prostatectomy	The prostate gland is removed through an incision made between the scrotum and anus.
Radical prostatectomy	The prostate gland and its capsule, seminal vesicles, and lymph nodes are removed through a retropubic or perineal incision; *this procedure is reserved for clients with prostatic cancer.*

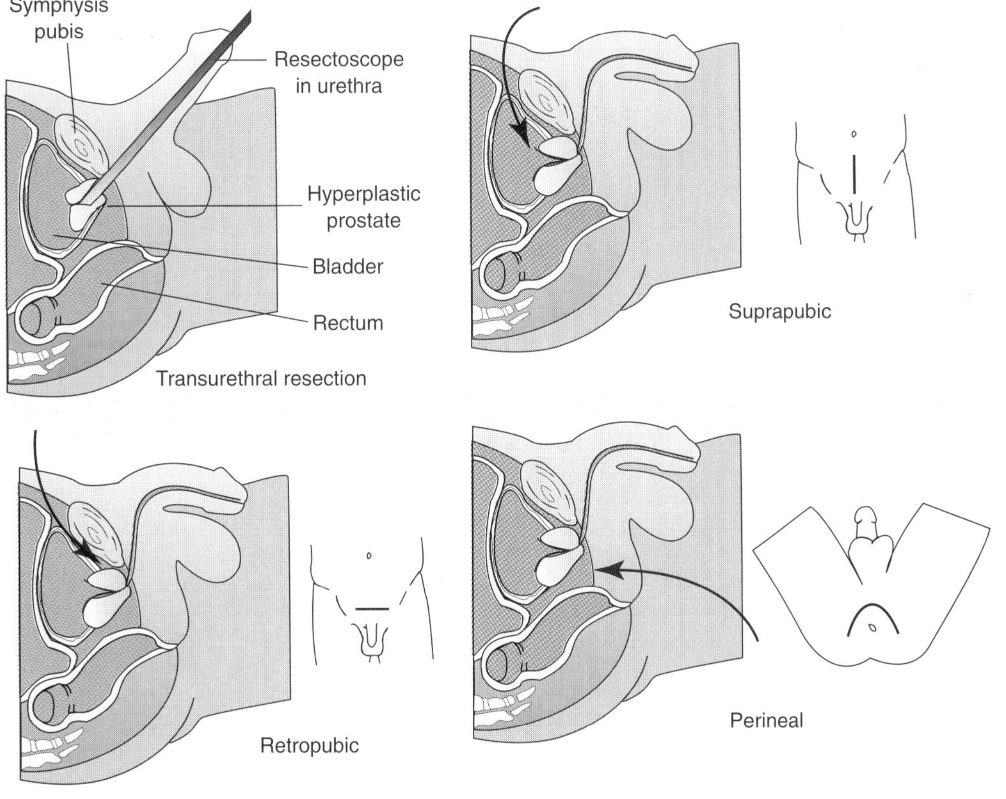

FIGURE 60-10. Examples of prostatectomy techniques.

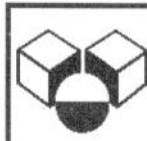

Nursing Guidelines 60-2

Teaching Optimal Bladder Function

- Tell the client to void often and assist bladder emptying by leaning forward on toilet and "bearing down" (Valsalva maneuver), or pressing down on the bladder while seated on the toilet (Credé's maneuver).
- Encourage frequent small volumes of oral fluids so that the bladder does not become extremely full at any one time.
- Review signs and symptoms of acute urinary obstruction and urinary infection such as distended bladder, lower abdominal discomfort, inability to urinate, small and frequent urination, fever and chills, and flank pain that indicate a need for medical attention.

geon's technical skill. Perineal surgical approaches often result in permanent impotence, although some nerve-sparing techniques are being developed.

NURSING MANAGEMENT

For the client who is not yet a candidate for surgery, the nurse provides education on how to maintain optimal bladder emptying (Nursing Guidelines 60–2).

The surgical client requires support and information to allay anxiety and promote a postoperative period that is free of complications. Teach deep breathing and leg exercises and explain that he will have continuous bladder irrigation for at least 24 hours after surgery.

Urethral catheterization before surgery will be necessary for clients with sudden or acute retention. If difficulty is encountered while inserting a urethral catheter, a coudé catheter, which has a curved tip, and instillable anesthetic lubricant are used to facilitate the procedure. If the catheter cannot be passed urethrally, a temporary suprapubic catheter will be required to relieve bladder distention. For care following a prostatectomy, see the nursing process section.

NURSING PROCESS
The Client Undergoing a Prostatectomy

Assessment
Preoperative

A complete medical, drug, and allergy history is obtained. The client is questioned about the symptoms and the length of time the symptoms have been present. When taking the history, it is important to determine if the client has had an acute, sudden episode of urinary retention because this problem may require immediate attention. Vital signs are taken and the client is weighed.

Diagnosis and Planning

The nursing care plan includes, but is not limited to, the following:

Nursing Diagnoses and Collaborative Problems	Nursing Interventions
Risk for Hemorrhage related to inadequate hemostasis	Monitor vital signs frequently until stable.
Goal: Bleeding will be managed and minimized.	Assess color of urine and status of dressing, if there is one, at least every 4 hours. Report if the color of urine changes from burgundy to bright red like catsup.
	Maintain traction on the urinary catheter to support hemostasis by keeping it taped to the leg for at least 6 hours following surgery.
	Discourage straining to have a bowel movement or other activities that increase blood pressure such as attempting to void with the catheter in place and lifting heavy objects.
Risk for Anemia related to postoperative bleeding	Assist with administering whole blood or packed cells as prescribed by the physician
Goal: Anemia will be managed and minimized.	
Risk for Urinary Retention related to obstruction of urinary catheter with tissue debris and blood clots or urethral stricture	Instill bladder irrigation solution at a rate to maintain light pink or clear urine (see Clinical Procedure 60-1).
Goal: Catheter will remain patent.	Palpate bladder and assess true urine volume every 4 hours or whenever patient complains of pain or if there is urine leaking around catheter.
	Avoid dependent loops and kinks in the urinary catheter, never clamp the urinary catheter, and do not allow the client to lay on the drainage tubing; keep drainage bag below the level of the bladder.
Risk for Hyponatremia related to absorption of bladder irrigation solution	Analyze if there is a realistic relationship between the amount of instilled irrigation solution and the drainage volume.
Goal: Hyponatremia will be managed and minimized.	Monitor and report if the client develops weakness, muscle cramps, nausea, vomiting, confusion, seizures, or elevated blood pressure.

Nursing Diagnosis	Interventions
	Slow or interrupt the bladder irrigation if hyponatremia or fluid excess is suspected.
Pain related to tissue injury or bladder spasms **Goal:** Pain will be controlled within the client's level of tolerance.	Check that catheter is patent and draining before administering medication. Administer a prescribed antispasmodic, such as belladonna and opium suppositories, for bladder spasms or an analgesic for incisional pain. Explain that the large balloon holding the catheter in place, traction on the catheter, and the volume of instilling irrigant tend to produce the urge to void, but an effort to do so contributes to discomfort. Use nursing measures such as changing position, diversion, guided imagery, and relaxation techniques to enhance response to drug therapy.
Risk for Infection related to impaired tissue and potential contamination of catheters and incisional drains **Goal:** The client will be free of infection as evidenced by progressive wound healing, no fever, no purulent drainage, white blood count within level expected, urine free of bacteria.	Practice conscientious handwashing before providing nursing care. Keep ports used for emptying drainage clean. Reinforce or change moist dressings using surgical asepsis. Keep perineum clean after a bowel movement for clients with a perineal prostatectomy. Report tenderness, unusual drainage, foul odor, and fever.
Risk for Impaired Skin Integrity related to leaking urine from suprapubic catheter	Clean skin around suprapubic catheter with mild soap and water; dry skin thoroughly afterwards (Refer to Nursing Guidelines 60-3 on managing a suprapubic catheter). Apply and change drain gauze around suprapubic catheter as it becomes moist. Enclose the suprapubic catheter within an ostomy appliance to keep the skin dry. Consult an enterostomal therapist on substances, such as karaya, that can be moisture resistant and protect the skin.
Urge or Total Incontinence related to altered urinary sphincter or nerve damage secondary to surgical procedure if nerves have been spared	Provide absorbent pads or underwear. Teach pelvic floor strengthening exercises (Nursing Guidelines 60-4).
Goal: Client will disguise incontinence or regain continence.	Suggest using a penile clamp (Fig. 60-11) to control incontinence.
Sexual Dysfunction related to structural changes secondary to surgical procedure **Goal:** Sexual activity will be satisfactory.	Provide information on support groups (see "Additional Resources" at the end of this chapter). Clarify information concerning potential sexual consequences of the specific surgical procedure.
Risk for Ineffective Management of Therapeutic Regimen related to lack of knowledge about care following discharge **Goal:** Client will refer to written instructions that correlate with drug teaching, wound and catheter care, and medical follow-up.	Emphasize ongoing medical care Explain drug action, frequency of administration, and side effects of medications that will be taken after discharge. Demonstrate and have client return demonstration for catheter and wound care. Identify when client can resume activity, including sexual intercourse. Explain the goal for 10–12 glasses of oral fluid daily and methods for preventing constipation by increasing dietary fiber and moderate activity. List signs of infection to report immediately such as pain in the pelvis or perineum, cloudy or bloody urine, or fever or chills.

Evaluation and Expected Outcomes

- Urine is light pink, clear, or amber.
- Hemoglobin is $\geq$ 10 g/dL.
- Urine drains freely from catheter or with spontaneous voiding.
- Serum sodium is within 135–145 mEq/L.
- Pain and discomfort are relieved.
- No evidence of infection; vital signs are normal.
- Skin remains intact or wound heals normally.
- Resumes sexual activity, if desired, or adapts to sexual changes.
- Demonstrates understanding of perineal exercises, medication schedule, activities to avoid, when to contact physician, and wound care.

Malignancies of the Male Reproductive System

Cancer of the Prostate

Prostatic cancer is most common in men older than 50. In fact, it is the third most common cause of death from cancer in men of all ages and is the most common cause of death from cancer in men over 75 years of age.

ETIOLOGY AND PATHOPHYSIOLOGY

The cause of prostatic cancer is unknown, but there seems to be a relationship with increased testosterone levels and a diet that is high in fat. Most prostatic carcinomas occur in the periphery of the gland. As it enlarges, it causes genitourinary symptoms that are similar to a variety of other conditions (eg, BPH and cystitis). If untreated, tumor cells spread by way of the bloodstream and lymphatics to the pelvic lymph nodes and bone, particularly the lumbar vertebrae, pelvis, and hips.

ASSESSMENT FINDINGS

Signs and Symptoms

At first, no symptoms occur, and none may occur for years. When the tumor grows large enough, it compromises urinary flow and causes frequency, nocturia, and dysuria (difficult or painful urination). The first symptoms of metastases may be back pain or pain down the leg from nerve sheath involvement. When pain develops, the disease is often in an advanced stage.

Diagnostic Findings

Rectal examination detects a prostatic nodule. A PSA greater than 4 ng/mL is the basis for performing more definitive diagnostic procedures and a PSA above 10 ng/mL indicates a prostatic malignancy. A PSA greater than 80 ng/mL indicates advanced metastatic disease. Transrectal ultrasound confirms the presence of a mass. The definitive diagnosis is made by biopsy and microscopic examination of tissue. Sometimes the malignancy is detected after microscopic examination of tissue removed during a TURP or open prostatectomy for BPH.

Pelvic or spinal radiographs, bone scan, and magnetic resonance imaging (MRI) or computed tomography (CT) scanning detect metastasis to the bone. An elevated serum acid phosphatase is associated with bone metastasis. Intravenous pyelogram (IVP) and other renal function studies detect kidney damage

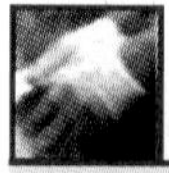

Clinical Procedure 60-1
Continuous Bladder Irrigation

PURPOSE	EQUIPMENT
• To maintain patency of indwelling catheter • To remove blood clots and tissue debris • To control bleeding • To instill diluted medication	• 1 or 2 liter bags of irrigating solution • Tubing • IV pole or electronic infusion device • Medication label • Bedside intake and output record • Clean gloves

Nursing Action	Rationale
ASSESSMENT	
Check the medical orders.	Collaborates nursing activities with medical treatment
Read and compare the print on the bag of irrigation solution with the medical order or medication administration record.	Prevents errors
Check for any documented allergies if the solution contains a medication	Ensures safety
Determine how much the client understands about the purpose and technique for the procedure.	Provides an opportunity for health teaching
Inspect the urethral catheter to determine that it contains three lumens: one through which the catheter balloon is inflated, one through which urine drains, and one through which the irrigating solution will infuse.	Verifies there is appropriate equipment for instilling and draining solution

continued

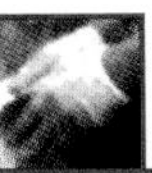

Clinical Procedure 60-1
Continued

Nursing Action	Rationale

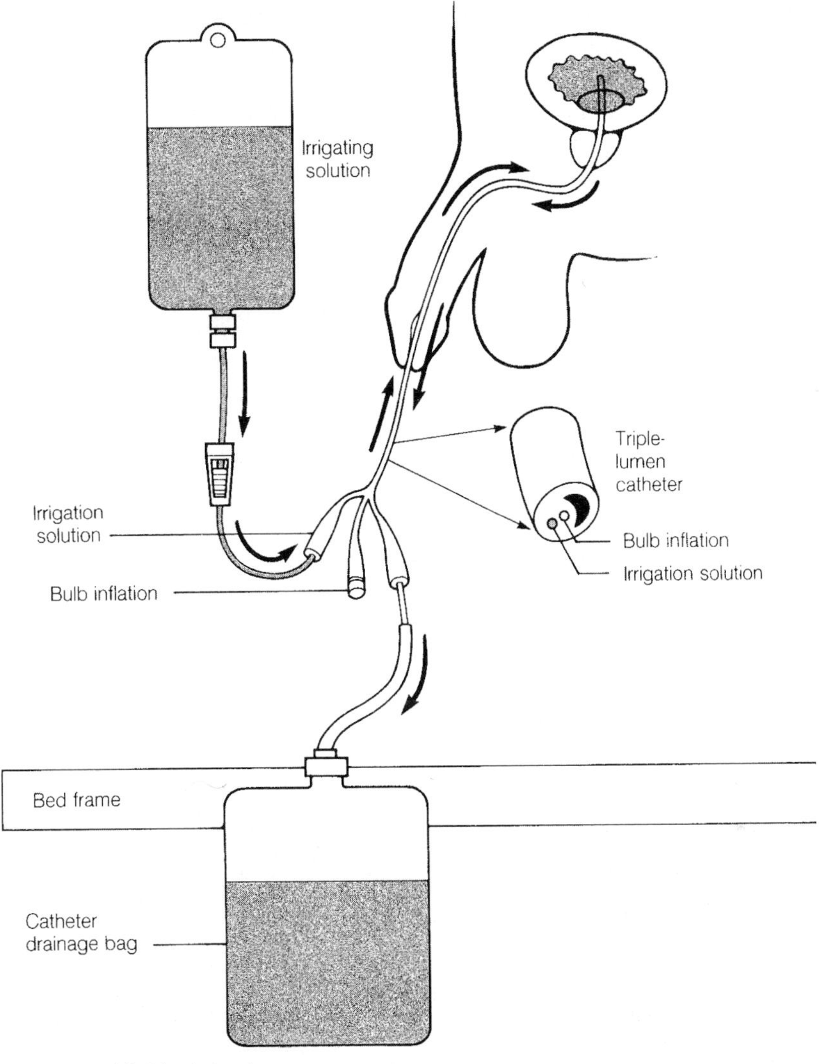

Continuous bladder irrigation.

Nursing Action	Rationale
Observe the appearance and volume of urine that has collected in the gravity drainage bag.	Provides data for future comparisons
PLANNING	
Obtain the necessary equipment.	Prevents unnecessary delays in the plan of care
Attach a label to the solution identifying the client's name, date and time, and your initials.	Facilitates following standards for infection control
IMPLEMENTATION	
Check the client's identification.	Prevents errors
Wash your hands.	Reduces the transmission of microorganisms

continued

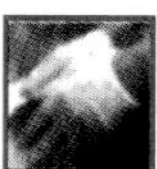

Clinical Procedure 60-1
Continued

Nursing Action	Rationale
Hang the bag of solution from the IV pole or hanger on an electronic infusion device approximately 24 to 36 inches above the client's bladder.	Uses the principle of gravity for instilling the solution
Open the tubing wrapper and tighten the roller clamp on the tubing.	Prohibits the solution from gushing from the tubing once the spike is inserted
Remove the protective cover from the spike on the tubing and insert it into the port of the solution.	Facilitates the flow of solution
Squeeze the drip chamber to fill it approximately half full.	Helps in monitoring the rate of infusion
Open the roller clamp and purge the air from the tubing.	Prevents instilling air into the bladder
Tighten the roller clamp while keeping the free end of the tubing from being contaminated.	Avoids loss of fluid and ensures aseptic technique
Don clean gloves.	Acts as a barrier against contact with body fluids containing blood-borne pathogens
Connect the free end of the tubing to the unused lumen of the catheter.	Completes the circuit for administering the irrigation
Discard gloves and wash your hands.	Removes transient pathogens
Open the clamp on the irrigation solution until it is instilling approximately 1 mL/min by gravity or 60 mL/hr with an electronic infusion device.	Begins initial administration
Monitor the appearance of the drainage from the urinary catheter, not the collection bag.	Provides the most current assessment data
Adjust the rate, faster or slower, so as to maintain clear or light pink drainage from the catheter.	Permits a flexible rate according to the client's response
Don clean gloves and empty the collection bag as it becomes half full.	Promotes continuous drainage without overfilling the collection bag
Record the volume of solution that instills and the volume of drainage at least every 8 hours; the urinary output is the difference between the two sums.	Ensures accurate intake and output records
Replace the solution bag as it becomes empty or change the solution after 24 hours.	Provides continuous bladder irrigation and supports standards for infection control
Document the type and rate at which the solution is instilling and each time the rate is changed, the appearance of the drainage, intake and output, and the client's level of comfort.	Aids in communicating the implementation of care and evaluating the client's response

caused by long-standing urethral obstruction and urinary retention (if present).

MEDICAL AND SURGICAL MANAGEMENT

The tumor size, microscopic characteristics, and presence or absence of metastases are used to establish the stage, which in turn determines treatment (Table 60–4). The client's age and general health status are also considered when planning treatment. Treatment regimens include observation, surgery, radiation, hormone therapy, or a combination of these.

Surgery

If the nodule is localized, an open suprapubic prostatectomy is the treatment of choice. A radical prostatectomy, performed through a perineal or retropubic approach, is the surgical preference if the tumor is large enough to be palpated or if it has spread to adjacent tissue.

When a radical prostatectomy is performed, the entire prostate, its capsule, and the seminal vesicles

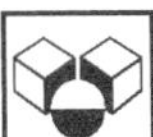

Nursing Guidelines 60-3

*Managing the Care of a Client With a Suprapubic Catheter**

PURPOSE: To drain urine from the bladder through a catheter that is inserted through the anterior abdominal wall and anchored with external skin sutures. The client may or may not have a urethral (Foley) catheter as well.

- Stabilize the catheter by taping it to the skin of the abdomen.
- Keep the catheter connected to a sterile drainage system.
- Keep the drainage system below the level of the insertion site.
- Empty the urine from the bag periodically to reduce tension on the catheter and skin.
- Record the urine output from the suprapubic catheter separate from voided urine output or output from another catheter.
- Keep the skin clean and dry at the insertion site to avoid skin irritation and compromised skin integrity.
- For "trial voiding":

  Clamp the catheter for 4 hours.
  Have the client void naturally.
  Unclamp the suprapubic catheter.
  Measure the residual urine.

- Collaborate with the physician on removing the suprapubic catheter when the residual urine is repeatedly ≤100 mL.
- To remove the catheter

  Offer an analgesic 30 minutes before proceeding
  Wash hands and don gloves
  Empty the urinary drainage and record amount
  Remove gloves, rewash hands
  Position the client on his back
  Free the tape from the skin
  Open a package of sterile gloves and suture removal kit
  Remove the skin sutures
  Pull gently on the catheter until it is free
  Place a sterile dressing over the insertion site
  Remove gloves and wash hands
  Change the dressing when it becomes moist until the site heals in approximately 2 days.

**A suprapubic catheter also may be called a cystostomy tube.*

are removed. The bladder neck is sutured to the membranous urethra over an indwelling urethral catheter, which is left in place for 10 to 14 days. Potential complications of this surgery include a 25% to 50% chance of impotence, difficulty with urinary control, and genital and lower extremity edema. A TURP may be done if the client has urethral obstruction and

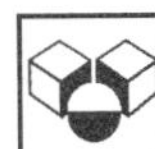

Nursing Guidelines 60-4

Teaching Pelvic Floor Strengthening Exercises

- Squeeze the pelvic floor muscles (those used to stop urination and hold back a bowel movement) for as long as possible up to 10 seconds—*longer is not better.*
- Relax completely for 10 seconds—*less is not better.*
- Repeat sequence as many times as possible in 5 minutes or a cycle of 15 contractions followed by relaxation.
- Interrupt exercises when muscles can no longer be contracted tightly.
- Perform exercises in the morning and evening.
- Perform shorter pelvic floor exercises four or five times during the day:

  Squeeze pelvic floor muscles and hold for one second.
  Relax for 1 second.
  Repeat five times in succession within 2 minutes.

- Continue long and short exercises for 3 to 4 months or until continent.

Adapted from the Pelvic Floor Retraining Team, Incontinence Clinic, Beth Israel Hospital, Boston, MA, and The Prostate Cancer Infolink (1995).

his physical status is not amenable to treatment. Occasionally, permanent suprapubic drainage may need to be established.

A bilateral **orchidectomy** (surgical removal of the testes) may be performed to eliminate the production

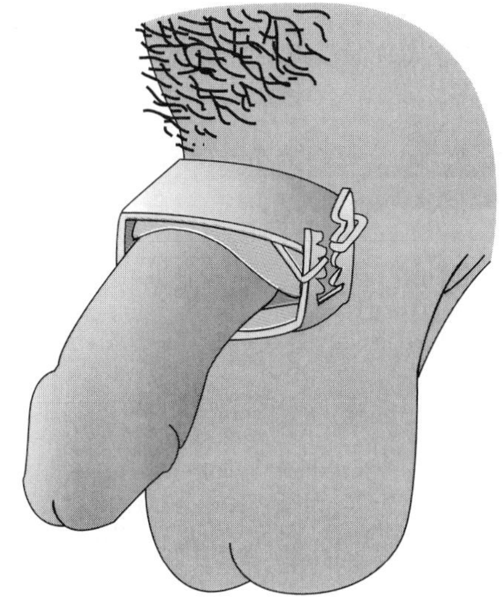

FIGURE 60-11. Penile clamp. Clamp is molded to comfortably fit penis and gently compress urethra.

TABLE 60-4 **Staging and Treatment of Prostate Cancer**

Stage	Treatment	5-Year Survival Rate
Stage A1: Cancer is found incidentally with <5% malignant cells	Observation	98%
Stage A2: Tumor is not palpable, biopsy is positive	Observation, surgery, or radiation therapy	90%
Stage B: Tumor is palpable, confined to prostate	Surgery or radiation therapy	77%
Stage C: Local extension of tumor but no distant metastasis	Radiation therapy or combination of surgery, radiation and hormone therapy	60%
Stage D: Distant metastasis	Medical therapy	26%

of testosterone in men with advanced prostatic carcinoma (stage D). Permanent side effects are impotence, loss of libido, hot flashes, and possible psychological disturbances. Many men do not accept surgical castration and low levels of testosterone are achieved with hormone therapy.

Radiation Therapy

Radiation therapy (see Chap. 19) may be used alone or in conjunction with other treatment modalities especially when there is local metastasis. Possible side effects include impotence, diarrhea, and urinary frequency and urgency.

Hormone Therapy

Men with stage D carcinoma of the prostate are candidates for hormone therapy (Table 60–5). With the use of antiandrogenic (male) hormones or estrogenic hormones, the progression of the malignancy may be retarded and there may be a prolonged period of palliation (comfort). Estramustine (Emcyt), is a combination of estrogen and an antineoplastic drug that also is used for palliative treatment.

Feminizing side effects occur with hormone therapy. The client's voice may become higher, hair and fat distribution may change, and breasts may become tender and enlarged. Libido and potency are also diminished. When estrogens are used in lower doses, the client may not experience these problems.

NURSING MANAGEMENT

Refer to Chapter 24 for general preoperative and postoperative standards of care. Radical prostatectomy is similar to other prostatectomy procedures and the same immediate postoperative nursing diagnoses and interventions apply.

Client and Family Teaching

As the client recovers, the nurse promotes increased self-care, and provides instructions for home management. The discharge plan of care includes, but is not limited to, the following:

TABLE 60-5 **Hormonal Drug Therapy for Prostatic Cancer**

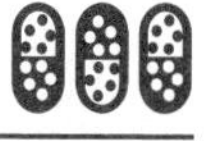

Drug Category/Example	Side Effects	Nursing Considerations
diethylstilbestrol (DES) Synthetic estrogen that reduces testosterone levels	Breast enlargement, nausea, vomiting, photosensitivity elevates blood sugar	Offer small frequent meals to offset nausea. Monitor blood sugar especially of those with diabetes mellitus. Recommend using a sunscreen or wearing protective clothing.
flutamide (Eulexin) Blocks androgens	Breast enlargement, impotence, diarrhea, anemia, leukopenia, thrombocytopenia, jaundice	Instruct clients that periodic blood tests are required. Observe if urine is dark yellow.
goserelin acetate (Zoladex) Inhibits pituitary gonadotropin secretion, which reduces testosterone to castration levels	Hot flashes, impotence, loss of libido	Administer as a monthly injection or subcutaneous implant. Use a local anesthetic prior to administering injection. Repeat injection every 28 days. Drug resistance occurs after 2 to 3 years of therapy.

Nursing Diagnoses and Collaborative Problems	Nursing Interventions
Risk for Infection related to home care of Foley catheter Goal: No infection occurs as evidenced by clear urine without the presence of bacteria or white blood cells.	Tell the client to use soap and water to clean around the urethral meatus and several inches of the catheter at least twice a day. Demonstrate and have the client return the demonstration for keeping the connection between the catheter and leg bag clean when changing and replacing leg bags for routine cleaning. Tell the client or caregiver to clean the leg bag by using soap and water and then rinse it with a 1:7 solution of vinegar and water.
Incontinence related to surgical compromises to internal and external urinary sphincter muscles Goal: Urinary control will be reestablished within 3 months after surgery or client will use equipment to collect urine.	Teach pelvic floor retraining exercises (see Nursing Guidelines 60-4) if incontinence is not permanent. For permanent incontinence, show the client how to apply a penile clamp or an external catheter connected to a leg bag.
Sexual Dysfunction related to temporary impotence when pudendal nerve (responsible for erection and orgasm) is spared Goal: Client will use alternatives other than intercourse for sexual pleasure until potency resumes.	Explain to the client and spouse or sexual partner that it may take from 3 to 12 months for sexual potency to return. See interventions for impotence for additional suggestions.
Impotence related to pudendal nerve damage secondary to nonnerve-sparing radical perineal prostatectomy Goal: Client and sexual partner will adapt to expressing sexual feelings despite the man's erectile dysfunction.	Recommend demonstrating sexual feelings in ways other than intercourse. Discuss the use of manual stimulation or the use of a mechanical vibrator to promote female orgasm, if it does not compromise the sex partner's moral values.
Possible metastasis Goal: Reoccurrence or metastasis will be identified early.	Explain that the PSA level will decrease after prostatectomy; a subsequent rise indicates the cancer has reoccurred. Clarify that repeat lymph node biopsies may be part of the surgical follow-up. Inform the client that blood tests for measuring serum acid phosphatase are used to monitor evidence of bone metastasis.

Cancer of the Testes

Cancer of the testes is a rapidly metastasizing malignancy that is seen in young men between the ages of 18 and 40. Although this cancer is relatively rare, it is the most common type that occurs in men between the ages of 15 and 34 and is the leading cause of death from cancer in men between 25 and 34 years of age. However, significant advancement in treatment in recent years has resulted in a high cure rate even in clients with metastatic disease.

ETIOLOGY AND PATHOPHYSIOLOGY

The incidence is higher among men with a history of cryptorchidism whether or not an orchiopexy was performed. Although the exact etiology is unknown, one possible explanation is that the cells in the undescended testis(es) degenerate earlier than occurs with natural aging. The degenerative process then leads to abnormal cellular changes. In most cases, only one testicle is affected, but the other may become cancerous if the tumor is not diagnosed early.

Nearly all testicular tumors involve the sperm-forming germ cells. Those that are comprised of immature germ cells are called *seminomas*; *nonseminomas* develop among more mature, specialized germ cells. Nonseminomas grow more rapidly and tend to metastasize at a faster rate and, therefore, treatment is more aggressive.

ASSESSMENT FINDINGS

Signs and Symptoms

Gradual or sudden swelling of the scrotum or a lump felt on palpation always deserves prompt medical attention. The tumor generally presents as a hard, nontender nodule of the testis with additional coexisting symptoms (Box 60–1). Unless discovered early through testicular self-examination, the first symptoms may be those of tumor metastasis. They may include abdominal pain, general weakness, and aching in the testes.

Diagnostic Findings

Tumor markers include elevated levels of AFP and bHCG. An IVP may show lymph node enlargement that displaces the ureters. Lymphangiography also is used to detect lymph node involvement. A CT scan or MRI can detect metastases. Because biopsy risks

BOX 60-1 Signs and Symptoms of Testicular Cancer

- Testicular lump that is hard or granular
- Increase in the size of one testicle
- Heavy or dragging feeling in the scrotum
- Dull ache in the groin or above the pubis
- Diminished sensitivity to testicular pressure

spreading the highly malignant tumor cells, surgery is recommended immediately.

MEDICAL AND SURGICAL MANAGEMENT

Treatment of testicular tumors depends on the stage of the disease (Table 60–6) and includes surgery, chemotherapy, and radiation. An autologous (self-donated) bone marrow transplantation may be recommended for recurrent disease or for clients who are resistant to drug therapy. Before medical or surgical treatment, however, the topic of sperm banking should be discussed. Locating a sperm bank and then collecting and banking sperm, which may take as long as 12 to 24 days, is omitted if the outcome of treatment is jeopardized by the delay.

Surgery

A *radical inguinal orchiectomy* (removal of the testis) and ligation of the spermatic cord is performed. Clients with nonseminomas usually undergo a *radical retroperitoneal lymph node dissection* as well. If only one testis is removed, sexual activity, the libido, and fertility are usually unaffected. After a radical lymph node dissection, libido and erections are preserved, but surgical disruption of nerve pathways results in impaired ejaculation. New nerve-sparing techniques are being developed that preserve ejaculatory function, and therefore, fertility, in most clients.

Chemotherapy

A multiple antineoplastic drug regimen usually is instituted after surgery. The types of drugs, the frequency of their administration, and the duration of therapy depend on the type of tumor and if metastasis has occurred. Chemotherapy, which is generally aggressive initially, is modified as the tumor markers show a response. Sperm tend to be destroyed or mutated when exposed to toxic cancer drugs, but spermatogenesis eventually resumes.

Radiation

Seminomas are sensitive to radiation and most clients receive radiation to the retroperitoneal lymph nodes. For clients with nonseminomas, radiation is considered an adjunct to lymphadenectomy and chemotherapy.

NURSING MANAGEMENT

Preoperative Period

One of nursing's chief concerns is responding to the client's emotional distress over having a life-threatening diagnosis, being unfamiliar with the surgical experience, and confronting alterations in body image and sexuality. All clients are understandably concerned over the potential change in their sexual image and fertility; however it may be of even greater concern to men in this age group. The nurse provides private opportunities for the client to ask questions and uses therapeutic communication techniques to encourage the client to verbalize his feelings.

Postoperative Period

Refer to Chapter 24 for postoperative standards of care. After an orchiectomy a scrotal support is applied. If drains have been inserted, they are connected to closed (Jackson-Pratt) or open (machine) suction. Prophylactic antibiotics are given to prevent infection. Pain, which may be severe after a radical lymph node dissection, is managed with narcotic analgesics. If pain is not relieved, and nursing measures to augment their effect are inadequate, the nurse collaborates with the physician so that modifications in drug therapy are made.

As the client's comfort improves, the nurse may discuss the impact of the diagnosis and treatment and again provide opportunities for the safe expression of anxiety, fear, and grief. The nurse advises the client that a testicular prosthesis can be inserted at a later date if he desires and that fertility may be regained in 2 to 3 years after drug therapy is discontinued and sooner when surgery or radiation is used. The nurse provides the client with names of local support groups and encourages him to contact them for emotional support after discharge.

TABLE 60-6 **Staging and Treatment of Germ Cell Tumors of the Testis**

Stage	Treatment	Survival Rate
Stage I: Tumor confined to the testis	Orchiectomy, retroperitoneal lymph node dissection	95%
Stage II: Involvement of testis plus retroperitoneal nodes	Orchiectomy, retroperitoneal lymph node dissection, possible chemotherapy	93%
Stage III: Distant metastasis	Orchiectomy, retroperitoneal lymph node dissection, four cycles of chemotherapy, surgery to resect residual masses	70%

Client and Family Teaching

Develop a teaching plan that includes the following:

- Drink plenty of fluids and eat a well balanced diet to avoid constipation.
- Obtain adequate rest; avoid fatigue and heavy lifting.
- Wash the incision with warm soap and water. Report any redness, drainage, pain, or swelling of the incision or scrotum.
- Take any prescribed medication exactly as directed.
- Perform self-examination of the remaining testicle every month and immediately report any changes.
- Seek care if any of the following occur: fever, chills, adverse drug effects, weight loss, or anorexia.
- Assure the client who has banked sperm that normal pregnancies have occurred with sperm stored up to 10 years.
- Identify other pregnancy alternatives for clients for whom treatment has proceeded without collecting and storing sperm, such as donor insemination or adoption.
- Suggest contacting the department of social services to become foster parents.
- Recommend volunteering as a Big Brother or to lead a scout troop or youth group to compensate for the inability to raise biologic children.

Cancer of the Penis

Penile cancer is rare and occurs more often in men who are uncircumcised. The cause is unknown but it is thought that chronic irritation leads to a precancerous skin lesion that eventually undergoes malignant changes. Medical attention is sought when the lesion, which typically has been present for years, becomes infected. Biopsy confirms the existence of malignant cells and lymphangiography identifies if the lymph nodes are involved. The tumor is staged using MRI and CT scanning.

Treatment includes tumor excision, chemotherapy, external or interstitial radiation therapy, or all three. In some cases, the penis is partially or completely amputated and the scrotum and testes excised. Full amputation of the penis requires the insertion of a permanent drainage tube in the perineal tissue to empty the bladder. The 5-year survival rate for cancer of the penis is less than 50% (Gordon, Brendon, Wyble, & Ivey, 1997).

Elective Sterilization

A **vasectomy** is a minor surgical procedure done in a physician's office or clinic. It involves the ligation of the vas deferens and results in permanent sterilization by interrupting the pathway that transports sperm. On occasion, the client may complain of impotency, although the procedure has no effect on erection or ejaculation. It may take several weeks or more after surgery before the ejaculatory fluid is free of sperm, and the client is informed to use a reliable method of contraception until sperm are no longer present. The client may wish to consider banking sperm before undergoing the procedure. Some men feel ambivalent about having this procedure and the nurse provides the client with an opportunity to express these feelings.

A *vasovasostomy* is a surgical attempt to reverse a vasectomy by restoring patency and continuity to the vas deferens; a *vasoepididymostomy* connects the stump of the vas deferens directly to the epididymis (Fig. 60–12). It may take from 3 to 6 months after

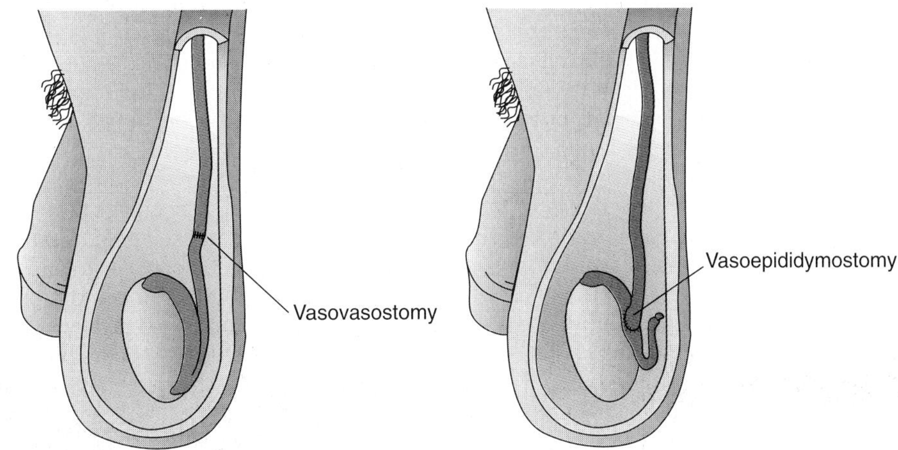

FIGURE 60-12. Vasectomy reversal procedures.

reversal procedures before sperm counts and motility are normal. Lack of success is generally due to either scar formation or sperm leakage from the surgical connection.

Client Teaching

The nurse reinforces the following important information for home care after a vasectomy:

- Expect some bruising and incisional soreness after the local anesthetic wears off.
- Apply ice packs to the scrotum to reduce swelling; remove the cold application after 20 minutes and replace again after the tissue rewarms.
- Take a mild analgesic, such as aspirin or acetaminophen, for discomfort.
- Wear an athletic support for several days for comfort.
- Resume usual activities in 2–3 days, but avoid strenuous exercise for up to 5 days.
- Resume sexual activity when comfort allows, which is usually in a week.
- *Use a reliable method of contraception until the physician indicates that sperm are no longer present,* which may be determined after 10 or more ejaculations.
- Report severe pain, fever, or swelling at the top of the testicle(s).

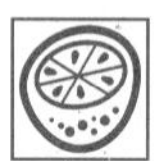

General Nutritional Considerations

Studies show a high-fat diet may increase the risk of prostate cancer by 30% to 50%. Other risk factors include living an inactive lifestyle and being overweight.

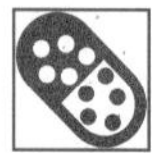

General Pharmacologic Considerations

Platinum-based drugs such as cisplatin (Platinol) are very effective in treating certain forms of testicular cancer. It is almost always used in combination with other antineoplastic drugs.

Other drugs used in combination with cisplatin in treating testicular cancer include etoposide (VePesid) and bleomycin (Blenoxane). Bleomycin can cause pulmonary toxicity in those taking high doses of the drug or in those over the age of 70. Some patients taking bleomycin for testicular cancer have developed Raynaud's phenomenon (see Chap. 32).

Cisplatin is extremely nephrotoxic and the patient must be kept well hydrated. Administration of at least 3,000 mL of fluid per 24 hours is necessary if the client's condition permits. Report any evidence of fluid retention such as edema, weight gain, difficulty breathing, or bubbly lung sounds. Irreversible ototoxicity can occur. Audiometric testing is recommended before the first dose and before each subsequent dose. Ototoxicity can occur after a single dose.

Chemotherapy for cancer increases the risk for infection, anorexia and vomiting, and hair loss.

Drugs such as epoetin (Epogen) and filgrastin (Neupogen) can stimulate the development of red and white blood cells whose production has been suppressed with antineoplastic drugs.

Administration of antiemetic drugs before chemotherapy can reduce or eliminate the incidence of nausea and vomiting. However, some chemotherapeutic agents, such as cisplatin, can cause severe nausea and vomiting that does not respond well to antiemetics and that can persist for up to 7 days after treatment.

Certain medications such as antihypertensive drugs (eg, methyldopa, spironolactone), antidepressants, narcotics, and cimetidine can cause sexual dysfunction in men. If impotence or sexual dysfunction occurs, a thorough drug history should be obtained to determine if the sexual dysfunction is an adverse reaction to a drug and could be corrected by the use of a different medication.

All chemotherapeutic agents are capable of causing an anaphylactoid reaction. Report any of the following symptoms to the primary health care provider: any skin rash, hives, difficulty breathing, wheezing, tachycardia, or hypotension.

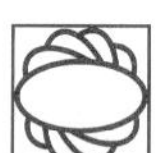

General Gerontologic Considerations

When an older man develops a varicocele when none existed before, the congestion of blood may be due to pressure from a urologic tumor.

Impotence increases as men age; 15% to 25% experience impotence by age 65. Over half of all men 75 years or older are chronically impotent.

There is a gradual decrease in sperm and testosterone production as men age. This phenomenon is possibly due to degenerative changes in the vascular system within the testes.

There are greater numbers of older than middle-aged men who are uncircumcised because many were born at home and the procedure was not performed. Therefore, the incidence of phimosis, paraphimosis, balanoposthitis, and penile cancer is more common in older men.

Along with decrease in sperm production, the volume and viscosity of seminal fluid decreases with age. A loss of muscular tone causes the scrotum to become more pendulous. As the scrotum drops, there is an increased risk of trauma and injury to this area.

Impotence in the male is not a normal part of aging. If impotence occurs, other causes should be explored such as adverse reactions to medication, atherosclerosis, or psychological problems.

SUMMARY OF KEY CONCEPTS

- The penis and scrotum are external male reproductive structures. Internal structures are the testes, epididymides, vas deferens, and seminal vesicles. Together with the prostate gland and bulbourethral glands, they form a complex secretory and ductal system.
- Disorders that affect the male reproductive system or their treatment can compromise urinary elimination, fertility, and sexuality.
- Examples of structural disorders that affect the male reproductive system include cryptorchidism; torsion of the spermatic cord; phimosis and paraphimosis; and hydrocele, spermatocele, and varicocele.
- Monthly testicular self-examinations are performed by rolling each testicle between the thumb and index finger to detect abnormal masses that may be cancerous.
- Some infectious and inflammatory disorders that affect the male reproductive system, such as prostatitis, epididymitis, and orchitis, may be the result of the transfer of bowel organisms like *E. coli* or sexually transmitted pathogens.
- Two erectile disorders, priapism and impotence, can damage self-esteem and affect fertility.
- Impotence can be managed with drug therapy or the surgical implantation of a penile prosthesis.
- Following surgical correction of impotence, the nurse relieves the client's pain, reduces swelling, monitors for unusual bleeding, assesses for urinary retention, follows aseptic principles to prevent infection, reports signs of skin damage, preserves the client's self-esteem, and provides teaching that promotes restoration of sexuality and prevention of postoperative complications.
- Enlargement of the prostate gland narrows the urethra, which causes more effort to initiate voiding, retention of urine, nocturia, and the potential for cystitis.
- Besides standard perioperative nursing activities after a prostatectomy, nursing measures include performing a continuous bladder irrigation and teaching pelvic floor strengthening exercises to facilitate control of urination.
- Cancer of the testes tends to occur in young adult males; cancer of the prostate and penis are more common in older males. Cancer of the prostate is the most common of the three male reproductive cancers; cancer of the penis is the rarest. The most desirable outcomes occur when cancer is diagnosed in its earliest stages.
- After a vasectomy, men are taught to expect some bruising and soreness, relieve swelling with cold applications to the surgical area, take a mild analgesic for discomfort, protect the genitalia with an athletic support, and continue practicing reliable birth control measures until sperm are permanently absent from semen.

CRITICAL THINKING EXERCISES

1. Compare and contrast the sexual implications that may result in two clients, one who is 60 and undergoing a TURP, and the other who is 23 and undergoing a radical inguinal orchiectomy with retroperitoneal lymph node dissection for testicular cancer.
2. Assume you are attending a team conference to plan the care of a client who is having a suprapubic prostatectomy. What nursing interventions are appropriate for managing the client's care?
3. Describe the typical client who acquires prostatic hypertrophy versus one who develops testicular cancer.

Suggested Readings

Brodsky, M. S. (1995). Testicular cancer survivors impression of the impact of the disease on their lives. *Qualitative Health Research, 5*(1), 78–96.

Bullock, B. L. (1996). *Pathophysiology: Adaptations and alterations in function* (4th ed.). Philadelphia: Lippincott-Raven.

Churchil, J. A. (1997). Transurethral prostatectomy–New trends. *Geriatric Nursing, 18*(2), 78–80.

Gordon, I. G., Brendan, J. A., Wyble, J. C. & Ivey, C. L. (1997). When the diagnosis is penile cancer. *RN 60*(3), 41–44.

Hawkins, C., & Miaskowski, C. (1996). Continuing education. Testicular cancer: A review. *Oncology Nursing Forum, 23*(8), 1203–1213.

Kelley, W. N. (1997). *Textbook of internal medicine* (3rd ed.). Philadelphia: Lippincott-Raven.

Memmler, R. L., Cohen, B. J. & Wood, D. L. (1996). *The human body in health and disease* (8th ed.). Philadelphia: Lippincott-Raven.

Sherwood, L. (1995). *Fundamentals of physiology: A human perspective* (2nd ed.). St. Paul: West Publishing.

Additional Resources

American Cancer Society
website: http://www.cancer.org

Support groups for prostate cancer:

Man to Man, Inc.
910 Contento St.
Sarasota, FL 34242–1816
(813) 349–1719
Fax (813) 365–3256

Us Too
930 North York Road
Suite 50
Hinsdale, IL 60521–2993
(800) 80-US-TOO
Fax (708) 323–1003

Prostate Information Hot Line
(800) 543–9632

Recovery of Male Potency (ROMP)
c/o Harper Hospital
27177 Lahser Road
Suite 101
Southfield, MI 48034
(801) 357–1314

Cancer InfoService, sponsored by the National Cancer Institute
(800) 4-CANCER

Chapter 61

Caring for Clients With Sexually Transmitted Diseases

KEY TERMS

Autoinoculation
Chancre
Chancroid
Charcot's joints
Chlamydia
Condylomas
Epidemiology
Genital herpes
Gonorrhea
Granuloma inguinale
Herpes simplex virus
Human papillomavirus
Lymphogranuloma venereum
Neuropathic joint disease
Syphilis
Tabes dorsalis
Venereal diseases

LEARNING OBJECTIVES

On completion of this chapter, the reader will:

- Name five common sexually transmitted diseases (STDs) and identify which ones are curable.
- List seven STDs that by law must be reported.
- Give two reasons why statistics on reportable STDs are not totally accurate.
- Discuss several reasons that contribute to the transmission of STDs.
- Give two reasons why women acquire STDs more often than men.
- Name the most common and fastest spreading STD.
- Explain two ways STDs are spread.
- Discuss methods that are helpful in preventing STDs.
- Discuss information that is important to teach clients about using condoms.
- Give the classification of the infectious microorganism that causes each of the common STDs.
- Identify complications that are common among clients who acquire each of the most common STDs.
- Name drugs that are used to treat the common STDs.• Discuss the general nursing management of clients with STDs.

Sexually transmitted diseases (STDs), also known as **venereal diseases**, are a diverse group of infections spread through sexual activity with an infected person and represent a significant public health problem. Some, such as acquired immunodeficiency syndrome (AIDS; see Chap. 42), hepatitis (see Chap. 54), and skin infestations with lice and mites (see Chap. 68), are spread by additional routes as well. The pathogens that cause STDs include bacteria, fungi, parasites, protozoans, and viruses. Besides AIDS, the five most common STDs include clamydia, gonorrhea, syphilis, and genital herpes and genital warts. Of these, clamydia, gonorrhea, and syphilis are easily cured with early and adequate treatment. Social, sexual, and biologic factors contribute to the high incidence of venereal disease and include:

- Ignorance of how STDs are transmitted or prevented
- Asymptomatic sex partner(s)
- Casual sex with partner(s) about whom little is known
- Sex with high-risk partner(s), like those who use intravenous drugs, are bisexual, or have sex with prostitutes
- Multiple concurrent or sequential sex partner(s)
- Failure to use contraceptive techniques that also reduce the risk for acquiring STDs
- Sexual contact during the period between infection and the manifestation of symptoms
- Failure to seek early treatment
- Noncompliance with treatment or instructions to refrain from sexual contact until treatment is complete
- Mutation and resistance of microorganisms to antimicrobial drug therapy

Epidemiology

Epidemiology is the study of the occurrence, distribution, and causes of human diseases. The Centers for Disease Control and Prevention (CDC) has the awesome task of gathering disease statistics such as the incidence of STDs. It is difficult to determine the exact incidence of these diseases because only a few are reportable by law (Box 61–1), and some go untreated, treated and unreported, or misdiagnosed or undiagnosed. Women acquire STDs more often than men probably because the moist, warm vaginal environment is conducive to microbial growth and because the vagina, as a receptive orifice, is more readily traumatized during sexual activity. Table 61–1 lists common STDs and their estimated incidence in the U.S.

Obtaining a sexual history (Nursing Guidelines 61–1) is a crucial component of assessment of clients presenting with signs or symptoms of an STD and it is important to ask questions nonjudgmentally. In addition to curing the infection when possible (some STDs are not curable), treatment consists of education and counseling to reduce the client's risk for contracting an STD in the future (Nursing Guidelines 61–2), and screening, counseling and, if indicated, treating their sexual partner(s).

TABLE 61-1. **Common STDs and Estimated Incidence in the United States**

STD	Number of Cases/Year
Chlamydia	4,000,000
Condyloma acuminata	500,000–1,000,000
Gonorrhea	800,000
Genital herpes	200,000–500,000
Syphilis	101,000
AIDS	90,000
Hepatitis	53,000

Adapted from Centers for Disease Control and Prevention, Division of STD/HIV Prevention annual report, 1994.

Common Sexually Transmitted Diseases

Chlamydia

Chlamydia is the most common and fastest spreading STD in the United States. The number of new cases and reinfections amount to as many as 4 million annually.

ETIOLOGY AND PATHOPHYSIOLOGY

The causative microorganism is a bacterium, *Chlamydia trachomatis*, which lives inside the cells it infects. The disease is spread by sexual intercourse or genital contact without penetration.

The microorganism invades the reproductive structures (see pelvic inflammatory disease [PID] in Chap. 58), the urethra in women, and the urethra and epididymis in men (see nongonoccocal urethritis in Chap. 63). The irritated tissue, which may be permanent despite successful eradication of the bacteria, puts those with chlamydial infections at greater risk for acquiring other STDs, such as AIDS. Untreated chlamydia can cause sterility in infected women; infected pregnant women can transmit the microorganism to their infants during birth.

Chlamydial infections also can be spread to the eyes by **autoinoculation** (self-transmission to another area of the body) usually via unwashed hands. Ophthalmic infections, which are more common in underdeveloped countries where flies are the vector for transmitting the microorganism, can cause granulation of the cornea and blindness.

ASSESSMENT FINDINGS

Signs and Symptoms

As many as 75% of all infected women and 25% of all infected men are asymptomatic. Symptoms, if they

BOX 61-1. Reportable STDs

By federal law, the following STDs must be reported to the Department of Public Health:

- Gonorrhea
- Syphilis
- Chlamydia
- Chanroid
- Granuloma inguinale
- Lymphogranuloma venereum
- Acquired immunodeficiency syndrome

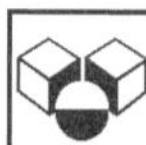

Nursing Guidelines 61-1

Obtaining a Sexual History from the Client With an STD

- Has the client had new or multiple sexual partners in recent weeks?
- Was a condom used during sexual activity?
- Is there a past history of STD?
- Has the client engaged in vaginal, anal, or oral sex?
- Was the client the receptive partner in anal or oral sex?
- Is there a history of infection with human immunodeficiency virus?
- Is there a history of employment as a sex worker?
- Are drugs and alcohol used?
- Is there a possibility of pregnancy?

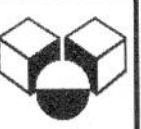

Nursing Guidelines 61-2

Methods for Reducing the Risk for STDs

- Abstain from sexual activities.
- Have monogamous sex with an uninfected partner.
- Use latex condoms with nonoxynol-9 (a spermicide) when having oral, vaginal, or anal intercourse.
- Combine the use of male condoms with a spermicide when having vaginal intercourse or use a female condom.
- Urinate and wash the genital and perineal areas before and immediately after having sexual intercourse.
- Wash your hands and any areas where there has been direct contact with semen or vaginal mucus.
- Refuse or terminate sexual activity that causes trauma to the genitals, internal reproductive structures, anus, and elsewhere.
- If infected, report the information to all sexual partners and encourage them to seek medical diagnosis and treatment.
- Avoid unprotected sex until you and sex partners have completed treatment.

occur, may appear 1 to 3 weeks after infection. They include a sparse, clear urethral discharge, redness and irritation of the infected tissue, burning on urination, lower abdominal pain in women, or testicular pain in men.

Diagnostic Findings

Diagnosis is made by microscopic examination and culture of secretions. A test kit is available that identifies the microorganism in approximately 15 minutes. It is common practice to test clients for chlamydia, gonorrhea, and syphilis because it is not unusual for clients to have concurrent infections with more than one STD.

MEDICAL MANAGEMENT

Antimicrobial drugs, such as doxycycline (Vibramycin), the tetracyclines, erythromycin, clarithromycin (Biaxin), and azithromycin (Zithromax) are used for treatment.

NURSING MANAGEMENT

The nurse sensitively obtains a sexual history, follows precautions for preventing infection transmission, assists in collecting a specimen for microscopic analysis, explains the course of treatment, and discusses methods for preventing transmission and reinfection (see Nursing Care Plan 61–1 and Nursing Guidelines 61–3).

For more specific nursing management, refer to Nursing Care Plan 61–1.

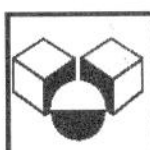

Nursing Guidelines 61-3

Educating the Client With an STD

- Take prescribed medication according to label directions for the full length of time that it is prescribed.
- Stop having sex until retesting indicates that the infection is gone.
- Urge any and all sex partners to be examined and follow through with concurrent treatment.
- Use a *condom*, a contraceptive barrier device, consistently and correctly (see Nursing Guidelines 61-4) before any and all sexual contact after completing medical treatment.
- Do not assume that successful treatment means there is any permanent immunity; reinfection can and does occur if preventive sexual practices are not implemented.
- Seek treatment as soon as possible if the symptoms continue or if they recur following successful treatment.

Gonorrhea

Gonorrhea is a common STD with the highest incidence in the 15- to 24-year-old age group. Many women are asymptomatic, a factor that contributes to the spread of the disease.

ETIOLOGY AND PATHOPHYSIOLOGY

The infection is caused by a bacteria, *Neisseria gonorrhoeae,* which can be transmitted hetero- or homosexually. The microorganism invades the urethra, vagina, rectum, or pharynx depending on the nature of sexual contact; it can spread throughout the body.

In untreated men, the localized infection may spread to the prostate, seminal vesicles, and epididymis. Urethral strictures may develop, requiring periodic dilatation of the urethra or, possibly, reconstructive urethral surgery. In women the infection may progress upward to the cervix, endometrium, and fallopian tubes and symptoms of PID (see Chap. 57) may develop. Gonorrhea can also be transmitted to an infant's eyes at the time of birth.

ASSESSMENT FINDINGS

Signs and Symptoms

In men, symptoms usually appear 2 to 6 days after infection. Urethritis with a purulent discharge and pain on urination are the most common signs and symptoms. A small proportion of men are asymptomatic. More than half of infected women experience no symptoms. When symptoms do occur, women have a white or yellow vaginal discharge, intermenstrual bleeding

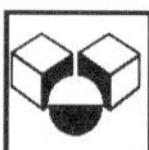

Nursing Guidelines 61-4

Teaching Clients How to Use a Condom

- Purchase condoms that are made in the United States because they are of high quality and have been tested for reliability.
- Select condoms that are lubricated with a spermicide or silicone.
- Natural-membrane condoms are porous and although they act as a barrier to sperm, viruses may pass through.
- Discard condoms beyond their expiration date or that are more than 5 years old.
- Never unroll or examine a condom before its use or use one that appears to have deteriorated.
- Unroll the condom over the erect penis while pinching the space at the condom tip.

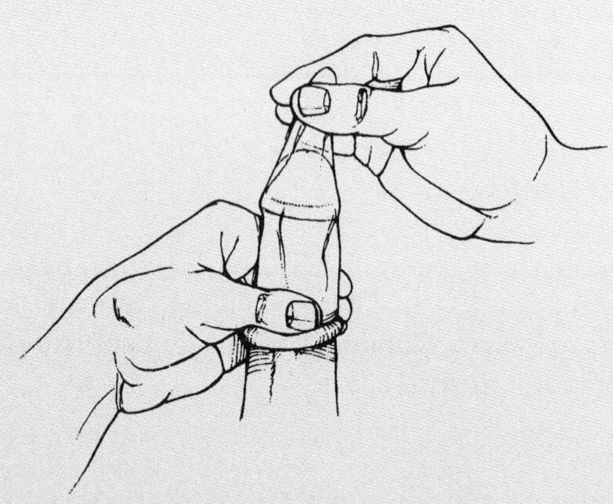

- Remove the condom at the base of the penis during its removal from the vagina before the penis becomes limp.
- Apply a new condom for each sex act.
- Breakage and slipping rates may be higher during anal sex.
- Condom breakage rate can be reduced by using a silicone-based lubricant; silicone does not deteriorate latex.

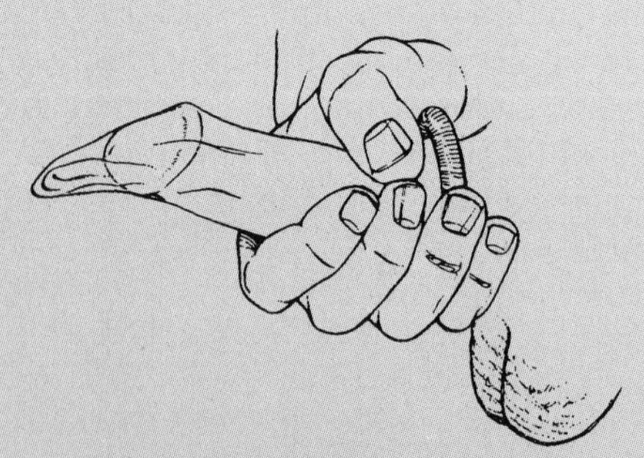

Adapted from CDC National Training Bulletin #138, 1995.

due to cervicitis, and painful urination. An anal infection is accompanied by painful bowel elimination and a purulent rectal discharge; the throat is sore when the pharynx is infected. If the microorganism disseminates (scatters) throughout the body, the client may manifest a skin rash, fever, and painful joints.

Diagnostic Findings

Specimens of drainage from infected tissue are examined microscopically immediately after they are collected or are inoculated on a culture medium and incubated to reveal the causative organism.

MEDICAL MANAGEMENT

Due to the increasing resistance of *N. gonorrhoeae* to penicillin, gonorrhea is now treated with a single intramuscular dose of ceftriaxone (Rocephin) or a single oral dose of ciprofloxacin (Cipro). Coinfection with chlamydia is common and clients are also given oral doxycycline (Vibramycin) for 7 to 10 days. Clients with complicated gonococcal infections, as in PID or disseminated infection, are hospitalized and treated with intravenous, multiple drug therapy. Repeat therapy with different antibiotics may be required.

NURSING MANAGEMENT

The nursing management and client teaching are similar to that provided clients with chlamydia. However, when a culture is collected from a woman, the vaginal speculum is moistened with water rather than lubricated, which may destroy the gonococci and cause inaccurate test results. (Also, see Nursing Care Plan 61–1.)

Syphilis

Syphilis is a curable STD that can also be transmitted from the blood of an infected person or across the placenta to an unborn infant. The incidence of syphilis in the United States has reached epidemic proportions and has risen dramatically in certain groups particularly young African American men and women. Surprisingly, there were fewer cases reported in 1995 than any year since 1960 (Division of STD Prevention, 1996).

ETIOLOGY AND PATHOPHYSIOLOGY

The spirochete *Treponema pallidum* is the causative microorganism of syphilis. The time between infection and the first occurrence of symptoms is about 21 days. If untreated, syphilis progresses through three distinct stages: primary, secondary, and tertiary.

Syphilis is infectious only during the primary and secondary stages. In the third stage, the client becomes demented and dies from complications involving other organ systems.

ASSESSMENT FINDINGS

Signs and Symptoms

In the primary (early) stage, a **chancre** (painless ulcer) appears on the genitals, anus, cervix, or other parts of the body (Fig. 61–1). At first the lesion resembles a small papule, which later ulcerates. The chancre heals in several weeks and, if treatment has not been initiated, the client progresses to the secondary stage of syphilis.

Symptoms of secondary stage syphilis include fever, malaise, rash, headache, sore throat, and lymph node enlargement. Late, or tertiary, syphilis is noninfectious because the microorganism has invaded the central nervous system (CNS) as well as other organs of the body. Symptoms of tertiary syphilis include **tabes dorsalis** (a degenerative condition of the CNS that results in loss of peripheral reflexes and of vibratory and position senses), ataxia, and **neuropathic joint disease** also called **Charcot's joints.** Cardiovascular complications include aortic aneurysm and aortic valve insufficiency.

Diagnostic Findings

Diagnosis is made by detecting the spirochete in microscopic examination of scrapings from the chancre, by a positive Venereal Disease Research Laboratory (VDRL) test on blood serum, and a positive fluorescent treponemal antibody absorption test (FTA-ABS). Occasionally the FTA-ABS test is falsely positive in clients with systemic lupus erythematosus (SLE), a connective tissue disease.

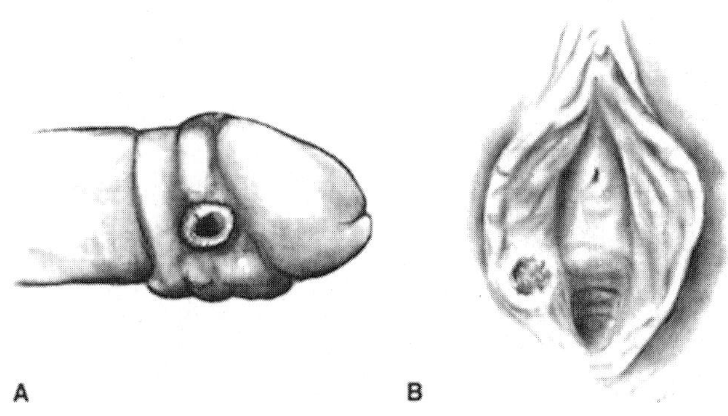

FIGURE 61-1. Syphilitic chancres. (A) Penile chancre. (B) Vulvar chancre.

MEDICAL MANAGEMENT

Penicillin is used to treat primary and secondary syphilis. Clients who are allergic to the penicillins are given tetracycline or doxycycline. Follow-up examinations and laboratory tests are recommended 3, 6, and 12 months after initial treatment. Those with tertiary syphilis require larger doses of penicillin. The response is poor in those with cardiovascular syphilis.

NURSING MANAGEMENT

The nurse gathers health information and a sexual history, asks about the client's allergy history in anticipation of antibiotic treatment, prepares the client for diagnostic laboratory tests, supports the client emotionally at the time the diagnosis is confirmed, and informs the client that case-finding is reported to the department of public health. (See Nursing Care Plan 61–1 for more on nursing management.)

Herpes Infection

Herpes infection is a highly contagious STD that is controllable but not curable. It increases the risk for cervical cancer and infection with human immunodeficiency virus (HIV).

ETIOLOGY AND PATHOPHYSIOLOGY

Although **herpes simplex virus** type 2 (HSV-2), also known as **genital herpes,** is primarily responsible for genital and perineal lesions, herpes simplex virus type 1 (HSV-1), associated with cold sores around the nose and lips, can also cause anogenital lesions. Transmission of these viruses is either by direct contact with oral or genital secretions from a person during an active stage of the disease, sexual contact during periods of asymptomatic viral shedding, or by autoinoculation. Either virus may be introduced into the eye, the mouth, the genital area, or a skin site.

Genital herpes increases the risk for cervical cancer and HIV infection. Transmission can also occur from mother to infant during a vaginal birth and carries a neonatal mortality rate of 50% (Reeder, Martin, & Koniak, 1992).

Herpes recurs because after the initial infection, the virus remains dormant in the ganglia of the nerves that supply the area. Symptoms are generally more severe with the initial outbreak. Subsequent episodes are usually shorter and less intense. When the virus is active, shedding viral particles are infectious.

Most victims have at least one outbreak per year and many clients report 5 to 10 outbreaks per year. Some clients note that stress, emotional situations, exposure to sunlight, menstruation, and fever reactivate the disease.

ASSESSMENT FINDINGS

Signs and Symptoms

After a short incubation period, HSV-2 causes single or multiple vesicles on the penis, prepuce, buttocks, thighs, introitus, or cervix (Fig. 61–2). The HSV-2 lesions burn and itch before becoming fluid-filled blisters. The vesicles rupture in 1 to 3 days and are followed by painful reddened ulcers that scab over and eventually disappear. The outbreak may be accompanied by swelling of the inguinal lymph nodes, flu-like symptoms, and headache.

The initial attack lasts 3 to 4 weeks; subsequent attacks usually last 10 days.

Diagnostic Findings

Diagnosis of HSV-1 and HSV-2 is tentatively made by inspecting the lesions. Smears and scrapings from the lesions are examined microscopically using special stains to confirm the clinical impression.

MEDICAL MANAGEMENT

Because an outbreak of HSV-1 is often self-limiting, treatment may be unnecessary. If treated, either type of HSV responds to the antiviral drug acyclovir (Zovirax) (Table 61–2). Intravenous acyclovir is used if there is a severe episode of HSV-2 or if the client is immunocompromised. Acyclovir shortens subsequent active episodes and tends to reduce the frequency of outbreaks. Cesarean delivery is performed on pregnant women with active lesions.

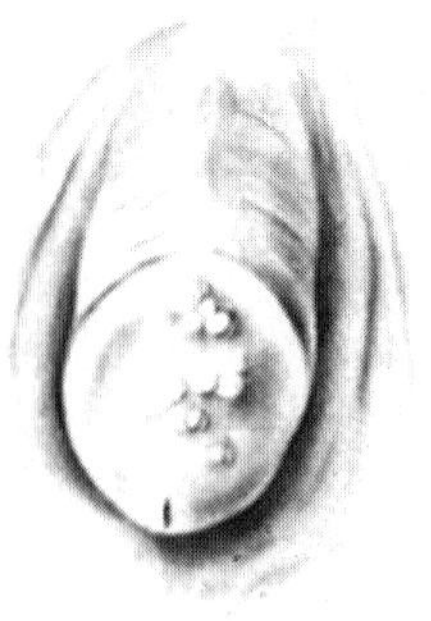

A

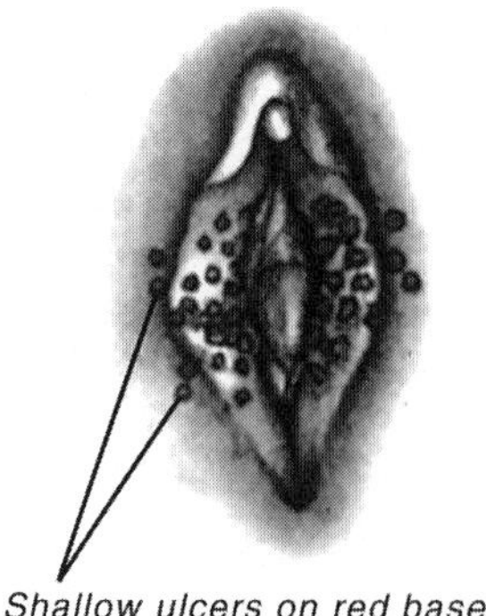

B

FIGURE 61-2. Herpes genitalis lesions. (A) Penile lesions. (B) Vulvar lesions.

NURSING MANAGEMENT

The nurse collects appropriate health and sexual data, uses Standard Precautions when inspecting lesions, obtains specimens, and provides related health teaching.

More on nursing management appears in Nursing Care Plan 61–1.

Client Teaching

Clients with HSV-2 infections are instructed to:

- Inform all potential sexual partners of the HSV infection, even if it is in an inactive state.
- Use a condom during sexual activity even if the disease is dormant.
- Avoid sexual contact if there is any question that the infection is active; condoms will not protect skin and mucous membrane that is left exposed.
- Keep lesions dry using alcohol, peroxide, witch hazel, and warm air from a hair dryer.
- Check with the physician about taking warm baths with Epsom salts or baking soda to relieve discomfort.
- Wear loose clothing that promotes air circulation about the genitals.
- Perform thorough handwashing after direct contact with lesions, and keep any personal hygiene articles like a towel, separate from the inadvertent use by others.
- Use a separate towel to pat lesions dry and another when drying other body parts to avoid autoinoculation.
- Have annual Pap smears to detect cervical cancer.
- Investigate stress management strategies because reducing stress tends to decrease the frequency of outbreaks.

Venereal Warts

Venereal (genital) **warts,** also called **condylomas,** are an STD that tends to recur even after treatment. Anyone can become infected with venereal warts, but people with AIDS as well as others with an immunodeficiency are particularly susceptible. One-fourth of the people in the United States carry the virus, are infectious, but do not manifest symptoms.

ETIOLOGY AND PATHOPHYSIOLOGY

Venereal warts are caused by the **human papillomavirus** (HPV). It is transmitted by genital–genital, genital–anal, or genital–oral contact with an infected person and is contagious as long as the warts are

TABLE 61-2. **Drug Therapy for STDs**

Drug/Use	Side Effects	Nursing Considerations
Antibiotics	Allergy, anaphylaxis (applies to all antibiotics listed below)	Inquire about allergies and past reactions to medications. Be aware that clients allergic to cephalosporins may also be allergic to penicillin antibiotics. Inform client to seek treatment if rash, hives, fever or difficulty breathing occur.
Penicillin G: syphilis, gonorrhea	Allergy, stomatis, nausea, vomiting, diarrhea, rash, fever, wheezing, pain at injection site	Give intramuscularly into gluteus maximus only. Massage site. Have client wait for 30 min after injection in case allergic reaction occurs.
Erythromycin: syphilis, gonorrhea, chlamydia, chancroid, lymphogranuloma venereum, prophylactically to prevent eye infection in newborns	Allergy, abdominal cramps, diarrhea, vomiting, rash, emotional lability, altered thinking, ototoxicity, hepatitis	Reassure client that emotional and cognitive side effects, should they occur, are temporary. Report tinnitus and jaundice.
Doxycycline: syphilis, gonorrhea, granuloma inguinale, lymphogranuloma venereum	Allergy, anorexia, nausea, vomiting, diarrhea, sensitivity to light, liver failure, discoloration of developing teeth, liver damage	Suggest taking with meals if gastrointestinal upset occurs. Inform client to report dark-colored urine or light-colored stools. Use a sunscreen. Strongly encourage client to return for all follow-up visits to ensure that organism has been eradicated.
Ceftriaxone: gonorrhea	Allergy, anorexia, nausea, vomiting, diarrhea, rash fever, decreased hematocrit, disulfiram-like reaction with alcohol	Avoid alcohol during and for 3 days after drug therapy. Inform client of possible side effects and to report unusual fatigue.
Tetracycline: syphilis, gonorrhea, chlamydia	Allergy, nausea, vomiting, diarrhea, discoloration of developing teeth, phototoxicity, superinfections	Take on an empty stomach. Avoid antacids, dairy products, and iron supplements. Do not use outdated drugs because they are nephrotoxic. Use a sunscreen. Report appearance of oral or vaginal yeast infections.
Ciprofloxacin: gonorrhea	Headache, dizziness, nausea, diarrhea, vomiting	Take on an empty stomach and avoid antacids within 2 hrs of antibiotic dose. Drink plenty of water. Report any side effects.
Antivirals		
Acyclovir: decreases severity and frequency of herpes outbreaks	Transient burning at application site	Apply with a rubber glove or finger cot. Inform client that drug does not cure the disease. Clients should avoid sexual activity during outbreaks and wear a condom at other times.
Caustics		
Podophylium resin: venereal warts	Peripheral neuropathy, thrombocytopenia and leukopenia when absorbed systemically, irritation of normal tissue	Highly toxic and should be applied only by the physician. Surrounding skin may be protected with petroleum jelly. Use minimal amount possible. Warn client that local irritation may occur in 12–48 h.

Strongly encourage all clients to return for all follow-up visits to ensure that organism has been eradicated.

present. Sexual penetration is not necessary to transmit the virus and the warts can also be spread to other body areas by autoinoculation. The virus is contagious as long as the warts are present. Warts can grow in the mouth and throat of infants infected at birth. There is an increased risk of cancer of the vulva, vagina, and cervix in women with genital warts.

ASSESSMENT FINDINGS

Signs and Symptoms

Genital warts usually are painless and appear as a single lesion or cluster of soft, fleshy growths on the genitalia (Fig. 61–3), cervix, within the vagina, on the perineum, anus, throat, or mouth. Sometimes the warts are so small that they are inconspicuous. However, they

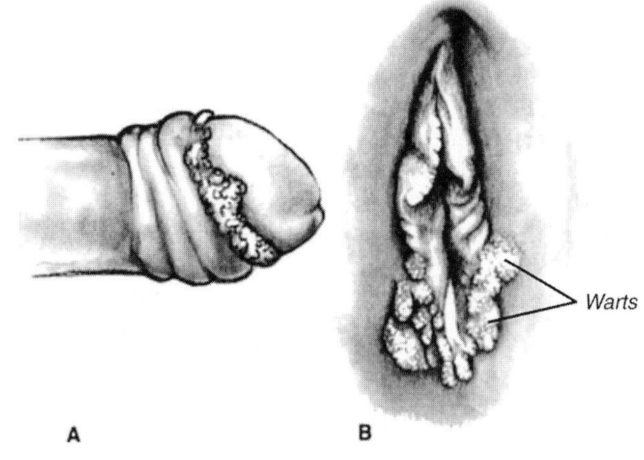

FIGURE 61-3. Venereal warts. (A) Penile warts. (B) Vulvar warts.

can become large and raised—resembling a cauliflower. Large venereal warts may narrow or obstruct the urethra, vagina, anus, or throat.

Diagnostic Findings

Venereal warts turn white when vinegar is applied to the lesion. The highlighted tissue is then examined with a magnifying glass.

MEDICAL AND SURGICAL MANAGEMENT

Warts are removed in various ways: laser therapy, electrocautery (heat), cryosurgery (freezing), or by treating them with chemicals. Three major drugs are used to eradicate the warts: trichloroacetic acid, podophyllin solution in tincture of benzoin, and fluorouracil (5-FU). Eradication does not mean the condition is cured; the person is temporarily noncontagious once the warts are destroyed.

NURSING MANAGEMENT

Nurses provide information about STD transmission to sexually active people and prepare affected individuals for medical examination, diagnosis, and treatment.

Nursing management is discussed further in Nursing Care Plan 61–1.

Client Teaching

The nurse tells clients with venereal warts to:

- Avoid intimate contact until the warts are removed.
- Advise all sexual contacts to be examined and treated.
- Seek treatment at an STD clinic or with a private physician when, and if, the warts return.
- Use a condom even when the lesions are absent, and suggest that the sex partner wash his or her genitals or other skin areas immediately after intimate contact.
- Provide information about the diagnosis and treatment in future health histories, especially if a pregnancy occurs.
- Avoid stress and genital trauma, which appear to be factors in reactivating the virus (Porth, 1994).
- Obtain yearly examinations for the possibility of reproductive cancers.

Other Sexually Transmitted Diseases

Granuloma Inguinale

Granuloma inguinale, or donovanosis, is caused by *Calymmatobacterium granulomatis* and is relatively uncommon in the United States. The infection is characterized by lesions in the genital, inguinal, and anal areas; it is treated with antimicrobials, usually tetracycline or sulfisoxazole (Gantrisin).

Chancroid

Chancroid is caused by the *Haemophilus ducreyi* bacillus. The infection is characterized by the appearance of a macule, followed by vesicle–pustule formation and, finally, a painful ulcer. It is treated and cured with erythromycin or tetracycline.

Lymphogranuloma Venereum

Lymphogranuloma venereum, caused by a strain of *C. trachomatis,* is characterized by a small erosion or papule and enlargement of adjacent lymph nodes. The affected lymph nodes can become necrotic. The usual site of infection is the genital area. The infection is treated with tetracycline.

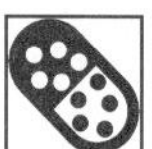

General Pharmacologic Considerations

An allergy history is obtained before administration of any antimicrobial agent. The physician is informed of an allergy to any antimicrobial agent, so that a different drug can be ordered.

The prescribed drug regimen is explained to the client. Information includes the number of capsules or tablets per dose, the time of day the drug is to be taken, food restrictions (if any), and possible adverse effects. Emphasis is placed on the importance of completing a course of therapy.

Both doxycycline and azithromycin are contraindicated during pregnancy.

Clients receiving penicillin are monitored for at least 30 minutes after a parenteral injection to watch for a possible allergic reaction. Symptoms of an allergic reaction include pruritus, difficulty breathing, hypotension, sweating, and tachycardia.

Observe the client closely for an allergic reaction, which can occur at any time during antibiotic administration. If an allergic reaction occurs, contact the primary health care provider immediately.

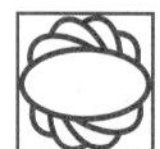

General Gerontologic Considerations

Nurses must abandon biases that older adults are sexually inactive. Therefore, when taking a health history, questions about sexuality and behaviors that put them at risk for STDs are not ignored.

NURSING CARE PLAN 61-1
Nursing Management of the Client with an STD

Potential Problems and Nursing Diagnosis	Nursing Management	Outcome Criteria
Risk for Infection Transmission related to infectious drainage and viral shedding	Follow Standard Precautions prior to diagnosis and contact precautions after diagnosis is confirmed. Advise to have sexual partners tested and treated. Identify methods for preventing STD transmission such as abstinence, using barrier and chemical types of contraceptives, washing following intercourse. Recommend early prenatal care to women who are infected with diseases that can be transmitted during childbirth. Explain how to manage articles used for personal hygiene or items to avoid sharing with noninfected people. Direct the client to take medications as prescribed and return for medical follow-up to verify that the disease is responding to treatment or has been cured.	Infection transmission is prevented.
Risk for Noncompliance and **Ineffective Management of Therapeutic Regimen** related to lack of knowledge or abandoning recommendations	Provide specific client teaching appropriate for the particular STD. Stress completing the duration of drug therapy to cure the STD, relieve symptoms, or put the disease in a latent stage. Provide a hot-line telephone number where the client can receive objective, authoritative information. Schedule an appointment for follow-up care.	The client complies with treatment regimen.
Pain and Altered Comfort related to inflammation and changes in the skin and mucous membranes.	Consult with the physician about recommending a nonprescription analgesic. Advise regular bathing and patting rather than rubbing the skin dry. Recommend wearing loosely woven underclothing and full cut, nonconstricting outer clothing. Tell the client that comfort depends on completing a full course of medical treatment.	The client is comfortable; symptoms are reduced or relieved.
Impaired Skin Integrity and **Altered Mucous Membranes** related to inflammation of local tissues secondary to infectious process	Provide information on appropriate hygiene and local applications that help to restore the integrity of the tissue. Reinforce compliance with medical treatment.	Lesions heal integrity of skin and mucous membrane is restored.
Anxiety related to possible consequences of STD.	Explain the cause of the STD and how potential consequences or complications can be avoided. Instruct the client infected with carcinogenic (cancer-causing) viruses to have regular cancer screening examinations.	Anxieties are relieved with realistic information.
Situational Low Self-Esteem related to shame or guilt about infection	Avoid being judgmental. Affirm the client's good judgment to seek treatment. Assure the client that medical information is confidential and though some diseases are reported, access to that information is carefully guarded. Refer the client to a support group for people who have acquired STD.	Self-esteem is restored.
Altered Sexuality Patterns related to shame about revealing STD risk to sexual partner(s)	Role play situations in which STD status is communicated to a significant other, and suggest that sex partner(s) consult with a physician or public health nurse about sexual practices that reduce the potential for STD transmission.	Relationships continue with modified sexual practices to avoid disease transmission.

Older clients who are sexually active have the same risks of acquiring an STD as other age groups.

Some older clients have limited knowledge about STDs and therefore may not recognize the symptoms or seek treatment.

Older adults who are not in monogamous relationships may not understand that barrier and chemical contraceptives are appropriate for preventing STDs.

Approximately 10% of heart disease in those over 50 years of age is caused by syphilis. The most frequently seen valvular disorder as the result of syphilis is aortic insufficiency. Damaged valves may need to be replaced with a ball-valve prosthesis.

Some older adults with an STD are embarrassed and may not seek medical attention. Careful assessment is necessary to help the older adult obtain medical treatment as quickly as possible.

SUMMARY OF KEY CONCEPTS

- Besides AIDS, five common STDs include chlamydia, gonorrhea, syphilis, herpes infections, and venereal warts. Of these, chlamydia, gonorrhea, and syphilis are curable.
- Despite the fact that there are many STDs, public health statistics are kept on only seven: chlamydia, gonorrhea, syphilis, chancroid, granuloma inguinale, lymphogranuloma venereum, and AIDS.
- Statistics on the reportable STDs are somewhat inaccurate because some diseases are untreated and some that are treated are not reported.
- Several factors contribute to the spread of STDs: ignorance of how STDs are transmitted and prevented, sex partners who can be asymptomatic yet infectious, failure to seek early treatment, noncompliance with the treatment regimen, and resistance of curable STDs to antimicrobial therapy, to name just a few.
- Women acquire STDs more often than men because the vaginal environment is warm and moist–conditions that favor microbial growth, and because the female reproductive tract, the usual receptive orifice for sex, is more susceptible to infection when traumatized and subsequently inflamed.
- The most common and fastest spreading STD is chlamydia.
- STDs are spread by direct contact—genital to genital or skin to skin, but they may also be spread by autoinoculation.
- STDs can be prevented in a number of ways. Some examples include: sexual abstinence, having monogamous sex with an uninfected partner, using barrier and chemical contraceptive techniques, avoiding intercourse with anyone who has symptoms of an STD or who has not completed medical treatment.
- Some information that is important to provide when explaining the use of a condom include: use condoms manufactured and tested in the United States, discard old or deteriorated condoms, unroll a fresh condom over the erect penis, remove the condom before the penis becomes limp, and use a new condom for each sex act.
- Not all STDs are caused by the same infectious microorganism. Chlamydia is caused by a bacterium, *C. trachomatis*; gonorrhea is caused by the bacterium, *N. gonorrhoeae*; syphilis is caused by a bacterial spirochete, *T. pallidum*, and herpes infections and venereal warts are caused by two different viruses.
- Serious complications can result from STDs in both men and women. Having any one STD predisposes to acquiring others, especially AIDS. Chlamydia and gonorrhea can extend to other urinary and reproductive structures sometimes leading to sterility. All of the common STDs, including AIDS, can be transmitted to infants at the time of birth. Untreated syphilis can cause damage to the nervous and cardiovascular systems. HSV and HPV predispose to reproductive cancers in women.
- Several drugs are used to treat STDs, including penicillin, doxycyline, ceftriaxone, acyclovir, fluorouracil, and podophyllin.
- Nursing management of clients with STDs includes obtaining a sexual history, following Standard Precautions for preventing infection transmission, assisting in collecting a specimen for microscopic analysis, providing the physician with the forms for reporting certain diseases, and explaining the course of treatment and methods for preventing transmission and reinfection. Other aspects of nursing care are to implement measures for restoring integrity to the skin and mucous membranes, relieving pain and discomfort, alleviating fears through education, supporting the client's self-esteem, offering suggestions for modifying sexual practices, and reinforcing compliance with the therapeutic regimen.

CRITICAL THINKING EXERCISES

1. Discuss STD information that is appropriate to provide for a person who confides that he or she is having unprotected sexual intercourse with more than one person.
2. Explain information a person should know who has never used a condom before.

Suggested Readings

Division of STD Prevention. (1996, September). *Sexually transmitted disease surveillance, 1995.* U.S. Department of Health and Human Services, Public Health Service. Atlanta, GA: Centers for Disease Control and Prevention.

Bolus, J. (1996, July/August). Straight talk about condoms. *Office Nurse*, 36–39.

Frugate, K. A., & McCloskey, M. M. (1996). Impact of sexually transmitted diseases on fertility. A review of the literature and nursing opportunities. *Infertility and Reproductive Medicine Clinics of North America*, 7(3), 521–534.

Porth, C. M. (1994). *Pathophysiology, concepts of altered health states* (4th ed.). Philadelphia: J. B. Lippincott.

Reeder, S. J., Martin, L. L., & Koniak, D. (1992). *Maternity nursing: Family, newborn, and women's health care* (17th ed.). Philadelphia: J. B. Lippincott.

Sharts-Hopko, N. S. (1997). STDs in women: What you need to know. *American Journal of Nursing 97*(4), 46–53.

Additional Resources

American Social Health Association
P.O. Box 13827
Research Triangle Park, NC 27707
(800) 783–9877

Centers for Disease Control and Prevention (CDC)
Department of Health and Human Services
Public Health Information Service
1600 Clifton Road, NE
Atlanta, GA 30333
(404) 639–3311

Centers for Disease Control and Prevention
http://www.cdc.gov/cdc.html

CDC National STD Hotline
(800) 227–8922

American Foundation for the Prevention of Venereal Disease, Inc.
799 Broadway, Suite 638
New York, NY 10003
(212) 759–2069

Sex Information and Education Council of the United States (SIECUS)
130 West 42nd Street
Suite 2500
New York, NY 10036
(212) 819–9770

15

Caring for Clients With Urinary and Renal Disorders

Chapter 62

Introduction to the Urinary Tract

KEY TERMS

Blood urea nitrogen
Costovertebral angle
Creatinine
Creatinine clearance test
Cystogram
Cystometrogram
Cystoscope
Cystoscopy
Excretory urogram
Intravenous pyelogram
Post void residual
Renal arteriograms
Retrograde pyelogram
Ultrasonography
Urinalysis
Urine protein test
Urine specific gravity
Urodynamic studies
Uroflowmetry
Urography
Voiding cystourethrogram

LEARNING OBJECTIVES

On completion of this chapter, the reader will:

- Name the five parts of the urinary system.
- Name the primary functions of the kidney and other structures in the urinary system.
- List eight tests performed for the diagnosis of urinary and renal system diseases.
- Name four laboratory tests performed for the diagnosis of urinary and renal system diseases.
- Discuss the nursing management for a client undergoing diagnostic evaluation of the urinary tract.

The urinary system consists of the kidneys, renal pelves (sing. pelvis), ureters, urinary bladder, and urethra. The kidneys have four primary functions: (1) to excrete excess water and the nitrogenous waste products of protein metabolism; (2) to assist in maintaining the acid–base balance of the body and the equilibrium of plasma electrolytes; (3) to produce the enzyme renin, which acts to raise the blood pressure, and (4) to produce the hormone erythropoietin, which regulates red blood cell production. The remainder of the urinary system is involved in the transport (ureters and pelves), storage (bladder), and excretion (urethra) of urine.

Urologic nursing assessment centers on changes in urine production, transport, storage, and elimination. Urologic nursing as it involves the reproductive systems is discussed in Chapters 58 and 60.

Anatomy and Physiology

The upper urinary tract is composed of the kidneys, renal pelves, and ureters; the lower urinary tract consists of the bladder, urethra, and pelvic floor muscles (Fig. 62–1**A**). Each of the two kidneys is enclosed in a thin, fibrous capsule and separated from the abdominal cavity anteriorly by the peritoneum. The blood supply to each kidney consists of a renal artery and renal vein. The renal artery arises from the aorta and the renal vein empties into the vena cava (Fig. 62–1**B**). Twenty-five percent of the total cardiac output is received by the kidneys.

The cross-section of the kidney (see Fig. 62–1**B**) helps to illustrate the inner structures. The two main areas are the renal pelves and the parenchyma. The parenchyma is made up of a cortex (outer layer) and a medulla (inner core). Within each cortex are microscopic nephrons that carry out the functions of the kidneys. Each kidney contains about 1 million nephrons. The *nephron* is the smallest functioning unit of the kidney. It consists of the *glomerulus, afferent arteriole, efferent arteriole, Bowman's capsule, distal* and *proximal convoluted tubules,* the *loop of Henle,* and the *collecting tubule* (Fig. 62–1**C**). The medulla contains calyces (pyramids), cone-shaped structures that open to the pelvis, a large funnel-like structure in the center of the kidney. The renal pelvis then empties into the ureter, which carries urine to the bladder for storage.

The bladder, urethra, and pelvic floor muscles form the urethrovesical unit. The urinary bladder is a hollow, muscular organ; its shape and size vary with the amount of urine it contains as well as the age of the person. The urethra is a hollow tube that begins at the bladder neck and ends at the external *meatus*. It serves as a conduit during urination and has a sphincter mechanism to prevent urine leakage. The male urethra extends approximately 24 cm (10 inches) from the bladder neck through the prostate and the penile shaft to the glans penis. The female urethra extends about 4 cm (1½–2 inches) from the bladder neck to the external meatus. The pelvic floor muscles constitute the final part of the urethrovesical unit. These muscles form a sling that supports the bladder and urethra, rectum, and some reproductive organs.

The first step in urine formation is the filtration of plasma by the glomerulus (Fig. 62–1**D**). Once the filtrate enters Bowman's capsule, it moves through the tubular system of the nephron and is either reabsorbed (placed back into the systemic circulation) or excreted as urine. The formed urine drains from the collecting tubules, into the renal pelves, and down each ureter to the bladder.

The desire to urinate comes from the feeling of bladder fullness. A nerve reflex is triggered when approximately 150 mL of urine accumulates. During urination, the bladder muscle contracts and the sphincter muscles relax, forcing urine out of the bladder and urethra through the urethral meatus. If there is any interference or abnormality of these muscles, the bladder may not empty completely or empty uncontrollably (incontinence).

Assessment

History

Obtain information about general health, childhood and family illnesses, past medical history, allergies, sexual and reproductive health, exposure to toxic chemicals or gas, and history of present complaint (Box 62–1).

Physical Examination

Ask the client to void before the examination. Inspect the abdomen for scars, symmetry, abdominal movements, and pulsations. Examine the back and note any bulging, bruising, or scars. The experienced examiner will auscultate the abdomen for bruits (abnormal vascular sounds heard over a blood vessel). Percuss the area over the bladder beginning 2 inches above the symphysis pubis and percuss toward the base of the bladder (Fig. 62–2). Percussion usually produces a tympanic sound. A dull sound is produced if the bladder is filled. Palpate the suprapubic area but note that the bladder can only be palpated if it is moderately distended. Assess the kidneys for tenderness or pain by lightly striking the fist at the **costovertebral angle** (CVA), which is the area where the lower ribs meet the vertebrae (Fig. 62–3). Normally, the client experiences a dull thud; pain or tenderness may indicate a renal disorder. Assess for signs of electrolyte and water imbalance (see Chap. 21).

Evaluate the client's general health and other symptoms such as periorbital edema (swelling around the eyes), edema of the extremities, signs of cardiac failure, and mental changes, all of which may indicate urinary tract disorders. Obtain vital signs and weight.

Diagnostic Tests

In the male client, diseases and disorders of the reproductive system also affect the urinary system. In addition to the diagnostic tests discussed below, additional tests may be performed on the male client and are discussed in Chapters 60 and 61.

Radiography

An x-ray of the abdomen, referred to as a KUB (kidney–ureter–bladder), is performed to show the size and position of the kidneys, ureters, and bony pelvis as well as the presence of radiopaque urinary *calculi* (stones), abnormal gas patterns (indicative of renal mass), and anatomic defects of the bony spinal column (indicative of neuropathic bladder dysfunction). A radiograph of the pelvis, chest, or other area may reveal metastatic bone lesions that could be a result of renal or bladder tumors.

Ultrasonography

Renal **ultrasonography** identifies the kidney's shape, size, location, collecting systems, and adjacent tissues. Other uses include identification of renal cysts or obstruction sites, assistance in needle placement for renal biopsy or nephrostomy tube placement, and drainage of a renal abscess. There are no contraindications for this procedure. It is not invasive, does not require the injection of a radiopaque dye, and does not require fasting or bowel preparation for renal or bladder sonogram.

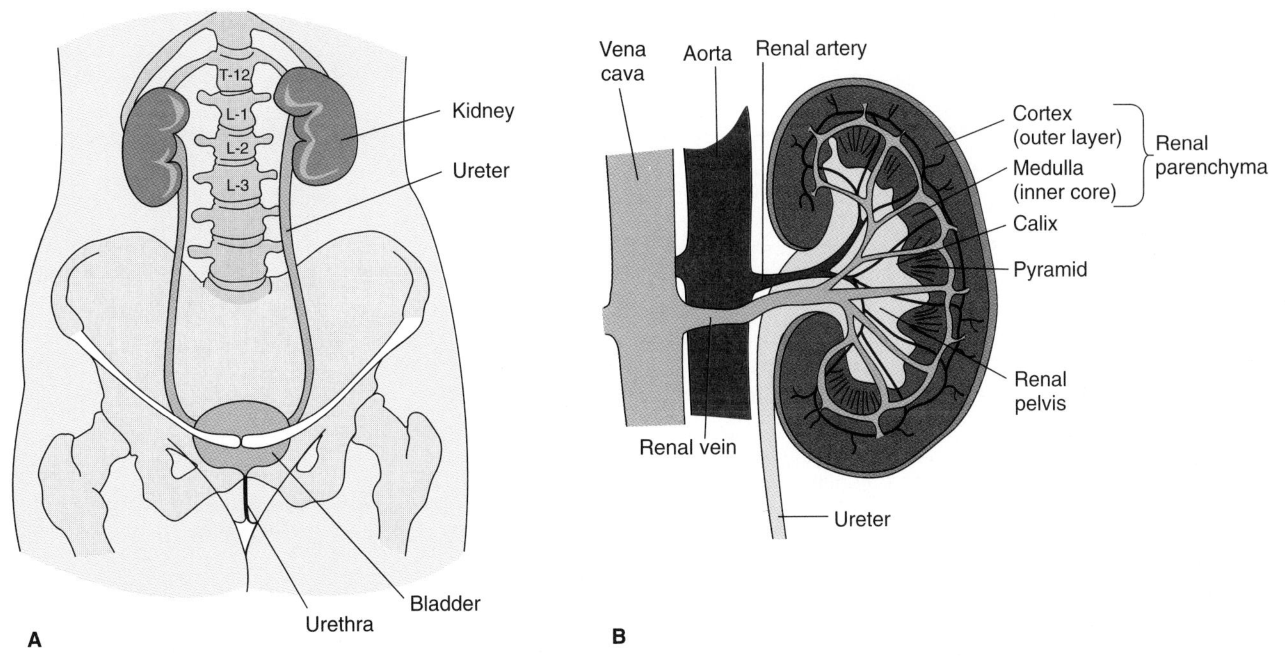

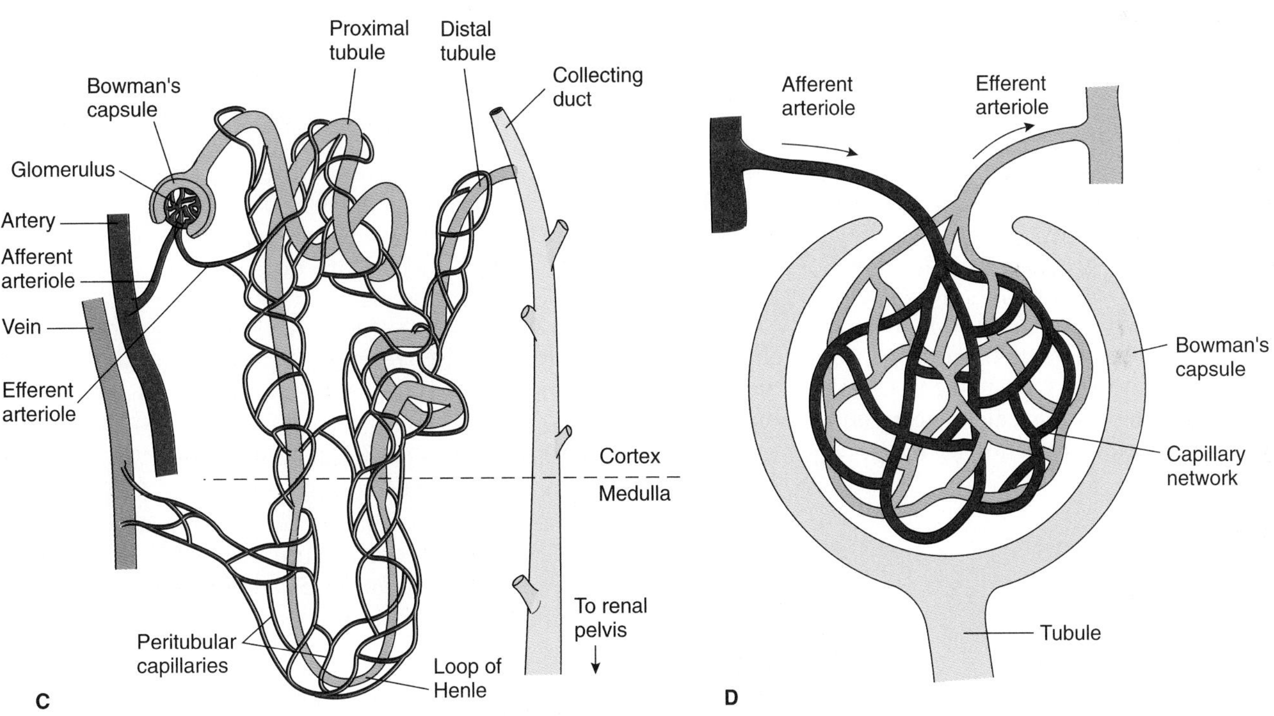

FIGURE 62-1. (*A*) Structures of the urinary tract. (*B*) Cross-section of the kidney. (*C*) Schematic view of a single nephron. (*D*) The glomerulus.

BOX 62-1 Assessing the Chief Complaint

- Voiding changes or disturbances
- Urine volume changes
- Irritative voiding symptoms (frequency, urgency, nocturia, dysuria)
- Obstructive voiding symptoms (hesitancy, straining, residual urine, retention, urinary stream force and size)
- Urinary incontinence (total overflow, stress, urge, functional)
- Urine characteristics changes (color, hematuria, clarity, odor, pH)
- Systemic manifestations (fever, weight loss)
- Gastrointestinal systems (nausea, vomiting, diarrhea, abdominal cramping, distention)
- Pain (type, location, severity, local, referred, colic, spasms)
- Masses of the flank, abdomen, or genital areas (polycystic kidneys, hydronephrosis, renal cell carcinoma)
- Abnormal abdominal or genital appearance
- Sexual or reproductive dysfunction

Computed Tomography Scan and Magnetic Resonance Imaging

A computed tomography (CT) scan or magnetic resonance image (MRI) of the abdomen and pelvis may be obtained to diagnose renal pathology, determine kidney size, and evaluate tissue densities with or without contrast material. An iodine-based contrast medium may be injected intravenously (IV) after the initial scan to enhance the images, especially when vascular tumors are suspected. The CT scan is also useful in identifying calculi, congenital abnormalities, obstruction, infections, and polycystic disease.

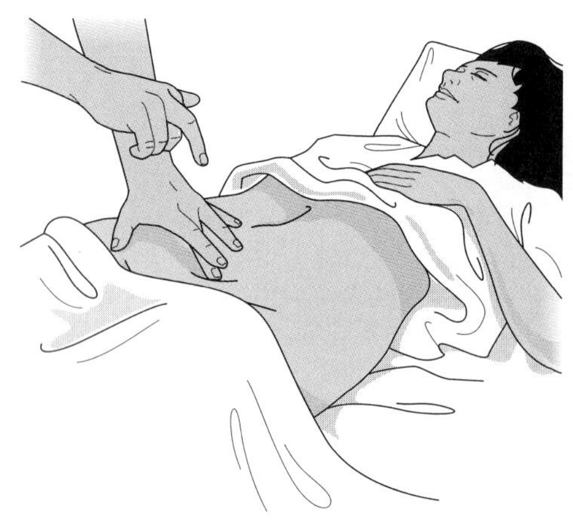

FIGURE 62-2. Bladder percussion.

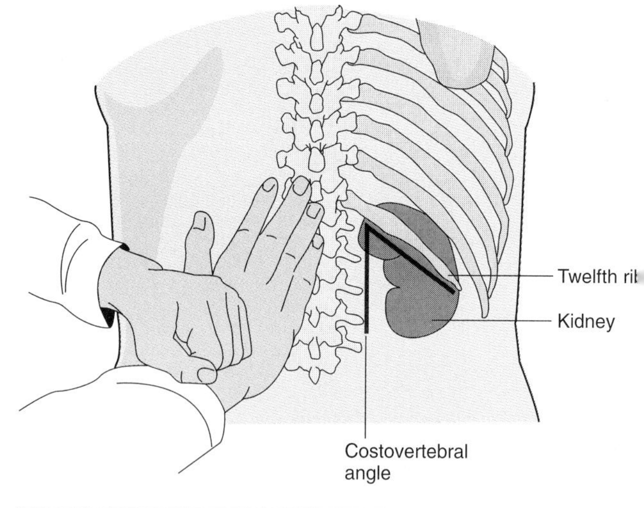

FIGURE 62-3. Assessing for CVA tenderness.

An MRI produces sharp images of the kidneys and can delineate the renal cortex from the medulla. It is also useful in identifying bladder tumors, staging renal cell carcinoma, and imaging the vascular system.

Angiography

A renal angiogram (**renal arteriogram**) provides details of the arterial supply to the kidneys, specifically the location and number of renal arteries (multiple vessels to the kidney are not unusual) and the patency of each renal artery. A catheter is passed up the femoral artery into the aorta to the level of the renal vessels. Contrast medium is then injected into the catheter and serial radiographics are taken. The radiopaque dye first outlines the aorta in the area of the renal artery then enters the renal artery and the kidney. A series of radiographs are taken. The catheter tip also may be passed into each renal artery for additional images. The procedure lasts 30 to 90 minutes. This procedure is contraindicated if a client is allergic to iodine contrast material.

NURSING MANAGEMENT

Ask the client about allergy to iodine or seafood, and any previous dye reactions. Review pertinent laboratory tests (blood urea nitrogen [BUN], creatinine) to assess renal function. Record vital signs and assess peripheral pulses. Have the client void before the procedure. Administer a sedative, if ordered, to promote relaxation before the procedure. After the procedure, the physician applies a pressure dressing to the femoral area; it is left in place for several hours. Palpate the pulses in the legs and feet at least every 1 to 2 hours for signs of arterial occlusion. Check the pressure dressing for frank bleeding or hematoma formation; notify the physician immediately if either condition occurs. Assess for hypersensitivity responses to contrast material. Maintain bed rest for 4 to 8 hours. Assess and document intake and output. Nursing Guidelines 62–1 offer client education points.

Cystoscopy

Cystoscopy is the visual examination of the inside of the bladder using an instrument called a **cystoscope.** When the urethra is examined, the procedure is called cystourethroscopy. The cystoscope consists of a lighted tube with a telescopic lens. Cystoscopy is used to identify the cause of painless hematuria, urinary incontinence, or urinary retention. It is useful in the evaluation of structural and functional changes of the bladder. The cystoscope is inserted through the urethra into the bladder. Local anesthesia is usual; however, spinal or general anesthesia may also be used. The procedure lasts 30 to 45 minutes. The size of the cystoscope is graded in the French (F) scale; usually, one that is 20 to 24 F is used in adults. Biopsy samples (tissue examination), cell washings (cytologic analysis), and urine samples may be obtained.

NURSING MANAGEMENT

Preoperative sedatives or antispasmodics may be ordered. Any abnormality of the urinary tract may be aggravated by a cystoscopy. A urine culture should be obtained before testing. If a urinary infection was present before the cystoscopy, chills, fever, and possibly septicemia may occur. Observe the client for these and other symptoms and report findings to the physician. Administer anti-infective agents after a cystoscopy. Record vital signs before and after the procedure. If general anesthesia is used, vital signs should be monitored every 15 to 30 minutes until the client is stable. Significant prostatic obstruction may result in pain and complete urinary retention following a cystoscopy. Administer medications for pain or bladder spasms postprocedure as ordered.

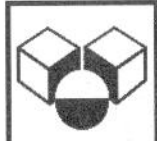

Nursing Guidelines 62-1

Care of the Client Undergoing Renal Angiography

- Explain the procedure and its purpose (need to lie still during test, various equipment to be used).
- Tell the client to drink extra fluids on the day before the test; no food or fluids (per protocol) before testing; IV fluids will be given before, during, and after the test; medication will be given to promote relaxation; local anesthesia is administered.
- Inform the client to expect a burning sensation or feeling of heat, pain, or nausea while contrast material is injected. Reassure client that these reactions are normal and transient.
- Instruct the client to remain on strict bed rest for 4 to 8 hours or more as per protocol. A urinal or bedpan must be used in the meantime.
- Encourage extra fluid intake (2,000–3,000 mL over the 24-hour postprocedure period).

Intravenous Pyelogram and Retrograde Pyelogram

An **intravenous pyelogram** (IVP) is a radiographic study used to evaluate the structure and function of the kidneys, ureters, and bladder. It locates the site of any urinary tract obstructions and is helpful in the investigation of the causes of flank pain, hematuria, or renal colic. It is based on the ability of the kidneys to excrete a radiopaque dye (also called a contrast medium) in the urine. The intravenous radiopaque dye outlines the kidney pelves, ureters, and bladder as the blood containing the dye passes through the urinary tract. Synonymous terms for this procedure are **excretory urogram** (EUG) and IV **urography** (IVU, IUG). After the IV injection of contrast material, radiographs of the urinary tract are taken after 1 minute (kidney visualization), at 3 to 5 minutes (renal collecting system visualization), at 10 minutes (ureters visualization) and at 20 to 30 minutes (bladder filling visualization). A postvoiding film shows the emptying of the bladder.

Because radiopaque dye usually contains iodine, the physician may inject a minute amount of the radiopaque dye IV and observe the client for 5 to 10 minutes to determine whether an allergy to iodine is present. Radiopaque dyes that do not contain iodine, called nonionic contrast agents, are available and produce fewer allergic reactions.

A **retrograde pyelogram** may be performed if better visualization of the complete ureter and renal pelvis is needed. A flexible radiopaque ureteral catheter is inserted in each ureteral orifice (opening at the terminal end of the ureter), which lie on the lower posterior wall of the bladder. This is done during a cystoscopy. Visualization of the ureters and renal pelves is possible after sterile contrast medium is instilled into the renal collecting system. This procedure is also used to evaluate ureteral stent or catheter placement. Retrograde pyelography carries a risk of sepsis and severe urinary tract infection.

NURSING MANAGEMENT

Schedule the IVP before any barium test or gallbladder series that uses contrast material (iodine). If the client is already scheduled for barium studies of the upper or lower gastrointestinal tract, these diagnostic tests will probably be delayed until urologic studies are completed. It may take several days for barium to be removed from the gastrointestinal tract, and its presence can distort IVP findings. Nursing Guidelines 62–2 provide information on the care of the client undergoing a pyelogram.

After the IVP or retrograde pyelogram, provide adequate fluid intake, continue the IV fluid replacement, and observe for urinary output of at least 30 mL/hour. Clients who are dehydrated are at high risk for renal failure due to the toxic effect of the contrast medium on the kidney tissues. Document vital signs. If additional radiographic films are to be taken in the next 24 hours (if the excretory function of the kidney is abnormal), follow instructions by the department of radiology or the physician regarding the food and fluid intake.

The client undergoing a retrograde pyelogram may experience a dull ache caused by distention of the renal pelves with the radiopaque dye. Observe for signs and symptoms of pyelonephritis (see Chap. 63) 24 to 48 hours postprocedure due to instrumentation and injection of material. Report any symptoms to the physician and obtain urine for culture and analysis. Anti-infective agents are administered as directed.

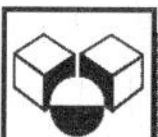

Nursing Guidelines 62-2

Care of the Client Undergoing Intravenous or Retrograde Pyelogram

- Check the client's allergy history especially to intravenous contrast dye (iodine) or seafood. Inquire about previous reactions to x-ray studies that used contrast media. Report allergies to the physician or radiology department personnel.
- Instruct the client to fast from food for 8 to 12 hours before the pyelogram. Fluid is permitted.
- Cleanse the bowel so that there is no interference with visualization of the kidneys on the radiographic film. It is important that the bowel preparation is effective because poor cleansing of the intestinal tract may require that the test be repeated. Clients with a peptic ulcer or ulcerative colitis usually require modification of the bowel-cleansing preparation.
- Document baseline vital signs.
- Explain the procedure and its purpose. Tell clients that a series of x-rays will be taken after injection or instillation of IV contrast material and that the entire test requires 1 to 1.5 hours to complete.
- Caution clients that they may experience burning, hot flushing sensations, unpleasant (metallic) taste in the mouth, or nausea or vomiting as the contrast is given. Half the clients will experience nausea or vomiting. Reassure clients that these reactions are transient.
- Encourage adequate fluid intake postprocedure and voiding within 8 hours postprocedure. A burning sensation on voiding and small amounts of blood-tinged urine are normal and should disappear after the third voiding.
- Advise the use of warm tub baths to decrease urethral discomfort or spasms after a retrograde pyelogram. These reactions should disappear within 24 hours.
- Instruct the client to abstain from alcohol 48 hours postprocedure to avoid irritating the bladder.
- Discuss taking antibiotics for 1 to 3 days postprocedure. Teach the client to report flank pain, chills, fever, dysuria, or bleeding. Advise client to notify physician should symptoms present.

Biopsy

Biopsies of urinary tract tissue are taken to diagnose cancer, assess prostatic enlargement, diagnose and monitor progression of renal disease, and assess and evaluate treatment of renal transplant rejection. Bladder biopsies are obtained during cystoscopy. Information about prostate biopsy can be found in Chapter 60. Table 62–1 describes renal biopsy techniques. Renal biopsy carries the risk of postprocedure bleeding because the kidneys receive up to 25% of the cardiac output each minute.

NURSING MANAGEMENT

Reassure the client undergoing a renal biopsy and explain the procedure and its purpose. Record vital signs and review pretest coagulation studies, urinalysis, IVP, and renal scan. After the procedure, maintain the client on bed rest and check for hematuria. Assess the dressing frequently for signs of bleeding, monitor vital signs, and evaluate the type and severity of pain; severe pain in the back, shoulder, or abdomen can indicate bleeding. Notify the physician of these signs and symptoms immediately. Assess for difficulty voiding. Encourage adequate fluid intake after the biopsy. If the client is to be discharged the following day, instruct him or her to:

- Maintain limited activity for several days to avoid bleeding.
- Complete prophylactic anti-infective therapy as indicated.
- Report signs of systemic infection (fever, malaise), urinary tract infection (*dysuria*, frequency, discolored urine, malodorous urine), or bleeding (hema-

TABLE 62-1 **Techniques for Renal Biopsy**

Type of Biopsy	Description
Needle biopsy	• Minimally invasive • Renal tissue is removed through a needle • Useful when CT or MRI findings are inconclusive
Fine needle aspiration biopsy	• Minimally invasive • Performed under local anesthesia in the operating room • Needle placement guided by fluoroscopy
Open biopsy	• Small incision made into flank • Usually performed if needle biopsy tissue samples are not satisfactory

turia, light-headedness, flank pain, or rapid pulse). Advise the client to notify the physician immediately should symptoms occur.

Cystogram and Voiding Cystourethrogram (VCUG)

A **cystogram** evaluates abnormalities in bladder structure and filling through the instillation of contrast dye and radiography. A **voiding cystourethrogram** (VCUG) is similar to a cystogram except the client is instructed to void (the urine contains the radiopaque dye), and a rapid series of radiographs are taken. Urinary tract infection is a contraindication for a cystogram or VCUG.

Urodynamic Studies

Urodynamic studies evaluate bladder and urethral function and are performed to assess causes of reduced urine flow, urinary retention, and urinary incontinence. Two of the main tests are uroflowmetry and cystometrogram.

Uroflowmetry (determination of the urinary flow rate) is performed to evaluate bladder and sphincter function. This noninvasive procedure measures the time and rate of voiding, the volume of urine voided, and the pattern of urination. The results are compared with normal flow rates and urinary patterns. Results vary by age and gender. See Table 62–2 for normal uroflowmetry values. The client is usually catheterized afterward for the post void residual. A **post void residual** is the amount of urine left in the bladder after voiding and provides information about bladder function. Normal post void residual is 0 to 30 mL; however, retention of up to 100 mL may be acceptable in the older adult.

A **cystometrogram** (CMG) evaluates the bladder tone and capacity. A retention catheter is inserted into the bladder after the client voids. The bladder is slowly filled with sterile saline and the client indicates at what point the first urge to void is felt and when the bladder feels full. These measurements indicate whether or not the client's bladder capacity is normal. Most clients feel a mild urge to void at approximately 120 mL and a strong urge to void at about 250 mL. By comparison, clients with a neurogenic bladder (see Chap. 64) may not feel an urge to void till 500 mL or more has been instilled; in many instances the client with a neurogenic bladder will never feel an urge to void and instillation is terminated at this point. The client is assessed for bladder contractions that he or she cannot control, leakage around the catheter, or leakage of urine when asked to cough. Pressures within the bladder are also assessed. The client may be given antibiotics for a day or two after a CMG.

Laboratory Tests

Urinalysis

Much information about systemic diseases and the condition of the kidneys and lower urinary tract can

TABLE 62-2 **Normal Urine Flow Rates**

Gender	Young Adult	Middle-Aged Adult	Older Adult
Male	21 mL/second	12 mL/second	9 mL/second
Female	18 mL/second	15 mL/second	10 mL/second

be learned by **urinalysis**, a study of the components and characteristics of the urine. Urinalysis is also useful in monitoring the effects of treatment of known urinary or renal conditions. The characteristics of normal urine and possible causes contributing to abnormal results are listed in Table 62-3. A clean-catch midstream specimen from the first voiding of the morning is preferred. See Nursing Guidelines 62–3 for instructing the client how to collect a clean-catch specimen.

URINE CULTURE AND SENSITIVITY

When infection is suspected, a urine specimen may be taken for culture by collecting a clean-catch midstream specimen or by urinary catheterization. It is important that the urine specimen is not contaminated by skin bacteria. Label the container with the client's name along with the time and date of the voiding. To prevent the growth of bacteria in the urine and decomposition, deliver the urine specimen immediately to the laboratory or refrigerate promptly until it can be taken to the laboratory.

24-HOUR URINE COLLECTION

Sometimes the entire 24-hour volume of urine is collected, for example, for a 24-hour urine for 17-ketosteroids. The client is instructed to void and discard the urine. The collection bottle is marked with the time the client voided. Thereafter, all the urine is collected for the entire 24 hours. The last urine is voided at the same time the test originally began. Refrigerate the entire specimen to prevent bacterial growth. To

TABLE 62-3 **Urinalysis Characteristics**

Characteristic and Normal Value	Abnormal Findings	Possible Causes
Color: yellow	Colorless	Overhydration, diabetes insipidus, chronic renal disease, diuretic therapy, diabetes mellitus
	Red, pink	Hematuria, foods (beets, rhubarb, blackberries), drugs (phenothiazines, rifampin)
	Dark yellow or orange	Bilirubin, dehydration, drugs (multiple vitamins, pyridium, azo gantrisin)
	Green	Pseudomonas infection, bilirubin, drugs (methylene blue, amitriptyline, vitamin B complex)
	Brown	Dehydration, urobilinogen, drugs (Cascara, Flagyl)
	Dark brown to black	Melanin, drugs (Macrodantin, Quinine, Methyldopa)
Clarity: clear	Cloudy	Phosphaturia
	Turbid	Pyuria, bacteriuria, parasitic disease
	Hazy	Mucus
	Smoky, milky	Prostatic fluid, sperm, lipids
	Pinkish precipitates	Hyperuricemia
Specific gravity: 1.003–1.029	Dilute (1.001–1.010) or concentrated (1.029–1.030)	Low: diabetes insipidus, kidney disorders High: false reading due to pus, albumin, protein, glucose, or dextran in urine
pH: 4.5–7.5	> 7.5	Urinary tract infection, metabolic acidosis, Cushing's syndrome; low protein diet with large vegetable intake; high dairy and citrus fruit diet; drugs (sodium bicarbonate, thiazides)
Ketones: none	Ketonuria	Starvation; fasting abnormal carbohydrate metabolism, diabetes mellitus pregnancy, pernicious vomiting; high-protein diet
Protein: none	Proteinuria	Cancer, severe heart failure, renal disease, glomerulonephritis, nephrotic syndrome; trauma, fever, heavy exercise
Glucose: none	Glycosuria	Diabetes mellitus, gestational diabetes
Red blood cells: 0–3 RBCs/high-power field	> 3 RBCs/high-power field	Renal disorders (glomerulonephritis, calculus, cancer, trauma, cysts), systemic disease (lupus, sickle cell, hypertension)
White blood cells: 0–4/high-power field	> 4/high-power field	Urinary tract infection (acute pyelonephritis, cystitis, urethritis), renal disease, urinary stones
Bilirubin: none	Bilirubinuria	Hepatitis, biliary obstruction
Urobilinogen: <1 mg/dL	>1 mg/dL	Hepatitis, cirrhosis, congestive heart failure, hemolytic anemia
Casts: 0–2 hyaline casts/low-power field	>2/low-powered field	Granular casts (glomerulonephritis, renal disease); fatty casts (nephrotic syndrome); cellular casts (glomeruli or tubule infection); hyaline casts (fever, strenuous exercise, congestive heart failure)
Crystals: none to few	Many	Urolithiasis, chronic renal failure, gout, urinary tract infection
Bacteria: negative per high-power field	Positive	

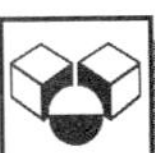

Nursing Guidelines 62-3

Instructing the Client on Obtaining a Clean-Catch Midstream Specimen

Tell the client to:

- Wash hands and remove the lid from the specimen container without touching the inside of the lid.
- Open antiseptic towelette package and cleanse the urethral area. Tell the female client to hold labia apart with one hand and wipe down one side of the urethra with the first towelette and discard, wipe down the other side with the second towelette and discard, and wipe down the center with the third towelette and discard. Emphasize wiping one time only, from front to back. Tell the male client to retract foreskin if uncircumcised and to clean the urethral meatus in a circular motion using each towelette one time.
- Instruct the client to begin voiding into the toilet, urinal, or bedpan; tell the female client to continue to hold labia apart while voiding.
- Tell the client to void 30 to 50 mL of the midstream urine into the collection container and then finish urinating into the toilet, bedpan, or urinal. Emphasize not contaminating the container.
- Tell the client to carefully replace the lid, dry the container if necessary, and wash his or her hands.

prevent any part of the specimen from being lost or contaminated, tell the client to use separate receptacles for voiding and defecation. If any urine is discarded by mistake or lost while defecating, stop the test; loss of even a small amount of urine can invalidate the test.

URINE SPECIFIC GRAVITY

Urine specific gravity is a measurement of the kidney's ability to concentrate and excrete urine. The specific gravity measures urine concentration by measuring the density of urine and comparing it with the density of distilled water. The density of distilled water is 1.000 (1 mL of distilled water weighs 1 g). The number, weight, and size of urine solutes (particles) determine its specific gravity (density). Normally, the specific gravity is inversely proportional to urine volume. On a hot day, a person who is perspiring profusely and taking little fluid has urine with a high specific gravity. Conversely, a person who has a high fluid intake and who is not losing excessive water from perspiration, diarrhea, or vomiting has copious urine with a low specific gravity. When the kidneys are diseased, the ability to concentrate urine may be impaired and the specific gravity remains relatively constant, no matter what the water needs of the body are or how much the client drinks.

URINE PROTEIN

The **urine protein test** is used to identify renal disease. Normally, protein is minimally present in the urine. An increase in urine protein levels may also be seen with salt depletion, strenuous exercise, fever, or dehydration. Proteinuria on an individual urine specimen may be detected by dipping a test reagent stick (dipstick method) in the urine and comparing color changes with the provided color chart.

CREATININE CLEARANCE TEST

A **creatinine clearance** test is used to determine kidney function and creatinine excretion. Creatinine is a substance that results from the breakdown of phosphocreatine (amino acid waste product), which is present in muscle tissue. It is filtered by the glomeruli and is excreted at a fairly constant rate by the kidney. The total amount of excreted creatinine is called creatinine clearance. The renal tubules increase creatinine secretion with any decrease in glomerular filtration (renal failure). Muscle necrosis and atrophy greatly increase urinary creatinine due to accompanying protein catabolism. For this test a 4-, 12-, or 24-hour urine specimen and a sample of blood (serum creatinine) are collected. The blood sample is obtained either midpoint or at the beginning and end of urine collection (varies per protocol). Both urine and blood samples are sent to the laboratory.

Blood Chemistries

When the nephrons fail to remove waste products efficiently from the body, the blood chemistry is altered. Deterioration in renal function is manifested by rises in the **blood urea nitrogen** (BUN) and **creatinine** values, both of which are protein breakdown products. Table 62–4 shows normal values of common blood studies performed on clients with signs and symptoms of a urinary system disorder as well as renal implications regarding abnormal results. A moderate decrease in renal function occurs, however, before these values rise.

Nursing Management

Clients undergoing diagnostic testing are often anxious and worried; clients having urologic testing may feel embarrassed and afraid that the testing will be

TABLE 62-4 **Normal Serum Values and Renal Disease**

	Normal Value	Change Seen in Renal Disease
Calcium	8.8–10 mg/dL	Decreased in renal failure
Carbon dioxide combining power	23–30 mmol/L	Decreased in acute renal failure
Magnesium	1.3–2.1 mEq/L	Decreased in chronic renal disease
Phosphate, inorganic phosphorus	2.7–4.5 mg/dL	Increased in renal failure
Potassium	3.5–5.0 mEq/L	Increased in renal failure
Total protein	6.0–8.0 g/dL	Increased in poor renal function; decreased in nephrotic syndrome
Sodium	135–148 mmol/L	Decreased in severe nephritis; increased in renal disease
Blood urea nitrogen	7–18 mg/dL	Increased in renal disease and urinary obstruction
Creatinine	Male: 0.7–1.3 mg/dL Female: 0.6–1.1 mg/dL	Increased in renal disease or insufficiency
Albumin	> 60 years: 3.4–4.8 g/dL < 60 years: 3.5–5 g/dL	Decreased in renal failure
Chloride	98–107 mEq/L	Decreased in renal failure (onset)
Uric acid	Male: 4.5–8 ng/dL Female: 2.5–6.2 ng/dL	Increased in renal failure

painful. Provide privacy, reassurance, and information. Maintain a professional and empathic attitude.

The nursing management of a client undergoing diagnostic evaluation of the urinary tract includes, but is not limited to, the following:

Nursing Diagnoses and Collaborative Problems	Nursing Interventions
Anxiety and **Fear** related to uncertainty of outcomes of diagnostic testing and the undertaking of an unfamiliar experience **Goal:** The client will verbalize a reduction in feelings of apprehension about diagnostic testing.	Assess client's level of anxiety. Explain or reexplain the test, diagnostic procedure, equipment, tubes, or drains to be used. Use simple language with client or significant others especially with outpatient procedures or tests. Answer questions about testing or consult with other health team members in matters that involve their expertise. Acknowledge appropriateness of client's feelings; correct any misinterpretations. Avoid false reassurances. Encourage the client to verbalize thoughts and feelings. Ask client to describe in detail what is causing anxiety or fear (any previous negative experiences). If particular stressors are identified, explore ways to minimize them. For generalized, nonspecific threats, provide feedback about reality of current situation. Stay with the client when apprehensive feelings are expressed. Maintain calm and tolerant environment. Provide positive reinforcement as needed and be empathic. Encourage the client's significant other to remain with the client. Assist the client to develop problem-solving abilities. Administer sedative medications as ordered.
Knowledge Deficit related to diagnostic procedures, tests, and pre- and postprocedure care **Goal:** The client will be able to demonstrate or verbalize an understanding of diagnostic procedure, test, and pre- and postcare.	Provide for physical comfort and quiet atmosphere for the client (or significant other) without disruptions to allow for concentration on topic. Assess the client's knowledge base, explain the purpose of and discuss the procedure or test. Move from general to specific details (ie, radiologic site, required medications, equipment, IV lines, anesthesia, pre- and postcare, catheters or drains used). Discuss home care (ie, fluid intake, medication usage, signs and symptoms of genitourinary infection) and postprocedure conditions requiring physician follow-up (ie, frank bleeding, inability to urinate, increased pain, or fever posttest). Discuss concerns about radiographic exposure or refer concerns to the physician or radiologist. Encourage questions, repetition of information, return demonstration (as appropriate) from the client or significant other.

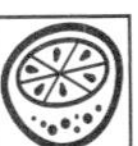

General Nutritional Considerations

Dietary intake can affect urine characteristics as well as urinary tract disorders and their management. An acid ash or basic ash diet may be ordered in conjunction with drug therapy to help alter urine pH. Drug therapy is a more effective and consistent means of altering urinary pH.

A high-protein, low-carbohydrate diet can cause ketonuria. Megadoses of vitamin C can interfere with certain lab tests, such as for glycosuria and fecal occult blood. Asparagus has a weak diuretic action and produces a pungent urine odor.

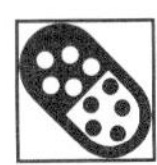

General Pharmacologic Considerations

Nephrotoxicity may occur with the administration of certain drugs and is potentially serious because it decreases urinary excretion of the drug and increases the risk of drug toxicity.

Some drugs may have an effect on the outcome of urinary tract tests as well as the appearance of the urine. For example, nitrofurantoin may color the urine brown and methylene blue may color the urine a pale blue-green. Contamination of urine with povidone-iodine can cause a false-positive hematuria result (dipstick method). Other drugs can affect urine pH such as ammonium chloride and mandelic acid, which both can cause acidic urine; whereas, sodium bicarbonate, thiazide diuretics, acetazolamide, and potassium citrate promote alkaline urine.

Aminoglycosides such as gentamicin can result in increased levels of blood urea nitrogen (BUN) and serum creatinine, indicating nephrotoxicity. Signs of nephrotoxicity may not occur until the client has received 5 or more days of therapy. Nephrotoxicity from the use of the aminoglycosides is reversible if the drug is discontinued as soon as the symptoms appear.

Diuretic therapy can result in increased sodium, chloride, and magnesium levels with 24-hour urine electrolyte testing.

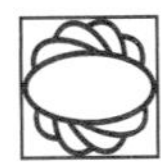

General Gerontologic Considerations

The older client may have difficulty following directions when collecting a 24-hour urine specimen. The directions may need to be repeated and the client supervised at frequent intervals.

Age-related changes in kidney function, for example, decreased GFR and thickening of the renal tubules, can alter the excretion of drugs in older adults, increasing the risk of drug toxicity.

Nephrotoxicity is more likely to occur in older adults than in younger adults receiving prolonged or high doses of nephrotoxic drugs. It is important for the nurse to identify and report signs of nephrotoxicity (increased BUN or serum creatine levels, oliguria, or proteinuria).

SUMMARY OF KEY CONCEPTS

- The urinary system consists of the kidneys, renal pelves, ureters, urinary bladder, and urethra.
- The kidneys have four primary functions: (1) to excrete excess water and the nitrogenous waste products of protein metabolism; (2) to assist in maintaining the acid–base balance of the body and the equilibrium of plasma electrolytes; (3) to produce the enzyme renin, which acts on certain plasma constituents to form angiotensin I, which enters the circulation and in the lungs is converted to angiotensin II (this compound that raises the blood pressure); and (4) to produce the hormone erythropoietin, which regulates red blood cell production.
- Tests performed for the diagnosis of urinary and renal system diseases include radiographs, IV pyelogram/urogram, cystoscopy, cystoscopy with retrograde pyelograms, voiding cystourethrogram, computed tomography, magnetic resonance imaging, biopsy, renal angiography, ultrasonography, and uroflowmetry. Specific procedures may require pretest preparation and posttest follow-up.
- Laboratory tests used in the diagnosis of urinary and renal system diseases include urinalysis, blood chemistries, urine concentration test, urine protein, and creatinine clearance test.
- The nursing management of clients undergoing diagnostic evaluation of the urinary tract includes relieving anxiety and fear and providing teaching and information to decrease any knowledge deficit related to diagnostic procedures and tests.

CRITICAL THINKING EXERCISES

1. A client is scheduled for a cystoscopy and retrograde pyelograms. He is very nervous and asks many questions about the procedure. What could you do to try to decrease his anxiety?
2. A client has possible renal disease and is scheduled for many tests on her upper and lower urinary tract and gastrointestinal tract. What would you do to be sure one test does not interfere with another test?

Suggested Readings

Brunzel, N. A. (1994). *Fundamentals of urine and body fluid analysis.* Philadelphia: Saunders.

Bullock, B. L., & Rosendahl, P. P. (1992). *Pathophysiology: Adaptations and alterations in function* (3rd ed.) Philadelphia: J. B. Lippincott.

Daly-Gawenda, D. (Ed.). (1997). *Manual of medical-surgical nursing.* Boston: Little, Brown.

Fischbach, F. T. (1992). *A manual of laboratory diagnostic tests* (4th ed.). Philadelphia: J. B. Lippincott.

Gray, M. (1992). *Genitourinary disorders.* St. Louis: Mosby.

Karlowicz, K. A. (Ed.). (1995). *Urologic nursing: Principles and practice.* Philadelphia: Saunders.

King, M., & Lambert, L. (1996). Understanding culture and sensitivity reports. *Nursing, 26*(9), 36–37.

Kuhn, M. (1996). Laboratory analysis. *Critical Care Nurse, 16*(5), 74–76.

Melillo, K.D . (1993, February). Interpretation of abnormal laboratory values in older adults, part 2. *Journal of Gerontological Nursing, 19*, 35.

Memmler, R. L., Cohen, B. J., & Wood, D. L. (1992). *The human body in health and disease* (7th ed.). Philadelphia: J. B. Lippincott.

Nagle, G. M. (1997). *Genitourinary surgery.* St. Louis: Mosby.

Ouslander, J. G., Schapira, M., & Schnelle, J. F. (1995). Urine specimen collection from incontinent female nursing home residents. *Journal of the American Geriatrics Society, 43*(3), 278– 281.

Welford, K. (1994). Testing lower urinary tract function. *Nursing Standard, 9*(7), 27–30.

Wozniak-Petrofsky, J. (1997). Urodynamic tests: Client preparation, assessment, and follow-up. *American Journal of Primary Health Care, 22*(3), 70–71, 77–79, 83–84.

Zanderer, B. (1996). Age-related changes in renal function. *Critical Care Nursing, 19*(2), 34–40.

Chapter 63

Caring for Clients With Disorders of the Kidneys and Ureters

KEY TERMS

Acute renal failure
Acute tubular necrosis
Anasarca
Anuria
Arteriovenous fistula
Arteriovenous graft
Azotemia
Bruit
Calciuria
Calculus
Casts
Chronic renal failure
Colic
Dialysate
Dialysis
Dialyzer
Disequilibrium syndrome
End-stage renal disease
Extracorporeal shock wave lithotripsy
Glomerulonephritis
Hematuria
Hemodialysis
Hydronephrosis
Nephrectomy
Nephrolithiasis
Nephrostomy tube
Nocturia
Oliguria
Osteodystrophy
Periorbital edema
Peritoneal dialysis
Pyelonephritis
Pyeloplasty
Pyuria
Thrill
Uremia
Uremic frost
Ureteral stent
Ureterolithiasis
Ureteroplasty
Urolithiasis

LEARNING OBJECTIVES

On completion of this chapter, the reader will:

- Differentiate between pyelonephritis and glomerulonephritis.
- Name three problems the nurse manages when caring for clients with glomerulonephritis.
- Explain the pathophysiology of polycystic disease and name three associated renal complications.
- Give three examples of conditions that predispose to renal calculi.
- Identify methods for eliminating small renal calculi and methods used for larger stones.
- Discuss the nursing management of a client with a nephrostomy tube.
- List examples of conditions that cause a ureteral stricture.
- Name the classic triad of symptoms associated with renal cancer.
- List problems managed by the nurse when caring for a client with a nephrectomy.
- Explain the difference between acute and chronic renal failure.
- List at least five pathophysiologic problems associated with chronic renal failure.
- Give three sources of organs for kidney transplantation.
- Identify at lest three nursing methods for managing pruritus.
- Explain the purpose of dialysis and name two methods for performing the procedure.
- Discuss nursing assessments performed when caring for clients undergoing dialysis.

The most common urologic disorders are infectious and inflammatory conditions. Those that affect the kidneys are extremely dangerous because damage to the nephrons can result in permanent renal dysfunction. The same is true of other upper urinary tract disorders such as kidney and ureteral stones and tumors. The consequences can lead to acute or chronic renal failure.

Infectious and Inflammatory Disorders of the Kidney

Infectious and inflammatory disorders of the kidney affect structures such as the renal pelvis, the nephrons, or both.

Pyelonephritis

Pyelonephritis is an acute or chronic bacterial infection of the kidney and the lining of the collecting system (kidney pelvis). Acute pyelonephritis presents with moderate to severe symptoms that usually last 1 to 2 weeks. If the treatment of acute pyelonephritis is not successful and the infection recurs, it is termed chronic pyelonephritis.

ETIOLOGY AND PATHOPHYSIOLOGY

Bacteria ascend to the kidney and kidney pelves by way of the bladder and urethra. Normal fecal flora such as *Escherichia coli, Klebsiella pneumoniae, Proteus mirabilis, Streptococcus fecalis, Pseudomonas aeruginosa,* and *Staphylococcus aureus* are the most common bacteria that cause acute pyelonephritis. *E. coli* accounts for about 85% of infections. Additional risk factors such as urinary obstruction and reflux (Fig. 63–1) are listed in Table 63–1.

In acute pyelonephritis, the inflammation causes the kidneys to grossly enlarge. The cortex and medulla develop multiple abscesses. The renal calyces and pelvis also can become involved. Resolution of the inflammation results in fibrosis and scarring. Chronic pyelonephritis occurs after recurrent episodes of acute pyelonephritis. The kidneys develop irreversible degenerative changes and become small and atrophic. If extensive numbers of nephrons are destroyed, renal failure develops. Renal dysfunction may not occur for 20 or more years after the onset of the disease. About 10% to 15% of clients with chronic pyelonephritis require dialysis.

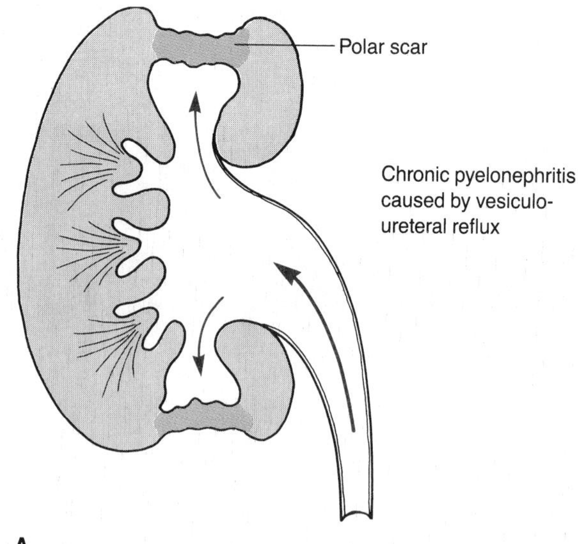

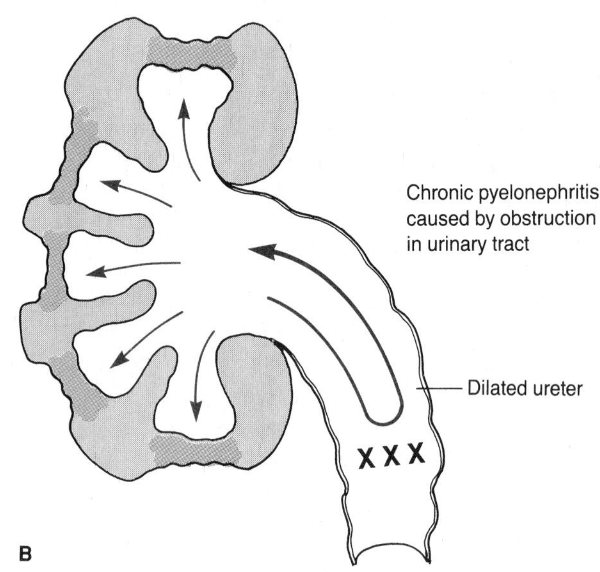

FIGURE 63-1. Causes of chronic pyelonephritis.

ASSESSMENT FINDINGS

Signs and Symptoms

Flank pain or tenderness, chills, fever, and malaise occur in clients with acute pyelonephritis. Frequency and burning on urination are present if there is an accompanying cystitis (bladder infection). Some clients with chronic pyelonephritis are asymptomatic; others have a low-grade fever and vague gastrointestinal complaints. Polyuria and nocturia develop when the tubules of the nephrons fail to reabsorb water efficiently.

Diagnostic Findings

A urinalysis demonstrates multiple abnormalities—chief of which is **pyuria,** pus—a combination of bacteria and leukocytes, in the urine (Table 63–2). A urine culture identifies the causative microorganism. A cystoscopy, or intravenous or retrograde pyelogram, demonstrates obstruction or damage to structures of the urinary tract. A radiograph of the kidneys, ureters, and bladder (KUB) may reveal calculi, cysts, or tumors in the kidney or other urinary structures. The diagnosis of chronic pyelonephritis is based on a history of repeated acute pyelonephritis. Serum creatinine and blood urea nitrogen (BUN) levels, if elevated, indicate impaired renal function.

TABLE 63-1 **Risk Factors for Pyelonephritis**

Acute Pyelonephritis	Chronic Pyelonephritis
• Instrumentation of the urethra and bladder (catheterization, cystoscopy, urologic surgery) • Inability to empty the bladder • Pregnancy • Urinary stasis • Urinary obstruction (tumors, strictures, calculi, prostatic hypertrophy) • Diabetes mellitus • Other renal disease (polycystic kidney disease) • Neurogenic bladder (stroke, multiple sclerosis, spinal cord injury) • Women with increased sexual activity, diaphragm, spermicide use, failure to void after intercourse, history of recent urinary infection • Men who perform anal intercourse, infection with human immunodeficiency virus	• Recurrent episodes of acute pyelonephritis • Chronic obstruction (eg, strictures and stones) • Reflux disorders that allow urine to flow backward up the ureters

MEDICAL AND SURGICAL MANAGEMENT

Treatment of acute pyelonephritis includes relieving the fever and pain and prescribing antimicrobial drugs such as trimethoprim-sulfamethoxazole (Septra) or ciprofloxacin (Cipro) for 14 days. Antispasmodics and anticholinergics such as oxybutynin (Ditropan) and propantheline (Pro-Banthine) are additional pharmacologic interventions that relax smooth muscles of the ureters and bladder, promote comfort, and increase bladder capacity. Symptoms usually disappear within a few days of antibiotic therapy. Four weeks of drug therapy is prescribed for clients who have a history of frequent relapsing infections with the same microorganism.

The aim of treatment for chronic pyelonephritis is to prevent progressive kidney damage. When possible, any urinary tract obstruction is relieved. An effort is made to improve the client's overall health. A **nephrectomy**, the surgical removal of a kidney, is performed if severe hypertension develops and if the other kidney is adequately functional.

NURSING MANAGEMENT

Obtain a complete medical, drug, and allergy history. Assess vital signs and report abnormal findings such as an elevation in temperature and blood pressure. Continue to monitor vital signs on a regular basis for evidence of changes. Perform a physical examination to determine the location of discomfort and any signs of fluid retention such as peripheral edema and shortness of breath. Observe and document the characteristics of the client's urine. Collect a clean-catch urine specimen for urinalysis and urine culture. Measure intake and output. Provide a liberal fluid intake of approximately 2,000 to 3,000 mL to flush the infectious microorganisms from the urinary tract. Administer prescribed medications. Review laboratory test results such as BUN, creatinine, serum electrolytes, and urine culture to evaluate the client's response to therapy. If chronic pyelonephritis develops, the treatment is often lengthy. Poor health and prolonged medical therapy are discouraging. Advocate that the client follow the recommendations of the physician and adhere to the prescribed medication regimen.

TABLE 63-2 **Urinalysis Results With Pyelonephritis**

Acute Pyelonephritis	Chronic Pyelonephritis
• Bacteria and bacterial casts • Leukocytes (large) • Casts (leukocytes, granular, renal tubular) • Red blood cells (few) • Low specific gravity • Slightly alkaline pH • Proteinuria (minimal to mild) • Urine culture: organism colony count of > 100,000 organisms/ mm^3 urine	• Leukocytes (increased) • Proteinuria (absent, minimal, or intermittent) • Bacteria • Casts (in early stages present and absent in late stages) • Low specific gravity

Client and Family Teaching

Discuss the following with the client and family:

- Explain the disease, its cause, related risk factors, treatment, and preventive measures.
- Discuss the purpose, dosage, side effects, and toxic effects of all prescribed medications.
- Instruct the client to complete the entire regimen of antimicrobial therapy as indicated, even if symptoms abate.
- Reinforce the importance of consuming a large volume of oral fluids on a daily basis.
- Suggest consuming acid-forming foods such as meat, fish, poultry, eggs, grains, corn, lentils, cranberries, prune, plums, and their juices to prevent calcium and magnesium phosphate stone formation.
- Recommend avoiding alcohol and caffeine products if bladder spasms are present or until a clinical response to therapy is verified.
- Explain the purpose and protocols for diagnostic procedures.
- Teach the client how to collect a clean-catch urine specimen for subsequent medical follow-up at 2 weeks and 3 months after treatment.
- Refer the client to resources where his or her blood pressure can be monitored from time to time.
- Identify the signs of recurring or worsening pyelonephritis or lower urinary tract infection (frequency, urgency, burning, cloudy urine, and fever) and emphasize the need to consult the primary care provider.
- Discuss methods to prevent reinfection. Women should wipe from front to back after defecation and wear cotton undergarments. Tell clients of both genders to void every 2 to 3 hours when awake and before and after intercourse.

Acute Glomerulonephritis

The term nephritis describes a group of inflammatory but noninfectious diseases characterized by widespread kidney damage. **Glomerulonephritis** is a type of nephritis that occurs most frequently in children and young adults; however, it can affect individuals at any age. The exact incidence of the disease is unknown, but it occurs twice as often in men as in women. Most recover spontaneously or with minimal therapy without sequelae. Some develop chronic glomerulonephritis.

ETIOLOGY AND PATHOPHYSIOLOGY

Symptoms of acute glomerulonephritis appear about 1 to 2 weeks after a group A beta-hemolytic streptococci upper respiratory infection. The relationship between the infection and acute glomerulonephritis is not clear; microorganisms are not present in the kidney when symptoms appear, but the glomeruli are acutely inflamed. Most believe that the inflammatory response is due to antigen–antibody stimulation within the glomerular capillary membrane. The disruption of membrane permeability causes red blood cells and protein molecules to filter from the glomeruli into Bowman's capsule and eventually become lost in the urine.

ASSESSMENT FINDINGS

Signs and Symptoms

About 50% of clients with glomerulonephritis are symptom free. Early symptoms may be so slight that the client does not seek medical attention. Occasionally the onset is sudden with pronounced symptoms such as fever, nausea, malaise, headache, generalized edema, or **periorbital edema,** puffiness around the eyes. Some clients experience pain or tenderness over the kidney area and mild to moderate hypertension. In some instances, the disorder is discovered during a routine physical examination. More often, the client or family notices that the person's face is pale and puffy and that slight ankle edema occurs in the evening. The appetite is poor, and **nocturia** (urination during the night) may be present. Irritability and shortness of breath also develop. As the condition progresses, the client develops **hematuria** (blood in the urine), anemia (due to hematuria), convulsions associated with hypertension, congestive heart failure, **oliguria** (low urine output of 100–500 mL/day), and perhaps **anuria** (< 100 mL of urine per 24-hour period). Fluid retention and hypertension contribute to visual disturbances, often due to papilledema or hemorrhage in the eye, and epistaxis (nosebleeds).

Diagnostic Findings

Gross or microscopic hematuria gives the urine a dark, smoky, or frankly bloody appearance. Laboratory findings include proteinuria (primarily as albumin in the urine), and an elevated antistreptolysin O titer (ASO titer) due to a recent streptococcal infection. There is decreased hemoglobin, slightly elevated BUN and serum creatinine levels, and an elevated erythrocyte sedimentation rate (ESR). If renal insufficiency develops, serum electrolyte levels indicate hyperkalemia, hypermagnesemia, hypocalcemia, and dilutional hyponatremia. Percutaneous renal biopsy reveals cellular changes characteristic of an antigen–antibody response and the extent of damage that has already occurred.

MEDICAL MANAGEMENT

No specific treatment exists for acute glomerulonephritis and treatment is guided by the symptoms and their underlying abnormality. Treatment may consist of bed rest, a sodium-restricted diet (if edema or hypertension is present), and antimicrobial drugs to prevent a superimposed infection in the already inflamed kidney. Penicillin may be used to abolish any remaining streptococci from the recent infection. Diuretics to reduce edema and antihypertensive agents for severe hypertension may be necessary. Vitamins are added to the diet to improve general resistance and oral iron supplements may be needed to counteract anemia. A trial of corticosteroids may be given to attempt to control the inflammatory process. Any increase in hematuria, proteinuria, or blood pressure is an indication for aggressive treatment (Table 63–3). The client is not considered cured until the urine is free of protein and red blood cells for 6 months. Return to full activity usually is not permitted until the urine is free of protein for a month.

NURSING MANAGEMENT

Maintain bed rest when the blood pressure is elevated and edema is present. Collect daily urine specimens to assist with evaluating the client's response to treatment. Assess the blood pressure every 4 hours or as ordered. Encourage adequate fluid intake and measure intake and output. Although the diet may be restricted in sodium and protein, encourage carbohydrate intake to prevent the catabolism of body protein stores.

Client and Family Teaching

Provide teaching based on the following guidelines:

- Identify the specific amount of sodium that is allowed in the client's case and sources of sodium to avoid.
- Explain the purpose of diuretic therapy or other prescribed medications, the dosing regimen, and side effects.
- Recommend blood pressure monitoring on a regular basis.
- Caution to avoid contact with persons who have infections.
- Emphasize compliance with medical appointments and the necessity for repeated urinalyses.
- Advise the client to contact the physician if urinary volumes diminish, if weight is unexplainedly gained, and if headaches or nosebleeds occur.

Chronic Glomerulonephritis

Chronic glomerulonephritis is a slowly progressive disease characterized by inflammation of the glomeruli that causes irreversible damage to the kidney nephrons. The course of the disease is highly variable. Some live for years with only occasional symptomatic episodes or none at all, or the disease may be rapidly fatal unless renal failure is treated with dialysis.

ETIOLOGY AND PATHOPHYSIOLOGY

A small number of those with chronic glomerulonephritis are known to have had acute glomerulonephritis, but many give no such history. Complications of connective tissue disorders that are autoimmune in nature such as lupus erythematosus (see Chap. 66) and Goodpasture's syndrome, may also cause chronic glomerulonephritis.

The chronic inflammation leads to ever-increasing bands of scar tissue that replace nephrons, the vital functioning units of the kidney. Decreased glomerular filtration can eventually lead to renal failure. Chronic glomerulonephritis accounts for approximately 40% of people on dialysis.

ASSESSMENT FINDINGS

Signs and Symptoms

Some experience no symptoms of this disorder until renal damage is severe. Generalized edema known

TABLE 63-3 **Treatment for Rapidly Progressive Glomerulonephritis**

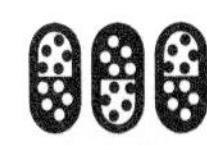

Drug Category	Mechanism of Action	Nursing Considerations
Methylprednisolone pulse therapy	Acts by reducing the inflammatory process and preventing damage to the glomerulus	Patients must be hemodynamically stable, have normal serum electrolytes, and not be taking diuretics. The usual dosage is 30 mg/kg per day to a maximum of 3 g given IV over 30 minutes given every other day with prednisone 1–2 mg/kg on alternate days. This regimen is tapered over 3–6 months.
Plasma exchange therapy	Removes antibodies from the circulation	Involves 3–4 liters of plasma exchange through vascular access daily or on alternate days. This therapy can take several weeks. Concommitant steroid and cytotoxic therapies are used.

as **anasarca** is a common finding. Anasarca is due to the shift of fluid from the intravascular space to interstitial and intracellular fluid locations. The fluid shift is due to depletion of serum proteins, albumin in particular, which is lost in the urine. Clients remain markedly edematous for months or years. The client may feel relatively well, but the kidney continues to excrete albumin. The fluid burden and subsequent renal failure contribute to fatigue, headache, hypertension, dyspnea, and visual disturbances.

Diagnostic Findings

Low red blood cell volume is detected through complete blood counts. Its underlying cause is the excretion of erythrocytes in the urine and a reduction in production of erythropoietin. **Azotemia,** accumulation of nitrogen waste products in the blood, is evidenced by elevated BUN, serum creatinine, and uric acid levels. The urine contains protein (albumin), sediment, **casts** (deposits of minerals that break loose from the walls of the tubules), and red and white blood cells. The urinary creatinine clearance is reduced. Serum electrolyte changes indicate nephron dysfunction.

A chest radiograph and electrocardiogram (ECG) evaluate cardiac size because enlargement is often the case. A percutaneous kidney biopsy may be performed in the early stage to confirm the diagnosis and to determine the severity of the disorder. In late stages, the kidneys are too small to safely perform a biopsy.

MEDICAL MANAGEMENT

Treatment is nonspecific and symptomatic. Management goals include (1) controlling hypertension with medications and sodium restriction, (2) correcting fluid and electrolyte imbalance, (3) reducing edema with diuretic therapy, (4) preventing congestive heart failure, and (5) eliminating urinary tract infections with antimicrobials. Renal failure may eventually necessitate dialysis or kidney transplantation, which is discussed later in this chapter.

NURSING MANAGEMENT

The nursing plan of care for clients with chronic glomerulonephritis includes, but is not limited to, the following:

Nursing Diagnoses and Collaborative Problems	Nursing Interventions
Fluid Volume Excess related to decreased glomerular filtration **Goal:** The client will maintain a fluid volume within normal limits as evidenced by urine output >500 mL/day, systolic blood pressure <140 mm Hg, reduced proteinuria, and absence of crackles or gurgles and S_3 heart sound.	Weigh daily at the same time on the same scale while wearing similar clothing. Measure intake and output. Proportionately distribute restricted fluid volumes within waking hours. Monitor blood pressure, heart rate, lung and heart sounds each shift; notify the physician of significant changes. Assess for pitting edema, tight rings or shoes, clothes that do not fit comfortably. Request that the dietitian instruct the client on sodium restriction and adequate caloric intake. Suggest herbs or spices that increase the palatability of food. Administer prescribed diuretics.
Fatigue and **Activity Intolerance** related to anemia and generalized edema	Avoid clustering nursing tasks and physical activities. Provide periods of rest and promote uninterrupted sleep at night. Facilitate an adequate nutritional intake that includes some complete protein and iron-rich foods. Eliminate any activities of daily living that are not necessary. Assist the client with activities when evidence of tachycardia or dyspnea is present.

Client and Family Teaching

Evaluate the client's ability to manage home care and maintenance or the support system that is available to the client before discharge plans are developed. If the client lacks a support system from the family or extended family members, consult with the physician; referral to a social agency or home health care agency may be necessary. Develop a teaching plan based on the following:

- Follow the diet and fluid regimen recommended by the physician and as outlined by the dietitian.
- Take medications exactly as directed on the container label. Do not omit or discontinue any medication unless ordered to do so by the physician. Do not take nonprescription drugs unless their use is approved by the physician.
- Monitor and record temperature and weight daily. (In some instances, clients may be asked to monitor their blood pressure.)

- Follow the physician's recommendations as to physical activity and exercise. Take frequent rest periods if fatigue occurs.
- Contact the physician with any question about the medication, if symptoms become worse, or if fever, chills, blood in the urine, weight gain, swelling of the arms or legs or periorbital edema, difficulty in breathing, difficulty in thinking, severe fatigue, excessive sleepiness, constipation, loss of appetite, or an upper respiratory infection occurs.
- Emphasize that frequent follow-up visits and laboratory tests are necessary to monitor response to treatment.

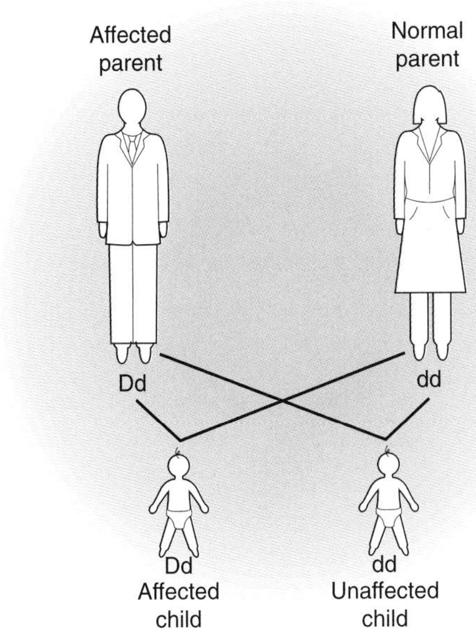

FIGURE 63-2. Inheritance of an autosomal dominant disorder.

Congenital Kidney Disorders

Individuals may be born with a variety of malformations of renal structures. Most of these are unpredictable because they are the result of errors in fetal development. However, polycystic disease is a disorder that has a familial tendency.

Polycystic Disease

The two manifestations of polycystic disease are the infantile and adult forms. The infantile form is rare. It may cause fetal death (before delivery), early neonatal death, or renal failure during childhood. The adult form has its onset between 30 to 50 years of age and insidiously progresses to renal insufficiency. Once renal failure develops, polycystic disease is usually fatal within 4 years, unless the client receives dialysis treatment or organ transplant. Women and men are affected equally. Death is usually due to renal failure or the complications of hypertensive cardiovascular disease.

ETIOLOGY AND PATHOPHYSIOLOGY

Adult polycystic kidney disease is the result of autosomal dominant inheritance. This means that the gene for the disease is passed from an affected parent to his or her children. Each child has a 50:50 chance of acquiring the defective gene (Fig. 63–2) as opposed to a recessive gene in which there is a 25% chance of being affected.

As the name implies, this disorder is characterized by the formation of multiple bilateral kidney cysts (Fig. 63–3). The cysts interfere with kidney function and eventually lead to renal failure. The fluid-filled cysts cause enormous enlargement of the kidneys from normal fist size to as much as the size of a football. As the cysts enlarge, they compress the renal blood vessels and cause chronic hypertension. Bleeding into cysts causes flank pain. Individuals with polycystic disease are much more susceptible to kidney infections and kidney stones. Besides renal failure, other complications include cysts on the pancreas and liver, an enlarged heart, mitral valve prolapse, and brain aneurysm.

ASSESSMENT FINDINGS

Signs and Symptoms

Hypertension is present in approximately 75% of affected individuals at the time of diagnosis. Other symptoms, such as pain from retroperitoneal bleeding, lumbar discomfort, and abdominal tenderness, are due to the size and effects of the cysts. **Colic** (acute spasmotic pain) is experienced when there is ureteral passage of clots or calculi.

Diagnostic Findings

A family history of affected members is a presumptive diagnostic indicator. Urinalysis shows mild proteinuria, hematuria, and pyuria. A complete blood count (CBC) may show decreased or increased red blood cells and hematocrit because sometimes erythropoietin production is accelerated. Abdominal ultrasound, computed tomography (CT) scan, magnetic resonance imaging (MRI), and IVP reveal enlarged kidneys with indentations caused by cysts. Laboratory tests such as a BUN and serum creatinine indicate the degree of current kidney dysfunction.

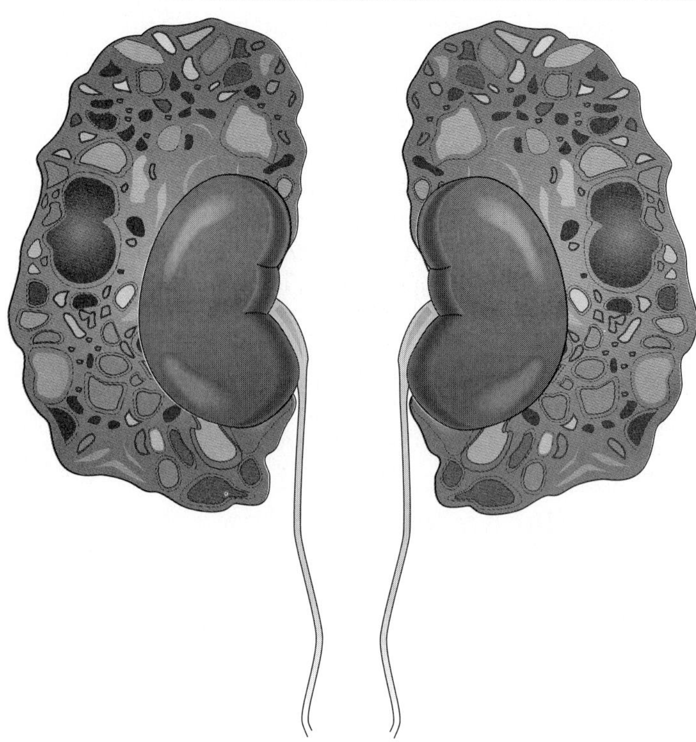

FIGURE 63-3. Normal kidneys in comparison with polycystic kidneys.

MEDICAL AND SURGICAL MANAGEMENT

Polycystic disease has no cure, but some interventions reduce the rate of progression. Hypertension is treated with antihypertensive drugs, diuretic medications, and sodium restriction. Despite these interventions, the hypertension is difficult to control. When and if urinary infections develop, they are treated promptly with antibiotics. Low red blood cell counts are treated with iron supplements, injections of erythropoietin (Epogen), or blood transfusions. Nephrotoxic medications, such as nonsteroidal anti-inflammatory drugs and cephalosporin antibiotics, are avoided at all costs.

Dialysis substitutes for kidney function when renal failure occurs and while the client awaits an organ transplant. Surgical removal of one or both kidneys may be required. Animal research is currently being conducted using the antineoplastic drug, paclitaxel (Taxol), steroids such as methylprednisolone (Depo-Medrol), and an antihyperlipidemic agent, lovastatin (Mevacor), to evaluate if these drugs slow the rate of disease progression.

NURSING MANAGEMENT

Many clients with polycystic disease are treated as outpatients by primary care physicians or nephrologists, physicians who specialize in the diagnosis and treatment of renal diseases. When hospitalization is necessary, assess vital signs, especially blood pressure, and report any significant elevations. Monitor laboratory test results for indicators of renal function. Observe the urine for signs of bleeding or infection. Measure intake and output. Report any decrease in or absence of urine output. Refer to the nursing management of the client with kidney stones, renal failure, and dialysis for the care of clients with complications or advanced stages of this disease.

Obstructive Disorders

Kidney and Ureteral Stones

A stone (**calculus;** pl. calculi), is a precipitate of mineral salts that ordinarily remain dissolved in urine. About 80% of renal calculi in the United States are composed of calcium oxalate. Others are composed of urate crystals (uric acid), cystine, xanthine, and magnesium ammonium phosphate, or struvite. Stones may be smooth, jagged, or staghorn shaped (Fig. 63–4).

Calculi can occur anywhere in the urinary tract from the kidney pelvis and beyond. When a stone forms, the condition is called **urolithiasis. Nephrolithiasis** refers to the presence of a kidney stone, the size of which may range from microscopic to several centimeters in diameter. **Ureterolithiaisis** is a stone within the ureter. Ureteral stones are usually small; some may be no larger than a grain of sand.

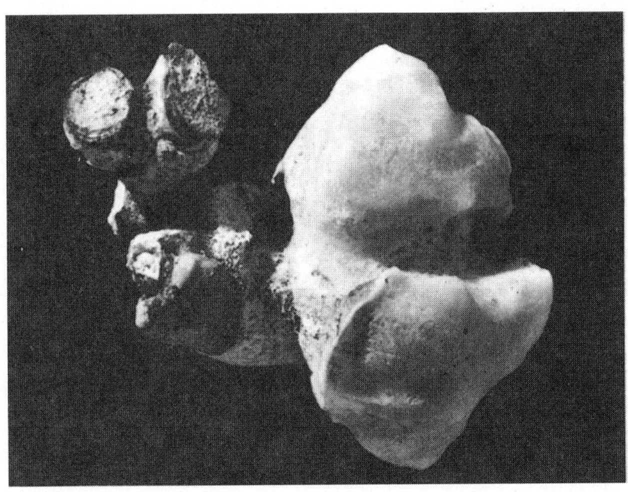

FIGURE 63-4. Example of a large staghorn kidney stone.

ETIOLOGY AND PATHOPHYSIOLOGY

The reason urinary calculi form is not fully understood. Predisposing factors include:

- **Calciuria,** excessive calcium in the urine, as may occur with hyperparathyroid disease, administration of calcium-based antacids, and excessive intake of vitamin D
- Dehydration
- Urinary tract infection with urea-splitting organisms such as *P. mirabilis,* which makes urine alkaline, a condition that promotes precipitation of calcium
- Obstructive disorders, such as an enlarged prostate gland, which foster urinary stasis,
- Metabolic disorders such as gout in which uric acid crystallizes
- Osteoporosis in which bone is demineralized
- Prolonged immobility from paralysis secondary to spinal injuries or other incapacitating conditions that result in sluggish emptying of urine from the urinary tract

Calculi traumatize the walls of the urinary tract and irritate the cellular lining, causing pain as violent contractions of the ureter develop to pass the stone along. But the ureteral spasms may just as easily hold a stone in place. If a stone totally or partially obstructs the passage of urine beyond its location, pressure increases in the area above the stone. The pressure contributes to pain and urinary stasis promotes secondary infection. The retained urine distends the renal pelvis, a condition called **hydronephrosis.** Eventually, there may be compression of the glomeruli and tiny arterioles that supply blood to the kidney, which can result in permanent kidney damage.

ASSESSMENT FINDINGS

Signs and Symptoms

Symptoms of a kidney or ureteral stone vary with size, location, and cause of the calculi. Small stones may pass unnoticed. However, sudden, sharp, severe flank pain that travels to the suprapubic region and external genitalia is the classic symptom of urinary calculi. The pain is accompanied by renal or ureteral colic, painful spasms that attempt to move the stone. The pain comes in waves that radiate to the inguinal ring, the inner aspect of the thigh, and to the testicle or tip of the penis in men, or the urinary meatus or labia in women. The severity of the pain is generally inversely proportional to the size of the stone; smaller stones travel more rapidly down the ureter causing more forceful ureteral spasm and, therefore, greater pain. The severity of the pain can cause nausea, vomiting, and shock.

If an infection develops, the client may experience chills, fever, and serious hypotension. Urinary retention or dysuria may accompany obstruction. The kidney pelvis and ureter may become markedly enlarged as a consequence of urinary obstruction, and a mass may be palpated. Renal tenderness may be present.

Diagnostic Findings

Urinalysis shows evidence of gross or microscopic hematuria from trauma as the calculus tears at tissue as it moves downward. In addition, the urinalysis may show a pH conducive to stone formation, increased specific gravity, mineral crystals, and casts. Leukocytes in the urine and an elevated white blood cell count indicate the presence of an infectious process. A urine culture identifies specific infectious microorganisms.

Most translucent kidney stones are identified by radiography. But if visualization is inconclusive, an

IVP shows dye-filling defects caused by the presence of a stone. The dye stops at a certain point in the ureter and demonstrates an enlarged ureter above the obstruction. A kiney ultrasonography also detects obstructive changes. Depending on the length of time the stone has been present, some blood chemistry values, such as serum creatinine, BUN, and serum uric acid may be elevated. Analysis of the stone content is useful in preventing recurrence.

MEDICAL MANAGEMENT

Small calculi are passed naturally with no specific interventions. If the stone is 5 mm or less in diameter, moving, the pain is tolerable, and no obstruction is present, the client is managed medically with vigorous hydration, analgesics, antimicrobial therapy, and drugs that dissolve calculi or eventually alter conditions that promote their formation (Table 63–4).

For larger stones, **extracorporeal shock wave lithotripsy** (ESWL), a procedure that uses 800 to 2,400 shock waves aimed from outside the body toward dense stones (Fig. 63–5) may be used. The stones are shattered into smaller particles that are passed from the urinary tract. ESWL is administered with the client in a water bath or surrounded by a soft cushion while under light anesthesia or sedation. Stones can also be pulverized with laser lithotripsy. To do so, a fine wire, through which the laser beam passes, is inserted into the ureter by means of a cystoscope. Repeated bursts of the laser reduce the stone to a fine powder, which is then passed in the urine.

Other stone removal procedures are performed with ureteroscopic approaches in which the endoscope is inserted from the urethra into the upper urinary tract under anesthesia to grasp, crush, and remove stones from the kidney pelvis or ureter. Afterward, a catheter or **ureteral stent,** a slender supportive device, is left in place for 3 days to splint the ureter or divert the urine past any possible tear in the ureteral wall (Fig. 63–6). If the stone cannot be removed, a ureteral catheter is left in place for 24 hours to dilate the ureter in the hope that the stone will pass through it or that it will be pulled into the bladder when the catheter is removed.

SURGICAL MANAGEMENT

Calculi that are large, complicated by obstruction, ongoing urinary tract infection, kidney damage, or constant bleeding require surgical removal. Surgical options include a percutaneous nephrolithotomy, or uretero-, pyelo-, nephrolithotomy. Drainage of urine from the affected kidney is accomplished with a nephrostomy tube during the postsurgical healing process.

A **nephrostomy tube,** which is also called a pyelostomy tube, is a catheter that is inserted through the skin into the renal pelvis. A nephrostomy tube is used to manage any obstruction to urine flow above the bladder. The tube is kept in place with a suture through the skin. Unlike the bladder, the kidney pelvis can only hold approximately 5 to 8 mL of urine. If urinary drainage through the tube is impaired for even a short time from a blood clot or kinking or compression of the tubing, hydronephrosis and damage to surgically repaired tissue can result. The client will complain of pain if the renal pelvis becomes distended with urine.

Percutaneous Nephrolithotomy

A percutaneous nephrolithotomy is an endoscopic procedure. A nephroscope is tunneled into the kidney through a tiny skin incision while the client is under general anesthesia (Fig 63–7). Ultrasound is used to crush the stone. The fragments are removed through the endoscope.

Ureterolithotomy, Pyelolithotomy, Nephrolithotomy

With the patient anesthetized, a suprapubic abdominal or flank incision is made and the stone is removed under direct visualization. A **pyeloplasty,** surgical repair of the ureteropelvic junction or other anatomic anomalies, may be performed at the same time. The additional surgery is done to correct conditions that contribute to the development of stones and prevent their recurrence. A **nephrectomy,** surgical removal of a kidney, is indicated if a stone has permanently and severely damaged a kidney beyond adequate function. The other kidney must be fully functional.

NURSING PROCESS
Care of the Client with Renal Calculi

Assessment

Obtain a complete history, including a drug and allergy history, family history, history of immobility, episodes of dehydration, urinary tract infections, and diet. Assess pain intensity and location and associated symptoms such as nausea and vomiting. Monitor vital signs and assess all urine for stones by straining it through a gauze or wire mesh and closely inspecting it. Save any solid material for laboratory analysis.

Diagnosis and Planning

The nursing management of a client with renal calculi includes, but is not limited to, the following:

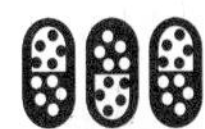

TABLE 63-4 **Drug Therapy for Pyelonephritis**

Drug Category	Drug Action	Nursing Considerations
Antispasmodics oxybutinin chloride (Ditropan) flavoxate (Urispas), belladonna and opium suppositories	Inhibits the action of acetylcholine and relaxes smooth muscle of the ureters and bladder.	Side effects include dizziness, drowsiness, blurred vision, dry mouth, constipation, increased heart rate, and delirium. Should not be used in clients with closed-angle glaucoma or hypotension.
Anticholinergics propantheline (Pro-Banthine), hyoscyamine (Levsinex), tincture of belladonna	Reduces spasms and smooth muscle contractions by inhibiting the effects of acetylcholine, thereby increasing bladder capacity	Side effects are the same as for antispasmodics.
Oral Antibiotics trimethorprim-sulfamethoxazole (Bactrim, Septra), ciprofloxacin (Cipro)	Inhibits bacterial growth and destroys microorganisms	Use for up to 14 days. Clients do not require hospitalization unless nausea, vomiting, or signs of septicemia develop.

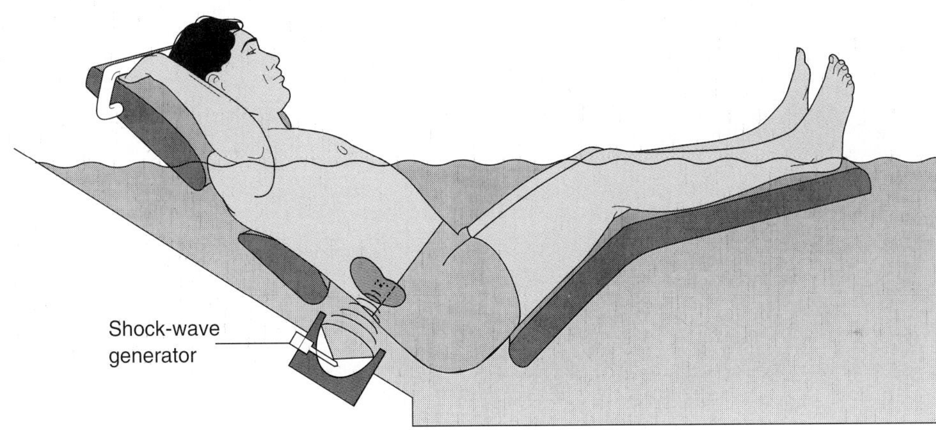

A

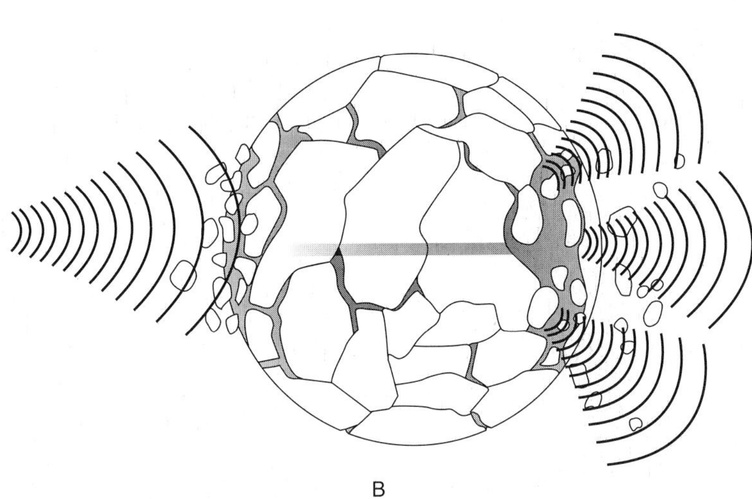

B

FIGURE 63-5. (*A*) Extracorporeal shock wave lithotripter aimed at kidney. (*B*) Shock waves disrupt front and rear surfaces while fracturing the center of the calculus.

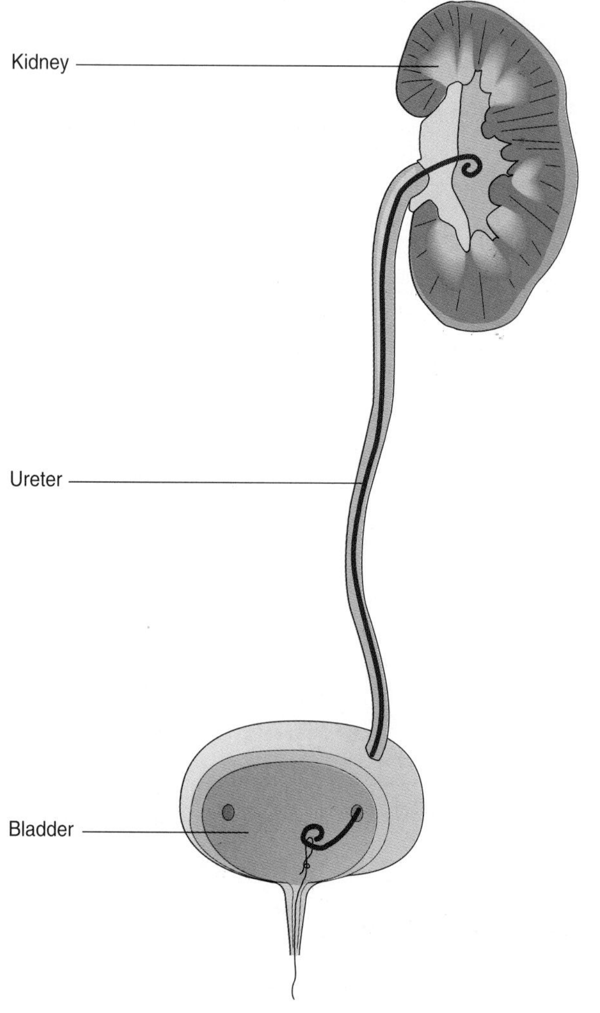

FIGURE 63-6. Example of a ureteral stent, in this case a double J stent.

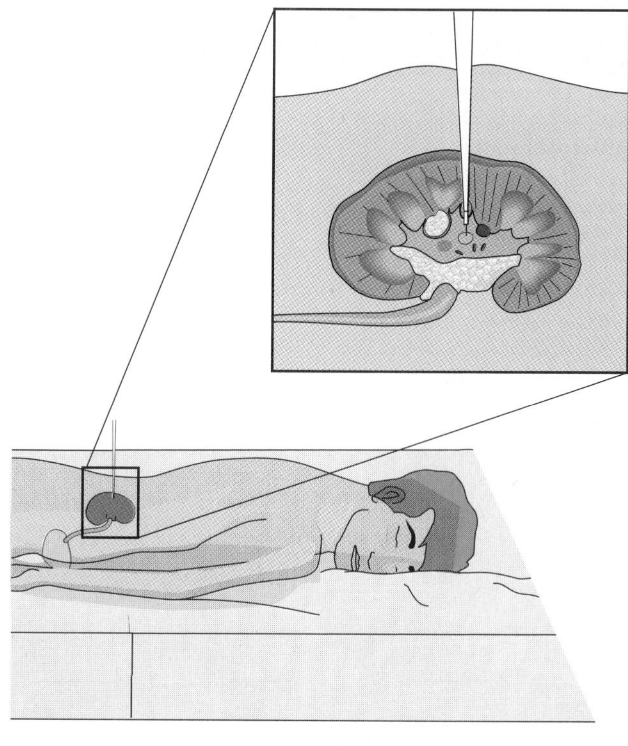

FIGURE 63-7. A nephroscope is inserted through a surgically created tunnel when a percutaneous nephrolithotomy is performed.

Nursing Diagnoses and Collaborative Problems	Nursing Interventions
Pain related to increased pressure in the renal pelvis or renal colic	Administer prescribed narcotic analgesic.
Goal: Pain will be less in 30 minutes after a nursing measure than original assessment.	Provide nonpharmacologic interventions such as a comfortable position, guided imagery, and distraction as supplements to analgesia.
	Encourage ambulation and liberal fluid intake when the client is comfortable.
	Consult with the physician about reducing the rate of IV fluid administration during periods of renal colic.
PC: Hydronephrosis related to ureteral obstruction	Monitor intake and output.
Goal: Hydronephrosis will be managed and minimized.	Palpate the costovertebral angle (CVA) where the last rib joins the vertebra, to detect tenderness or a mass that increases in size.
	Manage a nephrostomy tube by following the Nursing Guidelines 63-1.
Risk for Infection related to urinary stasis	Administer antimicrobial therapy as prescribed.
Goal: Urinary tract infection will not develop as evidenced by urine free of pus and microorganisms, normal temperature and white blood cell count.	Encourage fluid intake to 3,000 mL/day unless contraindicated.
	Offer cranberry, plum, or prune juices that acidify the urine and inhibit bacterial growth.
	Maintain patency of all catheters or encourage to void every 2 to 3 hours.
	Follow aseptic principles when changing dressings or urinary drainage equipment.
Risk for Altered (Renal) Tissue Perfusion related to increased fluid pressure in ureter and kidney pelvis	Monitor laboratory and diagnostic test results.
Goal: Kidney will remain adequately perfused with blood as evidenced by normal serum creatinine, BUN, and distribution of radiopaque dye following IVP.	Prepare the client safely but quickly for treatment measures that promote urinary drainage if it becomes apparent that kidney function is compromised.

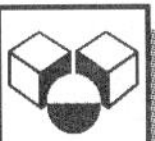

Nursing Guidelines 63-1

Managing a Nephrostomy Tube

- Connect the nephrostomy tube to a closed drainage system.
- Have a second nephrostomy tube available at the bedside for the physician's use in case the present one is displaced.
- Secure the tube to the client's flank with tape to ensure that it does not become dislodged.
- Keep the urine collection bag below the level of insertion.
- *Never* clamp the nephrostomy tubing.
- Check that the nephrostomy and drainage tubing are not kinked or that the client is not compressing the tubing.
- Use no more than 5 to 8 mL of sterile normal saline to maintain patency if an irrigation is medically ordered.
- Record the urine output from the nephrostomy tube separately from other urinary volumes.
- Assess the tube insertion site for bleeding and drainage.
- Change the dressing around the nephrostomy tube if and when it becomes damp; apply a skin barrier ointment around the incision to prevent excoriation.
- Notify the physician immediately if the nephrostomy tube becomes dislodged or if there is an absence of urinary drainage.

Evaluation and Expected Outcomes

- The client's pain is reduced.
- Urine output is adequate; urine is clear.
- The client is afebrile.
- Urine and blood tests indicate adequate renal function.

For clients undergoing surgical procedures, explain the procedure and follow standards for perioperative care in Chapter 24. After lithotripsy, endoscopy, or surgery, assess vital signs, measure fluid intake and output, and inspect the color of urine, which may be grossly bloody for a time. After ESWL, inspect the flank for ecchymosis, which is expected, and record the location of discoloration. Administer analgesics for postprocedural discomfort.

If a ureteroscopy is performed and a urethral catheter is in place, attach the catheter to a closed drainage system. Pink-tinged urine may be seen, but immediately contact the physician if frank blood appears in the urine or the client complains of severe abdominal pain. If a ureteral stent is present, check for the presence of the suture that extends from the urinary meatus, which is used for its removal. Continue to provide a total daily fluid volume of approximately 3,000 mL.

Client and Family Teaching

Consider the following recommendations when teaching the client and family:

- Explain the causes and methods for preventing renal calculi.
- Recommend drinking plenty of liquids; water is one of the best.
- Provide a list of foods (Box 63–1) that are restricted to small amounts if the stone(s) are composed of calcium oxalate.
- Review the self-administration of antimicrobial and analgesic drugs, and antigout medications, if prescribed. Discuss the purpose for the medications, dosing schedule, and side effects to report.
- Discuss catheter or nephrostomy tube care.
- Teach the client how to strain urine if the stone or its fragments have not been passed.
- Advise the client to report signs of acute obstruction immediately, such as inability or difficulty in voiding or pain.
- Identify signs of infection such as fever, chills, dysuria, frequency, urgency, and cloudy urine. Review the relationship between urinary calculi and infection.
- Provide discharge teaching following a treatment procedure that includes activity level, hygiene measures, dietary modifications, goals for oral fluid intake, and wound care.
- Emphasize consulting with the physician before self-administering any over-the-counter medications.

Ureteral Stricture

A stricture is a narrowing of a lumen; in this case the ureter is narrowed.

ETIOLOGY AND PATHOPHYSIOLOGY

A stricture of the ureter is relatively rare, but the incidence is higher among those with chronic ureteral stone formation. The recurrent inflammation and infection cause scar tissue to accumulate within the ureter. Other conditions that can interfere with urine passing through the ureter are congenital anomalies

BOX 63-1 Sources of Calcium and Oxalate

Apples	Cheese	Grapes	Spinach
Asparagus	Chocolate	Ice cream	Swiss chard
Beer	Cocoa	Milk	Rhubarb
Beets	Coffee	Oranges	Tea
Berries	Cola	Parsley	Turnips
Black pepper	Collards	Peanut butter	Vitamin C
Broccoli	Figs	Pineapples	Yogurt

or conditions that mechanically compress the ureter such as pregnancy and tumors within the abdomen or upper urinary tract.

In many instances the ureter is only partially narrowed. Symptoms develop over time as the area of the ureter above the stricture dilates with urine (hydroureter) and the kidney pelvis slowly enlarges. Stasis of urine promotes an upper urinary tract infection.

ASSESSMENT FINDINGS

Signs and Symptoms

Flank pain or discomfort and tenderness at the costovertebral angle (CVA) due to enlargement of the renal pelvis often develop. The client experiences back or abdominal discomfort. The discomfort tends to increase during periods when fluid intake is higher.

Diagnostic Findings

A voiding cystourethrogram and ultrasonography help to identify structural changes consistent with impaired passage of urine.

MEDICAL AND SURGICAL MANAGEMENT

Various measures are used to treat strictures. Management depends on the location, the density, and the length of the stricture. The ureter can be stretched by inserting a dilator called a filiform or urethral sound, a curved metal rod, followed by others that are sequentially larger.

If the obstruction persists, the physician performs a **ureteroplasty,** removal of the narrowed section of ureter and reconnection of the patent portions. This is the preferred procedure for a midureteral stricture. A ureteral stent is placed in the ureter to provide support to the walls of the ureter, relieve the obstruction, and maintain the flow of urine through the ureter and into the bladder. Lower ureteral strictures are treated by removing the narrowed portion of the ureter and reimplanting the remaining section into the bladder wall.

Besides correcting strictures, ureteral surgery is performed to remove tumors, repair accidental ligation of the ureter during abdominal surgery (the highest incidence is seen in hysterectomies), and to extricate a ureteral stone that cannot be removed by other means.

NURSING MANAGEMENT

Follow standards of care for the perioperative client if the client undergoes surgery (see Chap. 24). If a ureteral catheter is inserted preoperatively, measure the urine output from the catheter hourly. Immediately report if there is no urine output from the ureteral catheter.

On return from surgery, all urinary drainage tubes and catheters are connected to a closed drainage system or to the type of drainage ordered by the physician. The main complication associated with ureteral surgery is failure of the ureter to transport urine from the kidney to the bladder. Contact the physician if signs of shock appear, urinary output from the ureteral catheter is decreased or absent, or if the client complains of significant abdominal pain, which may indicate leakage of urine into the peritoneal cavity. Notify the physician if signs of a urinary tract infection develop, such as fever and chills or if the urine is cloudy or has a foul odor.

Client and Family Teaching

Depending on the surgical procedure, the client may need instruction in the care of the ureteral or urethral catheter(s), the type and management of the drainage collection system, incision care, and a review of the prescribed diet and medication schedule.

Tumors of the Kidney

A hypernephroma (renal adenocarcinoma) is the most common malignant tumor of the kidney in adults. Squamous cell tumors are second. Men are affected more than women.

ETIOLOGY AND PATHOPHYSIOLOGY

The cause of kidney tumors is unknown. The incidence is higher in older adults, which suggests chronic exposure to a carcinogen whose metabolites involve renal excretion. Because bladder cancer (see Chap. 64) is associated with the carcinogenic effects of long-term cigarette smoking, perhaps renal tumors are similarly initiated via this mechanism or some other environmental toxin (eg, asbestos) or volatile solvents (eg, gasoline).

Because the kidneys are deeply protected in the body, tumors can become quite large before causing symptoms. As the tumor enlarges, it occupies space, extends into adjacent renal structures, and interferes with urine outflow. Tumor cells tend to metastasize by way of the renal vein and vena cava to the lungs, bone, lymph nodes, liver, and brain. Lung metastases predominate. Sometimes, the first symptom occurs when the hypernephroma has metastasized to other organs.

ASSESSMENT FINDINGS

Signs and Symptoms

The classic triad of renal cancer is *painless* hematuria, flank pain, and the presence of a palpable mass.

Additional symptoms include weight loss, malaise, and unexplained fever. Later, there is colic-like discomfort during the passage of blood clots.

Diagnostic Findings

An abdominal mass found on a routine physical examination or on radiographic examination for other purposes suggests the presence of a kidney tumor. An IVP, cystoscopy with retrograde pyelograms, ultrasonography, MRI, renal angiogram, and CT scan are used to locate the tumor. Sequential urine samples contain red blood cells as well as malignant cells.

MEDICAL AND SURGICAL MANAGEMENT

Nephrectomy, including removal of the surrounding perinephric fat, is the treatment for a malignant renal tumor. When a tumor arises within the collecting system or in the ureter, a complete nephroureterectomy (removal of the kidney and ureter) is done. A cuff of bladder tissue is removed as well because the recurrence rate in any stump of ureter left behind is high. Surgery may be followed with radiation therapy, chemotherapy, or both while the client is still in the hospital or on a postdischarge basis. If extensive metastases are found, only palliative treatment is given. When medical management is limited to palliative treatment because of metastases, the physician explains that the treatment measures are not curative.

NURSING MANAGEMENT

In addition to the standard preoperative preparations, carry out other prescribed procedures that facilitate the postoperative assessment and recovery of the client such as inserting a urethral catheter and nasogastric tube. Connect a water manometer, if ordered, to the IV tubing infusing parenteral fluid through a central venous catheter. The water manometer is used to monitor to measure central venous pressure (CVP).

On the client's return from surgery, assess vital signs frequently. Inspect and identify the type and location of drains or catheters that are present. Place an indwelling (Foley) catheter drainage system *below* the level of the bed. Drains within or around the incision may drain by closed negative pressure (ie, Jackson-Pratt) or low mechanical suction.

The postoperative plan of nursing care includes, but is not limited to, the following:

Nursing Diagnoses and Collaborative Problems	Nursing Interventions
PC: Internal Hemorrhage related to bleeding from the ligated renal artery or vein **Goal:** Hemorrhage will be managed and minimized.	Monitor blood pressure and pulse rate every 1 to 4 hours for the first 24 to 48 hours after surgery. Report a decrease in blood pressure, rise in pulse, restlessness, or sudden onset of flank pain; death can occur in a short time unless the client is immediately returned to surgery to control the bleeding. Administer IV fluids and blood transfusions as ordered. Note the color of drainage from each tube and catheter and record assessment findings for further comparison. Follow the physician's orders concerning postoperative positioning; some prefer to keep the client from lying on the operative side to avoid interfering with wound drainage. Contact the surgeon if there is any sudden decrease in urine output or presence of frank bleeding; pink tinged drainage is normal for several days after surgery.
Pain related to tissue trauma and pressure from urinary obstruction **Goal:** The client's pain will be relieved to within a tolerable level within 30 minutes of an intervention.	Keep drainage catheters unclamped, unkinked, and below the level of insertion. Secure all tubings to reduce movement at the site of insertion or displacement. Encourage oral fluids as soon as allowed and tolerated without causing nausea or vomiting; fluids dilute the urine and prevent catheter obstruction from sediment or small blood clots. Irrigate tubings following the physician's orders as to volume of irrigant. Administer prescribed analgesia and supplement drug therapy with nursing measures that promote comfort. Splint the incision when repositioning the client or during efforts to cough and deep breathe.
Risk for Ineffective Breathing Pattern related to incisional pain and restricted positioning; **Risk for Ineffective Airway Clearance** related to weak cough secondary to incisional pain	Encourage the client to breathe deeply and cough every 2 hours. Use an incentive spirometer to evaluate effectiveness.

Goal: The client's breathing rate and depth will be sufficient to maintain a SpO_2 at 90% or above; secretions will be raised; lung sounds will be clear in all lobes.	Use two hands to apply firm support of the incision when the client is coughing or performing deep breathing exercises. Auscultate the lungs daily and notify the physician if abnormal breath sounds or absence of breath sounds develop.
Risk for Infection related to impaired skin integrity and stasis of urine **Goal:** The client will be free of infection as evidenced by normal temperature, urine culture, and white blood cell count.	Monitor temperature every 4 hours. Contact the physician if the client has a temperature higher than 101°F (38.3°C) or if chills, purulent drainage, or redness, swelling, warmth, at the incision is noted. Use aseptic technique when changing the surgical dressing or managing the catheter and drainage systems. Administer antibiotic therapy as prescribed.

Client and Family Teaching

Clients who have had a nephrectomy usually have the drains (if any) removed before discharge. A dressing over the incision may or may not be required. If the physician orders a dressing applied and changed at home, show the client and family how to change the dressing and provide a list of the necessary materials for dressing changes. Develop a teaching plan based on the following:

- Change the dressing as ordered by the physician; wash hands *thoroughly* before and after each dressing change.
- Drink plenty of fluids and follow the diet recommended by the physician.
- Avoid exposure to others who have possible infections.
- Take prescribed medication as directed on the container. Do not omit a dose.
- Contact the physician immediately if pain, fever, or chills occurs or if the urine becomes bloody, cloudy, or foul smelling.

Renal Failure

Renal failure is the inability of the nephrons within the kidneys to maintain fluid, electrolyte, and acid–base balance, excrete nitrogen waste products, and perform regulatory functions such as maintaining calcification of bones and producing erythropoietin.

There are two types of renal failure: acute and chronic. **Acute renal failure** (ARF) is characterized by a sudden and rapid decrease in renal function. ARF is potentially reversible with early, aggressive treatment of its contributing etiology. **Chronic renal failure** (CRF) is characterized by progressive and irreversible damage to the nephrons. It may take months to years for CRF to develop.

Acute Renal Failure

ETIOLOGY AND PATHOPHYSIOLOGY

Renal failure can occur as a consequence of prerenal, intrarenal, and postrenal disorders (Table 63–5). Prerenal disorders are nonurologic conditions that disrupt renal blood flow to the nephrons, affecting their filtering ability; intrarenal conditions are conditions within the kidney itself that destroy nephrons; and postrenal disorders are generally obstructive problems in structures below the kidney(s) that have damaging repercussions to the nephrons located above.

Acute renal failure progresses through four phases:

- Initiation phase
- Oliguric phase
- Diuretic phase
- Recovery phase

Initiation Phase

The initiation phase begins with the onset of the contributing event. It is accompanied by a reduction in blood flow to the nephrons to the point at which there is acute tubular necrosis (ATN). **Acute tubular necrosis** refers to the death of cells within the collecting tubules of the nephrons where reabsorption of water, electrolytes, and excretion of protein wastes and excess metabolic substances occurs (Fig. 63–8).

Oliguric Phase

The oliguric phase is associated with the excretion of less than adequate urinary volumes. This phase begins within 48 hours after the initial cellular insult and may last for 10 to 14 days or longer (Porth, 1994). Fluid volume excess develops, which leads to edema, hypertension, and cardiopulmonary complications. Azotemia, marked accumulation of urea and other nitrogenous wastes such as creatinine and uric acid in the blood, creates a potential for neurologic changes such as seizures, coma, and death.

Currently, there is better treatment of many prerenal causes of ARF; consequently, some clients excrete urinary volumes greater than 500 mL/day. However, the urine has a very low specific gravity because it lacks normal amounts of excreted substances such as excess potassium and hydrogen ions, to maintain homeostasis. Consequently, hyperkalemia, metabolic

TABLE 63-5 **Causes of Renal Failure**

Prerenal	Intrarenal	Postrenal
Hypovolemic shock Cardiogenic shock secondary to congestive heart failure Septic shock Anaphylaxis Dehydration Renal artery thrombosis or stenosis Cardiac arrest Lethal arrhythmias	Ischemia Nephrotoxicity secondary to drugs such as aminoglycosides Acute and chronic glomerulonephritis Polycystic disease Untreated prerenal and postrenal disorders Myoglobinuria secondary to burns Hemoglobinuria secondary to transfusion reaction	Ureteral calculi Prostatic hypertrophy Ureteral stricture Ureteral or bladder tumor

acidosis, and **uremia,** a toxic state caused by the accumulation of nitrogen wastes, develop regardless of the excreted water volume.

Diuretic Phase

Diuresis begins as the nephrons recover. Despite an increase in the water content of urine, the excretion of wastes and electrolytes continues to be impaired. The BUN, creatinine, potassium, and phosphate levels remain elevated in the blood.

Recovery Phase

It may take one or more years of recovery while normal glomerular filtration and tubular function are restored. Some clients recover completely; others develop varying degrees of permanent renal dysfunction.

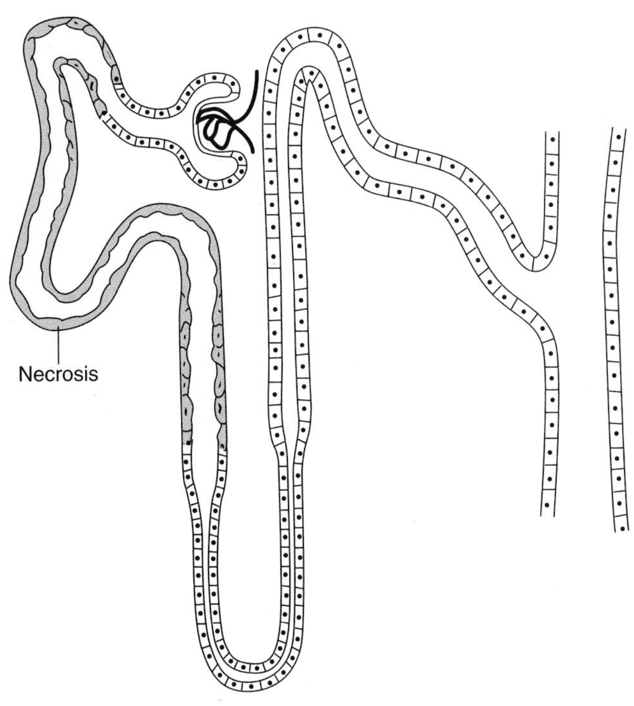

FIGURE 63-8. Acute tubular necrosis.

Chronic Renal Failure

ETIOLOGY AND PATHOPHYSIOLOGY

Chronic renal failure is more often associated with intrarenal conditions or it is a complication of systemic diseases such as diabetes mellitus and disseminated lupus erythematosus. In CRF, the kidneys are so extensively damaged that they do not adequately remove protein by-products and electrolytes from the blood and do not maintain acid–base balance. **End-stage renal disease** (ESRD) is the term given for the point at which a regular course of dialysis or kidney transplantation is necessary to maintain life.

Because damage to the nephrons occurs slowly, declining renal function is not as apparent until the end-stage. The BUN and serum creatinine levels gradually rise. Hyponatremia is a reflection of diluted sodium ions in an excess volume of water in the blood. Actual electrolyte imbalances include hyperkalemia, hyperphosphatemia, hypermagnesemia, and hypocalcemia. The skin becomes the excretory organ for the substances the kidney usually clears from the body. A precipitate, referred to as **uremic frost**, may form on the skin.

Metabolic acidosis develops because the tubules cannot convert carbonic acid in the blood to water and bicarbonate ions. Erythropoietin production is inadequate, causing anemia. Susceptibility to infection increases due to a deficient immune system, particularly cellular immunity (see Chap. 40), as well as a decrease in the white blood cell count. Edema and hypertension are consequences of impaired urinary elimination. **Osteodystrophy,** a condition in which the bones become demineralized, occurs due to hypocalcemia and hyperphosphatemia. The parathyroid glands secrete greater amounts of parathormone to raise blood calcium levels.

ASSESSMENT FINDINGS

Signs and Symptoms

In both ARF and CRF, the client has an elevated blood pressure and weight gain. Urine output is generally decreased. Those with CRF develop other symptoms as the disease worsens. Facial features appear puffy due to fluid retention. The skin is pale; ulceration and bleeding of the gastrointestinal tract may occur. The oral mucous membranes bleed, and blood may be found in the feces. There are reports of vague symptoms such as lethargy, headache, anorexia, and dry mouth. Later, other problems develop such as pruritus and dry scaly skin. The client's breath and body may have an odor characteristic of urine. Muscle cramps, bone pain or tenderness, and spontaneous fractures can develop. Mental processes are progressively slowed as electrolyte imbalances become marked and nitrogenous wastes accumulate. Seizures may be experienced. Table 63–6 lists the systemic manifestations of CRF.

Diagnostic Findings

Laboratory blood tests reveal elevations in BUN, creatinine, potassium, magnesium, and phosphorus. Calcium levels are low. The red blood cell count, hematocrit, and hemoglobin are decreased. The pH of the blood is on the acidotic side. Urinalysis reveals a decreased specific gravity. An IVP provides evidence of renal dysfunction. In clients with severe renal failure, dye excretion is generally delayed. A percutaneous renal biopsy shows destruction of nephrons. Radiography and ultrasonography demonstrate structural defects in the kidneys, ureters, and bladder. Renal angiography identifies obstructions in blood vessels.

MEDICAL MANAGEMENT

In ARF, measures are taken to quickly remedy the primary cause of renal failure. Renal damage can be limited by aggressive administration of parenteral fluids to increase plasma volume, giving vasodilating and diuretic drugs, and infusing dopamine (Intropin) to improve cardiac output and perfuse the renal arteries.

To reduce complications and keep the client alive during the 2 or 3 weeks while the tubules are regenerating, hemodialysis (discussed later), a technique in which the blood is filtered externally with a machine, is performed. When hemodialysis is a temporary measure, the blood is removed and returned through a double-lumen or twin central venous catheters (Fig. 63–9). Another option is peritoneal dialysis, a much slower process (discussed later), in which fluids and electrolytes are removed by osmosis and diffusion across the peritoneum, which acts as a semipermeable membrane.

Fluid and dietary restrictions that include low protein, high calories, low sodium, and low potassium are required as the client is stabilized. Sodium polystyrene sulfonate (Kayexalate), an ion-exchange resin, is prescribed for oral or rectal administration to remove excess potassium when hyperkalemia occurs. An IV infusion of glucose and insulin also facilitates movement of potassium within the cell. Acid–base balance is restored by administering IV sodium bicarbonate if renal function is insufficient to do so.

The medical management of CRF is similar to that for ARF except the period of treatment is lifelong or until a kidney transplant is performed. Rather than

TABLE 63-6 **Systemic Complications of Chronic Renal Failure**

Body System	Complication
Cardiovascular	Congestive heart failure, hypertension, cardiac arrhythmias, edema
Metabolic	Electrolyte imbalance, metabolic acidosis
Respiratory	Shortness of breath, pulmonary edema
Gastrointestinal	Malnutrition, vitamin deficiencies, anorexia, nausea, bleeding
Integumentary	Dry skin, pruritus
Neurologic	Lethargy, confusion, depression, seizures, coma
Sensory	Peripheral neuropathies
Musculoskeletal	Bone demineralization, muscle cramps, joint pain
Immunologic	Impaired immune function, decreased antibody production, increased incidence of hepatitis B and other infections

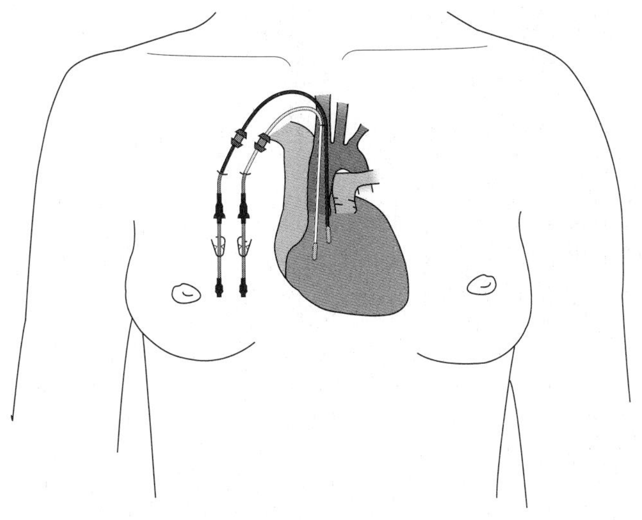

FIGURE 63-9. Twin catheters used for emergency hemodialysis.

administer blood transfusions to correct chronic anemia, epoetin alfa (Epogen) is administered to stimulate bone marrow production of red blood cells.

SURGICAL MANAGEMENT

Some clients in the end-stage of CRF are candidates for a kidney transplant. One healthy kidney can perform the work of two. Donors for a transplant are selected from compatible living donors who may or may not be relatives or from organ donors who are brain dead and whose next of kin give permission for harvesting organs. Any potential donor with a history of hypertension, malignant disease, or diabetes is excluded from donation. To facilitate matching a recipient with a donor, a client is placed on a national computerized transplant waiting list. Whenever an organ becomes available, the computer searches for the recipient who is the best match.

When a transplant is performed, the donor kidney is inserted through an abdominal incision and the nonfunctioning kidneys are left in place unless the client is extremely hypertensive. The blood vessels from the donor kidney are sutured to the iliac artery and vein and the ureter is implanted in the bladder (Fig. 63–10).

Even a perfect match does not guarantee that a transplanted organ will not be rejected. Ironically, even some less than perfectly matched transplanted organs are successful primarily because of immunosuppressive drugs such as azathioprine (Imuran), cyclosporine (Sandimmune), and muromonab-CD-3 (Orthoclone OKT3). If rejection occurs, the client resumes hemodialysis and waits for another transplant.

NURSING MANAGEMENT

Before conducting an initial interview and physical assessment, learn the cause (if known), type (acute versus chronic), and prognosis of the client's renal disorder. Clients may be unable to give an accurate history because of the effect of renal failure on the thought process or because they are acutely ill. It may be necessary to obtain information from the family.

Depending on the collected data, the nursing plan for care includes, but is not limited to, the following:

Nursing Diagnoses and Collaborative Problems	Nursing Interventions
Fluid Volume Excess related to impaired renal function **Goal:** The urinary output will be 500 mL/day or greater.	Weigh the client daily at the same time, with the same type of clothing, on the same scale. A gain of 1 kg (2.2 lb) is the equivalent of 1 liter of fluid.
	Record output accurately; as a rule of thumb, allow 500 mL of intake (the equivalent of insensible fluid losses) and the volume of excreted urine per day. For some patients this may be 500 mL/day.
	Assess lung and heart sounds. Report abnormal sounds. Inspect for jugular vein distention.
	Administer prescribed diuretics and monitor their effectiveness.
	Prepare the client for dialysis if that becomes necessary.
Risk for Altered Oral Mucous Membranes related to restricted oral intake and increased nitrogenous wastes in body fluids like saliva **Goal:** The oral mucosa and lips will remain moist and intact.	Inspect the mouth for evidence of inflammation, ulceration, or bleeding.
	Provide oral care after each meal and at bedtime or every 4 hours while awake.
	Encourage the client to swish, but not swallow water as frequently as desired.
	Provide a lanolin-based lip balm for use as needed.
Risk for Constipation related to fluid restrictions and inactivity **Goal:** The client will pass moist stool regularly.	Administer stool softener as medically prescribed.
	Promote activity within the client's level of tolerance.
	Provide full fluid allotment.
PC: Hypertension	Assess blood pressure every 4 hours.
	Maintain fluid restrictions.

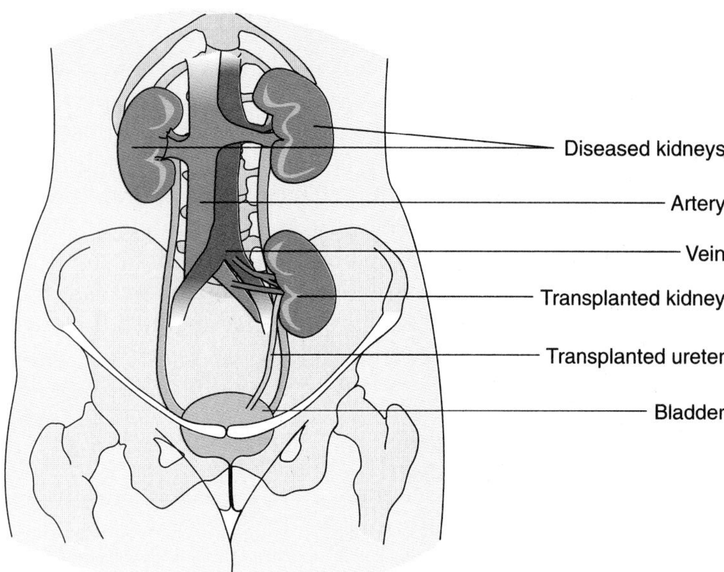

FIGURE 63-10. Transplanted kidney and ureter.

Goal: Diastolic blood pressure greater than 90 mm Hg or systolic blood pressure of 140 mm Hg or more will be managed and minimized.	Administer prescribed antihypertensive drugs and diuretic therapy.
PC: Azotemia **Goal:** Elevated serum levels of nitrogen wastes will be managed and minimized as evidenced by BUN and creatinine levels at normal or near normal levels	Restrict protein foods to those of high biologic value (complete proteins that contain all the essential amino acids) within the amounts prescribed by the physician. Provide sufficient calories from carbohydrates and fats to prevent catabolism of muscle and body stores of protein.
PC: Electrolyte Imbalances (hyperkalemia, hypernatremia, hypocalcemia, hypermagnesemia, hyperphosphatemia) **Goal:** Electrolyte imbalances will be managed and minimized as evidenced by normal or near normal serum levels.	Monitor serum electrolyte results and report critical levels. Monitor cardiac rhythm and report elevated T waves (hyperkalemia) or other dangerous arrhythmias. Restrict sources of potassium that are generally found in fresh fruits and fresh vegetables. Administer prescribed dosages of sodium polystyrene sulfonate (Kayexalate). Be prepared to administer glucose and regular insulin (250 U/250 mL) to promote transfer of potassium from extracellular to intracellular locations. Restrict sodium intake according to the physician's specifications. Give calcium containing antacids like Tums™ or calcium carbonate (OsCal) to increase serum calcium; give supplements of vitamin D. Limit phosphorous-containing foods like milk, cheese, dried beans, and soft drinks; administer aluminum hydroxide (Amphogel) to bind with phosphorus. Withhold any sources of magnesium-like laxatives such as magnesium citrate, milk of magnesia, etc.
Risk for Impaired Skin Integrity related to scratching secondary to pruritus **Goal:** The client's skin will remain intact and free of crystals.	Limit bathing or showering to less than ½ hour; use lukewarm water and apply soap only to areas such as the axilla and anogenital areas. Add oil or colloidal oatmeal to bathwater or use an emollient like petrolatum, lanolin, or mineral oil to the skin two to three times a day. Keep the environment humidified. Use cotton flannel bedding; wear loose clothing made from other than harsh or rough fabrics. Apply firm pressure or vibration to skin areas that itch rather than scratching; cut the fingernails short to prevent traumatizing skin.
Risk for Infection related to compromised immune defenses **Goal:** The client will not acquire an infection as evidenced by normal temperature and absence of infectious symptoms.	Monitor temperature every shift and signs of infection such as chills, malaise, sore throat, redness, or drainage. Restrict contact with family, friends, or staff that may have an infectious disorder.

	Practice good medical asepsis techniques such as handwashing and keeping the environment clean.
PC: Anemia; Activity Intolerance related to reduced production of erythropoietin **Goal:** Anemia will be managed and minimized as evidenced by normal red blood cell and hemoglobin levels; the client will tolerate activities of daily living.	Administer prescribed iron supplement or Epogen. Provide periods of rest between activities. Give assistance if the client is unable to complete a task.
Risk for Altered Thought Processes related to encephalopathy secondary to rising BUN; **Risk for Injury** related to encephalopathy and osteodystrophy **Goal:** The client will be oriented and free of injuries throughout period of nursing care.	Assess mental status every shift. Reorient the client verbally and provide environmental cues like a large-sized calendar. Locate the client in a room close to the nursing station where the client can be closely observed. Place an electronic bed monitor under the mattress. Keep the signal light attached to the bed and remind the client to call for assistance. Keep the bed in a low position.

CLIENT AND FAMILY TEACHING

The discharge teaching plan depends largely on the type and degree of renal failure, the client's condition, prognosis, and the postdischarge treatment plan. If medications are prescribed, review the dose regimen and adverse drug effects with the client and family. If a special diet is recommended, ask the dietitian to review the prescribed diet and provide written information.

Develop a teaching plan based on the following:

- Follow the diet and fluid intake recommended by the physician. Do not use salt substitutes (which often contain potassium) unless allowed by the physician.
- Take medications exactly as prescribed by the physician.
- Do not use any nonprescription drug unless use has been approved by the physician.
- Measure and record fluid intake and urine output. Limit fluids as recommended.
- Avoid exposure to those with any type of infection (eg, colds, sore throats, flu).
- Monitor blood pressure as recommended by the physician.
- Keep skin clean and dry. Take brief showers with tepid water, pat skin to dry, use moisturizing lotions or creams like Eucerin™, Nivea™, Alpha Keri™, or Lubriderm™. Avoid scratching.
- When doing laundry, use a mild laundry detergent. Use an extra rinse cycle to remove all detergent or add 1 tsp of vinegar per quart of water to the rinse cycle to remove detergent residue.
- Keep a record of daily weight, and report any rapid weight gain to the physician.
- Take frequent rest periods; avoid heavy exercise.
- If any of the following occurs, contact the physician immediately: inability to urinate, slow decrease in daily urine output, weight gain (more than 5 lb or amount recommended by physician), chills, fever, sore throat, cough, blood in the urine or stool, easy bleeding or bruising, lethargy, extreme fatigue, persistent headache, nausea, vomiting, or diarrhea.

Dialysis

Dialysis is a procedure for cleaning and filtering the blood. It provides a substitute for kidney function when the kidneys are unable to remove the nitrogenous waste products and maintain adequate fluid, electrolyte, and acid–base balances.

During dialysis the client's blood is filtered by diffusion and osmosis (see Chap. 21). Substances such as urea, creatinine, and dangerously high levels of potassium, and water move *from* the blood through the semipermeable membrane *to* the **dialysate,** the solution used during dialysis that has a composition similar to normal human plasma. Dialysis is performed by hemodialysis and peritoneal dialysis. Either technique can be performed at home or in a dialysis center. Each type of dialysis has advantages and disadvantages (Table 63–7).

Hemodialysis

Hemodialysis requires transporting blood from the client through a **dialyzer,** a semipermeable membrane filter within a machine (Fig. 63–11). The dialyzer contains many tiny hollow fibers. Blood moves through the hollow fibers; water and wastes from the blood move into the dialysate fluid that flows around the fibers, but protein and red blood cells do not (Fig. 63–12). The filtered blood is returned to the client. The entire cycle takes 4 to 6 hours and is performed three times a week.

There are several methods for facilitating the removal and return of the client's dialyzed blood. One

TABLE 63-7 **Comparisons of Hemodialysis and Peritoneal Dialysis**

Type of Dialysis	Advantages	Disadvantages
Hemodialysis	Rapid removal of solutes and water Takes less time No risk for peritonitis Personnel perform procedure in a dialysis center	Bulge from fistula or graft is obvious Risk for vascular complications, infection, distal ischemia, carpal tunnel syndrome, hypotension, and disequilibrium Strict fluid and dietary restrictions Lifestyle cycles around dialysis appointments Home hemodialysis requires space for the machine and training to use it
Peritoneal	Simple to perform Facilitates independence Easier access No anticoagulation Fewer problems with hypotension or disequilibrium Less rigid dietary and fluid restrictions More flexibility in lifestyle activities	More time consuming Weight gain from glucose in the dialysate Peritonitis is a potential complication Requires training and motivation

technique using tunneled central venous catheter access has already been described. Two others that are more commonly created for clients with CRF are (1) an arteriovenous (AV) fistula, and (2) an AV graft.

ARTERIOVENOUS FISTULA

An **arteriovenous fistula** is a surgical anastomosis (connection) of an artery and vein lying in close proximity (Fig. 63–13). The vessels usually joined are the cephalic vein and the radial artery or the cephalic vein and brachial artery. Fistulae are preferred over grafts because they have a better record of remaining patent and have fewer complications, such as thrombosis and infection, compared with other access options. However, they require from 1 to 4 months to mature before being used. Consequently, some fistulae are created prematurely so they are ready when a client eventually requires dialysis.

At the time of dialysis, two venipunctures are performed at either end of the fistula (Fig. 63–14). The distal venipuncture is used to remove blood that is transported to the machine. The proximal needle puncture is used to return the dialyzed blood. When dialysis is completed, the needles are removed and pressure dressings are applied for several hours.

Blood samples are taken before and after dialysis. The client's predialysis and postdialysis weights are compared. Sometimes as much as 10 lb of fluid is removed. Examples of postdialysis laboratory studies include BUN, creatinine, sodium, potassium, chlorides, and hematocrit. These are used as indicators of the efficiency of dialysis.

ARTERIOVENOUS GRAFT

An **arteriovenous graft** is a type of vascular access method that uses a tube of synthetic material (eg, Gortex™) or polytetrafluoroethylene to connect a vein and artery in the upper or lower arm (Fig. 63–15). The graft pulsates with blood flow. AV grafts can be used 14 days after their insertion. Although the graft reseals after each needle puncture, the expected life of the graft is 3 to 5 years with repeated use.

NURSING MANAGEMENT

Assess and record vital signs before and after hemodialysis. Weigh the client and obtain blood for laboratory testing. To prepare for vascular access:

- Inspect the skin over the fistula or graft for signs of infection.
- Palpate for a **thrill** (vibration) over the vascular access; listen for a **bruit,** a loud sound caused by turbulent blood flow (Fig. 63–16). If absent, postpone further use and report findings.
- Note the color of skin and nailbeds and mobility of fingers.
- Wash the skin over the fistula or graft with soap and water or antiseptic.
- Avoid puncturing the same site that was used previously.
- After dialysis is completed, do not administer injections for 2 to 4 hours. This allows time for the metabolism and excretion of heparin, which is administered during dialysis, to reach safe levels. Before discharging the client, observe for disequilibrium syndrome.

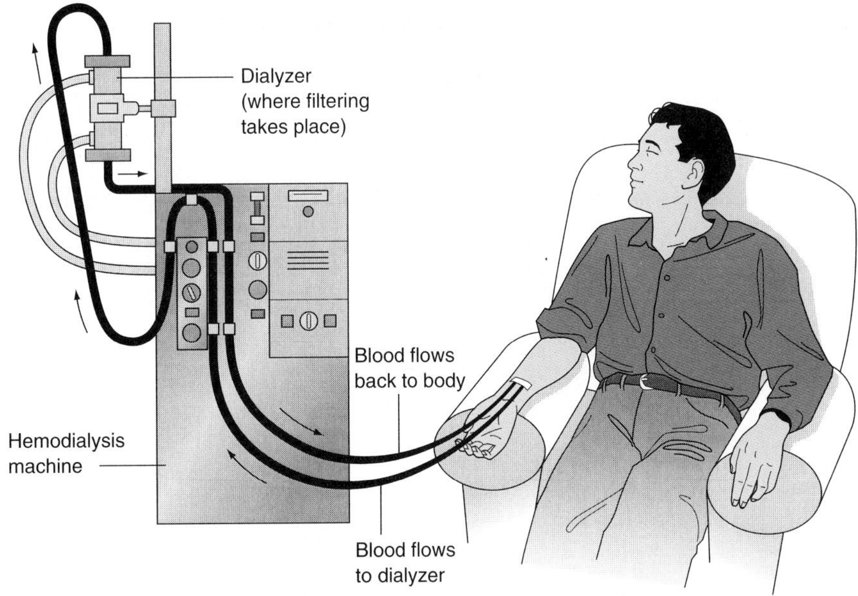

FIGURE 63-11. Hemodialysis machine and dialyzer.

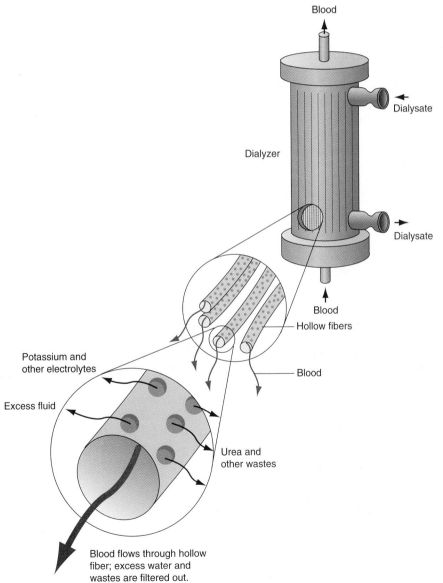

FIGURE 63-12. Osmosis and diffusion through a dialyzer.

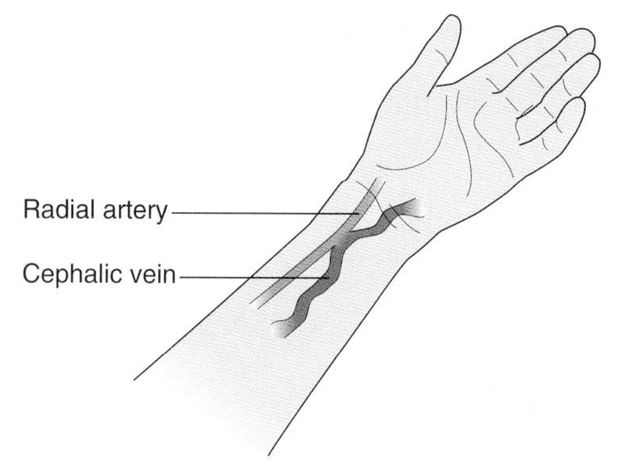

FIGURE 63-13. An arteriovenous fistula.

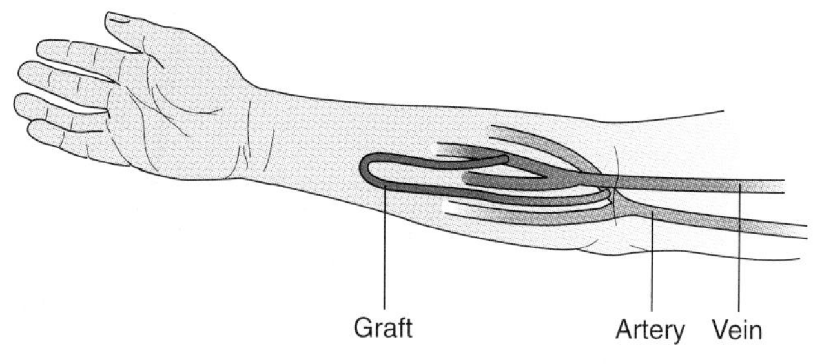

FIGURE 63-15. An arteriovenous graft is looped between an artery and a vein.

Disequilibrium syndrome is a neurologic condition believed to be caused by cerebral edema. The shift in cerebral fluid volume occurs when the concentrations of solutes within the blood are lowered rapidly during dialysis. Decreasing solute concentration lowers the plasma osmolality. Water then floods the brain tissue. The syndrome is characterized by headache, disorientation, restlessness, blurred vision, confusion, and seizures. The symptoms are self-limiting and disappear within several hours after dialysis as fluid and solute concentrations equalize. The syndrome can be prevented by slowing the dialysis process to allow time for gradual equilibration of water.

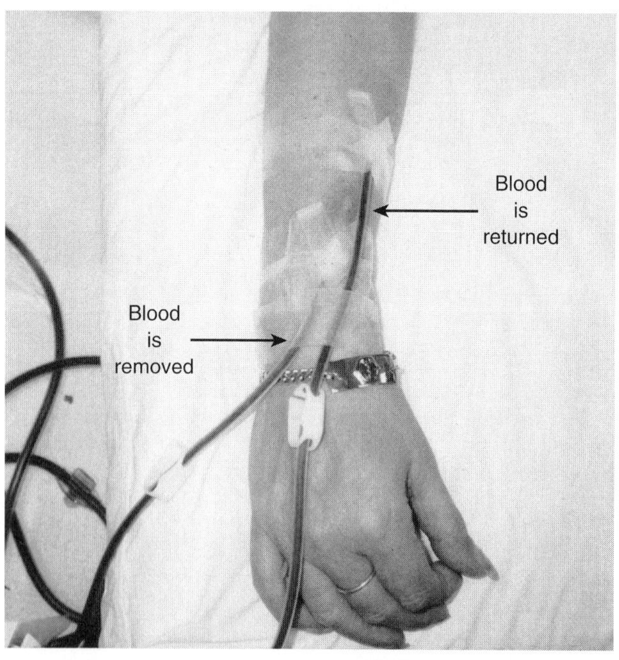

FIGURE 63-14. Blood circulates in a loop from the distal venipuncture to the dialysis machine and back through the proximal venipuncture.

Client and Family Teaching

Teach the client undergoing hemodialysis the following:

- Avoid carrying heavy items in the arm with the fistula or graft.
- Wear clothing with loose sleeves or made of fabrics that will not obstruct blood flow.
- Do not sleep on the vascular access arm.
- Do not permit venipunctures, injections, or blood pressures in the arm with the vascular access.
- Wash the skin over the vascular access daily.
- Assess for a thrill or bruit daily.
- Report signs of an infection or signs of impaired blood flow to dialysis personnel or physician immediately.

Peritoneal Dialysis

Peritoneal dialysis uses the peritoneum, the semipermeable membrane lining of the abdomen, to filter fluid, wastes, and chemicals (Fig. 63–17). The dialysate is instilled and drained from the abdominal cavity by means of a catheter. Substances pass from the tiny blood vessels in the peritoneal membrane into the dialysate. The catheter, which has many perforations, is sutured in place and a dressing is applied. There are three types of peritoneal dialysis: (1) continuous ambulatory peritoneal dialysis (CAPD), (2) continuous cyclic peritoneal dialysis (CCPD), and intermittent peritoneal dialysis (IPD).

CONTINUOUS AMBULATORY PERITONEAL DIALYSIS

When CAPD is performed, approximately 2,000 mL of dialysate is instilled by gravity through the catheter in 30 to 40 minutes. The catheter is clamped and the solution dwells for 4 to 6 hours. The instillation bag is lowered below the level of the catheter and unclamped for 30 to 40 minutes to allow time for

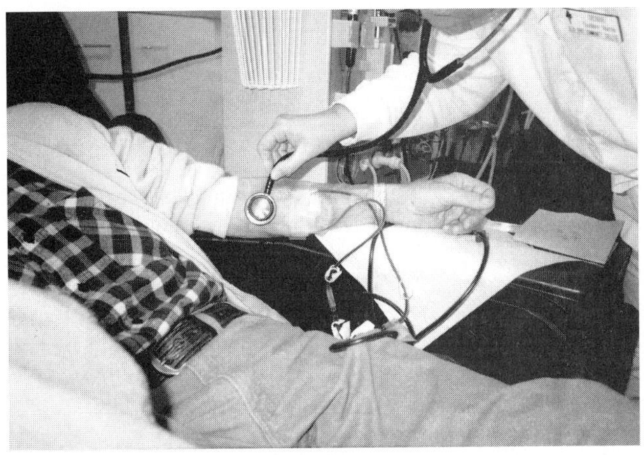

FIGURE 63-16. A nurse auscultates the bruit in the client's fistula.

gravity drainage. The process is then repeated about four times a day on a continuous basis.

CONTINUOUS CYCLIC PERITONEAL DIALYSIS

In CCPD, a machine is connected to the dialysis catheter. It automatically fills and drains dialysate from the abdomen when the person sleeps. CCPD is performed during a 10- to 12-hour time period. The peritoneum is filled with solution during the daytime, but it allows the client to go about activities during the day without performing exchanges of dialysate solutions.

INTERMITTENT PERITONEAL DIALYSIS

Treatments for IPD are performed with the same type of machine as that used for CCPD. However, the process occurs periodically with perhaps several days between dialysis treatments. When IPD is done, sessions may last 24 hours. The sum total of IPD is between 36 and 42 hours per week.

NURSING MANAGEMENT

Obtain and review laboratory test findings before dialysis. Record vital signs and weight. If the client is acutely ill, use a bed scale; it may be necessary to weigh the client as often as every 8 hours while the procedure is in progress. Peritonitis is a major complication of peritoneal dialysis. Observe and report fever, nausea, vomiting, severe abdominal pain, rigidity, or tenderness before, during, or after dialysis.

Instillation

Warm the dialysate solution to approximately body temperature. Add prescribed drugs such as an antibiotic to the dialysate. Attach the bag of dialysate and administration tubing to the abdominal catheter. Instill the solution and clamp the tubing. If the infusion is slow, reposition the client from side to side. If this maneuver is unsuccessful, the physician may need to reposition the catheter. Pain in the left shoulder, if it occurs, may be due to diaphragmatic irritation caused by the high concentration of glucose.

Record the instillation time, the volume and type of dialysate, plus any medications added. Monitor and record blood pressure and pulse frequently. A

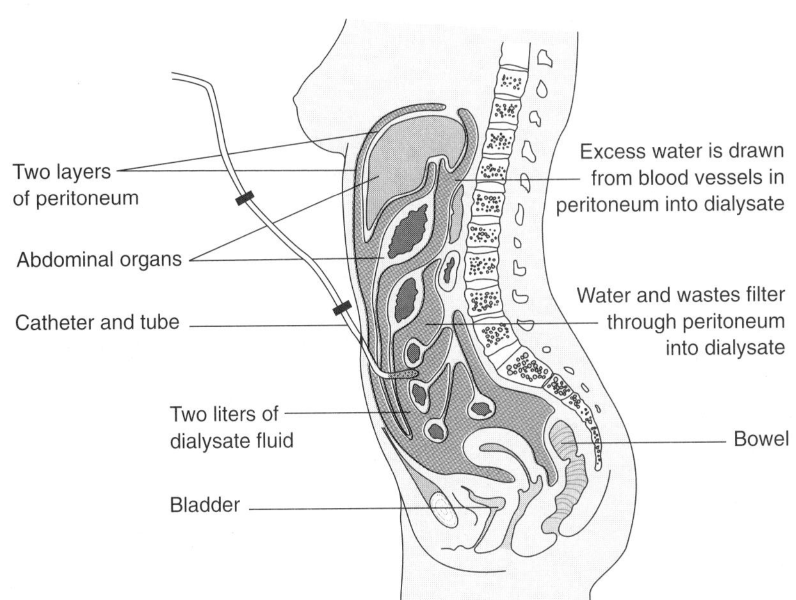

FIGURE 63-17. Peritoneal dialysis.

drop in blood pressure and increased pulse rate are associated with rapid shifts in fluid that may happen because the dialysate has a high concentration of glucose. As long as the client is stable, he or she can change positions, eat, and drink.

Drainage

At the end of the dwell time, lower the empty bag used for instilling the solution and open the clamp. Observe the appearance of the siphoned fluid; it should be relatively clear. Report drainage that is cloudy or tinged with blood. Abdominal pain that occurs at the end of the drainage period may be relieved by the next instillation. Notify the physician if pain is accompanied by marked abdominal distention. Delay the next dialysis cycle until the client is examined.

Measure the difference between the volume instilled and the volume removed. If there is a drainage deficit, notify the physician before instilling more fluid. Weigh the client after the last cycle of drainage.

Client and Family Teaching

When a client performs peritoneal dialysis at home, provide the following information:

- Keep dialysis supplies in a clean area away from children and pets.
- Avoid using any dialysate solutions that are expired and look cloudy, discolored, or contain sediment.
- Wash hands before handling the catheter.
- Prevent infection by using sterile gloves during cleaning and exchanges of dialysate.
- Wear a mask when performing exchanges if you have an upper respiratory infection.
- Clean the catheter insertion site daily with an antiseptic such as povidone iodine (Betadine).
- Inspect the catheter insertion site for signs of infection.
- Keep the catheter stabilized to the abdomen above the beltline to avoid constant rubbing.
- Avoid using scissors during dressing changes to prevent puncturing or cutting the catheter.
- Report if a fever develops; redness, pain, or pus drains around the catheter; if the external length of the catheter increases; or if nausea, vomiting, or abdominal pain develop.

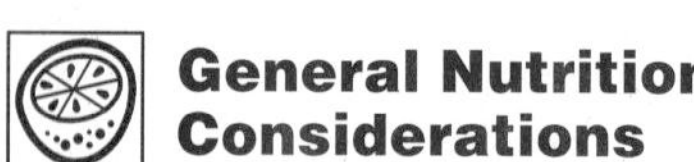

General Nutritional Considerations

The objectives of dietary intervention for renal disorders are to reduce serum nitrogen levels, reduce hypertension and edema, prevent body catabolism, improve renal function, and prevent or delay the onset of complications. Dietary interventions are frequently adjusted according to the client's laboratory values and clinical symptoms.

Debate continues over whether lowering protein intake prevents or delays the onset of renal failure. Because a low-protein diet is noninvasive, lessens kidney workload, and has the potential to be beneficial, protein restriction remains the cornerstone of dietary treatment for renal insufficiency.

The recommended protein intake for adults with renal insufficiency is 0.6 to 0.8 g/kg, at or slightly below the RDA for protein (0.8 g/kg). However, because most Americans consume almost twice as much protein as needed, the diet is often viewed as unrealistically restrictive. The majority of protein should be from animal sources, which generally have a higher biologic value than plant proteins. Pure sugars and pure fats are used liberally for calories to spare body and dietary protein.

Multiple and complicated restrictions in protein, sodium, potassium, and fluid, compounded by anorexia and taste alterations in chronic renal failure, make dietary compliance difficult to achieve and maintain. Factors that appear to improve dietary adherence include strong social support, frequent self-monitoring of protein intake, the use of specially formulated low-protein foods, and adequate guidelines for increasing calorie intake.

Renal diet food lists, called "choices" to distinguish them from diabetic "exchanges," are used to simplify meal planning. Foods are grouped into lists according to their protein, sodium, and potassium content; phosphorus and fluid may also be considered. Portion sizes are specified so that all servings within a list have approximately the same amount of protein, sodium, and potassium. An individualized meal plan specifies the number of choices allowed from each list for each meal and snack; any item may be chosen within a list, but items from one list cannot be substituted for another. The complexity and composition of choice lists vary greatly among institutions.

Once dialysis begins, protein restrictions are liberalized to 1.2 g/kg to 1.5 g/kg to account for nutritional losses through the dialysate. Calorie requirements decrease for clients receiving peritoneal dialysis because, on average, 680 cal/day are absorbed from peritoneal dialysate. Potassium, sodium, and fluid allowances are determined on an individual basis.

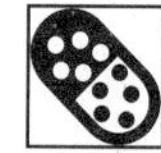

General Pharmacologic Considerations

Nephrotoxic drugs are not administered to a client with renal disease unless the client's life is in danger and no other therapeutic agent is of value.

Drugs excreted by the kidney are given with caution to those with renal disease. If the drug is deemed necessary, it may be given in lower than normal doses; the client is observed closely for any changes in renal status if normal doses are necessary. The nurse pays special attention to the client's urinary output because this method is a way to determine a change in renal status.

Sodium bicarbonate (baking soda), usually in tablet form, may be used to alkalize the urine of clients with kidney stones to prevent stone recurrence.

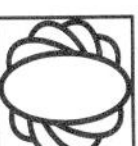

General Gerontologic Considerations

Acute glomerulonephritis in the older adult usually occurs in those with preexisting chronic glomerulonephritis. Symptoms in the older adult are subtle and may go undetected.

Urinary obstruction is the most common cause of pyelonephritis in the older adult. When present, the older adult may not experience the fever and difficulty voiding that is common in younger adults.

The older adult is at high risk for acute renal failure because of a decline in the glomerular filtration rate, loss of nephrons, and a reduced number of glomeruli. Although the aging kidney can recover from acute renal failure, survival rates are only approximately 50%.

Elderly clients often have slightly abnormal renal function tests. Mild abnormalities are due to the aging process and are usually of no clinical significance.

Elderly clients usually are not considered candidates for kidney transplants but may be able to use CAPD. Supervision of the procedure by a family member may be necessary. More frequent monitoring of the client's progress is required when this technique is used.

SUMMARY OF KEY CONCEPTS

- Pyelonephritis is an acute or chronic bacterial infection of the kidney and the lining of the collecting system (kidney pelvis); glomerulonephritis is an inflammatory but noninfectious disease characterized by widespread kidney damage.
- When caring for a client with glomerulonephritis, the nurse implements measures to reduce or eliminate such problems as fluid volume excess, fatigue, and activity intolerance.
- Polycystic disease is an inherited disorder that causes the kidneys to enlarge and become nonfunctional. The disorder is associated with hypertension, hematuria, pain, infection, kidney stones, renal failure, and complications affecting other organs.
- Renal calculi are precipitates of mineral salts that ordinarily remain dissolved in urine. Some factors that predispose to their formation include excessive calcium in the urine, urinary tract infections, and urinary stasis.
- Small calculi are managed medically with vigorous hydration, analgesics, antimicrobial therapy, and drugs that dissolve calculi or eventually alter conditions that promote their formation. Larger stones are crushed with lithotripsy procedures or removed by endoscopic retrieval or percutaneous and open surgical techniques.
- When caring for a client with a nephrostomy tube, the main concern is to maintain urinary drainage. Consequently, the nurse ensures that the catheter is patent at all times, that no more than 5 to 8 mL of irrigant is used when necessary, and that the physician is notified immediately if it becomes displaced.
- Ureteral strictures are associated with scar tissue that forms as a consequence of chronic infection and inflammation secondary to chronic stone formation. Other etiologies include congenital anomalies or conditions that mechanically compress the ureter such as pregnancy and tumors within the abdomen or upper urinary tract.
- The classic triad of renal cancer is *painless* hematuria, flank pain, and the presence of a palpable mass.
- When caring for a client with a nephrectomy for whatever reason, the nurse implements nursing measures for monitoring and managing internal hemorrhage, pain, risk for ineffective breathing and ineffective airway clearance, and the client's risk for infection.
- Acute renal failure is a sudden, rapid decrease in renal function that is potentially reversible. Chronic renal failure is a progressive and irreversible condition that eventually requires lifesaving treatment measures such as dialysis or a kidney transplant in end-stage disease.
- Acute renal failure progresses through four phases: (1) initiation phase, (2) oliguric phase, (3) diuretic phase, and (4) recovery phase, which occur over a matter of months to years.
- Chronic renal failure is associated with multiple physiologic problems some of which include hypervolemia, electrolyte and acid–base imbalances, azotemia, anemia, and osteodystrophy.
- Some clients in the end-stage of chronic renal failure undergo a kidney transplant if a match can be found among living related or nonrelated donors or those who are brain dead.
- Clients with chronic renal failure are particularly bothered by pruritus. Some nursing measures that relieve pruritus include limiting bathing time, using tepid water, applying soap sparingly, applying skin emollients, and substituting pressure or vibration rather than scratching the skin.
- Dialysis is a technique for cleaning and filtering the blood; there are two different methods: hemodialysis and peritoneal dialysis.
- When caring for dialysis patients, it is essential to monitor laboratory test results, take vital signs, weigh the client, inspect the access site for signs of infection, palpate and auscultate arteriovenous access sites to validate blood flow, observe the characteristics of peritoneal dialysate, and assess mental status especially at the termination of a dialysis treatment.

CRITICAL THINKING EXERCISES

1. A client with a ureteral stone is experiencing severe pain. Another nurse believes the client has a low pain tolerance. What action is appropriate at this time and why?
2. A client who had a left nephrectomy is having discomfort when coughing, deep breathing, and changing positions. What nursing measures could relieve her discomfort?
3. If you had chronic renal failure and must decide to have either hemodialysis or peritoneal dialysis when end-stage disease develops, explain which choice you would make and the reasons for that choice.

Suggested Readings

Arlanian-Engoren, C. (1997). Balancing calcium and phosphorus in chronic renal failure patients. *Dimensions in Critical Care Nursing, 16*(6), 282–291.

Atwill, W. H., Graham, R. W., & Wood, N. L. (1993). The laparoscopic approach to urologic surgery. *Journal of Urologic Nursing, 12*(2), 421–433.

Bullock, B. L. (1996). *Pathophysiology: Adaptations and alterations in function* (4th ed.). Philadelphia: Lippincott-Raven.

Harris, F. (1996). A new way of life...renal failure...transplantation. *Nursing Times, 92*(8), 52, 54.

Karlowicz, K. A. (1995). *Urologic nursing: Principles and practice.* Philadelphia: Saunders.

King, B. A. (1994). Detecting acute renal failure. *RN, 57*(3), 34.

Lines, V. (1997). Renal transplant care in the home. *Caring, 16*(6), 26–28, 30–32, 34.

McConnell, E. A. (1998). Myth & facts...about end-stage renal disease. *Nursing, 28*(1), 17.

McKinney, B. (1996). When this rare cancer strikes...renal cell carcinoma. *RN, 59*(12), 36–41, 51.

Pahl, J., Conrad, D., & Dunagen, C. (1997). Management of dialysis catheters. *Journal of Intravenous Nursing, 20*(5), 230–232.

Porth, C. M. (1994). *Pathophysiology: Concepts of altered health states* (4th ed.). Philadelphia: J. B. Lippincott.

Ruth-Sahd, L. A. (1995). Renal calculi. *American Journal of Nursing, 95*(11), 50.

Segal, S. (1996). Nursing rounds: Radical nephrectomy. *American Journal of Nursing, 96*(7), 37.

Wood, J. M., & Bosley, C. L. (1995). Acute postrenal failure. *Nursing, 25*(3), 48–50.

Additional Resources

National Kidney Foundation
600 South Federal
Suite 201
Chicago, IL 60605
(312) 663–3103
http://www.nkfi.org/

Polycystic Kidney Research Foundation
4901 Main Street
Suite 200
Kansas City, MO 64112
(800) PKD-CURE
http://www.kumc/pkrf/research.html

American Foundation for Urologic Disease
300 West Pratt Street
Baltimore, MD 21201–2463
(800) 242–2383

National Institute of Diabetes and Digestive and Kidney Diseases
Building 31, Room 9A04
9000 Rockville Pike
Bethesda, MD 20892
(301) 496–3583
http://www.niddk.nih.gov/PG_

Chapter 64

Caring for Clients With Disorders of the Bladder and Urethra

KEY TERMS

Cystectomy
Cystitis
Cystostomy
Diverticulum
Fulguration
Ileal conduit
Incontinence
Interstitial cystitis
Kock pouch
Litholapaxy
Neurogenic bladder
Residual urine
Retention
Stricture
Ureterosigmoidostomy
Urethritis
Urethroplasty
Urinary diversion

LEARNING OBJECTIVES

On completion of this chapter, the reader will:

- Differentiate urinary retention and urinary incontinence.
- Discuss the nursing management of a client with urinary retention and incontinence.
- Describe the pathophysiologic changes seen in cystitis, interstitial cystitis, and urethritis.
- Discuss the cause and treatment of urethral strictures.
- Identify the most common early symptom of a malignant tumor of the bladder.
- Describe various types of urinary diversion procedures.
- Identify components of a teaching plan for a client who is having a urinary diversion procedure.

Disorders of the bladder and urethra are common and can be the source of severe problems that become chronic, altering a client's lifestyle. Many disorders affecting the bladder and urethra are treated on an outpatient basis, but the more serious disorders require hospitalization.

Voiding Dysfunction

Urinary retention and urinary incontinence are voiding dysfunctions. Urinary **retention** is the inability to urinate or effectively empty the bladder. Urinary **incontinence** is the inability to control the voiding of urine. Clients experiencing either retention or incontinence face temporary or permanent alterations in their ability to urinate normally. These conditions require individualized approaches to solving the problem and sensitivity to the client's needs, both physiologic and psychosocial.

Urinary Retention

ETIOLOGY AND PATHOPHYSIOLOGY

Urinary retention may be either acute or chronic. Acute urinary retention is seen in complete urethral obstruction, after general anesthesia, or with the administration of certain drugs such as atropine or a phenothiazine. Chronic urinary retention is often seen in clients with disorders such as prostatic enlargement or neurologic disorders that result in a **neurogenic bladder** (a bladder that does not receive adequate nerve stimulation).

The client with acute urinary retention usually is not able to void at all. The client with chronic urinary retention may be able to void but does not completely empty the bladder (retention with overflow) and has a large residual volume. The **residual urine** is urine retained in the bladder after the client voids. The amount may vary from 30 mL to several hundred milliliters.

ASSESSMENT FINDINGS

Signs and Symptoms

Symptoms of acute urinary retention are sudden inability to void, distended bladder, and severe lower abdominal pain and discomfort. Chronic urinary retention may produce no symptoms because the bladder has stretched over time and accommodates large volumes without producing discomfort. The overstretched bladder does not contract effectively and the client is unaware that the bladder is not emptying completely. If the amount of residual urine is large, the client may void frequently in small amounts. Signs of a bladder infection (eg, fever, chills, pain on urination) and dribbling of urine may also be present.

Diagnostic Findings

Urinalysis may show an increased number of white blood cells, indicating an acute or chronic bladder infection. Catheterization or ultrasound can determine post void residual volume.

MEDICAL AND SURGICAL MANAGEMENT

Acute urinary retention requires immediate catheterization. If a catheter cannot be inserted through the urethra, special urologic instruments that dilate the urethra may also be used.

Chronic retention is managed by permanent drainage with a urethral catheter, suprapubic **cystostomy** tube (a catheter inserted through the abdominal wall directly into the bladder), or clean intermittent catheterization (CIC). Permanent catheterization of the bladder carries the risk of bladder stones, renal disease, bladder infection, and urosepsis, a serious systemic infection from microorganisms in the urinary tract invading the bloodstream. Because the incidence of complications is less, CIC is the preferred treatment. Other methods, particularly for clients who have lost nervous system control secondary to disease or injury, are to use Credé voiding or abdominal strain (Valsalva voiding). Box 64–1 describes these methods. CIC may not be possible for clients who lack the mobility or cognitive functioning to perform the procedure. Some male clients who cannot perform CIC can avoid the complications of permanent indwelling catheters by undergoing surgery to release the urethral sphincters. Urine then drains freely out the urethra and the client wears a condom catheter. Clinical Procedure 64–1 describes the application of a condom catheter. If it is possible to remove the cause, such as excising excess prostatic tissue, surgery is performed; however, surgery does not always result in restoration of normal voiding.

External collection systems for women are available but proper fit is a problem. Women who cannot accomplish CIC are usually treated with a permanent indwelling catheter.

BOX 64-1 Credé or Valsalva Voiding

Credé

Apply gentle downward pressure to the bladder during voiding. This maneuver may be done by the client or family member. The client may also do this by sitting on the toilet and rocking back and forth gently.

Valsalva

Instruct the client to bear down as with defecation. Do not teach this method to a client with cardiac problems or who may be adversely affected by a vagal response (heart rate slows).

NURSING MANAGEMENT

The conscious client is able to verbalize the pain and discomfort associated with urinary retention. Other clients with Alzheimer's disease or psychiatric disorders, or the comatose, anesthetized, or spinal cord-injured client may unable to communicate or feel the pain and discomfort associated with acute urinary retention. An important nursing responsibility is measuring intake and output, palpating the abdomen for a distended bladder, promoting complete urination, and monitoring the voiding pattern of clients.

Acute Urinary Retention

Acute retention that is likely to resolve quickly (eg, after anesthesia) will probably be treated by intermittent catheterization. Clients with acute retention unlikely to resolve without surgical intervention (such as retention caused by an enlarged prostate) will have an indwelling catheter.

Collaborate with the physician to determine (1) if the catheter is to be left in place or removed after the bladder is emptied, and (2) the size and type of catheter to be used. Catheters are sized according to the French system, for example, 14F to 24F. The higher the number, the larger the diameter of the catheter. Examples of the various types of catheter tips are shown in Figure 64–1.

Clients with an obstruction may be more easily catheterized with a coudé catheter; the curved tip slides over obstructing tissue more readily than the straight-tipped catheter. Select the appropriate catheter and insert it under sterile conditions. Note the characteristics and volume of urine returned. If the volume of urine is large (> 700 mL), it may be necessary to clamp the catheter before the bladder has emptied com-

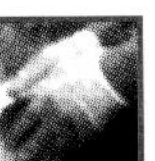

Clinical Procedure 64-1
Applying a Condom Catheter

PURPOSE

- To provide passage of urine from the urinary meatus to a collection bag
- To prevent skin breakdown

EQUIPMENT

- Cleansing supplies—cleanser or soap and towel
- Condom catheter with packaged adhesive strips or Velcro device for securing the catheter
- Drainage tubing
- Collection bag
- Disposable gloves

Nursing Action	Rationale
ASSESSMENT	
Assess the penis for swelling or skin breakdown.	Provides a data base for future comparison, or provides a basis for selecting another method for urine collection
Determine how much the client understands about the application and use of an external catheter.	Provides an opportunity for health teaching
Verify the client's willingness to use a condom catheter.	Respects the client's right to participate in making decisions
PLANNING	
Gather supplies listed above.	Promotes organization and efficient time management
Provide privacy.	Demonstrates respect for dignity
Place the client in a supine position and cover him with a bath blanket or sheet.	Facilitates application of the condom catheter
IMPLEMENTATION	
Wash your hands and don clean gloves.	Reduces the transmission of microorganisms and follows the guidelines for Standard Precautions
Wash and dry the penis well.	Promotes skin integrity
Wrap the adhesive strip in an upward spiral about the penis, taking care not to wrap it tightly.	Reduces the potential for restricting blood flow
Roll the wider end of the sheath toward the narrow catheter tip (some condom catheters are packaged this way).	Facilitates the application of the condom catheter to the penis
Hold approximately 1 to 2 inches (2.5 to 5 cm) of the lower sheath below the tip of the penis and unroll the sheath upward.	Leaves space below the urethra to prevent irritation of the meatus
Secure the upper end of the unrolled sheath to the skin with a second strip of adhesive or a Velcro strap, but not tightly as to interfere with circulation.	Ensures that the catheter will remain in place
Connect the catheter drainage tip to a drainage bag.	Collects urine
Keep the penis positioned in a downward position.	Promotes urinary drainage
Assess the penis at least every two hours.	Ensures prompt attention to signs of impaired circulation
Check that the catheter has not become twisted.	Maintains catheter patency
Empty the leg bag, if one is used, because it becomes partially filled with urine.	Ensures that the catheter will not be pulled from the penis by the weight of the collected urine
Remove and change the catheter daily or more often as it becomes loose or tight.	Maintains skin integrity
Substitute a waterproof garment during periods of nonuse.	Provides a mechanism for absorbing urine
Wash the catheter and collection bag with mild soap and water and rinse with a 1:7 vinegar and water solution.	Extends the use of the equipment and reduces offensive odors

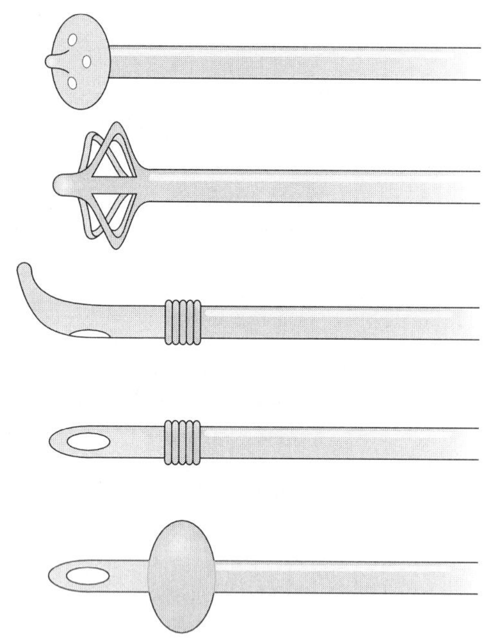

FIGURE 64-1. Catheter tips (*top to bottom*): de Pezzer catheter, Malecot catheter, coudé catheter, Foley catheter, Foley catheter with balloon inflated. The de Pezzer and the Malecot catheters are inserted by the physician with a stylet that temporarily straightens the tip. The Foley and coudé catheters are retained by inflating the balloon.

pletely to prevent bladder spasms or loss of bladder tone. This practice varies so check agency policy.

If the client is going to be managed by CIC, establish the schedule. Clients are catheterized every 4 to 6 hours depending on the amount of urine obtained and the fluid intake. The bladder should not be allowed to get distended beyond 350 mL because bladder overdistention results in loss of bladder tone, decreased blood flow to the bladder, and reduction in the layer of mucin that protects the bladder mucosa. CIC continues until the post void residual volume is less than 30 mL. To obtain accurate residual volumes, it is important that clients have the opportunity to void first and that catheterization occur immediately after the attempt. Record both the volume voided (even if it is zero) and the volume obtained by catheterization. Postoperative urinary retention usually resolves within 24 to 48 hours.

Chronic Urinary Retention

Chronic urinary retention may go unrecognized. Ask all clients during an initial health assessment about voiding frequency, the amount (eg, small, moderate, large) of urine passed each time, the presence of pain or discomfort in the lower abdomen, pain or discomfort on voiding, and difficulty in starting the urinary stream. Gently palpate or percuss the lower abdomen to determine if the bladder is distended. Obtain a complete medical, drug, and allergy history. Report suspected chronic urinary retention to the physician.

INTERMITTENT CATHETERIZATION. Intermittent catheterization performed in the hospital setting is a sterile procedure. When performed by clients or family members in the home, clean rather than aseptic technique is used. A commercially prepared straight catheterization kit is available in hospitals that includes a straight-tipped catheter, sterile gloves, lubricant and a sterile collection container. At home the client uses a red rubber catheter that can be washed and reused for 2 to 3 months before replacing; gloves are not required but clients must wash their hands thoroughly before and after the procedure. The client can drain the urine into a clean container or directly into the toilet bowl. The schedule is usually three to four times per day, although the frequency can be increased depending on residual volume. If more than 400 mL is returned, the client should be catheterized more often. Client education in technique, catheter care, and follow-up care is an important function of the nurse both in the acute and home care settings.

INDWELLING CATHETERS. A urethral indwelling catheter is one route for permanent bladder catheterization. A cystostomy tube, also called a suprapubic catheter, is an alternative that is inserted through an abdominal incision into the bladder. Clients require catheter care including careful cleansing of the urethral meatus or cystostomy site and proximal catheter, maintenance of the integrity of the closed drainage system, proper anchoring of the tube to avoid tension and promote drainage (Fig. 64–2), and scheduled changes of the catheter and drainage system according to facility policy. Nursing Guidelines 64–1 offers additional general management points.

Urinary Incontinence

Urinary incontinence affects many clients and is a major health care concern. It is estimated that 30% of older adults living in the community and 50% of older clients in institutions suffer from incontinence (Eliopoulos, 1997). Not only is incontinence a psychosocial problem, it is also a physical problem in that skin breakdown and urinary tract infection may result from incontinence. Table 64–1 describes the different types of incontinence.

ETIOLOGY AND PATHOPHYSIOLOGY

Urinary incontinence may result from either bladder or urethral dysfunction (or both). The bladder can

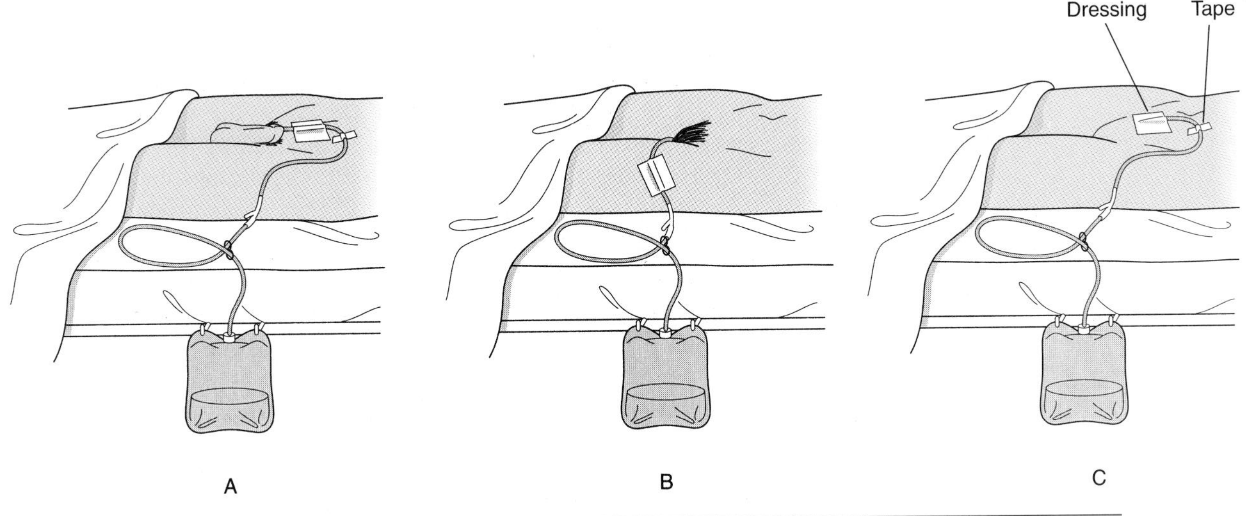

FIGURE 64-2. Catheter tubing correctly anchored and attached to closed drainage system. (*A*) Male; (*B*) Female; (*C*) Suprapubic.

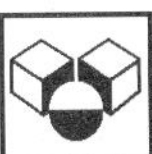

Nursing Guidelines 64-1

General Principles of Catheterization and Catheter Care

The following general principles apply to the insertion and maintenance of urethral or suprapubic catheters:

- Aseptic technique is always used for insertion.
- The urethral meatus is thoroughly cleansed before insertion of a catheter.
- An adult urethra usually takes a size 14F to 18F indwelling catheter; a smaller size may be used for intermittent (straight, single) catheterization.
- When an indwelling catheter is inserted, the balloon is tested before insertion.
- The catheter is lubricated with a sterile water-soluble lubricant and inserted.
- Never force a catheter if resistance is felt.
- An indwelling catheter that accidentally becomes dislodged is never reinserted but is replaced by a new sterile catheter.
- Catheters are connected to a sterile closed drainage system.
- Keep the drainage bag lower than the catheter.
- Indwelling urethral catheters are changed according to the physician's orders or agency policy.
- Provide urethral catheter care twice a day and after bowel movements.
- Inspect the cystostomy tube site for leakage of urine around the catheter, bleeding, or signs and symptoms of infection.
- Change the cystostomy dressing once per shift or more often if necessary.
- If a permanent vesicocutaneous (bladder to skin) fistula forms and the size of the cystostomy tube may need to be increased to prevent leakage of urine.
- Unless contraindicated by heart failure or renal disease, clients should be encouraged to drink plenty of fluids (2,000–3,000 mL) especially those that acidify the urine, such as cranberry juice.
- Monitor the client for signs and symptoms of urinary tract infection: fever, chills, hypotension, and confusion.
- Monitor fluid balance and laboratory tests that measure kidney function.

contract without warning, fail to accommodate adequate volumes of urine, or fail to empty completely and become overstretched, resulting in overflow incontinence. These conditions result from neurologic disease, prostatic enlargement, bladder outlet obstruction, or trauma in all clients, and bladder prolapse or low estrogen levels in women.

Another cause of incontinence is failure of the urethral sphincters to hold urine in the bladder. This may result from trauma, prostate surgery, or relaxed pelvic muscles. Impingement of the spinal nerves, such as in tumors of the spinal cord, herniated disk, or spinal cord injuries, can interfere with the impulse conduction to the brain, resulting in a neurogenic bladder and incontinence. A neurogenic bladder may be spastic, causing incontinence, or it may be flaccid, causing retention.

ASSESSMENT FINDINGS

Signs and Symptoms

Clients complain of urgency, frequency, leaking small amounts when coughing or sneezing, or com-

TABLE 64-1 **Types of Urinary Incontinence**

Type of Incontinence	Symptoms	Cause
Stress incontinence	Involuntary loss of urine from intact urethra; results from sudden increase in intra-abdominal pressure, such as with sneezing or coughing.	Decreased pelvic muscle tone, primarily seen in women, and associated with multiple pregnancies, obstetric injuries, obesity, menopause, or pelvic disease
Urge incontinence	Client experiences urge to void, but cannot control voiding for a sufficient time to reach a toilet.	Bladder irritation related to urinary tract infections, bladder tumors, or radiation therapy, enlarged prostate, or neurologic dysfunction
Total incontinence	Continuous loss of urine from the bladder. Bladder is overdistended and does not empty normally or completely.	Neurologic abnormalities, such as spinal cord lesions or tumors, or obstruction to urine output, such as tumors, enlarged prostate, or urethral strictures
Functional incontinence	Client has intact function of the lower urinary tract but is unable to identify the need to void or ambulate to the toilet.	Cognitive impairments, such as brain injury or Alzheimer's disease, or physical limitations, such as rheumatoid arthritis or musculoskeletal injuries
Reflex incontinence	Uninhibited bladder contractions; involuntary reflexes producing spontaneous voiding, partial or complete loss of sensation of bladder fullness or urge to void.	Impaired conduction of impulses above reflex arc level secondary to spinal cord injury, tumor, or infection.

plete inability to control urine, depending on the underlying cause.

Diagnostic Findings

Tests such as a urine culture and sensitivity, cystoscopy, or urodynamics are used to determine the type of incontinence.

MEDICAL AND SURGICAL MANAGEMENT

Treatment is aimed at correcting the disorder causing incontinence (when possible), providing medication to control incontinence, correcting the situational problems that contribute to functional incontinence, or instituting a bladder retraining program. Pharmacologic agents that can improve bladder retention, emptying, and control include drugs such as oxybutynin chloride (Ditropan), which reduces bladder spasticity and involuntary bladder contractions, and phenoxybenzamine hydrochloride (Dibenzaline), which may be useful in treating problems with sphincter control. Sometimes medication to control incontinence results in retention and must be discontinued. Occasionally clients who can easily perform CIC may opt for medication-induced retention and CIC because it allows them to stay dry.

Surgeries to improve urinary control include bladder augmentation, a procedure that increases the storage capacity of the bladder; implantation of an artificial sphincter that can be inflated to prevent urine loss and deflated to allow urination (Fig. 64–3); surgeries to provide better support for urinary structures; and urethroplasty, surgery to repair structures damaged by trauma.

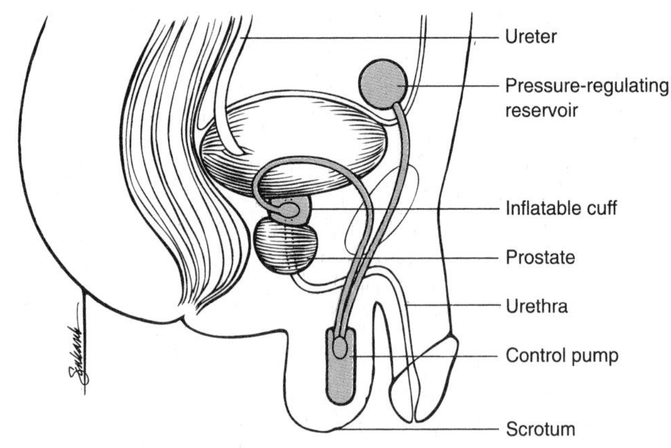

FIGURE 64-3. Artificial urinary sphincter. An inflatable cuff is inserted surgically around the urethra or bladder neck. To empty the bladder, the cuff is deflated by squeezing the control pump located in the scrotum.

NURSING MANAGEMENT

Goals when caring for a client with urinary incontinence include maintaining continence as much as possible, preventing skin breakdown, reducing anxiety, and initiating a bladder training program. Determine if the client is truly incontinent or if situations prevent the client from getting to the bathroom. Such situations include impaired mobility, physical restraints, and use of sedatives. In addition to assessing for functional causes of incontinence, obtain details regarding the pattern of incontinence and use of medications that may play a role in the problem. Assess for skin breakdown and determine methods the client has used to manage incontinence.

Instruction centers on exercises to increase muscle tone and voluntary control (Kegel exercises), techniques to assist bladder emptying, and bladder training. Refer to Nursing Guidelines 64–2 for teaching Kegel exercises. Success of a bladder retraining program depends not only on the cause of incontinence but also on the motivation of the client and the amount of skillful help and encouragement received from the health care team.

Bladder Training

One method of bladder training for the client with an indwelling urethral catheter is to alternately clamp and unclamp the catheter. The clamping and unclamping of the catheter begins to re-establish normal bladder function and capacity. In the beginning, the catheter may be unclamped for 5 minutes every 1 or 2 hours. Gradually lengthen the interval to every 3 or 4 hours, giving the bladder a chance to fill more completely. When possible, teach the client to release the clamp at scheduled times. The catheter later is removed.

At this point, or when training clients who have not had an indwelling catheter, instruct the client to try to void every hour. Usually the client is not able to retain urine longer than an hour, and frequent voiding is necessary to prevent incontinence. Gradually lengthen the interval between voidings to 2, 3, or 4 hours. At first many clients do not empty the bladder and they must be catheterized after voiding to remove residual urine. When the client is catheterized for residual urine, record the amount removed.

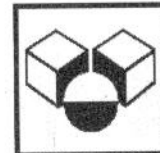

Nursing Guidelines 64-2

Teaching Kegel Exercises

Initial Instructions

- Sit or stand with legs slightly apart.
- Draw in perivaginal muscles and anal sphincter as when controlling voiding or defecating.
- Hold this position of contraction for 5 seconds (instruct client to count or time with a watch).
- Relax contraction for at least 10 seconds
- Repeat exercises 5 to 6 times, increasing slowly to 25 times.
- Repeat the sequence of exercises 3 to 4 times a day.
- Gradually do the exercises for a total of 200 repetitions.

Advanced Instructions

- Sit on the toilet and begin to urinate.
- Stop the flow of urine by doing a Kegel exercise.
- Hold this position for 5 seconds.
- Relax and begin voiding.
- Repeat this sequence 5 times with each voiding.

When a client is unable to control the storage and passage of urine or when a bladder training program fails, clients may exhibit varying degrees of anxiety and depression. Offer constant encouragement throughout the bladder training program. Anxiety may be reduced once the client notes the effort, concern, and interest of the health care team. If an accident occurs, change the bed linen promptly and assure the client that accidents are to be expected during the retraining process. Reducing anxiety may, in some instances, contribute to the success of a bladder training program.

Barrier Garments and External Collection Devices

If it is not possible to establish a voiding routine and incontinence persists, work with the client to devise a system of collecting the urine. Male clients can use a condom catheter over the penis and connect the tubing to a closed drainage system or disposable urinary drainage bag. External drainage systems are available for women, but it is difficult to get the devices to fit securely. Male and female clients may choose to wear protective pants with a plastic outside layer and absorbent material inside. These pants can be pinned or snapped in place. Liners also are available and are worn next to the skin. They are nonabsorbent and thus the urine passes through them to the absorbent layer. For this reason the liners dry quickly and leave the skin dry and free of urine, even though the absorbent material is soaked.

Clients who are incontinent may have problems with odor and maintaining skin integrity. Urea-splitting microorganisms, such as *Micrococcus ureae*, cause the urea in urine to react with water, creating ammonia and causing urine odor, skin breakdown, and ammonia dermatitis. One way to protect the skin is to avoid any contact with urine. When contact is unavoidable, use soap and water after each episode to thoroughly clean the skin. Dry the skin completely and apply a skin barrier or moisture sealant to protect the skin. When possible, expose the affected area to air.

Client and Family Teaching

Encourage clients to actively participate in whatever methods used to empty the bladder. Demonstrate procedures as needed for the client and family to understand. Develop a teaching plan based on the client's individual needs to include one or more of the following:

- Control odors by frequent cleansing of the perineum, changing clothes and incontinence briefs (eg, Attends, Depends) when they become wet, and using an electric room deodorizer; avoid using perfume or scented powders, lotions, or sprays. Mixing a perfumed scent with a urine odor may intensify the odor, irritate the skin, or cause a skin infection.

- Wash garments as soon as possible in warm, soapy water.
- Use plastic to cover objects, such as a mattress and chairs, to prevent staining and lingering odors. The plastic must be washed with mild soapy water daily or more often if needed. Instruct the client to place a sheet or blanket between the skin and the plastic.
- Follow the recommendations of the physician about clamping and unclamping the catheter (when this method is prescribed) or changing the catheter or cystostomy tube.
- Keep a record of fluid intake. Drink plenty of fluids during waking hours. Drink most of the required fluids in the morning and early afternoon hours and decrease the intake toward evening.
- Follow the recommended bladder training program. Time is required to achieve success.
- Contact the physician if any of the following occurs: increased discomfort, rash around the perineal area, pain in the lower abdomen, fever, chills, or cloudy urine.

Infectious and Inflammatory Disorders

Infections and inflammations of the bladder and urethra are common. Although generally able to be treated on an outpatient basis, they are a potential source of more complex problems requiring invasive treatment.

Cystitis

ETIOLOGY AND PATHOPHYSIOLOGY

Cystitis is an inflammation of the urinary bladder. The inflammation is usually caused by a bacterial infection. Bacteria can invade the bladder from an infection in the kidneys, lymphatics, and urethra (Fig. 64–4). Because the urethra is short in women, ascending infections or microorganisms from the vagina or rectum are more common. Causes of cystitis include urologic instrumentation (eg, cystoscopy, catheterization), fecal contamination, prostatitis or benign prostatic hyperplasia, indwelling catheters, pregnancy, and sexual intercourse.

The lining of the bladder provides a natural resistance to most bacterial invasions by preventing an inflammatory reaction from occurring. However, if bacteria do survive in the bladder, they adhere to the mucosal lining of the bladder and multiply. The surface of the bladder becomes edematous and reddened and ulcerations may develop. When urine contacts these irritated areas, the client experiences pain and urgency, which is magnified in the presence of even slight bladder distention.

ASSESSMENT FINDINGS

Signs and Symptoms

The symptoms of cystitis include urgency (feeling a pressing need to void although the bladder is not full), frequency, low back pain, dysuria, perineal and suprapubic pain, and hematuria, especially at the termination of the stream (terminal hematuria). If bacteremia is present, the client also may have chills and fever. Chronic cystitis causes similar symptoms, but usually they are less severe.

Diagnostic Findings

Microscopic examination of the urine reveals an increase in the number of red and white blood cells. Culture and sensitivity studies are used to identify the causative microorganism and appropriate antimicrobial therapy. If repeated episodes occur, intravenous pyelogram (IVP) or cystoscopy with or without retrograde pyelograms may be needed to identify the possible cause, such as chronic prostatitis or a bladder **diverticulum** (weakening and outpouching of the bladder wall), which encourages urinary stasis and infection.

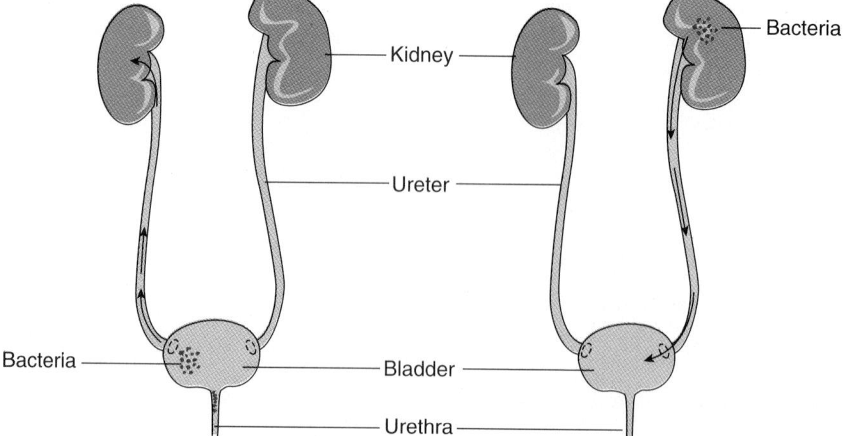

FIGURE 64-4. Urinary tract infection. (*A*) Microorganisms invade the bladder and ascend to the ureter and kidney. (*B*) Microorganisms in the kidney descend the ureter to the bladder.

MEDICAL MANAGEMENT

Medical management includes antimicrobial therapy and correction of contributing factors. Examples of drugs that may be used include trimethoprim-sulfamethoxazole (Septra) and sulfisoxazole (Gantrisin). Cranberry juice or vitamin C may be recommended to keep the urine acidic and enhance the effectiveness of drug therapy. When there is a partial urethral obstruction, no treatment of cystitis is fully effective until adequate drainage of urine is restored by the removal of the obstruction (see discussion of urethral strictures). In some instances, treatment may be prolonged and may need to be repeated.

NURSING MANAGEMENT

Advise the client to drink extra fluids. Cranberry juice helps to acidify the urine and provides a less favorable climate for bacterial growth. Emphasize the importance of finishing the prescribed course of therapy. Instruct the client in the prevention of repeated cystitis (Nursing Guidelines 64–3).

Interstitial Cystitis

ETIOLOGY AND PATHOPHYSIOLOGY

Interstitial cystitis (IC) is a chronic inflammation of the bladder mucosa. It is more common in women than men. The bladder wall contains multiple pinpoint hemorrhagic areas that join and form larger hemorrhagic areas that may progress to fissuring and scarring of the bladder mucosa. Superficial erosion of the bladder mucosa (Hunner's ulcer) may develop. Eventually the bladder shrinks from scarring. The cause of IC is unknown but it has been suggested that there may be a hormonal link because flare-ups appear to occur before menstruation. Another theory is that IC may be an autoimmune disorder or part of a systemic condition because some persons have a history of migraine headaches, ulcerative colitis, endometriosis, or chronic fatigue syndrome.

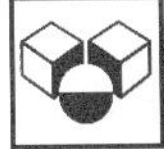

Nursing Guidelines 64-3

Preventing Cystitis

Tell clients with recurrent cystitis to:

- Increase fluid intake to 2 to 3 liters a day.
- Avoid coffee, teas, colas, and alcohol.
- Shower rather than bathe in a tub.
- Cleanse perineum after each bowel movement with front to back motion.
- Avoid irritating substances such as bubble bath, bath salts, perineal lotions, vaginal sprays, nylon underwear, scented toilet paper.
- Wear cotton underwear.
- Void every 2 to 3 hours while awake.
- Empty bladder completely with each voiding.
- Void after sexual intercourse.
- Notify physician if the following symptoms occur:
    - Urgency
    - Frequency
    - Burning with urination
    - Difficulty urinating
    - Blood in the urine
- Take medication exactly as prescribed.

ASSESSMENT FINDINGS

Signs and Symptoms

Symptoms mimic other disorders such as cystitis, bladder cancer, or a sexually transmitted disease (STD). Frequent, painful urination and passing a small volume of urine are the most common symptoms. The pain may be described as searing or burning. The client reports an onset of pain and the need to void as soon as a small amount of urine is present in the bladder.

Diagnostic Findings

A cystoscopy reveals a markedly inflamed bladder mucosa with pinpoint hemorrhages and a bladder capacity that is smaller than normal. Filling the bladder during cystoscopy to improve visualization usually results in severe pain.

A voiding cystourethrogram also demonstrates a small bladder capacity. A urinalysis is usually normal but if cystitis is present, an increase in the number of red and white blood cells may be seen; urine cultures are negative. A record of the number of voidings and the amount voided over a 2- or 3-day period, along with the symptoms, help to confirm the diagnosis. A biopsy of the bladder mucosa reveals an inflammatory process with scarring and hemorrhagic areas and confirms the diagnosis.

MEDICAL AND SURGICAL MANAGEMENT

There is no single effective specific therapy for IC. Antidepressant drugs may relieve pain as well as treat the depression that accompanies the disorder. Other therapies include bladder instillation of DSMO (dimethyl sulfoxide) or silver nitrate. Elmiron (pentosan polysulfate) is an *orphan drug* (a drug that is used for treatment of a disease affecting a small number of persons) that is taken orally. It appears to help in restoration of the bladder mucosa. A more recent treatment uses a laser, inserted into the abdominal cavity with a laparoscope, to sever the sensory (pain) fibers of the bladder. This procedure is used to relieve the severe pain associated with IC. Severe IC can be incapacitating and a urinary diversion procedure (see later discussion) may offer the only relief of symptoms for a selected group of clients.

NURSING MANAGEMENT

Advise the client to avoid spicy and acidic foods because they may contribute to pain and discomfort. Psychological support is necessary because many times IC has gone undiagnosed and the client told that there is nothing wrong. Clients with IC often have their lives severely disrupted by pain and frequent trips to the bathroom, sometimes several times an hour. Some are unable to hold jobs due to the severity of symptoms. Sexual activity is avoided because of fear of pain, straining their relationships and interfering with intimacy. Clients should be referred to a chronic pain center to cope with the pain and an IC support group.

Urethritis

ETIOLOGY AND PATHOPHYSIOLOGY

Urethritis (inflammation of the urethra) is seen more commonly in men than in women. Urethritis caused by microorganisms other than gonorrhea is called nongonococcal urethritis. Gonorrhea, an STD, is a specific form of infection that can attack the mucous membrane of a normal urethra (see Chap. 61).

In women, urethritis may accompany cystitis but also may be secondary to vaginal infections. Soaps, bubble baths, sanitary napkins, or scented toilet paper may also cause urethritis.

In men, a common cause of urethritis is *Chlamydia trachomatis*, which causes an STD. The distal portion of the normal male urethra is not totally sterile. Bacteria that are normally present cause no difficulty unless these tissues are traumatized, usually after instrumentation such as catheterization or cystoscopic examination. Under such conditions, bacteria may gain a foothold to cause a nonspecific urethritis. Other causes of nonspecific urethritis in men include irritation during vigorous intercourse, rectal intercourse, or intercourse with a woman who has a vaginal infection.

ASSESSMENT FINDINGS

Signs and Symptoms

Infection of the urethra results in discomfort on urination varying from a slight tickling sensation to burning or severe discomfort and urinary frequency. Fever is not common, but fever in the male client may be due to further extension of the infection to areas such as the prostate, testes, and epididymis.

Diagnostic Findings

The client's history and symptoms often provide a tentative diagnosis. In men, a urethral smear is obtained for culture and sensitivity to identify the causative microorganism. In women, a urinalysis (clean-catch specimen) may identify the causative microorganism.

MEDICAL MANAGEMENT

Treatment includes appropriate antibiotic therapy, liberal fluid intake, analgesics, warm sitz baths, and improvement of the client's resistance to infection by a good diet and plenty of rest. If urethritis is due to an STD, it is treated with appropriate antibiotic therapy (see Chap. 61). Failure to seek treatment for gonococcal urethritis may result in a urethral stricture in men.

NURSING MANAGEMENT

Reinforce the need to complete antibiotic therapy, drink plenty of fluids, and take warm sitz baths and analgesics for pain.

Urethritis may be seen in clients with indwelling urethral catheters. To prevent or decrease urethritis, exercise gentleness when it is necessary to change catheters. Give frequent perineal care, especially if the client is incontinent of feces. In addition to washing around the anus and buttocks, also clean the meatus and labia of the female client. When cleaning the anal area, wipe away from the urethra. If cotton pledgets are used, wipe from the urethral meatus to the anus in a single stroke and discard the pledget.

The nurse's responsibilities, when caring for a client with an inflammation or infection of the bladder or urethra, include but are not limited to the following:

Nursing Diagnoses and Collaborative Problems	Nursing Interventions
Pain related to inflammation of the bladder and or/urethra **Goal:** The client will express relief of pain and discomfort.	Assure the client that pain and discomfort will decrease with treatment. Administer analgesics and antispasmodics as indicated. Encourage the client to use warm sitz baths two or three times a day to relieve discomfort.

	Encourage the client to increase daily fluid intake.
Anxiety related to pain, discomfort, and frequent urination **Goals:** The client will verbalize anxiety related to symptoms. The client will state self-care measures to relieve anxiety.	Implement above measures. Encourage the client to talk about her/his symptoms and fears related to the disorder. Provide information that assists in alleviating fears. Teach the client measures to prevent future occurrences.
Altered Urinary Elimination related to inflammation and irritation **Goals:** The client will resume normal voiding patterns. The client will adhere to treatment regimen as prescribed.	Administer antibiotics as ordered. Administer analgesics and antispasmodics as indicated. Encourage the client to increase fluid intake to two to three liters per day, not including caffeine or alcohol. Instruct the client to void at regular intervals, even if uncomfortable.
Knowledge Deficit regarding inflammation and infection of the bladder and urethra related to disease process and treatment **Goal:** The client will verbalize understanding of condition, prognosis, and treatment. The client will participate in the treatment regimen.	Review the treatment plan. Instruct the client about medications, dosage, frequency, expected effects, and possible side effects. Emphasize the need to complete the entire course of medications, even after symptoms have subsided. Teach the client the importance of increased fluid intake. Review the client's hygiene practices. Teach the client methods to prevent future infections.

Client and Family Teaching

Most cases of cystitis and urethritis are treated in the physician's office. Develop a teaching plan to include the following:

- Take the medication as directed on the container. Do not stop taking the medication even though symptoms have disappeared. It is important that the entire course of therapy be completed.
- Take warm tub baths if discomfort is severe.
- Drink at least 8 large glasses of fluids per day. Include one or more glasses of cranberry juice in the daily fluid intake.
- Fluids include water, cranberry juice, clear carbonated beverages, or any food (eg, flavored gelatin, ice cream) that is liquid at room temperature. If on a special diet (eg, low-sodium or diabetic diets), check with the physician about drinking juices or beverages or eating foods that are liquid at room temperature. Some of these liquids either must be considered part of the daily dietary allowances or may not be allowed because they contain substances that must be eliminated from the diet. In some diets, a limited amount of certain liquids may be allowed.
- Notify the physician if symptoms persist after the course of drug therapy is completed, if the symptoms become worse, or if fever or chills occur.
- Follow recommendations preventing future episodes of infection or inflammation.

Obstructive Disorders

Obstruction of the lower urinary tract is a blockage in the bladder or in the urethra. Many obstructions are related to congenital anomalies, but in adults, obstructions occur from stones that block the passage of urine, or from a narrowing that occurs as a result of a trauma, inflammation, or infection. Box 64–2 lists general signs of an outflow obstruction.

Bladder Stones

ETIOLOGY AND PATHOPHYSIOLOGY

Stones may form in the bladder or originate in the upper urinary tract and travel to and remain in the bladder. Large bladder stones develop in those with chronic urinary retention and urinary stasis. Clients who are immobile (eg, the unconscious client or those with paraplegia or quadriplegia) also may have a tendency to form bladder stones.

ASSESSMENT FINDINGS

Signs and Symptoms

Symptoms of bladder stone formation include hematuria, suprapubic pain, difficulty starting the

BOX 64-2 Signs of Obstructed Urine Flow

- Straining to empty bladder
- Feeling that bladder does not empty completely
- Hesitancy
- Weak stream
- Frequency
- Overflow incontinence
- Bladder distention

urinary stream, symptoms of a bladder infection, and a feeling that the bladder is not completely empty. Some clients may have few or no symptoms.

Diagnostic Findings

Cystoscopy, a kidney–ureter–bladder (KUB) study, IVP, or ultrasound studies detect the presence of bladder stones. Blood chemistries and 24-hour urine collection for serum calcium and uric acid may identify the possible cause of stone formation.

MEDICAL AND SURGICAL MANAGEMENT

Bladder stones may be removed through the transurethral route, using a stone-crushing instrument (lithotrite). This procedure, called a **litholapaxy,** is suitable for small and soft stones and is performed under general anesthesia. Larger, noncrushable stones must be removed through a surgical (suprapubic) incision into the bladder.

When it is possible to determine the chemical composition of stones that have been passed or removed, dietary treatment may be attempted to adjust the pH of the urine to keep the urinary salts in solution and thus prevent the formation of stones. These diets, however, are not fully effective. Uric acid stones may be prevented by a low-purine diet. Oral sodium bicarbonate may be used to raise the pH of the urine to approximately 6.0 to 6.5. Increased fluid intake and the administration of sodium bicarbonate may prevent the formation of cystine stones. Clients with a history of calcium stone formation may have to limit their intake of milk and milk products. Despite dietary changes and urine pH regulation, some clients continue to form stones in the urinary tract.

NURSING MANAGEMENT

Obtain a complete medical, drug, and allergy history. Ask the client to describe the symptoms, including the type and location of the pain. Determine if the client is allergic to iodine or seafood because iodine-containing radiopaque substances may be used during diagnostic tests to locate the obstruction. Monitor vital signs every 4 hours or as ordered. Notify the physician if the client's temperature is higher than 101°F (38.3°C) orally. Measure intake and output and note the color of the urine.

Report any evidence of gross hematuria immediately. Encourage the client to drink fluids (unless contraindicated by heart failure or renal disease) because extra fluids help pass stones and reduce the chance of infection or inflammation. Filter the urine for stones by straining all urine through gauze or wire mesh. If solid material is found, send it in a labeled container to the laboratory for analysis. If the client has moderate to severe pain, administer a narcotic analgesic as ordered. Notify the physician if the analgesic fails to relieve at least some of the pain or if the pain becomes worse despite administration of an analgesic. Provide details regarding medical or surgical procedures.

If a litholapaxy successfully removes the stone, a urethral catheter may be left in place to keep the bladder continuously empty for 1 to 2 days after the procedure. Give antibiotics as ordered. Once oral fluids are tolerated, encourage the client to drink extra fluids to reduce inflammation of the bladder mucosa. Monitor the urine output and voiding pattern. If open removal is required, the bladder is incised and the stone removed. A urethral catheter may be left in place for a week or more to keep the bladder empty and prevent tension on the bladder sutures. In addition to standard postoperative care (see Chap. 24), nursing management involves providing the same care as for the client having a suprapubic prostatectomy (see Chap. 60). Closely monitor the client's voiding once the catheter is removed to prevent urinary retention.

Client and Family Teaching

Teach the client to:

- Strain urine and send any stone found to the laboratory for examination.
- Follow the dietary recommendations.
- Take the prescribed medications as directed.
- Contact the physician if symptoms return.
- Drink plenty of fluids (at least 10 large glasses each day) and exercise regularly.
- Contact the physician if hematuria, burning, chills, fever, or pain occurs.

Urethral Strictures

ETIOLOGY AND PATHOPHYSIOLOGY

Strictures of the urethra are caused by infections such as untreated gonorrhea or chronic nongonococcal urethritis. Other causes include trauma to the lower urinary tract or pelvis, such as accidents, childbirth, intercourse, or surgical procedures. Urethral strictures may be congenital.

A **stricture** (narrowing) in the urethra obstructs the flow of urine and can cause complications in the bladder or upper urinary tract. The kidney pelves can become distended with the backflow of urine. The bladder distends when the urethra is obstructed and a diverticulum (outpouching) of the muscular bladder wall may form (Fig. 64–5). In some instances more than one diverticulum may be seen. Urine becomes trapped in the diverticulum, stagnates, and becomes a culture medium for bacteria. For this reason, infection occurs often and is difficult to control until the obstruction is corrected. Men experience urethral stricture more frequently than women, secondary to the anatomic differences and the length of the urethra. A urethral stricture may result in acute or chronic urinary retention.

ASSESSMENT FINDINGS

Signs and Symptoms

Symptoms include a slow or decreased force of stream of urine, hesitancy, burning, frequency, nocturia, and the retention of residual urine in the bladder, which may lead to bladder distention and infection. The client may be able to pass more urine after voiding and waiting a few minutes. The final quantity of urine comes from the diverticulum and may be malodorous.

Diagnostic Findings

The stricture may be seen on cystoscopy, retrograde pyelogram, and IVP. A voiding cystourethrogram also may show the stricture as well as the presence of a bladder diverticulum.

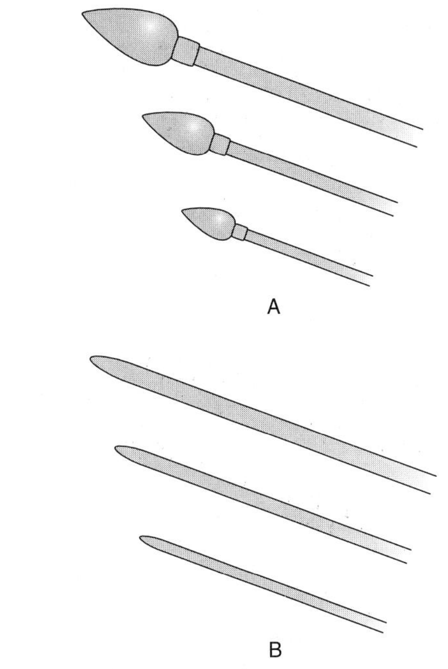

FIGURE 64-6. Bougies (*A*) and filiforms (*B*) are used to dilate the urethra.

MEDICAL AND SURGICAL MANAGEMENT

Urethral strictures are treated by dilatation, which is the use of specially designed instruments called bougies, sounds, filiforms, and followers (Fig. 64–6) that are passed gently into the urethra. Although done gently, the procedure is usually painful. Because forceful stretching of the urethra may cause bleeding and further stricture formation, dilatation begins with a 6F or 8F urethral dilator. During subsequent treatments, the physician increases the size of the dilator until a 24F or 26F can be tolerated. Depending on the cause of the stricture and the response to the therapy, the condition may subside after one or two treatments. However, periodic dilatations are usually required indefinitely or until the condition is corrected surgically.

If dilatation is unsuccessful, a **urethroplasty** (surgical repair of the urethra) may be attempted. The urine is diverted from the urethra by a cystostomy tube until the urethra has been repaired. In one method of reconstructing the urethra, the constricted area is resected, and a mucosal graft (which may be taken from the bladder) is inserted to restore the continuity of the urethra. After surgery, the client has a splinting catheter in the urethra that remains until healing has occurred. This operation may be performed in two stages: urinary diversion at the first operation and plastic repair at the second.

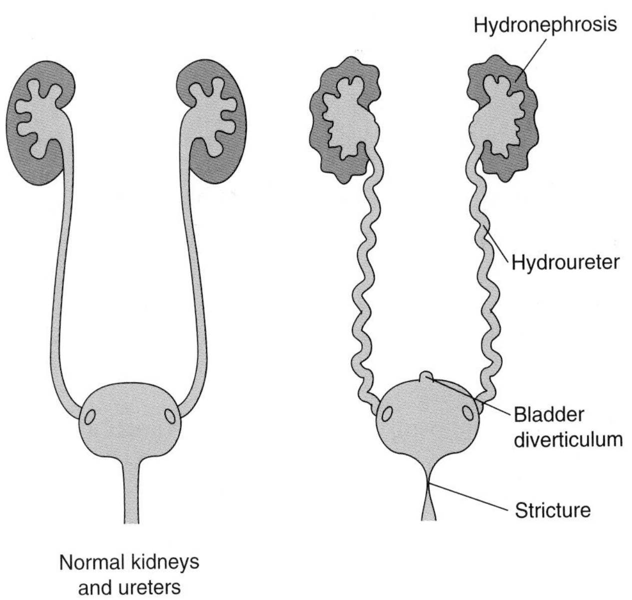

FIGURE 64-5. Urethral stricture can result in hydroureters, hydronephrosis (dilation of the ureters and kidney), and bladder diverticulum.

NURSING MANAGEMENT

Advise the client that the urine may be blood tinged following urethral dilatation and that it may burn when voiding. Suggest sitz baths and nonnarcotic analgesics to relieve discomfort. Tell the client to drink extra fluids for several days after the procedure. Encourage the client to keep appointments for follow-up dilatations and not to wait until there is a marked reduction in the urinary stream or other symptoms of obstruction to return. Instruct the client to take all of the antibiotics and to contact the physician if difficulty voiding or frank bleeding occurs.

If a urethroplasty is performed, it is most important that the urethral catheter remains in place and securely anchored. Following surgery, turning and repositioning requires special attention to prevent excessive tension on the urethral catheter.

Malignant Tumors of the Bladder

Malignant tumors of the bladder are frightening for clients. Bloody urine is often the first sign of problems and is the reason that clients seek medical attention.

ETIOLOGY AND PATHOPHYSIOLOGY

Malignant tumors of the bladder are the most common tumors in the urinary system. They occur more frequently in men than women and usually affect clients 50 years of age and older. Environmental and occupational health hazards are thought to be associated with bladder tumors. These hazards include:

- Exposure to industrial dyes, paint, or rubber
- Occupational exposure to sewage
- Coal gas
- Cigarette smoking and second-hand smoke
- Coffee drinking
- Use of artificial sweeteners

The most common type of bladder tumor is a transitional cell carcinoma. It develops in the epithelial lining of the bladder. The tumors are classified as papillary or nonpapillary. Papillary lesions are superficial tumors that extend outward from the mucosal layer. Nonpapillary tumors are solid growths that grow inward, deep into the bladder wall. This type is more likely to metastasize, usually to the lymph nodes, liver, lungs, and bone. Other types include squamous cell carcinoma and adenocarcinoma.

ASSESSMENT FINDINGS

Signs and Symptoms

The most common first symptom of a malignant tumor of the bladder is painless hematuria. Additional early symptoms include urinary tract infection with symptoms such as fever, dysuria, urgency, and frequency. Later symptoms are related to metastases and include pelvic pain, urinary retention (if the tumor blocks the bladder outlet), and urinary frequency due to occupation of bladder space by the tumor. If bleeding has been present for a period of time, the client also may have symptoms of anemia (fatigue, shortness of breath) caused by blood loss.

Diagnostic Findings

The tumor is usually seen by cystoscopic examination and confirmed by microscopic biopsy of the lesion. A retrograde pyelogram may be obtained to detect any kidney damage, if the tumor is obstructing one of the ureteral orifices. A computed tomography scan and radiographs of the pelvis may show a tumor shadow or bony metastases. Ultrasonography may also show tumor size and location. Routine laboratory tests may be performed to evaluate kidney function and determine the degree of anemia due to persistent hematuria.

MEDICAL MANAGEMENT

Treatment varies according to the grade and stage of the tumor. Metastases usually have not occurred as long as the muscle wall of the bladder has not been penetrated by the tumor. Small, superficial tumors may be removed by cutting (resection) or coagulation (**fulguration**) with a transurethral resectoscope (the same instrument used in a transurethral resection of the prostate). Bladder tumors removed in this manner have a high incidence of recurrence; consequently, a cystoscopic examination is performed every 2 to 3 months. Clients having no recurrence of the tumor for at least a year require cystoscopic examinations every 6 months for the rest of their lives so that recurrence of the tumor or a new malignant growth can be detected early.

Topical application of an antineoplastic drug may be used after resection and fulguration of a tumor. The drug, in liquid form, is instilled into the bladder by means of a catheter (intravesicular injection). Fluid intake usually is limited before and during this procedure so that the drug remains concentrated and in contact with the bladder mucosa for about 2 hours. The client then voids and is given extra oral fluids to flush the drug from the bladder.

Intravesicular injection of BCG (bacillus Calmette-Guérin) Live, a weakened strain of *Mycobacterium bovis*, may also be used. It appears that BCG causes an inflammatory reaction in the bladder wall that in turn destroys malignant cells. Another form of therapy includes the administration of interferon alfa-2a (Roferon-A) injected intravenously (IV) or directly into the bladder. Interferon appears to stimulate the production of lymphocytes and macrophages that may destroy malignant cells.

Photodynamic therapy also may be used in the treatment of bladder cancer. This experimental treatment involves the IV injection of a photosensitizing agent that is absorbed in concentration by malignant cells. A laser, inserted through a cystoscope, is used to destroy those cells that have a high concentration of the photosensitizing agent.

SURGICAL MANAGEMENT

A **cystectomy** (surgical removal of the bladder) and a urinary diversion procedure are often necessary when the tumor has penetrated the muscle wall. When a cystectomy is performed, the bladder and lower third of both ureters are removed. If the tumor has extended through the bladder wall, the surgeon may perform a radical cystectomy.

In women, a radical cystectomy usually includes removal of the bladder, lower third of both ureters, uterus, fallopian tubes, ovaries, anterior vaginal wall, and urethra. In men, a radical cystectomy usually includes removal of the bladder, lower third of both ureters, prostate, and seminal vesicles.

Once a cystectomy is performed, urine must be diverted to another collecting system. This is called a **urinary diversion.** Although urinary diversion procedures are used for the treatment of bladder tumors, they also are used for extensive pelvic malignancies and severe traumatic injury to the bladder. Some urinary diversions require external ostomy bags to collect the urine; other types create a reservoir within the body and the reservoir is catheterized to drain the urine. In some instances the urine is diverted to the colon and the client voids rectally. The more common types of urinary diversion procedures are described in Table 64–2. Each of the procedures has advantages and disadvantages. The type of procedure used depends on many factors, such as the age and physical condition of the client, the procedure that can produce the best results for the client, and the extent of metastases.

NURSING MANAGEMENT

Preoperative Period

Obtain a complete medical, drug, and allergy history on admission. Ask the client or family member to describe all of the symptoms. Evaluate the client's general physical and emotional status. Take vital signs and weigh the client.

Caring for a client during the preoperative period includes reducing anxiety and increasing understanding of the preparations for surgery and postoperative care. The client may display a variety of emotional responses before surgery. Some may appear depressed, others show a mixture of anxiety and depression. The client faces drastic changes in the manner of excreting urine from the body, the diagnosis of cancer, and the changes in body image. Encourage the client to talk about the surgery and the changes that will occur. Suggest a visit from a member of a local ostomy group to provide emotional support as well as information. The enterostomal therapist should meet with the client to discuss placement of the stoma and collection devices. Photographs or drawings are useful in showing the placement of the stoma and urostomy pouch.

Determine the client's ability to manage stoma care or self-catheterization by assessing manual dexterity, level of understanding, and vision. Assess the client's social support and resources including whether insurance will cover ostomy supplies. Explain all preoperative preparations to the client and family and give them time to ask additional questions about the surgery, preparations for surgery, and management after surgery.

Depending on the extent and type of surgery, preoperative preparations may include insertion of a nasogastric tube, IV and central venous pressure lines; cleansing enemas; and a low-residue diet several days before surgery. Laxatives and enemas and a drug such as kanamycin (Kantrex) or neomycin (Mycifradin) may be given if a ureterosigmoidostomy is to be performed. These agents decrease the number of microorganisms in the bowel and lessen the possibility of infection as a complication of connecting the ureters to the bowel. Clients scheduled for an ileal conduit or continent ileal urinary diversion procedure also may have the bowel prepared in this manner.

Postoperative Period

Clients undergoing urinary diversion are subject to the same conditions and complications as any surgical client. Refer to Chapter 24 for nursing diagnoses and interventions for managing standard postoperative care. Management issues related specifically to urinary diversion procedures include observing for leakage of urine or stool from the anastomosis, maintaining renal function, assessing for signs and symptoms of peritonitis, maintaining integrity of the urinary diversion and urine collection devices, maintaining skin and stomal integrity, promoting a positive body image, and teaching the client how to manage the diversion.

Check the client's chart for information regarding the type and extent of surgery and orders for connection of catheters or drains, IV fluids, and analgesics. Clients will have multiple drainage tubes, ureteral stents, and a nasogastric tube. Label all urinary drainage tubes, and measure and record the urine output from *each* catheter or stoma every hour. Record each measurement separately.

TABLE 64-2 **Types of Urinary Diversions**

Urinary Diversion	Description	Advantages	Disadvantages
Ileal Conduit (ileal loop) Stoma Ileal conduit	A small segment of ileum is resected from the intestines; proximal end is closed to form a pouch; distal end is brought out as a stoma; ureters are anastomosed to this pouch.	Technically easy to perform	Complications include ureteroileal obstruction requiring reoperation, stomal stenosis requiring reoperation, upper urinary tract deterioration secondary to reflux and infection, kidney stones, electrolyte imbalances. Not recommended for younger clients due to long-term complications
Continent Urinary Diversion (**Kock pouch,** Indiana pouch, Mainze pouch) 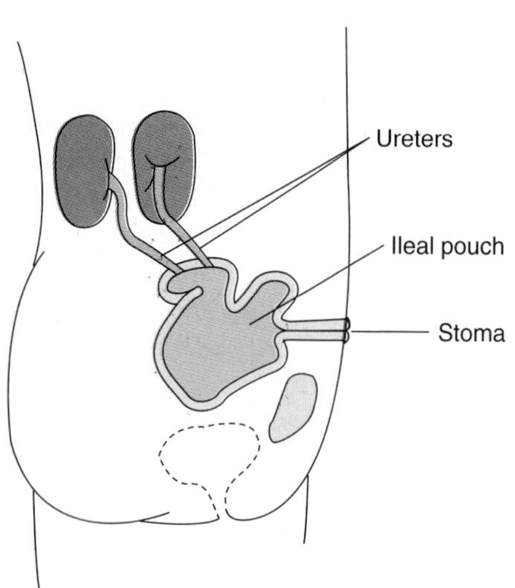 Kock pouch	Ureters are anastomosed to isolated segment of ileal pouch with a nipple-like one-way valve; urine is periodically drained with a catheter.	Client does not have to wear an external collection bag; upper urinary tract deterioration, kidney stones, and electrolyte imbalances are rare.	Technically challenging procedure; may require reoperations to correct leakage or sliding nipple valve. Not recommended for older or poor-risk clients

(continued)

TABLE 64-2 *(Continued)*

Urinary Diversion	Description	Advantages	Disadvantages
Ureterosigmoidostomy	Ureters attached to the sigmoid colon; urine flows through the colon, which becomes the reservoir. The client voids and defecates through the rectum.	No external collection bag; no need to self-catheterize; technically easy to perform	Electrolyte imbalances, increased risk of colon cancer, recurrent upper urinary tract infection requiring long-term antibiotic therapy

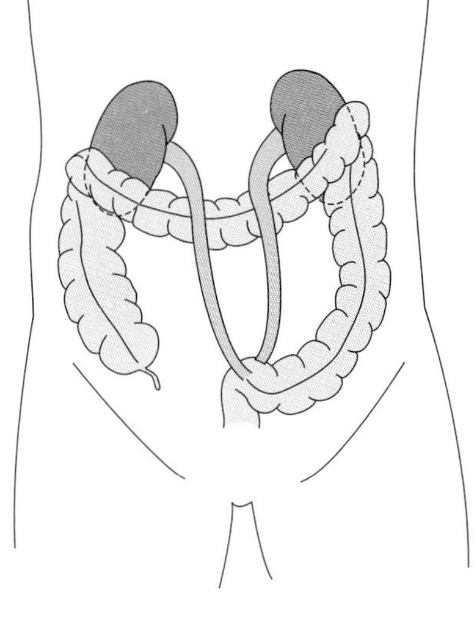

Ureterosigmoidostomy

Maintaining accurate intake and output measurements during the postoperative period is important because it indicates both renal function and the integrity of the urinary diversion structures. Obstruction of urine flow can severely damage the kidneys; if urinary drainage stops or decreases to less than 30 mL/hour, or if the client complains of back pain, notify the physician immediately. Inspect the urine for color, clarity, and presence of blood. Immediately report concentrated, cloudy, or bloody urine to the physician. Ureteral stents will remain in place for several days after surgery.

Connect the nasogastric tube to low intermittent suction. This prevents distention and pressure on the suture line due to the collection of gas in the bowel. The nasogastric tube is removed once peristalsis has returned and the diet can be advanced. Review all laboratory reports as soon as they are received and report abnormalities to the physician promptly. The following text addresses management issues specific to the most common procedures.

ILEAL CONDUIT. Apply a transparent ostomy bag over the stoma to make stomal assessment easier (Fig. 64–7). Contact the physician immediately if there is excessive bleeding, changes in the color of the stoma (eg, from a normal to a cyanotic color), or separation of the stoma edges from the surrounding skin. Clean mucus away from the stoma with gauze pads. Because the intestinal anastomosis can leak fecal material or the ileal conduit may leak urine into the peritoneal cavity, observe for and promptly report symptoms of peritonitis (eg, abdominal tenderness or distention, fever, severe

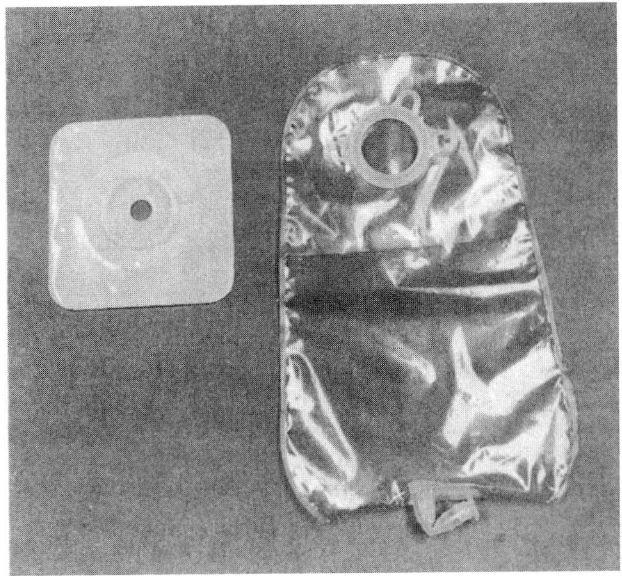

FIGURE 64-7. Urostomy pouch and stomadhesive wafer.

pain). Management of the urinary stoma is similar to management of a fecal stoma (see Chap. 53). The skin needs protection, the surgical dressings are changed promptly when they become wet, and the appliances need care and cleansing. Each time a temporary drainage bag is changed, inspect the skin around the stoma for signs of infection and skin breakdown.

CONTINENT URINARY DIVERSION (KOCK POUCH, INDIANA POUCH, MAINZ POUCH). Inspect the stoma for bleeding or cyanosis. Irrigate the pouch, if ordered, to prevent mucous plugs or blood clots. Teach the client how to perform intermittent self-catheterization (Fig. 64–8). Initially this will be done every 1 to 2 hours but eventually will be performed every 4 to 6 hours.

URETEROSIGMOIDOSTOMY. A catheter is inserted in the rectum to continuously drain urine. Check the amount and color of drainage from the rectal catheter every 1 or 2 hours. Inspect the anal and gluteal areas for signs of early skin breakdown. The catheter is removed when peristalsis returns. Because urinary constituents are reabsorbed by the sigmoid colon, clients are prone to fluid and electrolyte imbalances throughout the postoperative period (as well as for the rest of their lives). Observe for signs of electrolyte losses. Teach the client exercises to improve sphincter control. Once good control is achieved, instruct the client to void (rectally) every 2 hours to prevent reabsorption of fluid and electrolytes. Clients must never have enemas, suppositories, or laxatives.

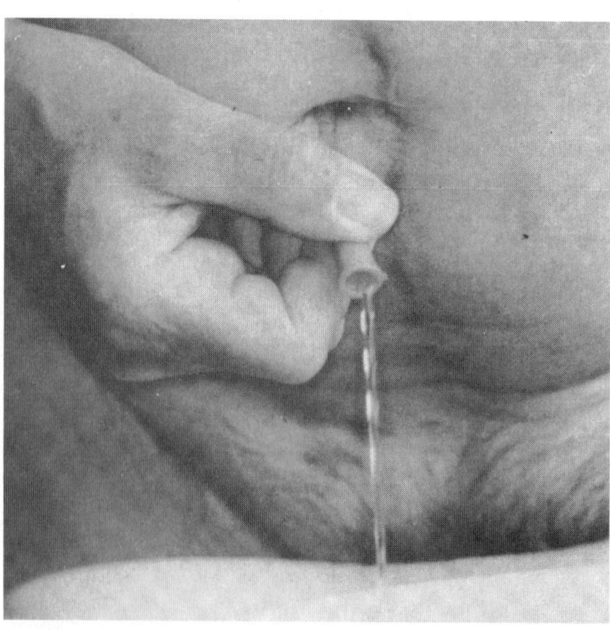

FIGURE 64-8. Self-catheterization of a continent urinary diversion through the stoma.

NURSING PROCESS
Psychosocial Nursing Care of the Client Undergoing Urinary Diversion

Assessment

Assess the client's knowledge about the effects of surgery on sexual function. Up to 85% of men are impotent after urinary diversion; women may have painful intercourse and lack lubrication. Discuss the client's current level of social activity and what changes he or she thinks will occur after surgery. Assess the client's understanding of long-term postoperative care.

Diagnosis and Planning

Psychosocial care of the client includes, but is not limited to, the following:

Nursing Diagnoses and Collaborative Problems	Nursing Interventions
Risk for Altered Sexuality Patterns related to impotence (male) or dyspareunia (female) **Goal:** The client will regain erectile function or ease painful intercourse.	Provide an opportunity to discuss sexuality issues by tactfully asking if the client has any questions. Discuss alternatives to sexual intercourse such as closeness and giving pleasure to a partner. Discuss penile prosthesis for men and water-soluble lubricants for women. Inform women that Kegel exercises may ease painful intercourse.
Body Image Disturbance related to change in appearance and function **Goal:** The client will accept altered appearance and perform self-care.	Assess the client's willingness to look at the stoma. Accept the client's response, reinforce that anxiety is normal. Reassure the client that nursing staff will provide care until he or she is ready. Discuss change in function and let client know what to expect when recovery from surgery is complete. Suggest a visit from an ostomate who can provide valuable personal information, support, and resources. Help the client gain independence by reinforcing that self-care is quite manageable and providing time for practice.
Risk for Social Isolation related to fear of accidents or urine odor **Goal:** Client will maintain social relationships.	Explain that odor-proof pouches or pouches with carbon filters are available. Suggest avoiding odor-producing foods, such as asparagus. Teach the client to care for the pouch and to change it every 3 days if it is a one-piece pouch or every 4 to 7 days if it is a two-piece pouch.

	Tell the client to empty the bag before it gets half full to prevent tension on the adhesive wafer and to eliminate source of odors. Inform the client to carry a spare pouch in case adhesive loosens while out. Suggest drinking cranberry juice or using an appliance deodorant. Suggest that client contact the urostomy association for suggestions and additional support in alleviating anxiety. Instruct the client with a ureterosigmoidostomy to avoid gas-forming foods.
Risk for Ineffective Management of Therapeutic Regimen related to inadequate knowledge about stomal care **Goal:** The client will demonstrate ability to change ostomy pouch.	Explain procedure for removing the old pouch, and fitting and applying a new one. Tell the client to change the pouch in the morning before consuming liquids and to insert a tampon or rolled gauze into the stoma to absorb urine during appliance change. Make sure the appliance fits well and the skin is completely dry when applying adhesive wafer. Picture frame the wafer with paper tape to seal edges. Show the client how to empty the pouch and attach it to an overnight drainage system. Teach the client to inspect the periostomal skin each time the pouch is changed. Advise using a liquid skin barrier to protect the skin. If abdominal skin must be shaved, use an electric razor.
Risk for Ineffective Management of Therapeutic Regimen related to inadequate knowledge about intermittent catheterization of continent urinary diversions (Kock pouch, Indiana pouch, Mainze pouch) **Goal:** The client will demonstrate ability to catheterize pouch.	Identify need for continuous drainage and frequent catheterizations in early postoperative period. Explain need for irrigations (to flush mucus and prevent plugging of catheter). Teach client to self-catheterize by lubricating catheter, inserting it into pouch, and allowing urine to drain into the toilet bowl.

Evaluation and Expected Outcomes

- The client discusses methods for resuming sexual activity and alternatives to sexual intercourse.
- The client states methods to avoid accidents and control urine odor.
- The client verbalizes a willingness to maintain social activity.
- The client correctly changes ostomy appliance.
- The client successfully self-catheterizes continent pouch.

Client and Family Teaching

The material included in a client teaching plan varies according to the type of surgery or the physician's specific discharge orders. In addition to the points discussed above, consider the following when preparing a teaching plan:

- Clients with a ureterosigmoidostomy must know the signs of fluid and electrolyte imbalances. To ensure understanding, give the client a written or printed list of the symptoms.
- Closed collection containers should always be below the level of the stoma. The tubing that connects the catheter or collection appliance to the closed drainage system must be kept straight so that urine does not collect in a curve of the tube. Avoid kinks that prevent the drainage of urine.
- Adequate fluids are necessary. Note the color of the urine. If the urine appears darker than usual, more fluids may be needed. Dark urine, despite an adequate fluid intake, is brought to the attention of the physician.
- Medications are taken as prescribed by the physician. Do not omit or stop taking the drugs. Do not take or use any nonprescription drug without first checking with the physician. Those with a ureterosigmoidostomy must not use laxatives or enemas.
- Odors can be controlled with cranberry juice, yogurt, or buttermilk. Avoid foods that may impart an odor to the urine, such as asparagus or onions.
- The enterostomal therapist will recommend skin care techniques. The skin *must* be kept clean. When the adhesive wafer (to which the urostomy collection bag is attached) is changed, all remaining adhesive is removed before application of a new wafer.
- The continent urostomy should be drained four times a day or as directed by the physician.
- The urinary collection pouch needs to be washed thoroughly after changing; rinse with or soak in a solution of vinegar and water if crystals form in the pouch.
- The physician is contacted if any of the following occur:

  - Fever
  - Chills
  - Blood in the urine
  - Failure of a stoma or catheter to drain urine
  - Skin problems around the stoma
  - Weight loss (> 5 lb)
  - Loss of appetite (more than a few days)
  - Inability to insert the catheter in the continent urostomy
  - Pain in the flank (kidney area or lower abdomen)
  - Signs of fluid or electrolyte imbalance
  - Any unusual symptom or problem

Trauma

Trauma to the bladder or urethra are potentially harmful and frequently require surgical intervention.

ETIOLOGY AND PATHOPHYSIOLOGY

Various types of injury can affect the urinary tract. Gunshot and stab wounds, crushing injuries, and forceful blows can result in tears, hemorrhage, or penetration of one or more parts of the urinary tract. Some penetrating bladder injuries are small, whereas others are large with a rapid collection of urine in the peritoneal cavity. Injuries to the kidney area may result in bruising or tearing of the kidney and its capsule. Depending on the severity of the injury, blood and urine may leak into the peritoneal cavity.

ASSESSMENT FINDINGS

Signs and Symptoms

Symptoms vary according to the area affected and the type of injury. Anuria, hematuria, pain in the abdomen (which may indicate bleeding or leakage of urine into the abdominal cavity), pain in the bladder or kidney areas, and symptoms of shock may be indicators of urinary tract injury. During treatment of a client with extensive injury, an indwelling catheter may be inserted, and hematuria or lack of urine output may be the first sign that a traumatic injury to the urinary tract injury has occurred. Certain other types of injuries, such as stab or gunshot wounds, may be immediately identified because of outward signs of injury (eg, entry wounds on the skin surface).

Diagnostic Findings

Injury to the urinary tract may be initially overlooked when the client has incurred widespread, massive injuries. Abdominal radiographs, cystoscopy, IVP and exploratory surgery may be used to identify the type and location of the injury.

SURGICAL MANAGEMENT

Treatment depends on the type, location, and extent of injury as well as on the condition of the client. For example, a stab wound in the kidney area may require emergency exploratory surgery. Once the kidney is exposed, the physician needs to determine if the trauma to the kidney can be repaired or if the kidney must be removed immediately. Examples of surgeries that may be performed for urinary tract trauma include cystostomy (temporary or permanent), nephrectomy, insertion of a nephrostomy tube, repair (reanastomosis) of the ureter, and cystectomy.

NURSING MANAGEMENT

The most important nursing task is recognition of abnormal findings. Lack of urinary output, diffuse and severe abdominal pain, and hematuria are examples of signs and symptoms that may be indicative of an injury to the urinary tract. In some instances, the injury may be such that symptoms do not appear for several hours or days after the initial trauma.

Other nursing management depends on the surgical interventions performed and the symptoms the client experiences. In addition, focus on the client's physical and emotional needs related to the trauma.

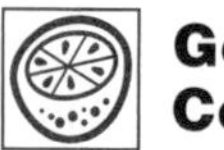

General Nutritional Considerations

Cranberry Juice Cocktail sold in grocery stores is only about 25% cranberry juice; the amount needed to acidify the urine is too large to be of practical value. However, cranberry juice may be effective against urinary tract infections by preventing bacteria from adhering to the lining of the urinary tract, thus promoting their excretion. Not all bacteria are sensitive to the juice, and protection lasts only as long as the juice is consumed regularly.

Clients with bladder stones should be encouraged to drink 8 ounces of fluid hourly during waking hours, or at least 2 liters of fluid daily.

Clients with calcium oxalate stones should limit calcium intake to 1000 mg/day or less (3 cups of milk or less daily). Because fiber interferes with the absorption of oxalate from the GI tract, a high fiber diet is recommended. High intakes of protein and sodium are avoided because they promote urinary calcium excretion.

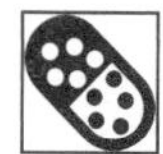

General Pharmacologic Considerations

Antibiotics and sulfonamides are drugs commonly used to treat urinary tract infections. Other drugs used are furan derivatives, nitrofurantoin microcrystals (Macrodantin) and nitrofurantoin (Furadantin), and acids, methenamine mandelate (Mandelamine) and nalidixic acid (NegGram). An azo dye, phenazopyridine (Pyridium), may be ordered for its soothing effect on bladder mucosa and is often used in conjunction with urinary antimicrobial drugs.

Clients who receive drugs for urinary tract infections are instructed to finish the course of therapy even though they may feel improved and be symptom free after several days of therapy. A *completed* course of therapy is essential to be sure the infection is under control.

Clients must be advised to follow the instructions of their physician about the medication and any instructions specific to that medication, such as drinking extra fluids.

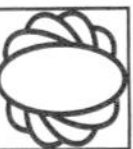

General Gerontologic Considerations

The older adult may have some form of incontinence. In some, involuntary leakage of urine may occur when the client coughs or sneezes, whereas others may be completely incontinent.

Some older adults may be unable to follow the instructions of a bladder rehabilitation program; others may have involuntary relaxation of the bladder sphincter, making rehabilitation extremely difficult.

Older clients with continence problems must not be treated like infants or scolded for their behavior (eg, bed-wetting, soiling clothes). The nurse must make every effort to help rehabilitate the client. If bladder rehabilitation is not successful, other methods to keep the client clean, dry, and odor free must be tried.

The cause of incontinence must be carefully assessed in the older adult. Older adults may be incontinent simply because environmental or physical conditions prevent them from maneuvering quickly enough to get to the bathroom before urination occurs. In these situations a change in the environment or an assistive device may alleviate the incontinence.

If the elderly client is incontinent, the perineal area is particularly susceptible to skin breakdown.

Clients must not be made to feel isolated when they have a problem with urinary continence. Planned exercise and social activities should be a part of a bladder rehabilitation program.

SUMMARY OF KEY CONCEPTS

- Urinary retention is defined as an inability to urinate when the bladder is full, or to completely empty the bladder. Urinary incontinence is the inability to retain urine and control the voiding of urine. Nursing management includes assessment, catheterization, and client education.
- Nursing management of clients with urethral or suprapubic catheters includes always using aseptic technique to insert the catheter, providing catheter care, maintaining the integrity of the closed drainage system, encouraging fluids, and monitoring for signs and symptoms or urinary tract infection.
- Cystitis is an inflammation of the urinary bladder. The inflammation is usually caused by a bacterial infection. Nursing management includes teaching clients how to prevent cystitis.
- In interstitial cystitis the bladder wall contains multiple pinpoint hemorrhagic areas that join and form larger hemorrhagic areas that may progress to fissuring and scarring of the bladder mucosa. Superficial erosion of the bladder mucosa (Hunner's ulcer) may be seen. Most treatments are only temporarily effective. Clients need referral to a support group.
- Urethritis caused by microorganisms other than gonorrhea is called nongonococcal urethritis. Treatment includes antibiotic therapy, liberal fluid intake, analgesics, warm sitz baths, and improvement of the client's resistance to infection.
- Symptoms of bladder stone formation include hematuria, suprapubic pain, difficulty starting the urinary stream, symptoms of a bladder infection, and a feeling that the bladder is not completely empty. Some clients may have few if any symptoms.
- Strictures of the urethra may occur after infections such as untreated gonorrhea or chronic, long-standing, nongonococcal urethritis. They also may be congenital. Urethral strictures may be treated by dilatation or by a urethroplasty.
- The most common first symptom of a malignant tumor of the bladder is painless hematuria. Treatment may include cutting or fulguration of the tumor, topical application of an antineoplastic drug, intravesicular injection of BCG Live, administration of interferon alfa-2A (Roferon-A) injected IV or directly into the bladder, photodynamic therapy followed by destruction of the tumor by a laser, and cystectomy with a urinary diversion procedure.
- The more common types of urinary diversion procedures include ileal conduit, continent urinary diversion, and ureterosigmoidostomy. Nursing management includes standard postoperative care, careful assessment of urine output, maintenance of urinary drainage systems, client education in self-care and follow-up care, and psychosocial support.
- The teaching plan for a client with a urinary diversion focuses on self-catheterization, importance of maintaining the medication regimen, care and cleaning of the skin and pouch, and self-monitoring for complications.

CRITICAL THINKING EXERCISES

1. A client has recurrent cystitis and her physician wants to perform a cystoscopy and retrograde pyelograms. She asks you why she needs these tests because the medication she took in the past cured her problem. What explanation would you give the client?
2. Discuss the possible psychosocial impact of interstitial cystitis.
3. A client has a ureterosigmoidostomy. What teaching will you do regarding long-term follow-up and care?

Suggested Readings

Bullock, B. L. (1996). *Pathophysiology: Adaptations and alterations in function* (4th ed.). Philadelphia. Lippincott-Raven.

Carpenito, L. J. (1997). *Nursing care plans and documentation: Nursing diagnoses and collaborative problems.* Philadelphia. Lippincott-Raven.

Dickson, C. (1995). The bladder: Cystectomy and ileal conduit to treat cancer. *Nursing Times, 91*(42), 34–35.

Dudek, S. G. (1993). *Nutrition handbook for nursing practice* (2nd ed.). Philadelphia: J. B. Lippincott.

Eliopoulos, C. (1997). *Gerontological nursing* (4th ed.). Philadelphia: Lippincott-Raven.

Karlowicz, K. A. (1997). Pharmacologic therapy for acute cystitis in adults: A review of treatment options. *Urologic Nursing, 17*(3), 106–116.

Kaufman, M. W. (1997). Caring for the patient with interstitial cystitis. *MEDSURG Nursing, 6*(4), 203–208.

Kelly, L. P., & Miaskowski, C. (1996). An overview of bladder cancer: Treatment and nursing implications. *Oncology Nursing Forum, 23*(3), 459–470.

Khoury, J. M., & Webster, G. D. (1997). *Urinary incontinence in women: A guide for women.*

Rosenberg, A. G., Jensen, J. K., Morell, P., & Ratner, V. (1996). *Interstitial cystitis: Understanding your painful bladder condition* (No. 1683). Krames-Communications.

Smeltzer, S. C., & Bare, B. G. (1996). *Brunner and Suddarth's textbook of medical-surgical nursing* (8th ed.). Philadelphia: Lippincott-Raven.

Valerius, A. J. (1997). Quality of life tools for assessment of urinary incontinence. *Urologic Nursing, 17*(3), 104–105.

Valerius, A. J. (1997). The psychosocial impact of urinary incontinence on women aged 25 to 45 years. *Urologic Nursing, 17*(3), 96–103.

Additional Resources

National Association for Continence (NAFC)
P.O. Box 8310
Spartanburg, SC 29305–8310
(800) BLADDER
www.nafc.org

Bladder Health Council
American Foundation for Urologic Disease
1128 North Charles Street
Baltimore, MD 21201
www.access.digex.net/~afud/bladhc.html

Interstitial Cystitis Association
P.O. Box 1553
Madison Square Garden Station
New York, NY 10159
(212) 979–6057
www.ichelp.com

United Ostomy Association, Inc.
19772 MacArthur Boulevard
Suite 200
Irvine, CA 92612–2405
(800) 826–0826
www.uoa.org

Urology Page
www.urolog.nl/uropage/uroeng.htm

16

Caring for Clients With Musculoskeletal Disorders

Chapter 65

Introduction to the Musculoskeletal System

KEY TERMS

Arthrocentesis
Arthrogram
Arthroscopy
Bone scan
Bursa
Calcification
Cancellous bone
Cartilage
Cortical bone
Diaphyses
Epiphyses
Joint
Ligament
Ossification
Osteoblasts
Osteoclasts
Osteocytes
Periosteum
Red bone marrow
Resorption
Skeletal muscles
Tendon
Yellow bone marrow

LEARNING OBJECTIVES

On completion of this chapter, the reader will:

- Describe major structures and functions of the musculoskeletal system.
- Discuss elements of the nursing assessment of the musculoskeletal system.
- Identify common diagnostic and laboratory tests used in the evaluation of musculoskeletal disorders.
- Discuss the nursing management of clients undergoing tests for musculoskeletal disorders.

The musculoskeletal system supports the body and facilitates movement. Other functions include calcium storage, blood cell production in the bone marrow, and protection and support to the body organs, such as the lungs, heart, and brain. The musculoskeletal system consists of bones, muscles, joints, tendons, ligaments, cartilage, and bursae. Injury or disease to any part of the system can cause pain, immobility, or disability and potentially affect the quality of life.

Anatomy and Physiology

Bones

The human body has 206 bones. The bones of the skeleton are classified as:

- Short bones, such as those in the fingers and toes
- Long bones, such as the femur and ulna
- Flat bones, such as the sternum
- Irregular bones, such as the vertebrae

There are two types of bony tissue. The first is **cancellous** bone, or spongy bone, which is light and contains many spaces. The second is **cortical bone**, or compact bone, which is dense and hard. Both types are found in varying amounts within all bones. Cancellous bone is found at the rounded, irregular ends, or **epiphyses,** of long bones. Cortical bony tissue covers bones and is found chiefly in the long shafts, or **diaphyses,** of bones in the arms and legs. The combination of the two types of bony tissue provides strength and support, yet keeps the skeleton light to promote endurance during activity.

Bone is composed of cells, protein matrix, and mineral deposits. The three types of bone cells are osteo*blasts*, osteo*cytes*, and osteo*clasts*. Cells that build bones are called **osteoblasts.** These cells secrete bone matrix (mostly collagen) in which inorganic minerals, such as calcium salts, are deposited. This process of **ossification** and **calcification** transforms the blast cells into mature bone cells called **osteocytes,** which are involved in the maintenance of bone tissue.

During times of rapid bone growth or bone injury, osteocytes function as osteoblasts to form new bone. **Osteoclasts** are the cells involved in the destruction, resorption, and remodeling of bone.

During growth, bones primarily lengthen. However, the diameter also increases when osteoclasts break down previously formed bone, making the central canal wider. At the completion of skeletal growth, the osteoclasts, which are part of the mononuclear phagocyte system (blood cells involved in ingesting particulate matter—or recycling old cells), continue with the remodeling of bones by balancing bone **resorption** with new bone cell replacement. Bone formation and resorption continue throughout life. The greatest activity occurs from birth through puberty. Factors that affect bone growth are reviewed in Table 65–1.

A layer of tissue called **periosteum** covers the bones (but not the joints). The inner layer of the periosteum contains the osteoblasts necessary for bone formation. The periosteum is rich in blood and lymph vessels and supplies the bone with nourishment.

Inside bones there are two types of bone marrow: red and yellow. **Red bone marrow,** found primarily in the sternum, ileum, vertebrae, and ribs, manufactures blood cells and hemoglobin. Long bones have **yellow bone marrow,** which consists primarily of fat cells and connective tissue. If the blood cell supply becomes compromised, the yellow marrow may take on the characteristics of red marrow and begin producing blood cells.

Muscles

There are three kinds of muscles: skeletal, smooth, and cardiac. **Skeletal muscles** are voluntary muscles; their function is controlled by impulses that travel from efferent nerves of the brain and spinal cord. The skeletal muscles promote movement of the bones of the skeleton. Examples of skeletal muscles are the biceps in the arms and the gastrocnemius in the calf of the leg.

Skeletal muscle is composed of muscle fibers that contain several myofibers. Sliding filaments called sarcomeres make up myofibers. They are the contractile units of skeletal muscle. Impulses from the central nervous system cause the release of acetylcholine at the motor end plate of the motor neuron that innervates the muscle. As a result, calcium ions are released, and the release stimulates actin and myosin in the sarcomeres to slide closer together, resulting in contraction of the muscle. When calcium is depleted, the actin and myosin fibers move apart, causing relaxation of the sarcomeres, and thus the muscle.

Smooth and cardiac muscles are involuntary muscles; their activity is controlled by mechanisms within their tissue of origin and by neurotransmitters released from the autonomic nervous system. Smooth muscles are found mainly in the walls of certain organs or cavities of the body, such as the stomach, intestine, blood vessels, and ureters. Cardiac muscle is found only in the heart.

TABLE 65-1 **Factors That Affect Bone Formation**

Bone Formation Facilitators	Bone Formation Retardants
Calcium	Estrogen/androgen deficiency
Phosphorus	Vitamin deficiency
Estrogen	Starvation
Testosterone	Diabetes
Calcitonin	Steroids
Vitamins D, A, C	Inactivity/immobility
Growth hormone	Heparin
Exercise	Excess parathyroid hormone
Insulin	

From Bullock, B. L. (1996). *Pathophysiology: Adaptation and Alterations in Function* (4th ed., p. 853). Philadelphia: Lippincott-Raven.

Joints

A **joint** is the junction between two or more bones. Joints are classified in Table 65–2. Free moving joints, or diarthrodial joints, make up most skeletal joints. They allow certain movements. Terms related to diarthrodial joint movement are presented in Box 65–1. The surfaces of diarthrodial joints are covered with hyaline cartilage, which reduces the friction during joint movement. The space between is the joint cavity, which is enclosed by a fibrous capsule lined with synovial membrane. This membrane produces synovial fluid, which acts as a lubricant.

Tendons

Tendons are cordlike structures that attach muscles to the periosteum of the bone. A muscle has two or more attachments. One is called the origin and is more fixed. The other is called the insertion and is more movable. When a muscle contracts, both attachments are pulled, and the insertion is drawn closer to the origin. An example of this can be found in the biceps of the arm, which has two origin tendons, attached to the scapula, and one insertion tendon, attached to the radius. When the biceps contracts, the lower arm (with the insertion tendon) moves toward the upper arm (with the origin tendon).

TABLE 65-2 **Types of Joints**

Type	Characteristic	Example
Synarthrodial joints	Immovable	At the suture line of skull between the temporal and occipital bones
Amphiarthrodial joints	Slightly movable	Between the vertebrae
Diarthrodial joints (also called synovial joints)	Freely movable	Gliding joint: fingers Hinge joint: elbow Pivot joint: ends of radius and ulna Condyloid joint: between the wrist and forearm Saddle joint: between the wrist and metacarpal bone of the thumb Ball and socket joint: hip

BOX 65-1 Glossary of Diarthrodial Movement

Adduction

Abduction

Abduction: Movement away from midline of the body
Adduction: Movement toward the midline of the body

Flexion: Bending of a joint
Extension: Return movement from flexion
Hyperextension: Extension beyond straight or neutral position

Flexion
extension
hyperextension

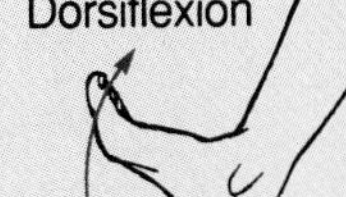

Dorsiflexion: Movement that flexes hand back toward body or foot toward leg

Rotation: Turning or movement of a part around its axis
Internal (inward) rotation: Movement toward the center
External (outward) rotation: Movement away from the center

Rotation:
outward
inward

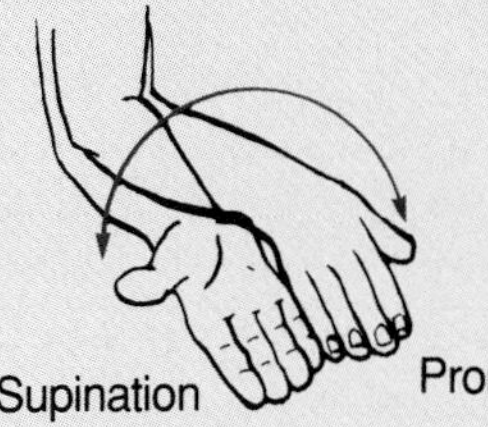

Pronation: Rotation of forearm so that palm of hand is down
Supination: Rotation of the forearm so that palm of hand is up

Ligaments

Ligaments consisting of fibrous tissue connect two adjacent freely movable bones. They help protect the joints by stabilizing the joint surfaces and keeping them in proper alignment. In some instances, ligaments completely enclose a joint.

Cartilage

Cartilage is a firm, dense type of connective tissue that consists of cells embedded in a substance called the matrix. The matrix is firm and compact, thus enabling it to withstand pressure and torsion. Its primary functions are to reduce friction between articular surfaces, absorb shocks, and reduce stress on joint surfaces.

Hyaline or articular cartilage covers the surface of movable joints, such as the elbow, and acts as a protection for the surface of these joints. Other types of cartilage include costal cartilage, which connects the ribs and sternum, semilunar cartilage, which is one of the cartilages of the knee joint, fibrous cartilage, which is found between the vertebrae (intervertebral discs), and elastic cartilage, found in the larynx, epiglottis, and outer ear.

Bursae

A **bursa** is a small sac filled with synovial fluid. Bursae reduce friction between areas, such as tendon and bone and tendon and ligament. Inflammation of these sacs is called bursitis.

Assessment

Health History

The focus of the initial history depends on whether the client has a chronic disorder or whether there has been a recent injury. If the disorder is long-standing, obtain a thorough medical, drug, and allergy history. If the client is injured, find out when and how the trauma occurred. Compile a list of symptoms that includes information about the onset, duration, and location of discomfort or pain. Determine whether activity makes the symptoms better or worse. Also identify associated symptoms, such as muscle cramping or skin lesions. Ask the client if the problem interferes with activities of daily living. If the client has an open wound, determine when the client last received a tetanus immunization.

Obtain a history of past disorders and medical or surgical treatments as soon as possible. Attention to chronic or concurrent disorders, such as diabetes mellitus, is essential. Also obtain a family history, especially when relatives have had similar symptoms, and an occupational history.

Physical Examination

For a general musculoskeletal assessment, observe the client's ability to ambulate, sit, stand, and to perform activities requiring fine motor skills, such as grasping objects. General inspection includes examining the client for symmetry, size, and contour of extremities, and random movements. A spinal inspection includes identifying spinal curvatures (Fig. 65–1):

- Scoliosis—lateral curvature of the spine
- Kyphosis—exaggerated convex curvature of the thoracic spine (humpback)
- Lordosis—excessive concave curvature of the lumbar spine (swayback)

Palpate the muscles and joints to identify swelling, degree of firmness, local warm areas, and any involuntary movements. Test the client's muscle strength by applying force to the client's extremity as the client pushes against that force. Perform a neurovascular assessment (Table 65–3). Assess range of motion for the joints, taking care not to force movement. Note any abnormal muscle movements such as spasms or tremors. Make the following observations of the affected area:

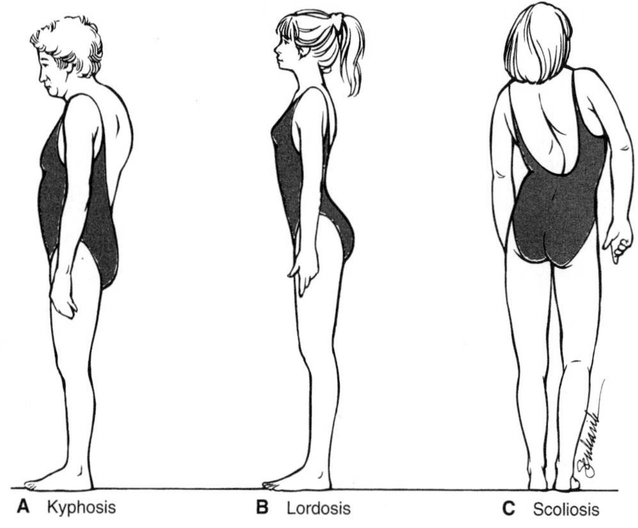

FIGURE 65-1. Common spinal curvatures.

TABLE 65-3 **Neurovascular Assessment Findings in Musculoskeletal Assessment**

Assessments	Normal Findings	Abnormal Findings
Circulation		
Distal pulses	Present and strong	Absent or weak
Capillary refill	Color returns to compressed nailbed in ≤ 3 seconds	Nailbed stays blanched ≥ 3 seconds
Skin color	Similar to color in other body areas	Pale or dusky
Skin temperature	Warm	Cold
Local edema	Absent	+1 to +4 swelling
Sensation		
Arm injury	Can identify pressure applied to the tip of the index finger (median nerve) and the fifth finger (ulnar nerve), web between the thumb (radial nerve)	Numb to touch; or feels abnormal sensation like tingling or burning
Leg injury	Can identify pressure applied to great toe (peroneal nerve), and sole of the foot at the base of the toes (posterior tibial nerve) without observing the stimulus	Same as above
Mobility		
Arm injury	Can spread fingers on affected hand (ulnar nerve)	Weak or unable to move fingers
	Able to press thumb to last digit on affected hand (median nerve)	Cannot approximate thumb to finger
	Demonstrates the "hitch-hiker's sign" with affected hand, can flex and extend wrist (radial nerve)	Unable to extend thumb Wrist drop is apparent
Leg injury	Can flex and extend ankle (peroneal and posterior tibial nerve)	Footdrop is apparent
Pain	Proportional to injury but relieved with analgesia or nursing interventions	Constant or increased despite implementation of pain-relieving techniques

- Look for abnormal size or alignment and symmetry; compare one side to the other.
- Inspect and palpate for pain, tenderness, swelling, and redness.
- Observe the degree of movement and range of motion, but never persist beyond the point of pain.
- Test for muscle strength.
- Inspect for muscle wasting.

Depending on the symptoms and findings, additional assessments may include looking for changes in gait and body posture, favoring one side over the other, and the client's ability to bend and twist the trunk, head, and extremities.

If the client has a traumatic injury, physical assessment begins with taking vital signs. Further assessment depends on the type and area of injury. Maintain standard precautions. Cut the clothing from around an injured area if there is no other way to examine the client. Compare structures and assessment findings on one side of the body with those on the opposite side. Be gentle but thorough; the assessment technique may increase the client's pain. The examination includes the following:

- Observe for swelling, external bleeding, or bruising.
- Palpate the peripheral pulses.
- Evaluate peripheral circulation, assessing peripheral pulse (rate and character), skin coloration (pink, gray, pale, ashen), temperature, capillary refill time.
- Check the sensation of the injured part.
- Look for broken skin, open wounds, superficial or embedded debris in or around the wound, protrusion of bone or other tissue from the wound.
- Look for injury beyond the original area; for example, auscultate the chest and abdomen if an abdominal or thoracic injury occurred. Check the pupils and mental status if a head injury occurred.
- Look for malalignment of the injured limb.
- Assess for pain; note the type and location.

The physician needs to examine the client before open wounds are touched, cleaned, or disturbed and before the injured extremity is moved.

Diagnostic and Laboratory Procedures

Radiography, Computed Tomography, and Magnetic Resonance Imaging

Radiographic films, computed tomography (CT), or magnetic resonance imaging (MRI) help to identify traumatic disorders, such as fractures and dislocations, and other bone disorders, such as malignant bone lesions, joint deformities, calcification, degenerative changes, osteoporosis, and joint disease.

Arthroscopy

Arthroscopy is the internal inspection of a joint by means of an instrument called an arthroscope. The most common use of arthroscopy is visualization of the knee joint, a common site of injury. After administering a local or general anesthetic, the physician inserts a large-bore needle into the joint and injects sterile normal saline solution to distend the joint. After inserting the arthroscope, the examiner inspects the joint for signs of injury or deterioration. Joint fluid may be removed and sent to the laboratory for examination. Depending on the findings, the physician can sometimes use the arthroscope to perform therapeutic procedures, such as removing bits of torn or floating cartilage.

Afterward, the client's entire leg is elevated without flexing the knee. A cold pack is placed over the bulky dressing covering the site where the arthroscope was inserted. A prescribed analgesic is administered as necessary. Nursing management strategies for a client undergoing arthroscopy appear in Nursing Guidelines 65–1.

Arthrocentesis

Arthrocentesis is the aspiration of synovial fluid. The client is given local anesthesia just before this procedure. The physician inserts a large needle into the joint and removes the fluid. Synovial fluid may be aspirated to relieve discomfort caused by an excessive accumulation in the joint space or to inject a drug, such as a corticosteroid preparation. The removed synovial fluid may be sent to the laboratory for microscopic examination or for culture and sensitivity studies. Arthrocentesis may also be performed at the time of an arthrogram or arthroscopy.

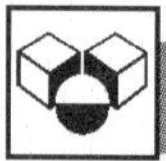

Nursing Guidelines 65-1

Assisting the Client Through Arthroscopy

Before the Procedure

- Explain procedure.
- Ensure that informed consent form is signed.
- Verify that client has been NPO for at least 6 hours.
- Administer preoperative medications, if ordered.

After the Procedure

- Instruct the client to report unusual pain, bleeding, drainage, or swelling at the arthroscopic site.
- Advise the client to resume usual diet as tolerated.
- Review discharge instructions with the client and explain medication regimen.
- Inspect dressing before discharge.

Arthrogram

An **arthrogram** is a radiographic examination of a joint, usually the knee or shoulder. The physician injects a local anesthetic and then inserts a needle into the joint space. Fluoroscopy may be used to verify correct placement of the needle. The synovial fluid in the joint is aspirated and sent to the laboratory for analysis. A contrast medium is then injected, and x-ray films are taken. After arthrography, the client is informed that crackling or clicking noises may be heard in the joint for up to 2 days. Noises continuing beyond this time are abnormal and should be reported.

Synovial Fluid Analysis

Synovial fluid is aspirated and examined to diagnose disorders such as traumatic arthritis, septic arthritis (which is caused by a microorganism), gout, rheumatic fever, and systemic lupus erythematosus. Normally, synovial fluid is clear and nearly colorless. Laboratory examination of synovial fluid may include microscopic examination for blood cells, crystals, and formed debris that may be present in the joint space following an injury. If an infection is suspected, culture and sensitivity studies are ordered. A chemical analysis for substances such as protein and glucose may also be performed.

Bone Scan

A **bone scan** uses the intravenous injection of a radionuclide to detect the uptake of the radioactive substance by the bone. A bone scan may be ordered to detect metastatic bone lesions, fractures, and certain types of inflammatory disorders. The radionuclide is taken up in areas of increased metabolism, which occurs in bone cancer, metastatic bone disease, and osteomyelitis (bone infection).

Biopsy

A biopsy is done to identify the composition of bone, muscle, or synovium. The specimen may be removed with a needle or excised surgically while the client is under general anesthesia. Afterwards, observe the site for signs of bleeding or swelling. Assess the client for pain. Apply ice to the site and administer analgesics as indicated.

Blood Tests

A complete blood count (includes a red blood cell count, hemoglobin level, white blood cell count, and differential) may be ordered to detect infection, inflammation, or anemia. Examples of other diagnostic blood tests and findings of various musculoskeletal disorders include:

- Elevated alkaline phosphatase level: bone tumors and healing fractures
- Elevated acid phosphatase level: Paget's disease (a disorder characterized by excessive bone destruction and disorganized repair) and metastatic cancer
- Decreased serum calcium level: osteomalacia, osteoporosis, and bone tumors
- Increased serum phosphorus level: bone tumors and healing fractures
- Elevated serum uric acid level: gout (treated or untreated)
- Elevated antinuclear antibody level: lupus erythematosus, a connective tissue disorder

Urine Tests

When ordered, collect 24-hour urine samples for analysis to determine levels of uric acid and calcium excretion. In gout, the 24-hour excretion of uric acid is elevated. Elevated calcium levels are found in metastatic bone lesions and in clients with prolonged immobility.

Nursing Management

Some diagnostic tests are performed while the client is being assessed in the emergency department, on an outpatient basis, or after admission for treatment of the disorder. The nurse implements protocols necessary to prepare the client for the diagnostic examination, identifies and sends collected specimens to the laboratory, and manages the client's safe recovery after invasive procedures.

If the client has a chronic disorder, a general medical history and a description of the current symptoms are obtained. Drug and allergy histories are compiled. An allergy to iodine and seafood may be a contraindication for performing an arthrogram or other test in which a contrast medium is instilled.

No special care is required after most laboratory tests, general radiography, or a bone scan. If the client has had an invasive joint examination, the area is inspected for swelling and bleeding or serous drainage. Any dressing is reinforced or changed as needed. If the client has severe pain in the area, the physician is informed. The physician may order the application of ice and an analgesic for pain or discomfort.

In the case of a traumatic injury, obtain information regarding the injury from the client, the individual accompanying the client, or paramedics and ambulance personnel. Vital signs are taken at the time of the initial examination and at frequent intervals until the client's condition stabilizes. Keep the client calm and promote comfort; for example, if the client has an injury of the arm, prepare a sling to ease pain until treatment can be initiated (Clinical Procedure 65–1).

NURSING PROCESS
The Client With a Musculoskeletal Injury

Assessment

Assess the client's injury in terms of the location and nature of the injury and the impact on the client's mobility. Determine the circulatory status to the injured area—check circulation, sensation, and mobility, if it is not contraindicated. Assess the client's level of pain. Monitor the client's vital signs and closely observe the client for signs of shock.

Diagnosis and Planning

Nursing management of the client with an orthopedic injury includes, but is not limited to, the following:

Nursing Diagnoses and Collaborative Problems	Nursing Interventions
Pain related to tissue injury **Goal:** Client will have relief from pain.	Minimize or avoid moving the painful body part. If the client must be moved from a stretcher, wheelchair, or an examination table, request sufficient help and support the joints above and below the area of discomfort during transfer. Support an acutely or chronically inflamed joint in a comfortable position. Elevate a swollen extremity as long as this does not potentiate the trauma from an injury, or cradle a painful arm in a sling when the client is up and about.

	Observe for signs of shock if administering a prescribed narcotic analgesic for pain relief to a client with a traumatic injury.
	Notify physician, if pain increases or is unrelieved.
Risk for Impaired Tissue Perfusion related to swelling, inflammation or inactivity imposed by injury	Keep a swollen body part above the level of the heart to promote venous circulation and relieve edema.
Goal: Client will maintain tissue perfusion in the injured area as evidenced by normal neurovascular assessment findings.	Consult with the physician about applying a cold pack if an injury is recent.
	Elevate the head slightly while keeping the neck in a neutral position if a head injury has occurred.
	Report the absence of a peripheral pulse and severe pain immediately because this may indicate ischemia.
Anxiety related to pain and injury, its treatment, and the potential for altered mobility	Relieve discomfort as much as possible to reduce at least one aspect of the client's concerns.
Goal: Client's anxiety will be reduced as evidenced by vital signs within normal range, no signs of being overly alert or easily startled.	Call the client by name; be empathic and attentive.
	Instill confidence by demonstrating technical skill and competence in explanations or preparations for tests or treatments.
	Speak quietly in simple sentences that the client can understand.
	Allow a supportive family member to stay with the client if possible.

Client and Family Teaching

Provide a brief, broad overview of the diagnostic tests or treatments because comprehension of details is difficult when a client is anxious. Tell the client and family how long the test or examination will take, where it will be done, and what preparations (if any) are necessary. Allow the client an opportunity to ask questions or make comments as the information is processed. Before carrying out any preliminary activities prior to a diagnostic test, describe what is about to be done.

Invasive procedures, such as an arthroscopy, and treatment procedures require the client to sign a consent form. It is the responsibility of the physician to explain the purpose for the procedure, the risks, benefits, and available alternatives available. Repeat or clarify the physician's explanations. After an outpatient procedure, the physician often gives the client special instructions for self-care. However, because recalling information from memory can lead to confusion or injury, provide the client with written discharge instructions as well. Information that may be identified includes:

- Signs or symptoms that need reporting such as excessive pain or throbbing, prolonged or fresh bleeding, swelling, skin color changes, decrease in sensation, or purulent drainage
- Any special body position that must be maintained
- When bathing and activity may be resumed
- How soon the client may return to work
- Purpose of prescribed drugs, how they are to be taken, and side effects that may be experienced
- Approximate date for a follow-up appointment with the physician, if one is required
- How to remove and reapply dressings, and how to apply an immobilizer or sling, if one is used
- If the client is required to use crutches temporarily, provide instructions and demonstrations of the crutch-walking gait to use and how to ensure safety.

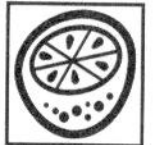

General Nutritional Considerations

Although bone formation and resorption are continuous throughout life, net bone loss exceed net bone gain in all people after peak bone mass is attained, sometime between the ages of 30 to 35. An adequate calcium intake prior to that time helps maximize peak bone mass; the denser the bones, the less susceptible they are to fracture.

Because most Americans do not eat enough calcium to protect against bone loss, the Institute of Medicine of the National Academy of Sciences has issued new calcium recommendations that are higher than the previous RDAs for almost all age groups. Adults under age 50 are advised to consume 1000 mg of calcium daily; those over 50 need 1200 mg daily, which translates to about four servings from the milk group each day. Clients who are not able or willing to consume ample dairy products are not likely to meet their calcium requirement through diet alone.

Nondairy sources of calcium include green leafy vegetables, sardines, canned salmon with bones, broccoli, and calcium-fortified orange juice. With the exception of calcium-fortified orange juice, the calcium from nondairy sources is not absorbed well.

Vitamin D protects against bone loss and decreases the risk of fracture by facilitating the absorption of calcium from food and supplements. Without adequate vitamin D, calcium is excreted, not absorbed, even if calcium intake is adequate. Many people do not consume enough vitamin D because dietary sources are limited to fatty fish and vitamin D-fortified milk and cereals. Skin makes vitamin D when exposed to sunlight, but older skin makes less, and sun exposure does not produce vitamin D during the winter in people living in northern climates.

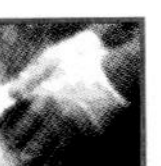

Clinical Procedure 65-1
Applying an Arm Sling

PURPOSE	EQUIPMENT
• To elevate, cradle, and support the arm following an injury • To reduce arm pain	• Commercial (canvas) sling or triangular muslin cloth • Safety pin if needed to secure triangular sling

Nursing Action	Rationale
ASSESSMENT	
Check the medical orders	Coordinates nursing activities with medical treatment
Assess the color, skin temperature, capillary refill time, and amount of edema. Verify peripheral pulse in injured arm.	Provides objective baseline data for future comparisons
Ask the client to describe how the fingers or arm feel, and to rate the pain, if it is present, on a scale of 1 to 10.	Provides baseline subjective data for future comparisons
Determine if the client has ever required an arm sling in the past.	Indicates the level and type of health teaching needed
PLANNING	
Explain the purpose of the sling.	Adds to the client's understanding
Obtain a canvas or triangular sling, whichever is available or prescribed for use.	Complies with medical practice
IMPLEMENTATION	
Have the client sit or lie down.	Promotes comfort and facilitates applying the sling
Position forearm across the client's chest with the thumb pointing upward.	Flexes the elbow
Avoid more than 90° of flexion, especially if the elbow has been injured.	Facilitates circulation

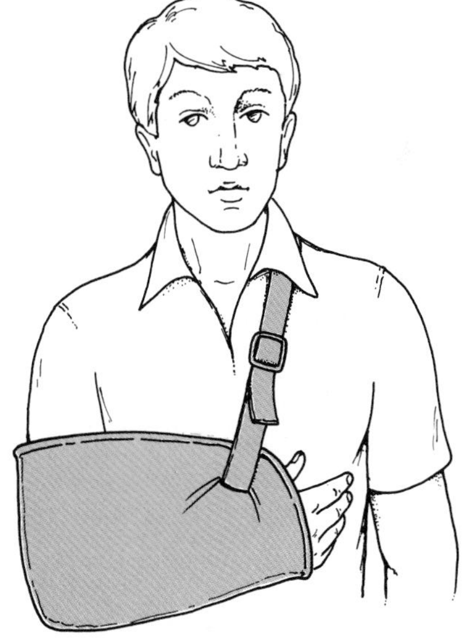

Commercial arm sling.

Nursing Action	Rationale
Slip the flexed arm into the sling so that the elbow fits flush with the corner of the sling.	Encloses the forearm and wrist
Bring the strap around the opposing shoulder and fasten it to the sling.	Provides the means for support
Tighten the strap sufficiently to keep the elbow flexed and the wrist elevated.	Promotes circulation

continued

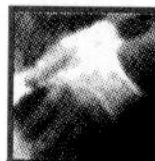

Clinical Procedure 65-1
Continued

Nursing Action	Rationale
Triangular sling	
Place the longer side of the sling on the chest (opposite the injured arm) from shoulder to the waist.	Positions the sling where length is needed

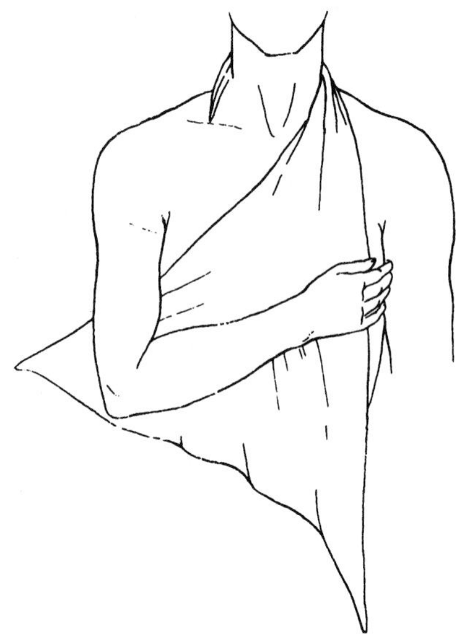

Positioning a triangular sling.

Nursing Action	Rationale
Position the apex or the point of the triangle under the elbow.	Facilitates making a hammock for the arm
Bring the points together at the neck and tie them.	Encloses the injured arm
Keep the knot to the side of the neck.	Avoids pressure on the vertebrae

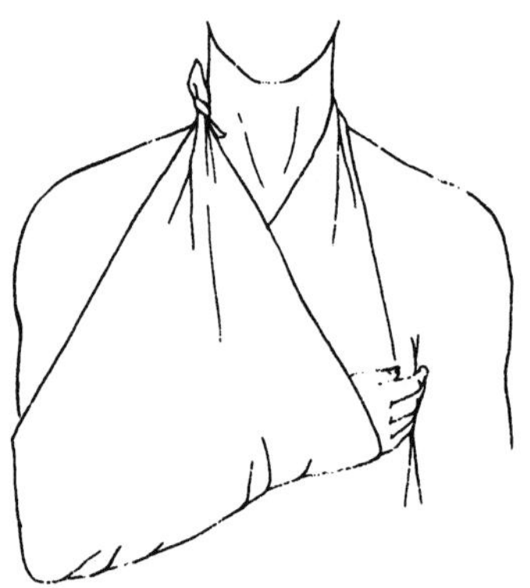

Completed sling.

Nursing Action	Rationale
Fold and secure excess fabric at the elbow; a safety pin may be necessary.	Keeps the elbow enclosed
Inspect the condition of the skin at the neck, and the circulation, mobility, and sensation of the fingers at least once every 8 hours.	Provides comparative data
Pad the skin at the neck with soft gauze or towel material, if the skin becomes irritated.	Reduces pressure and friction
Instruct the client to report any changes in sensation or level of pain.	Indicates developing complications

Sunscreen, smog, and clothing block the ultraviolet light that makes vitamin D.

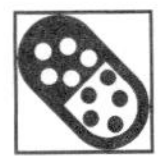

General Pharmacologic Considerations

Oral calcium preparations containing vitamin D are better absorbed than those without vitamin D.

Oral calcium preparations should not be taken with other oral drugs because absorption of the other drugs may be altered or blocked. For example, calcium decreases absorption of tetracycline and phenytoin. Take other drugs 1 to 2 hours after calcium carbonate.

Oral calcium should be taken with meals to enhance absorption as well as to minimize gastric distress.

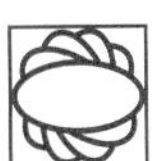

General Gerontologic Considerations

Women over age 45 have a 9% or 10% decrease in cortical bone per decade.

Older adults are more prone to skeletal fractures because bone resorption occurs more rapidly than bone formation.

Maintaining an active lifestyle delays the decline in muscle strength and bone mass among older adults.

With age the fibrocartilage of intervertebral disks become thinner and drier, causing compression of the disks of the spinal column and leading to a loss of height amounting to as much as 1.5 to 3 inches (3.75 to 7.5 cm).

Estrogen deficiency, which occurs at menopause, is considered the leading factor in osteoporosis among aging women.

With age, the water content of joint cartilage decreases, leading to a loss of height, which amounts to as much as 1.5 to 3 inches (3.75–7.5 cm).

SUMMARY OF KEY CONCEPTS

- The musculoskeletal system consists of bones, muscles, joints, tendons, ligaments, cartilage, and bursae. Collectively these structures are responsible for locomotion, the storage of calcium, production of blood cells, and protection and support for many organs.
- When assessing a client with an orthopedic disorder, it is important to determine the client's chief complaint, which is often pain, and other current signs and symptoms that are being experienced. A thorough history of the client's medical disorders, surgical treatment, and drug and allergy history are also obtained. The client is physically assessed with a focus on examining the area of discomfort and identifying changes in appearance, such as color, size, alignment, weakness, and restricted range of motion. If trauma has occurred, the nurse looks for signs of skin impairment, swelling, bleeding, impaired circulation, and sensation. Signs of internal injuries in the area of trauma also are investigated.
- The client's musculoskeletal disorder is often confirmed from diagnostic tests, such as x-rays, CT scans, MRI, arthroscopy, arthrocentesis, arthrogram, bone scan, and biopsy.
- Laboratory tests used to detect orthopedic and musculoskeletal disorders include a complete blood count, alkaline and acid phosphatase levels, serum calcium and phosphorus, uric acid, antinuclear antibodies, and 24-hour urine collection.
- When a client is having diagnostic tests, the nurse promotes the client's comfort, uses techniques for relieving anxiety, explains the procedures that will be implemented, carries out the pre-examination procedures, identifies and sends specimens to the laboratory, manages the client's safe recovery after invasive procedures, and provides instructions that the client can follow for self-care following discharge.

CRITICAL THINKING EXERCISES

1. A client you are caring for in a nursing home falls. Describe what assessments you would make.
2. What signs and symptoms would indicate to the nurse that the tissue in an injured extremity is not being adequately perfused?

Suggested Readings

Bove, L. A. (1996). Calcium and phosphorus. *RN, 3*, 47–51.

Bullock, B. L. (1996). *Pathophysiology: Adaptations and alterations in function* (4th ed.). Philadelphia: Lippincott-Raven.

Fischbach, F. T. (1996). *A manual of laboratory and diagnostic tests* (5th ed.). Philadelphia: J. B. Lippincott.

Roberts, A. (1992, January 8–14). Bone and bones, part 2. *Nursing Times, 88*, 47.

Roberts, A. (1992, February 12–18). Bone and bones, part 3. *Nursing Times, 88*, 53.

Roberts, A. (1992, March 11–17). Joints, part 1. *Nursing Times, 88*, 39.

Roberts, A. (1992, April 8–14). Joints, part 2. *Nursing Times, 88*, 61.

Roberts, A. (1992, May 13–19). Muscle, part 1. *Nursing Times, 88*, 43.

Roberts, A. (1992, June 10–16). Muscle, part 2. *Nursing Times, 88*, 57.2.

Roberts, A. (1992, July 8–14). Muscle, part 3. *Nursing Times, 88*, 43.

Smeltzer, S. C., & Bare, B. G. (1996). *Brunner and Suddarth's textbook of medical-surgical nursing* (8th ed.) Philadelphia: Lippincott-Raven.

Timby, B. K. (1996). *Fundamental skills and concepts in patient care* (6th ed.). Philadelphia: Lippincott-Raven.

Chapter 66

Caring for Clients With Orthopedic and Connective Tissue Disorders

KEY TERMS

Ankylosing spondylitis
Ankylosis
Arthritis
Arthrodesis
Arthroplasty
Avascular necrosis
Avulsion fracture
Bouchard's nodes
Bursitis
Callus
Carpal tunnel syndrome
Cast
Closed reduction
Compartment syndrome
Contusion
Degenerative joint disease
Dislocation
Ecchymosis
Epicondylitis
External fixation
Fasciotomy
Fibrous ankylosis
Fracture
Gout
Heberden's nodes
Hallux valgus
Hammertoe
Hyperuricemia
Internal fixation
Involucrum
Lupus erythematosus
Lyme disease
Open reduction
Osseous ankylosis
Osteomalacia
Osteomyelitis
Osteoporosis
Osteotomy
Paget's disease
Palsy
Pannus
Rheumatoid arthritis
Rheumatic disorder
Sequestrum
Sprain
Strain
Subluxation
Synovectomy
Synovitis
Tophi
Traction
Volkmann's contracture

LEARNING OBJECTIVES

On completion of this chapter, the reader will:

- Differentiate strains, contusions, and sprains.
- Describe the signs and symptoms of a fracture and the common treatments.
- Identify the principles for maintaining traction.
- Discuss the complications associated with a fractured hip.
- Describe the difference between rheumatoid arthritis and degenerative joint disease.
- Describe the positioning precautions following a total hip replacement.
- State the pathophysiology of gout, bursitis, and ankylosing spondylitis.
- Explain the inflammatory process associated with Lyme disease.
- Identify the causes of osteomyelitis.
- Discuss the multisystem involvement associated with systemic lupus erythematosus.
- Describe methods to prevent or reduce low back pain due to poor posture and body mechanics.
- State who is at risk for developing osteoporosis.
- Differentiate between bunions and hammer toe.
- Explain the cause of carpal tunnel syndrome.
- Discuss characteristics of malignant bone tumors.
- Identify reasons that orthopedic surgery may be done.
- Describe four principles followed when wrapping a stump.
- Discuss the nursing management for a client with a sprain, dislocation, or cast; who is in traction or undergoing orthopedic surgery; or with an amputation.

The musculoskeletal system consists of structures the body uses for support and movement. It also protects body organs. Disorders affecting the musculoskeletal system affect an individual's ability to perform activities of daily living (ADL) and to remain active, mobile, and physically fit.

Traumatic Injuries

Strains, Contusions, and Sprains

A **strain** is an injury to a muscle when it is stretched or pulled beyond its capacity. A **contusion** is a soft tissue injury resulting from a blow or blunt trauma. **Sprains** are injuries to the ligaments surrounding a joint.

ETIOLOGY AND PATHOPHYSIOLOGY

A strain results from excessive stress, overuse, or overstretching. Small blood vessels within the muscle rupture and the muscle fibers sustain tiny tears. The client experiences inflammation, local tenderness, and muscle spasms.

In contusions, injury is confined to the soft tissues and does not affect the musculoskeletal structure. Many small blood vessels rupture, causing bruises (**ecchymosis**) or a hematoma (collection of blood). Applying cold packs helps alleviate the symptoms of local pain, swelling, and bruising. A contusion generally resolves within 2 weeks.

Areas most subject to sprains are the wrist, elbow, knee, and ankle. A sprain of the cervical spine is commonly called a whiplash injury. Sprains result from sudden, unusual movement or stretching about a joint, common with falls or other accidental injuries. The force twists the joint in a direction that it was not designed to move to or displaces it beyond its normal range of motion (ROM) by partially tearing or rupturing the attachment of ligaments. The damage is usually confined to the ligaments and adjacent soft tissue. However, in severe traumatic sprains, a chip of bone to which the ligament is attached may become detached. At this point, the injury becomes an **avulsion fracture.** A hematoma that may develop subsequently contributes to the pain because the mass exerts additional pressure on nerve endings in the area.

ASSESSMENT FINDINGS

Signs and Symptoms

The injured area becomes painful immediately, and swelling usually follows. The person typically avoids full weight-bearing or use of the injured joint or limb. Later, ecchymoses may appear. In cases of extensive ligamental tearing, the joint may be unstable until healing occurs.

Diagnostic Findings

In most cases, diagnosis is made by examination of the affected part and symptoms. Radiographic films may show a larger than usual joint space and rule out or confirm an accompanying fracture. Arthrography demonstrates asymmetry in the joint due to the damaged ligaments or arthroscopy may disclose trauma within the joint capsule.

MEDICAL AND SURGICAL MANAGEMENT

Treatment consists of applying ice or a chemical cold pack to the area to reduce swelling and relieve pain for the first 24 to 48 hours after the injury. Elevation of the part and compression with an elastic bandage also may be recommended. After 2 days, when swelling is no longer likely to increase, applying heat reduces pain and relieves local edema by improving circulation. Full use of the injured joint is discouraged temporarily. Nonsteroidal anti-inflammatory drugs (NSAIDs) ease the discomfort of the injury.

Continued trauma during the healing period may result in a permanently unstable joint or the formation of fibrous adhesions that may limit full ROM. Occasionally, a removable splint or light cast is applied for several weeks. A soft cervical collar limits motion if the client has a neck sprain. When sufficient healing has occurred, progressively active exercises are prescribed.

Dislocations

Dislocations occur when the articular surfaces of a joint are no longer in contact. The shoulder, hip, and knee are commonly affected. A partial dislocation is referred to as a **subluxation.**

ETIOLOGY AND PATHOPHYSIOLOGY

In adults, trauma generally causes dislocations. Occasionally diseases of the joint result in dislocations when the ligaments supporting a joint are torn, stretched, or relaxed.

Separation of adjacent bones from their articulating joint interferes with normal use and produces a distorted appearance. The injury may disrupt the local blood supply to structures such as the joint cartilage, causing degeneration, chronic pain, and restricted movement. **Compartment syndrome** (a condition in which a structure such as a tendon or nerve is constricted within a confined space) may also develop. Nerve innervation is affected, leading to a subsequent **palsy** (decreased sensation and movement). If insufficient collagen is deposited during the repair stage, the ligaments may have reduced tensile strength and future instability leading to recurrent dislocations of the same joint.

ASSESSMENT FINDINGS

Signs and Symptoms

The client often reports hearing a "popping" sound when the dislocation occurs. Another common complaint is that the joint suddenly "gave out," implying that it became unstable or nonsupportive. If the dislocation results from trauma, the client usually experiences considerable pain from the injury or the resultant muscle spasm.

On inspection, the structural shape is altered. A depression may be noted about the circumference of the joint, indicating that the bone above and below are no longer in alignment. If the dislocation affects an extremity, the arm or leg may be shorter than its unaffected counterpart due to the displacement of one of the articulating bones. ROM is limited. Evidence of soft tissue injury includes swelling, coolness, numbness, tingling, and pale or dusky color of the distal tissue.

Diagnostic Findings

Radiographic films show intact yet malpositioned bones. Arthrography or arthroscopy may reveal damage to other structures within the joint capsule.

MEDICAL AND SURGICAL MANAGEMENT

The physician manipulates the joint until the parts return to normal position, then immobilizes the joint with an elastic bandage, cast, or splint, for several weeks. This allows the joint capsule and surrounding ligaments to heal. The client may receive a local or general anesthetic before the manipulation is performed. Some dislocations may require surgery, either to correct the dislocation or to repair damage caused by the injury.

NURSING MANAGEMENT

Relieve the client's discomfort by administering prescribed analgesics, elevating and immobilizing the affected limb, and applying cold packs to the injury. Perform neurovascular assessments every 30 minutes for several hours and then at least every 2 to 4 hours for the next 1 or 2 days to detect complications such as compartment syndrome. See Chapter 65 (Table 65–3) for more information.

Fractures

A **fracture** is a break in the continuity of a bone. Tissues or organs in close proximity to the bones may be affected also. Fractures are classified according to type and extent (Table 66–1 and Fig. 66–1).

ETIOLOGY AND PATHOPHYSIOLOGY

When force applied to a bone exceeds maximum resistance, the bone breaks. Most fractures are caused by sudden direct force from a blow or fall. However, some may occur from indirect force—for example, a

TABLE 66-1 **Classifying Fractures**

Type of Fracture	Description
Open (compound)	The broken bone protrudes through the skin.
Closed (simple)	The broken bone is contained within intact skin.
Displaced	The broken bone is malaligned.
Greenstick	The bone bends and splits, but it does not break completely; common in children.
Complete	The break line goes completely through the bone.
Comminuted	The bone splinters into many small fragments at the fracture site.
Impacted	One portion of the bone is driven into another.
Depressed	Bone is driven inward; common in the skull.
Compression	The bone is compacted together.
Transverse, oblique, longitudinal, spiral	The break line occurs in the described direction.
Avulsion	A fragment of bone chips off when an attached ligament or tendon is injured.
Stress (fatigue)	A break occurs when the bone cannot withstand repeated impact, even that delivered at levels of submaximal force; common among athletes.
Complicated	The fracture involves injury to the surrounding tissues, such as blood vessels, nerves, muscles, tendons, joints, or internal organs.
Pathologic (spontaneous)	The bone breaks with normal activity or minor force after being weakened by a disease process.

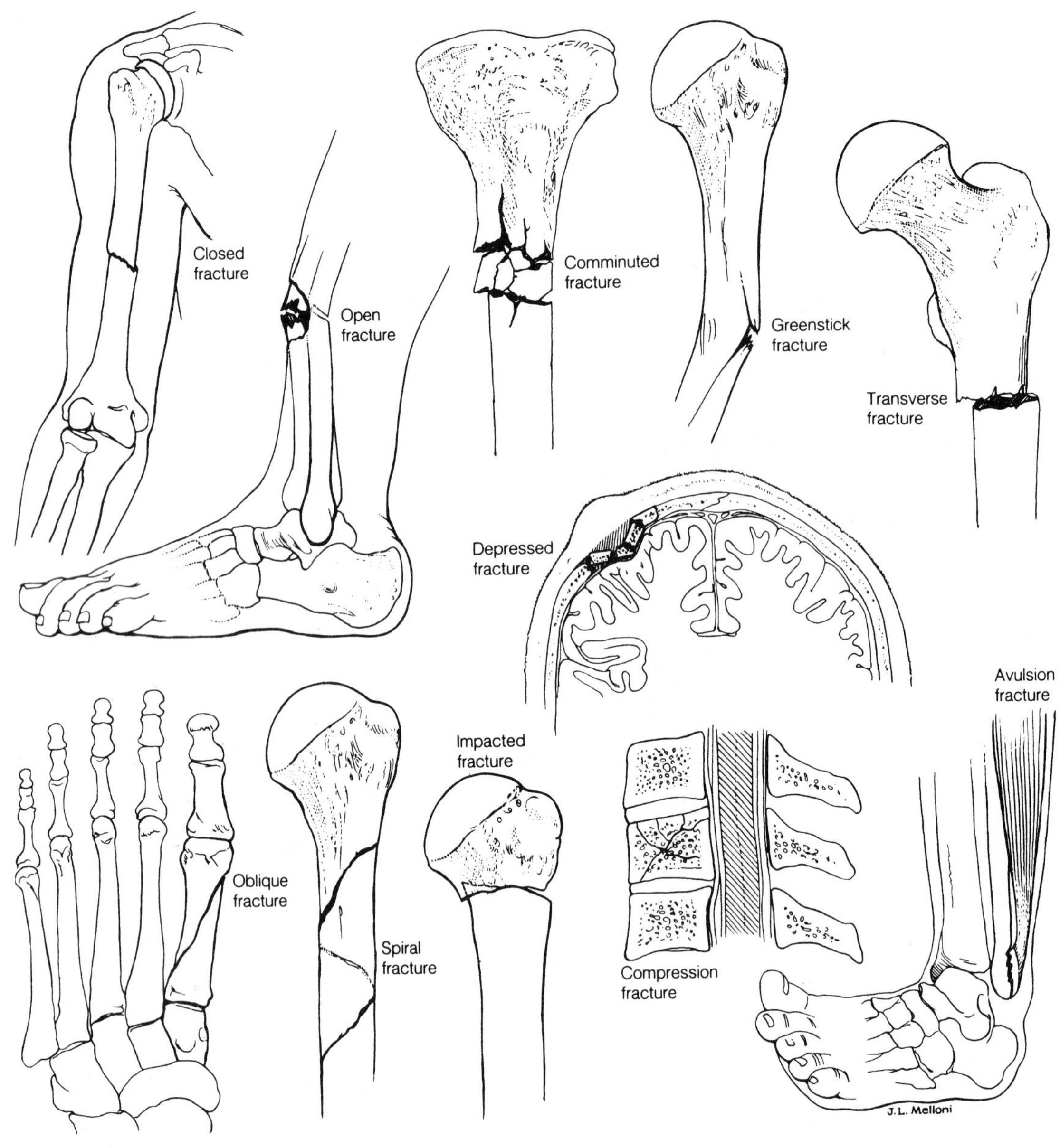

FIGURE 66-1. Types of fractures.

strong muscle contraction, such as that which occurs in a seizure. A few fractures result from an underlying weakness created by bone infections, bone tumors, or more bone resorption than production as occurs in individuals who are inactive or aging.

For 10 to 40 minutes after a bone breaks, the muscles surrounding the bone are flaccid. Then they go into spasm, often increasing deformity and interfering with the vascular and lymphatic circulations. The tissue surrounding the fracture swells from hemorrhage and edema. Healing begins (Fig. 66–2) when blood in the area clots and a fibrin network forms between the broken bone ends. The fibrin network changes into granulation tissue. Osteoblasts, which proliferate in the clot, increase the secretion of an enzyme that restores the alkaline pH. As a result, calcium is deposited and true bone forms. The healing mass is called a **callus.** It holds the ends of the bone together, but cannot endure strain. Bone repair is a local process. About a year of healing occurs before bone regains its former structural strength, becomes well consolidated and remodeled (re-formed), and possesses fat and marrow cells.

Although fractures are a common occurrence, they are associated with a variety of complications, particularly if the fracture is very complex. Table 66–2 briefly describes the types of complications that can occur. Complications of a fracture include compartment syndrome, thromboembolism, fat embolism, delayed healing, nonunion, malunion, infection, and

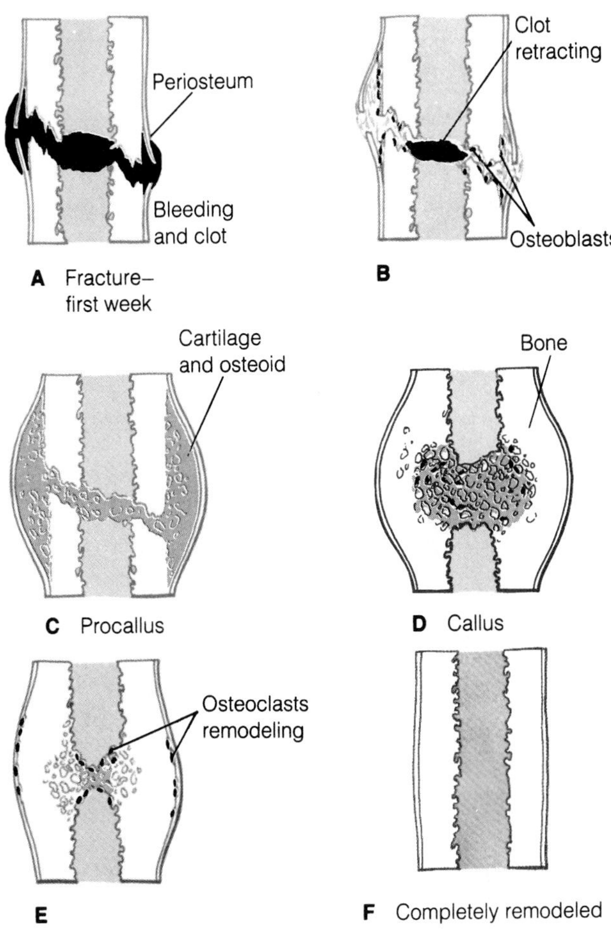

FIGURE 66-2. Process of bone healing. (*A*) Immediately after a bone fractures, blood seeps into the area and a hematoma (blood clot) forms. (*B*) After 1 week, osteoblasts form as the clot retracts. (*C*) After about 3 weeks, a procallus forms and stabilizes the fracture. (*D*) A callus with bone cells forms in 6 to 12 weeks. (*E*) In 3 to 4 months, osteoblasts begin to remodel the fracture site. (*F*) If the fractured bone has been accurately aligned during healing, remodeling will be complete in about 12 months.

avascular necrosis (death of bone due to insufficient blood supply). In addition, any client who is inactive during convalescence is prone to pneumonia, thrombophlebitis, pressure sores, urinary tract infection, renal calculi, constipation, muscle atrophy, weight gain, and depression.

ASSESSMENT FINDINGS

Signs and Symptoms

The signs and symptoms of a fracture vary, depending on the type and location of the fracture. They include:

- Pain—One of the most consistent symptoms of a fracture is pain. It may be severe and is increased by attempts to move the part and by pressure over the fracture.
- Loss of function—Skeletal muscular function depends on an intact bone.
- Deformity—A break may cause an extremity to bend backward or to assume another unusual position.
- False motion—Unnatural motion occurs at the site of the fracture.
- Crepitus—The grating sound of bone ends as they move over one another may be heard (this term also refers to a popping sound caused by air trapped in soft tissue).
- Edema—Swelling usually is greatest directly over the fracture.
- Spasm—Muscles near fractures involuntarily contract. Spasm, which accounts for some of the pain, may result in the shortening of a limb when a long bone is involved.

If sharp bone fragments tear through sufficient surrounding soft tissue, there will be bleeding and black and blue discoloration of the area. If a nerve is damaged, paralysis may result.

Diagnostic Findings

One or more radiographic views of the area almost always demonstrate an alteration in the structure of the bone. Stress fractures may not be apparent radiographically for a couple of weeks. A bone scan can usually identify a nondisplaced or stress fracture before radiographic changes become evident. In some instances, a computed tomography (CT) scan or magnetic resonance imaging (MRI) may be necessary.

MEDICAL AND SURGICAL MANAGEMENT

The aim of treatment is to re-establish functional continuity of the bone. Treatment of fractures includes one or a combination of methods: traction, closed or open reduction, internal or external fixation, or a cast application. The method of treatment depends on many factors, including the first aid given, the location and severity of the break, and the age and overall physical condition of the client.

Traction

Traction is a method of pulling structures of the musculoskeletal system. For traction to achieve its purpose, it requires countertraction, a force opposite to the mechanical pull, that is usually supplied by the client's own weight. Traction is used to relieve muscle spasm, align bones, and maintain immobilization. The two most common types are skin traction and skeletal traction.

Skin traction is achieved by applying devices to the skin that indirectly affect the muscles or bones. An ex-

TABLE 66-2 **Complications of Fractures**

Complication	Description	Nursing Implications
Shock	Hypovolemic shock related to blood loss and loss of extracellular fluid from damaged tissue. If untreated, the client's condition will deteriorate.	Administer blood and fluid volume replacements as prescribed to prevent further losses.
Fat embolism	Fat globules released following fractures of pelvis or long bones, or after multiple injuries or crushing injuries. Globules combine with platelets to form emboli. Onset is rapid, with client experiencing respiratory distress and cerebral disturbances.	Monitor client for symptoms, which usually occur within 48–72 hours. To prevent fatty emboli, provide early respiratory support, ensure rapid immobilization of fracture, and observe client closely for signs of respiratory and nervous system problems.
Pulmonary embolism	Thromboembolism may occur after fracture or surgery to repair fractures. These lead to pulmonary emboli in some clients and can be fatal.	Promote circulation and prevent venous stasis to avoid pulmonary embolism. Administer low-dose heparin subcutaneously as prescribed to prevent clot formation.
Compartment syndrome	Tissue perfusion in the muscle compartment (muscle covered by inelastic fascia) is compromised secondary to tissue swelling, hemorrhage, or a cast that is too tight. If circulation is not restored, ischemia and tissue anoxia lead to permanent nerve damage, muscle atrophy, and contracture.	Monitor client for signs and symptoms of compartment syndrome such as unrelenting pain, unrelieved by analgesics. Elevate the extremity, apply ice, and perform neurovascular checks to help prevent this complication. As indicated, relieve pressure by loosening cast or preparing the client for a **fasciotomy** (surgical incision of fascia and separation of muscles).
Delayed bone healing	Bone fails to heal at the expected rate. Delayed healing may result from nonunion, characterized by the ends of the fractured bone failing to unite and heal, or it may result from malunion, characterized by the ends of the fractured bone healing in a deformed position.	Delayed union may require surgical intervention to promote bone growth, and correct the incorrect union. If necessary, prepare the client for use of electrical stimulation measures that promote bone growth or for a bone graft.
Infection	The potential for infection increases with compound fractures, application of skeletal traction, or surgical procedures.	Perform careful assessments and maintain aseptic technique to prevent infections. Monitor for early signs of infection because early detection promotes early correction of the problem.
Avascular necrosis	This condition occurs from interruption of the blood supply to the fracture fragments after which the bone tissue dies; most common in the femoral head.	Be alert for client reports of pain and decreased function of the affected limb. If necessary, prepare the client for surgery, such as bone graft, bone prosthesis, joint replacement, joint fusion, or amputation.

ample of skin traction is Buck's traction; another example is Russell traction (Fig. 66–3). Skeletal traction is applied directly to a bone by using a wire (Kirschner), pin (Steinmann), or cranial tongs (Crutchfield). General or local anesthesia may be used when inserting these devices. The pull is achieved by connecting the attachment from the client to a system of ropes, pulleys, and weights on an orthopedic bed frame. A Thomas splint with a Pearson attachment is often used to suspend a leg in traction. This is referred to as balanced suspension traction. Figure 66–4 presents an example of skeletal traction with balanced suspension. The principles for maintaining effective traction are discussed in Box 66–1. Nursing care measures for a client in traction are presented in Nursing Guidelines 66–1.

Closed Reduction

In a **closed reduction,** the bone is restored to its normal position by external manipulation. The area is then immobilized with a bandage, cast, or traction, and x-ray films are made to be sure the bone is correctly aligned. Depending on the site and type of fracture, the client receives a local (nerve block) or general anesthetic for this procedure.

Open Reduction

In an **open reduction,** which is performed in the operating room, the bone is surgically exposed and realigned. Usually the client receives a general or spinal anesthetic. Radiographic studies, taken while the client is still anesthetized, show whether realignments are needed.

Internal Fixation

If **internal fixation** is needed to stabilize the reduced fracture, the surgeon secures the bone with metal screws, plates, rods, nails, or pins. A cast or other method of immobilization is then applied. Open reduction is required when:

- Soft tissue, such as nerves or blood vessels, are caught between the ends of the broken pieces of bone.
- The bone has a wide separation.

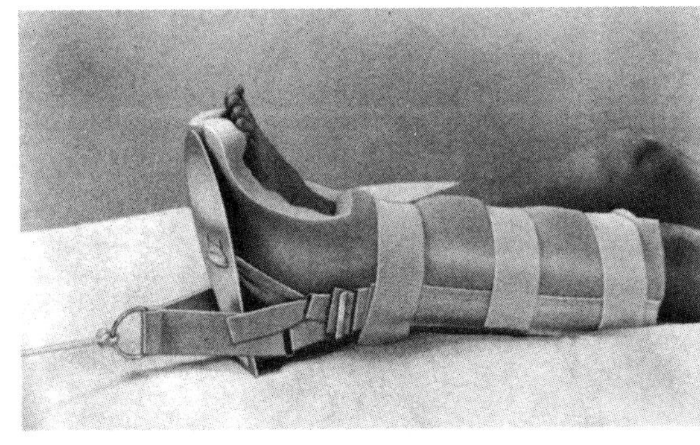

A

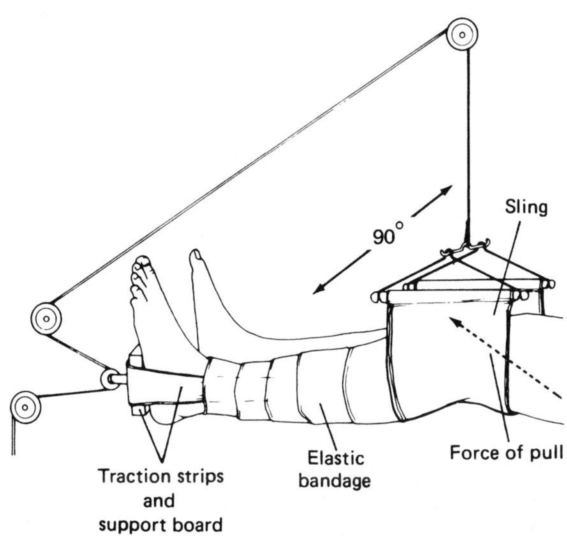

B

FIGURE 66-3. Two examples of skin traction: (*A*) Buck's traction. (*B*) Russel traction.

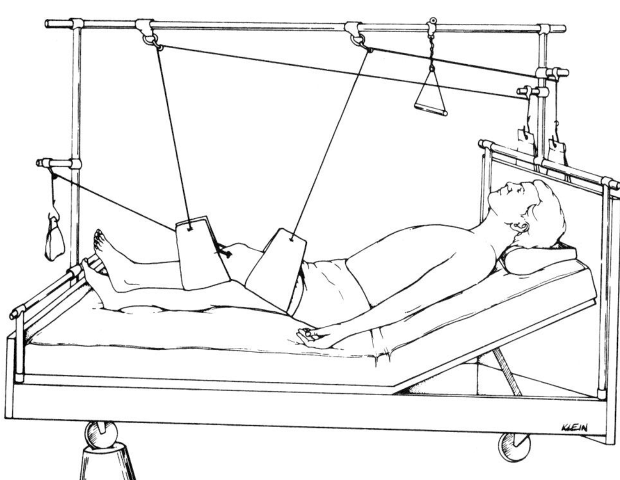

FIGURE 66-4. Skeletal traction with balanced suspension.

BOX 66-1 Principles of Effective Traction

- Ensure continuous traction.
- Maintain countertraction.
- See that the pull of traction and countertraction are in opposite directions but in straight alignment.
- Suspend splints and slings without interference.
- Be sure that ropes move freely through each pulley.
- Apply the exact amount of weight prescribed.
- Make sure that the weights hang free.

- Comminuted fractures are present.
- Patella and other joints are fractured.
- Open fractures are evident.
- Wound debridement is necessary.
- Internal fixation is needed.

External Fixation

In **external fixation,** the surgeon inserts metal pins into the bone or bones from outside the skin surface and then attaches a compression device to the pins. Some complex or comminuted fractures may require an external fixation device, to stabilize and position the bone. Because the pin sites are an entry for infection, monitor for redness, drainage, and tenderness (Clinical Procedure 66–1 discusses pin care).

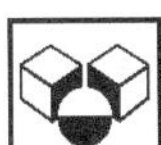

Nursing Guidelines 66-1

Managing the Care of the Client in Traction

- Assess the client's neurovascular status frequently. Compare assessment findings in the affected limb to those in the unaffected limb.
- Check traction equipment for:
  - Proper alignment (position client so that the body is in an opposite line to the pull of traction)
  - Correct attachment
  - Prescribed amount of weight
  - Freely hanging weights and freely moving ropes over unobstructed pulleys
  - Maintenance of countertraction
- Monitor client for signs of pressure areas.
- Encourage client to be as mobile as possible and to perform exercises as indicated.
- If traction is applied to the lower extremity, observe foot position and prevent footdrop.
- If skeletal traction is applied, follow procedure for pin care.
- Cover tips of any protruding metal pins or rods with corks or other protective material.

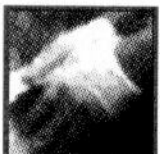

Clinical Procedure 66-1
Providing Pin Care

PURPOSE

- To prevent localized infection at the pin sites
- To prevent systemic infection and osteomyelitis

EQUIPMENT

- Prescribed cleansing agent
- Gloves
- Cotton-tipped applicators

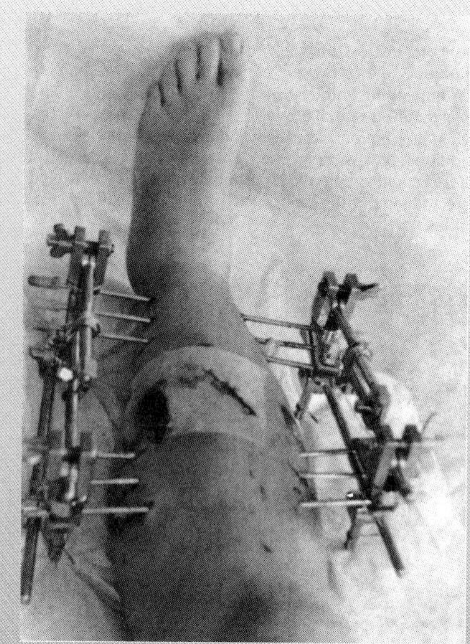

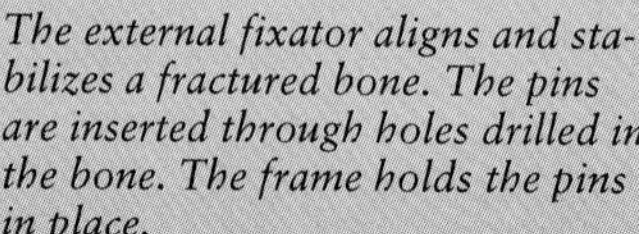

The external fixator aligns and stabilizes a fractured bone. The pins are inserted through holes drilled in the bone. The frame holds the pins in place.

Nursing Action	Rationale
ASSESSMENT	
Check the medical orders.	Integrates nursing activities and medical treatment
Assess the area around the pin site for redness, swelling, increased tenderness, and drainage.	Provides baseline data for future comparisons
Examine pin for signs of breakage, bending, or shifting.	Identifies potential problems with maintaining traction or the fixator
PLANNING	
Explain the purpose of pin care.	Adds to the client's understanding
Assemble the necessary equipment in one place.	Contributes to organization and efficient time management
Remove cap from prescribed cleansing solution.	Prepares non-prepackaged items and promotes asepsis
IMPLEMENTATION	
Wash your hands.	Removes colonizing organisms
Place bed at appropriate height.	Prevents back strain
Open cotton-tipped applicator packages; use at least one applicator per pin.	Provides access to supplies and maintains sterility
With gloved hands, clean pin site from the pin outward, using the cotton-tipped applicators and the cleansing agent.	Prevents microorganisms from being introduced into the pin sites
Gently remove crusted areas.	Removes medium for microbial growth and reduces contamination at pin site
Use separate applicator for each pin site or if one site needs to be more thoroughly cleaned.	Prevents cross-contamination
Avoid application of ointment to pin sites unless medically prescribed. Obtain culture if purulent drainage is present.	Ointment occludes drainage, keeps site moist, and increases risk for microbial growth; all are undesirable
Teach the client not to touch the pin sites.	Prevents contamination of pin sites
Discard soiled supplies, remove gloves, wash hands.	Ensures asepsis

Casts

A **cast** is a rigid mold that immobilizes an injured structure while it heals. There are basically three types of casts. A cylinder cast encircles an arm or leg, leaving the fingers or toes exposed. A body cast is a larger form of a cylinder cast that encircles the trunk from about the nipple line to the iliac crests. A hip spica cast surrounds one or both legs and the trunk. It may be strengthened by a bar that spans a casted area between the legs (Fig. 66–5). This type of cast is trimmed open in the anal and genital areas to facilitate elimination.

To keep aligned bone fragments from becoming displaced, the cast is applied from the joint above the break to the one below it. The joint is slightly flexed to decrease stiffness. Some fractures (eg, a stress fracture) do not require surgical reduction or manual manipulation to realign the bone because the fractured bone still remains perfectly aligned. If a closed or open reduction is required, the client receives an analgesic or a general or local anesthetic to relieve pain.

CAST COMPOSITION. Casts are usually made of fiberglass, polyester, or thermoplastic material. Plaster of Paris is still used in some circumstances. Plaster casts require several hours for drying, whereas the other materials dry rapidly. A client with a synthetic cast may bear weight soon after the cast is applied.

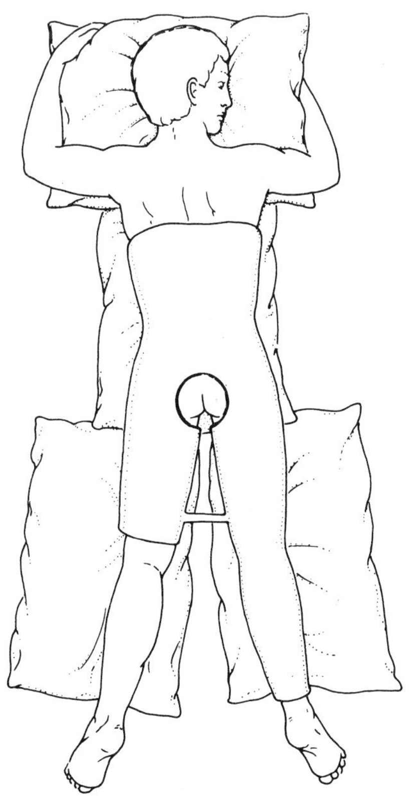

FIGURE 66-5. Spica cast. This client with a spica cast is resting on pillows until the cast dries. His feet are positioned so that they support the desired body alignment. Note the bar ensuring adequate space between the casted legs.

When applying the cast, the physician positions the client in a way that ensures the proper alignment of the part to be immobilized. The client's buttocks may be supported on a casting frame when a body cast or spica cast is applied so the casting material can be wrapped around the client's trunk. A nurse or an assistant holds the arm or leg in place when a cylinder cast is applied (Box 66–2). If the client is awake, explain that the cast material will feel warm during its application as a result of being mixed with water.

Keep a wet cast uncovered so that water can evaporate. Most physicians prefer natural evaporation, but may order a cast dryer to speed evaporation. Never use intense heat. Not only is there a danger of burning the client, there is danger of cracking the outside of the cast while leaving the inside damp and hospitable to mold. Support the drying cast on pillows. If necessary, reposi-

BOX 66-2 Applying a Cast

In general, the physician or nurse practitioner applies a cast as follows:

- Clean and dry the skin surface.
- Cover the skin with stockinette, a tubular knitted material.
- Wrap padding around the limb, especially over bony prominences.
- Apply rolls or strips of cast material over the stockinette and padding.
- Smooth the layers and edges of the cast.
- Fasten the stockinette in cufflike fashion to the outside of the cast.
- Arrange for an x-ray study after casting to check bone alignment.

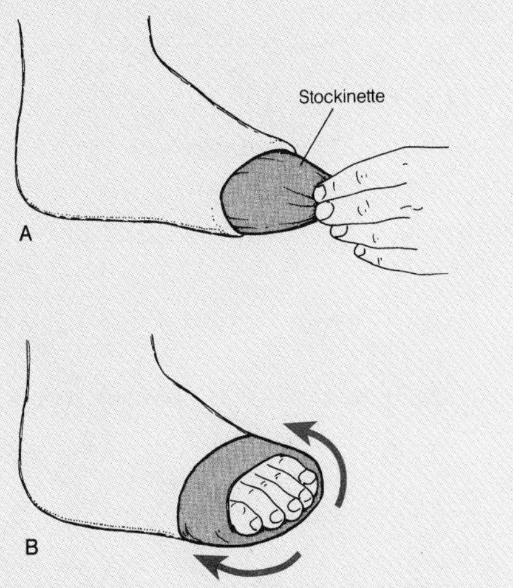

The edges of this cast are made smooth by (*A*) pulling the stockinette and (*B*) fastening it to the outside of the cast.

tion the casted arm or leg with the palms of the hands. Using the fingertips or compressing the cast on a hard surface can lead to a pressure sore later.

CAST WINDOWS. After the cast dries, a cast window, or opening, may be cut. This is usually done when the client reports an area of discomfort under the cast or has a wound that requires a dressing change. The window permits direct inspection of the skin, a means for checking the pulse in a casted arm or leg, or a way to change a dressing. Once a window is cut, the solid piece of cast is replaced in its original site and secured with adhesive tape or a roller bandage. Leaving the window open may allow the skin and soft tissue to bulge through the opening.

BIVALVE CASTS. Once a cast has been applied, it may be bivalved, or cut into two pieces (Fig. 66–6). This may be necessary if the arm or leg swells, causing the rigid cast to compress the tissue and interfere with its blood supply. A bivalved cast also may be used for a client who is being weaned from a cast, when a sharp x-ray is needed, or as a splint for immobilizing painful joints when a client has arthritis.

CAST REMOVAL. Casts are removed with a mechanical cast cutter. Cast cutters are noisy and frightening, and the client needs reassurance that the machine will not cut into the skin. Once the cast is off, the skin appears mottled and may be covered with a yellowish crust composed of accumulated body oil and dead skin. This residue is usually shed within a few days. Lotions and warm baths or soaks may help to soften the skin and remove debris.

The now uncasted limb feels surprisingly light, and the client may report weakness and stiffness. For some time, the limb will need support. An elastic bandage may be wrapped on a leg, the client may use a cane, and an arm may be kept in a sling until progressive active exercise and physical therapy help the client regain normal strength and motion.

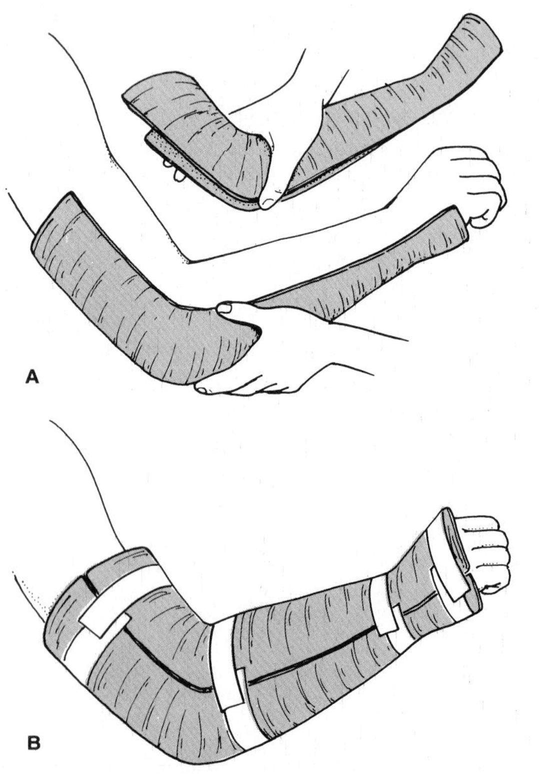

FIGURE 66-6. (*A*) A bivalved cast. (*B*) The two halves are rejoined.

NURSING MANAGEMENT

For information about managing fractures and problems related to casting, refer to Nursing Guidelines 66–2. For information about nursing care for clients with specific fractures, such as those affecting the clavicle or knee, refer to Table 66–3.

NURSING PROCESS
The Client With a Fracture

Assessment

When caring for the client with a fracture, assess for neurovascular and systemic complications, administer analgesics and provide comfort measures, assist with ADL, prevent constipation, promote physical mobility, prevent infection, maintain skin integrity, and prepare the client for self-care. Nursing responsibilities include, but are not limited to, the following:

Nursing Diagnoses and Collaborative Problems	Nursing Interventions
Pain related to tissue and bone trauma, swelling, skeletal traction, or cast pressure **Goal:** The client will report relief of pain after analgesics and comfort measures are administered.	Administer prescribed analgesics. Elevate extremity. Apply ice pack to site of injury as indicated. Change client's position within prescribed limits.
Risk for Altered Tissue Perfusion related to venous stasis, arterial insufficiency, and swelling **Goal:** The client will maintain intact circulation, sensation, and mobility.	Perform neurovascular assessments frequently, reporting any compromise immediately. Prevent interference with arterial and venous circulation. Encourage the client to actively move toes, fingers, and unaffected extremities. Apply elastic stockings if indicated.
Impaired Physical Mobility related to pain, swelling, surgical procedure, or immobiliza-	Assess level of mobility.

tion from traction, cast, or splint **Goals:** The client will regain or maintain maximum mobility and optimal functional position. The client will experience increased strength and function in the affected limb.	Instruct client in active and passive ROM exercises for affected and unaffected extremities, within physical and medical restrictions. Teach client how to turn safely, adhering to restrictions. Assist client in the use of mobility aids—wheelchair, walker, crutches, or canes. Instruct client as needed. Encourage self-care activities.
Self-Care Deficit: Feeding, Hygiene, Dressing, Toileting related to immobility secondary to traction or casts **Goal:** The client will maintain the maximum level of self-care.	Assist client to meet self-care needs as indicated. Instruct client to perform self-care activities as much as possible. Provide assistive devices as indicated. Allow client to plan self-care that best meets ongoing needs.
Impaired Tissue Integrity related to puncture wound, compound fracture, presence of pins, wires, or screws, or other surgical intervention, or to physical immobility **Goals:** The client will demonstrate adequate wound healing without infection. The client will maintain intact skin.	Provide pin care. Report any signs of infection in the pin care sites, wounds, or surgical incisions. Administer antibiotics as indicated. Protect bony prominences from pressure by using pressure-relieving techniques under elbows, heels, and coccyx. Massage bony prominences and skin surfaces subjected to pressure unless they remain red when pressure is relieved. Reposition client frequently as indicated. Assess traction frequently to ensure proper alignment and to prevent pressure areas. Petal cast edges with waterproof tape.
Risk for Constipation related to immobility and change in toileting methods **Goal:** The client will experience normal bowel elimination.	Encourage client to drink more fluids. Assist client to be as mobile as possible. Instruct client to select foods that are higher in fiber content. Administer nonnarcotic analgesics as soon as possible. Provide a fracture bedpan as indicated. Administer stool softeners, suppositories, or low-volume enemas as ordered.

Evaluation and Expected Outcomes

- The client's pain is reduced or relieved.
- The client's circulatory status supports tissue perfusion.
- The client regains mobility and function and achieves the maximum level of self-care.
- The client's wounds heal without infection and the skin is intact.
- The client reports normal bowel elimination.

Client and Family Teaching

Because the client may be discharged shortly after an immobilization device or a cast is applied, review care with the client and family. In addition, reinforce instructions regarding exercise and ambulatory activities.

If a client is in traction, provide simple and direct explanations about the traction and its purpose. Point out activities that are allowed or contraindicated, and identify the approximate length of time for the restrictions. When the traction is discontinued, prepare the client for further treatment, such as casting (see Nursing Guidelines 66–2), and the appearance of the affected area—skin and muscles. Reassure the client that with gradual exercise and use, the muscles will regain strength and tone, and joints will be flexible.

Fractured Femur

A fracture of the femur commonly occurs in automobile accidents, but may occur in falls from ladders or other high places or in gunshot wounds. Fractures of the femur often are accompanied by multiple injuries because they usually occur with severe trauma.

ASSESSMENT FINDINGS

Signs and Symptoms

Severe pain, swelling, and ecchymosis may be seen. The client usually cannot move the hip or knee. If a compound fracture has occurred, an open wound or a protrusion of bone is seen.

Diagnostic Findings

Radiographic films show the type and location of the fracture.

MEDICAL AND SURGICAL MANAGEMENT

Fractures of the femur are usually treated initially with some form of traction to prevent deformities and soft tissue injury. Skeletal traction or an external fixator is used to align the fracture in preparation for future reduction if the fracture occurred in the lower two-thirds of the femur. Once the femur is aligned, a

continued on page 1027

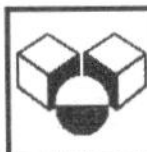

Nursing Guidelines 66-2

Caring for the Client With a Cast

Before Cast Application

- Inspect the condition of the skin that will be covered with a cast.
- Assess circulation, sensation, and mobility to establish a baseline.
- Evaluate the client's pain level.
- Remove clothing that will be difficult to remove after the cast is applied.
- Explain the procedure to the client. Remember to tell the client that the cast will feel warm—even hot—as it is applied, but that it will not burn the skin.

After Cast Application

- Leave the cast uncovered.
- Assess circulation, sensation, and mobility in exposed fingers and toes every 1 to 2 hours.
- Monitor for signs of complications related to cast application. Report abnormal findings immediately.
- Handle wet cast with the palms of the hands, not the fingers.
- Elevate casted extremity so that it is higher than the heart.
- Reposition the client frequently while cast is drying so that the cast dries as evenly as possible.
- Apply ice packs to the cast where surgery was performed.
- Circle areas where blood seeped through and write the time on the circle.
- Petal cast edges with strips of adhesive tape to prevent chipping and to cover any remaining rough areas.
- Replace windows in the hole from which they were cut to prevent tissue from bulging through the opening.
- Ambulate client as soon as indicated.

Discharge Teaching

- Elevate casted extremity for 24 to 48 hours following cast application, and as indicated.
- If the client has a leg cast, show him or her how to ambulate safely.
- Exercise joints proximal and distal to the cast as indicated to prevent muscle atrophy, weakness, and loss of joint mobility.
- Keep the cast clean and dry. A damp cloth may be used.
- Explain that the skin under the cast may feel itchy, and caution client not to insert objects like straws, combs, eating utensils, knitting needles, and the like.
- Report the following to the physician or nurse: unusual and sudden pain, painful or decreased movement, or persistent pain; fever, foul odors, or increased warmth of extremity; drainage from under the cast; changes in circulation, mobility, or sensation (burning, numbness, tingling, or cold).

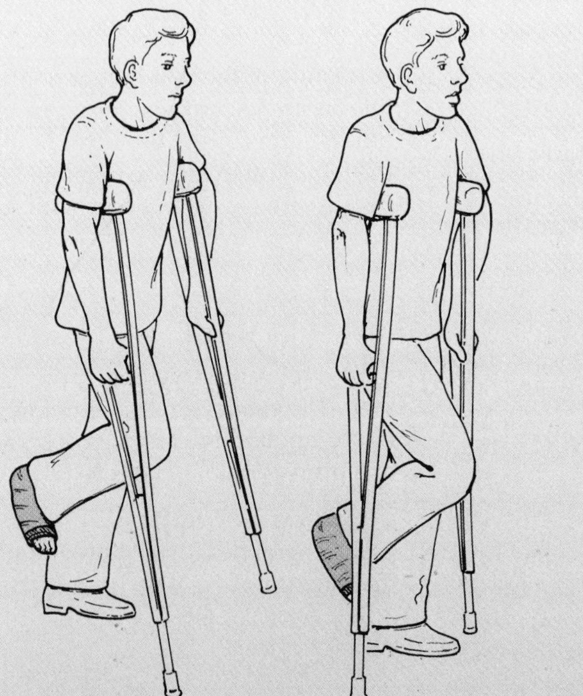

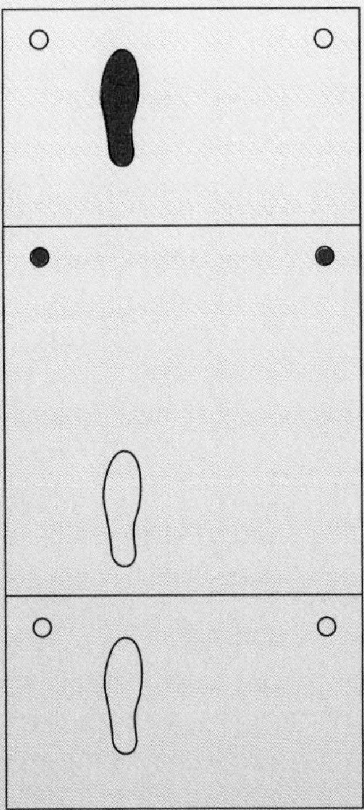

Crutch-walking using the three-point, non–weight-bearing gait pattern (three blocks at right). At left the client positions himself at the bottom of a triangle composed of each crutch and the unaffected leg. In the center the client advances his unaffected leg forward by supporting himself on the hand grips of the crutches and swinging his hips and the unaffected leg through the crutch opening.

TABLE 66-3 **Nursing Care for Specific Fractures**

Site of Fracture	Signs and Symptoms	Treatment	Nursing Management
Mandible	Inability to close mouth after trauma to jaw Chin displaced from midline Teeth absent, loose, or broken Lacerations to mouth and tongue Oral pain, swelling, bruising, and bleeding	Fractures are surgically reduced and immobilized with wire loops to stabilize the lower jaw to the upper jaw. Broken teeth are repaired or removed. Oral lacerations are sutured.	Ensure that wire cutters are easily accessible at the client's bedside. Be familiar with how to cut wire loops if client vomits or chokes. Administer antiemetics to treat nausea and prevent vomiting. Administer liquid or semiliquid diet. Assist client to thoroughly clean mouth after each meal and every 2 hours.
Clavicle	After fracture or dislocation, arm on the affected side held close to the chest to reduce pain Affected shoulder appears to slope downward and droop inward Motion restricted Muscle spasm common	Motion can be limited with a sling or clavicular strap. Displaced fractures are immobilized with a figure 8 or Velpeau bandage. 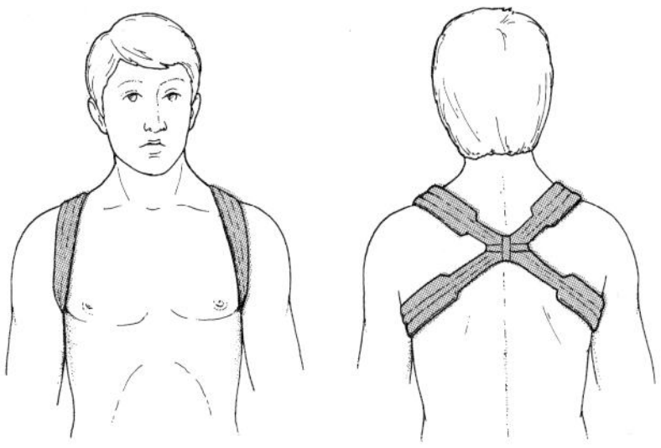 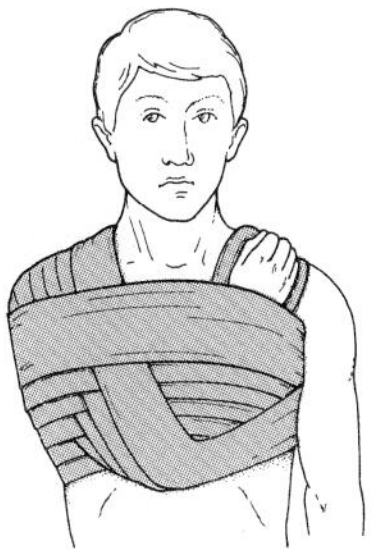 Velpeau bandage.	Use a layer of stockinette or soft, porous material between skin surfaces. Teach client how to assess circulation, sensation, and mobility frequently. Instruct client to abduct arms or rest elbows on table or chair to relieve axillary pressure.
Rib	Additional injuries—to the lungs, subclavian arteries or veins, liver, or spleen Severe chest pain on inspiration and shallow respirations. The client has other symptoms if other injuries are present	Clients are treated for the pain that accompanies fractured ribs, especially when breathing. A rib belt or elastic bandage is used to support the injured rib cage although this restricts chest movement and may cause further lung problems.	Assess for signs and symptoms of pneumonia and atelectasis (collapsed lung) secondary to shallow respirations. Encourage deep breathing. Administer pain medications as indicated.
Upper extremity (fractures ranging from uncomplicated to complex and involving the bone ends, joints,	Pain Compartment syndrome, common complication of forearm fractures, possibly leading to **Volkman's contracture,**	Extent of injury determines treatment: • Cast with or without closed reduction • Open reduction with internal fixation • Hanging cast heavy cast that pulls a fractured humerus into alignment	Assess neurovascular status frequently. Report abnormal findings immediately. Implement measures to relieve pain and swelling.

(continued)

TABLE 66-3 *(Continued)*

Site of Fracture	Signs and Symptoms	Treatment	Nursing Management
tendons, and ligaments)	a clawlike deformity of the hand	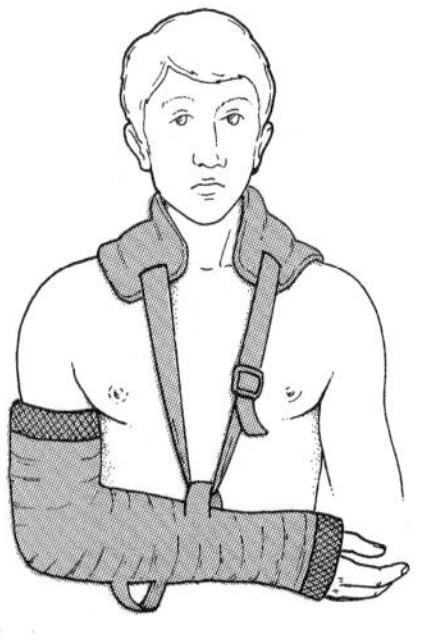 Hanging arm cast.	Pad skin around neck if the client has a hanging cast.
Wrist, hand, or finger	Typically results from a fall May involve only the lower radius (eg, a Colles' fracture in which the distal end of the radius breaks off and becomes displaced) Pain and swelling in the affected area Deformed-looking hand, wrist or finger	Closed reduction with a cast Open reduction with internal fixation Splints applied to fractured fingers	Show client how to use a sling. Teach client how to do active ROM exercises in fingers of affected hand.
Spine	May follow severe injury; if compression fracture, may result from osteoporosis Pain radiating to the leg Tenderness at injury site Muscle spasms Deformity of spinal column Neurologic deficits	Bed rest for an uncomplicated fracture Spinal brace Laminectomy with fusion Cast Head traction: halo brace with rigid vest that allows client to move but immobilizes vertebrae	Teach client to log roll if on bed rest, and as indicated. Assess client's sensation, mobility, and strength in the extremities. Administer pin care if client has a halo brace.
Pelvis (fractures range from minor to severe or crushing injuries)	Tenderness, swelling, and ecchymoses, or more severe symptoms if internal injuries accompany fracture Severed nerves Loss of lower limb function Internal bleeding	Minor fractures: bed rest and comfort measures Severe injuries: multiple system approach related to the nature of the injuries Pelvic slings, spica casts, or open reduction with internal or external fixation	Assess circulation, sensation, and mobility in the lower extremities. Monitor elimination patterns. Insert an indwelling catheter as necessary. Provide a fracture bedpan. Administer suppositories or small volume enemas as indicated. Assess skin frequently for signs of breakdown. Provide frequent skin care. Administer pain medications as prescribed.
Knee (involving kneecap or the ends of the femur or tibia; injuries to the ligaments or tendons)	May follow falls or blows or athletic competition (particularly tears of the cruciate ligaments) Pain, swelling, ecchymoses Inability or limited ability to move or bend the joint	Immobilization with a leg splint 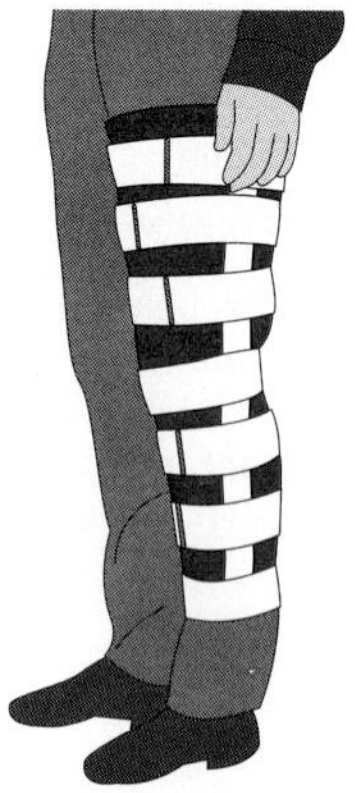 Leg immobilizer.	Assist client to use ambulatory aids, such as crutches or walker. Teach client to perform active ROM exercises within limitations.

(continued)

TABLE 66-3 *(Continued)*

Site of Fracture	Signs and Symptoms	Treatment	Nursing Management
		Arthroscopic surgery to remove bone fragments or to repair ligament tears Open reduction and insertion of wire sutures Removal of patella if fragmented extensively Skeletal traction	
Lower leg (fibula fracture usually occurs with tibial fracture)	Generally results from fall or trauma Pain and swelling Inability to bear weight Ecchymoses and possible deformity Bleeding and protrusion of bone fragments (in compound fractures)	Closed reduction with cast Open reduction with internal fixation	Assess signs and symptoms of compartment syndrome. Urge client to perform active and passive ROM exercises frequently. Assist client to use ambulatory aids.
Ankle	Severe pain Difficulty bearing weight Swelling Protruding bone fragments (severe fractures)	Cast or splint Open or closed reduction and internal fixation followed by casting	Administer pain medications as prescribed. Implement methods to reduce swelling. Assist client to use ambulatory aids. Assess for signs and symptoms of compartment syndrome.
Feet and toes (can occur alone or with other lower extremity fractures)	Pain, swelling, ecchymosis, and difficulty bearing weight Inability to wear shoe Protrusion of small bones (in crushing injuries)	Casting Open reduction with internal fixation Fusion (bones with multiple fractures) Supportive measures: analgesics, cold applications, elevation of foot, and loose-fitting shoes	Assess neurovascular status frequently. Provide cast care as needed. Assist client to use ambulatory aids. Instruct client in safety measures to prevent additional injuries (using nightlights, avoiding narrowed pathways, removing throw rugs, clearing stairways).

spica cast may be used to maintain the corrected position.

NURSING MANAGEMENT

Because the client is confined to bed, implement measures to prevent complications of immobility and inactivity. Position the client in line with the pull exerted by the traction. Clean pin sites with a prescribed cleansing agent to prevent infection (see Clinical Procedure 66–1).

Fractured Hip

Usually a hip fracture affects the proximal end of the femur (Fig. 66–7). This type of fracture commonly results from a fall and occurs more frequently in older adults with osteoporosis. Usually the falls are not that traumatic, but the client's condition contributes to the resulting fracture. Fractures may occur in the femoral neck (intracapsular or within the hip joint capsule), between the trochanters (intertrochanteric-extracapsular or outside the hip joint capsule), or below the trochanters (subtrochanteric-extracapsular). The elderly client is prone to complications after a hip fracture. Some die as a result of associated complications.

ASSESSMENT FINDINGS

Signs and Symptoms

The client reports severe pain that increases with movement of the leg. The pain frequently radiates to the knee, and the client may have a sensation of pressure in the outer aspect of the hip. Discontinuity of the bone and muscle spasm cause shortening and external rotation of the leg. Subtrochanteric and intertrochanteric fractures may be accompanied by a

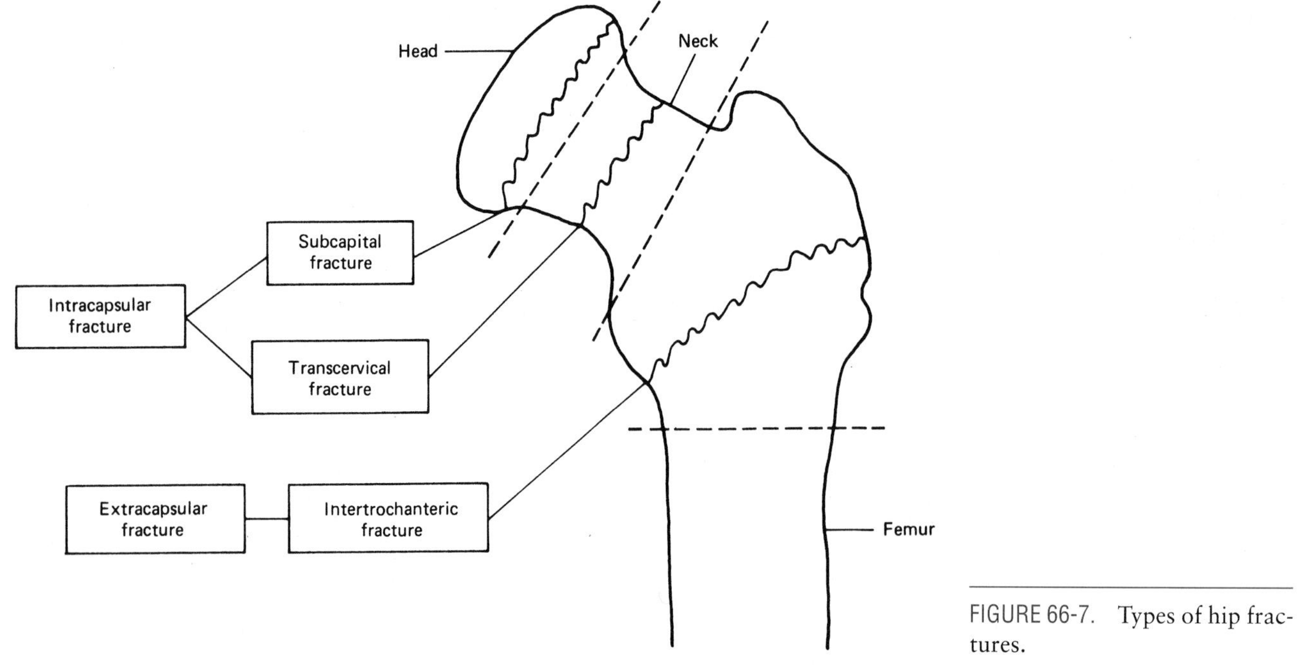

FIGURE 66-7. Types of hip fractures.

large blood loss, leading to hypovolemic shock. With these fractures extensive bruising and swelling in the hip, groin, and thigh occur. Femoral neck fractures are intracapsular, so the bleeding is more likely to be contained within the joint capsule.

Diagnostic Findings

Radiographic studies reveal the exact location of the fracture, which may be within or outside the joint capsule.

MEDICAL AND SURGICAL MANAGEMENT

Buck's extension or other skin traction may be applied to relieve muscle spasm and pain until surgery is performed. Open reduction internal fixation (ORIF), accomplished with a nail or an intramedullary rod (a rod inserted into the center of the bone with wires around the bone for stabilization), is most commonly done for fractures of the hip, particularly extracapsular fractures. Examples of internal fixation devices include the Jewett nail, the Richardson hip screw, the Moe intratrochanteric plate, and the Smith-Petersen nail. Intracapsular hip fractures are prone to nonunion and avascular necrosis due to the disruption of blood supply. Therefore, the fractured head and neck may be removed and replaced with a metal device such as an Austin-Moore or Thompson prosthesis. This procedure is referred to as hemiarthroplasty. A total hip arthroplasty is discussed later in the chapter.

The bone heals around the metallic device, which in the meantime holds the bone together. Thus, the bone is united immediately, and clients are mobilized much earlier than they are with traction. Plates, bands, screws, and pins may be removed after the bone has healed. More often, they are left in place permanently. The precautions with hemiarthroplasty are greater because the surgeon must dislocate the hip to replace the femoral head.

NURSING MANAGEMENT

Most clients with a fractured hip are elderly and are prone to complications. Postoperatively, the nurse implements measures to prevent skin breakdown, wound infection, pneumonia, constipation, urinary retention, muscle atrophy, and contractures. The client generally has a wound drain in place for 2 days after surgery. Monitor the drainage and administer antibiotics as prescribed.

Show the client how to use the overhead trapeze safely for independent movement and activity. While the client is recumbent, place a trochanter roll or long, covered sandbag beside the hip to maintain a neutral position so that the repaired hip stays in place. Abductor pillows are placed between the legs when turning the client from side to side.

If a hip prosthesis has been inserted, instruct the client to avoid adduction of the affected leg until healing occurs. Abductor pillows are used at all times. Soon after surgery, assist the client to transfer from the bed to a chair. The chair must have an elevated seat, either with its structure or with pillows, so that the client does not flex the hips beyond 90 degrees. The client usually requires much encouragement and assistance. Eventually the client progresses to ambulating with a walker. Before discharge, explore ways to ensure safety in the client's home to avoid future injuries and falls.

Inflammatory and Infectious Disorders

Arthritis is a general condition characterized by inflammation and degeneration of a joint. **Rheumatic disorders** include more than 100 different types of recognized inflammatory disorders, making this collective group the most common orthopedic problem. These disorders involve inflammation and degeneration of connective tissue structures, especially joints. Infectious disorders may also affect the musculoskeletal system, causing temporary or chronic problems with musculoskeletal function. Inflammatory and infectious disorders have the potential to interfere with mobility and ADL. Clients with inflammatory and infectious disorders may need assistance with tasks that most people take for granted in independent self-care. These disorders affect a client's physical, psychological, and social functions.

The discussion in this chapter is limited to rheumatoid arthritis, osteoarthritis, gout, bursitis, ankylosing spondylitis, Lyme disease, osteomyelitis, and lupus erythematosus. Many clients with inflammatory and infectious disorders affecting the musculoskeletal system are treated on an outpatient basis. A few may require hospitalization in the acute phase of the disorder, or for surgery on a degenerative joint, or for other medical or surgical therapies.

Rheumatoid Arthritis

Rheumatoid arthritis (RA) is a systemic inflammatory disorder of connective tissue characterized by chronicity, remissions, and exacerbations. The potential for disability with rheumatoid arthritis is great and is related to the effects on joints, as well as the systemic problems.

ETIOLOGY AND PATHOPHYSIOLOGY

The nature of RA, a crippling disease, is not fully understood. Its cause is unknown, although it is believed to be an autoimmune disease. Genetic predisposition and other factors may be involved. RA strikes in the most productive years of adulthood, usually in the 20- to 40-year-old group. The disorder also can be found in young children and older adults. Young adult women appear to be affected more than men, but the incidence equalizes as adults age. Typically small joints are affected early, whereas large joint involvement occurs later (Bullock, 1996).

Initially, the immune system produces antibodies, called rheumatoid factor (RF), that attack and destroy joint structures. The destruction occurs as follows:

1. The synovium of the joint first experiences pathologic changes, resulting in **synovitis** (inflammation of the synovial membrane surrounding a joint) and excess synovial fluid, which causes edema (swelling).
2. Surrounding articular cartilage and tendons and ligaments are affected.
3. Chronic congestion and thickening of the synovium produce **pannus,** or granulation tissue.
4. The pannus, which leads to further erosion of the articular cartilage, invades the joint capsule.
5. The destruction continues, affecting bone and connective tissue.
6. The pannus is replaced by fibrous connective tissue that fills the joint cavity; this condition is called **fibrous ankylosis** (joint immobility).
7. The fibrous tissue calcifies, causing **osseous (bony) ankylosis** (fusion) of the joint.
8. Fusion results in pain, deformity, and limited mobility or immobility.

In essence, when the restricting band of tissue calcifies, the joint no longer exists. This process from nonspecific synovitis to complete ossification of the joint may take years, and it may occur at different rates in different joints in the same person (Fig. 66–8).

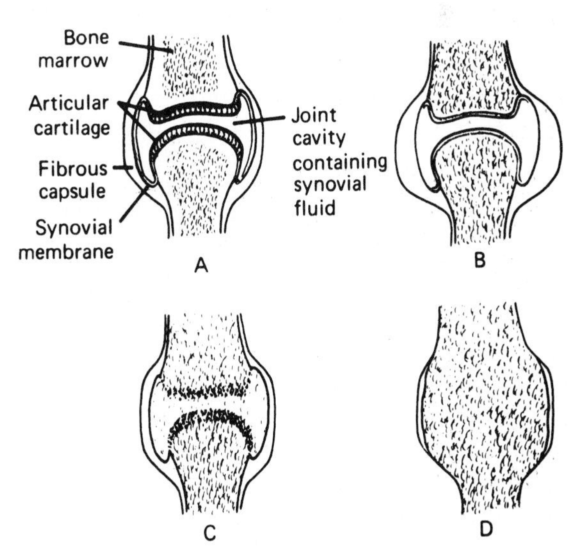

FIGURE 66-8. Pathologic changes in rheumatoid arthritis. (*A*) Normal ball-and-socket joint. (*B*) Same joint, showing acute inflammation and progressive destruction of cartilage. (*C*) Inflammation subsided; fibrous ankylosis. (*D*) Bony ankylosis: the joint is immobile.

ASSESSMENT FINDINGS

Signs and Symptoms

In most clients, the onset of symptoms is acute. Joint involvement is usually bilateral and symmetrical. Localized symptoms include:

- Joint pain, swelling, and warmth
- Erythema
- Mobility limitation
- Spongy tissue on joint palpation
- Fluid aspirated from joint

Over several weeks, more joints become involved. Swelling and pain comes and goes. Fatigue, malaise, anorexia, and weight loss are common. Fever may develop. Tolerance for any kind of stress decreases, as does tolerance for environmental temperature changes. Although dietary iron intake is adequate, clients characteristically have persistent anemia resulting from the effect of RA on the blood- forming organs. Other systemic features include vasculitis, neuropathy, scleritis, pericarditis, splenomegaly, and Sjögren's syndrome (dry eyes and dry mucous membranes).

In some clients subcutaneous nodules, known as rheumatoid nodules, develop. Appearing in more advanced stages of RA, they are usually nontender and movable and evident over bony prominences, such as the elbow or the base of the spine.

Muscles weaken and atrophy (shrink), partially from disuse. Connective tissue and neurovascular changes lend a smooth, glossy appearance to the extremities, which may be cold and clammy. Flexion contractures are common.

As the disease progresses, muscle wasting around affected joints accentuates the appearance of swelling. The proximal finger joints swell the most and demonstrate classic deformities (Fig. 66–9), which include:

- Swan neck deformity—hyperextension of the proximal interphalangeal joint with fixed flexion of the distal interphalangeal joint
- Boutonniere deformity—persistent flexion of the proximal interphalangeal joint with hyperextension of the distal interphalangeal joint
- Ulnar deviation—fingers deviate laterally toward the ulna

Whether resting or moving, clients in this stage of the disease have considerable chronic pain. Typically, the pain is more severe in the morning after a night's rest. The symptoms may subside suddenly for no apparent reason. Inflammation leaves joints that were sore and red; the client is not stiff, has no fever, and the pain is gone. Yet the symptoms almost invariably return after the client has had a symptom-free period. Inflammation causes more joint damage, followed by another remission. The pattern of remissions and exacerbations can continue for years.

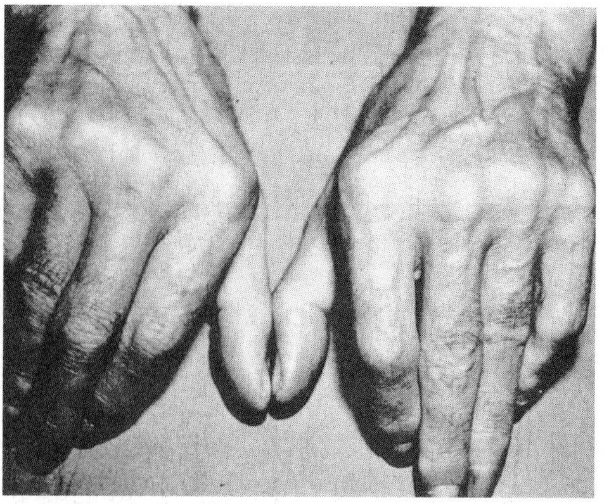

FIGURE 66-9. Typical appearance of arthritic hands. The joints are sore, swollen, and deformed.

Without treatment, and sometimes with it, joint destruction may be total. As bony growth replaces the synovial space, the joint loses motion. Once the joint becomes immobile, the pain of the inflammation decreases, but discomfort continues because of contractures and immobility.

Diagnostic Findings

Radiographic films show characteristic joint changes and the extent of damage. The synovial fluid may be aspirated (the client receives a local anesthetic) for microscopic examination. In RA, the synovial fluid usually appears cloudy and dark yellow and may contain white blood cells. Arthroscopic examination also may be carried out to visualize the extent of joint damage as well as to obtain a sample of synovial fluid.

A positive C-reactive protein test, low red blood cell count and hemoglobin levels in later stages, and positive RF are laboratory findings that support the diagnosis. The erythrocyte sedimentation rate (ESR) may be elevated, particularly as the disease progresses. A serum protein electrophoresis may disclose an increase in levels of gamma and alpha globulin but a decrease in albumin level.

MEDICAL AND SURGICAL MANAGEMENT

Although RA cannot be cured, much can be done to minimize damage. Treatment aims include decreasing inflammation of the joint before bony ankylosis occurs, relieving discomfort, preventing or correcting deformities, and maintaining or restoring function of affected structures. Early treatment gives the best results.

Optimal health conditions must be maintained because supporting the resistance of the body to the inflammation is one of the few truly therapeutic steps that medicine has to offer. Rest, systemic and local, is balanced carefully with exercise. Unless the client has other medical complications, such as diabetes or hypertension, the diet need not be modified from that of a normal individual.

Local applications of heat and cold are used concurrently with drug therapy to relieve swelling and pain. Drug therapy is not curative but helps relieve pain and, in some instances, suppresses the inflammatory process (Table 66–4). Drug dosages are generally quite high, and because of the long-term nature of this disorder, narcotic analgesics are avoided.

Therapeutic doses of salicylates (aspirin) or NSAIDs, such as indomethacin, are frequently used first for their anti-inflammatory and analgesic effects. Corticosteroids, such as prednisone, can alleviate inflammation and, therefore, pain. Azathioprine (Imuran), an immunosuppressant, may be used in clients with severe classic RA that does not respond to more conventional therapies. Methotrexate (Mexate), an antineoplastic agent, and captopril (Capoten), an antihypertensive drug, also are tried for clients who do not respond to other drug therapies.

Several surgical techniques may be performed to minimize or correct the joint deformities of RA (Box 66–3). Many individuals with various types of arthritis undergo an **arthroplasty,** or reconstruction of the joint, using an artificial joint that restores previously lost function and relieves pain. Reconstructive joint surgery is discussed more fully with the surgical management of degenerative joint disease.

NURSING MANAGEMENT

Nursing management involves teaching clients about the disease and providing information about maintaining general health, relieving pain, reducing stress, decreasing the inflammatory process, and preserving joint mobility. The nurse also instructs clients about the medication regimen—and particularly about effects and side effects. Other nursing activities may center on how to apply heat and cold packs locally to relieve pain or how to use a transcutaneous electrical nerve stimulation (TENS) unit to relieve pain in a particular joint. A TENS unit has electrodes that are applied to the skin from a portable stimulation unit that the client learns to operate.

Nurses collaborate with occupational therapists to provide equipment, utensils, and instruction regarding energy conservation and maintenance of joint alignment. Physical therapists plan an appropriate exercise regimen. Home care planning involves providing nursing assistance for ADL and ensuring that the home environment is safe. Out of consideration for the typical pain and morning stiffness, the nurse teaches the nursing assistant to allow extra time for completing hygiene or other procedures.

When joints are severely inflamed, active motion may be reduced with the use of a splint, but motion is not totally eliminated. Even during an acute episode, the client can be encouraged to move affected parts gently to help lessen the possibility of ankylosis, muscle wasting, osteoporosis, and the debilitating effects of prolonged rest. Positions of flexion are avoided.

The nurse continues to urge the client to eat nutritious, well balanced meals despite anorexia. As joints become deformed and destroyed, the techniques and equipment used to perform ADL may require modification. Clients will need assistance to deal with chronic pain, changes in function, changes in appearance, and related depression and feelings of helplessness. Education about the disease is essential because many people spend large sums of money on unscientific treatments in hopes of a cure.

Degenerative Joint Disease

Degenerative joint disease (DJD), sometimes referred to as osteoarthritis, is the most common form of arthritis. It is also known as the wear and tear disease, and typically affects the weight-bearing joints. It is characterized by a slow and steady progression of destructive changes in weight-bearing joints and those that are repeatedly used for work. Unlike RA, DJD has no remissions and no systemic symptoms, such as malaise and fever. It usually is limited to one or two joints that may start as early as the middle thirties, but is mainly associated with aging.

ETIOLOGY AND PATHOPHYSIOLOGY

A lifetime of repeated trauma leads to degenerative joint changes. Hips, knees, the spine, and the distal interphalangeal joints in the hands are commonly affected. Obese people, whose joints must bear heavy weight, are more likely to develop symptoms earlier than lean people. Genetic predisposition to arthritis also may be a factor in the disease.

The degenerative process begins when the cartilage that covers the bone ends becomes thin, rough, and ragged. Malacia or soft spots develop. The cartilage no longer springs back into shape after normal use. As the cartilage wears away, the joint space decreases, so that the bone surfaces are closer and rub together. In an attempt to repair the damaged surface, new bone develops in the form of bone spurs, bone cysts, or osteophytes, which are extended margins of the joints. The joint becomes deformed, and the client

TABLE 66-4 **Drug Therapy for Rheumatoid Arthritis**

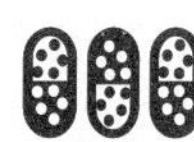

Drug Category	Drug Action	Nursing Considerations
Salicylates		
aspirin	Relieves mild to moderate pain Interferes with the inflammatory response	Give with food or milk. Monitor for ringing in the ears, gastrointestinal (GI) distress, unusual bleeding or bruising, dark-colored stools.
Nonsteroidal Anti-inflammatory Drugs (NSAIDs)		
indomethacin (Indocin)	Relieves moderate to severe pain Interferes with the inflammatory response	Give with food or milk. Monitor blood counts and urinalysis reports. Advise the client not to take aspirin or other anti-inflammatory drugs unless approved by the physician.
Corticosteroids		
prednisone (Meticorten)	Anti-inflammatory and immunosuppressant	Give with food or milk. Decrease the dose and frequency of administration gradually when discontinuing long-term steroid therapy. Monitor for GI distress, hyperglycemia, edema, poor wound healing, fat redistribution, thinning of skin, muscle weakness, visual changes, personality changes, pathologic fractures. Protect from acquiring infections. Recommend reducing salt intake. Suggest that the client wear a Medic Alert bracelet, be examined regularly by an ophthalmologist, and be followed closely by the prescribing physician.
Pyrazolones		
phenylbutazone (Butazoladin)	Relieves severe inflammation and related pain that does not respond to salicylates	Give with food or milk. Expect that the drug will be prescribed for short-term use. Inspect the skin for petechiae or rash. Monitor laboratory test results for drops in blood cell counts. Inspect the urine for signs of hematuria or low volume. Report any signs of an infection such as slight fever, sore throat. Reduce salt consumption and monitor blood pressure.
Gold Salts		
auranofin (Ridaura)	Temporarily arrests the progression of rheumatoid arthritis	Administer oral forms on an empty stomach and withhold food, milk, antacids, or other drugs for 1 hour afterward. Expect that drug therapy will be long and the response may be delayed up to 3 months. Monitor for blood cell and urine abnormalities. Caution the client to take the drug as prescribed; when the drug is discontinued, it is done gradually.
4-Aminoquinolines		
hydroxychloroquine (Plaquenil)	Reduces inflammation; used to treat rheumatoid arthritis and lupus erythematosus	Give with food or milk. Monitor blood counts. Consult before administering to clients with ophthalmic, neurologic, hepatic, or GI disorders. Do not give with gold compounds or other anti-inflammatory drugs. Contraindicated for children, pregnant or nursing women, and those with a glucose-6-phosphate dehydrogenase deficiency. Inform the client that the urine will appear brown. Monitor for muscle weakness, visual changes, skin lesions, hypotension, and electrocardiographic changes.
Antirheumatic penicillamine (Cuprimine)	Suppresses immune response, by lowering IgM associated with the rheumatoid factor	Give on an empty stomach and withhold all food and drugs for 1 hour. Do not administer during pregnancy. Assess for a fever during the second or third week of therapy. Taste may be diminished. Use cautiously in those with an allergy to penicillin; they may also be sensitive to penicillamine. Monitor for a rash or other skin changes, and depression of blood cells, liver, or renal function. Anticipate improvement in about 3 months.

BOX 66-3 Surgical Procedures for Rheumatoid Arthritis

Arthrodesis: Fusion of a joint (most often the wrist or knee) for stabilization and pain relief
Arthroplasty: Total reconstruction or replacement of a joint (most often the knee and hip) with an artificial joint to restore function and relieve pain
Osteotomy: Cutting and removal of a wedge of bone (most often the tibia or femur) to change the bone's alignment, thereby improving function and relieving pain
Synovectomy: Removal of enlarged and hypertrophied synovium to prevent the formation of pannus and delay destruction within the joint (most often the fingers, wrist, elbow, and knee)

experiences pain and limited joint movement. Ankylosis does not occur, but the joint may become partially dislocated by the resulting deformity.

ASSESSMENT FINDINGS

Signs and Symptoms

Early symptoms are brief joint stiffness and pain following a period of inactivity. The pain generally increases with heavy use and is relieved by rest. Later, even rest may not adequately relieve the pain. Eventually the joint undergoes enlargement and increased limitation of movement. When the hands are afflicted with DJD, the fingers frequently develop painless bony nodules on the dorsolateral surface of the interphalangeal joints: **Heberden's nodes** (bony enlargement of the distal interphalangeal joints) and **Bouchard's nodes** (bony enlargement of the proximal interphalangeal joints). Crepitus may be heard and felt when the joint is moved. The ROM of the affected joint becomes progressively limited, and stiffness and pain increase.

Diagnostic Findings

Radiographic films demonstrate disruption of the joint cartilage and bony changes. Some clients have a slightly elevated ESR.

MEDICAL AND SURGICAL MANAGEMENT

Systemic anti-inflammatory drugs, such as aspirin and NSAIDs, are first used in treating DJD. Although these drugs do not prevent or cure this disorder, they may decrease the severity of joint destruction. Corticosteroids may be injected into acutely inflamed joints with limited success. However, when possible, long-term use of these agents is avoided. Use of narcotics is deferred because of the chronic nature of the disorder.

Local rest of the affected joints is advised more so than total body rest. Heat applied to the painful part may afford some relief. Weight loss is recommended for obese clients. Splints, braces, canes, or crutches may reduce discomfort, relieve pain, and prevent further joint destruction of the affected joints. An exercise program helps to preserve joint ROM and strength. Clients should not engage in activity that places excessive stress on affected joints. A TENS unit may help reduce joint pain.

Reconstructive joint surgery is performed when the client's mobility and quality of life are compromised. The two joints most frequently replaced are the knee and the hip. Other joints that may be replaced are the elbow, ankle, wrist, and finger joints. Total joint replacement is not strictly for clients with DJD. This type of procedure may also be done for individuals with RA, trauma, hip fracture, or a congenital deformity.

The materials used in an artificial joint are metal and high-density polyethylene (Fig. 66–10). Special bone cement or a specialized coating on the prosthesis pieces, which promotes bone growth on the implant, hold the prosthesis parts in place. Postoperative complications include hemorrhage, subluxation or dislocation of the artificial hip, infection, thromboembolism, and avascular necrosis. A cemented prosthesis may loosen many years later.

Some clients may want to predonate their own blood for use if a transfusion is needed. Anticoagulant therapy and early ambulation are implemented to prevent clot formation. Clients with a knee or hip replacement may use a continuous passive motion (CPM) machine postoperatively. This machine promotes healing and flexibility within the knee or hip joint and increases circulation to the operative area. The physician orders the amount of extension and flexion produced by the machine as well as the frequency of use. The amount of flexion and frequency of movement are increased daily for clients with knee replacements. By discharge, the client's goal is the ability to bend the knee 90 degrees. The amount of flexion for clients with hip replacements should never exceed 30 degrees in a CPM machine.

NURSING MANAGEMENT

The nurse instructs the client about the purpose of drug therapy, administration times, and the drug effects and side effects. Because aspirin and NSAIDs can cause gastric bleeding, instruct clients to take the medication with food. Encourage moderate activity. The client needs to understand how to regulate the type, vigor, and frequency of exercise according to the

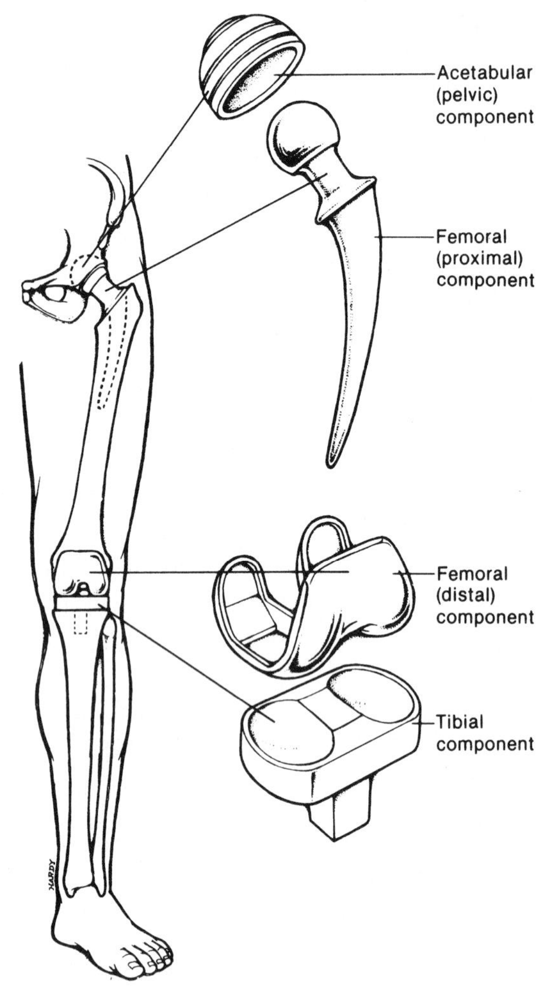

FIGURE 66-10. Artificial hip and knee joints.

symptoms experienced. Explain dietary changes that promote weight loss. If appropriate, gently remind the client to assume good posture to avoid unusual stress on a joint. If ambulatory aids such as crutches, a cane, or a walker are required, arrange a referral to a physical therapist for fitting and practice.

For the client being treated surgically, withhold aspirin preoperatively to reduce the risk for excessive bleeding. Monitor the complete blood count, prothrombin time, and bleeding and clotting times to make sure that the client's ability to control bleeding is not compromised. Also advise the client of the possibility of using a CPM machine.

When the client returns from surgery, review the physician orders concerning movement, turning, or positioning of the extremities (Box 66–4). Usually, keep the head of the bed at 45 degrees or less. Position the legs of clients with a hip replacement in abduction and extension because the opposite positions of adduction and flexion can dislocate the prosthetic femoral head from the acetabulum. Make sure that clients sit in an elevated chair or on a seat raised by pillows, so that the flexion is less than 90 degrees. Apply ice packs to the incisional site (particularly after knee surgery).

If CPM devices are prescribed to promote gentle flexion and extension of the knee, increase the flexion as indicated up to the goal of 90 degrees. If CPM devices are used after hip surgery, do not exceed 30 degrees of flexion.

BOX 66-4 Precautions for Clients After Total Hip Replacement

To avoid dislocating the new hip, the following precautions are advised:

- Keep legs abducted at all times.
- Use pillows or abductor pillow to maintain abduction.
- Limit hip flexion to 90 degrees or less.
- Do not elevate head of bed more than 45 degrees.
- Sit only on a raised chair and toilet seat.
- Do not bend over to pick up objects from the floor and do not flex the hip to dress or undress.

Gout

Gout, a painful metabolic disorder involving an inflammatory reaction within the joints, usually affects the feet (especially the great toe), hands, elbows, ankles, and knees.

ETIOLOGY AND PATHOPHYSIOLOGY

Gout is characterized by **hyperuricemia** (accumulation of uric acid in the blood), caused by alterations in uric acid production or excretion, or a combination of both. Hyperuricemia occurs from one or a combination of the following pathologies:

- Abnormal purine metabolism
- Increased rate of protein synthesis with overproduction of uric acid or underexcretion of uric acid
- Excessive ingestion of purines (organ meats, shellfish, sardines)
- Increased cellular turnover, as in leukemia, multiple myeloma, and other cancers
- Altered renal tubular function related to using diuretics and salicylates and excessive alcohol intake

Urate (a salt of uric acid) crystallizes in body tissues and is deposited in soft and bony tissues, causing local inflammation and irritation. Collections of urate crystals, called **tophi,** are found in the cartilage of the outer ear (pinna), joints, ligaments, bursae, and tendons. As these deposits accumulate, they destroy the joint, producing a chronically swollen, deformed appearance. The uric acid also may precipitate in urine, causing renal stones.

The disorder tends to be inherited and affects more men than women. Gout may occur secondarily to other diseases marked by decreased renal excretion of uric acid. It has also been identified among organ transplant clients treated with the antirejection drug cyclosporine.

ASSESSMENT FINDINGS

Signs and Symptoms

A gout attack is characterized by a sudden onset of acute pain and tenderness in one joint. The skin turns red and the joint swells so that it is warm and hypersensitive to touch. Fever may be present. Tophi may be palpated around the fingers or earlobes, particularly if the client has chronic and severe hyperuricemia. The attack may last for 1 or 2 weeks, but moderate swelling and tenderness may persist beyond that time. A symptom-free period is usually followed by another attack, which may occur at any time. Repeated episodes in the same joint may deform the joint.

Diagnostic Findings

Diagnosis is usually based on the obvious clinical signs and hyperuricemia. Synovial fluid aspirated from the joint during arthrocentesis contains urate crystals. The urate deposits may also be identifiable with a radiographic examination. Elevated serum uric acid levels and urinalysis on 24-hour specimens correlate with gout, but these findings are common to other disorders as well.

MEDICAL AND SURGICAL MANAGEMENT

Although gout cannot be cured in the sense of removing the basic metabolic difficulty of constant or recurrent hyperuricemia, the attacks usually can be controlled so that they no longer occur. The aim of treatment is to decrease the amount of sodium urate in the extracellular fluid so that deposits do not form.

Two main treatment approaches involve (1) using uricosuric drugs that promote renal excretion of urates by inhibiting the reabsorption of uric acid in the renal tubules and (2) decreasing ingestion of purine. The regimen is individualized and may be changed in response to the changes in the course of the disease.

Pain during a severe acute attack may require NSAIDs, such as ibuprofen and indomethacin. Acute attacks of gout may be treated with colchicine or phenylbutazone. Colchicine is administered every 1 or 2 hours until the pain subsides or nausea, vomiting, intestinal cramping, and diarrhea develop. When one or more of these symptoms occur, the drug should be stopped temporarily. Drugs used for long-term gout management include colchicine, allopurinol (Zyloprim), probenecid (Benemid), indomethacin (Indocin), and sulfinpyrazone (Anturane). To prevent future attacks, drug therapy continues after the acute attack subsides (Table 66–5). Salicylates inactivate uricosurics. Clients with a history of gout should not use them.

It is now known that purines can be synthesized and thus there is less emphasis on strict diet restriction than on the use of uricosuric drugs. The prescribed diet includes adequate protein with limitation of purine-rich foods to avoid contributing to the un-

TABLE 66-5 **Selected Antigout Medications**

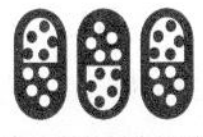

Medication	Description	Nursing Implications
colchicine	Lowers the deposition of uric acid and interferes with leukocytes and kinin formation, thus reducing inflammation. Does not alter serum or urine levels of uric acid. Used in acute and chronic management.	*Acute management:* Administer when attack first begins. Dosage is increased until pain is relieved or diarrhea develops. *Chronic management:* Prolonged use may decrease vitamin B_{12} absorption. Causes gastrointestinal upset in most clients.
probenecid (Benemid)	Uricosuric agent Inhibits renal reabsorption of urates and increases the urinary excretion of uric acid. Prevents tophi formation.	Be alert for nausea, rash, and constipation.
allopurinol (Zyloprim)	Xanthine oxidase inhibitor Interrupts the breakdown of purines before uric acid is formed. Inhibits xanthinoxidase because it blocks uric acid formation.	Be alert for side effects, including bone marrow depression, vomiting, and abdominal pain.

derlying problem. The diet prescription is also relatively high in carbohydrates and low in fats because carbohydrates increase urate excretion and fats retard it. Clients who are overweight are encouraged to lose weight. A high fluid intake will help increase excretion of uric acid. Alcohol is restricted because it can trigger an attack.

Surgery may be performed to remove the large tophi of advanced gout. Surgery also may be used to correct crippling deformities that may result from treatment delays or to fuse unstable joints and increase their function.

NURSING MANAGEMENT

Place a bed cradle over the affected joint to protect it from the pressure of the bed linen. If colchicine is prescribed, provide an explanation about the hourly administration until side effects occur or the acute pain subsides. Instruct the client to report gastrointestinal (GI) symptoms. Measure intake and output, especially when diarrhea occurs with colchicine therapy for acute gout. Provide clear explanations of long-term drug and diet therapy before discharge.

Bursitis

Bursitis is an inflammation of the bursa, a fluid-filled sac that cushions bone ends to enhance a gliding movement. The elbow, shoulder, and knee are common sites of bursitis.

ETIOLOGY AND PATHOPHYSIOLOGY

Trauma is the most common cause of acute bursitis. Other causes include infection and secondary effects of gout and RA. Typical of any inflammation, pain and swelling occur with compromised function.

ASSESSMENT FINDINGS

Signs and Symptoms

Painful movement of a joint, such as the elbow or shoulder, is the most common symptom. A distinct lump may be felt. If the bursa ruptures, tissue in the area may become edematous, warm, and tender.

Diagnostic Findings

An x-ray study may reveal a calcified bursa, and aspiration of fluid may demonstrate:

- A few leukocytes in transparent fluid if the etiology is trauma
- A large collection of leukocytes if the cause is sepsis
- Colonies of staphylococcal or streptococcal microorganisms
- Urate crystals in bursitis secondary to gout
- Cholesterol crystals, common in clients with bursitis and RA, which may cause the fluid from the bursa to appear cloudy

MEDICAL AND SURGICAL MANAGEMENT

Joint rest is usually recommended. Salicylates or NSAIDs may be prescribed. If the problem persists, a corticosteroid preparation may be injected into the joint to reduce inflammation. After pain and inflammation are reduced, ongoing therapy involves mild ROM exercises.

NURSING MANAGEMENT

Review the prescribed medication and exercise regimens with the client and allow time for questions and answers. Advise the client not to traumatize or overuse the recovering joint but to use it normally. Failure to use the joint after pain and inflammation are controlled may result in partial limitation of joint motion.

Ankylosing Spondylitis

Ankylosing spondylitis, or Marie-Strumpell disease, is a chronic, connective tissue disorder of the spine and surrounding cartilaginous joints, such as the sacroiliac joints and soft tissues around the vertebrae. Characteristics include spondylosis and fusion of the vertebrae.

ETIOLOGY AND PATHOPHYSIOLOGY

Ankylosing spondylitis generally begins in early adulthood and is more common in men. The etiology is unknown although some theorize that an altered immune response occurs when T-cell lymphocytes mistake human cells for similar-appearing bacterial antigens. There is also a strong familial tendency for some affected individuals. Once the inflammation begins, it continues causing progressive immobility and fixation (**ankylosis**) of the joints in the hips and ascends up the vertebrae of the spine. Respiratory function may be compromised if kyphosis (a hunchback-like spinal curve) develops. In a few cases, there may be extra-articular (nonjoint) manifestations, such as aortitis (inflammation of the aorta), iridocyclitis (inflammation of the iris and ciliary body of the eye), and pulmonary fibrosis.

ASSESSMENT FINDINGS

Signs and Symptoms

The most common symptoms are low back pain and stiffness. As the disease progresses, the spine and hips become more immobile, thus restricting movement. The lumbar curve of the spine may flatten. The neck can be permanently flexed. Aortic regurgitation or atrioventricular node conduction disturbances may occur. Lung sounds may be reduced, especially in the apical areas.

Diagnostic Findings

Evidence of inflammation is demonstrated by an elevated ESR. However, a culture of synovial fluid is negative for causative microorganisms. Elevations of alkaline phosphatase and creatinine phosphokinase levels usually occur. A human leukocyte antigen (HLA) test, used for determining inherited tissue markers for immune functions, demonstrates the presence of HLA-B2 in 90% of individuals with this disorder. X-ray films or CT scans show erosion, ossification, and fusion of the joints in the spine and hips.

MEDICAL AND SURGICAL MANAGEMENT

Treatment of this disorder is supportive, the major goal being to maintain functional posture. Aspirin, indomethacin, phenylbutazone, or NSAIDs usually are prescribed for relieving inflammation and pain. Sleeping on a firm mattress (preferably without a pillow) and following a prescribed exercise program may help delay or prevent spinal deformity, especially if begun in the early stages of the disease. A back brace also may be prescribed for some clients. Severe hip involvement may be treated with a total hip replacement.

NURSING MANAGEMENT

Administer prescribed drugs and clarify information about the disease. Encourage the client to perform ADL as much as possible. Teach the client to perform mild exercises that reduce stiffness and pain. Provide emotional support, recognizing that the client must deal with pain, skeletal changes, and impaired mobility.

Lyme Disease

Lyme disease (*Lyme borreliosis*) gained large recognition in the 1970s when residents of Lyme, Connecticut, experienced an epidemic of progressive symptoms, beginning with a characteristic rash and progressing to cardiac, neurologic, and musculoskeletal involvement.

ETIOLOGY AND PATHOPHYSIOLOGY

Typically Lyme disease is prevalent during warmer months, when ticks are abundant, but it may occur at any time. It occurs most commonly in the northeast and other northern areas of the United States. Deer ticks and similar ticks carry a spirochetal bacterium named *Borrelia burgdorferi*. When ticks bite humans, they transmit the bacteria, which results in a chronic inflammatory process and multisystem disease.

ASSESSMENT FINDINGS

Signs and Symptoms

Three stages of the disease process usually occur, if the disease is untreated. Early stage 1 symptoms for about one-third of clients include a red macule or papule at the site of the tick bite, characteristic bull's eye rash with round rings surrounding the center, headache, neck stiffness, and pain. Secondary pruritic lesions may occur along with fever, chills, and malaise. The initial papule may not develop until 20 to 30 days after the bite. Some clients experience nausea, vomiting, and sore throat.

Midstage symptoms occur as the organism proliferates throughout the body and cardiac and neurologic involvement becomes evident. Cardiac problems include dysrhythmias and heart block. Neurologic symptoms such as facial palsy, meningitis, and encephalitis may occur. Some clients have problems with weakness, pain, and paresthesia (abnormal sensations).

Later symptoms (at least 4 weeks after the bite) include arthritis and other musculoskeletal problems. Joints, particularly knees, become warm, swollen, and painful. Joint erosion may occur as a result of the inflammatory process.

Diagnostic Findings

Diagnosis is based on the presenting signs and symptoms. The Lyme disease diagnosis is assisted by serologic studies for immunoglobulin G antibodies for *Borrelia*, which can be detected 6 weeks after the tick bite.

MEDICAL AND SURGICAL MANAGEMENT

Treatment includes administering antibiotics and supportive measures. If the disease is treated early, the prognosis is favorable. Permanent multisystem problems may occur if treatment is delayed.

NURSING MANAGEMENT

Nursing management involves teaching the client and family about the disease and its treatment. Educate clients about avoiding Lyme disease (Box 66–5).

Osteomyelitis

Osteomyelitis is an infection of the bone. Limited blood supply, inflammation and pressure of the tissue, and formation of new bone around devitalized bone tissue make osteomyelitis a difficult and challenging condition to treat. In adults, osteomyelitis may become chronic, greatly affecting quality of life and possibly resulting in the loss of an extremity (Smeltzer & Bare, 1996).

ETIOLOGY AND PATHOPHYSIOLOGY

Staphylococcus aureus and *Streptococcus pyogenes* are common causes of bone infections. Acute osteomyelitis results from bacteria reaching the bone via the bloodstream. Acute localized osteomyelitis occurs when bone is contaminated directly by trauma, such as penetrating wounds or compound fractures. Occasionally, surgical contamination or direct extension of bacteria from an infected area adjacent to the bone, such as the pin sites of skeletal traction, can cause osteomyelitis.

Microorganisms appear to migrate to the area just below the epiphysis of a long bone where the blood supply is more generous, but circulation through the area is limited. As the microorganisms multiply, they spread down to the bone shaft. The pressure from the collecting exudate elevates the periosteum. New bone cells (**involucrum**) are deposited on the periosteum while the underlying bone becomes necrotic. The pocket of necrotic bone (**sequestrum**) may remain sequestered for years or eventually drain by forming a sinus tract through to the skin. The infection tends to linger in a chronic state because it is difficult to penetrate the infected tissue by administering systemic antibiotic drugs.

In its weakened condition, the infected bone is prone to pathologic fracture. The diseased bone may lengthen as bone growth is stimulated, or it may shorten because of the destruction of the epiphyseal plate. Other complications of osteomyelitis include septicemia, thrombophlebitis, muscle contractures, pathologic fractures, and nonunion of fractures.

ASSESSMENT FINDINGS

Signs and Symptoms

Evidence of an acute infection occurs suddenly: high fever, chills, rapid pulse, tenderness or pain over the affected area, redness, and swelling. Chronic infection may be characterized by a persistent draining sinus.

Diagnostic Findings

With acute osteomyelitis, laboratory tests usually show an elevated leukocyte count, an elevated ESR, and possibly a blood culture positive for infective organisms. Identification of the causative organism may require an aspiration of subperiosteal pus for culture and sensitivity. Radiographic findings may be inconclusive in the early stages of infection, but later studies demonstrate irregular bone decalcification, bone necrosis, elevation of the periosteum, and new bone formation. Bone scans and MRI are useful in definitive diagnoses.

Radiographic studies for chronic osteomyelitis show large cavities, sequestra or dense bone formations, and raised periosteum. Areas of infection are delineated by bone scan. Blood studies reveal normal leukocyte count and ESR and possible anemia (Smeltzer & Bare, 1996).

MEDICAL AND SURGICAL MANAGEMENT

Management of osteomyelitis includes:

- Immobilization with a cast or immobilizer to decrease pain and prevent fracture. The cast may be windowed to provide access for wound care.
- Application of warm saline soaks to the affected area for 20 minutes several times a day to increase circulation to the affected area
- Identification of the causative organism to initiate appropriate and ongoing antibiotic therapy for infection control
- Surgical debridement of the necrotic tissue and sequestrum to remove the infected areas

BOX 66-5 Tips for Avoiding Lyme Disease

- When walking or hiking in areas that are likely to harbor ticks—high grass, wooded sites, and dense underbrush—wear long-sleeved shirts, long pants, and cover the head.
- Tuck pant legs into socks or boots.
- Inspect skin daily for ticks. Deer ticks are extremely small and may be mistaken for a new dark freckle.
- Check pets and children daily for ticks.
- Remove the entire tick with tweezers. Inspect the result to make sure that the whole tick was retrieved.
- Place ticks in a sealed container to be disposed of appropriately.

- Closed irrigation with saline or an antibiotic solution and low suction to the affected area to flush away necrotic tissue
- Bone grafts for the debrided cavity to stimulate bone growth
- Muscle flaps grafted to the affected area to enhance blood supply

NURSING MANAGEMENT

Clients with osteomyelitis experience pain, inflammation, swelling, and impaired mobility because of pain and the inability to bear weight. Handle the arm or leg or related area gently to prevent additional pain or fracture. Protect the infected area from injury. Instruct the client to keep the area elevated and to bear weight only as indicated. Protect skin from breakdown. Administer the prescribed antibiotics and pain medications and inform the client about the expected therapeutic effects and possible side effects. Clients with chronic osteomyelitis require extensive emotional support, related to the long-term nature of this illness.

Lupus Erythematosus

Lupus erythematosus is a diffuse connective tissue disease. There are two major types: systemic lupus erythematosus (SLE) and discoid lupus erythematosus (DLE). SLE, as the name implies, affects multiple body systems such as the skin, joints, kidney, serous membranes of the heart and lungs, lymph nodes, and GI tract. DLE affects only the skin. The most common type of lupus erythematosus is SLE, but clients with DLE may ultimately develop the systemic form of the disease.

ETIOLOGY AND PATHOPHYSIOLOGY

Lupus erythematosus is more common in women than in men. Most clients have this disorder in the third or fourth decade of life, but it may be seen in young children as well as in middle-aged and older adults. It is believed to be an autoimmune disease, but the triggering mechanism is still unknown. There is a strong familial tendency suggesting that certain inherited cellular antigenic markers confuse the ability of T cells to distinguish self from nonself. By mistake, helper T cells alert B cells to produce antibodies against normal cells, or suppressor T cells may be ineffective in controlling a B-cell response once it has been initiated. However, the disease may have periods during which it is in a subacute form or even in remission. Exposure to ultraviolet light is a factor in reactivating the disease.

Antibodies destroy connective tissues of the body. Affected structures undergo inflammation, fibrosis, scarring, and dysfunction. The nuclei of attacked cells are engulfed by polymorphonuclear leukocytes (neutrophils). Laboratory studies confirm this finding, which is considered diagnostic.

ASSESSMENT FINDINGS

Signs and Symptoms

The earlier signs and symptoms of SLE may include fever, weight loss, pain in the joints (arthralgia), malaise, muscle pain, and extreme fatigue. These symptoms are vague and may persist for several months to 2 years before more prominent symptoms develop and the client seeks medical advice.

A prominent sign of this disorder is a red butterfly-shaped rash on the face over the bridge of the nose and the cheeks. The word *lupus* means wolf. The term may have been used as a description for the facial rash that, to some, resembled the mask of reddish brown fur on a wolf.

Clients may also exhibit behavioral disturbances (confusion, hallucinations, irritability), chest pain (due to involvement of the pleura or pericarditis), fluid retention, proteinuria, and hematuria (due to renal involvement), progressive weight loss, nausea and vomiting, and in women, irregular or heavy menses. Other signs of the disease include:

- Nonspecific electrocardiographic changes
- A pericardial friction rub
- Pulmonary changes see on radiographic studies
- Enlargement of the spleen and lymph nodes
- Raynaud's phenomenon (vasospasm of the smaller vessels of the hands and feet resulting in blanching of the skin, and at times, pain and cyanosis of the extremities)

The symptoms of DLE are related only to the skin, the most prominent symptom being the appearance of the facial rash. Skin manifestations of the disorder also may be found on the forehead, earlobes, and scalp. Scalp involvement usually results in patchy loss of hair (alopecia). These symptoms also may be seen in people with SLE.

Diagnostic Findings

Diagnosis of SLE is based on presenting symptoms and blood tests. Blood studies show anemia, thrombocytopenia, leukocytosis or leukopenia, and positive antinuclear antibodies (ANA). Other laboratory studies may indicate multisystem involvement, such as an elevated creatinine level with kidney involvement. Additional tests, such as a renal biopsy and urinalysis, may be performed to determine the effect of the disorder on other body systems.

MEDICAL AND SURGICAL MANAGEMENT

There is no specific treatment for this disorder. Medical management is aimed at producing a remission and preventing or treating acute exacerbations of the disorder. High doses of corticosteroids are used initially. Those with severe disease or for whom steroid-related side effects are problematic may be treated with cytotoxic drugs such as azathioprine (Imuran) and cyclophosphamide (Cytoxan). Simple analgesics such as aspirin or an NSAID may be prescribed for fever and joint discomfort. Topical corticosteroids may be used for skin manifestations. Renal impairment may be treated with dialysis or kidney transplantation. Cardiac, GI, and central nervous system complications are treated symptomatically.

NURSING MANAGEMENT

Nursing management focuses on measures to minimize exacerbations of disease and to alleviate symptoms. The nurse administers prescribed medications and monitors for side effects. Before discharge, client education efforts involve reminding the client of the need for close medical follow-up and thorough medication instruction (eg, never to abruptly discontinue taking a prescribed corticosteroid without consulting the physician and to follow the dosage regimen exactly, particularly if the drug dose is being decreased gradually). Because the disease and drugs alter body image, assist the client to verbalize feelings and implement effective coping mechanisms. If the client desires, arrange a referral to the Lupus Foundation of America, which is dedicated to providing information about the disease, or to a local support or self-help group.

NURSING PROCESS
The Client With Systemic Lupus Erythematosus

Assessment

Review the medical record and diagnostic findings to evaluate the stage of disease and interventions that are appropriate. Assess the client's understanding of the nature of the disorder, its treatment, and limitations imposed by the disease process. Inspect the skin for rashes, purpuric lesions and other skin changes. Ask about the client's degree of sensitivity to sunlight. Also inspect for ulcerations in the mouth and throat (signs of GI involvement).

Listen to the heart for pericardial friction rub and the lungs for abnormal sounds suggesting pleural involvement.

Diagnosis and Planning

When caring for a client with lupus erythematosus, the nurse plans and implements care to help the client meet individual needs. This plan of care includes, but is not limited to, the following:

Nursing Diagnoses and Collaborative Problems	Nursing Interventions
Pain, Chronic related to inflammation and progressive disease activity	Administer prescribed analgesic and anti-inflammatory medications.
Goals: The client will experience relief from pain and discomfort.	Review the rationale for adhering to the prescribed regimen.
The client will adhere to the prescribed pharmacologic regimen.	Elevate swollen and painful joints and apply heat or cold as indicated.
The client will demonstrate use of alternative methods to reduce pain.	Monitor the client if braces or splints are used.
	Balance activity with rest periods.
	Provide utensils that can assist client to reduce pain associated with performing ADL.
	Move painful joints gently and slowly while supporting the extremity above and below the joint.
	Avoid heavy blankets or clothing that will increase pressure and, therefore, pain.
Impaired Physical Mobility related to inflammation, joint problems, pain, or decreased muscle strength.	Assist the client to maintain appropriate body alignment and neutral positioning during periods of inactivity.
Goals: The client will maintain maximal physical function within limitations.	Encourage moderate and progressive exercise as indicated.
The client will increase muscle strength in affected areas or in areas that compensate for physical limitations.	Advise client to use moist heat before performing ROM exercises.
The client will retain function with limitation of contractures.	Urge client to wear supportive shoes and to use assistive devices for ambulation as needed.
	Recommend sitting in elevated chairs that have arm rests that can help client to stand up.
	Encourage client to maintain erect posture when sitting, standing, and walking.
Self-Care Deficit (specify areas) related to exacerbation of disease, inflammation, and decreased mobility	Modify clothing so that it is easily put on and taken off (eg, use Velcro fasteners instead of buttons, front fasteners rather than back zippers, elastic shoe laces, cardigan sweaters instead of pullovers).

Goals: The client will perform self-care activities at highest possible level. The client will identify methods that assist her or him to meet self-care needs.	Pad handles for easy grasping. Suggest an electric toothbrush that is easier to handle. Provide cooking and eating utensils that are designed to promote a good grip, particularly useful for clients with hand deformities. Identify equipment resources and dealers for wheelchairs, elevated commode seats, and the like.
Body Image Disturbance related to change in appearance and inability to perform tasks and activities **Goals:** The client will verbalize increased confidence when dealing with changes in appearance and functional abilities. The client will establish realistic goals for the future.	Accept the client without reservation. Avoid nonverbal messages that convey impatience with the client's disabilities. Assist client only as needed or requested. Do not overprotect the client or increase dependency. Focus on what the client can do rather than not do. Assist the client to identify strengths. Encourage client to express fears, misgivings, or other concerns. Acknowledge feelings of grief and hostility. Refer client for counseling if client withdraws, shows signs of denial, or otherwise exhibits maladaptive behavior.
Ineffective Coping related to depression associated with lifestyle changes secondary to chronic illness **Goal:** The client will demonstrate adequate coping methods to deal with the chronicity of the disease.	Encourage the client to discuss feelings. Do not discourage crying or other expressions of emotion. Acknowledge emotions as real. Explore with the client options for resolving problems and dealing with dilemmas. Identify groups that provide support for individuals with the disease.

Evaluation and Expected Outcomes

- The client reports relief of pain and discomfort, adheres to prescribed drug therapy, and uses alternative methods to reduce pain.
- The client demonstrates maximal physical function within limitations, showing evidence of increased muscle strength function.
- The client can perform self-care at the highest possible level and has a plan for meeting future self-care needs as independently as possible.
- The client reports self-confidence and acceptance in the face of altered physical appearance and function and states realistic future goals.
- The client copes realistically and well with the chronicity of the disease.

Client and Family Teaching

Because SLE is a chronic disease, treated mainly on an outpatient basis, much nursing management revolves around teaching. Clients and their families need accurate and complete information about the disease, its treatment and prognosis, and self-care measures to increase comfort and promote health. Client education typically includes:

- Explain the treatment plan and necessary lifestyle modifications related to musculoskeletal restrictions and systemic involvement. Because sunlight tends to exacerbate the disease, for example, instruct the client to avoid sunlight and ultraviolet radiation. When outdoors, the client should apply effective sunscreens with a sun protection factor (SPF) of 15 or higher and wear clothing that covers the arms and legs and a wide-brimmed hat to shade the face. Sunlamps and tanning booths are taboo.
- Because fatigue is a major issue for clients with SLE, assist the client to pace activities, allowing for adequate rest along with regular activity to promote mobility and prevent joint stiffness. Discourage activities that cause severe pain or discomfort.
- Discuss additional lifestyle concerns. Topics may focus on dietary requirements and illness prevention.
- Teach the client how to maintain a well balanced diet and increased fluid intake to raise energy levels and promote tissue healing and to prevent infections by avoiding crowds when possible and people with known infections, such as colds.
- Periodically review the medication program, particularly the effects and adverse effects of medications and related signs and symptoms that require attention and should be reported to the physician (increased severity of symptoms, involvement in other joints or areas of the body, weight loss, prolonged anorexia, nausea, vomiting, fever, cough, shortness of breath, difficult urination, infection, or any other unusual occurrence).
- Advise the client to take medications exactly as directed and not to stop taking the medication if symptoms are relieved unless advised to do so by the physician.
- If symptoms become worse, avoid increasing the dosage unless advised to do so by the physician. Do not use over-the-counter drugs unless a physician approves their use.
- Explore the client's proactive role in meeting her or his needs and managing pain and discomfort.

- Identify nonpharmacologic comfort measures. For instance, using a moist form of heat may relieve joint stiffness. Advise the client to use warm, not hot, soaks, wraps, or towels hot from the clothes dryer and to take care not to burn the skin.
- Inform other physicians and dentists of current therapy before any treatment, surgery, or drugs are prescribed.
- Identify available community groups and other resources focused on supporting the client with lupus erythematosus.

Low Back Pain

The occurrence of low back pain is common and accounts for many of the lost working hours in the United States. Low back pain may be acute or chronic and involves the lumbar or sacral areas.

Etiology and Pathophysiology

Causes of low back pain include muscle strain, osteoarthritis involving the spine, lumbar or sacral disk herniation or degeneration, metastatic bone lesions, obesity, poor posture, lack of exercise, and some uterine or menstrual disorders. Occupations that require prolonged sitting or standing, heavy lifting, vibrations from drilling equipment, or prolonged driving contribute to problems with lower back pain.

The spinal column consists of the vertebrae, which are rigid, and the intervertebral disks, which are flexible. Ligaments and paravertebral muscles join the vertebrae and intervertebral disks together. This construction allows the spinal column to absorb shocks as a person engages in running, jumping, and other activities. Abdominal and thoracic muscles assist in lifting activities. Disuse of these muscles, along with contributing factors listed above, can lead to back pain.

When injury occurs within or around the spinal column, released neurotransmitters travel over sensory pathways in the spinal cord to pain receptor sites in the brain. This results in the sensation of pain or discomfort.

ASSESSMENT FINDINGS

Signs and Symptoms

Pain is totally subjective. Only the client can describe its onset, characteristics, location, radiation, intensity, duration, and activities that relieve or worsen it. Some clients with low back pain have a limited ROM. Some guard the spine against being moved. Gait or posture may be altered.

Clients with low back pain frequently limit their activity. They complain of pain that radiates to the legs (sciatica). Numbness and tingling (paresthesia) can also occur along with muscle spasms. The straight leg test (lifting leg straight up while flexing the foot 90 degrees) is a positive sign if the client experiences pain while doing this.

Diagnostic Findings

Radiography, CT scanning, MRI, and myelography are methods that determine the source of the low back pain. A gynecologic examination may indicate a tumor of the uterus, which may be the source of the low back pain.

Medical Management

Treatment depends on the cause (if known) and the severity of the disorder. Mild symptoms usually respond to the application of heat or cold and analgesics or muscle relaxants. The client is encouraged to avoid activities that cause further discomfort until pain is relieved. The physician may prescribe bed rest for several days.

Other therapies include an exercise program, physical therapy, weight loss, and a back brace. Intermittent pelvic traction may be necessary for those who do not respond to symptomatic treatment. Short-term use of back supports and braces may be prescribed.

Nursing Management

When the cause of low back pain is poor posture and body mechanics, instruct the client to:

- Stand (or sit) straight and tall: contract the abdominal muscles, pull the buttocks in, hold the chest up, square the shoulders, and look straight ahead.
- Keep the feet slightly separated for a broad base of support.
- Bend the knees and keep the back straight when lifting.
- Use the long, strong muscles in the legs and hips.
- Carry heavy objects close to the body near the center of gravity.
- Push, pull, or roll objects rather than lift them.
- Sleep on a firm mattress or use a bed board.
- Wear sturdy, supportive shoes; repair the heels when they wear down.
- Engage in active exercise regularly to maintain muscle tone, strength, and stamina.

Structural Disorders

Structural disorders of the musculoskeletal system involve metabolic conditions that alter bone structure. These alterations result in pain, bone deformity, and fracture.

Osteoporosis

Osteoporosis, a loss of bone density, occurs principally in older adults and affects more women than men.

ETIOLOGY AND PATHOPHYSIOLOGY

Normally the processes of bone formation and bone resorption occur at an even rate. In osteoporosis, loss of bone substance exceeds the rate of bone formation. The total bone mass is reduced, resulting in bones that become progressively porous, brittle, and fragile. Compression fractures of the vertebrae are common. Aging contributes to osteoporosis (the loss of bone mass) in the following ways:

- Calcitonin levels, which inhibit bone resorption and promote bone formation, decrease with aging.
- Estrogen levels, which inhibit bone breakdown, decrease in postmenopausal women.
- Parathyroid hormone levels, which increase bone resorption, increase with aging.

Other causes of osteoporosis, which may occur in any age group and both sexes, include Cushing's syndrome, prolonged use of high doses of corticosteroids, prolonged periods of immobility, hyperthyroidism, hyperparathyroidism, and dietary deficiency of vitamin D and calcium. Some medications interfere with the body's ability to use and metabolize calcium, including thyroid supplements, anticonvulsants, isoniazid, tetracycline, and heparin.

ASSESSMENT FINDINGS

Signs and Symptoms

Clients with osteoporosis frequently complain of lumbosacral pain or thoracic back pain or both. The bone pain or tenderness results from tiny compression fractures occurring in the vertebrae. There is an accompanying loss of height.

Diagnostic Findings

Radiographic examination of the bones shows a loss of bone when there is at least a 25% loss. Bone deformities (especially in the spine), such as kyphosis and lordosis, and pathologic fractures in long bones also may be seen in x-ray studies. Laboratory studies are usually normal but may be performed to rule out other disorders such as multiple myeloma, hyperparathyroidism, or metastatic bone lesions. Bone densimetry measures bone loss of less than 3% and may be used to assess and monitor bone loss and to serve as a guide to therapy.

MEDICAL AND SURGICAL MANAGEMENT

Osteoporosis cannot be treated directly, but medical management can slow the rate of bone resorption. Bone pain or tenderness may respond to mild analgesics such as aspirin. Oral calcium preparations (calcium gluconate, calcium lactate, calcium carbonate, or dibasic calcium phosphate) may be recommended to supplement dietary calcium. Some of these preparations also contain vitamin D, which is needed for absorption of calcium in the intestine. New medications, such as biphosphonate-alendronate sodium (Fosamax) inhibit bone resorption. Administration of calcitonin also inhibits bone resorption. Hormone replacement therapy for postmenopausal women as well as adequate rest and exercise, especially weight-bearing exercise such as walking, are part of the treatment regimen.

NURSING MANAGEMENT

In providing care for clients with osteoporosis, the nurse emphasizes the need for a nutritious, well balanced diet that is high in calcium, vitamin D, and protein—all recommended to delay or prevent osteoporosis. Women especially are advised to drink 4 to 6 glasses of milk daily or eat other dairy products to acquire approximately 1,000 to 1,500 mg of calcium; those who smoke cigarettes may require more. Orange juice fortified with calcium is a nutritious alternative. If the client takes antacids, suggest those containing calcium. Recommend activity that promotes bone formation, such as regular, aerobic exercise (eg, walking).

Osteomalacia

Osteomalacia, a metabolic bone disease, is characterized by inadequate mineralization of bone.

ETIOLOGY AND PATHOPHYSIOLOGY

New bone has decreased deposits of calcium and phosphorus. The bone mass is structurally weaker and bone deformities occur. Poor calcium absorption or excessive loss of calcium contributes to osteomalacia. Additional risk factors are identified in Box 66–6.

Signs and Symptoms

Clients with osteomalacia experience bone pain and weakness. They also complain of tenderness if the bones are palpated. Bone deformities, such as kyphosis and bowing of the legs, occur as the disease advances. Clients exhibit a waddling type of gait, putting them at risk for falls and fractures.

Diagnostic Findings

Radiographic studies demonstrate demineralization of the bone. Serum levels of calcium and phosphorus are low. Alkaline phosphatase levels are typically elevated.

MEDICAL AND SURGICAL TREATMENT

Treatment is aimed at correcting the underlying cause of the osteomalacia. This includes supplements of calcium, phosphorus, and vitamin D; adequate nutrition; exposure to sunlight; and progressive exercise and ambulation. Bone deformities may require braces or surgery for correction.

NURSING MANAGEMENT

The nurse is in a primary role of educating the client about the disease and its treatment and, therefore, includes teaching in the care plan. Teach the client about methods and medications used to relieve pain and discomfort. Allow the client to verbalize self-concept issues related to deformities and activity restrictions.

BOX 66-6 Risk Factors for Osteomalacia

- Dietary deficiencies
- Malnutrition, particularly low calcium intake
- Malabsorption
- Gastrectomy
- Chronic renal failure
- Anticonvulsant therapy (phenytoin, phenobarbital)
- Insufficient vitamin D (no supplements in food and lack of sunlight)
- Poverty
- Food fads
- Lack of nutritional knowledge

(Adapted from Smeltzer, S. C., & Bare, B. G. [1996], *Brunner and Suddarth's textbook of medical-surgical nursing* [8th ed., p. 1894.]. Philadelphia: Lippincott-Raven.)

Paget's Disease

Paget's disease (osteitis deformans) is a chronic bone disorder characterized by abnormal bone remodeling. Adults over age 60 years of age are affected. The most common areas of involvement are the long bones, spine, pelvis, and skull.

ETIOLOGY AND PATHOPHYSIOLOGY

In Paget's disease, some skeletal bones are unaffected; other bones are marked by a disturbance in the ratio between bone formation and resorption. The excessive osteoclastic activity causes the bones to become soft and bowed initially. Later the bones thicken when compensatory osteoblastic activity resumes. The process of bone turnover continues to occur, resulting in a classic mosaic pattern of bone matrix development. The new bone has high mineral content but is not well formed. This causes the bones to be weak and prone to fracture.

Although the cause of Paget's disease is unknown, the process by which individuals with this disorder deposit collagen, a protein in connective tissue, is thought to be defective. This is based on the fact that the affected bones are high in mineral content but poorly constructed. A family history of the disorder is not uncommon. Additional findings indicate a possible link between the disease and a previous viral infection.

Complications include pathologic fractures, paralysis from spinal cord compression, cranial nerve damage, such as deafness from compression of the skull, and kidney stones. Occasionally, the lesions undergo malignant changes.

ASSESSMENT FINDINGS

Signs and Symptoms

Some clients are asymptomatic with only some mild skeletal deformity. Other clients have marked skeletal deformities, which may include enlargement of the skull, bowing of the long bones, and kyphosis (hunchback). Bone pain and tenderness on pressure may be elicited. Paget's disease may go undiscovered until an x-ray for another problem reveals the disorder.

Diagnostic Findings

Radiographic examination discloses bones in various stages of resorption and remodeling with a mosaic appearance to the bone structure. Pathologic fractures appear and the bones are curved and enlarged. Bone scans are usually done. Elevated serum alkaline phosphatase level and increased urinary hydroxyproline (an amino acid found in collagen) excretion are common.

MEDICAL AND SURGICAL MANAGEMENT

Clients without symptoms usually do not need treatment. Those with symptoms may benefit from drug therapy. Pain usually can be controlled with analgesics such as aspirin or NSAIDs. Those with moderate to severe pain may benefit from treatment with calcitonin (Calcimar), a hormone that appears to block the resorption of bone by reducing the number of osteoclasts and decreasing the rate of bone turnover. Treatment with calcitonin usually results in a drop in the serum alkaline phosphatase level and urinary excretion of hydroxyproline, followed by regression of the lesions. Although not an analgesic, calcitonin reduces pain because it seems to promote the regression of lesions. However, the client may still require analgesics until bone pain is relieved.

A drug used in advanced disease is EHDP or etidronate disodium (Didronel, Didronel IV), given orally or intravenously (IV). This drug reduces normal and abnormal bone resorption and secondarily reduces bone formation that is coupled to bone resorption. When other drugs prove unsuccessful, mithramycin (Mithracin), an antibiotic usually used in cancer treatment for its cytotoxic effect, may be administered.

Surgery may be performed to repair pathologic fractures or relieve neurologic complications.

NURSING MANAGEMENT

Implement prescribed drug therapy and monitor for side effects. If self-care is limited, assist the client with ADL. Client safety is a priority because strength and balance may be compromised. As appropriate, teach the client how to use ambulatory aids (eg, a walker or cane), self-administer prescribed drugs, and implement measures to reduce falls within the home. For nursing management of a client who requires surgery refer to the nursing process discussion for clients undergoing orthopedic surgery.

Disorders of the Feet

Many foot disorders are treated on an outpatient basis or encountered by nurses when caring for clients with other disorders. Foot disorders that commonly affect clients and for which surgery may be performed are bunions and hammertoes.

Hallux Valgus (Bunions) and Hammertoe

Hallux valgus, also called bunions, is a deformity of the great (large) toe at its metatarsophalangeal joint (Fig. 66–11**A**). **Hammertoe** is a flexion deformity of the interphalangeal joint and may involve several toes (Fig. 66–11**B**).

ETIOLOGY AND PATHOPHYSIOLOGY

Bunions are associated with heredity, arthritis, or improperly fitting shoes. Women tend to be affected more than men. The first metatarsal bone enlarges on the medial side. The metatarsal bone protrudes at an acute angle toward the midline of the body while the great toe points laterally. There is an overgrowth of soft tissue (bursa), which is actually the bunion. The foot widens and the arch flattens. The malalignment results in pain from the stress on the joint, improper support and distribution of body weight, and inflammation of the bursa.

Like bunions, hammertoe also results from wearing poorly fitting shoes. Toes are pulled upward by the shoe, as the ball of the foot is pulled down. Corns (small, round, elevated overgrowths of epidermis) usually develop on top of the toes. Calluses (wide, thickened layer of skin) form under the metatarsal area.

ASSESSMENT FINDINGS

Signs and Symptoms

The malalignment typical of bunions results in pain from the stress on the joint, improper support

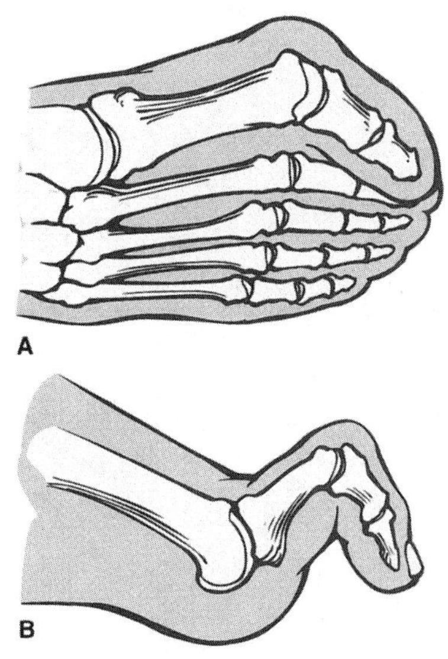

FIGURE 66-11. Common foot problems: (*A*) Bunion; (*B*) Hammertoe.

and distribution of body weight, and inflammation of the bursa. The client complains of pain on walking or flexing the foot, tenderness, and redness of the joint. The typical appearance of the foot deformity is obvious. In hammertoe, the foot deformity is evident. Corns and calluses are easily seen. The client complains of discomfort with ambulation.

Diagnostic Findings

Radiographic films of the foot reveal the degree of joint deformity.

MEDICAL AND SURGICAL MANAGEMENT

No treatment is necessary for bunions if pain is not severe and the client has little or no difficulty. Low-heeled, properly fitted shoes are recommended. A bunionectomy, the surgical procedure to remove the bunion and correct the deformity, may be performed when the individual has pain and difficulty walking. Treatment of hammertoe includes exercises, wearing properly fitting or open-toed shoes, use of pads to protect the joints, and surgery to correct the malalignment. Both surgeries are performed on an outpatient or short-term admission basis, with the client discharged in the late afternoon or the following morning. Rest, elevation of the foot, and analgesics are prescribed.

NURSING MANAGEMENT

Nursing management of foot disorders includes relieving pain and discomfort, improving mobility, and instructing clients about the necessity for proper foot attire. Many clients are treated in an outpatient setting. Nurses in these settings are usually charged with teaching the client about the foot condition, treatment, medications, and postoperative care if the client had surgery. Refer to Nursing Guidelines 66–3 for specific nursing actions.

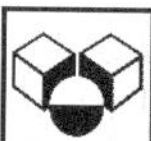

Nursing Guidelines 66-3

Instructions for a Client Following Foot Surgery

Pain Management—Methods to Reduce Pain

- Elevate foot
- Apply ice as instructed
- Take pain medications as prescribed
- Call physician for pain not relieved

Signs of Impaired Circulation to Report to Physician

- Change in sensation
- Inability to move toes
- Toes or foot cool to touch
- Toes or foot are pale or blue in color

Mobility

- Use assistive devices appropriately
- Adhere to weight-bearing restrictions
- Wear protective shoe over wound dressing

Wound Care

- Keep dressing or cast clean and dry
- Report signs of wound infection—pain, drainage, fever
- Take antibiotics as prescribed

(Adapted from Smeltzer, S.C., & Bare, B.G. [1996]. Brunner and Suddarth's textbook of medical-surgical nursing *[8th ed.]. Philadelphia: Lippincott.)*

Disorders of the Upper Extremity

Frequent sites of injury and pain in the upper extremity include the shoulder, elbow, and wrist. Among disorders frequently encountered are painful shoulder syndrome, epicondylitis, ganglion, and carpal tunnel syndrome.

Shoulder, Elbow, and Wrist Problems

The shoulder is frequently a site of injury and pain. Common conditions include tendonitis, tears and rupture of the rotator cuff, and bursitis. These result in painful shoulder syndrome.

Epicondylitis (tennis elbow) is a painful inflammation of the elbow. A ganglion is a cystic mass that develops near tendon sheaths and joints of the wrist. **Carpal tunnel syndrome** is a term for a group of symptoms located in the wrist where the carpal bones, carpal tendons, and median nerve pass through a narrow, inelastic canal.

ETIOLOGY AND PATHOPHYSIOLOGY

The primary causes of shoulder injuries are trauma and repeated stress. Injury is also responsible for epicondylitis, which occurs when the tendons of the medial or lateral radial and ulnar epicondyles sustain damage. The injury typically follows excessive pronation and supination of the forearm, such as that which occurs when playing tennis, pitching ball, or rowing. Ganglion cysts form through defects in the tendon sheath or joint capsule and occur most commonly in women under age 50.

Carpal tunnel syndrome results from repetitive wrist motion that traumatizes the tendon sheath or ligaments in the carpal canal. The trauma produces swelling that compresses the median nerve against the transverse carpal ligament. Those affected tend to be in occupations that perform repetitive hand movements such as cashiers, typists, musicians, and assemblers.

Signs and Symptoms

Shoulder injuries are marked by pain and inflammation, which can spread to surrounding tissues. In epicondylitis, clients report pain radiating down the dorsal surface of the forearm and a weak grasp. Clients with ganglion cysts experience pain and tenderness in the affected area.

Clients with carpal tunnel syndrome describe pain or burning in one or both hands, which may radiate to the forearm and shoulder in severe cases. The pain tends to be more prominent at night and early in the morning. Shaking the hands may reduce the pain by promoting movement of edematous fluid from the carpal canal. Sensation may be lost or reduced in the thumb, index, middle, and a portion of the ring finger. The client may be unable to flex the index and middle fingers to make a fist. Flexion of the wrist usually causes immediate pain and numbness.

Diagnostic Findings

In general, x-ray studies are used to identify abnormalities and rule out fracture and other problems. In carpal tunnel syndrome, results of electromyography, which relies on a mild electrical current to stimulate the nerve, show a delay in motor response in muscles innervated by the median nerve.

MEDICAL AND SURGICAL MANAGEMENT

Shoulder treatment includes applications of cold (ice) and heat, exercise, anti-inflammatory medications, local injection of corticosteroids, analgesics, NSAIDs, and rest. Surgical intervention may be necessary to repair tears and ruptures. In many cases, clients with injuries of the shoulder or other portions of the upper extremity are referred for physical therapy.

Treatment for epicondylitis is similar to that for shoulder injuries and splinting is added to rest and support the joint structures. Corticosteroids may be injected locally. Treatment of the ganglion cyst includes aspiration of the ganglion, corticosteroid injection, and surgical excision.

Carpal tunnel treatment involves resting the hands when possible and splinting the hand and wrist. NSAIDs and periodic injections of a corticosteroid preparation may relieve the inflammation and discomfort. If conservative treatment fails, surgery to release the pressure of the ligament on the median nerve may be performed.

NURSING MANAGEMENT

Provide the client with information about medications. If the client is taking NSAIDs, stress that these medications should be taken with food. If corticosteroid injections are ordered, explain what the client can expect and mention that the injection itself may cause some discomfort.

Show clients how to use and care for prescribed splints and braces and how to perform related ROM exercises. Some clients find that hand exercises are less painful if performed with the hand under warm water. Additional management activities involve exploring ways to perform ADL or alter job responsibilities to relieve stress and reduce injury to joints.

Client and Family Teaching

Key teaching points include:

- Rest the joint in a position that reduces stress.
- Support the affected arm joint on pillows while sleeping.
- Apply cold for the first 24 to 48 hours to reduce swelling and pain.
- Gradually increase joint movement.
- Avoid working or lifting above shoulder level. Do not push objects with the arm joint, particularly the shoulder.
- Perform ROM and strengthening exercises as prescribed by the physician or physical therapist

Bone Tumors

Bone tumors may be malignant or benign. Malignant tumors are primary, originating in the bone, or secondary, originating from elsewhere in the body (ie, breast, lung, prostate, or kidney) and traveling to the bone (metastasis). Secondary or metastatic bone tumors are more common than primary bone tumors. Benign tumors of the bone are also more common than malignant bone tumors.

Benign Bone Tumors

Benign bone tumors have the potential to cause fractures of bones. However, they are not life-threatening and usually present few symptoms.

ETIOLOGY AND PATHOPHYSIOLOGY

Benign tumors are usually the result of misplaced or overgrown clusters of normal bone or cartilage cells that cause the structure to enlarge and impair local function. They grow slowly and do not metastasize. Their growth can weaken the bone structure by compressing or displacing the normal tissue.

ASSESSMENT FINDINGS

Signs and Symptoms

Clients with benign bone tumors experience pain that worsens when bearing weight. The bone appears deformed and swelling may appear over the involved area. If the tumor is in a bone of the extremities, movement may be decreased and pathologic fractures occur easily.

Diagnostic Findings

Radiography, bone scans, and biopsy of the tumor determine the diagnosis.

MEDICAL AND SURGICAL MANAGEMENT

Medical management includes treating pain and preventing fractures. Surgery is performed if the tumor does not stop growing, bone deformity is present, or if the pain is interfering with ADL and mobility.

Curettage (scraping) or local excision is the usual procedure. Bone grafts may need to be done to promote bone growth and healing. Splints or casts are applied until the bone heals. Clients require close monitoring after surgery because benign bone tumors can recur.

NURSING MANAGEMENT

Providing adequate explanations to the client and alleviating anxiety are key nursing responsibilities. Provide adequate explanations to the client, emphasizing the nature of the tumor, prognosis, and treatment. Allow time for questions and expressions of fear and anxiety. Administer pain medications as indicated. Teach the client methods to reduce pain and swelling. Encourage the client to elevate the affected extremity.

Malignant Bone Tumors

Malignant bone tumors are abnormal osteoblasts or myeloblasts (marrow cells) that exhibit rapid and uncontrollable growth.

ETIOLOGY AND PATHOPHYSIOLOGY

Prior exposure to radiation and toxic chemicals has been associated with the genesis of some malignant bone tumors. A hereditary link in which a tumor suppressor gene may be absent or impaired also is suspected because the same type of tumor may appear among siblings in the same family. Primary tumors include osteosarcoma, Ewing's sarcoma, and chondrosarcoma.

Malignant bone tumors are usually located around the knee in the distal femur or proximal fibula; a few are found in the proximal humerus. As the tumor expands, it lifts the periosteum in much the same way as osteomyelitis. Metastasis occurs via the circulatory or lymphatic system. Metastasis to the lungs is common.

ASSESSMENT FINDINGS

Signs and Symptoms

A pathologic fracture may be the event that leads the client to seek treatment. Clients with malignant tumors of the bone complain of persistent pain, swelling, and difficulty in moving the involved extremity. A limp or abnormal gait may be noted when the client walks. However, by the time symptoms are experienced, the tumor has usually spread beyond its primary site.

Diagnostic Findings

The bone appears abnormal on radiographic examination, MRI, or bone scan. Abnormal cells are identified by biopsy. A malignancy of the skeletal system is associated with an elevated serum alkaline phosphatase level.

MEDICAL AND SURGICAL MANAGEMENT

Treatment of primary malignant bone tumors involves surgical removal of the tumor by amputating the extremity or by wide local resection. Radiation therapy and chemotherapy may be used as well. Chemotherapy after surgery aims to destroy tumor cells that escape from the original tumor site.

NURSING MANAGEMENT

Clients with malignant bone tumors require extensive emotional support and information about the disease, treatment, and prognosis. Implement preoperative and postoperative measures for clients who are having surgery. Refer to the section on amputations for specific nursing care for amputees. As in other orthopedic surgeries, general nursing responsibilities include keeping the affected extremity elevated to reduce swelling, assessing neurovascular status frequently (see Chap. 65), and monitoring closely for complications if the affected limb is immobilized postoperatively.

Orthopedic Surgery

Orthopedic surgery may be performed for various reasons: to correct a deformity, remove a primary bone tumor, align fractured bones (open reduction), repair or replace a joint, insert a bone graft to promote bone healing, or stabilize a bone internally (using rods, pins, screws, nails, or wires).

Preoperative Nursing Management

ASSESSMENT

Preoperatively obtain a complete medical, drug, and allergy history from the client or a family member. Assess the client's physical condition and mental status at the time of the initial interview. Review the client's chart, noting the diagnosis, type of surgery to be performed, and any previous treatments, such as traction or drug use. If the client's disorder was treated previously, determine whether any complications or problems occurred because of or during treatment.

Client goals in the preoperative period focus on helping the client to experience reduced pain; continue to be active, mobile, and injury free; practice measures to reduce the potential for postoperative wound infection; control anxiety at manageable levels; understand instructions; and comprehend the procedures and rationale of postoperative management (Nursing Guidelines 66–4).

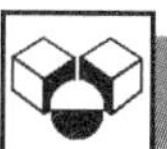

Nursing Guidelines 66-4

Ensuring Complete Care for Clients Before Orthopedic Surgery

- Review the operation and the reason for it.
- Administer prescribed analgesics.
- Relieve the client's discomfort through positioning and joint immobilization.
- Support painful joints and be gentle when moving the client.
- Allow ample time for physical activities because the client with a musculoskeletal disorder needs more time to carry out preoperative routines. Allow the client to use any ambulatory aid that was brought from home.
- Demonstrate use of the overbed trapeze and encourage its use.
- Demonstrate and have the client perform necessary postoperative activities, such as coughing and deep breathing exercises.
- Provide preoperative skin care as indicated by agency policy and procedure. If the client has initiated skin preparation at home, check to be sure the procedures were performed.
- Obtain adequate help when transferring a sedated client who is not in traction from the bed to the surgical stretcher. However, keep a client who is in traction in the hospital bed. Then, without lifting or removing the traction weights, transport the bed to the operating room.
- Administer the IV prophylactic antibiotic if ordered before surgery. (Although laminar airflow in the operating suite has reduced the incidence of postoperative infection, a great risk for infection remains for every client having orthopedic surgery. The number of personnel in the operating room may need to be limited to reduce a potential reservoir of infecting microorganisms.)

Postoperative Nursing Management

Ideally, postoperative nursing management begins preoperatively with demonstrations of deep breathing and coughing exercises and descriptions and demonstrations of the incentive spirometer (if that is likely to be used after surgery). Even if the client will have physical therapy postoperatively, explain and help the client practice active and isometric leg exercises. Describe other devices that may be used postoperatively such as IV infusions of fluid and blood, oxygen, a wound drain, elastic stockings, or roller bandages. Discuss the possible use of traction or the CPM machine.

NURSING PROCESS
The Client Undergoing Orthopedic Surgery

Assessment

When the client returns from surgery, review orders in the chart regarding immobilization, movement or turning, and positioning of the arm or leg. Inspect the dressing over the incision. If a wound drain is present, assess the patency of the drain and the type and amount of drainage in the collection receptacle. Assess the neurovascular status of the affected extremity. Monitor vital signs frequently until they stabilize and thereafter on a routine basis. Maintain the infusing IV fluids as ordered. Assess the client's respiratory status. Encourage the client to identify pain levels and the effectiveness of analgesics.

Within the first 24 to 72 hours after orthopedic surgery, complications, such as a fat embolus, may occur (see Table 66–2). The symptoms of a fat embolus are similar to those of a pulmonary embolus. In addition, petechial hemorrhages may appear on the skin of the chest. Report severe chest pain or incisional pain that is unrelieved to the physician immediately. Additional nursing management includes, but is not limited to, the following:

Nursing Diagnoses and Collaborative Problems	Nursing Interventions
Risk for Ineffective Breathing Pattern related to mucus and inability to mobilize secretions from the airway **Goal:** The client will demonstrate effective respiratory rate and depth with clear breath sounds.	Have the client do deep breathing and coughing exercises every 2 hours until the client can ambulate. Use an incentive spirometer to motivate and evaluate the client's efforts. Change the client's position to facilitate lung expansion and encourage activity within prescribed limits. Auscultate the lungs every 4 hours. If the client has thick secretions or if lung sounds are diminished or breath sounds abnormal or the client experiences fever, cough, chills, or other signs of a respiratory problem, implement measures to reduce these problems, and inform the physician.
Pain related to surgery **Goal:** The client will report relief of pain after receiving comfort measures.	Be gentle when moving the client or adjusting positions. Administer analgesics as ordered. If a patient-controlled analgesia device is prescribed, show the client how to operate it. As pain subsides to a less acute level, collaborate with the physician and client about alternating or switching to a non-narcotic analgesic. Augment pain relief by changing positions and using elevation or cold applications to relieve swelling. Monitor pain level, duration, and location. Continued severe pain after the first several postoperative days requires investigation, as does pain in other than the affected area.
Risk for Disuse Syndrome related to immobility imposed by casting, traction, non–weight-bearing status and the like **Goal:** The client will be free of muscle atrophy, pressure ulcers, and other complications of immobility.	Assist the client to move in bed. Encourage the client to use the overhead trapeze. Unless the physician orders otherwise, perform active or passive exercises on limbs not affected by surgery to prevent muscle atrophy. Put unaffected joints through a full ROM several times a day. As healing progresses, implement activity and ambulation orders. Transfer the client to a wheelchair. Obtain sufficient assistance for the transfer and comply with orders for full, partial, or non–weight-bearing status. Transport the client to physical therapy for instruction and practice in using a walker or other ambulatory aid. Assist the client to practice using the ambulatory aid on the nursing unit for increasing distances.
Risk for Impaired Skin Integrity related to inadequate peripheral circulation imposed by surgery and resultant immobility. **Goal:** The client's skin will remain intact.	Change the client's position at least every 2 hours but avoid placing joints in a position of flexion. Use a turning sheet if the client cannot assist with movement. Avoid dragging the client across the sheets, which creates skin friction. Keep the sheets dry and free of wrinkles. Do not allow the client to sit for long periods. Provide pressure-relieving devices or a special mattress if bony prominences appear reddened. Massage reddened skin areas that blanch when pressure is relieved. Encourage the independent use of a trapeze to adjust body positions and relieve pressure briefly. Instruct the client to use the trapeze and upper body strength rather than pushing with the heel. For clients who are extremely prone to skin breakdown, such as those who are very thin, debilitated, or paralyzed, consider using one of a variety of therapeutic beds, such as the Clinitron bed, to reduce pressure on capillaries. Apply pressure-relieving devices beneath the client's body, under bony prominences or, in cases of amputation, underneath the stump.
Risk for Infection related to compromised skin integrity **Goal:** The client will not contract an infection.	Inspect pin or wire sites used in traction or external fixation devices, the surgical incision, or beneath a cast window for signs of infection.

	Perform conscientious handwashing.
	Reinforce moist dressings or change them completely using aseptic principles.
	Keep the drainage collection container below the level of the incision.
	Follow the physician's orders for irrigating and aspirating wound drainage tubing to maintain its patency.
	Encourage the client to eat a nutritious diet with adequate amounts of complete protein for wound healing.
	Administer prescribed antibiotics.
	Report purulent wound drainage, elevated temperature, chills, and increased white blood cell count to the physician.
Risk for Constipation or Diarrhea related to altered nutrition and activity status **Goal:** The client will maintain normal bowel elimination.	Encourage oral fluids, especially fruit juice, and a diet that contains whole grains, fresh fruits, and vegetables. Keep the client as active as possible.
	Advise the client not to ignore or control the stimulus to have a bowel movement.
	Use a fracture bedpan and provide privacy until the client can use a bedside commode or ambulate to the bathroom.
Self-Care Deficit: Bathing and Hygiene, Feeding, Dressing and Toileting **Goal:** The client gradually will perform ADL as independently as possible.	Collaborate with the client on tasks that may be performed independently. Encourage as much independence and participation as it is realistic to expect.
	Ask the client to provide information on how best to arrange equipment for its convenient use and document this information on the plan of care.
	Evaluate the client's strength and endurance daily.
	Progressively increase the client's involvement in self-care activities, striving for eventual independence.

Evaluation and Expected Outcomes

- The client has an unobstructed, mucus-free airway achieved by effective coughing and deep breathing.
- The client reports pain relief and can ambulate independently.
- The client's peripheral circulation is adequate to sustain tissue perfusion and skin is intact without signs of breakdown.
- The client is free of infection, has regular bowel elimination patterns, and can perform ADL independently.

Client and Family Teaching

Discuss with the client, family, and other significant caregivers the support system that will be available after discharge. Explore the kinds of assistance the client needs for moving and walking, preparing meals, getting to the physician's office or physical therapy department, and performing other household tasks. Try to identify modifications that will be necessary in the home environment such as relocating the bed to a ground floor level. Provide information about renting home care equipment, arranging for home delivery of meals through a community agency or church service group, scheduling transportation with an agency that has a medical van or hydraulic lift available, or referring the client to a home health care agency or extended care facility. Be sure to provide printed discharge instructions for future reference and cover the following general points:

- Follow the directions of the physician. Do not resume any activity that has been restricted until told to do so.
- Perform exercises exactly as prescribed by the physician and physical therapist.
- Use the recommended device (walker, cane, crutches) for walking.
- Wear supportive shoes when using crutches, walker, or cane.
- Eliminate safety hazards in the home, such as scatter rugs.
- Eat a nutritious diet and drink plenty of fluids.
- Take prescribed medications as directed; do not use or take any nonprescription drugs unless they have been approved by the physician.
- Notify the physician if the incision has unusual drainage or if fever, chills, sudden onset of pain, redness, or swelling occurs.

Amputation

Amputation is the removal of a limb. The amputation may occur as a result of trauma (traumatic amputation) or in an effort to control disease or disability (therapeutic amputation).

Etiology

The following are conditions for which an amputation may be performed:

- Malignant tumors
- Long-standing infections of bone and tissue that prohibit restoration of function
- Extensive trauma to an extremity
- Death of tissues from peripheral vascular insufficiency or from peripheral vasospastic diseases such as Buerger's and Raynaud's diseases
- Thermal injuries
- Deformity of a limb rendering it a useless hindrance
- Life-threatening disorders, such as arterial thrombosis and gas bacillus infections

Medical and Surgical Management

Unless surgery is performed on an emergency basis, the client is treated for any disorder that may influence healing, for example, uncontrolled diabetes mellitus, dehydration, infection, electrolyte imbalances, poor nutrition, and chronic respiratory disorders.

When it is decided that amputation must be performed as a lifesaving measure, the following factors help the surgical team decide at which level to amputate the arm or leg (eg, above or below the knee, above or below the elbow): the amount of tissue that must be removed to eliminate the disorder, the level at which the blood supply is adequate enough to preserve circulation to tissue that will remain, the number of joints that can be preserved, and the length of residual limb that will promote fitting a prosthesis, an artificial limb, for rehabilitation.

The levels of some commonly planned amputations include below the knee (BK), above the knee (AK), below the elbow (BE), and above the elbow (AE). The surgical objective is to create a gently tapering stump with muscular padding over the end. Occasionally, knee disarticulations (amputation through a joint), disarticulation at the ankle joint, and partial foot amputations are performed.

AMPUTATION METHODS

An amputation may be performed using an open or closed method. In an open amputation (guillotine amputation), the end of the residual limb, or stump, is temporarily open with no skin covering the stump. Open amputations are usually performed in the presence of infection. Skin traction is applied, and the infected area is allowed to drain. The traction must be continuous. The surgeon may arrange the traction so that the client can turn over in bed.

In the more common closed amputation (flap amputation), skin flaps cover the severed bone end. Clients with a closed amputation return from surgery with either a soft compression dressing or rigid plaster shell covering the residual limb. The compression dressing consists of gauze over which elastic roller bandages are wrapped to create pressure to control bleeding. There may be a walking pylon, a type of temporary prosthesis composed of a metal post and molded foot, attached to the rigid plaster shell (Fig. 66–12). It may be weeks before the postoperative client is referred to a prosthetist, a professional who creates and fits artificial limbs.

ARM AMPUTATION

The arms have highly specialized functions. Consequently, the amputation of an arm, particularly the arm with the dominant hand, requires great physical and emotional adjustment during the preoperative as well as the postoperative periods. Fortunately, most clients with arm amputations can be measured for a prosthesis shortly after the surgical scar heals.

Three types of prostheses are available for arm amputees: a shoulder harness with cables that attach to a mechanical terminal device, referred to as a hook; a

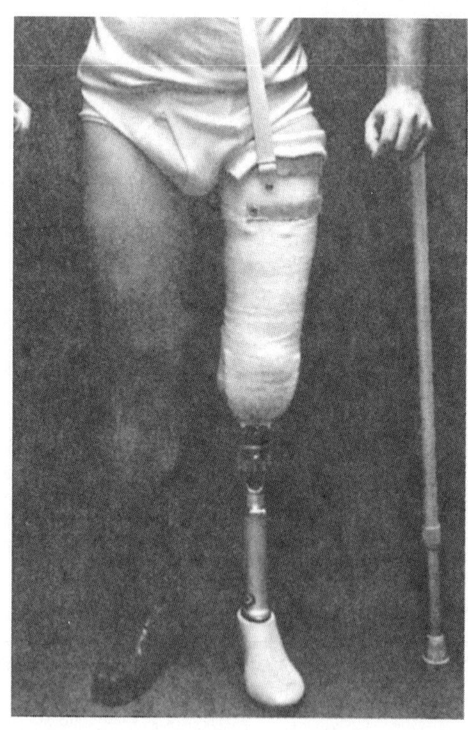

FIGURE 66-12. A rigid plaster shell has been applied postoperatively to the residual limb of this client with an above-knee amputation. The walking pylon facilitates early ambulation. (Courtesy of the Prosthetics Research Study, Veterans Administration Contract V663P-784)

semifunctioning cosmetic hand that can be substituted for the hook; and a myoelectric arm.

The hook performs the functions of the hand and fingers when the amputee moves the scapula and expands the chest activating the cables attached from a shoulder harness to the mechanical device. The mechanical terminal device is strong, sturdy, and functional. The cosmetic hand, which can be attached to the same cables as the hook, has the appearance of a natural hand, but it lacks the capacity for performing fine motor skills. The myoelectric arm has a realistic-looking hand that is activated by electrical impulses from muscles in the upper arm. The electrical activity is relayed from electrodes within the shell of the prosthesis to microcircuits in the prosthetic fingers. The myoelectric arm has three advantages: it eliminates the need to wear a harness, the terminal device looks natural, and it has somewhat better function than the cosmetic hand. Despite its advantages, the myoelectric arm is not rugged enough to do the work of the mechanical terminal device.

LEG AMPUTATION

Amputation of a leg is a more common operation than amputation of an arm. The AK amputation is more disabling than a BK amputation; therefore, unless evidence suggests that the knee cannot be saved, every attempt is made to amputate below the knee.

The trend is to have a temporary prosthesis attached to the plaster shell covering the residual lower limb immediately after surgery. It reduces psychological trauma for the client because it promotes a more intact sense of body image following surgery. Also, the walking pylon facilitates early ambulation. Almost immediately, the client is allowed to stand and place a limited amount of weight on the residual limb. As the stump heals and edema disappears, a second cast may be reapplied or a temporary socket made of lightweight polypropylene may be constructed. Ultimately, a conventional prosthesis is custom made to conform to the stump as well as to the client's needs. Leg prostheses may be held in place by means of a pelvic belt or suction.

COMPLICATIONS

Hematoma, hemorrhage, and infection are complications that occur in the immediate postoperative period. Complications that may occur late in the postoperative course include chronic osteomyelitis (after persistent infection) and, rarely, a burning pain (causalgia), the cause of which is unknown. Pain may result from a stump neuroma, which is formed when the cut ends of nerves become entangled in the healing scar. A neuroma is treated with injections of procaine, a local anesthetic, or reamputation.

PHANTOM LIMB AND PHANTOM PAIN

The surgeon informs the client of the potential phenomenon of phantom limb sensation, which is a feeling that the amputated portion of the limb still remains. It is a normal, frequently occurring, physiologic response after amputation. Phantom sensations can persist for months or decades or can come and go. Although clients are aware of phantom sensations, they usually learn to ignore the sensations.

Phantom pain is the presence of pain or other discomfort, such as burning, tingling, throbbing, or itching, in the missing limb. Pain felt from the phantom limb can be an extremely serious problem in relation to the emotional status of the client and the ability to use a prosthesis. Severe, prolonged phantom limb pain may require surgical removal of nerve endings at the end of the stump.

REHABILITATION

The success of the amputee's rehabilitation depends on variables such as age, type of amputation, condition of the stump, physical status, condition of the remaining limb, concurrent debilitating illness, visual motor coordination, motivation, acceptance, and cooperation. Clients vary greatly in their learning capacity and ability to master the use of a prosthesis. The period allotted for training also varies with each client. It is vital that the physician, the nurse, the physical and occupational therapists, the family, and the client maintain realistic expectations throughout the rehabilitation period.

Nursing Management

Nursing management of an amputee can be segmented into two key functions: those before surgery and those after surgery. In general, presurgical nursing management involves considerations for any surgery, specifically taking a complete medical, drug, and allergy history and evaluating the client for mental and emotional acceptance of the surgical procedure.

It is important to assess motor strength and joint flexibility of other joints to determine potential problems involving rehabilitation. If the client is acutely ill, for example with a gangrenous limb and related fever, disorientation, and electrolyte imbalances, monitor circulation in the limb for changes, such as severe pain, color changes, and lack of peripheral pulses. Inform the physician of problems as they occur because surgery may become an emergency.

Presurgical nursing management includes a reduction in pain and anxiety and support for the client as he or she begins to grieve the loss of the limb and adapt to potential changes. Narcotic analgesics are administered before surgery to clients with severe pain. Other comfort measures include handling the painful limb gently, elevating a swollen limb, encouraging family presence and support, being available especially at times when the client is alone, helping the client to express concerns, and clarifying misperceptions.

Before surgery explain all of the routine preoperative preparations. Reinforce what the physician has discussed with the client and family regarding the extent of physical disability; the psychological, aesthetic, social, and vocational implications; and the realistic possibilities for prosthetic restoration. Exercise care in answering questions about prosthetic devices and their use because it is always possible that the amputation may need to involve more of the limb than originally anticipated. Review the postoperative management, such as deep breathing, coughing, positioning, and routine exercises. Practice the exercises if time and the client's condition permit.

Clients vary in their reactions to the impending loss of a limb. The amount of grief is thought to be proportional to the symbolic significance of the part and the resultant degree of disability and deformity. Anger and depression are common emotions. Acknowledge the client's feelings. Remain objective and nonjudgmental as the client expresses negative emotional responses. Reassure the client that the reaction is normal. Do not shame, criticize, or trivialize the client's behavior.

How well the client can cope usually depends on prior experience and how the individual has dealt with previous losses. Protect the client from additional sources of stress. While the client is preoccupied with the potential loss, do not make unnecessary demands or expect full participation in the plan of care. Provide assistance with activities that at any other time the client could carry out independently. Promote adequate sleep. Discuss coping techniques that have been used successfully in the past and encourage their repetition. Foster communication with supportive family members or friends.

NURSING PROCESS
Caring for the Client After a Limb Amputation

Assessment

Monitor vital signs. Review the chart for the type and level of amputation. Inspect the dressing or plaster shell. At any dressing change, inspect the wound for signs of infection, excessive drainage, or separation of wound edges. Evaluate the client's level of discomfort and general condition. Assess pain and implement measures to relieve it. Institute measures to prevent infection, promote healing, and avoid skin breakdown.

Diagnosis and Planning

Nursing management involves all concerns addressed after any orthopedic surgery (discussed above) and also includes, but is not limited to, the following:

Nursing Diagnoses and Collaborative Problems	Nursing Management
Risk for Self-Care Deficit related to impediments imposed by amputation **Goal:** Client will participate in self-care and recuperative measures to the fullest extent possible.	Encourage clients with leg amputations to assume some of their own care 1 or 2 days after surgery. Assist clients with an arm amputation, especially an amputation on the dominant side, until they are able to use the opposite extremity. Exercise and position the client in ways that help prevent contractures after an amputation, maintain skeletal alignment, and promote active movement of the uninvolved limbs. Work with the physical therapist to implement a program of active and isometric exercises.
Risk for Disuse Syndrome related to altered mobility after amputation **Goal:** Client will become progressively mobile and independent.	Place the client with a leg amputation in the prone position several times a day to promote stump extension. Do not gatch the knees or keep the amputated stump elevated on a pillow after the first 48 hours. Discourage long periods of sitting. Use a trochanter roll to prevent external rotation of the hip and knee. Avoid placing pillows between the legs. Advise the client who is lying on the stomach to adduct the stump so it presses against the other leg. Help the client with a temporary prosthesis to sit on the edge of the bed and dangle the unaffected leg on the day of surgery. On the first or second postoperative day, assist the client to stand to regain a sense of bal-

ance. Stepping on the floor with the temporary prosthesis and weight-bearing of about 10% of body weight usually is permitted at this time.

Expect the client with a temporary prosthesis to progress to walking with crutches or a walker or in parallel bars 2 to 4 days after the amputation with a high degree of safety (full weight-bearing on the unaffected leg).

Risk for Dysfunctional Grieving related to loss of body part

Goal: Client will state that he or she is beginning to resolve loss and develop strategies for coping without an arm or leg.

Listen actively and empathetically.

Allow clients time to express their feelings and to talk about their loss, and feelings of grief, anger, depression, anxiety, and so forth.

Discuss each new challenge as it arises.

Allow the client time to process the information that is being provided.

Implement changes gradually.

Reinforce progress that has been made.

Remain available to the client for physical and emotional support.

Foster family involvement because their encouragement often helps motivate a client to face each new problem, accept failure, and develop a determination to overcome obstacles.

Ambulate the client with a leg amputation as soon as possible to dispel the doubt that permanent disability will prevail.

Support clients who have undergone an amputation to proceed at their own pace to fully integrate the experience.

Explore the possibility of a meeting with a rehabilitated amputee.

Body Image Disturbance related to loss of body part and function

Goal: Client will demonstrate progressive adjustment to the change in body image.

Keep in mind that the attitude of staff and family members has great bearing on how clients perceive themselves.

Do not treat the client as less than competent.

Avoid nonverbal implications that the client, the stump, or the prosthesis is repulsive.

Make a point to visit the client frequently, especially when no particular nursing activity must be performed.

Make eye contact during verbal interactions.

Sit close to the client's bedside and lean forward when talking to communicate a personal interest in the client.

Offer praise when a task is successfully accomplished to build self-esteem and self-confidence.

If appropriate, explore the client's reasons for refusing to use a prosthesis. If the problem is amenable to change, enlist the help of the surgeon, physical therapist, or prosthetist.

Evaluation and Expected Outcomes

- By discharge, the client reports reduced and manageable pain, no infection, and intact skin, and demonstrates optimal participation in self-care.
- The client experiences increasing mobility along with increasing resolution of grief, great self-acceptance and acceptance of current situation.
- The client does not withdraw from social situations, has a positive attitude about the future, and can demonstrate adequate independent self-care.

Client and Family Teaching

Client and family education begins before amputation surgery and extends beyond hospitalization.

After surgery, discharge teaching depends on many factors, including the length of hospitalization, the type and location of the amputation, the age and physical condition of the client, and the type of dressing or prosthesis the client wears. Explore factors related to the home environment and determine a plan for continued rehabilitation before discharge. Modifications in living arrangements, the use of a wheelchair, or other accommodations or changes may need to be made for some individuals.

If the client has to bandage the stump at home, teach both the client and the family how to apply the bandage and how to care for the stump (Nursing Guidelines 66–5). Instruct the client to wash the bandages, to rinse them well, and to lay them flat to dry because hanging tends to decrease the elasticity. When the bandages are dry, they must be rolled without stretching. Be sure to include the following general points in the discharge instructions:

- Follow the physician's recommendations regarding caring for the stump, applying a stump dressing, washing the stump, and elevating the stump when sitting.
- Do not apply nonprescription drugs (ointments, creams, topical pain relievers) to the stump unless

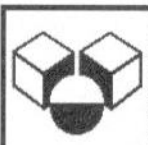

Nursing Guidelines 66-5

Stump Care and Bandaging

Stump Care

- Assess the covering over the stump frequently to determine the type and amount of drainage from the incision. Expect some oozing of blood but if a gauze dressing is used, it may need to be reinforced.
- Keep a tourniquet in plain view at bedside and if hemorrhage occurs, apply it and notify the physician.
- Generally, elevate the stump for the first 24 to 48 hours to prevent edema. In some cases, such as an AK amputation, a slight Trendelenburg position is preferred to elevating the stump on pillows because bending the hip promotes a flexion contracture. A bed board or a firm mattress provides skeletal support.
- If the client has a rigid plaster cast with walking pylon, loosen the harness, which suspends the cast from the waist, when the client is in bed. Slightly tighten the harness when the client is ambulatory.

Bandaging

Before a permanent prosthesis can be made, the stump must shrink and be shaped. This is done with elastic bandages that are wrapped about the stump. Unlike leg stumps, arm stumps do not need as massive a shrinkage over as long a period. Various bandaging techniques are appropriate but several principles are observed:

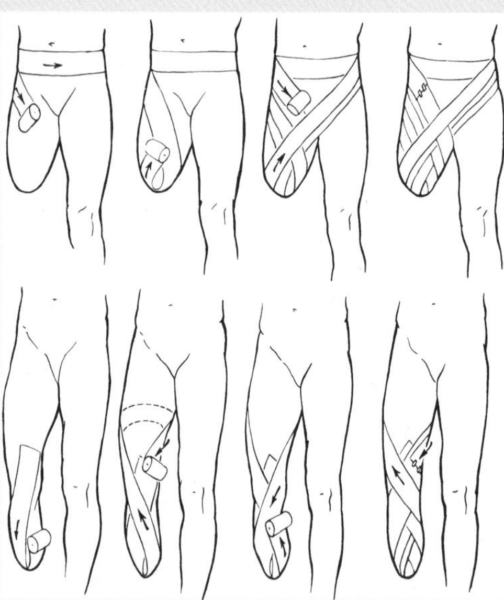

Stump bandaging technique for above-knee and below-knee amputations.

- Remove and rewrap the bandage at least twice during the day and before the client retires for the night.
- Bandage joints in a way that promotes a neutral or extended position.
- Avoid circular turns, which act like a tourniquet and interfere with blood flow.
- Wrap the stump in a distal to proximal direction to promote venous circulation.
- Apply compression evenly about the stump to prevent areas of localized edema.

use of a specific product has been approved by the physician.

- Adhere to the plan of scheduled exercises and complete each group of exercises as outlined by the physical therapist.
- Do not exceed the physician's recommendations regarding weight-bearing and joint flexion.
- Eat well balanced and nutritious meals or follow the diet recommended by the physician. Gaining excess weight must be avoided during the recovery period because weight gain may interfere with use of a leg prosthesis.
- Expect that phantom limb sensation, if present, may persist for a period of time, which is normal.
- Avoid injury to the stump, even though it appears to be healed. Report any skin impairment immediately.
- Continue deep breathing exercises until fully mobile.
- Contact the physician if fever, chills, productive cough, bleeding or oozing from the stump, purulent drainage from the incision, new or different pain in the stump, or any change in the appearance of the stump occurs.

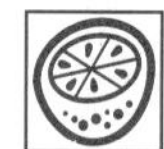

General Nutritional Considerations

Protein requirements increase during prolonged immobility to correct negative nitrogen balance, promote healing, and help prevent skin breakdown and infections. A protein intake of 1.2 g/kg body weight is recommended, and adequate calories are needed to spare protein. A high fiber intake helps prevent constipation.

To reduce the risk of renal calculi, a complication of prolonged immobility and gout, clients are advised to drink at least 2 quarts of fluid daily. Drinking fluid before bed and during the night helps keep the urine dilute.

There is no conclusive evidence that diet therapy can prevent or cure rheumatoid arthritis. However, some studies suggest that a small percentage of cases of rheumatoid arthritis may be caused by a food allergy, with milk and milk products, corn, cereals, citrus fruits, and tomatoes proposed as possible offenders. Other studies suggest that omega-3 fatty acids found in fatty fish (eg, mackerel, herring, salmon), and to a lesser extent in flaxseed, olive, and canola oils, may help relieve joint tenderness and fatigue, possibly by inhibiting the inflammatory response of certain prostaglandins. The use of fish oil supplements is not recommended, but eating more dietary sources of omega-3 fatty acids may be beneficial. Malnutrition is common among clients with rheumatoid arthritis; monitor weight changes. Discourage quack "cures" and self-prescribed supplements.

Gradual weight loss helps reduce serum uric acid levels in clients with gout. Clients should avoid fasting, low-carbohydrate diets, and rapid weight loss because they favor ketone formation, which inhibits uric acid excretion.

Excess fiber and protein, caffeine, alcohol, and smoking promote calcium excretion and thereby increase the risk of osteoporosis.

General Pharmacologic Considerations

Oral calcium preparations containing vitamin D are better absorbed than those without vitamin D.

Oral calcium preparations should not be taken with other oral drugs because absorption of the other drugs may be altered or blocked. For example, calcium decreases absorption of tetracycline and phenytoin. Take other drugs 1 to 2 hours after calcium carbonate.

Oral calcium may be taken with meals to enhance absorption and minimize gastric distress.

Arthritic clients should be warned about drugs, health foods, and certain food substances available in drug form and promoted as cures for arthritis.

Clients taking large doses of salicylates should be told of the signs of GI bleeding, salicylism, and the possibility of easy bruising and other bleeding tendencies. Signs of salicylism include headache, nausea, vomiting, tinnitus, increased pulse and respiratory rates, fever, mental confusion, and drowsiness.

Large doses of salicylates can interfere with the clotting mechanism of the blood. Clients taking these drugs are instructed to inform their physicians and dentists of their prolonged and high-dose ingestion of salicylates.

Clients with gout need detailed instructions about their medical regimens in relation to the drugs to be taken and the importance of increasing their fluid intake to reduce the possibility of urate stone formation in the urinary tract.

Clients with diseases of the bones and joints should be cautioned against discontinuing their drugs if and when they begin to feel improved.

Clients taking aspirin for arthritis should be instructed *not* to substitute buffered aspirin or enteric-coated aspirin for regular aspirin unless the physician approves the change. Aspirin cannot be used in clients with ulcers, a history of ulcers, or bleeding disorders.

The most common adverse effects of NSAIDs are related to the GI tract: nausea, vomiting, diarrhea, and constipation. GI bleeding, which in some cases is severe, has been reported with the use of these drugs.

Calcitonin may be used in the treatment of Paget's disease and is administered subcutaneously. Some of the adverse effects associated with calcitonin include nausea (with or without vomiting), inflammation at the injection site, increased urinary frequency, anorexia, diarrhea, and abdominal pain.

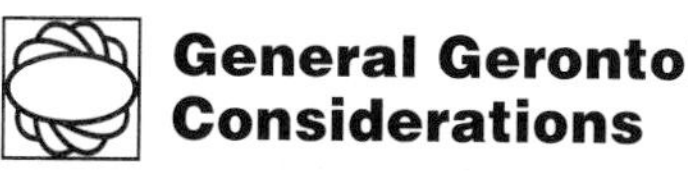

General Gerontologic Considerations

Women over age 45 have a 9% to 10% decrease in cortical bone per decade.

Older adults are more prone to skeletal fractures because bone resorption takes place more rapidly than bone formation.

Maintaining an active lifestyle delays the decline of muscle strength and bone mass among older adults.

With age the fibrocartilage of intervertebral disks becomes thinner and drier, causing compression of the disks of the spinal column and leading to a loss of height amounting to as much as 1.5 to 3 inches (3.75 to 7.5 cm).

Estrogen deficiency, which occurs at menopause, is considered the leading factor in osteoporosis among aging women.

SUMMARY OF KEY CONCEPTS

- Common traumatic injuries include strains—muscles stretched or pulled beyond capacity; contusions—injuries to soft tissue following a blow or blunt injury; sprains—the ligaments joining two bones are partially torn or ruptured; dislocations—the articular surfaces of a joint are no longer in contact; and fractures—broken bones.
- Frequent neurovascular assessment, including checking circulation, sensation, mobility, and pain in an injured limb, must be done with all orthopedic injuries before and after treatment.
- Compartment syndrome occurs when bone, muscles, and nerves are compressed due to swelling within a compartment surrounded by inelastic fascia. If unrelieved, permanent nerve damage, muscle atrophy, and contracture can result.
- The signs and symptoms of a fracture include pain after injury, loss of function, deformed appearance, false motion, crepitus, edema, and muscle spasm.
- A fracture may be treated by any one or a combination of the following: traction, closed reduction, open reduction that may include internal or external fixation, and cast application.
- Traction, a pull applied to the musculoskeletal system, may be attached to skin or directly to bone.
- When using traction, it is essential to (1) maintain continuous pull, (2) sustain countertraction, (3) preserve skeletal alignment in the line of pull, (4) keep splints and slings suspended, (5) ensure that ropes move freely through each pulley, (6) apply the prescribed amount of weight, and (7) keep weights hanging free.
- When a cast is applied it generally extends from the joint above to the joint below the injury. Joints enclosed in a cast are placed in neutral or a slightly flexed position. First the skin is cleaned and dried; then it is wrapped

with stockinette and bony prominences are padded. Layers of cast material are wrapped while the area is supported or suspended. To make sure the bone is aligned properly, an x-ray image is taken once the cast is applied.

- A cast window may be cut to permit assessment. A cast is bivalved to relieve pressure from swelling, to provide intermittent support and immobilization, to facilitate gradual active use of the arm or leg, or to facilitate a sharper x-ray image.
- Complications associated with fractured hips include skin breakdown, wound infection, pneumonia, constipation, urinary retention, muscle atrophy, and contractures.
- Inflammatory and infectious disorders of the musculoskeletal system are characterized by inflammation and degeneration of connective tissue structures, especially the joints. Some examples include rheumatoid arthritis, degenerative joint disease, gout, bursitis, ankylosing spondylitis, Lyme disease, osteomyelitis, and lupus erythematosus.
- Rheumatoid arthritis is a systemic inflammatory disorder of connective tissue, causing destruction of the joints and connective tissue and joint fusion leading to immobility. Degenerative joint disease is known as the wear and tear disease, mostly affecting weight-bearing joints.
- Joint replacement surgery is considered when joint pain and function no longer respond or improve with conservative treatment.
- Following a total hip replacement, the client must avoid adducting and flexing the hip until healing has occurred.
- Gout is a metabolic disorder that involves an inflammatory reaction within the joints, related to hyperuricemia. Bursitis is the inflammation of the bursa following trauma, infection, or related to arthritis or gout. Ankylosing spondylitis is a chronic connective tissue disorder of the spine, resulting in progressive immobility and fixation of the joints in the hips.
- Lyme disease is a chronic inflammatory disease that is transmitted by the bite of a tick.
- Osteomyelitis may be acquired either from a blood-borne pathogen, from direct contamination of an open orthopedic injury at the time of trauma, or from migration of microorganisms through compromised skin.
- Systemic lupus erythematosus affects multiple body systems such as the skin, joints, kidneys, serous membranes of the heart and lungs, lymph nodes, and GI tract. This occurs because antibodies destroy the connective tissues through inflammation, fibrosis, and scarring.
- Low back pain is a common outcome from poor posture or body mechanics. Clients need to keep the feet slightly separated when performing heavy work; bend from knees while keeping the back straight; use the strong muscles in the legs and hips; carry objects close to the body; push, pull, or roll heavy objects rather than carry them; sleep on a firm mattress; wear supportive shoes; and perform regular, active exercise.
- Individuals at greatest risk for developing osteoporosis are postmenopausal women and older adults who are generally inactive. However, this condition may also occur secondarily to drug treatment with corticosteroids, Cushing's syndrome, hyperparathyroidism, and inadequate dietary consumption of vitamin D and calcium.
- Clients with bunions and hammertoes are advised to purchase shoes on the basis of comfort rather than fashion. Low-heeled, wide-width shoes are recommended. Individuals with corns and calluses, who also have diabetes, peripheral vascular disease, or poor vision, are instructed to rely on professionals such as podiatrists for regular foot care.
- Carpal tunnel syndrome often occurs in individuals who perform repetitive hand and wrist movements, causing recurrent trauma to the tendon sheath or ligaments in the carpal canal. The swelling that accompanies the inflammation compresses the median nerve causing pain, numbness, and impaired mobility in the fingers and hand.
- Malignant bone tumors occur usually in long bones, grow rapidly, and have a high rate of metastasis.
- Orthopedic surgery may be performed to correct a deformity, remove a bone tumor, align fractured bones, replace a joint, repair damaged tendons and ligaments, graft a section of bone, or insert an internal fixation device.
- Amputation may be required for treatment of malignant bone tumors, chronic osteomyelitis, extensive trauma, arterial insufficiency, thermal injuries (eg, frostbite), or gangrene, or to remove a useless or deformed limb.
- A closed amputation, one that uses skin flaps to cover the severed bone, is the usual surgical approach. However, an open amputation, one in which the operative tissue is left exposed, may be performed in clients with sepsis.
- There is a trend to enclose a leg stump in a plaster cast and attach a temporary prosthesis during the surgical procedure. This approach reduces psychological trauma and promotes more rapid ambulation and rehabilitation.
- It is not uncommon for clients, who have undergone an amputation, to experience phantom limp sensation, a feeling that the removed limb is still attached and intact. A few clients also report phantom pain, discomfort that they perceive in the phantom limb.
- If a stump has not been enclosed in a rigid plaster cast postoperatively, it must be bandaged to shrink and mold it before a permanent prosthesis can be constructed. When wrapping the stump, the distal tip is covered, circular turns with the roller bandage are avoided, the stump is wrapped with even compression, and joint flexion is avoided.
- To promote mobility and avoid joint contractures following an amputation, it is best to use a firm mattress for skeletal support, promote skeletal alignment, and encourage active movement of uninvolved limbs.

CRITICAL THINKING EXERCISES

1. A male client had a total hip replacement 3 days ago and wants to use the toilet for a bowel movement. Explain how to assist this client.
2. A female client has just returned from the recovery unit after an AK amputation. Fresh blood has saturated the stump dressing. What actions should the nurse take at this time?
3. A young man with a fractured radius complains of increasing pain in his hand despite having received a nar-

cotic analgesic 30 minutes ago. What assessments are important to make at this time?

Suggested Readings

Abrams, A. C. (1998). *Clinical drug therapy: Rationales for nursing practice* (5th ed.). Philadelphia: Lippincott-Raven.

Altizer, L. (1996). Total hip arthroplasty. *Orthopaedic Nursing, 14*(4), 7–19.

Bove, L. A. (1996). Calcium and phosphorus. *RN, 3*, 47–50.

Bradley, C. F., & Kozak, C. (1995). Nursing care and management of the elderly hip fractured patient. *Journal of Gerontological Nursing, 21*(8), 15–22.

Bullock, B. L. (1996). *Pathophysiology: Adaptations and alterations in function* (4th ed.). Philadelphia. Lippincott-Raven.

Carpenito, L. J. (1995). *Nursing care plans and documentation: Nursing diagnoses and collaborative problems* (2nd ed.). Philadelphia: J. B. Lippincott.

Cunningham, M. E. (1994). Bursitis and tendonitis. *Orthopaedic Nursing, 13*(5), 13–16.

McConnell, E. A. (1993). Providing cast care. *Nursing, 23*(1), 19.

Morris, M. K. G. (1993). Evaluating serum calcium levels. *Nursing, 23*(2), 69.

Pellino, T. A. (1994). How to manage hip fractures. *American Journal of Nursing, 94*(4), 46–50.

Resnick, B. (1994). Die from a broken hip? *RN, 57*(7), 22–27.

Ribeiro, V. E. S., & Blakeley, J. S. (1997). Osteoporosis: Preventing and treating an insidious disease. *Canadian Nurse. 93*(8), 31–36.

Smeltzer, S.C., & Bare, B. G. (1996). *Brunner and Suddarth's textbook of medical-surgical nursing* (8th ed.). Philadelphia: Lippincott-Raven.

Tremblay, L., Mitsionis, G., & Sotereanos, D. G. (1997). Toe-to-thumb transplantation. *Orthopaedic Nursing, 16*(3), 17–27.

Additional Resources

Arthritis Foundation
http://www.arthritis.org/

Lupus Homepage
http://www.hamline.edu:80/~lupus/

Amputee Homepage
http://vanbc.wimsey.com/~igregson/index.html

Lyme Disease Information Resource
http://www.sky.net/~deporter/lymel.html

17

Caring for Clients With Integumentary Disorders

Chapter 67

Introduction to the Integumentary System

KEY TERMS

Apocrine glands
Debridement
Dermis
Eccrine glands
Epidermis
Integument
Keratin
Melanin
Pheromones
Pressure sores
Sebaceous glands
Sebum
Shearing
Skin tear
Stratum corneum
Subcutaneous tissue
Sweat glands

LEARNING OBJECTIVES

On completion of this chapter, the reader will:

- Name the structures that form the integument.
- List four functions of the integumentary system.
- Identify the purpose of sebum and melanin.
- Differentiate between eccrine and apocrine glands.
- Name at least three facts about the integument that are pertinent to document when obtaining a health history.
- Give the characteristics of normal skin.
- Discuss the criteria for staging pressure sores.
- List characteristics of hair assessed during a physical examination.
- Describe the characteristics of normal nails.
- Name three diagnostic tests performed to detect the etiology of skin disorders.
- Name seven medical and surgical techniques for treating skin disorders.

The **integument** includes structures that cover the exterior surface of the body. The primary structure is the skin, which contains sebaceous and sweat glands and sensory nerve endings (Fig. 67–1). The integument also includes accessory structures such as the hair and nails. The structures that make up the integument protect the body from environmental injuries, help to regulate body temperature, serve as sensory organs, and facilitate the synthesis of vitamin D.

Anatomy and Physiology

Skin

The skin is composed of two layers: the **epidermis,** the outermost layer, and the **dermis,** which lies below the epidermis. The epidermis contains an outer layer of dead skin cells, the **stratum corneum**, that form a tough protective protein called **keratin.** The epidermis is constantly shed and replaced with epithelial cells from the dermis. The dermis, or true skin, consists of connective tissue and contains elastic fibers, blood vessels, sensory and motor nerve fibers, sweat and sebaceous (oil) glands, and hair follicles (roots). The **subcutaneous tissue** is the layer of skin attached to muscle and bone and is primarily composed of connective tissue and fat cells. Skin has a tremendous capacity to stretch with little subsequent damage, as is evident following soft tissue injury and pregnancy.

The color of the skin is determined by a pigment called **melanin,** which is manufactured by melanocytes located in the epidermis. The production of melanin is under the control of the middle lobe (pars intermedia) of the pituitary gland, which secretes

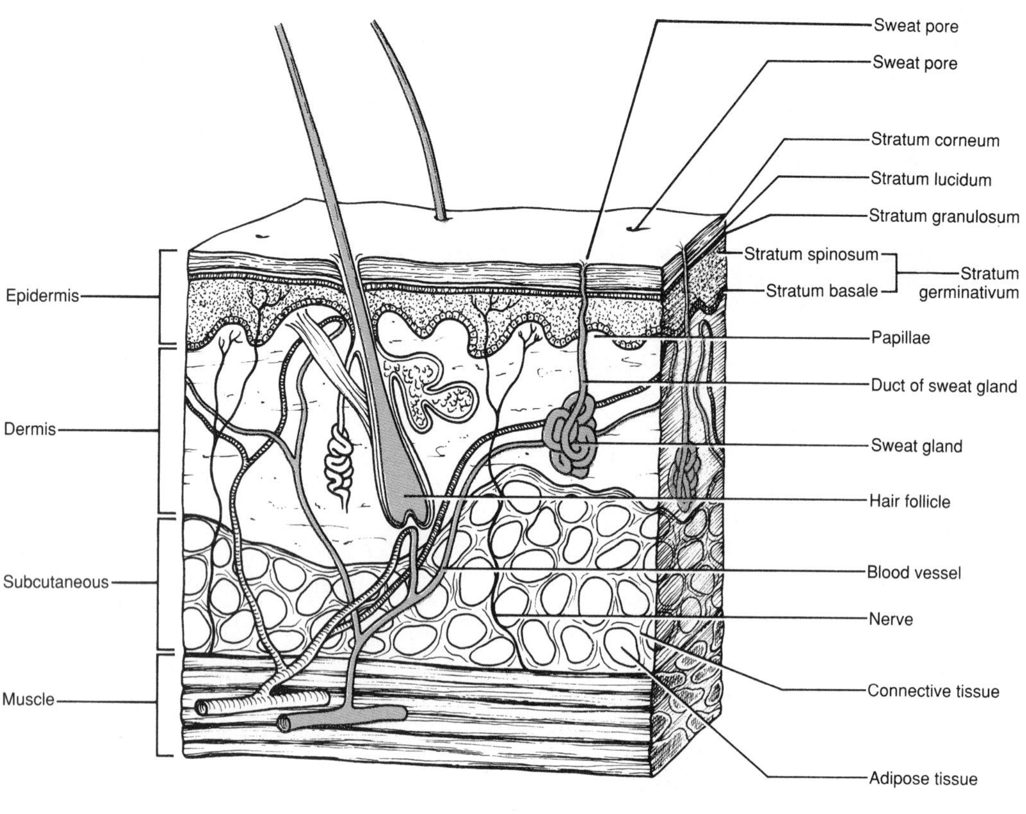

FIGURE 67-1. A cross-section of the skin.

melanocyte-stimulating hormone. The more melanin in the epidermis, the darker the skin color. Melanin production is temporarily stimulated by exposure to ultraviolet light whereupon it is used to absorb harmful radiation.

SKIN FUNCTIONS

The skin has four major functions: protection, temperature regulation, sensory processing, and chemical synthesis.

Protection

A primary function of the skin is the formation of a protective barrier between the outside world and underlying organs and structures of the body. The barrier it provides blocks microorganisms and other foreign substances from contact with the structures below the epidermis. It also prevents a loss of water from structures below the surface of the skin.

Temperature Regulation

To maintain an even body temperature, the skin heats or cools the structures below. Heat is continuously produced inside the body during cellular metabolism. To generate heat and prevent heat loss at the body's surface, erector muscles around shafts of hair contract. Elevation of skin hairs interferes with local air circulation and maintains the warmth of the skin.

Heat dissipates through the skin and respiration. Heat is lost by four methods: radiation, conduction, evaporation, and convection (Fig. 67–2).

- Radiation is the transfer of surface heat within the environment. An example of radiant heat loss is the escape of heat from the surface of warm skin into cooler air.
- Conduction is the transfer of heat through contact. An example of conductive heat loss is placing a cool cloth on warm skin.
- Evaporation is the loss of moisture or water. Water on the surface of the body is warmed. As the moisture vaporizes, the body is cooled. Evaporation occurs unnoticed (insensible loss) and when there is obvious perspiration.
- Convection is the transfer of heat by means of currents of liquids or gasses in which warm air molecules move away from the body. An example of convection is a cool breeze that blows across the body surface.

When the temperature and humidity outside the body rise, radiation, evaporation, and convection are

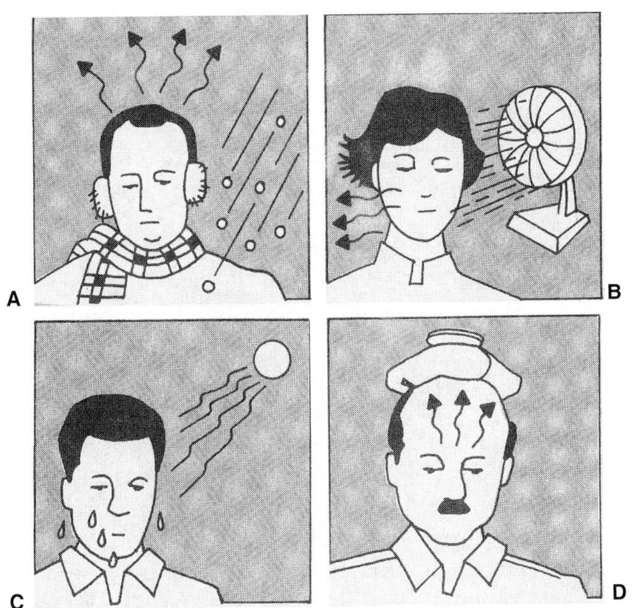

FIGURE 67-2. Methods of heat loss. (*A*) Radiation; (*B*) Convection; (*C*) Evaporation; and (*D*) Conduction.

ineffective. The only way heat is transferred under these conditions is by conduction. This is why exposure to warm temperatures and densely saturated moist air can raise the body temperature and result in heat stroke.

Sensory Processing

The skin serves as a means of monitoring the outside environment, as well as warning of danger. Specialized nerve endings in the skin respond to pressure, pain, heat, and cold.

Chemical Synthesis

The skin forms a chemical substance called 7-dehydrocholesterol, which facilitates the synthesis of vitamin D when the skin is exposed to ultraviolet light (sunlight). Vitamin D is necessary for healthy formation of bones and teeth. Dark-skinned individuals do not synthesize vitamin D as readily as light-skinned persons. Cloudy environments and the presence of air pollutants that block sunlight also interfere with vitamin D synthesis. Therefore, vitamin D is added to some food sources, such as milk.

Hair

Hair originates in the hair follicles within the dermis. It is formed from hundreds of strands of keratin linked together with amino acids. Melanin, produced by melanocytes within the hair root, influence hair color. There are three types of melanin: brown, black, and yellow. Types of melanin are genetically inherited, as are hair texture, shape, and rate of growth. Scalp hair grows more rapidly than any other. Illness, hormone levels, nutrition, aging, and other factors can affect hair growth and loss.

Hair covers all parts of the body except the palms, soles, dorsum of the fingers, lips, penis, labia, and nipples. In some areas, such as the pubis, axilla, and chest, the hair is more coarse than in other locations. Men of some ethnic groups (eg, Native Americans) have less facial and body hair than their Anglo-American counterparts.

Sebaceous and Sweat Glands

Sebaceous glands are connected to each hair follicle and secrete an oily substance called **sebum.** Sebum is a lubricant that prevents drying and cracking of the skin and hair. As sebum fills the glandular duct, it enters the hair follicle from where it is eventually released. During puberty, sebaceous glands in the forehead, nose, chest, and back become more active.

The two types of **sweat glands** are eccrine and apocrine. **Eccrine glands** release water and electrolytes, such as sodium and chloride, in the form of perspiration. The rate of perspiration is related to body temperature. As much as 3 liters can be produced by adults under extremely hot conditions (Bullock, 1996, p. 892). The pH of perspiration is slightly acidic, which helps in providing a hostile environment for microbial colonization. Frequent washing with alkaline soaps removes sebum and reduces the acid mantle of protection.

Apocrine glands are found around the nipples, in the anogenital region, in the eyelids (Moll's glands), in the mammary glands of the breast, and in the external ear canals—where the secretion is referred to as cerumen. In lower forms of animals, the apocrine glands release **pheromones,** hormone-like chemicals that communicate reproductive and social information among the species. For example, dogs and other animals release pheromones at the time of urination to mark their territory. The function of apocrine secretions in humans is unknown although the onset of secretion coincides with puberty. Some speculate that synchronization of menstruation among women in close living conditions such as a dormitory room is due to apocrine secretions (Arms, 1997).

Generally, perspiration, which includes secretions from both eccrine and apocrine glands, is odorless. However, an odor develops when perspiration mixes with bacteria on the skin.

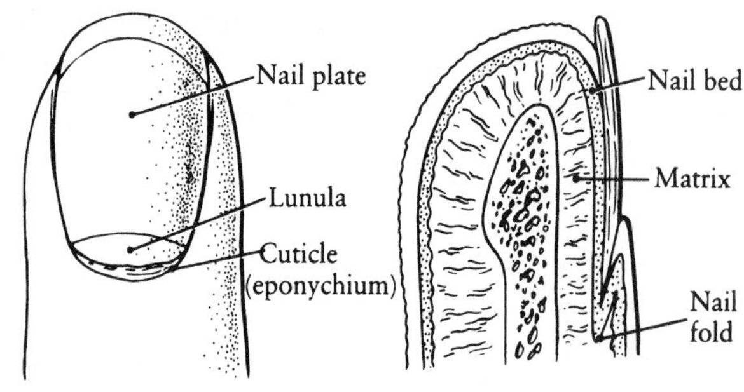

FIGURE 67-3. External and cross-sectional views of a nail.

Nails

Finger and toenails are layers of hard keratin that have a protective function. In primates and humans, the nails may be a biologic diversification of claws. Animal species that have claws use them to catch and tear prey, whereas primates and humans developed nails on their fingers and toes because they had a greater biologic need for grasping limbs and manipulating primitive tools or utensils.

The nail root lies buried beneath the nail's exposed surface in a fold of skin (Fig. 67–3). The nails have an abundant blood supply. Their semitransparent appearance facilitates circulatory assessment.

Assessment

Initial assessment of the client begins with a thorough history. The history is based on symptoms. The following questions are included:

- When did the disorder first begin and where did it first appear?
- Where are the lesions located?
- Have there been any changes in the disorder since it first appeared (an increase or decrease in symptoms; in appearance or color; in location)?
- Has the problem spread?
- What are the physical sensations pertaining to the disorder (pain, itching, burning, and intensity)?
- Are there other physical or emotional problems that appear to be associated with the disorder?
- Was a specific event associated with the onset of the disorder?
- What factors appear to make the condition better or worse?
- Do you or anyone in your family have known or suspected allergies?
- What prescription and nonprescription medications have you taken recently?
- Have you made changes in personal products, such as soaps, deodorants, and cosmetics?
- Have there been recent changes in your work or living environment, such as pets, plants, sprays, dust, and pollutants, that might have precipitated this problem?

Physical Assessment

During a physical assessment, the nurse inspects and palpates the structures of the integument.

Skin Assessment

Examine the skin on all areas of the body. This can be accomplished during the head-to-toe assessment or as a focused assessment. Good lighting is essential. The skin should be smooth, unbroken, of uniform color according to the person's ethnic or racial origin, warm, resilient, and feel neither wet nor unusually dry.

There are several possible causes for color deviations (Table 67–1). While examining the skin, the nurse may detect changes in its structure or integrity such as those listed in Box 67–1. The sites of any abnormalities are documented.

TABLE 67-1 **Common Skin Color Variations**

Color	Term	Possible Causes
Pale, regardless of race	Pallor	Anemia, blood loss
Red	Erythema	Superficial burns, local inflammation, carbon monoxide poisoning
Pink	Flushed	Fever, hypertension
Purple	Ecchymosis	Trauma to soft tissue
Blue	Cyanosis	Low tissue oxygenation
Yellow	Jaundice	Liver or kidney disease, destruction of red blood cells
Brown	Tan	Racial variation, sun exposure, pregnancy, Addison's disease

BOX 67-1 Terms for Various Skin Lesions

Type of Lesion	Description	Examples
Macule	Flat, round, colored	Freckles
Papule	Elevated, obvious raised border, solid	Wart
Vesicle	Elevated, round, filled with serum	Blister
Wheal	Elevated, irregular border, no free fluid	Hives
Pustule	Elevated, raised border, filled with pus	Boil
Nodule	Elevated solid mass, extends into deeper tissue	Enlarged lymph node
Cyst	Encapsulated, round, fluid-filled or solid mass beneath the skin	Tissue growth

Temperature is assessed by placing the dorsum of the hand on the surface of the skin. Moisture is detected with the palmar surface. The quality of skin turgor is determined by grasping the skin, for example, over the chest, between the thumb and forefinger. Normally the skin returns to its original position immediately after being released. Tight, shiny skin suggests fluid retention; loose dry skin may indicate dehydration.

STAGING PRESSURE SORES

Pressure sores, also known as decubitus ulcers, occur when capillary blood flow to the area is reduced. This often occurs when the skin over a bony prominence is compressed between the weight of the body and a hard surface for a prolonged period. Common locations include the skin over the coccyx and sacrum in the lower spine, the hips, heels, elbows, shoulder blades, ears, and back of head (Fig. 67–4). Prevention of pressure sores first involves identifying persons who are at greatest risk (Box 67–2).

Pressure sores are categorized into one of four stages (Fig. 67–5) depending on the extent of tissue injury.

Stage I

Stage I pressure sores are characterized by redness of the skin. The reddened skin of a beginning pressure sore fails to resume its normal color, or blanch, when pressure is relieved.

Stage II

A stage II pressure sore is red and is accompanied by blistering or a shallow break in the skin, some-

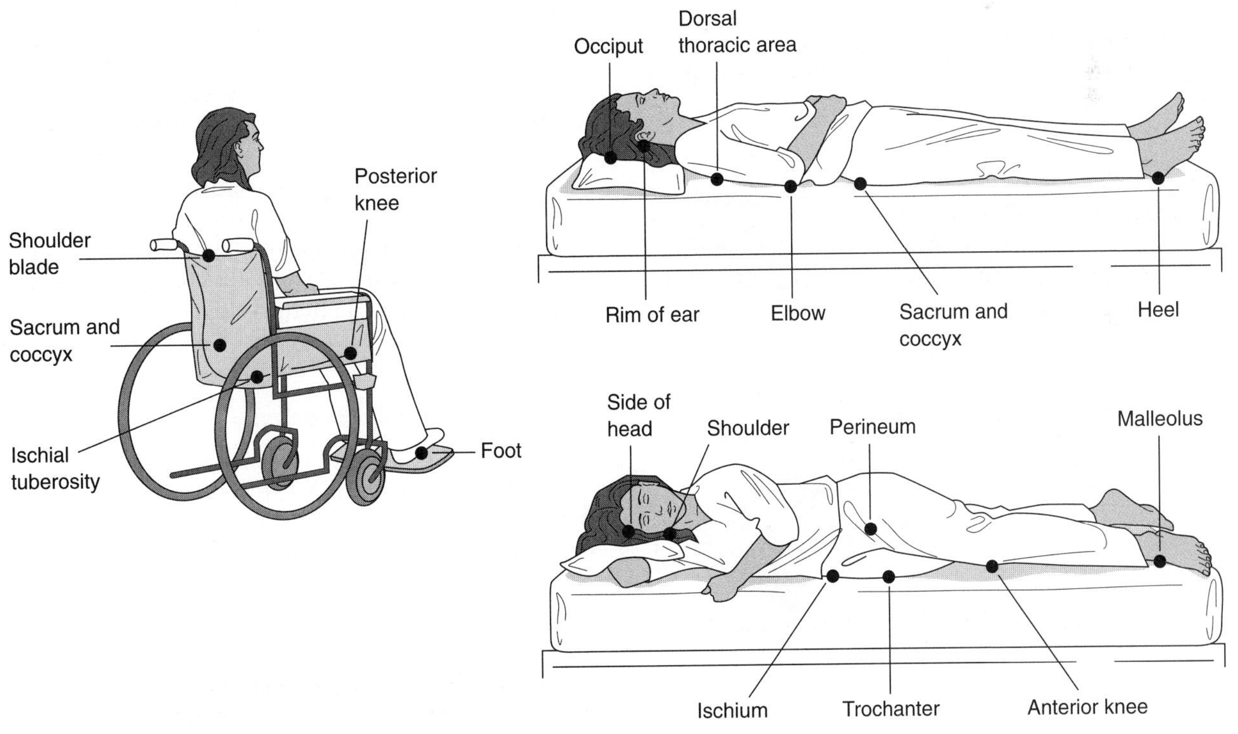

FIGURE 67-4. Common locations for pressure sores in supine, lateral, and sitting positions.

BOX 67-2 Risk Factors for Developing Pressure Sores

- Inactivity
- Immobility
- Malnutrition
- Emaciation
- Diaphoresis
- Incontinence
- Vascular disease
- Localized edema
- Dehydration
- Sedation

times described as a **skin tear.** Impairment of the skin leads to microbial colonization and infection of the wound.

Stage III

Pressure sores classified as stage III are those in which the superficial skin impairment progresses to a shallow crater that extends to the subcutaneous tissue. Stage III pressure sores may be accompanied by serous drainage from leaking plasma or purulent drainage (white or yellow-tinged fluid) caused by a wound infection. Although a stage III pressure sore is a significant wound, the area is relatively painless.

Stage IV

Stage IV pressure sores are the most traumatic and life-threatening. The tissue is deeply ulcerated, exposing muscle and bone (Fig. 67–6). The dead tissue produces a rank odor. Local infection, which is the rule rather than the exception, easily spreads throughout the body, causing a potentially fatal condition referred to as sepsis.

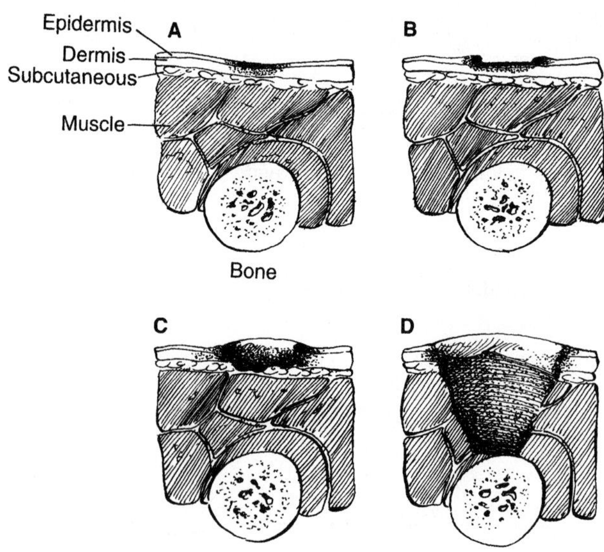

FIGURE 67-5. Pressure sore stages (*A*) Stage I; (*B*) Stage II; (*C*) Stage III; and (*D*) Stage IV.

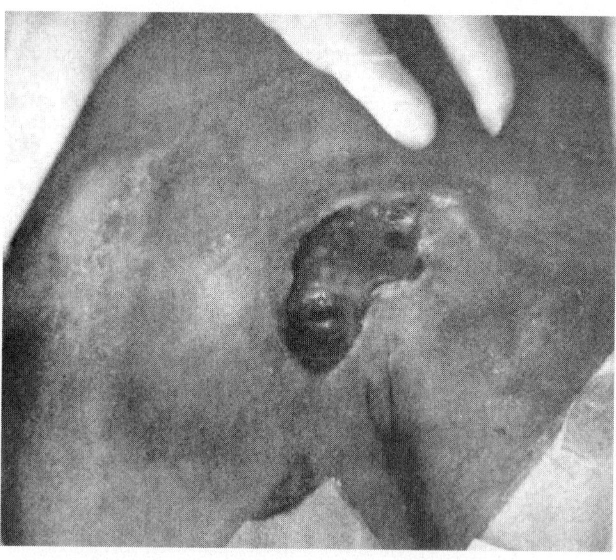

FIGURE 67-6. Example of stage IV pressure sore. (Courtesy of E. R. Squibb & Sons, Inc., Princeton, NJ.)

Once at-risk clients are identified, the nurse implements measures that reduce conditions under which pressure sores are likely to form. Some examples are:

- Turning and repositioning the client at frequent intervals
- Keeping the client's skin clean and dry
- Massaging bony prominences if the client's skin blanches with pressure relief
- Using a moisturizing skin cleanser rather than soap
- Applying pressure-relieving devices to the bed and chairs
- Padding body areas that are subject to pressure and friction
- Avoiding **shearing,** a physical force that separates layers of tissue in opposite directions, for example, when a seated client slides downward

Scalp and Hair Assessment

The scalp is assessed by separating the hair at random areas and inspecting the skin. The scalp is normally smooth, intact, and free of lesions.

Hair assessment not only applies to that which covers the head, but also to other locations such as the eyebrows, eyelashes, chest, arms, pubis, and legs. The color, texture, and distribution are noted, keeping gender and age-related variations in mind. Nits, eggs from a louse infestation, scales, and flaking skin are abnormal findings.

Nail Assessment

Normal nails appear slightly convex with a 160-degree angle between the nail base and the skin (Fig. 67–7). Concave-shaped nails, referred to as "spooning" because of their characteristic appearance, are a sign of iron deficiency anemia. Clubbing of the nails, evidenced by an angle greater than 160 degrees, suggests long-standing cardiopulmonary disease. Although the thickness of the nail varies from 0.3 to 0.65 mm (Fuller & Schaller-Ayers, 1994, p. 143), nails thicken when there is a fungal infection and poor circulation. There may be evidence of other nail abnormalities (Table 67–2).

Observe the color of the nailbeds. Pink nailbeds suggest adequate oxygenation; however, the nails may be darker in other than Anglo-American clients. To assess tissue perfusion, the nailbeds are compressed, causing them to blanch, and released. Color returns normally in 3 seconds or less. This assessment is called capillary refill time.

Diagnostic Tests

The diagnosis of a skin disorder is made chiefly by visual inspection. Some disorders may require additional testing, including:

- Biopsy—performed to identify malignant or premalignant lesions. A biopsy also is of value in helping to identify some skin disorders.
- Culture and sensitivity tests—performed on lesions that are suspected or known to contain microorganisms.
- Allergy tests—intradermal injection, the scratch test, and the patch test are used to confirm an allergy to one or more substances (see Chap. 41).

Medical and Surgical Treatment of Skin Disorders

Various types of therapies are used in the treatment or management of skin disorders. They include drug therapy, wet dressings, therapeutic baths, surgical excision, radiation therapy, photochemotherapy, hyperbaric oxygenation, and lifestyle changes.

Drug Therapy

Topical and systemic medications are used to treat skin disorders. Some examples are:

- Corticosteroids are applied topically or administered systemically (orally, intramuscularly, intravenously) to relieve inflammatory and allergic symptoms. When used systemically, corticosteroids can have serious toxic effects; therefore, they are used primarily to relieve acute problems. Continued use in long-term conditions brings greater risk and is justified only when the disease itself is serious and cannot be relieved by other treatments. Used as directed, topical application of a corticosteroid does not result in the pronounced adverse effects seen with systemic administration and can be used for longer periods of time.
- Antihistamines are frequently prescribed when allergy is a factor in causing the skin disorder. They relieve itching and shorten the duration of the allergic reaction.
- Antibiotic, antifungal, and antiviral agents are used to treat infectious disorders. They are applied topically or administered systemically.
- Scabicides and pediculicides are used in the treatment of infestations with the scabies mite and lice.
- Local (Topical) anesthetics are applied to relieve minor skin pain and itching.
- Emollients, ointments, powders, and lotions, which may be combined with other agents, soothe, protect, and soften the skin.
- Antiseborrheic agents are applied directly to the scalp or incorporated into shampooing products. They are used in the control of dandruff.
- Antiseptics are used to reduce the number of bacteria on the skin.
- Keratolytics dissolve thickened, cornified skin such as warts, corns, and calluses. Their action causes the treated area to soften and swell, facilitating removal.

Standard Precautions are used when applying any topical medication to impaired skin or changing dressings that cover an open lesion. Infected, drain-

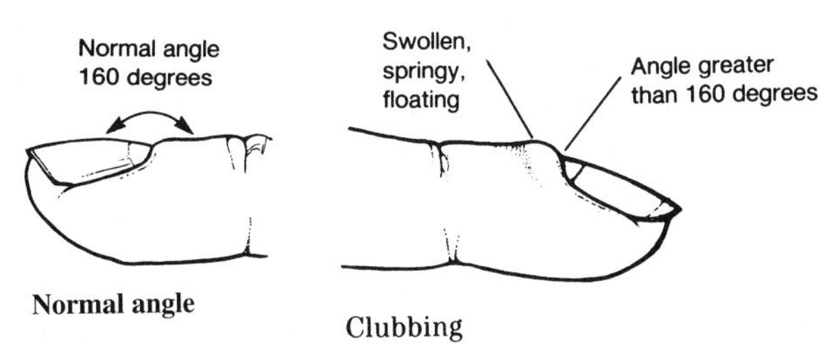

FIGURE 67-7. Normal nail angle and clubbed nail.

TABLE 67-2 **Nail Abnormalities**

Onychorrhexis

- Brittle, fragile, uneven nail edge
- Associated with malnutrition, overhydration, thyrotoxicosis, chemical damage, radiation, aging

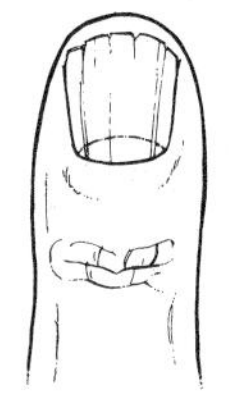

Onychorrhexis

Splinter Hemorrhages

- Blood streaks
- Associated with heart disease, hypertension, rheumatoid arthritis, neoplasms, trauma

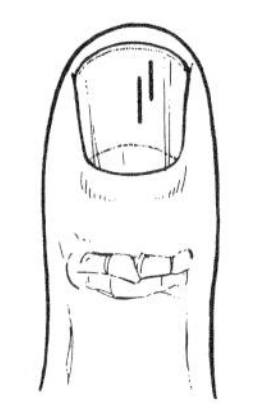

Splinter hemorrhage

Onychauxis

- Nail hypertrophy
- Associated with trauma, aging, fungal infections

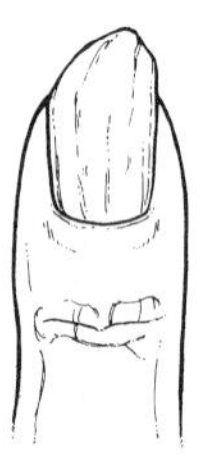

Onychauxis

Subungual Hematoma

- Blood clot
- Associated with trauma

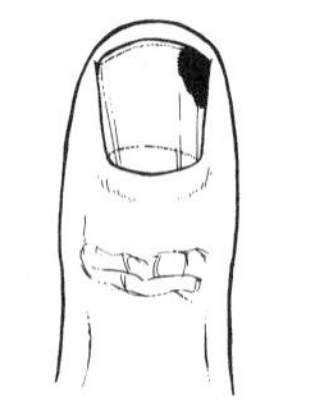

Subungual hematoma

Beau's Lines

- Transverse furrows in nail plate
- Associated with malnutrition, severe illness

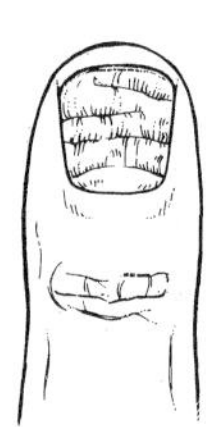

Beau's lines

ing, or weeping lesions may require contact precautions as well (see Chap. 18). It is important to apply topical medication as prescribed, such as a thin layer evenly spread over the area, or a thick layer dabbed on the area. Care is taken in applying medication so that lesions are not broken or the skin surfaces abraded.

Wet Dressings

Wet dressings are used to apply a solution to a skin lesion. They have a cooling and soothing effect. The nature of the skin lesion (open or intact) determines whether sterile technique is required. First, a dry dressing consisting of gauze or other porous material is applied to the area. Cotton is not used because of its tendency to stick to wound surfaces. The dressing is then saturated with the prescribed liquid. Dressings can be temporarily anchored with nonallergenic tape or roller gauze.

Some wet dressings are left in place until dry as a method of debridement. **Debridement** is a technique for removing damaged tissue from a wound. When the dried gauze is removed it generally contains bits of trapped debris within the gauze mesh. Removing dead and dying tissue provides an environment that fosters and promotes regeneration of healthy tissue and closure of the wound.

Therapeutic Baths

A therapeutic bath is one in which various solutions, powders, and oils, but no soap, are added to water into which the client's entire body or only a part is submerged. They are used to relieve inflammation and itching and to aid in the removal of crusts and scales. Examples of products that are used include corn starch, sodium bicarbonate (baking soda), oatmeal colloid bath preparations, and mineral oil.

The tub or container is filled with lukewarm water. The drug or product is then added and the water stirred so that the preparation mixes thoroughly. A washcloth or a compress is used to gently apply the solution without rubbing the face and any other parts not covered by the solution.

Surgical Excision

When it is necessary to remove a skin lesion, such as a benign or malignant growth, the tissue may be excised conventionally or with a laser, cryosurgery, or electrodesiccation. Surgical excisions are performed under local or general anesthesia.

LASER THERAPY

Laser stands for *L*ight *A*mplification by the *S*timulated *E*mission of *R*adiation. Lasers convert a solid, gas, or liquid substance into light. The energy of laser light vaporizes tissue and coagulates bleeding vessels. Lasers are also used to remove tattoos and pigmented skin lesions such as hemangiomas and nevi. When a laser procedure is performed, the eyes must be protected, taking precautions for preventing fires and burns from heated instruments, and removing vaporized fumes.

CRYOSURGERY

Cryosurgery is the application of extreme cold to destroy tissue. Liquid nitrogen circulates through a probe that is touched to the skin or inserted to the center of the lesion. Following application of extreme cold, the area thaws and becomes gelatin-like in appearance. A scab forms at the site. Healing takes approximately 4 to 6 weeks.

ELECTRODESICCATION

Electrodesiccation (or electrosurgery) is the use of electrical energy converted to heat, which destroys the tissue. Plantar warts and skin tumors are examples of disorders treated by this method.

RADIATION THERAPY

Radiation therapy is used to treat malignant skin lesions. For more information on radiation therapy, see Chapter 19.

PHOTOCHEMOTHERAPY

Photochemotherapy involves a combination of psoralen methoxsalen and ultraviolet A. It is one method used to treat psoriasis, a chronic skin condition (see Chap. 68). The psoralen methoxsalen is taken 1 to 2 hours before exposure to ultraviolet light A.

Lifestyle Changes

Some skin disorders grow worse when the person is tired or under emotional stress. Therefore, rest and sleep are an important part of treatment. Diet also is an important part of treatment because certain foods contribute to or aggravate skin disorders in some individuals and therefore must be eliminated from the diet.

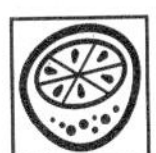

General Nutritional Considerations

Poor nutrition can lead to changes in skin integrity and turgor.

Nails may soften or develop abnormalities of shape and structure.

Hair may become brittle and thin due to poor nutritional status.

Depending on the stage of the pressure sore, protein requirements range from 1.0 g/kg to 1.6 g/kg to promote healing. Calories are increased to spare protein; small, frequent meals help maximize intake. Supplements of vitamins A, C, and zinc may be prescribed. Calorie counts help assess adequacy of intake.

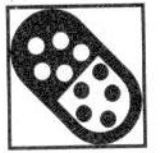

General Pharmacologic Considerations

Clients taking antibiotic, antiviral, or antifungal agents should be instructed to complete the entire prescription, even if the condition clears before all the medication is finished.

As with any medication, drug interactions may occur. If the client is taking medication for another disorder, all medications the client takes should be listed to rule out potential drug interactions.

The possibility of a drug allergy is suspected whenever the client has a skin rash.

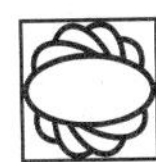

General Gerontologic Considerations

Melanin production decreases with the aging process; older adults develop gray hair.

Facial hair and sometimes chest hair appears in postmenopausal women due to a decrease in the production of estrogen.

Loss of skin elasticity and subcutaneous tissue causes wrinkles to form among older adults. Skin in the upper arms becomes fleshy and loose. The eyelids, cheeks, chin, and breasts tend to sag.

The skin becomes dry and flaked as sebum production is reduced.

Small brown, pigmented, benign lesions, known as liver spots or senile lentigines, form on the hands and forearms.

Small yellow or brown, raised lesions called senile keratoses appear on the face and trunk (refer to Color Plates 22 and 23). Senile keratoses are precancerous and require close observation by the nurse for any change in size, color, or form. These lesions may be removed by freezing, chemical peel, cauterization, or topical creams.

SUMMARY OF KEY CONCEPTS

- The integument broadly includes structures that cover the body—the skin, hair, and nails.
- The integument protects the body from environmental injuries, helps regulate body temperature, serves as a sensory organ, and participates in the synthesis of vitamin D.
- Sebum is an oily substance produced by sebaceous glands. It prevents drying and cracking of the skin and hair. Melanin is a skin pigment that absorbs ultraviolet radiation.
- Eccrine and apocrine glands are two types of sweat glands. Eccrine glands excrete water and electrolytes in the form of perspiration. Apocrine glands produce secretions, but their function in humans has not been determined. In lower animals, apocrine secretions communicate reproductive and social information among the species.
- When obtaining a health history, it is important to determine when a skin disorder began and how it first appeared, any physical changes that have occurred, associated discomfort, allergy history, and factors that make the disorder better or worse.
- Normal skin is smooth, unbroken, of uniform color according to the person's ethnic or racial origin, warm, resilient, and neither wet nor unusually dry.
- Pressure sores are categorized into one of four stages depending on the extent of tissue injury. Skin injury may range from as little as reddened skin that remains intact to deep cavitation that exposes muscle and bone.
- When the hair is assessed, the color, texture, and distribution are noted keeping gender and age-related variations in mind.
- Normal nails appear smooth, pink, thin, and slightly convex with a 160-degree angle between the nail base and the skin.
- Tissue biopsy, culture and sensitivity tests, and allergy tests are performed to detect the cause and appropriate treatment of skin disorders.
- Skin disorders are treated and managed with drug therapy, wet dressings, therapeutic baths, surgical excision, photochemotherapy, and lifestyle changes.

CRITICAL THINKING EXERCISES

1. A client has developed a rash over her arms and thorax. What additional data are important to obtain before contacting the physician?

Suggested Readings

Arms, K. (1997). *Biology: A journey into life* (4th ed.). Ft. Worth: Harcourt: Brace.

Bielan, B. (1996). What's your assessment? *Dermatology Nursing, 8*(2), 107–108.

Bullock, B. (1996). *Pathophysiology: Adaptations and alterations in function* (4th ed.). Philadelphia: Lippincott-Raven.

Fuller, J., & Schaller-Ayers, J. (1994). Health assessment: A nursing approach (2nd ed.). Philadelphia: Lippincott-Raven.

Geyer, N., & Naude, S. (1996). Diagnostic skills: Assessment of the skin, hair, and nails. *Nursing News, 20*(4), 38–39.

Hess, C. T. (1998). Keeping tabs on a pressure ulcer. *Nursing, 28*(1), 18.

Lamanna, L. (1996). Be on the lookout for skin cancer. *American Journal of Nursing, 96*(8), 16A, 16C–16D.

Talbot, L., & Curtis, L. (1996). The challenges of assessing skin indicators in people of color. *Home Healthcare Nurse, 14*(3), 167–173.

Titler, M. G., Pettit, D., Bulechek, G. M., et al. (1991). Classification of nursing interventions for care of the integument. *Nursing Diagnosis, 2*(2), 45–56.

Weiss, J. S. (1996). Sun damage and photoaging. *Women's Health Digest, 2*(3), 198–202.

Young, T. (1997). Skin assessment and unusual presentations. *Community Nurse, 3*(5), 33–36.

Chapter 68

Caring for Clients With Skin, Hair, and Nail Disorders

KEY TERMS

Acne vulgaris
Allograft
Alopecia
Autograft
Carbuncle
Closed method
Comedone
Debridement
Dermabrasion
Dermatitis
Dermatome
Dermatophytes
Dermatophytoses
Epithelialization
Erythema
Escharotomy
Eschar
Full-thickness graft
Furuncle
Furunculosis
Herpes zoster
Heterograft
Nits
Onychocryptosis
Onychomycosis
Open method
Pediculosis
Podiatrist
Pruritus
Psoriasis
Scabies
Shingles
Slit graft
Split-thickness graft

LEARNING OBJECTIVES

On completion of this chapter, the reader will:

- Define and name two types of dermatitis.
- Explain factors that lead to acne vulgaris.
- Differentiate between a furuncle, furunculosis, and carbuncle.
- Describe the appearance of psoriasis and the cause of the lesions.
- List a skin disorder caused by a mite, a fungus, and a virus.
- Discuss factors that promote skin cancer.
- Explain how the depth and percent of burns are determined.
- Name three life-threatening complications of serious burns.
- Differentiate between open and closed methods of burn wound care.
- Name three sources for skin grafts.
- List at least three priority nursing diagnoses for the care of a client with burns.
- Name two conditions characterized by hair loss and the etiology for each.
- Describe the appearance of head lice and nits.
- Explain how to remove head lice.
- Discuss factors that promote fungal infections of the nails.
- Name at least three techniques for preventing onychocryptosis, ingrown toenails.

Disorders of the skin, hair, and nails are common. Because self-image is inextricably related to how one looks, disorders that affect a person's appearance have personal and social consequences. Besides requiring medical or surgical treatment, individuals with disorders of the skin need empathic support while they cope with chronic conditions or acute and sometimes life-threatening conditions, such as burns.

Skin Disorders

Dermatitis

Dermatitis is a general term that refers to an inflammation of the skin. It is a common sign of many skin disorders that are accompanied by a red rash. An associated symptom is **pruritus,** or itching. Dermatitis and pruritus may be localized or generalized. Because both are nonspecific to any one disease, it is essential that the cause is diagnosed and definitively treated. Two common conditions include allergic and irritant dermatitis.

ETIOLOGY AND PATHOPHYSIOLOGY

Allergic contact dermatitis develops in individuals who are sensitive to one or more substances, such as drugs, fibers in clothing, cosmetics, plants (eg, poison ivy), and dyes (Fig. 68–1). Primary irritant dermatitis is a localized reaction that occurs when there is contact between the skin and a strong chemical such as solvents or detergents.

In allergic individuals, histamine is released by sensitized mast cells in the skin causing a red rash, itching, and localized swelling (see Chap. 42). Irritant dermatitis is not caused by an allergy, but rather by the caustic quality of the substance that damages the protein structure of the skin or eliminates secretions that protect it.

ASSESSMENT FINDINGS

Signs and Symptoms

The skin response is characterized by dilation of the blood vessels, causing redness and swelling, and sometimes by vesiculation (blister formation) and oozing. Itching is a prominent symptom. Primary irritant dermatitis may cause soreness or discomfort from irritation, itching, redness, swelling, and vesiculation.

Diagnostic Findings

Diagnosis is made by visual examination of the area. A detailed and thorough history helps in identifying the offending substances as well as the type of dermatitis. In difficult cases, a skin patch test may identify an allergic substance.

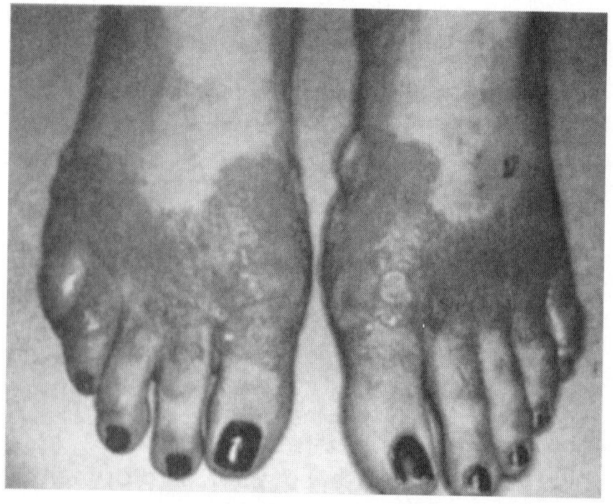

FIGURE 68-1. Contact dermatitis from shoe material.

Medical Management

Treatment of both types of dermatitis is to remove the substances causing the reaction. This is done by flushing the skin with cool water. Topical lotions, such as calamine, or systemic drugs, such as diphenhydramine (Benadryl) or cyproheptadine (Periactin), are prescribed to relieve itching. Moisturizing creams with lanolin restore lubrication. In more severe cases, wet dressings with astringent solutions, such as Burow's solution (aluminum acetate), are prescribed. Corticosteroids taken orally or applied topically also provide relief.

NURSING MANAGEMENT

Advise clients to wear rubber gloves when coming in contact with any substance such as soap or solvents, put all clothes through a second rinse cycle when laundering to remove soap residue, and avoid the use of cosmetics or any topical drug or substance until the etiology of the dermatitis is identified.

Client and Family Teaching

Measures that reduce itching or preserve the integrity of the skin include:

- Keep the nails short and clean.
- Use light cotton bedding and clothing that allow normal evaporation of moisture from the skin (avoid the use of wool, synthetics, and other dense fibers).
- Wear white cotton gloves if scratching occurs during sleep.
- Avoid regular soap for bathing; hypoallergenic or glycerin soaps can be used without causing skin irritation or itching.
- Use tepid bath water and pat rather than rub the skin dry.
- Inform the physician if the drug therapy fails to restore skin integrity or relieve itching.

Acne Vulgaris

Acne vulgaris, which tends to coincide with puberty, is an inflammatory disorder that affects the sebaceous glands and hair follicles. The severity of the condition varies from minimal to severe.

ETIOLOGY AND PATHOPHYSIOLOGY

Acne is believed to be related to the hormonal changes that occur when secondary sex characteristics are developing. It is aggravated by cosmetics as well as picking and squeezing blemishes that form. Any correlation with specific food items (eg, chocolate) is more myth than fact.

Sebum, keratin, and bacteria accumulate and dilate the follicle. The collective secretions form a **comedone,** or what most refer to as a "blackhead" (Fig. 68–2). The dark appearance is due to oxidation of the core material. The follicle becomes further distended and irritated causing a raised papule in the skin. If the follicular wall ruptures, the inflammatory response extends into the marginal areas of dermis. In serious cases, inflamed nodules and cysts develop. Severe acne, if neglected, leads to deep, pitted scars that leave the skin permanently pockmarked. Acne vulgaris improves after adolescence.

ASSESSMENT FINDINGS

Signs and Symptoms

Comedones and pustules appear on the face, chest, and back where the skin is excessively oily. Oiliness of the scalp often accompanies acne. Diagnosis is made by visual examination of the affected areas.

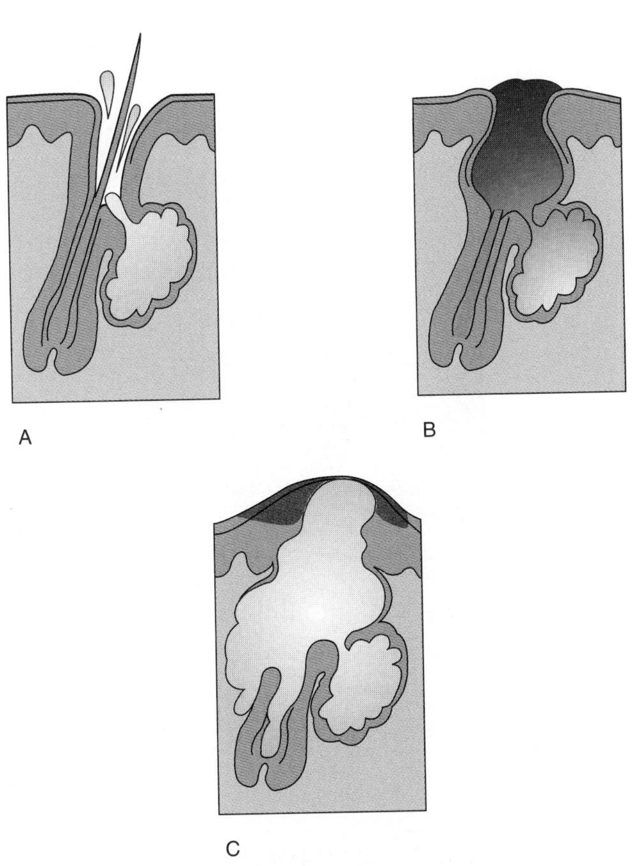

FIGURE 68-2. Acne vulgaris. (*A*) Normal sebaceous gland and hair follicle. (*B*) Comedone formation. (C) Pustule formation.

MEDICAL MANAGEMENT

Mild cases of acne improve with gentle facial cleansing and nonprescription drying agents containing benzoyl peroxide. Drug therapy includes the topical application of tretinoin (Retin-A) or oral administration of isotretinoin (Accutane). Topical and systemic antibiotics such as tetracycline and erythromycin, in low doses, also are used for severe acne and have produced good results. The comedones can be removed and the pustules drained with special instruments.

SURGICAL MANAGEMENT

Dermabrasion is a method for removing surface layers of scarred skin. It is useful in lessening scars such as the pitting from severe acne. The outermost layers of the skin are removed by sandpaper, a rotating wire brush, chemicals (chemical face peeling), or a diamond wheel. A local anesthetic, such as an ethyl chloride and freon mixture, is used during the procedure. Afterward, the skin looks and feels raw and sore, and some crusting from serous exudate occurs. Clients frequently say that the discomfort is much like that from a burn. The client is instructed not to wash the area until sufficient healing has occurred. Picking and touching the area must be avoided because this contact might cause infection or produce marking of the tissues.

NURSING MANAGEMENT

Advise the client to keep the face and hair clean and avoid the use of cosmetics that contribute to oily skin. Above all, explain that manipulating the lesions makes the condition worse. For female clients, discuss the risk of birth defects associated with oral isotretinoin. Women for whom this drug is prescribed must (1) have a negative pregnancy test 2 weeks before beginning therapy, (2) comply with contraceptive measures while taking the drug, and (3) continue reliable contraception for 1 month after therapy is discontinued.

Client and Family Teaching

Advise the person with acne to:

- Keep the hair short, clean, and away from the face and forehead.
- Wash the hair at frequent intervals; daily shampooing does not damage hair.
- Avoid the use of makeup, lotions, hair sprays, and skin care products unless their use is approved by the physician.

Furuncles, Furunculosis, and Carbuncles

A **furuncle** is a boil. **Furunculosis** refers to having multiple furuncles. A **carbuncle** is a furuncle from which pus drains.

ETIOLOGY AND PATHOPHYSIOLOGY

Furuncles and carbuncles are caused by skin infections with organisms that generally exist harmlessly on the skin surface. When the integrity of the skin is impaired due to an injury such as that caused by squeezing a lesion, microorganisms can enter and colonize within the skin. Furunculosis is also associated with diabetes mellitus because elevated blood sugar promotes microbial growth. Other factors that predispose to these conditions include poor diet and general health and any disorder that lowers resistance.

ASSESSMENT FINDINGS

Signs and Symptoms

The lesion, which may appear anywhere on the body, but especially around the neck, axillary, and groin regions, appears as a raised, painful pustule surrounded by erythema. The area feels hard to the touch. After a few days, the lesion exudes pus and later a core. The client may also experience a fever, anorexia, weakness, and malaise.

Diagnostic Findings

A culture of the exudate identifies the infectious organism.

MEDICAL AND SURGICAL MANAGEMENT

Hot wet soaks are used to localize the infection and provide symptomatic relief. It may be the only treatment necessary. Antibiotics are used in some instances especially when a fever is present, or if the lesion is a carbuncle. Surgical incision and drainage may be necessary.

NURSING MANAGEMENT

Follow strict aseptic technique when applying or changing a dressing to prevent the spread of the infection to other parts of the body or to others, and teach the client to do so also.

Client and Family Teaching

Inform the client to:

- Never pick or squeeze a furuncle because drainage is infectious and this practice favors spread of the infection to surrounding tissues or even to the bloodstream.
- Wash hands thoroughly before and after applying topical medications.
- Keep hands away from the infected areas.
- Use separate face cloths and towels than those used by others.
- Wash clothing, towels, and face cloths separately from family laundry in hot water and bleach.

Psoriasis

Psoriasis is a chronic, noninfectious inflammatory disorder of the skin. Both men and women are affected by psoriasis. Its onset occurs during young adulthood and middle life. Although there are many types of psoriasis, the most common is plaque psoriasis (Fig. 68–3). Periods of emotional stress, hormonal cycles, infection, and seasonal changes appear to aggravate the condition.

ETIOLOGY AND PATHOPHYSIOLOGY

The cause of psoriasis is unknown, but a genetic predisposition is likely because many report a family history of the disorder. Although the predisposition exists, the disorder seems to require a triggering mechanism such as systemic infection, injury to the skin, vaccination, or injection. This suggests that

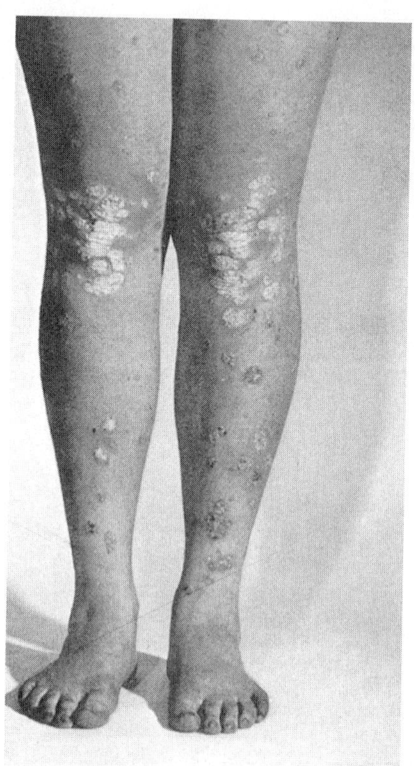

FIGURE 68-3. Typical psoriasis lesions.

there is also a link with the immune system. The hypothesis is further strengthened by the fact that the disorder goes through periods of exacerbation and remission.

In psoriasis, skin cells called keratinocytes behave as if there is a need to repair a wound. The cells of the epidermis proliferate at a faster rate than normal—so fast, in fact, that the upper layer of cells cannot be shed fast enough to make room for the newly produced cells. The excessive cells accumulate and form elevated, scaly lesions called "plaque." The area around the lesion becomes red due to the increased blood supply needed to nourish the rapidly developing skin cells.

ASSESSMENT FINDINGS

Signs and Symptoms

Psoriasis is characterized by patches of **erythema** (redness) covered with silvery scales, usually on the extensor surfaces of the elbows, knees, trunk, and scalp. Itching is usually absent or slight, but occasionally it is severe. The lesions are obvious and unsightly and the scales tend to shed.

Diagnostic Findings

Diagnosis is made by visual examination of the lesions. A skin biopsy reveals increased proliferation of epidermal cells.

MEDICAL MANAGEMENT

Psoriasis has no cure. Symptomatic treatment to control the scaling and itching includes the use of topical agents such as coal tar extract, corticosteroids, or anthralin. Anthralin, a distillate of crude coal tar, is applied to thick plaques; it tends to irritate unaffected skin areas. Topical corticosteroids have proved beneficial. Methotrexate, an antimetabolite used in the treatment of cancer, is prescribed for client with severe disease that does not respond to other forms of therapy. This drug inhibits the production of cells that divide rapidly (cancer cells, cells composing the skin and mucous membranes) and is capable of reducing plaque formation. Dosage is carefully individualized because the drug causes serious adverse effects.

Etretinate (Tegison) is related to retinoic acid and retinol (vitamin A) and is used to treat psoriasis that does not respond to other therapies. Its use is recommended only for those who are reliable in understanding and carrying out the treatment regimen, are capable of complying with mandatory contraceptive measures, and do not intend to become pregnant. Another method of treatment is the injection of triamcinolone acetonide (Kenacort), a corticosteroid, into isolated psoriatic plaques. This method of treatment is successful in some cases.

Photochemotherapy has also been used for severe, disabling psoriasis that does not respond to other methods of treatment. The extent of exposure is based on the client's skin tolerance. Treatments are given once every other day or less because phototoxic reactions may appear 48 hours or more after light exposure. Once the psoriasis clears, the client is placed on a maintenance treatment program.

Some clients respond well to treatment; others receive only minor relief. However, the condition tends to recur.

NURSING MANAGEMENT

Show acceptance of clients with skin lesions who need a great deal of understanding and emotional support. Explain that treatment is usually for a lifetime and the plan of therapy must be followed. Reassure clients who have had more than one form of treatment failure that other untried modalities may offer improved control of symptoms. Instruct the client receiving photochemotherapy to avoid exposure to sunlight for 8 hours after treatment because it takes this length of time for methoxsalen to be excreted from the body.

NURSING PROCESS
The Care of the Client With Psoriasis

Assessment

In a well lit area, inspect and evaluate the integrity of the skin. The nursing assessment should focus on the appearance of normal skin and the pathologic appearance of the affected skin. Elicit from the client whether there is a family history of psoriasis, and determine the onset, duration and possible triggering factors to the outbreak.

Nursing Diagnoses and Collaborative Problems	Nursing Interventions
Impaired Skin Integrity related to decreased protective function of epidermal tissue **Goal:** The client will achieve smoother skin with control of lesions and increased protective skin function.	Instruct client that repeat trauma to the skin (cuts, abrasions, sunburn) may exacerbate psoriasis. Advise client not to pick or scratch lesions. Inspect skin regularly for signs of infection. Wash affected area with warm water and pat dry. Apply moisturizing or medicated topical ointments as ordered.

Body Image Disturbance related to embarrassment of appearance of skin and self-perception of uncleanliness	Inform client that there is no permanent cure for psoriasis but the condition can usually be controlled or cleared.
Goal: The client will develop a sense of self-acceptance regarding disease.	Assist client in carrying out cosmetic efforts to decrease visibility of lesions.
	Encourage client to join support group to acknowledge that he or she is not alone.

Evaluation and Expected Outcomes

- Skin integrity and appearance improve.
- Itching is reduced or eliminated.
- The client understands clearly what the diagnosis of psoriasis means in terms of duration and length of treatment.
- The client copes effectively with altered appearance.

Client and Family Teaching

Explain that:

- Treatment is usually for a lifetime and the plan of therapy must be followed.
- Despite more than one form of treatment failure, other untried modalities may offer improved control of symptoms.
- Those receiving photochemotherapy must avoid exposure to sunlight for 8 hours after treatment because it takes this length of time for methoxsalen to be excreted from the body.
- It is prudent to be wary of advertised remedies that promise quick relief because they rarely do.

Scabies

Scabies is a fairly common infectious skin disease.

ETIOLOGY AND PATHOPHYSIOLOGY

Scabies is caused by infestation with the itch mite (*Sarcoptes scabiei*). Anyone can acquire this infection; it is erroneous to assume that infected individuals have poor personal hygiene. Outbreaks are common where large groups of people are confined such as nursing homes, military barracks, prisons, boarding schools, and child care centers.

The mites are spread by skin-to-skin contact. In rare cases, scabies is acquired from handling clothing and linen in recent contact with an infected individual. Scabies mites do not survive off the body more than 2 days.

ASSESSMENT FINDINGS

Signs and Symptoms

There is intense itching especially at night. The areas that are commonly affected include the webs and sides of fingers and around the wrists, elbows, armpits, waist, thighs, genitalia, nipples, breasts, and lower buttocks. The itching is accompanied by excoriation from scratching. Skin burrows are caused by the female itch mite that invades the skin to lay her eggs.

Diagnostic Findings

Diagnosis is made by examining the affected areas. However, scabies is often confused with other skin conditions. Therefore, the American Academy of Dermatology recommends an examination using mineral oil or ink. After dropping sterile mineral oil on the lesion, the skin is scraped onto a slide and examined microscopically to detect the mites, their eggs, or feces. The ink test is performed by applying a blue or black felt-tipped pen to the lesion, which highlights the burrows when the skin surface is wiped.

MEDICAL MANAGEMENT

Scabicides, chemicals that destroy mites, such as lindane (cream or lotion), permethrin cream, and crotamiton cream or lotion, are prescribed. The medication is applied to the skin from the neck down in a thin layer, left on for 8 to 12 hours, and then removed by washing. Thorough bathing, clean clothing, and the avoidance of contact with others who have scabies are essential in preventing recurrence.

NURSING MANAGEMENT

Before any treatment is started, advise the client to bathe thoroughly. Review the directions for applying the scabicide medication included with the product. Emphasize the importance of following the directions for complete eradication of the scabies mite. After bathing and applying the medication, instruct the client to don clean clothing and launder preworn clothing, towels, and bed linen in hot water as soon as possible. Tell the client to vacuum furniture and other unwashable items. Explain that itching may continue for 2 to 3 weeks after treatment.

Dermatophytoses

Dermatophytoses (tinea) are superficial fungal infections. There are many unscientific names for the conditions that develop. A common term for the skin infection is "ringworm," a misnomer because the infection is not caused by a worm. Many refer to foot infections as "athlete's foot," and those that appear in the groin are referred to as "jock itch."

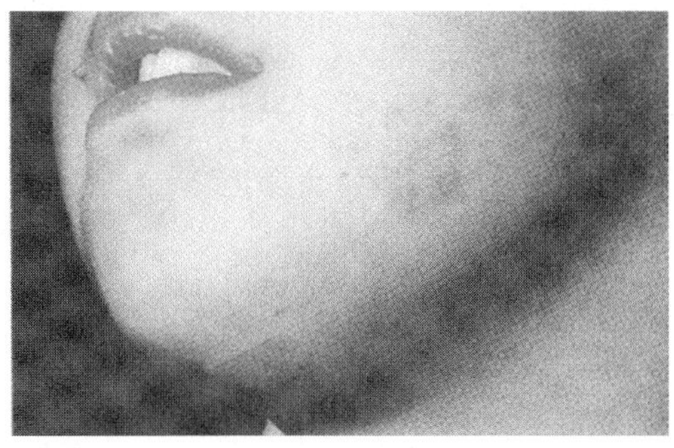

FIGURE 68-4. Tinea corporis of the face, commonly referred to as ringworm because of its circular appearance.

ETIOLOGY AND PATHOPHYSIOLOGY

Dermatophytes (also called tinea) are parasitic fungi that invade the skin, scalp, and nails (discussed later). The terms tinea pedis, tinea capitis, tinea corporis, and tinea cruris identify the skin areas of infection, namely, feet, head, body, and groin, respectively.

ASSESSMENT FINDINGS

Signs and Symptoms

Tinea corporis appears as rings of papules or vesicles with a clear center in nonhairy areas of the skin (Fig. 68–4). There may be several clusters of rings in the same general location. The affected skin often itches and becomes red, scaly, cracked, and sore. In tinea pedis, the infection begins in the skin between the toes and spreads to the soles of the feet. Tinea capitis, which is more common in children, invades the hair shaft below the scalp followed by breaking of the hair, usually close to the scalp.

Diagnostic Findings

Diagnosis is made by visual examination of the affected areas. The lesions are scrapped and examined microscopically. When a Wood's light is used, the affected areas fluoresce a green-yellow color.

MEDICAL MANAGEMENT

Treatment of tinea pedis includes the topical use of antifungal agents, such as benzoic and salicylic acids ointment (Whitfield's ointment), Burow's solution, undecylenic acid, and tolnaftate (Tinactin). Oral griseofulvin (Grisactin), a systemic antifungal agent, also is useful in treatment. The drug may be required for many weeks to eradicate the infection. Tinea capitis may be treated with oral griseofulvin, which is taken with meals. A topical antifungal agent also may be prescribed to destroy fungi present on the hair shafts above the surface of the scalp. Treatment of tinea corporis includes the use of topical antifungal agents for less severe infections. Oral griseofulvin is prescribed for more severe infections. Tinea cruris often responds to topical application of tolnaftate or miconazole (Micatin). Tinea onychomycosis (discussed later) may respond to oral griseofulvin but long-term therapy is usually necessary.

NURSING MANAGEMENT

If an oral or topical antifungal agent is prescribed, review the the directions for use. Explain that the infected person must use separate towels, washcloths, grooming articles, and clothing because the disorder is contagious. Stress that keeping the affected areas dry reduces its spread. After a bath or shower, recommend thoroughly drying all areas of the body, including the folds of the skin. Tinea cruris may be prevented by avoiding excessive heat and humidity, not wearing tight-fitting clothing or nylon next to the skin (in hot, humid weather), and keeping the skin as dry as possible.

To avoid acquiring or spreading a fungal infection of the feet, advise against sharing towels and slippers and going barefoot in locker rooms or community bathrooms. Recommend keeping the feet (particularly the area between the toes) dry, which increases resistance to the infection. Tell those whose feet perspire freely to apply powder between the toes, keep the area dry, wash and thoroughly dry the feet daily, and put on clean, dry socks and a different pair of shoes after coming home from work or school.

Shingles

Shingles, also known as **herpes zoster,** is a skin disorder that occurs years after a chickenpox (varicella) infection. The condition occurs more frequently in middle-aged to older adults, as well as those who are immunocompromised for other reasons.

ETIOLOGY AND PATHOPHYSIOLOGY

Herpes zoster is an acute reactivation of the varicella-zoster virus. The virus lies dormant in a nerve root. When the immune system becomes suppressed from aging, cancer, drugs, or acquired immunodeficiency syndrome, the virus migrates along one or more cranial or spinal nerve routes. Viral reactivation produces inflammatory symptoms in the **dermatome,** a skin area supplied by the nerve (Fig. 68–5). The inflammation is accompanied by raised, fluid-filled skin eruptions that are painful.

If the ophthalmic branch of the trigeminal nerve (third cranial nerve) is affected, corneal (eye) ulcerations may occur. Involvement of the vestibulococlear nerve (eighth cranial nerve) can lead to vertigo and

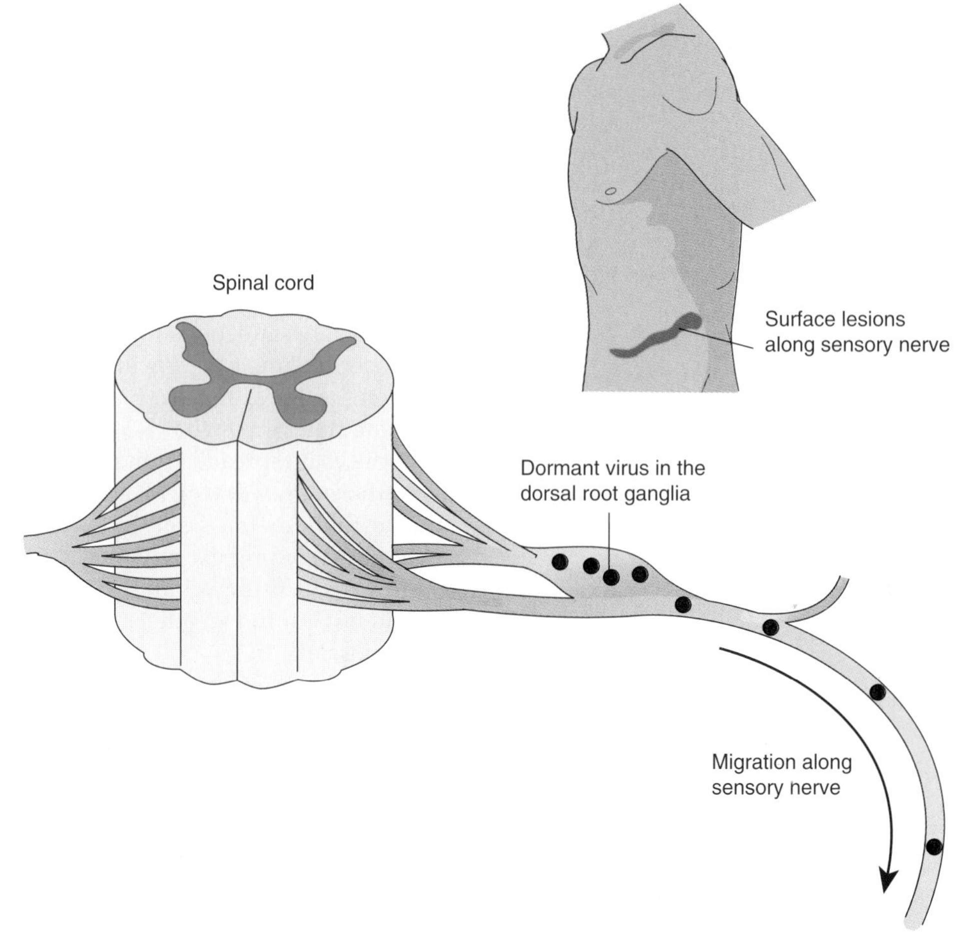

FIGURE 68-5. Reactivation of the varicella-zoster virus causing eruptions typical of shingles.

permanent hearing loss. Cerebral vasculitis (inflammation of cerebral vessels) is the most serious complication because involvement of the internal carotid arteries can result in a stroke. Rarely, the virus spreads to the brain, resulting in encephalitis.

Chickenpox can be acquired by susceptible individuals who are exposed to someone in the early stages of herpes zoster infection. The virus is contagious until the crusts from ruptured lesions have dried and fallen off the skin. Herpes zoster infection can recur.

ASSESSMENT FINDINGS

Signs and Symptoms

Initial symptoms include a low-grade fever, headache, and malaise. An area of skin along a dermatome develops a red, blotchy appearance that begins to itch or feel numb. In about 24 to 48 hours, vesicles appear on the skin along the nerve's pathway. Usually the eruptions are unilateral (one side) on the trunk, neck, or head. The eruptions become severely painful. The intense pain is soon followed by severe itching. Like chickenpox lesions, the vesicles rupture in a few days and crusts form. Scarring or permanent skin discoloration can occur. Pain (postherpetic neuralgia) and itching may persist for months or as long as 2 years or more. Secondary skin infections may occur from scratching the area.

Diagnostic Findings

Diagnosis is made primarily by examination of the lesions and symptoms.

MEDICAL MANAGEMENT

Oral acyclovir (Zovirax), when taken within 48 hours of the appearance of symptoms, reduces the severity of symptoms and prevents the development of additional lesions. Topical acyclovir also may be applied to the lesions. A brief course of corticosteroid therapy reduces pain. Lesions of the ophthalmic division of the trigeminal nerve require immediate examination and treatment by an ophthalmologist. Additional treatment is symptomatic. Analgesics and liquid preparations that have a drying or antipruritic effect are applied to the affected area once the crusts have fallen off. The skin may be so sensitive that any clothing or application of topical drugs may intensify pain or itching. A narcotic analgesic such as codeine is often necessary during the first few days to weeks.

NURSING MANAGEMENT

Reassign nursing personnel who have not had chickenpox so as to avoid contact with a client with herpes zoster. Instruct clients with crusted lesions to avoid contact with immunocompromised people and those who have not had chickenpox. Advise the client that pain and itching may be relieved by application of cool or warm compresses or warm showers; it may be necessary to experiment with both to determine which provides the most relief. Advise the client to wear loose clothing and avoid scratching the area. If oral acyclovir is prescribed, review the dose regimen, as printed on the prescription label.

Skin Cancer

Skin cancer is the most common type of cancer in the United States. It can involve any one of three types of cells in the epidermis: squamous cells that are flat and scaly; basal cells that are round; and melanocytes, cells that contain color pigment. One of every seven Americans acquires some form of skin cancer each year.

ETIOLOGY AND PATHOPHYSIOLOGY

Increased exposure to ultraviolet (UV) radiation, especially UVB and UVC, harmful components in the spectrum of sunlight, predisposes to malignant skin changes and other health risks including cataracts and premature aging of the skin. Fair-skinned individuals are more susceptible.

Several factors predispose to malignant changes in the skin:

- Thinning layer of ozone, a naturally occurring gas in the earth's atmosphere. Ozone absorbs UVB and UVC radiation (Fig. 68–6). Ozone depletion occurs primarily from the release of chlorofluorocarbons (CFCs) in refrigerants, aerosol propellants, and other industrial pollutants.
- Residence in high altitude areas where the atmosphere is thinner than at sea level or in areas with a regular cloud cover
- Decreased melanin in skin especially individuals who sunburn easily and tan minimally; black or brown-skinned people are rarely affected (Porth, 1994).
- Prolonged, repeated exposure to UV rays such as those who do farming, fishing, road construction, and so on, or those who frequent tanning salons and use sunlamps
- Prior radiation therapy for an unrelated form of cancer
- Ulcerations of long duration and scar tissue (both prone to malignant changes)

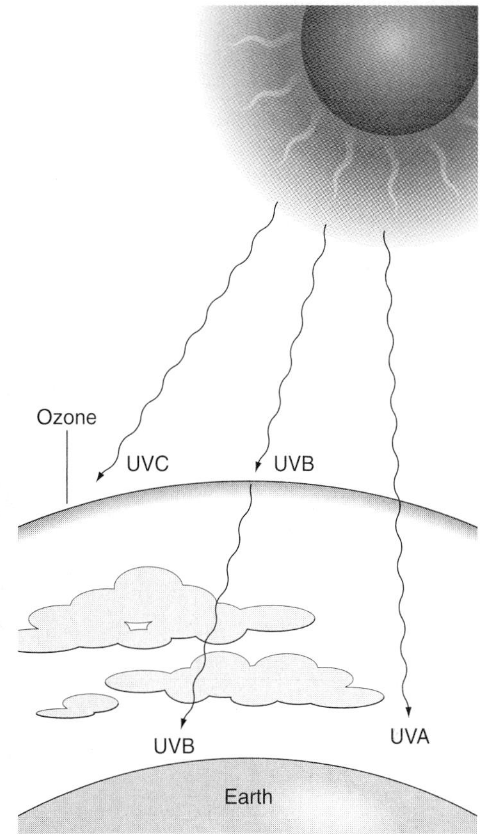

FIGURE 68-6. A layer of ozone shields or reduces the harmful spectrum of ultraviolet wavelengths known as UVC and UVB.

Malignant growths of the skin (Table 68–1) are usually primary lesions, that is, they originate in the skin. Their spread to other parts of the body or the tissues is prevented by prompt removal of the malignant tissue.

ASSESSMENT FINDINGS

Signs and Symptoms

Symptoms vary, but usually the new appearance of a growth or a change in color of the skin is the first symptom the client notices. The lesion can be smooth or rough, flat or elevated, feel itchy or tender, and even bleed.

TABLE 68-1 **Types of Skin Cancer**

Type	Incidence	Location	Appearance	Characteristics
Basal cell carcinoma	Most common especially in light-skinned individuals, increases with age	Sun-exposed areas	Small shiny, gray or yellowish plaque that undergoes central ulceration (see Color Plate 4)	Slow growing, rarely metastasizes; commonly recur
Squamous cell carcinoma	Second after basal cell in those with fair skin	Sun-exposed areas such as ears, nose, hands, scalp of bald persons	Scaly, elevated lesion with an irregular border; shallow large ulcerations form in untreated advanced lesions Squamous cell carcinoma.	Can metastasize through blood and lymph
Malignant melanoma	Increasing in incidence	Arise from preexisting moles anywhere on the body	Raised brown or black lesion (see Color Plate 3) in some cases, satellite lesions occur adjacent to the primary cancer	Poor prognosis due to distant metastases

Diagnostic Findings

Diagnosis is made by visual inspection and confirmed by biopsy.

MEDICAL AND SURGICAL MANAGEMENT

Depending on the size and the location of the lesion, treatment of squamous cell and basal cell carcinomas may involve electrodesiccation, surgical excision, cryosurgery, or radiation therapy. The client is followed at regular intervals for at least 3 to 5 years to be sure regrowth has not occurred.

The treatment of melanoma involves radical excision of the tumor and adjacent tissues, followed by chemotherapy. The administration of melphalan (Alkeran) and prednisone is an example of an initial antineoplastic therapy regimen. Interferon alfa-n3 (Alferon N) has controlled metastases in some persons. Clinical trials of other types of therapies are being conducted. In some instances skin grafting may be necessary to replace large areas of defect when a wide excision of the tumor is necessary.

NURSING MANAGEMENT

Examine and measure abnormal-appearing skin lesions, especially those in sun-exposed areas such as the face, nose, lips, and hands. Determine facts about the lesion, including when the lesion first was noticed, whether the lesion has undergone any recent changes, and, if so, what kind of changes.

Surgery for a malignant melanoma may involve structures of the head and neck, trunk, or extremities. The specific nursing management of those having radical surgery for this malignancy depends on the original site of the tumor and the extent of surgery. Give emotional support to those having disfiguring surgery.

Client and Family Teaching

Encourage all those with any type of skin change to seek medical attention. Advise those in high-risk groups for malignant skin lesions to examine all areas of their body and scalp for the appearance of new lesions or changes in moles or other growths or pigmented lesions. If any change is noted, make an appointment for a medical examination as soon as possible.

Educate individuals on measures to prevent skin cancer. Some measures include:

- Always use a sunscreen with a sun protection factor (SPF) of at least 15; higher SPFs are beneficial for individuals who sunburn easily.
- Reapply sunscreen at least every 2 hours or more often if swimming or perspiring.
- Use a lip balm with sunscreen.
- Wear a hat with a wide brim and cover the back of the neck.
- Stay in the shade when outdoors.
- Wear tightly woven, but loose-fitting clothing.
- Avoid prolonged sun exposure between 10:00 AM and 4:00 PM.
- Avoid artificial tanning.

Recommend that at-risk individuals consult the UV Forecast, a daily report that rates the UV conditions from 0 to 10+ in 30 metropolitan areas. The forecast is released by the United States Environmental Protection Agency and is broadcast during weather reports by radio and television stations as a public service. Depending on the numerical rating, called the UV Index, sun-sensitive individuals are advised to take protective measures (Fig. 68–7). A sensometer, a credit card-sized device, also is available to personally determine the UV level in one's immediate locale.

Burn Injuries

A burn is a traumatic injury to the skin and underlying tissues.

Etiology and Pathophysiology

Burn injuries are caused by heat, chemicals, or electricity. Burns caused by electricity are characteristi-

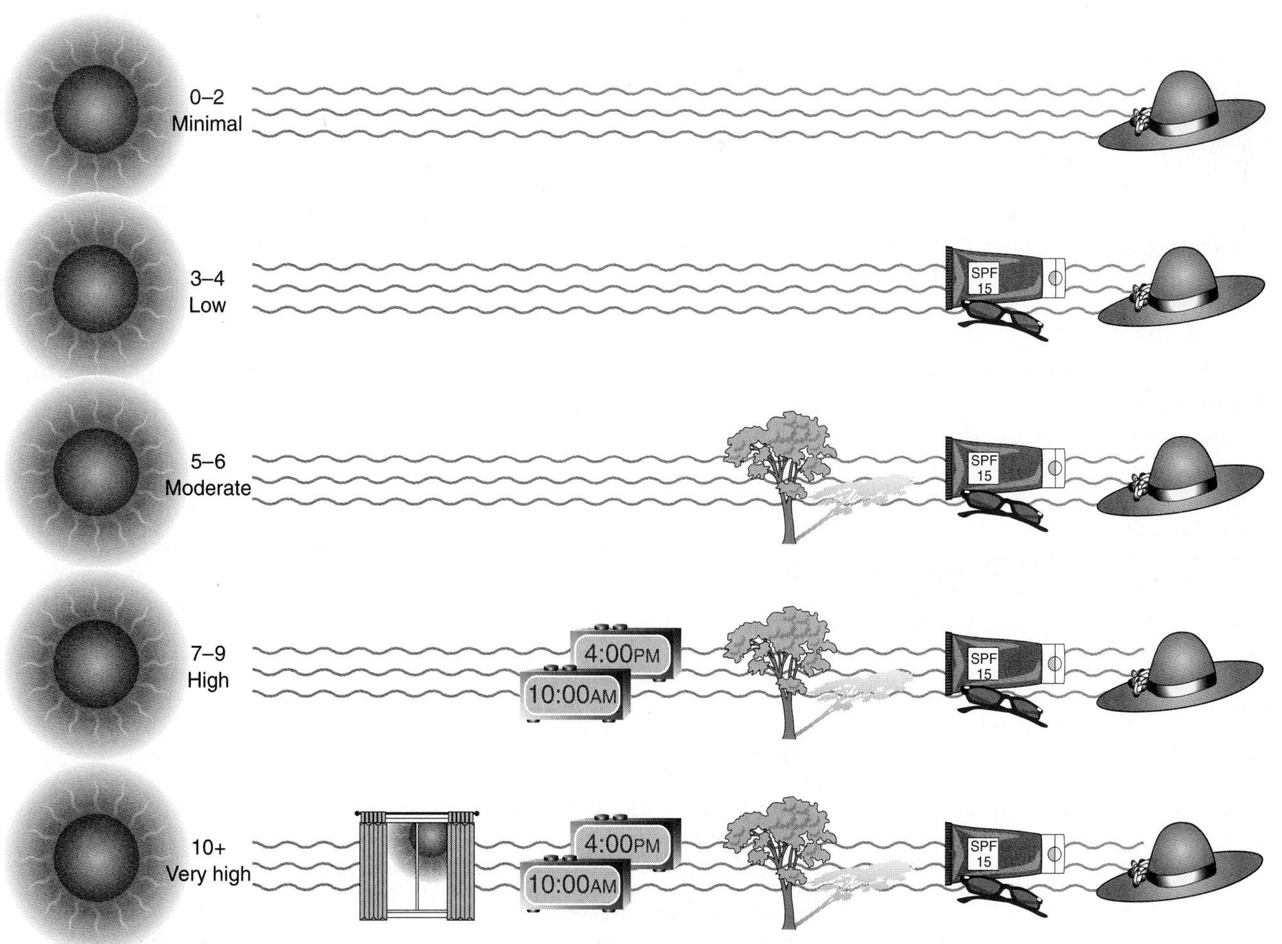

FIGURE 68-7. Sun protection measures based upon the UV index.

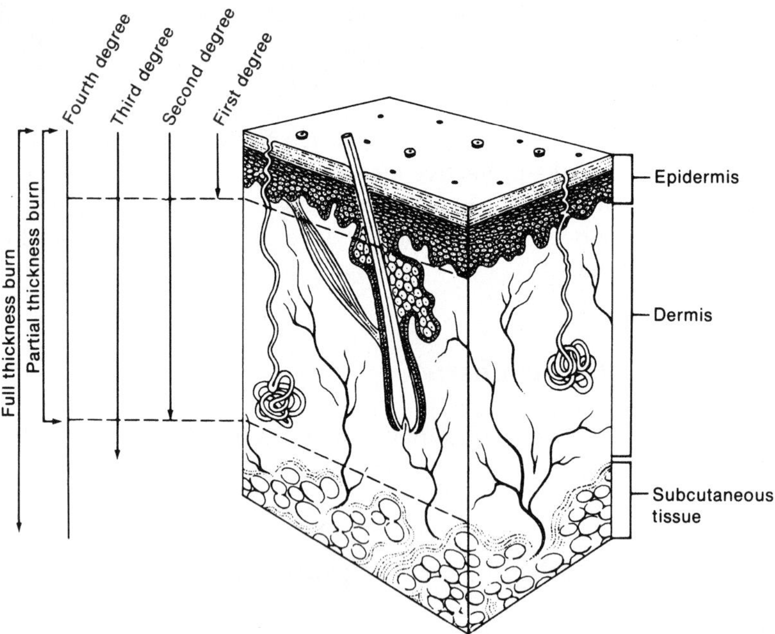

FIGURE 68-8. Depths of burn injury.

cally more severe because they are deep and the course of electricity moves about the body in an undetermined fashion from entrance to exit, causing major damage in its path.

The extent of damage is determined by (1) the depth of injury identified as superficial (first degree), partial thickness (second degree), and full thickness (third and fourth degree) (Fig. 68–8) and (2) the percent of the area of burn injury. Determining the depth of a burn (Table 68–2) is difficult because there are usually a combination of injury zones in the same location (Fig. 68–9). The "rule of nines" (Fig. 68–10) is a quick initial method of estimating how much of the client's skin surface is involved. Special charts and graphs, such as the one in Figure 68–11, provide more precise estimates for determining the percentage of the total body surface area that is burned.

After a burn, fluid from the body moves toward the burned area, accounting for edema at the burn site. Some of the fluid is then trapped in this area, is unavailable for use by the body, and therefore becomes fluid loss. Fluid also is lost from the burned area, often in extremely large amounts, in the forms of water vapor and seepage. A fall in blood pressure follows. If physiologic changes are not *immediately* recognized and corrected, irreversible shock can occur. These changes usually happen rapidly and may change from hour to hour, requiring that burned clients receive intensive care by skilled personnel.

Serum potassium increases as the ions move from the burned cells into the bloodstream. Once diuresis begins, potassium levels decrease and must be closely monitored. Decreased levels are as serious as in-

TABLE 68-2 **Depth of Burn Injuries**

Type	Depth	Characteristics
Superficial (first degree)	Epidermis and part of dermis	Painful, pink or red edema is present, but subsides quickly; no scarring
Partial thickness (second degree)	Epidermis and dermis, hair follicles intact	Mottled pink to red, painful, blistered or exude fluid, some scarring (see Color Plates 7 and 8)
Full thickness (third degree)	Epidermis, dermis, subcutaneous tissue	Red, white, tan, brown, or black; leathery covering (eschar); painless; (see Color Plate 9)
Full thickness (fourth degree)	Epidermis, dermis, subcutaneous tissue; may include fat, fascia, muscle, and bone	Black; depressed; painless; scarring

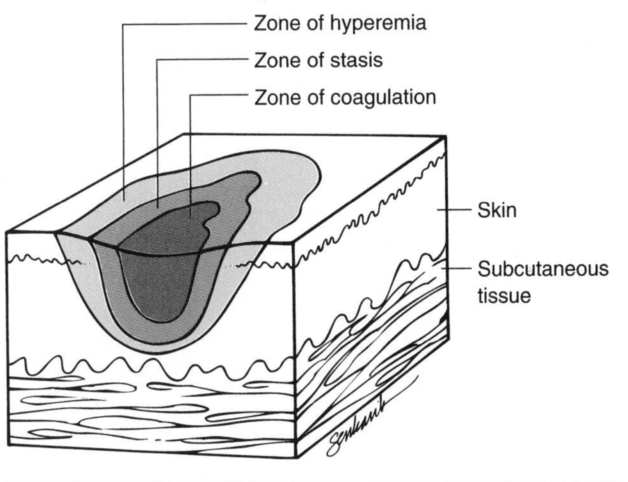

FIGURE 68-9. Zones of burn injury.

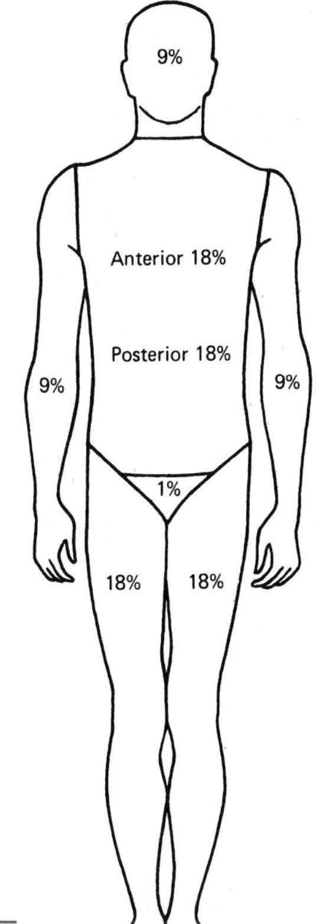

FIGURE 68-10. Rule of nines.

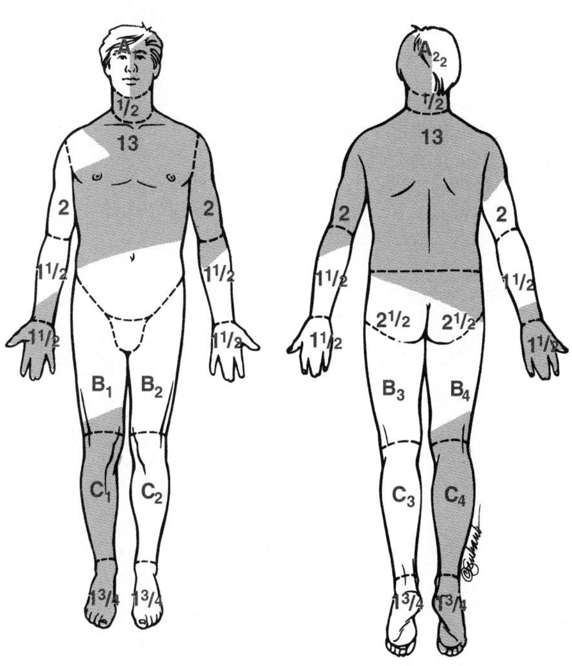

FIGURE 68-11. Sample chart for estimating percentage of body surface area burned (*indicated by shading*). (Courtesy of Crozer-Chester Medical Center, Upland, PA)

creased levels. Sodium levels may decrease initially as the ions leave the body along with the fluid lost from the burned area. Protein also is lost.

The burn victim experiences hemoconcentration when the plasma component of the blood is lost or trapped. The sluggish flow of blood cells through blood vessels results in inadequate nutrition of healthy body cells and organs.

ASSESSMENT FINDINGS

Signs and Symptoms

Skin color ranges from light pink to black depending on the depth of the burn. There may be edema or blistering. The client experiences pain in all but areas of full-thickness burns. Symptoms of hypovolemic shock, such as hypotension, tachycardia, oliguria, or anuria, may be present in clients with extensive burns. Breathing may be compromised. In electrical burns, there is generally an entrance and exit wound.

Diagnostic Findings

Diagnosis is made by physical inspection. Radiographs identify secondary injuries such as fractures or compromised lung function in inhalation injuries.

MEDICAL MANAGEMENT

The outcome of a burn injury depends on the initial first aid that is provided and the subsequent treatment in the hospital or burn center. Any one of three complications—inhalation injury, hypovolemic shock, and infection—can be life-threatening. Clients with major burns are transported to a regional burn center (Box 68–1).

Initial First Aid

At the scene of a fire, the first priority is to prevent further injury to the victim. If the clothing is on fire, the victim is placed in a *horizontal position* and rolled in a blanket to smother the fire. Laying the victim flat prevents the fire, hot air, and smoke from rising toward the head and entering the respiratory passages. The victim is taken to a hospital immediately thereafter for examination. During transport, individuals who have been burned around the face and neck or who may have inhaled smoke, chemicals, steam, or flames are observed *closely* for respiratory difficulty. When these substances are inhaled, the mucous membrane lining the respiratory passages may be damaged or extremely irritated, resulting in edema of the respiratory passages. In addition, there may be excessive mucous secretion, which also makes breathing difficult. Oxygen is administered and intravenous (IV) fluid therapy is begun en route.

Acute Care

When the burn victim arrives, the medical team works quickly to assess the extent of burn injury and additional trauma such as fractures, head injury, and lacerations. Several aspects of burn treatment, including maintaining adequate ventilation and initiating fluid resuscitation are implemented (Box 68–2). If the client has difficulty breathing or if there is edema of the face and neck, an endotracheal tube is inserted.

Blood samples are drawn. Fluid resuscitation is begun according to the severity of the burn injury (Table 68–3). IV analgesics are administered for pain, which often is severe. An indwelling urethral catheter is inserted and attached to a closed drainage system to facilitate evaluation of fluid resuscitation. Tetanus immunization and antibiotics are administered.

Wound Care

Staphylococcus aureus, *Pseudomonas aeruginosa*, and *Candida albicans* are the most common microorganisms causing infection in burned tissue. As soon as possible, all clothing is removed. The body hair around the perimeter of the burns is shaved because hair is a source of bacterial wound contamination.

BOX 68-1 Criteria for Major Burns

- Full-thickness burn greater than 10%
- Partial-thickness burn greater than 25%
- Burn in a critical location (face, eyes, ears, hands, perineum/genitalia, feet)
- Burn complicated by inhalation or electrical injury, fractures, or other major trauma
- Burn victim has preexisting medical disorder (eg, diabetes, heart disease)
- Age is less than 2 years or over 60 years
- Circumstances of burn suggest abuse (child abuse, spouse abuse)

BOX 68-2 Initial Management of the Burned Client

- Establish and maintain an adequate airway.
- Begin IV fluids; a cut down may be necessary.
- Administer IV analgesics for relief of pain.
- Withhold oral fluids.
- Insert indwelling urethral catheter.
- Give tetanus immune globulin, toxoid, or antitoxin, and antibiotics as ordered.
- Draw blood for laboratory studies.
- Give burned areas initial care.

TABLE 68-3 **Fluid Resuscitation Formulas**

Formula	Fluids	Amount*	Example for 220 lb Victim with 50% Burn
Brooke (modified)	Lactated Ringer's	2 mL/kg/% burn	10,000 mL†
	Second 24 hours	0.3–0.5 mL/kg/% burn	1,500–2,500 mL
	Colloid (plasma, albumin, dextran)	Approximate evaporative losses	2,000 mL (avg.)
	5% Glucose/water		
Parkland-Baxter	Lactated Ringer's	4 mL/kg/% burn	40,000 mL†
Evans‡	Saline	1 mL/kg/% burn	5,000 mL
	Colloid	1 mL/kg/% burn	5,000 mL
	5% Glucose/water	Approximate evaporative losses	2,000 mL (avg.)

*Goal: Establish urine output of 50 mL/hour.

†Half of fluid volume given in first 8 hours; remaining half in next 16 hours; time is calculated from time of burn injury not time fluid resuscitation begins.

‡Maximum of 10,000 mL over 24 hours if calculation exceeds this amount.

When the head, neck, and upper chest are burned, singed eyebrows and eyelashes are clipped, scalp hair shaved, the lips and mouth cleansed, and the lips lubricated. Eye ointments or irrigations are used to remove dirt and to lubricate the lid margins.

The burned areas are cleansed to remove debris. After cleansing, topical antimicrobial medications are applied. Wound management includes exposure to air or occlusive dressings and skin grafting.

OPEN METHOD. The **open method** (exposure method) exposes the burned areas to air. The client is placed in isolation, sterile linen is used, and health team members and visitors wear sterile gowns and masks. The skin of the burned client is sensitive to drafts and temperature changes; therefore, a bed cradle or sheets are placed over the client. The room is kept warm and humidified.

A hard crust forms over a second-degree or partial-thickness burn in 2 or 3 days, and **epithelialization** (regrowth of skin) is completed in about 2 or 3 weeks. At this time, the crust falls off, is debrided, or loosened by whirlpool baths. **Eschar,** a hard leathery crust of dehydrated skin, forms in areas of full-thickness burns. If the eschar constricts the area and impairs circulation, an **escharotomy** (an incision into the eschar) is done to relieve pressure on the affected area (see Color Plate 9). A dressing may be used to cover the exposed areas as the eschar is removed. New skin cannot grow beneath eschar.

CLOSED METHOD. When the **closed method** is used, the burn area is covered by occlusive dressings. Occlusive dressings are used most often when the arms, hands, feet, or legs are burned. Although there are variations, the burned area is covered with an ointment and gauze. Additional gauze, or a fluff dressing and gauze, is applied to cover the dressing adjacent to the skin.

DRUG THERAPY. Three major antimicrobials are used in the treatment of burns: silver sulfadiazine (Silvadene) 1% ointment, mafenide (Sulfamylon), and silver nitrate ($AgNO_3$) 0.5% solution (Table 68–4). Other drugs that are used are povidone-iodine (Betadine), gentamicin (Garamycin) 0.1% cream, and nitrofurazone (Furacin). Drugs have various advantages and disadvantages, and no one preparation appears to be superior to another. All drugs are applied using sterile technique. It also may be necessary to administer antibiotics systemically if an overwhelming infection occurs.

SURGICAL MANAGEMENT

Additional treatment modalities to promote healing include debridement and skin grafting. Wound **debridement** is the removal of necrotic tissue. Removal of dead tissue is accomplished in one of four ways:

1. Naturally as the nonliving tissue sloughs away from uninjured tissue
2. Mechanically when dead tissue adheres to dressings or is detached during cleansing
3. Enzymatically via the application of topical enzymes to the burn wound
4. Surgically with the use of forceps and scissors during dressing changes or wound cleansing

After dead tissue is removed, it is imperative that the healthy tissue be covered with a temporary biosynthetic covering, such as Biobrane™, a nylon-silicone membrane, artificial dermis made from a porous

TABLE 68-4 **Topical Antimicrobial Agents Used in Burn Care**

Drug	Characteristics	Nursing Implications
Silver sulfadizine (Silvadene)	Most widely used Fewest side effects Water-soluble cream Affects gram-negative and gram-positive bacteria and yeasts Prolonged use can produce resistant bacterial strains	Apply directly to wound with sterile gloved hands. Cover burn wound with 1⁄16 inch of ointment b.i.d. after thorough cleansing of previous application.
Mafenide acetate (Sulfamylon)	Available in cream or solution Antibacterial but little antifungal effect Good penetration into burn wound Painful during application and shortly thereafter Absorption can cause metabolic acidosis, compensatory hyperventilation, and diuresis. Can cause hypersensitivity reactions	Premedicate with an analgesic before application. Reapply cream every 12 hours; rewet dressing every 2–4 hours. Observe for rash in hypersensitive persons. Monitor acid–base balance.
Silver nitrate	Solution with good antimicrobial effects Nonallergenic No pain with application Depletes serum Na, K, Cl, and Mg Stains everything brown or black including normal skin; staining interferes with wound assessment.	Rewet dressings every 2–4 hours Monitor serum electrolytes.

collagen-chondroitin mat, or some type of natural skin graft.

SKIN GRAFTING. The purpose of a skin graft is to:

- Lessen the possibility of infection
- Minimize fluid loss by evaporation
- Prevent loss of function

Skin grafting is necessary for third-degree and fourth-degree burns because the skin layers responsible for regeneration have been destroyed. It may also be necessary for many second-degree burns. Unassisted healing, that is, healing without the use of temporary grafts, in second-degree burns can result in an overgrowth of granulation tissue. Some second-degree burns require grafting for cosmetic reasons and maintenance of function.

There are several sources for skin grafting. An **autograft** uses the client's own skin, which is transplanted from one part of the body to another. Only autograft or skin transplanted from one identical twin to another can become a permanent part of the client's own skin. An **allograft** or homograft is human skin obtained from a cadaver. Allografts temporarily cover large areas of tissue. Although allografts slough away after a week or more, they tide the client over the critical period until the client's own skin can be used for skin grafting. A **heterograft** or xenograft is obtained from animals, principally pig skin. Like allografts, heterografts are temporary and serve the same purposes. Some newer types of heterografts are made of synthetic and biosynthetic materials.

Skin grafting is done under general anesthesia. **Split-thickness** and **full-thickness grafts** are the two basic types of skin grafts. Split-thickness autografts vary in thickness (0.008–0.024 inch), size, and shape and are usually obtained from the buttocks or thighs. The skin is removed from the donor site by the use of a dermatome, a scalpel, or other special instrument. Full-thickness grafts, which may be 0.035 inch thick, are skin grafts that include subcutaneous tissue. This type of graft is used when the burned area is fairly small or when the hands, face, and neck are involved. A **slit graft** (also called a lace or an expansile graft) is used when the area available as a donor site is limited, as in clients with extensive burns. The skin is removed from the donor site and passed through an instrument that slits it; thus, a smaller piece of skin is stretched to cover a larger area (Fig. 68–12).

Pressure garments made of elasticized cloth or plastic are applied over the area once healing begins. These garments prevent scars and wound contractures. The client may need to wear a pressure garment for up to 2 years.

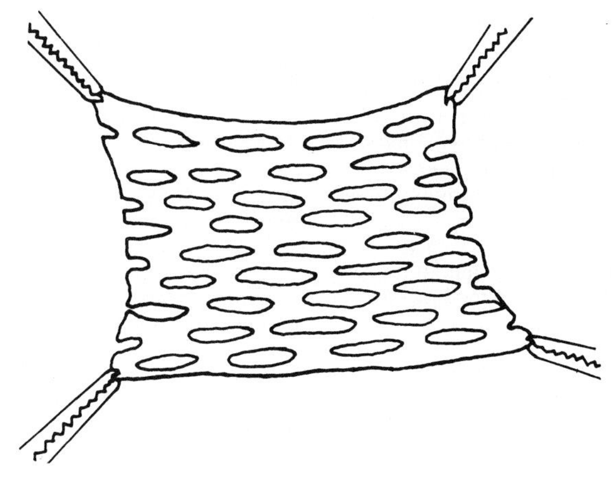

FIGURE 68-12. A slit graft. The slits allow for stretching to cover a larger area of tissue.

NURSING MANAGEMENT

Nursing assessment focuses on the major priorities, namely, respiratory and fluid status. Vital signs are taken either with a blood pressure cuff or a Doppler or Dynamapp device. Shock may be present and must be quickly recognized and efficiently treated.

Depending on the extent and degree of burns, some or all of the following nursing diagnoses may apply. Nursing diagnoses change as the client progresses through treatment and the stages of healing.

Nursing Diagnoses and Collaborative Problems	Nursing Interventions
Risk for Ineffective Airway Clearance related to increased airway secretions; **Risk for Impaired Gas Exchange** related to edema of airway and inhalation of carbon **Goal:** The client's airway will be patent and gas exchange adequate as evidenced by clear lung sounds, SpO_2 greater than 90%, PaO_2 greater than 80 mm Hg.	Monitor characteristics of respirations and lung sounds at frequent intervals.
	Measure SpO_2 with a pulse oximeter or analyze arterial blood gas results.
	Administer oxygen as prescribed.
	Suction airway cautiously if edema is present.
	Facilitate ventilation with artificial airways—ventilator, endotracheal tube, or tracheostomy.
PC: Hypovolemic shock **Goal:** Hypovolemia will be managed and minimized.	Monitor vital signs q 15 minutes.
	Measure intake and output hourly.
	Weigh the client daily at the same time with similar dressings.
	Administer fluids according to the fluid resuscitation formula.
	Report urine output of < 50 mL/hour.
	Reduce evaporation from the burn wound by humidifying the environment, preventing drafts, and keeping the burn wound covered with ointment or creams, gauze dressings, or skin grafts.
Pain related to tissue injury **Goal:** Pain will be within the client's level of tolerance.	Administer prescribed analgesia by IV routes or into sites that have not been burned.
	Give analgesics prophylactically 30 minutes before dressing change or debridements.
	Implement nonpharmacologic methods for pain relief such as imagery, self-hypnosis, and distraction.
	Place the client on a CircOlectric bed or other type of turning frame to facilitate turning and repositioning.
	Exercise caution and gentleness when removing and reapplying dressings.
Risk for Infection related to impaired skin integrity **Goal:** The burn will be free of infection or the infection will resolve.	Assess temperature every 4 hours; monitor results of blood counts and culture results.
	Use sterile or clean linen.
	Wear sterile or clean caps, gowns, and masks.
	Restrict infectious individuals from visiting or caring for client.
	Apply and administer prescribed antimicrobial and antibiotic therapy.
	Inspect burn areas for healing, drainage, formation of eschar, evidence of infection, and stability of the skin graft or wound covering, and accurately record all findings.
PC: Skin Graft Disruption **Goal:** Skin graft will establish adequate blood supply and consolidate with recipient tissue.	Avoid excessive pressure on the grafted area; keep movement to a minimum to promote vascularization.
	Assist the physician with dressing changes.
	Monitor bleeding and odor in the area of grafted tissue.
PC: Gastric and Intestinal Paresis (Hypomotility) related to stress	Assess for abdominal distention and status of bowel sounds.

PC: Stress-Related Peptic Ulcer **Goal:** Hypomotility will be managed and minimized. A stress ulcer will not develop.	Insert and connect a nasogastric tube to suction, if ordered, when nausea and vomiting develop. Administer histamine antagonists intravenously and drugs such as metoclopramide (Reglan). Instill antacid through nasogastric tube and clamp for 30 minutes before reconnecting to suction. Assess pH of gastric secretions q shift; report if pH is < 3.
Risk for Constipation related to fluid loss, absence of oral nutrition, inactivity, and side effect of narcotic analgesia **Goal:** Stool will be passed regularly and with ease.	Monitor bowel elimination. Administer prescribed stool softener or laxatives. Remove fecal impaction if one develops.
PC: Anemia related to destruction of red blood cells and blood loss from stress ulcer **Goal:** Anemia will be managed and minimized.	Monitor hemoglobin and hematocrit laboratory results. Check gastric secretions and stool for occult or frank blood. Administer whole blood or packed red blood cells as prescribed. Provide iron-rich food or supplements when it is safe to use the oral route.
Risk for Altered Nutrition: Less than Body Requirements related to increased caloric requirements and inability to ingest food orally **Goal:** Nutrition will be maintained.	Administer total parenteral nutrition until tube feedings or oral feedings can be initiated. Monitor weight loss or gain. Provide high-protein, iron-rich foods in small frequent feedings when oral nourishment is allowed.
Impaired Physical Mobility related to pain, bulky dressings, contracted skin secondary to scar formation **Goal:** Range of motion and muscle strength will be preserved or restored.	Keep the joints in burned areas in neutral positions—extended rather than flexed. Exercise uninvolved joints actively; exercise involved joints during hydrotherapy. Encourage the performance of activities of daily living, such as brushing teeth and eating.
Risk for Altered Thought Processes related to reduced mental stimulation sleep deprivation, social isolation, fluid and electrolyte imbalance, narcotic administration, and sepsis. **Goal:** The client will remain oriented and perceive the environment and situations realistically.	Assess mental status every shift. Reorient the confused client. Have a calendar and clock within the client's view. Discuss current events and encourage visits by family.
	Cluster nursing activities to facilitate a continuous period of sleep.
Risk for Ineffective Individual and **Family Coping** related to inadequate emotional resources for managing multiple stressors **Goal:** The client and family will adapt and learn methods for adequate coping.	Explain methods and reasons for treatment. Acknowledge signs of progress. Involve the client and family in long-range planning, physical therapy, and vocational rehabilitation. Refer the family to counseling for assistance.

Scalp and Hair Disorders

Some conditions are unique to the scalp and hair. They include inflammatory and noninflammatory scalp conditions and disorders that cause hair loss.

Seborrhea, Seborrheic Dermatitis, and Dandruff

Seborrhea and dandruff are noninflammatory conditions that generally precede or accompany seborrheic dermatitis. Seborrheic dermatitis has an inflammatory component.

ETIOLOGY AND PATHOPHYSIOLOGY

Seborrhea is a dermatologic condition associated with excessive production of secretions from the sebaceous glands. Although seborrhea is not always confined to the scalp, it is one of the primary sites. Seborrheic dermatitis presents as red areas covered by yellowish, greasy-appearing scales. Dandruff, on the other hand, is loose scaly material of dead, keratinized epithelium shed from the scalp in clients who may or may not have seborrheic dermatitis. Dermatologists believe that dandruff is caused by a tiny fungus known as *Pityrosporum ovale*. Most everyone harbors this fungus, yet only some individuals develop dandruff. Some possible factors for this phenomenon include excessive perspiration, inadequate diet, stress, and hormone activity.

Scalp conditions cause more of a cosmetic rather than health problem. The conditions come and go necessitating retreatment. They do not progress or become transformed into other serious skin disorders.

ASSESSMENT FINDINGS

Signs and Symptoms

Clients note that the hair is unusually oily. There may be red or scaly patches on the scalp. White flakes fall from the hair and become more obvious when they collect on the shoulders of dark clothing. The inflamed areas may itch.

Diagnostic Findings

No diagnostic testing is necessary unless the condition does not respond to treatment. In that case, a skin biopsy or laboratory blood work is performed to eliminate the possibility that the condition was misdiagnosed.

MEDICAL MANAGEMENT

Frequent shampooing with or without a medicated product helps to reduce the presence of scalp and hair oil. Effective medicated shampoos contain tar, zinc pyrithione, selenium sulfide, sulfur, and or salicylic acid. Some individuals require topical applications of corticosteroids.

NURSING MANAGEMENT

Explain the underlying cause of the client's problem. Review the directions for using medications and the frequency of use. Inform clients that the disorder may recur and that persistent treatment is necessary to keep the condition under control.

Alopecia

Alopecia means baldness. The condition affects the hair follicles and results in partial or total hair loss. It is normal to shed 50 to 100 hairs a day. The lost hair is normally replaced by a new one from the same hair follicle. However, in some conditions there is an excessive loss of hair, some of which may be temporary or permanent.

Alopecia is not life-threatening; however, whenever men or women lose their hair, most experience self-consciousness and a loss of self-confidence. Many spend great sums of money on unscientific methods for restoring hair growth. Although not everyone can be helped, several options are available to individuals with hair loss.

ETIOLOGY AND PATHOPHYSIOLOGY

Hair loss can develop for several reasons. Temporary hair loss is caused by medications such as antineoplastic drugs, inadequate diet, thyroid disease, tinea infection, improper application of hair care products, and hair styles that pull the hair tightly.

Alopecia areata and androgenetic alopecia are two conditions that are chronic and difficult to reverse. Alopecia areata is believed to be an autoimmune disorder characterized by patchy areas of hair loss about the size of a coin, but it can progress to total hair loss and even loss of hair from the entire body. Antibodies attack and destroy the hair follicle.

Androgenetic alopecia is a genetically acquired condition many refer to as male pattern baldness. The term is somewhat inaccurate because women also are affected, but to a milder degree. Androgenetic alopecia is inherited from either one's mother or father. When testosterone, an androgenic hormone, combines with an enzyme, 5-alpha-reductase (5-DHT), in the hair follicle, hair production stops. This condition begins in adolescence or early adulthood and progresses with age.

ASSESSMENT FINDINGS

Signs and Symptoms

Clients note that their hair is thinning or falling out in patches in several areas of the scalp. Those with a family history of baldness tend to lose hair in the lateral frontal areas or over the vertex of the head (Fig. 68–13). Women report thinning in the frontal, parietal, and crown regions. Primary hair loss is not associated with any other physical health problems.

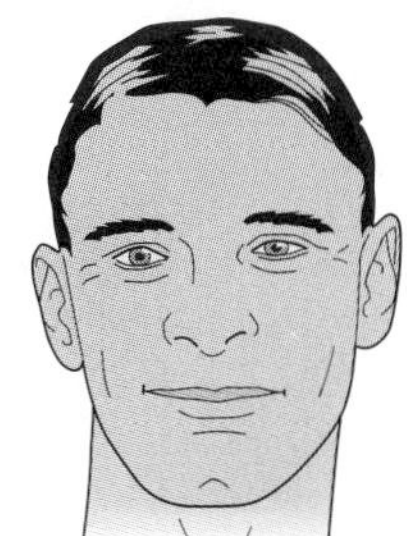

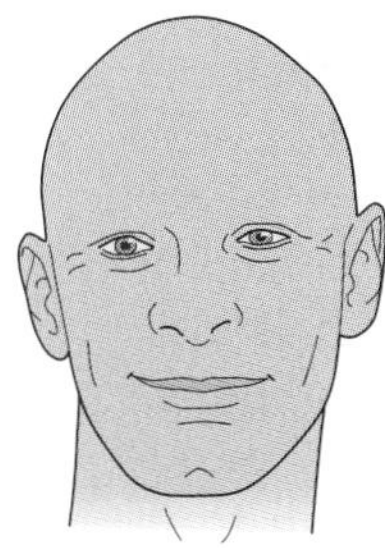

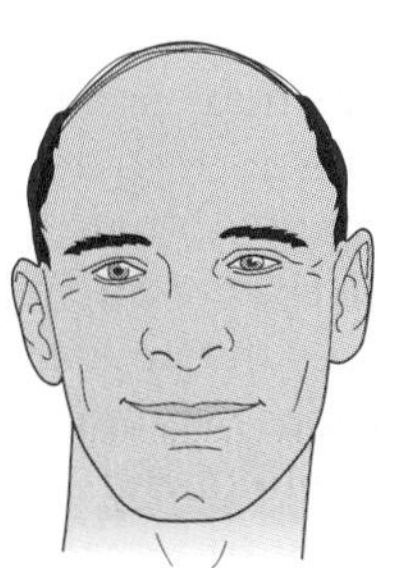

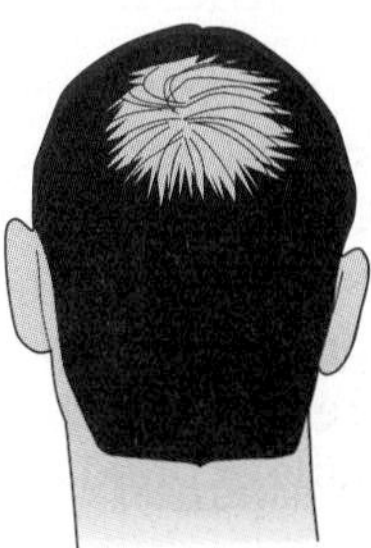

FIGURE 68-13. Patterns of hair loss. (*A* and *B*) Alopecia areata; (*C* and *D*) Androgenetic alopecia.

Diagnostic Findings

Diagnostic tests are performed to determine any physical disorder that is contributing to the hair loss. When these are negative, the family history and pattern of hair loss suggest hereditary baldness or an autoimmune disorder.

MEDICAL MANAGEMENT

If hair loss is caused by a medical disorder, relieving the cause generally restores hair growth. Some drugs can retard hair loss and promote hair growth. One drug is minoxidil (Rogaine); however, the hair growth that is stimulated has a downy texture. If the drug is discontinued, hair growth stops and baldness recurs. The best results are obtained by young individuals who begin drug therapy when their hair loss is minimal. A hair addition is a technique for giving the appearance of more hair by attaching extra hair to the client's natural hair.

SURGICAL MANAGEMENT

Some balding individuals prefer a more permanent solution with hair replacement surgery or other surgical techniques. Hair grafting is a technique for transplanting hair-bearing scalp from the back and sides of the head into bald areas. Each graft contains from 1 to 8 hairs. A bald area that is approximately 3 inches square requires approximately 500 to 600 hair grafts. Unfortunately, because of the progressive nature of androgenetic alopecia, transplanted hairs may not survive permanently.

A procedure that disguises hair loss is a scalp reduction that surgically removes a bald area. A scalp reduction is usually performed along with hair grafts. Another surgical technique is to transfer a skin flap. The flap transfers the greatest amount of hair in a short amount of time. But, the scalp may have to be expanded preoperatively to stretch the flap area because the flap remains attached in its original location at one end.

NURSING MANAGEMENT

Support clients who may not have the financial means for medical or surgical treatment. Reassure them that they can cope with hair loss. Suggest consulting a cosmetologist who can provide a haircut and style that minimizes the appearance of hair loss. Tell women to opt for loose styling rather than ponytails or braids. Recommend using a conditioner or detangler after shampooing to avoid pulling hair from the head and a wide-toothed comb or brush with smooth tips.

Head Lice

An infestation with lice is called **pediculosis.** Although lice can infest hairy parts of the body such as the pubic area, they are more likely to be found on and in the hair on the head.

ETIOLOGY AND PATHOPHYSIOLOGY

Lice are crawling brown insects about the size of sesame seeds; they do not fly or jump (Fig. 68–14). Nymphs look like moving dandruff, but they may appear red after feeding. Adult lice and nymphs creep over the skin and feed on human blood. The bites result in itching. Eggs, or **nits,** laid by adult females are tightly cemented to the side of hair shafts. They appear like small yellowish white ovals. Nits hatch in 7 to 10 days. Lice have a life span of approximately 30 days during which time one female can lay 100 to 400 nits. Researchers believe that lice are developing strains that resist chemical extermination.

Lice are transmitted from person to person through direct contact. They cannot survive longer than about 24 hours without blood. Sharing clothing, combs, and brushes promotes transmission. Anyone can acquire lice, but infestations among school children tend to be difficult to arrest. Many schools have a "zero tolerance" policy for lice infestation; that is, an infected child is barred from attending school until the hair and scalp are free of lice and nits.

ASSESSMENT FINDINGS

Signs and Symptoms

Itching of the scalp is the most common complaint. Intense scratching can lead to a secondary infection.

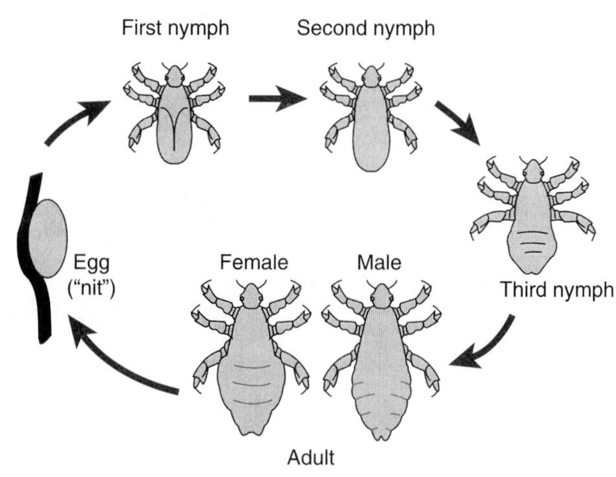

FIGURE 68-14. The life cycle of head lice.

The adult forms of lice are difficult to see because they quickly move away from light. The nits cling to hairs close to 1/20 to 1/4 inch from the scalp.

Diagnostic Findings

Diagnosis is made by scalp and hair inspection. Live lice are retrieved with tweezers or the adhesive side of tape.

MEDICAL MANAGEMENT

Nonprescription shampoos, gels, and liquids containing pediculocides are effective. One example is permethrin liquid (Nix), which kills adult forms of lice. Other over-the-counter products such as RID™, Pronto™, and A-200™ contain pyrethrin, a natural insecticide from the crysanthemum, and piperonyl butoxide. The National Pediculosis Association opposes the use of strong chemicals such as lindane (Kwell), which is neurotoxic, and those that contain benzene, which is carcinogenic, especially on children. Pediculocides are contraindicated for pregnant and nursing women, children under 2 years of age, and those who have health conditions such as open wounds, epilepsy, or asthma. Nits and live lice are removed mechanically with a fine-toothed combing tool such as one called the LiceMeister™.

NURSING MANAGEMENT

Train school volunteers and parents on how to detect and recognize lice and nits. Untrained or poorly trained individuals may mistake other hair and scalp conditions for lice and unnecessarily stigmatize children who are dismissed from school. Follow Nursing Guidelines 68–1 for removing nits and lice and teach the family to do likewise.

Teach the client or family to not shampoo or rinse with a conditioner before applying the pediculocide. Conditioner coats the hair and protects the nits. Instruct individuals to follow the label directions on the pediculocide; leaving the chemical(s) on for longer than 10 minutes or covering the head with a shower cap does not increase effectiveness and, in fact, may increase the potential for toxicity.

Client and Family Teaching

Nurses, especially those employed in school systems, can provide clients with important information on detection, elimination, and prevention of reinfestation. Some facts to include are:

- Anyone can become infected; infestation is not a reflection of hygiene or unsanitary living conditions.
- Perform hair inspection whenever there is an outbreak whether you or your child have symptoms or not.
- If everyone who is infested with lice follows the prescribed treatment, the outbreak can be controlled and eliminated.
- Pediculocides are contraindicated for pregnant and nursing women, children under 2 years of age, and those who have health conditions such as open wounds, epilepsy, or asthma.
- Never use a pediculocide on the eyebrows or eyelashes.
- There is no value in using a pediculocide prophylactically.
- Manual removal is one of the best and safest options for eliminating lice and nits.
- Do not use pediculocides on pets; pets do not harbor lice.
- Wash clothing and vacuum furniture, bedding, and carpets.

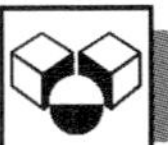

Nursing Guidelines 68-1

Removing Nits and Lice

- Cut long hair to make it more manageable.
- Apply the pediculocide to the hair.
- Seat the infested individual where there is good light.
- Comb the hair free of tangles while the hair is damp.
- Divide the hair into sections.
- Lift a 1-inch strand of hair from a hair section.
- Use a special lice comb that has narrow stainless steel teeth (available from the National Pediculosis Association).
- Start at the crown and comb firmly, deeply, and evenly away from the scalp to the end of the hair.
- Pin back or secure the combed strand and hair section before going to another area.
- Redampen the uncombed hair if it begins to dry.
- Dip the comb in water or wipe it with a paper towel periodically to remove dead lice and their eggs, or pull dental floss through the teeth of the comb.
- Deposit debris in a zip-lock plastic bag.
- Unfasten the sectioned hair and rinse the head thoroughly.
- Assume that some lice will be missed.
- Repeat combings on a daily basis until there is no longer any evidence of lice or nits.

Nail Disorders

The nails, especially toenails, are subject to disorders. Two that are common include fungal infections, known as onychomycosis, and ingrown toenails, technically called onychocryptosis.

Onychomycosis

Onychomycosis is a fungal infection of the fingernails or toenails. A fungus is a tiny plantlike parasite that thrives in warm, dark, moist environments. The fungi can spread unchecked from one nail to another. The toenails are more commonly affected because conditions inside shoes are perfect for breeding fungi.

ETIOLOGY AND PATHOPHYSIOLOGY

Onychomycosis and tinea pedis (athlete's foot) often occur together. The elderly and immunocompromised individuals are at greater risk for fungal infections. There has been an increased incidence in fungal fingernail infections among women who have artificial nails. Unsanitary cleansing of nail application utensils between customers in salons seems to be the mode of transmission.

The fungi locate themselves from the surrounding skin to beneath the nail plate. The fleshy portion underneath the nail becomes inflamed. The nail becomes elevated, thickens, loosens, and changes color. Eventually the nail plate is destroyed. The longer the infection is present, the more difficult it is to cure.

ASSESSMENT FINDINGS

Signs and Symptoms

One or more nails appears grossly different than normal. They are much thicker, causing them to be elevated and distorted. The nails are yellowed and friable. Because they are difficult to trim, the infected nail(s) may be long and jagged. The pressure and friction from thickened toenails can lead to pain because shoes do not fit comfortably and socks may wear through.

Diagnostic Findings

Diagnosis is made generally on the basis of appearance. However, microscopic examination of nail scrapings can confirm the diagnosis.

MEDICAL AND SURGICAL MANAGEMENT

Treatment involves prolonged systemic drug therapy with either of two antifungal agents: itraconazole (Sporanox) and terbinafine (Lamisil). Both drugs inhibit fungal enzymes that affect cell membrane permeability and result in fungal death. The medications are taken daily for 2 weeks for fingernail infections and for 3 weeks for toenail infections. Terbinafine can also be administered in a pulse-dosing regimen consisting of 1 week of medication followed by a 3-week rest period. Repeated pulse dosing is necessary to eradicate the infection. Drug therapy is more than 50% effective. Because nails grow slowly, it may take as long as 12 months before the nail appears normal.

A more radical solution involves removal of the infected nail. This is generally a last resort because it causes permanent cosmetic changes. Surgery is considered when the condition results in chronic pain or when it causes difficulty in wearing shoes.

NURSING MANAGEMENT

Reinforce the chronicity of the condition and the need to remain compliant with drug therapy for the duration of treatment. Explain the dosing regimen, side effects that may develop, and drug interactions. To prevent reinfection, remind clients to:

- Change to an alternate pair of shoes daily.
- Purchase leather shoes that promote evaporation of foot moisture.
- Never go barefoot.
- Wear footwear at communal pools or when showering in gyms or fitness centers.
- Avoid any damage to the skin around the nail which makes it easier for fungi to colonize.

Onychocryptosis

Onychocryptosis is the medical term for an ingrown toenail. This is a common condition that can affect anyone and everyone, although some are more predisposed than others. The inside edge of the great toe is usually affected. Recurrence tends to be a significant problem.

ETIOLOGY AND PATHOPHYSIOLOGY

Some people have an inherited trait that causes a curvature in the growing nail plate. These individuals have a higher incidence of ingrown toenails despite the fit of their shoes or methods for keeping the nails trimmed. The latter two factors along with fungal nail infections explain why most others acquire ingrown toenails. Athletes or those who are physically active seem to have repeated episodes once the condition develops due to recurring trauma.

When the nail curves during growth, a corner of the nail becomes trapped under the skin. As the the nail grows, it cuts into the flesh at the lateral border of the nail. The trauma causes local inflammation. The impaired skin provides an opportunity for bacteria to secondarily invade the traumatized tissue.

Color Plates

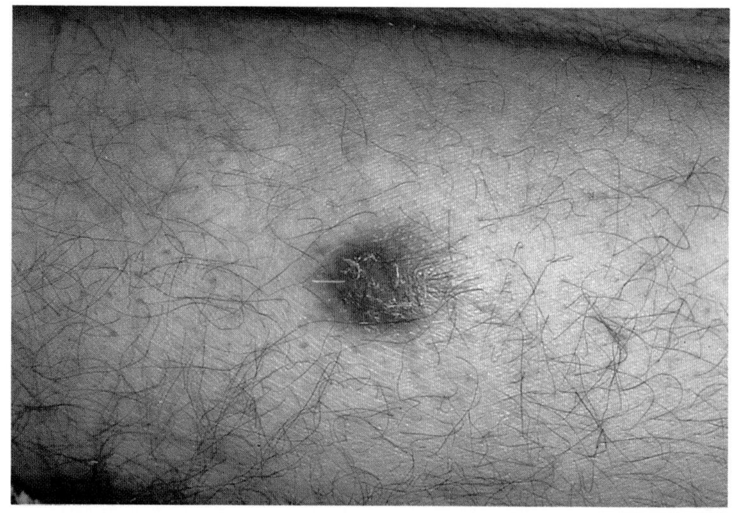

Color Plate 1. Kaposi's sarcoma, single lesion.

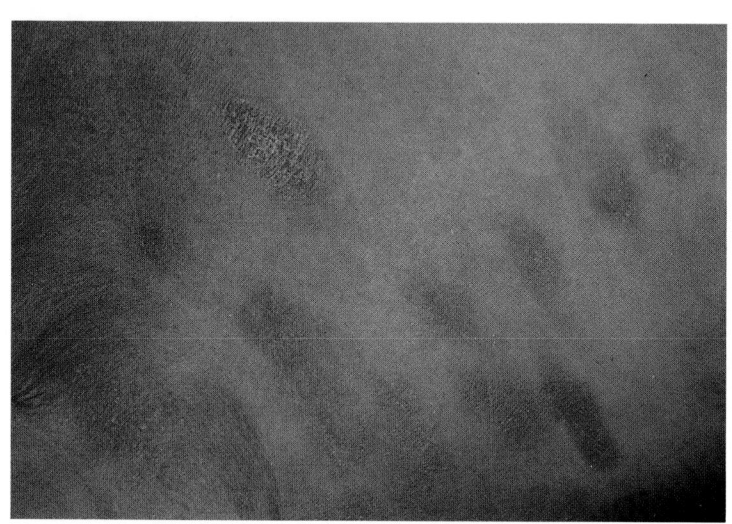

Color Plate 2. Kaposi's sarcoma, multiple lesions.

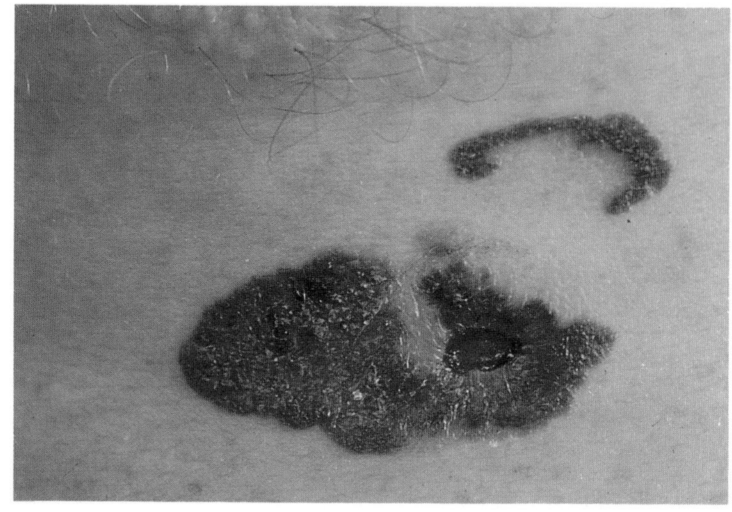

Color Plate 3. Melanoma.

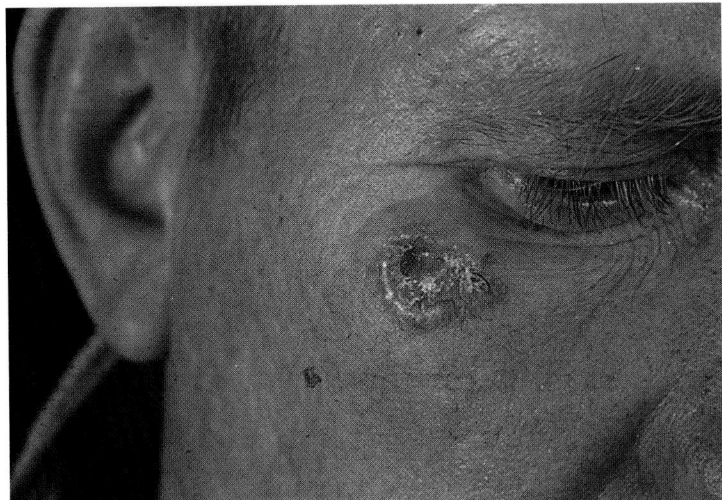

Color Plate 4. Epithelioma, basal cell cancer.

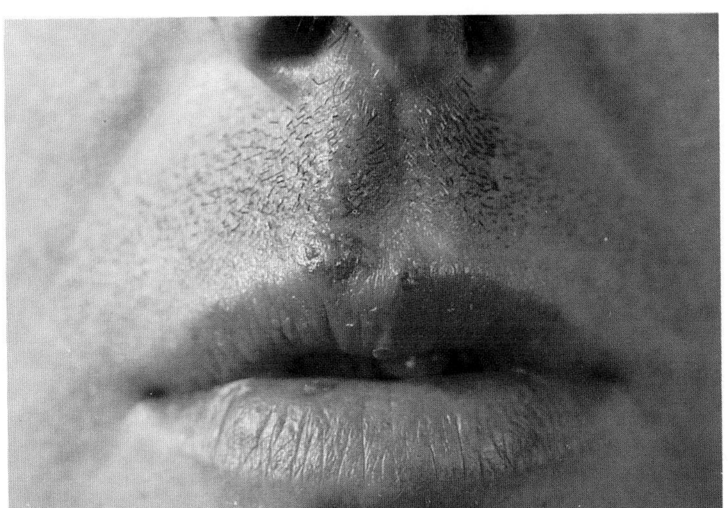

Color Plate 5. Herpes lesion.

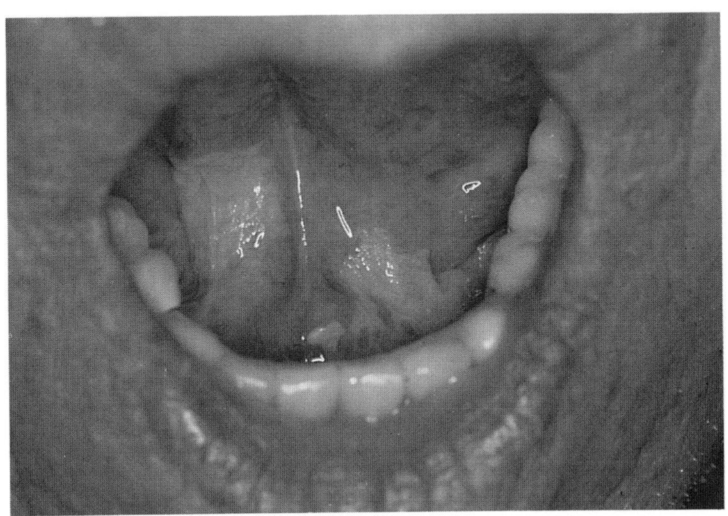

Color Plate 6. Leukoplakia.

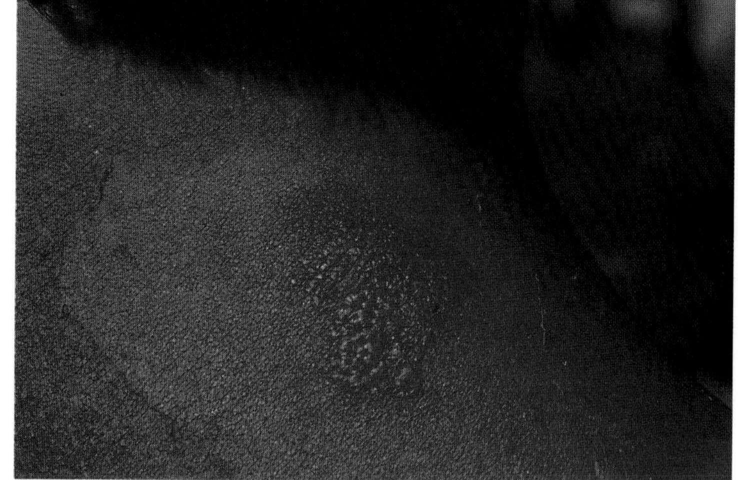

Color Plate 7. Sunburn, second degree.

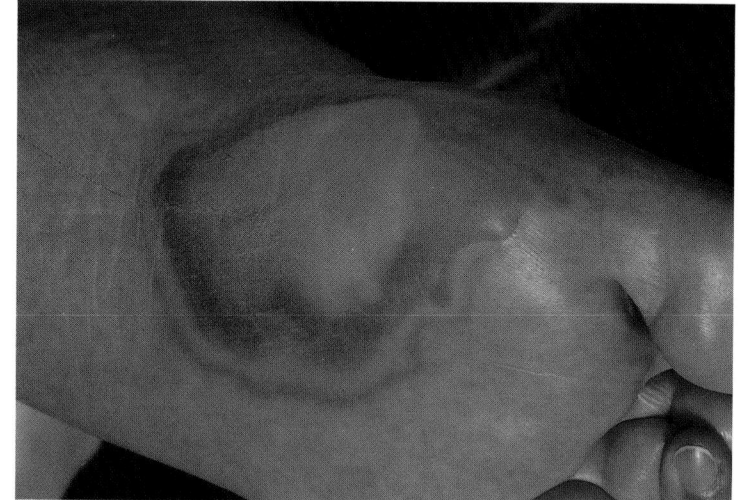

Color Plate 8. Second-degree burn.

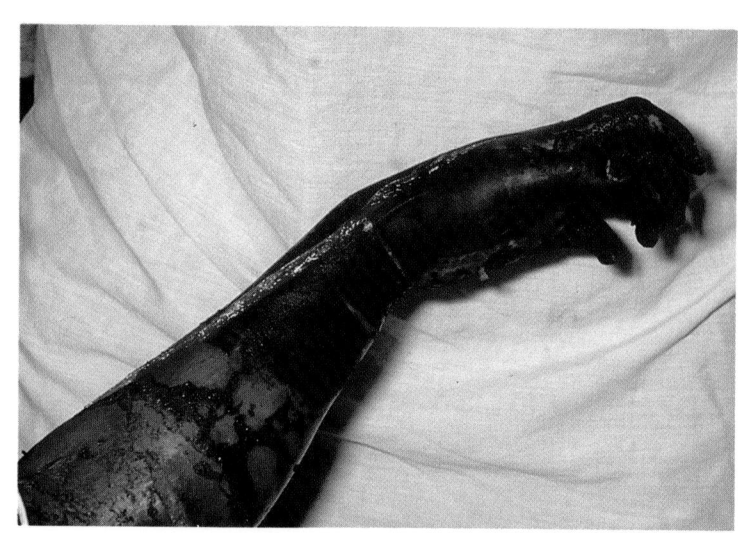

Color Plate 9. Third-degree burn.

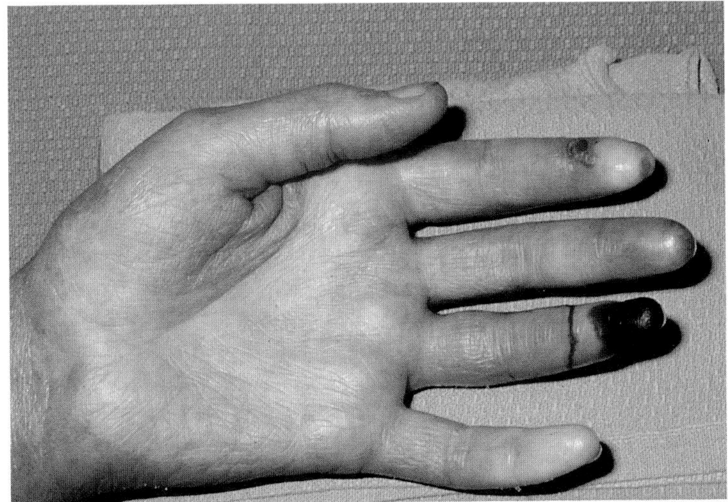

Color Plate 10. Gangrenous finger.

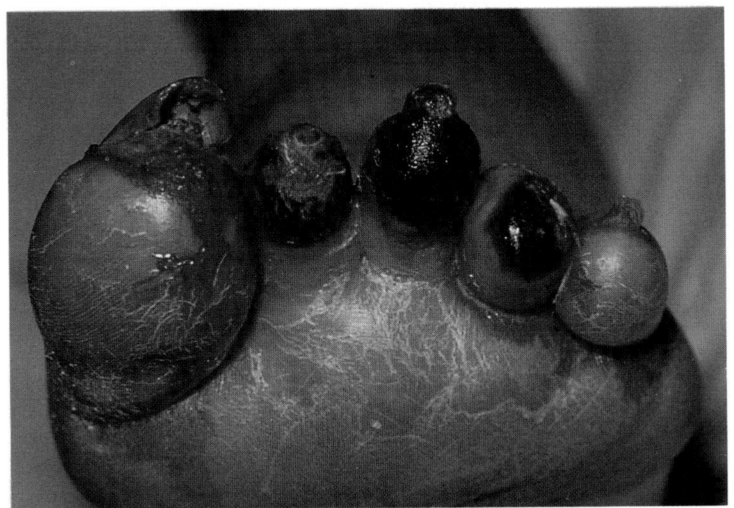

Color Plate 11. Gangrenous toes.

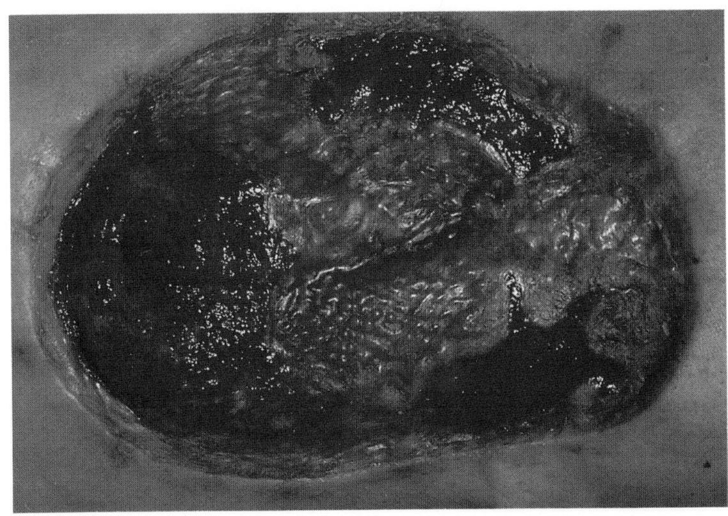

Color Plate 12. Red granulating tissue.

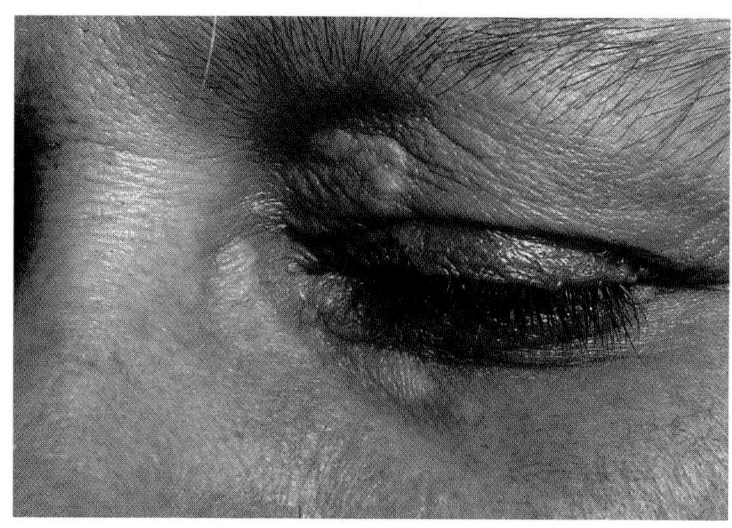

Color Plate 13. Xanthelasma.

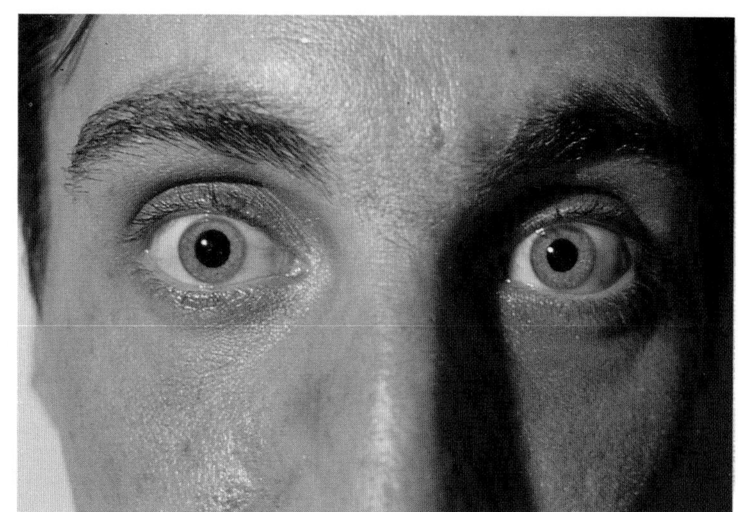

Color Plate 14. Jaundice.

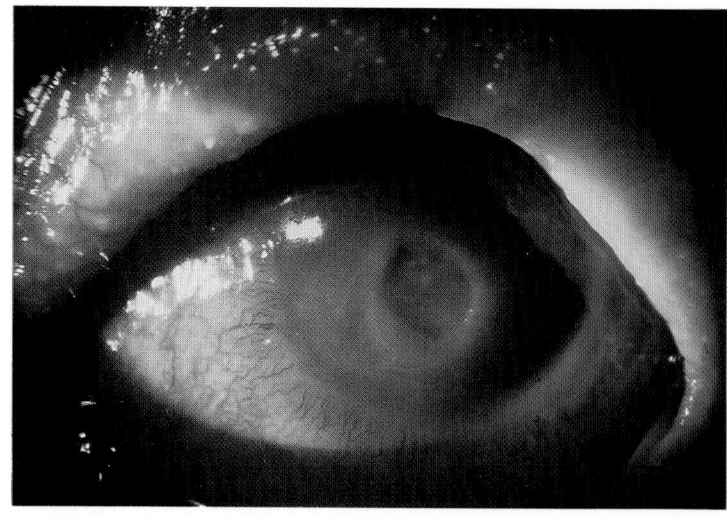

Color Plate 15. Corneal ulcer.

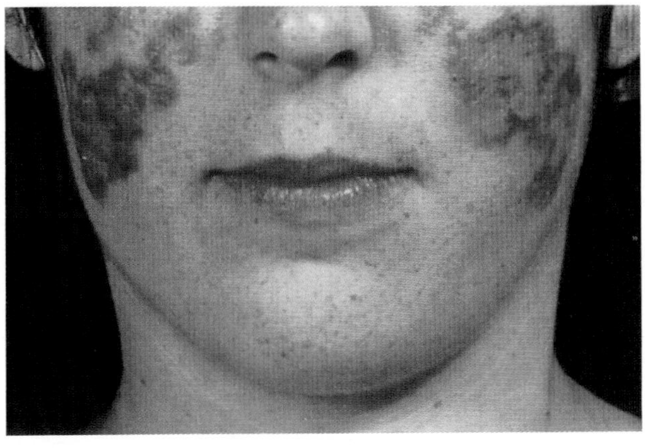

Color Plate 16. Lupus erythematosus.

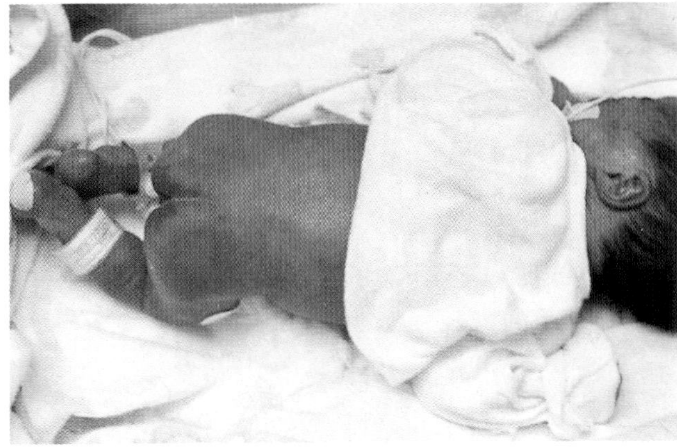

Color Plate 18. Mongolian spots.

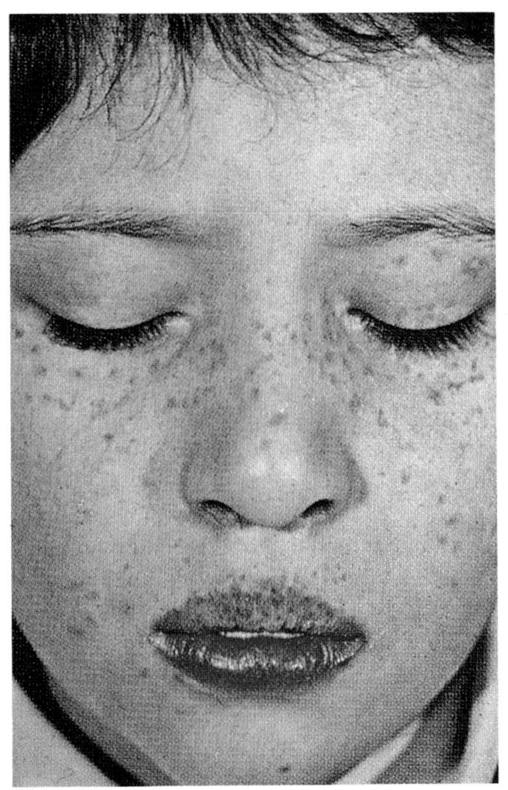

Color Plate 17. Petechiae.

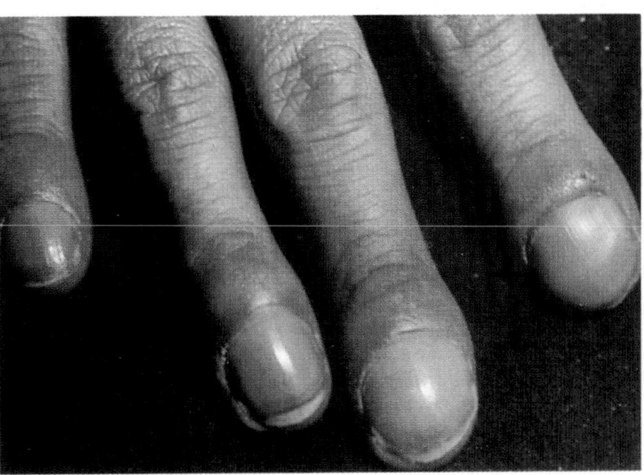

Color Plate 19. Clubbing and cyanosis of the fingernails.

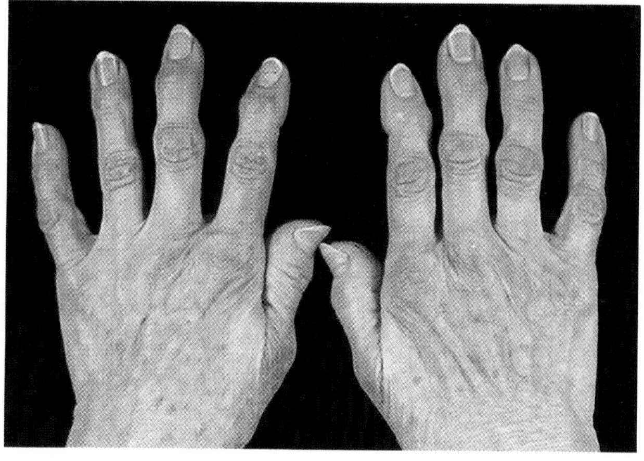

Color Plate 20. Heberden's nodes.

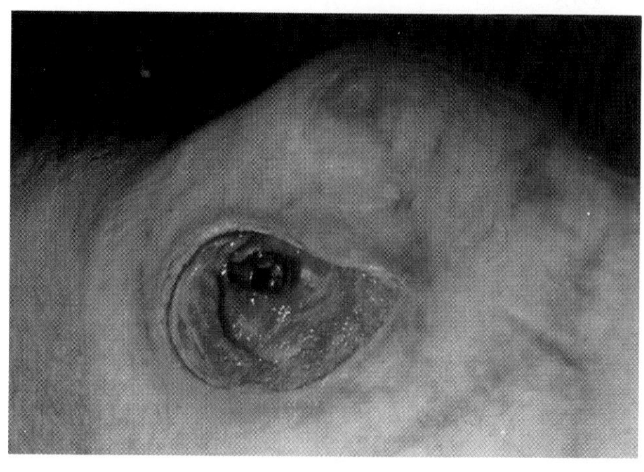

Color Plate 21. Pressure sore and Küntscher nail protruding.

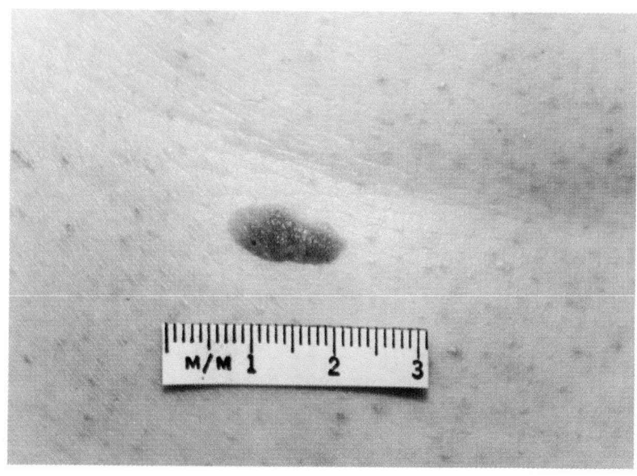

Color Plate 22. Senile keratosis (Courtesy of Ken Timby)

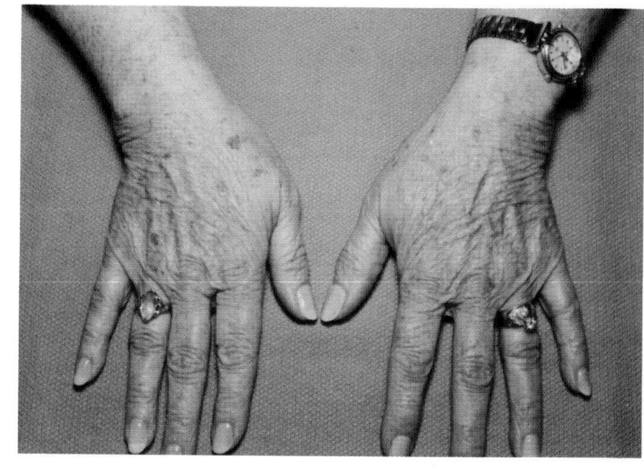

Color Plate 23. Senile lentigines (Courtesy of Ken Timby)

ASSESSMENT FINDINGS

Signs and Symptoms

The client feels local pressure from the abnormal nail growth. Redness, swelling, and pain occur where the nail pierces the adjacent tissue (Fig. 68–15). The corner of the upper nail is embedded in tissue. Purulent drainage and an odor are evident if the tissue is infected. Some people develop compensatory gait and postural changes in an effort to relieve the pain.

Diagnostic Findings

Physical examination is sufficient for diagnosis.

MEDICAL AND SURGICAL MANAGEMENT

Treating the infection, if present, is as important as correcting the nail disorder. Local or systemic antibiotic therapy is sometimes prescribed. Applications of hydrogen peroxide are used to loosen and remove exudate. To promote healing, the foot is soaked in warm water and Epsom salts followed by thorough drying. A wedge of cotton may be inserted to lift the corner of the nail. Clients with diabetes or peripheral vascular disease are referred to a podiatrist. A **podiatrist** is a person trained to care for feet. Older clients and those with chronic diseases are especially susceptible to traumatic complications that can impair circulation and necessitate amputation.

For persistent or recurrent ingrown toenails, surgery is indicated. Various techniques are used to remove the nail border, not the entire nail, and its root. Surgical procedures are done in the physician's office using local anesthesia or a laser to vaporize the abnormal tissue. Chemical cauterization controls bleeding and no sutures are required. The client may need to temporarily wear a slipper or shoe from which the toe has been cut out until the swelling and discomfort subside, but most activities can be resumed immediately.

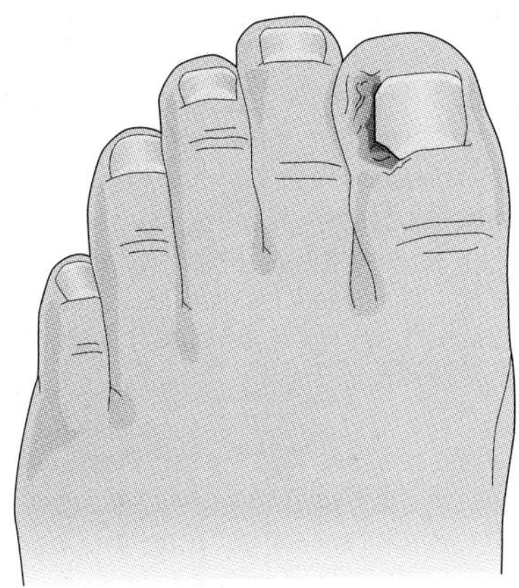

FIGURE 68-15. Infected ingrown toenail.

NURSING MANAGEMENT

Explain how to perform foot-soaking regimens and techniques for relieving the pressure around the ingrown nail. If surgery is performed, instruct the client on how to change the dressing, the frequency of dressing changes, and signs of infection or compromised circulation that must be reported immediately to the surgeon.

Client and Family Teaching

Provide the following information to affected individuals:

- Wear wide shoes and loose socks with sufficient room for the toes.
- Use nail clippers rather than scissors to trim toenails.
- Trim the toenails so that they are kept slightly longer than the end of the toes and do not round off the corners.
- Keep the feet clean and dry.
- Avoid physical activities that involve sudden stops, such as playing basketball, which jams the toes into the front of the shoe.
- Obtain regular foot and nail care from a podiatrist if there is a history of diabetes, diminished vision, or vascular problems.

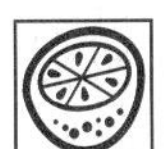

General Nutritional Considerations

Extensive burns are the most severe form of stress that a person can experience. Metabolism may increase as much as 100%; protein catabolism compromises wound healing and immunocompetence.

Weight loss and malnutrition increase morbidity and mortality unless aggressive nutritional support is initiated as soon as possible after fluid resuscitation.

Protein needs increase 2 to 4 times above the normal RDA; calorie needs may be 4000–5000/day.

Clients with adynamic ileus, impaired swallowing related to facial or neck burns, or bleeding related to a stress ulcer require enteral or parenteral nutritional support.

Large supplemental doses of vitamins and minerals, especially vitamin C, the B complex vitamins, iron, and zinc, are prescribed to promote healing and meet increased needs for metabolism.

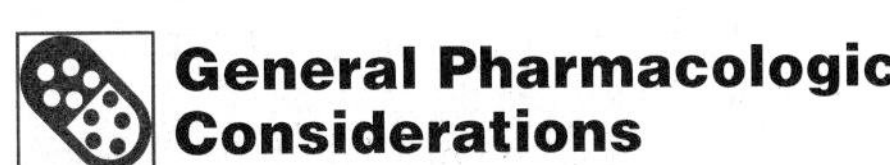

General Pharmacologic Considerations

Ointments, creams, and lotions prescribed for dermatologic disorders must be applied *exactly* as the physician directs (eg, sparingly or thick or thin coat covering the lesion). The client is reminded that unless the drug is applied exactly as ordered, it may not be of therapeutic value, and if an excessive amount is used, the drug is being wasted.

Drugs prescribed for dermatologic conditions may relieve symptoms but do not necessarily cure the disease. Skin disorders may require long-term therapy, often with a periodic change in prescriptions. This can be discouraging to the client. The nurse must encourage persistence in following the physician's instructions.

Individuals using acne preparations containing benzoyl peroxide are warned that this ingredient is an oxidizing agent and may remove the color from clothing, rugs, furniture, and so on. Thorough handwashing after drug use may not remove all the drug, and permanent fabric discoloration may still occur. Users of products containing benzoyl peroxide should wear disposable plastic gloves when applying the drug.

Clients receiving photochemotherapy for severe psoriasis must follow the physician's directions regarding the timing of taking the drug methoxsalen.

Isotretinoin (Accutane) is used in the treatment of severe acne. Dosage is determined by weight. Warn clients not to increase the dosage of the drug if the acne becomes worse or does not respond to treatment.

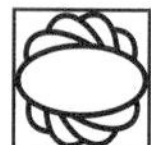

General Gerontologic Considerations

Advise the elderly client with any type of skin lesion to seek medical attention and caution against self-treatment. Early treatment of skin lesions helps prevent infection and complications.

Explain that excessive drying of the skin may result in pruritus and infection. Encourage older clients to apply creams and lotions to the skin, especially during winter or when living in a hot, dry climate. A daily bath is not necessary.

Burns can result in serious complications in the elderly because of diminished renal, cardiac, and respiratory functions associated with the aging process.

Older debilitated clients or clients with dementia must be carefully assessed for scabies and head lice. These individuals may be unable to inform the nurse of these problems or manifest the typical symptoms. Instead they may become confused, more confused, or agitated.

SUMMARY OF KEY CONCEPTS

- Dermatitis is a general term that refers to an inflammation of the skin. Two examples of dermatitis are allergic contact dermatitis and primary irritant dermatitis.
- Acne vulgaris is an inflammatory condition that develops during puberty when the sebaceous glands accumulate sebum, keratin, and bacteria within hair follicles. It is aggravated by cosmetics as well as picking and squeezing blemishes.
- A furuncle is a boil. Furunculosis refers to having multiple furuncles. A carbuncle is a furuncle through which pus drains.
- Psoriasis is characterized by patchy red areas covered with silvery scales. The cells of the epidermis proliferate so fast that the upper layer of cells cannot be shed fast enough to make room for the newly produced cells. The area around the lesion becomes red due to the increased blood supply.
- Several skin disorders involve an infecting agent: scabies is caused by an itch mite; parasitic fungi cause dermatophytoses in skin, scalp, and nails; and shingles is caused by a reactivated virus.
- Skin cancer, which is the leading type of cancer in the United States, is promoted primarily by exposure to UV radiation in sunlight. The intensity of UV radiation is increasing due to thinning of the ozone layer. Fair-skinned individuals are more susceptible because they do not have as many melanin-producing cells within their skin.
- The depth of a burn is determined by its characteristic appearance. The "rule of nines," and special body charts and graphs assist in determining the percentage of the total body surface area that is burned.
- Any one of three burn complications—inhalation injury, hypovolemic shock, and infection—can be life-threatening.
- Wound management following a burn includes exposure to air (open method), occlusive dressings (closed method), and skin grafting.
- Tissue for skin grafting is obtained from the client's own skin, from human cadavers, and from the skin of animals, principally pigs.
- When caring for clients with burns, nurses implement measures that prevent, reduce, or eliminate the following nursing diagnoses: *Risk for Impaired Gas Exchange, Pain, Risk for Infection*, and many other.
- Hair loss is an emotionally disturbing rather than life-threatening condition. Hair loss can be secondary to the side effects of chemotherapy and other conditions. Primary causes for baldness include an autoimmune disorder, known as alopecia areata, and that which is inherited, androgenetic alopecia.
- An infestation with lice is diagnosed by identifying the adult, nymph, and nits. Adult lice are crawling brown insects about the size of sesame seeds; they do not fly or jump. Nymphs look like moving dandruff, but they may appear red after feeding. Nits appear like small yellowish white ovals that are attached to shafts of hair.
- Head lice are destroyed chemically and removed manually with the help of a fine-toothed comb.
- Fungal nail infections thrive under conditions of a warm, dark, damp environment, as the inside of shoes. There has been an increase in fingernail infections due to unsanitary practices in salons where artificial nails are applied.
- Ingrown toenails, known as onychocryptosis, can be prevented or relieved by wearing wide shoes and socks, by leaving the nails slightly longer than the toes, and avoiding physical activities that jam the toes against the ends of the shoes.

CRITICAL THINKING EXERCISES

1. What health teaching is appropriate for keeping the skin, hair, and nails in healthy condition?
2. Name a skin disorder that is more common in younger adults and one that is more common in older adults. Discuss the factors that make these age groups particularly susceptible to the disorder.

Suggested Readings

Bjorgen, S. (1998). Herpes zoster. *American Journal of Nursing, 98*(2), 46–47.

Mantle, F. (1996). More than skin deep...complementary therapies have a valuable role to play in treating skin problems. *Nursing Times, 92*(36), 56–57.

Quillen, T. (1996). Myths and facts about psoriasis. *Nursing, 26*(10), 25.

Skewes, S. M. (1996). Skin care rituals that do more harm than good. *American Journal of Nursing, 96*(10), 33–35.

Venables, J. (1996). Skin graft...dermatology, liaison nursing. *Nursing Times, 92*(7), 42–43.

Wound care handbook. (1996). *Nursing, 26*(8), 42–45.

Additional Resources

American Academy of Dermatology
930 North Meacham Road
P.O. Box 4014
Schaumburg, IL 60168–4014

American Academy for Dermatologic Surgery
1567 Maple Avenue
Evanston, IL 60201
(847) 869–3954

American Academy of Cosmetic Surgery
401 North Michigan Avenue
Chicago, IL 60611–4267
(312) 527–6713

National Psoriasis Foundation
6600 SW 92nd Avenue
Suite 300
Portland, OR
(503) 244–7404

American Hair Loss Council
401 North Michigan Avenue
Chicago, IL 60611–4267
(312) 321–5128

National Pediculosis Association, Inc.
P.O. Box 610189
Newton, MA 02161
(617) 449-NITS
http://www.headlice.org/

Appendix A

Abbreviations

ACE angiotensin converting enzyme
ACTH adrenocorticotropic hormone
AD Alzheimer's disease
ADH antidiuretic hormone
ADL activities of daily living
AICD automatic implantable cardiac defibrillator
AIDS acquired immunodeficiency syndrome
ALS amyotrophic lateral sclerosis
AMA against medical advice
ANS autonomic nervous system
ARDS adult respiratory distress syndrome
AV atrioventricular
BMI body mass index
BMT bone marrow transplant
BPH benign prostatic hypertrophy
BSE breast self-examination
BUN blood urea nitrogen
CABG coronary artery bypass graft
CAD coronary artery disease
CAPD continuous ambulatory peritoneal dialysis
CEA carcinoembryonic antigen
CBC complete blood count
CHF congestive heart failure
CMV cytomegalovirus
CNS central nervous system
CO cardiac output
COPD chronic obstructive pulmonary disease
CPAP continuous positive airway pressure
CPPV continuous positive pressure ventilation
CPR cardiopulmonary resuscitation
CSF cerebrospinal fluid
CTcomputerized tomography (scan)
CVA cerebrovascular accident, costovertebral angle
CVP central venous pressure
D and C dilatation and curettage
DKA diabetic ketoacidosis
DNA desoxyribonucleic acid
DRG diagnostic related group
DVT deep vein thrombosis
ECG (also **EKG**) electrocardiogram
ECT electroconvulsive therapy
EEG electroencephalogram
ERT estrogen replacement therapy
ESR erythrocyte sedimentation rate
ESWL extracorporeal shock wave lithotripsy
FBS fasting blood sugar (glucose)
FSH follicle-stimulating hormone
FVD fluid volume deficit
FVE fluid volume excess
GH growth hormone
GI gastrointestinal
GU genitourinary
GVHD graft versus host disease
GYN gynecology, gynecologic
HCG human chorionic gonadotropin
HCl chemical abbreviation for hydrochloride
HIV human immunodeficiency virus
HMO health maintenance organization
HRT hormone replacement therapy
IABP intraaortic balloon pump
IC interstitial cystitis
ICP intracranial pressure
ICF intermediate care facility
IICP increased intracranial pressure
IOP intraocular pressure
IUD intrauterine device
IV intravenous
IVF in vitro fertilization
IVP intravenous pyelogram
JCAHO Joint Commission on the Accreditation of Healthcare Organizations
kg kilogram
KUB kidneys, ureters, and bladder
KVO keep vein open
laser *l*ight *a*mplification by *s*timulated *e*mission of *r*adiation
LH luteinizing hormone
LOC level of consciousness
LP lumbar puncture
LVEDP left ventricular end diastolic pressure
MAO monoamine oxidase
MAOI monoamine oxidase inhibitors
MCO managed care organization
MI myocardial infarction
mmHg millimeters of mercury
MRI magnetic resonance imaging
NSAIDS nonsteroidal antiinflammatory drugs
NANDA North American Nursing Diagnosis Association
NGU nongonococcal urethritis
NPO nothing by mouth
OTC over-the-counter (nonprescripton) drugs
PAP pulmonary artery pressure
Pap Papinocoloau test
PC potential complication
PCA patient-controlled analgesia
PCNL percutaneous nephrostolithotomy
PCP primary care provider; *Pneumocystis carinii* pneumonia
PCWP pulmonary capillary wedge pressure
PEEP positive end-expiratory pressure
PEG pneumoencephalogram; percutaneous endoscopic gastrostomy
PET positron emission tomography
PICC peripherally inserted central catheter
PID pelvic inflammatory disease
PMI point of maximal impulse
PMS premenstrual syndrome
PNI psychoneuroimmunology
PPO preferred provider organization
PPS prospective payment system
PSA prostatic specific antigen
PTCA percutaneous transluminal coronary angioplasty
PUL percutaneous ultrasonic lithotripsy
PVC premature ventricular contraction
RBCs red blood cells
REM rapid eye movements
RHD rheumatic heart disease
RNA ribonucleic acid
ROM range-of-motion (exercises)
SA sinoatrial
SPECT single-photon emission computed tomography
SSRI selective serotonin reuptake inhibitors
STD sexually transmitted disease
SVT supraventricular tachycardia
TCA tricyclic antidepressants
TNM Tumor, nodes, metastasis
TPN total parenteral nutrition
TSH thyroid-stimulating hormone
TUR transurethral resection
TURP transurethral resection of the prostate
UAP unlicensed assistive personnel
URI upper respiratory tract infection
UTI urinary tract infection
VAD ventricular assist device
WBCs white blood cells
WHO World Health Organization

Appendix **B**

Laboratory Values

Laboratory values vary somewhat in different references. Laboratory technique also may alter values. The nurse is responsible for checking reported laboratory values against the normal ranges provided by the laboratory.

ABBREVIATIONS	
cu	cubic
dL	decaliter (10 L)
dl	deciliter (100 mL)
g	gram
hpf	high powered field
IU	international unit
L	liter
LPF	low-power field
mcg	microgram
mEq	milliequivalent
mg	milligram
mm	millimeter
mmol	one-thousandth of a mole
mU	milliunit
μg	microgram
μL	microliter; also used for cubic millimeter
μm	micrometer
μU	microunit
na	nanogram (one billionth of a gram)
pg	picogram (one trillionth of a gram)
torr	measurement equivalent to 1 mm Hg
U	units

SYMBOLS

> greater than
< less than
/ per
μ micro (one-millionth)

COAGULATION TESTS	VALUES
Bleeding time (Ivy, Duke)	3–10 minutes
Partial thromboplastin time (PTT)	30–45 seconds
Activated partial thromboplastin time (APPT)	16–25 seconds
Prothrombin time (PT)	10–14 seconds or 70%–100% of control. Therapeutic range 2.0–3.0; high therapeutic range 3.0–4.5; over 4.5 critical
International normalized ratio (INR)	

HEMATOLOGY	VALUES
Platelet count	150,000–350,000/μL
Reticulocyte count	0.5%–2.5%
Sedimentation rate (ESR)	
Male	0–15 mm/hr
Female	0–20 mm/hr
Complete blood count (CBC)	
Hematocrit	
Male	40%–54%
Female	37%–47%
Hemoglobin	
Male	13.5–17.5 g/dl
Female	12–16 g/dl
Red cell count	
Male	4.6–5.4 million/μL
Female	3.6–5.0 million/μL
White cell count	5,000–10,000/μL
Neutrophils	60%–70% (3000–7000/μL)
Eosinophils	1%–4% (50–400/μL)
Basophils	0.5%–1% (23–100/μL)
Lymphocytes	20%–40% (1000–4000/μL)
Monocytes	2%–6% (100–600/μL)
Erythrocyte Indices	
Mean corpuscular volume (MCV)	87–103 μm^3
Mean corpuscular hemoglobin (MCH)	26–34 pg/cell
Mean corpuscular hemoglobin concentration (MCHC)	31%–37%

BLOOD VOLUME	
Plasma volume	30–45 mL/kg
Red cell volume	20–35 mL/kg (higher in men than in women)
Total blood volume	55–80 mL/kg

BLOOD CHEMISTRIES	VALUES
Alanine aminotransferase (ALT) (formerly SGPT)	7–24 U/L
Ammonia	14–45 μg/dl
Amylase	50–150 μ/L; 25–130 IU/L by enzymatic method
Aspartate aminotransferase (AST) (formerly SGOT)	6–20 μ/L
Bilirubin, total direct (conjugated)	0.2–1.0 mg/dl 0.0–0.2 mg/dl

BLOOD, CHEMISTRIES (Cont.)	VALUES
Bilirubin, indirect (unconjugated)	0.2–0.8 mg/dl
Anion gap (or R factor)	±12 mEq/L
Blood gases	
pH	7.35–7.45
$PaCO_2$	35–45 torr
$PvCO_2$	41–45 torr
SO_2	95% or higher arterial blood 70%–75% mixed venous blood
PaO_2	80 torr or greater
PvO_2	30–40 torr
Blood urea nitrogen (BUN)	7–18 mg/dl
Calcium (total)	8.8–10 mg/dl
Calcium (ionized)	4.4–5.4 mg/dl
Carbon dioxide (CO_2 content)	23–30 mmol/L
Carcinoembryonic antigen (CEA)	up to 2.5 ng/mL
Cephalin flocculation	negative to 1+
Chloride	98–106 mmol/L
Cholesterol	desirable range: 140–200 mg/dl
Coagulant factor assay	
Factor VIII	55%–145% of normal
Factor IX	60%–140% of normal
Creatine kinase (CK)	20–185 U/L
CK isoenzymes	
MM: 100%	
MB: 0%	
BB: 0%	
Creatinine	0.6–1.2 mg/dl
Ferritin	15–300 ng/mL
Folic acid (Folate)	3–17 ng/mL
Formiminoglutamic (FIGLU) Acid excretion test	<35 mg/day
Glucose (fasting, serum)	70–110 mg/dl
Glucose (postprandial)	<120 mg/dl
High-density lipoprotein (HDL)	35–85 mg/dl
Insulin	6–24 μU/mL
Ketone bodies	negative
Lactic acid dehydrogenase (LD)	95–200 mU/mL (results vary)
LD isoenzymes	
LD-1	14%–26%
LD-2	29%–39%
LD-3	20%–26%
LD-4	8%–16%
LD-5	6%–16%
Lipase	4–24 U/L
Low-density lipoproteins (LDL)	desirable: <130 mg/dl
Magnesium	1.3–2.1 mEq/L
Phosphatase, acid	0.15–0.65 BLB (Bersey, Lowry, Block) units
Phosphatase, alkaline	20–70 U/L
Phosphate, inorganic phosphorus	2.7–4.5 mg/dl
Potassium	3.5–5.0 mEq/L
Proteins, total	6.0–8.0 g/dl
Albumin	3.8–5.0 g/dl
Globulin	2.3–3.5 g/dl
Prostate-specific antigen (PSA)	0–4.0 ng/mL
Sodium	135–148 mmol/L
T_3 (free triiodothyronine)	230–660 pg/dL
T_4 (free thyroxine)	0.8–2.4 ng/dL

BLOOD, CHEMISTRIES (Cont.)	VALUES
Triglycerides	desirable: 35–160 mg/mL
Uric acid	3.5–7.2 mg/dL
Vitamin B_{12}	160–1300 pg/mL
Vitamin B_{12} (unsaturated binding capacity)	1000–2000 pg/mL

URINE	VALUES
Acetoacetic acid	negative
Acetone	negative
Albumin (quantitative)	negative
Aldosterone (24-hr specimen)	5–22 μg/24 hr
Bence-Jones protein	negative
Casts	rare/hpf
Color	pale yellow to dark amber
Creatinine clearance	
Male	<150 mg/24 hr
Female	<250 mg/24 hr
Glucose	negative to trace
17-hydroxycorticosteroid (as 17-ketogenic steroids or 17 KGS)	male: 3–10 mg/24 hr female: 2–6 mg/24 hr
17-ketosteroids	male: 8–20 mg/24 hr female: 6–15 mg/24 hr
Microscopic examination	RBC—0–1/hpf WBC—0–4/hpf casts—rare/hpf
pH	4.6–8.0
Protein	0–trace
Protein (24 hr)	10–140 mg/L in 24 hr
Specific gravity	1.003–1.035
Turbidity	usually clear (cloudiness not always abnormal)
Volume	600–1,600 mL/24 hr

CEREBROSPINAL FLUID	VALUES
Cell count	0–5 WBC/μL
Chloride	118–132 mEq/L
Color	clear, colorless
Glucose	40–70 mg/dl
Protein	15–45 mg/dl

SEROLOGY	VALUES
Antistreptolysin-O titer (ASLO)	<160 Todd units
Cold agglutins	<1:16
C-reactive protein (CRP)	<0.8 mg/dl
Fluorescent treponemal antibodies (FTA)	negative
Hepatitis-associated antigen (HAA or HBAg)	negative
Heterophile antibodies	<1:56
VDRL	nonreactive

DRUGS	VALUES
Ethanol	0.3%–0.4% marked intoxication 0.4%–0.5% alcoholic stupor >0.5% coma
Salicylates	<100 μg/mL therapeutic range >250 μg/dl toxic range
Digitoxin	14–26 ng/mL therapeutic range >35 ng/mL toxic range
Digoxin	0.5–2.0 ng/mL therapeutic range >2.5 ng/mL toxic range
Lidocaine	1.5–6.0 μg/mL therapeutic range >6 μg/mL toxic range

TESTS FOR AIDS	VALUES
ELISA (Enzyme-linked immunosorbent assay)	positive if antibodies to HIV present
Western blot (WB)	positive if antibodies to HIV present
P24 antigen	negative for HIV
PCR (polymerase chain reaction)	negative for HIV
Murex SUDS (single use diagnostic system) HIV-1 assay	negative (blue result is positive)
T-cell count	644–2201 cells/μL
T4 cells	493–1191 cells/μL
T8 cells	182–785 cells/μL
T4/T8 ratio	>1.0

Glossary

A

abduction. movement of the arms and legs away from the midline
abscess. localized collection of pus
acalculia. inability to do simple arithmetic
acceptance. according to Kübler-Ross, the last stage of the death and dying process
accommodation. adjustment of the lens of the eye to focus at various distances
acetylcholine. a neurohormone concerned with the transmission of nerve impulses
achlorhydria. absence of hydrochloric acid
acid. substance that releases hydrogen into fluid
acidosis. disturbance in the acid–base balance with an accumulation of acid
acquired immunodeficiency syndrome (AIDS). end stage of infection with human immunodeficiency virus (HIV)
acute retroviral syndrome. a cluster of signs and symptoms suggestive of infection with human immunodeficiency virus (HIV)
adduction. movement of the arms and legs toward the midline
adenohypophysis. the anterior lobe of the pituitary gland
adenoids. lymphoid tissue in the nasopharynx
adhesions. fibrinous tissue holding internal structures rigidly in place
administrative law. the branch of public law that creates governmental agencies with the power to develop rules and regulations.
adrenergic drugs. drugs that act like or mimic the action of the sympathetic nervous system
adrenocorticotropic hormone (ACTH). stimulates the adrenal cortex to secrete cortisol and other steroids
advocacy. ensuring that the client's rights are protected (see client advocate)
aerobic. needing oxygen to live
affect. external expression of the emotional state
affective learner. an individual who learns better when provided with information that appeals to his or her values or feelings
affective touch. touch that is used to demonstrate affection or concern
afferent. to or toward
afterload. resistive pressure against which the heart ejects blood
ageism. discrimination that characterizes older adults in a negative or stereotypical manner
agnosia. the inability to recognize familiar objects or other sensory stimuli
agranulocytes. white blood cells without visible granules
agranulocytosis. a decrease in the number of granulocytes
agraphia. loss of the ability to write words
albumin. protein found in blood and body tissues
albuminuria. presence of albumin in the urine
alcoholism. a disorder characterized by chronic alcohol dependence
aldosterone. a mineralcorticoid hormone secreted by the adrenal cortex
alexia. inability to understand written language
alkalosis. disturbance in acid–base balance with an accumulation of base
allergens. substances that cause an allergic reaction
allograft. a graft of tissue harvested from another person
alopecia. abnormal loss of hair; baldness
alpha-adrenergic receptors. structures in sympathetic neurons in which catecholamines produce excitatory effects
alpha-fetoprotein. a protein produced by the gastrointestinal tract and fetal liver; is elevated in liver cancer
alveolus. (pl., alveoli) structure in the lungs for gas diffusion
Alzheimer's disease. degenerative brain disease characterized by progressive mental deterioration
amenorrhea. absence of menses
anabolism. building up of body tissue; opposite of catabolism (adj., anabolic)
anaerobe. a microorganism that can survive and grow in the absence of oxygen (adj., anaerobic)
analgesic. a drug that relieves pain
analysis. determining significance of data
anaphylaxis. life-threatening allergic reaction
anastomosis. a joining, communication, or union (adj., anastomotic)
anasarca. generalized, massive edema
anecdotal note or record. an unofficial written report about an unusual event
anemia. a decrease in the number of red blood cells and a lower than normal hemoglobin (adj., anemic)
anesthesia. absence of sensation with or without the loss of consciousness
aneurysm. abnormal dilatation of a blood vessel caused by a defect or weakness in the vessel wall
anger. according to Kübler-Ross, the second stage of the dying process
angina pectoris. chest pain caused by myocardial ischemia
angioedema edema. acute swelling of the skin and mucous membranes
angiotensin. substance that increases blood pressure through vasoconstriction and stimulates release of aldosterone
angiotensin-converting enzyme (ACE) inhibitors. antihypertensive drugs that interrupt the renin-angiotensin-aldosterone mechanism
anion. negative ion
anion gap. the difference between sodium and potassium cation concentrations and chloride and bicarbonate anions in extracellular fluid
ankylosis. immobility of a joint

annuloplasty. repair of a cardiac valve
anorectal. pertaining to the anus and rectum
anorexia. loss of appetite (adj., anorectic)
anorexia nervosa. an eating disorder characterized by self-starvation
anoxia. lack of oxygen (adj., anoxic)
antiarrhythmics. class of drugs used to control cardiac arrhythmias
antibody. protein substance manufactured in response to a specific antigen
anticipatory grieving. dealing with a loss before it actually occurs
anticoagulant. a drug that interferes with blood-clotting
antidiuretic hormone. posterior pituitary hormone that promotes reabsorption of water in the nephrons
antiemetic. a drug used to treat or prevent nausea
antigen. a substance that induces the manufacture of antibodies
antihistamine. a drug that appears to compete with histamine receptor sites and is used in the treatment of allergy and motion sickness
anti-infective. against infection; an agent used to treat an infection
antimicrobial. an agent that destroys or stops the multiplication of microorganisms
antineoplastic. a drug used in the treatment of neoplasms, more specifically malignant diseases
antioxidants. substances that slow down the oxidation process of other substances
antipyretic. a drug that lowers an elevated body temperature
antiseptic. an agent that slows the multiplication of microorganisms
anuria. suppression of urine production
anxiety. a vague uneasy feeling
anxiety disorders. a group of psychobiologic illnesses that result from activation of the sympathetic division of the autonomic nervous system
aphasia. inability to use or understand spoken language
aphonia. loss of voice
aplasia. lack of development of tissue or an organ
apraxia. inability to accomplish activities of daily living (ADL), such as grooming, toileting, and eating, despite intact motor function
arrhythmia. abnormal heart rate or rhythm (syn., dysrhythmia)
arteriography. radiography of an artery after illumination with radiopaque dye
arteriole. distal end of an artery
arteriosclerosis. loss of arterial elasticity
artery. blood vessel that transports oxygenated blood
arthralgia. pain in a joint
arthritis. inflammation of the joints
arthrocentesis. aspiration of fluid from the joint space
arthrodesis. fusion of joint surfaces
artificially acquired active immunity. immunity that results from the administration of a killed or weakened microorganism or toxoid
ascites. fluid in the abdomen
assessment. systematic collection of data
asthma. a chronic obstructive lung disorder characterized by paroxysms of dyspnea, wheezing, and coughing, with production of thick, tenacious sputum
astigmatism. unequal curvature of the cornea
asymptomatic. without symptoms
asystole. without contraction
ataxia. motor incoordination; unsteady gait
atelectasis. partial or total collapse of lung tissue; airless area of lung tissue
atheroma. fatty plaque
atherosclerosis. fatty plaque within the intima layer of the artery
atrial fibrillation. quivering of the atria
atriovenous fistula. surgical anastomosis (connection) of an artery and vein
atriovenous graft. vascular access in which a tube of synthetic material connects a vein and artery
atrophy. decrease in size of an organ or tissue
attenuate. weaken
audiometry. measurement of hearing acuity
aura. a subjective sensation that precedes an epileptic seizure
auscultation. assess by listening
autograft. transplanted cells or tissue obtained from oneself
autoimmune disease. disorders in which the immune system attacks normal body cells
autoinoculation. self-transmitted to another area of the body
autologous. self-donated
automaticity. the ability of the heart to initiate its own electrical stimulus
automatism. behavior not under conscious control that occurs during a seizure
autonomic dysreflexia. exaggerated sympathetic nervous system response seen after spinal cord injury above the T6 level
autonomy. the right of clients to participate in and decide on questions concerning their health; personal self-determination. According to Erikson, autonomy is a developmental task of early childhood and refers to independence.
autophagocytosis. self-digestion of cells
autoregulation. the brain's ability to provide sufficient arterial blood flow despite rising intracranial pressure
avitaminosis. a deficiency of all vitamins
axon. a nerve process that conducts impulses away from the neuronal cell body
azotemia. an excess accumulation of nitrogen, creatinine, and uric acid in the blood

B

bacteremia. bacteria in the bloodstream
bacteria. single-celled microorganisms
bactericidal. an agent that kills bacteria
bacteriostatic. an agent that slows the duplication of bacteria
barbiturates. a group of drugs used as sedatives, hypnotics, and anesthetic agents; have addiction potential
bargaining. according to Kübler-Ross, the third stage of the dying process
base. substances that bind with hydrogen
Battle's sign. bruising of the mastoid process behind the ear
behavioral therapy. therapeutic techniques to promote or extinguish learned responses
benign. nonmalignant; not serious
benign prostatic hyperplasia. condition in which the prostate gland contains more than the usual number of normal cells
beta-adrenergic receptors. sites in sympathetic neurons that cause an increase in heart rate and constriction of bronchioles

bifurcate. to branch, having two branches
bigeminy. a cardiac arrhythmia characterized by repeated instances of premature ventricular contraction following each normal beat
biliary. pertaining to bile, the liver, and the gallbladder
binge eating disorder. an eating disorder characterized by the inability to control overeating
biofeedback. a technique for personally controlling physiologic functions such as heart rate, blood pressure, or brain waves
biologic variation. physical characteristics such as skin color and hair texture that vary according to race
biosynthesis. manufacture of substances by living organisms
biotherapy. the use of biologic response modifiers (BRMs) to stimulate the body's natural immune system to restrict and destroy cancer cells (syn., immunotherapy)
bipolar disorder. mood disorder characterized by episodes of depression and mania
blackouts. periods of amnesia experienced by alcoholics while drinking
blanch. to become pale
bleb. a blister filled with fluid
blindness. a legal term indicating the person has < 20/200 vision with best correction
blood products. components extracted from blood
board of nursing. state agency that administrates the state's nurse practice act
body mass index. a mathematical computation based on height and weight
bone scan. examination using a radioactive isotope
bowel resection. surgical removal of a portion of intestine
brachial plexus. a group of nerves in the lower part of the neck and axilla
bradyarrhythmia. slow abnormal heart rhythm
bradycardia. heart rate <60 beats per minute
bradykinesia. slow movement
brain mapping. a technique for comparing a client's brain activity patterns from an electroencephalogram or other electronic image with a computerized data base of electrophysiologic abnormalities
breast abscess. localized collection of pus in breast tissue
breast reconstruction. cosmetic surgery to give the appearance and feel of a natural breast after a mastectomy
breast self-examination. technique for self-assessing breast tissue for signs of cancer (compare to clinical breast examination)
bronchiole. terminal end of a bronchus
bronchus. (pl., bronchi) large airway in the lung
Brudzinski's sign. a neurologic sign in which flexion of the neck produces flexion of the knees and hips
bruit. abnormal purring sound in an artery
bulimarexia. an eating disorder characterized by both food restriction and purging
bulimia nervosa. an eating disorder characterized by food binges (rapid consumption of a large number of calories) followed by behaviors intended to prevent weight gain
bulla. (pl., bullae) a bleb filled with fluid and sometimes air when located in the lung
bursitis. inflammation of the bursa

C

cachexia. a state of wasting, emaciation (adj., cachectic)
calcification. process of hardening by depositing calcium salts
calcium channel blockers. drugs that block the influx of calcium through the cell membrane
calciuria. excessive calcium in the urine
calculus. (pl., calculi) stone
callus. fibrous tissue formed at ends of fractured bone; thickened layer of skin
cancellous bone. bone that is spongy
cancer. any of the various neoplastic diseases characterized by the overgrowth and metastasis of abnormal cells; fatal if untreated
cannula. a hollow tube
canthus. the angle formed by the upper and lower eyelids; "corner of the eye"
capillary. microscopic blood vessel connecting arterioles with venules
capitation. system of third-party reimbursement in which insurer pays the provider a set fee to provide all the necessary medical care required by the plan members
carbon dioxide. a colorless gas composed of carbon and oxygen; chemical symbol CO_2
carbuncle. skin infection composed of a cluster of boils
carcinoembryonic antigen (CEA). protein associated with intestinal tumors
carcinogens. agents capable of causing cancer (adj., carcinogenic)
carcinoma. a malignant tumor (syn., cancer)
carcinoma in situ. nonmetastasized cancer; still at its site of origin
cardiac arrest. sudden cessation of heart contraction
cardiac glycosides. drugs in the digitalis family
cardiac index. the cardiac output in relation to a person's body size
cardiac output. the volume of blood pumped per minute from the left ventricle
cardiac tamponade. constriction of the heart by fluid in the pericardial space
cardiogenic shock. shock caused by failure of the heart to act as an efficient pump
cardiomyopathy. general diagnostic term for conditions of diseased heart muscle
cardiopulmonary resuscitation (CPR). emergency measures taken to restore heart–lung function
cardiotonics. drugs that strengthen ventricular contraction
cardioversion. stopping the heart electrically to reestablish conduction by the sinoatrial (SA) node
carditis. inflammation of the layers of the heart
carpopedal spasm. spasm of the hands and feet
cartilage. fibrous connective tissue
case management. a system for controlling costs and quality by careful oversight and coordination of services
case method. a system for delivering nursing care in which one nurse is assigned to one client
casts. deposits of minerals that break loose from the walls of the renal tubules and appear in the urine
catabolism. breaking down of body tissue; opposite of anabolism (adj., catabolic)
catalyst. a substance capable of producing change in other substances without being changed itself
cataract. opacity of the lens in the eye causing impaired vision or blindness
catecholamines. a group of sympathomimetic neurochemicals (eg, norepinephrine, dopamine, and epinephrine)
catheterization. insertion of a catheter
cations. positively charged ions
-cele. a word ending indicating a swelling

cell-mediated response. immune response negotiated by T cells
centenarian. a person 100 years old or older
central venous pressure (CVP). pressure of fluid in the right atrium
cephalgia. headache
cerebellum. posterior section of the brain responsible for coordinating movement
cerebrovascular accident (CVA). bleeding in or loss of blood supply to part of the brain; lay term, "stroke"
cerebrum. the main portion of the brain
cervicitis. inflammation of the uterine cervix
chancre. painless ulcer
chancroid. a sexually transmitted disease, caused by *Haemophilus ducreyi bacillus*
Charcot's joints. a neuropathic joint disease
chemical dependence. the need to take a drug to avoid withdrawal
chemically impaired. decreased psychological or physiologic function resulting from drug use
chemotherapy. therapy using chemicals or drugs
Cheyne-Stokes respiration. shallow, rapid breathing that builds in intensity and depth and then decreases, followed by a period of apnea
chief complaint. current health problem
chlamydia. a sexually transmitted disease caused by *Chlamydia trachomatis*
cholecystitis. inflammation of the gallbladder
cholelithiasis. gallstones
cholesterol. a sterol contained in animal tissues
cholinergic blocking agent. a drug that inhibits the action of acetylcholine (eg, atropine)
chorea. involuntary muscle twitching
chronic disease. a disease that extends over a long period
chronic obstructive pulmonary disease. a broad, nonspecific term describing a group of pulmonary disorders with symptoms of chronic cough and expectoration, dyspnea, and an impaired expiratory airflow
chronotropic. action affecting heart rate
Chvostek's sign. spasm of the muscles innervated by the facial nerve when the nerve is tapped at a point anterior to the earlobe; indicates hypocalcemia
chyme. liquid mass of partly digested food
ciliated. hairlike projections that produce motion
circumoral paresthesia. numbness around the mouth
cirrhosis a degenerative disorder of the liver characterized by generalized cellular damage
cisternal puncture. insertion of a needle between the cervical vertebrae into the cisterna at the base of the brain to withdraw cerebrospinal fluid (CSF)
civil law. a source of law also called common law or private law
client. an active partner in nursing care
client advocate. one who protects the client's rights and helps the client obtain the best possible care
client data base. all subjective and objective data accumulated during initial assessment of a client
clinical breast examination. breast examination performed by a clinician
clonus. alternate contraction and relaxation of muscles that results in jerking movements and excessive thrashing of the arms and legs (adj., clonic)
closed question. a question that elicits a yes or no answer (see open-ended question)
coagulopathy. disorder of blood clotting mechanisms
code of ethics. written statements describing ideal behavior
cognitive learner. one who learns best by listening or reading
cognitive therapy. a type of psychotherapy that helps clients alter their irrational thinking, correct their faulty belief systems, and replace negative self-statements with positive ones
colectomy. excision of part or all of the colon
colic. spasm that causes pain; may be intestinal, uterine, renal, or biliary
collaborative problems. client complications that nurses manage with both nurse- and physician-prescribed interventions
collagen. fibrous protein found in connective tissue
collateral circulation. circulation in smaller blood vessels when a large vessel is occluded
colloid. a mixture of suspended particles that do not dissolve but remain distributed throughout the solvent
colostomy. an opening in the colon for the purpose of diverting fecal elimination
coma. a deep, stuporous, unresponsive state
comedo. (pl. comedones) a collection of sebum, keratin, and bacteria that dilates a hair follicle.
comfort zone. the area of personal space that when intruded does not create anxiety
commensals. microorganisms that live in a host and do not cause disease
commissure. where two tissue structures are joined together
commissurotomy. to incise or digitally disrupt the thickened cardiac valve leaflets
common law. a source of law also called civil law or private law
community-acquired infections. infections acquired outside of health care facilities (compare with nosocomial infections)
compensation. the body's ability to counterbalance deficiencies in structure or function
complete heart block. situation occurring when impulses initiated by the sinoatrial (SA) node do not depolarize the ventricles
compulsive overeating. eating when not hungry or regardless of feeling full
concussion. diffuse and microscopic injury to the brain
conductivity. the ability to transmit an electrical impulse
condyloma. a sexually transmitted disease caused by the human papillomavirus
congenital. present at birth
congestive heart failure (CHF). the accumulation of blood and fluid within organs and tissues due to impaired circulation
conization. removal of a cone-shaped piece of tissue
conjunctivitis. inflammation of the conjunctiva of the eye
connective tissue. fibrous tissue that supports and connects internal organs and bones
conscious sedation. the state of being free of pain, fear, and anxiety, and able to tolerate unpleasant procedures while maintaining independent cardiorespiratory function and the ability to respond to verbal commands and tactile stimulation
constitutional law. a type of public law concerned with federal, state, and local constitutions
contractility. the heart's ability to stretch as a single unit and recoil
contracture. shortening of muscles that results in a flexion deformity of the part and renders it resistant to movement
contrast medium. radiopaque dye
contrecoup injury. traumatic brain injury caused by the brain ricocheting from anterior to posterior areas of the skull

contusion. an injury in which the skin is not broken; a bruise
convulsion. involuntary muscle relaxation and contraction
coping mechanisms. unconscious tactics to protect the self from feeling inadequate or threatened
cor pulmonale. cardiac changes due to chronic lung disease
cordotomy. surgical interruption of sensory pathways in the spinal cord
coronary artery bypass graft (CABG). surgical technique for revascularizing the myocardium
coronary insufficiency. severe cardiac pain without necrosis
coronary thrombosis. occlusion of a coronary artery by a clot
cortex. outer portion of an organ
corticosteroid. any of the steroids manufactured by the cortex of the adrenal gland
coryza. a head cold with nasal congestion
countertraction. the force exerted opposite to the pull of mechanical traction
coup injury. brain injury that occurs when the head is struck directly
Credé's maneuver. placement of the hands on the abdomen and pressing firmly toward the lower abdomen
crepitation. a crackling or grating sensation or sound
criminal law. a type of public law concerned with the welfare and safety of the public
critical pathways. multidisciplinary plan of care that sequences care and expected outcomes over a specified time frame
critical thinking. an analytical approach to problem-solving that focuses on systematically gathering and analyzing information
cross-tolerance. reduced effect for analgesic-sedative-hypnotic drugs secondary to dependence on alcohol and other central nervous system depressant drugs
cryosurgery. use of extreme cold to produce cell destruction
cryptorchidism. failure of the testis(es) to descend into the scrotum
crystalloid. fluid containing dissolved substances
crystalluria. crystals in the urine
Cullen's sign. bluish gray discoloration to the skin about the umbilicus indicating bleeding of the pancreas
culture. the values, beliefs, and practices of a particular group; cultivation of bacterial growth
curettage. scraping
cutaneous. pertaining to the skin
cyanosis. a blue discoloration to the skin, nail beds, or mucous membranes caused by oxygen deficiency
cyclothymia. a mild mood disorder characterized by cycling between periods of depression and euphoria
cyst. a sac or capsule that contains fluid or semisolid material
cystitis. inflammation of the bladder
cystocele. protrusion of the bladder into the vagina
cystoscopy. visual examination of the inside of the bladder by use of a cystoscope
cystostomy. surgical opening into the bladder
cytokine. a substance that suppresses viral activity

D

data base. comprehensive collection of subjective and objective information
debridement. removal of foreign material or dead tissue from a wound
decalcification. loss of calcium from bone
decerebrate posturing. rigid extension of the arms and legs of a comatose client
decibel. measurement of the intensity of sound
decompression. removal of pressure in a body compartment
decorticate posturing. flexion of the arms and legs of a comatose client
defecation. act of eliminating stool
defibrillation. to stop fibrillation of the heart through use of electric current or drugs
defibrillator. a machine that delivers a specific amount of electric current to the heart; used to halt fibrillation of the heart
dehiscence. separation of wound edges without protrusion of organs
dehydration. excessive loss of water
delirium. a state of disorientation and confusion caused by interference with the metabolic processes of the brain
delusion. false belief that is maintained despite evidence to the contrary
dementia. loss of intellectual abilities
demyelinating disease. neurologic disorder characterized by destruction and degeneration of myelin (eg, multiple sclerosis)
dendrites. threadlike projections or fibers from neurons that conduct neural impulses to the cell body
deontology. an ethical doctrine holding that an act is either right or wrong independent of the consequences (compare with utilitarianism)
depolarization. transfer of positive ions to the inside of the cell membrane
depot injections. intramuscular injections of drugs in an oil suspension that are gradually absorbed over 2 to 4 weeks
depression. the fourth stage of the dying process, according to Kübler-Ross
depression, major. a disorder of mood characterized by profound sadness and a feeling of hopelessness
depression, reactive. a sad mood that occurs in reaction to situational events
dermabrasion. removing surface layers of scarred skin with sandpaper, a rotating wire brush, chemicals (chemical face peeling), or a diamond wheel
dermatitis. inflammation of the skin
dermatome. skin area supplied by a specific spinal nerve root; instrument used to remove skin for grafting
dermatophytes. parasitic fungi that invade the skin, scalp, and nails (syn., tinea)
dermis. the layer of skin that lies below the epidermis
desensitization. subcutaneous administration of gradually increasing doses of an antigen; a type of behavioral therapy that involves providing emotional support to a person with irrational fears while gradually exposing him or her to whatever it is that provokes anxiety
despair. a negative characteristic, according to Erikson, acquired during the developmental stage of older adulthood
detached retina. separation of the sensory layer from the pigmented layer of the retina
detoxification. the process of stabilizing a client with a sedative drug while alcohol or other substances are metabolized
development. the evolution of one's ability to perform physical, intellectual, social, and psychological tasks
developmental stage. a period of life during which unique physical and behavior changes occur
developmental tasks. work that needs to be done during a developmental stage

diagnosis. determining the nature of a specific disease condition through assessment of signs and symptoms

diagnosis, nursing. the identification of health problems that can be treated or prevented by independent nursing actions

diagnosis-related group (DRG). system of grouping clients according to major diagnoses for the purpose of standardizing reimbursement

dialysate. solution that is similar to plasma, used during dialysis

dialysis. removal of metabolic end products or other substances from the blood when the kidneys are nonfunctioning

diaphoresis. profuse perspiration (adj., diaphoretic)

diaphragm. large muscle that separates the abdominal cavity from the thoracic cavity

diaphysis. the shaft of long bones

diastole. relaxation of the atria and ventricles (adj., diastolic)

diastolic arterial pressure. the pressure within the vascular system during ventricular relaxation

diastolic filling volume. the volume of blood within the ventricles during diastole

diffusion. spontaneous movement of dissolved solutes and solvent from areas of high concentration to areas of low concentration until a state of equilibrium is attained

digital rectal examination (DRE). manual method by which the prostate gland is assessed

digitalization. administration of digitalis preparations to achieve a therapeutic blood level

dilation. stretching or widening

diplopia. double vision

dislocation. separation of the articular surfaces of a joint

dissecting aneurysm. separation of tunica intima from the tunica media with a collection of blood between the layers

distal. farthest from a point of reference; opposite of proximal

distress. excessive, ill-timed, or unrelieved stress

diuresis. excretion of large amounts of urine

diuretic. a drug capable of causing diuresis

diverticulitis. inflammation of diverticula

diverticulosis. the presence of diverticula (particularly in the colon) without inflammation

diverticulum. (pl., diverticula) a pouch in the mucous membrane

DNA. deoxyribonucleic acid; the primary genetic material of organisms

DNA replication. the duplication of DNA

dopamine. an intermediate compound in the synthesis of norepinephrine; also a neurotransmitter

Doppler ultrasound. a device that converts movement of blood cells to sound

doubt. a feeling of uncertainty; overcoming doubt is a developmental task of early childhood according to Erikson.

dumping syndrome. a cluster of symptoms that develops from the rapid emptying of the stomach into the jejunum

duodenal ulcer. erosion of the mucous membrane in the duodenum

duty. conduct expected and based on a moral obligation to another

dyscrasias. a group of blood diseases

dysmenorrhea. painful menstruation

dyspareunia. painful sexual intercourse

dyspepsia. epigastric discomfort

dysphagia. difficulty in swallowing

dysphasia. impairment in speech usually caused by a lesion of the brain

dyspnea. difficult breathing; air hunger (adj., dyspneic)

dysthymia. unremitting sad mood

dysuria. difficult or painful urination

E

eating disorders. any of the psychobiologic disorders marked by a distorted preoccupation with food, excessive or diminished intake of food, or purging of food

ecchymosis. bleeding into skin or mucous membrane that produces blue-black discolorations

ectopic. out of place; not in correct position

edema. swelling caused by the collection of fluid in the tissues

edentulous. without teeth

efferent. away from

effusion. accumulation of fluid between two tissue layers

ego identity. establishing self-identity, the developmental task of adolescence according to Erikson

ego integrity. a feeling of satisfaction that life has been happy and fulfilling, the developmental task of older adulthood

elder abuse. the emotional or physical abuse of an older adult, usually by a family member or caretaker

electrocardiogram (ECG, EKG). the electrical activity of the heart recorded on heat-sensitive paper

electroconvulsive therapy (ECT). treatment for mental illnesses, primarily depression, in which a generalized seizure is induced by applying low-voltage current to the brain

electroencephalogram (EEG). a record of the electrical activity of the brain

electrolyte. any compound that separates into charged particles (ions) when dissolved in water

element. a chemical substance, existing free or in combination with other elements, that cannot be further divided into substances different from itself (eg, oxygen, hydrogen, sodium)

embolectomy. surgical removal of an embolus

embolism. obstruction of a blood vessel with an embolus

embolus. (pl., emboli) a moving mass of either solid, liquid, or gas, in blood vessels or lymphatic tissue

embryonal. pertaining to an embryo

emmetropia. normal vision; light rays are bent to focus images precisely on the retina

emollient. skin softener

emphysema. chronic obstructive lung disease characterized by overdistention of alveolar sacs, rupture of alveolar walls, and destruction of the alveolar capillary bed

empyema. a collection of pus in a body cavity

emulsion. a mixture of two liquids, one of which is insoluble in the other, but when shaken is distributed throughout as small droplets

encephalopathy. dysfunction of the brain

encopresis. fecal incontinence

endarterectomy. removal of the lining of an artery

endogenous. arising or coming from within

endometriosis. the abnormal presence of endometrial tissue outside the uterus

endorphins. endogenous chemical substances that mimic morphine by binding to opioid receptor sites in the brain

endoscope. a tube that contains an optical system, often fiber optics, and a method of illumination

endoscopy. inspection of body cavities or organs by use of an endoscope

endotoxin. a toxin released by a bacterial cell
endotracheal. within the trachea
enema. introduction of fluid into the rectum
enkephalins. (see endorphins)
enteral. pertaining to the small intestine
enteric. pertaining to the small intestine
enteritis. inflammation of the intestines
enucleation. removal of the eye
enzyme. a complex protein produced by living cells that functions as a catalyst
enzyme-linked immunosorbent assay (ELISA). initial screening test for human immunodeficiency virus (HIV) infection
epidermis. the outer layer of skin
epididymitis. inflammation of the epididymis
epiglottis. cartilaginous structure that covers the larynx and trachea when swallowing
epilepsy. neurologic disorder characterized by seizures
epinephrine. sympathomimetic neurotransmitter and hormone
epiphysis. end of a long bone
epistaxis. nosebleed
epithelialization. regrowth of skin
Epstein-Barr virus. the virus that causes infectious mononucleosis
equianalgesic dose. an oral dose of analgesic that provides the same level of pain relief as that given by a parenteral route
erythema. redness of the skin
erythrocytes. red blood cells
erythropoiesis. the manufacture of red blood cells
erythropoietin. hormone secreted by the kidney that stimulates red blood cell production
eschar. a hard leathery crust of burned skin
esophageal varices. varicosities in the esophagus
estrogen. female sex hormone manufactured by the ovaries
ethics. the study of moral conduct
ethnicity. the bond or kinship a person feels with his or her ancestral country of origin
ethnocentrism. the belief that one's own ethnic heritage is superior to others'
etiology. the cause of disease or health problems
eustress. the amount of stress that helps individuals to pursue goals, learn to solve problems, or manage life's predictable and unpredictable crises
euthymia. mood state characterized by appropriate emotional responses
evaluation. determining the effectiveness of nursing care
evisceration. separation of wound edges with protrusion of organs; removal of the contents of the eye
exacerbation. an increase in intensity of symptoms or severity of a disease
excitability. the ability to respond to an electrical stimulus
excoriation. an abrasion of the outer layer of the skin
exenteration. removal of all structures in a cavity
exertional dyspnea. shortness of breath brought on by activity
exfoliated cells. dead cells shed from the skin, mucous membrane, or bone
exocrine gland. a gland whose secretions are transported through a duct
exogenous. coming or arising from outside the organism
expectorant. a drug that encourages raising of secretions from the lungs
external fixation. immobilization of a fracture with metal devices located outside the skin
extracellular. outside of cells
extracorporeal. outside of the body
extracorporeal circulation. method for oxygenating blood outside the body and recirculating it to body cells (eg, cardiopulmonary bypass, heart-lung machine)
extrapyramidal side effects. movement disorders associated with certain psychoactive drugs
extrasystole. (see premature ventricular contraction)
extravasation. the escape of fluid into surrounding tissues (synonym: infiltration)
exudate. fluid that usually contains pus, bacteria, and dead cells

F

family counseling. psychotherapy or counseling involving all family members
fasciculation. involuntary contraction of independent muscle fibers
fasciotomy. surgical incision of the fascia
fear. an emotional and physical reaction to real or imagined danger
fecalith. stonelike feces
feedback loop. a sensing mechanism for stimulating or suppressing function
feeding button. a device used for administering tube feedings through a healed gastrostomy
fertilization. the union of sperm and egg
fibrillation. a quivering of muscle fibers
fibrils. small fibers
fibrinolysis. the process of dissolving fibrin
fibroadenoma. benign tumor containing fibrous tissue
fibroblast. a cell from which connective tissue is developed
fibrocystic breast disease. formation of fluid-filled cysts in the breast
fibroid tumor. a uterine tumor having a fibrous structure (syn., leiomyoma)
fibrosis. formation of fibrous tissue
fibrous. containing fibers
fibrous ankylosis. restriction of movement by connective tissue
filtration. movement of fluid and some dissolved substances through a semipermeable membrane according to pressure differences
first-intention healing. healing that occurs when wound edges are approximated
fissure. a groove, crack, or slit
fistula. a passageway or connection from one area to another
flaccid. relaxed, weak, limp
flatus. intestinal gas
fluoroscopy. radiographic technique for real-time visualization of organs and tissues as they move and function
focus assessment. detailed data gathering
follicle-stimulating hormone (FSH). hormone produced by the anterior pituitary that stimulates the development of ova and sperm
fomites. nonliving reservoirs of an infectious agent
food binges. rapid consumption of a large number of calories in a short amount of time
footdrop. inability to maintain the foot in a normal position; a dragging of the foot
formal teaching. planned teaching (see informal teaching)
fracture. broken bone
free radicals. unstable atoms capable of damaging DNA
fulguration. destruction of tissue with an electric current

functional nursing. a method for delivering nursing care that assigns different tasks (functions) to different nurses
functional status. ability to perform activities of daily living (ADL)
fungus. (pl., fungi) a microorganism that belongs to the plant kingdom that lives on organic matter
furuncle. a skin infection commonly referred to as a boil

G

ganglion. a mass of nerve tissue
gangrene. necrosis of tissue almost always caused by a lack of blood supply to the affected part
gastrectomy. surgical removal of the stomach; may be total (all) or subtotal (part)
gastric bypass. a surgical procedure for treating obesity
gastric decompression. removing gas and fluids from the stomach
gastric intubation. insertion of a tube into the stomach
gastric ulcer. erosion of the mucosa within the stomach
gastritis. inflammation of the stomach
gastrocolic reflex. increased peristalsis after eating
gastroesophageal reflux. retrograde movement of stomach contents into the esophagus
gastroscopy. visualization of the stomach by means of an endoscope
gastrostomy. surgical opening into the stomach, usually for the purpose of feeding
gate-closing mechanism. nondrug techniques that interrupt pain transmission
gate-control theory. theory that suggests that "gates" in the spinal cord control the transmission of pain sensations to higher levels of the brain
gavage. to instill nourishment through a tube
gene therapy. in cancer treatment, replacing altered genes with normal genes, inhibiting defective genes, and introducing substances that cause genes or cancer cells to be destroyed
general adaptation syndrome (GAS). a series of physiologic responses to stressful stimuli that facilitates survival
generalization. a statement that is thought to be true in most instances
generalized infection. infection that has spread systemically from a local source in the body
generativity. a positive characteristic acquired during the developmental stage of middle adulthood according to Erikson
genital herpes. a sexually transmitted disease caused by the herpes simplex 2 virus
gerontology. the study of aging
gingivitis. inflammation of the gums
glomerulus. a tuft or cluster of blood vessels within each nephron
glaucoma. a condition that results from increased intraocular pressure
glossitis. inflammation of the tongue
glottis. the space between the vocal cords
glucagon. hormone manufactured by the pancreas; stimulates release of glucose by the liver
glucocorticoid. one of the adrenal cortical hormones
gluconeogenesis. conversion of glycogen to glucose
glycogen. a polysaccharide; starch
glycogenolysis. formation of glycogen from fats and proteins
glycosuria. presence of glucose in the urine
goal. the desired outcome of care
goal, long-term. a goal expected to be achieved over an extended period (weeks to months)
goal, short-term. a goal that can be achieved in a short time (days)
goiter. enlargement of the thyroid gland
gonorrhea. a sexually transmitted disease caused by *Neisseria gonorrhoeae*
Good Samaritan laws. laws designed to protect rescuers from prosecution
gout. metabolic disorder that causes a type of arthritis
gram positive. bacteria that retain the violet color of a Gram stain; opposite of gram negative, those bacteria that do not retain the Gram stain
granulation tissue. tissue formed during the repair and healing of wounds
granulocytes. white blood cell with visible granules when stained
granuloma. a fibrinous mass
granuloma inguinale. a sexually transmitted disease caused by the bacteria known as *Calymmatobacterium granulomatis*
group psychotherapy. therapeutic technique in which group dynamics are used to gain insight into behavior
growth. gradual development to maturity
guilt. a feeling of having done something wrong; a negative characteristic acquired during the developmental stage of the preschool child according to Erikson
gynecomastia. breast enlargement in a man

H

habituation. the repeated use of a drug
hallucination. sensory experiences that occur without any basis in fact
hardiness. a coping style characterized by having meaningful commitments, a sense of control, and a sense of being challenged rather than threatened
head-to-toe method. method of performing a physical examination (compare with systems method)
health beliefs. ideas about what causes illness and how one stays healthy
health care delivery system. the services, structures, and personnel who provide health care
health care services. the full range of assistance offered by the health care delivery system including primary, secondary, tertiary, and long-term care
health care team. all of the specially trained individuals who work together to provide clients with health care
health–illness continuum. the concept that health can shift back and forth from various levels of wellness and illness over an individual's lifetime
health maintenance. preventing illness
health maintenance organization (HMO). provides all of insured's healthcare for a fixed fee
health practices. activities that must occur for health to be maintained or restored
health promotion. improving health
Heberden's nodes. bony enlargement of the distal interphalangeal joints
helminth. a parasitic worm or wormlike organism
hematemesis. vomiting of blood
hematocrit. a measurement of the volume of red blood cells in a given amount of blood
hematogenic shock. shock caused by blood loss
hematoma. a swelling that contains blood
hematopoiesis. the production or development of blood cells

hematopoietic. blood cell producing
hematuria. blood in the urine
hemianopia. visual defect or blindness of half the visual field in one or both eyes
hemiplegia. paralysis of one side of the body
hemoconcentration. high ratio of blood components in relation to plasma
hemodialysis. the removal of chemical substances by passing blood through a system of tubes surrounded by a dialysate
hemodilution. reduced ratio of blood components to plasma
hemodynamic monitoring. assessing the fluid status within the circulatory system
hemoglobin. the oxygen-carrying pigment of red blood cells
hemolysis. destruction of red blood cells
hemoptysis. spitting up of blood from the respiratory tract
hemorrhoid. dilated veins about the internal and external anal sphincter
hemostasis. controlled bleeding; stagnation of blood in one area
hemothorax. blood in the pleural cavity
hepatitis. inflammation of the liver
hepatoma. primary malignant liver tumor
hepatomegaly. enlargement of the liver
hepatorenal syndrome. renal failure secondary to cirrhosis
hepatotoxic. toxic to the liver
hernia. protrusion of structures through a weakened muscle wall
herpes simplex virus. the virus that causes herpes type 1 infection
herpes zoster. a reactivation of herpes-varicella (chickenpox) that causes neuralgic pain; also known as "shingles"
heterogeneous. dissimilar characteristics
heterograft. a graft taken from another person
hiatal hernia. an enlarged opening in the diaphragm where the esophagus passes through
hip spica cast. rigid mold that surrounds one or both legs and the trunk
histocompatible cells. cells whose antigens match the individual's own genetic code
history, allergy. list of all drugs, foods, or environmental substances to which a person has had an allergic reaction and a description of the reaction
history, drug. list of all current prescribed and nonprescribed drugs the client takes
history, past health. all of the health problems a client has experienced from childhood to present
history, psychosocial. description of the client's social support systems and psychological state
histrionic. displaying dramatic, attention-seeking behavior
holism. the theory that humans cannot be viewed simply from a biologic perspective; psychosocial and spiritual perspectives must be included as well
Homans' sign. pain in the calf on dorsiflexion of the foot
home heath care. care provided in the client's home
homeostasis. term used to describe a dynamic state of equilibrium of the body
homeostatic mechanism. activities that restore equilibrium
homogeneous. of uniform or similar characteristics
hormone. a chemical substance secreted by an endocrine gland and carried to another area by the bloodstream
hormone replacement therapy. prescription of estrogens with or without progestins after menopause
hospice. an organization that provides care for dying clients
host. an animal or plant that harbors another organism
human immunodeficiency virus (HIV). the retrovirus that causes acquired immunodeficiency syndrome (AIDS)
human papillomavirus. the virus that causes warts in humans
humor. the ability to perceive or express what is funny or amusing
humoral response. immune response negotiated by B cells
hydronephrosis. distention of the kidneys with urine due to distal obstruction
hyperaldosteronism. excess production of aldosterone, an adrenal hormone
hypercalcemia. an excess of calcium in the blood
hypercalciuria. an excess of calcium in the urine
hypercapnia. increased carbon dioxide in the blood
hypercarbia. increased carbon dioxide in the blood (syn., hypercapnia)
hypercholesterolemia. excessive amount of cholesterol in the blood
hyperemia. congested with blood
hyperextension. extreme extension of a part
hyperglycemia. an excess of glucose in the blood
hyperinsulinism. excessive secretion of insulin
hyperkalemia. an excess of potassium in the blood
hyperlipidemia. elevated blood lipids
hypermagnesemia. an excess of magnesium in the blood
hypernatremia. an excess of sodium in the blood
hyperopia. farsightedness; seeing distant images more clearly
hyperphagia. increased appetite
hyperplasia. extra growth of normal tissue; increase in the number of cells
hypertension. sustained elevation of arterial pressure
hypertensive cardiovascular disease. elevated blood pressure accompanied by heart and vascular pathology
hypertensive heart disease. elevated blood pressure accompanied by cardiac abnormality
hypertensive vascular disease. elevated blood pressure with vascular damage without heart involvement
hyperthermia. elevation of body temperature; fever
hypertonia. increased tone of muscles or arteries (adj., hypertonic)
hypertonic solution. a solution with a greater osmotic pressure than another solution
hypertrophy. increase in size of an organ or structure (adj., hypertrophied)
hyperuricemia. accumulation of uric acid in the blood
hypervolemia. increased volume of fluid including circulating blood; opposite of hypovolemia (adj., hypervolemic)
hypnotic. a drug used to produce sleep
hypocalcemia. decrease in blood calcium below normal level
hypocapnia. decrease in carbon dioxide in the blood
hypochloremia. decrease in the chloride content of the blood
hypochlorhydria. reduced amounts of hydrochloric acid in the stomach
hypochromic. lighter than normal in color
hypoglycemia. decrease in blood glucose below normal level
hypokalemia. decrease in potassium in the blood below normal level

hypomagnesemia. decrease in magnesium in the blood below normal level
hypomania. mood state similar to mania but of a lesser intensity
hyponatremia. decrease in sodium in the blood below normal level
hypophysis. the pituitary gland
hypoproteinemia. decrease in the amount of protein in the blood
hypostatic pneumonia. pneumonia that results from failure to cough, move, and breathe deeply
hypotension. low blood pressure
hypothalamus. region of the brain that controls the pituitary gland and homeostasis
hypothermia. below normal body temperature
hypotonia. loss of or decrease in muscle tone (adj., hypotonic)
hypotonic solution. a solution with less osmotic pressure than another solution
hypovolemia. diminished volume of fluid including circulating blood; opposite of hypervolemia (adj., hypovolemic)
hypoxemia. reduced oxygen in the blood
hypoxia. inadequate oxygen at the cellular level (adj., hypoxic)
hysterectomy. removal of the uterus

I

iatrogenic. adverse effects of medical treatment
idiopathic. of unknown cause
ileal conduit. a urinary diversion using ileum to create the stoma
ileostomy. surgically created opening between the ileum and abdominal wall
illusion. an inaccurate interpretation of stimuli within the environment
imagery. visualizing positive physiologic processes
immune response. body's response to destroy foreign or harmful substances
immunizations. vaccines that stimulate the body to produce antibodies against a specific disease organism
immunocompromised. a state of being unable to develop immunity to one or more specific antigens
immunodeficient. decreased ability to develop immunity to one or more specific antigens
immunogen. another term for antigen
immunoglobulin. protein substance manufactured by the body in response to the presence of a specific antigen (synonym: antibody)
immunopeptides. substances that relay messages throughout the immune system and to the brain
implementation. carrying out the plan for care
impotence. inability to achieve or sustain an erection
incident report. a written description of an unusual event
incontinence. inability to control stool and/or urine elimination
industry. earnest and sustained effort; the developmental task of the school-age child according to Erikson
infarction. area of necrosis; death of tissue
infectious disorders. infections and infectious diseases caused by microorganisms
infectious process cycle. the cycle that describes the mechanism of infection; includes a portal of entry, the infectious agent, the host, a reservoir, exit route, and mode of transmission
inferiority. a feeling of inadequacy; a negative characteristic acquired during the developmental stage of the school-age child according to Erikson
infiltration. the collection of fluid within tissues (usually subcutaneous tissue) when the needle or catheter is out of the vein
inflammation. the body's response to cell injury
informal teaching. teaching that occurs spontaneously
initiative. ability to think or act without being prodded; a positive characteristic acquired during the developmental stage of the preschool child according to Erikson
inotropic action. affecting force of myocardial contraction
insensible fluid loss. fluid lost through the skin and lungs that is not measurable
insight-oriented therapy. therapeutic approach that helps clients understand the cause and relationship between their emotional distress and physical symptoms
inspection. assess by looking
insulin. hormone secreted by the pancreas; necessary for the metabolism of glucose
integrated delivery system (IDS). a health care organization that provides the full range of services from wellness programs to hospice care
integument. the structures that cover the exposed surfaces of the body
intentional torts. a violation of civil law in which a person consciously harms another
intercostal. between the ribs
interferon. a protein substance manufactured by white blood cells and probably other body cells in response to a viral infection
intermittent claudication. pain in the legs brought on by activity
interstitial. between cells
intertrigo. dermatitis within skinfolds
interventions. nursing actions designed to treat, alleviate, or prevent client health problems
intimacy. the state of being involved in very close relationships; a positive characteristic acquired during the developmental stage of young adulthood according to Erikson
intimate space. a 6-inch zone of personal space reserved for private communication
intra-aortic balloon pump. a device that acts as a secondary pump supplementing ineffectual contraction of the left ventricle
intracellular. within cells
intracerebral. within the brain
intractable pain. pain that cannot be controlled by analgesic medications or nursing management
intradermal. within the skin; between the epidermis and the dermis
intramedullary rod. metal device inserted into the center of a bone
intraocular lens implant. artificial lens placed within the eye
intraocular pressure (IOP). force within the eye
intrathecal. injection site within the subarachnoid space of the spinal cord
intrathoracic. within the thorax
intravascular. within blood vessels
intravenous. injection or infusion into a vein
introductory phase. the initial period of the nurse–client relationship
intussusception. telescoping of a portion of the intestine into the immediately adjoining section

ion. one or more atoms carrying a positive or negative electrical charge (eg, Na^+, OH^-)
ionization. the separation of molecules into their constituent ions
irritable bowel syndrome (IBS). a paroxysmal motor disorder of the colon characterized by alternating periods of constipation and diarrhea
ischemia. inadequate blood supply to a part
isoenzyme. one of several forms of the same enzyme
isolation. the state of being alone; a negative characteristic acquired during the developmental stage of young adulthood
isotonic. having the same tone; also, a solution having the same osmotic pressure as the solution being compared with it
isotope. any one of a series of chemical elements that has the same atomic number but a different atomic weight

J

jaundice. a yellowish color to the skin or sclera of eyes caused by excess bile pigment

K

keloid. elevated, thick, ropelike scars common among African Americans
keratin. any of the proteins that are the main constituents of the epidermis, hair, and nails
keratitis. inflammation of the cornea
keratoconjunctivitis. inflammation of the cornea and conjunctiva
keratotic lesions. elevated, darkly pigmented skin plaques
Kernig's sign. inability to extend the leg when the thigh is flexed on the abdomen; a sign of meningitis
ketoacidosis. acidosis caused by excess accumulation of ketones
ketone bodies. chemical intermediate products in the metabolism of fat; beta-hydroxybutyric acid, acetoacetic acid, acetone
ketonemia. presence of ketone bodies in the blood
ketonuria. presence of ketone bodies in the urine
ketosis. an accumulation of ketone bodies in the body
kinesics. body language
Kock pouch. a continent ileal reservoir with a valve created from intussusception of ileum
Kussmaul breathing. deep, rapid respirations; characteristic of metabolic acidosis
kyphosis. abnormal curvature of the thoracic spine

L

la belle indifference. inappropriate nonchalance toward one's symptoms or condition
lactic acid. an acid produced during anaerobic metabolism
Laennec's cirrhosis. fibrotic scarring of the liver due to malnutrition, alcoholism, or exposure to hepatotoxic chemicals
laminectomy. removal of the posterior arch of the vertebra
lanugo. fine hair covering the skin
laparotomy. an abdominal surgical opening
laryngospasm. spasmodic closure of the larynx
larynx. the voice box
latent. hidden
lavage. to wash out
learning capacity. the ability to receive, remember, analyze, and apply new information
learning needs. the information or skills the client must acquire
learning readiness. the period in which the client can best learn new information
learning style. an individual's preferred method for learning new information
left-sided heart failure. inefficient pumping by the left ventricle
lentigines. small, brown-pigmented macules
lethargy. sluggishness, stupor (adj., lethargic)
leukemia. a malignant disease of the bone marrow characterized by an abnormal production of white blood cells
leukocyte. a white blood cell
leukocytosis. excessive number of leukocytes
leukopenia. deficit of leukocytes
leukoplakia. patches of white, thickened tissue in the mouth or mucous membrane; often considered to be a forerunner of cancer
leukorrhea. a white or yellow-white vaginal discharge
liability. legally responsible
libido. sexual desire
ligament. band of fibrous tissue that supports a joint and connects bone or cartilage
ligation. tying off; application of a ligature (suture) to a part
life review. the process of examining one's life
limbic system. a network within the brain that contains structures involved in emotional behavior
lipofuscin. a brown substance that forms cells undergoing deterioration and oxidation
listening. giving attention to what another says
lithiasis. formation of stones
lithotripsy. crushing of a stone in the urinary system or gallbladder
living will. an informal document describing a person's wishes if terminally ill
lobectomy. removal of a lobe
localized infection. a confined infection
long-term care. chronic care and restorative services
lumbar puncture. insertion of a needle into the subarachnoid space of the spine
lumen. the inner space or diameter of a tube or tubular organ
lumpectomy. removal of a palpable lesion of tissue
luteinizing hormone (LH). hormone produced by the anterior pituitary that stimulates ovulation in females and testosterone production in males
lymph. fluid found in the lymphatic system
lymphedema. chronic edema of one or more extremities as a result of obstruction of lymph
lymphocytes. agranular white blood cell
lymphogranuloma venereum. a sexually transmitted disease caused by *Chlamydia trachomatis*
lymphokine. a substance that enhances the actions of phagocytic cells
lymphoma. a tumor of lymphoid tissue
lysozyme. chemical that destroys substances within the cell

M

macrophage. a large phagocytic white blood cell
macule. a small, colored spot on the skin
maintenance dose. the amount of drug needed to sustain a desired blood level

malaise. a feeling of fatigue; lack of energy
malignant. harmful; capable of producing death
malignant hypertension. dangerously elevated blood pressure accompanied by neurologic changes
malignant hyperthermia. rapid and progressive rise in body temperature
malingering. feigning illness to avoid responsibilities
malpractice. professional actions that deviate from the standard expected of others with similar education and experience
mammography. radiography of the breast
mammoplasty. plastic surgery of the breast
managed care organization (MCO). an umbrella term that refers to insurance systems that carefully monitor the costs and quality of care provided
mania. mood characterized by elation, excitability, hyperactivity, rapid speech, and disconnected thoughts (flight of ideas)
mast cells. a connective tissue cell that contains histamine and heparin
masticate. to chew
mastitis. inflammation of mammary glands
mastopexy. surgical procedure to elevate pendulous breasts
matrix. the basic substance of a structure
meatus. opening
mediastinum. the tissues and organs that occupy the space between the two lungs
medulla. inner portion of a gland or organ; a portion of the brain stem
melanin. brown pigment in the epidermis
melatonin. a hormone synthesized by the pineal gland that influences the regulation of sleep, mood, puberty, and ovarian cycles
melena. tarry stools
memory cells. cells that on reexposure to a specific antigen effect a more rapid immunologic response
menarche. the start of menstruation; usually occurs between ages 10 and 14
meninges. the membranous coverings of the brain and spinal cord: the dura mater, pia mater, and arachnoid
menopause. the period when menstruation begins to wane and finally ceases
menorrhagia. heavy or prolonged menstrual periods
menstrual diary. record of menstrual periods and associated symptoms
menstruation. cyclic discharge of blood and tissue from the nonpregnant uterus
mental status examination. an array of observations and questions that elicit information about a person's cognitive and mental state
mentation. mental activity
metabolic acidosis. an acid–base imbalance occurring from a loss of base and a gain in an acid; the blood pH is < 7.35
metabolism. the sum total of the physical and chemical changes and reactions that occur in the body
metastasis. spread; the spread of disease from one part of the body to another (adj., metastatic; v., metastasize)
methadone maintenance therapy. therapy used to help the heroin addict avoid withdrawal symptoms
metrorrhagia. uterine bleeding at times other than menstruation
microcytic. smaller than normal cell
microorganism. microscopic organisms including bacteria, viruses, fungi, and protozoa
microphage. a small phagocyte
micturition. urination
mid-life crisis. a sense of anxiety about relationships, values, and self-identity that some adults experience in mid-life
mineralocorticoid. hormone produced by the cortex of the adrenal glands
miotic. a drug that constricts the pupil
mistrust. lack of confidence or trust in others; a negative characteristic acquired during the developmental stage of infancy according to Erikson
mode of transmission. any of the various ways an infectious disease is spread
modified radical mastectomy. procedure for treating breast cancer in which the breast, some lymph nodes, the lining over the chest muscles, and the pectoralis minor muscle are removed
Monilia. same as Candida, a genus of yeastlike fungus
monoamine hypothesis. a theory that suggests that depression is the result of a deficiency in one or more of the monoamine neurotransmitters
monocyte. a type of white blood cell
Montgomery straps. adhesive strips that do not require removal each time a dressing is changed
mood. an individual's overall feeling state
morbidity. incidence of disease within a population
moribund. dying, near death
morphology. study of shape without regard to function
mortality. death rate
motivation. the quality of having a purpose for accomplishing something
mucolytic. a drug that thins mucus
mucopurulent. consisting of pus and mucus
multidrug resistance. microbial insensitivity to many different antibiotics
mycoplasmas. microorganisms smaller than bacteria and lacking a true cell wall
mydriatic. a drug used to dilate the pupil; usually applied topically
myelin. fatty material that covers and insulates axons of some nerves
myocardial infarction (MI). death of the muscle layer (myocardium) of the heart; lay term, "heart attack"
myopia. nearsightedness

N

narcotic. class of drugs capable of relieving pain and producing stupor and sleep
nasoenteric tube. a tube passed through the nose into the small intestine
nasogastric tube. a tube passed through the nose into the stomach
nasopharynx. the section of the pharynx above the soft palate
natriuretic factor. a hormone produced by the heart that affects blood pressure
naturally acquired active immunity. immunity acquired as a direct result of infection by a specific microorganism
nebulizer. device that produces a fine mist to deliver medication within the lungs
necrosis. death of tissue (adj., necrotic)
negative symptoms. in schizophrenia, impoverished speech and an inability to enjoy relationships or express emotions
negligence. unreasonable or careless action that results in injury or failure to act to prevent injury
neoplasm. new growth (adj., neoplastic)

nephrolithiasis. kidney stones
nephron. the functional unit of the kidney
nephrostomy tube. tube placed in the kidney to drain urine externally
nephrotoxic. toxic to the kidney
neuralgia. pain in a nerve
neurilemma. membrane that covers certain myelin fibers
neuritic plaques. deposits of beta-amyloid and degenerating nerve cells found in the brain cells of those with Alzheimer's disease
neurobiologic theory. a theory that suggests that mood disorders are a result of biochemical changes in the brain's chemistry
neurofibrillary tangles. twisted bundles of nerve fibers found in the brain cells of those with Alzheimer's disease
neurogenic bladder. bladder dysfunction due to inadequate nerve stimulation
neurohormone. a chemical substance found in the nervous system that affects nervous system function
neurohypophysis. the posterior lobe of the pituitary gland
neuroma. a benign tumor composed of nerve tissue
neuromuscular. involving nerves and muscles
neuron. the conducting cell of the nervous system
neuropeptide. a type of neurotransmitter that chemically relays biologic information
neurotransmitters. neurochemicals released during the transmission of nerve impulses
neutrophils. phagocytic granular white blood cell
nocturia. urination during the night
nodular. having or resembling nodules
nodule. a small node
nomogram. a chart based on height and weight that determines body surface area
nonpathogens. microorganisms that are generally harmless to healthy humans
nonverbal communication. the exchange of information without using words
norepinephrine. a neurohormone produced by the adrenal medulla
normal eating. ingesting sufficient amounts of nutrients to maintain ideal body weight, nourish and repair tissues.
normotensive. normal blood pressure
normovolemia. a normal blood volume (adj., normovolemic)
nosocomial infection. an infection acquired during hospital treatment
nuchal rigidity. pain and stiffness of the neck
nurse–client relationship. the therapeutic relationship established between the nurse and the client to achieve health care goals
nurse practice acts. statutes regulating the practice of nursing
nursing. the diagnosis and treatment of human responses to actual or potential health problems
nursing diagnosis. a health problem capable of being solved or prevented by independent nursing actions
nursing process. a method for identifying and solving health problems
nutritional therapy. providing nourishing meals, supplemental vitamins and minerals, intravenous fluids and electrolytes, tube feedings, or total parenteral nutrition
nystagmus. involuntary movement of the eyes

O

objective data. information obtained by observation and testing
occlusion. blockage of a passage
occult bleeding. hidden bleeding; not obvious to the naked eye
ocular therapeutic system. method for administering a sustained-release form of eye medication
oculogyric crisis. a sudden involuntary rolling downward or upward of the eyes
odynophagia. pain on swallowing
olfactory. pertaining to sense of smell
oligomenorrhea. scant or infrequent menstrual flow
oliguria. decrease in urinary elimination
oophorectomy. removal of the ovaries
open-ended questions. interview questions that encourage verbalization
opisthotonos. extreme hyperextension of the head and arching of the back; indicates meningeal irritation
opportunistic infections. infections caused by microorganisms that normally do not produce an infection unless the immune system is impaired
orchiectomy. excision of the testes
orchiopexy. surgery to secure the testis within the scrotum
orchitis. inflammation of the testes
orifice. entrance; opening
oropharyngeal airway. an airway inserted in the mouth and extending as far as the oropharynx
oropharynx. the section of the pharynx between the soft palate and the epiglottis
orthopnea. breathing facilitated by sitting upright
orthostatic hypotension. hypotension occurring when suddenly changing position or standing in one position for a prolonged period of time (see postural hypotension)
osmosis. movement of water through a semipermeable membrane
osmotic pressure. fluid pressure created by the concentration of solutes
osseous ankylosis. loss of joint mobility due to calcification
ossification. formation of bone
osteoarthritis. a chronic degenerative disease of the joints, especially the weight-bearing joints
osteoblasts. cells that build bones
osteoclasts. cells involved in the destruction, reabsorption, and remodeling of bone
osteocytes. mature bone cells
osteodystrophy. defective bone formation
osteolytic. bone destruction
osteomalacia. inadequate mineralization of bone
osteomyelitis. infection of the bone
osteoporosis. loss of calcium from bone
osteotomy. surgical cutting of a bone
ostomate. a person with an ileostomy or colostomy
ostomy. a surgical opening (eg, colostomy, ileostomy)
otorrhea. discharge from the ear
otoscope. an instrument used for examining the external auditory canal and eardrum (tympanic membrane)
ova. unfertilized eggs
ovulation. cyclic release of ova from the ovaries
oxidation. the process of combining with oxygen
oxytocin. hormone released by the anterior pituitary that stimulates contraction of pregnant uterus

P

pacemaker. the sinoatrial (SA) node; an artificial pacemaker is an electrical device that substitutes for the heart's own pacemaker

packed cells. blood product that has most of the plasma removed
pain. the sensation of physical or mental suffering or hurt that usually causes distress or agony
pain, acute. pain of recent onset, symptomatic of injury, specific, responds well to analgesics, diminishes, and resolves
pain, chronic. remote onset, uncharacteristic of primary injury, nonspecific, persists beyond healing stage, does not respond well to analgesics
pain, intractable. pain that does not respond to analgesic medications, noninvasive measures, or nursing management
pain management. techniques used to prevent, reduce, or relieve pain
pain, neuropathic. pain with atypical characteristics often experienced days, weeks, or months after the source of the pain has been treated and resolved (also called functional or psychogenic pain)
pain perception. the conscious experience of discomfort
pain, referred. discomfort perceived in a general area of the body, but not in the exact site where an organ pathology is anatomically located
pain, somatic. pain generated from deep connective tissue structures such as muscles, tendons, and joints
pain threshold. the point at which the pain-transmitting neurochemicals reach the brain causing conscious awareness
pain tolerance. the amount of pain a person endures once the pain threshold has been reached
pain, visceral. pain arising from internal organs; tends to be referred or poorly localized
palliative. promotes comfort without curing the disease
palpation. assess by feeling
palsy. decreased sensation and movement
pancytopenia. a decrease in erythrocytes, leukocytes, and platelets
pannus. inflammatory exudate
Papanicolaou's smear (Pap test). cytologic examination of exfoliated cells
papilledema. swelling of the optic nerve at its point of entrance into the eye
papule. a red, elevated area on the skin
paracentesis. removal of fluid from the abdominal cavity
paradoxical pulse. a pulse that weakens on deep inspiration
paralanguage. vocal sounds that convey a message but are not actually words
paralytic ileus. paralysis of the intestines and absence of peristalsis
paraphimosis. retracted foreskin that causes swelling of the glans
paraplegia. paralysis of both legs
parathormone. parathyroid hormone
parenchyma. the essential parts of an organ (adj., parenchymal)
parenteral therapy. the giving of fluids or other substances by routes other than the alimentary canal
paresthesia. numbness, prickling, tingling sensation
parietal cells. cells in the stomach that produce hydrochloric acid and the intrinsic factor
paroxysm. a sudden spasm; a sudden recurrence of symptoms
paroxysmal nocturnal dyspnea. being awakened by breathlessness
pars intermedia. the intermediate lobe of the pituitary gland
partial mastectomy. surgical treatment for breast cancer; the tumor, some breast tissue, and some lymph nodes are removed
passive immunity. that which results from receiving antibodies made by another person or animal
patent. open (n., patency)
pathogen. a microorganism that produces harm or disease (adj., pathogenic)
pathophysiology. the physiology of disordered function
patient-focused care. a system of hospital-based health care delivery that brings services to the client
pelvic inflammatory disease. inflammation and infection of the organs and structures of the female pelvis
peptic ulcer. an ulcer in the lower esophagus, stomach, or duodenum
percussion. assess by tapping
percutaneous. through the skin
perfusion. the passage of fluid (ie, blood) through the vessels of a specific organ
pericarditis. inflammation of the pericardium
periosteum. connective tissue covering the shaft of bones
peripheral. outer edge
peripheral resistance. opposition to blood flow
peristalsis. wavelike movements of hollow organs such as the intestine, esophagus, and ureter
peritonitis. inflammation of the peritoneum
persistent vegetative state. living with only primitive brain stem function
personal space. the area around an individual from 6 inches to 4 feet away
pet therapy. using animals to improve mood of depressed and isolated clients
petechiae. tiny hemorrhagic spots on the skin (adj., petechial)
pH. the degree of alkalinity or acidity. A pH of 7.0 is neutral (eg, neither acidic nor alkaline); a pH <7.0 is acidic and a pH >7.0 is alkaline
phagocytosis. to engulf or eat
pharynx. the passageway between the the mouth, posterior nares, larynx, and esophagus
phimosis. constriction of the opening of the foreskin preventing retraction
phlebitis. inflammation of a vein
phlebography. injection of contrast media into a vein to visualize the venous system
phlebothrombosis. presence of clots in a vein with little or no inflammation
phlebotomy. an opening into a vein
phonocardiogram. a graphic recording of heart sounds
photocoagulation. use of a laser beam for surgical coagulation
photophobia. sensitivity to light
physical assessment. obtaining objective data through examination of body structures
pica. eating of nonfood items
pigmentation. coloration caused by a deposit of pigments (colored material)
pitting edema. indentations left when compression displaces fluid in tissue
pituitary gland. endocrine gland located near and controlled by the hypothalamus; releases hormones that control other glands
placebo effect. the phenomenon whereby clients feel improvement with inactive substances
planning. actions that include identifying goals and selecting nursing actions
plaque. an elevated deposit

plasma. liquid portion of blood
plasma expander. nonblood solutions that pull fluid into the vascular space
platelet. cell fragment that plays a role in blood clotting
platelet aggregation. forming a clump of platelets
pleural effusion. escape of fluid into the pleural cavity
plexus. a network of blood vessels or nerves
pneumonia. inflammation of the lungs with consolidation
pneumothorax. air in the pleural cavity
poikilothermy. a condition seen in spinal shock in which body temperature reflects that of the environment
point of maximum impulse (PMI). the point on the chest at which the cardiac impulse can be most readily seen or felt
polarization. state in which positive ions align outside a cell membrane while negative ions align inside
polyarthritis. inflammation of more than one joint
polycythemia vera. an abnormal increase in red blood cells
polydipsia. drinking a great deal of water; excessive thirst
polydrug abuse. abuse of more than one substance
polyp. a tumor or growth attached by a pedicle (stem)
polyphagia. increase in the intake of food
polyuria. excessive secretion of urine; increased urination
pons. area of the brain that connects the cerebellum to the rest of the central nervous system
portal hypertension. elevated pressure within the portal vein and its collateral vessels
portal of entry. the way in which a disease-causing organism enters the body
portal of exit. the route by which an infectious agent escapes from the reservoir
portal system. collective term for the gastric, mesenteric, splenic veins that drain into the portal vein
positive symptoms. in schizophrenia, delusions, hallucinations, and fluent but disorganized speech
postpartum. after childbirth
postural hypotension. a feeling of weakness, dizziness, or faintness when assuming an upright position (see orthostatic hypotension)
post void residual. the amount of urine retained in the bladder after voiding
precordial. over the heart
preferred provider organization (PPO). insurance reimbursement plan that covers a greater share of health care costs when plan members use specified physicians and health care agencies
preload. the volume of blood entering the heart
premature ventricular contraction (PVC). a ventricular ectopic beat
premenstrual syndrome. syndrome of physical and emotional discomfort occurring 2 weeks before menstruation
presbycusis. loss of hearing as a result of aging
presbyopia. loss of visual accommodation as a result of aging
pressure sores. skin impairment that occurs when capillary blood flow to an area is reduced; also called decubitus ulcers
priapism. a sustained and painful erection in the absence of sexual stimulation
primary care. the first health resource a client contacts
primary condition. one that develops independently of any other
primary nursing. a method of nursing care delivery in which a nurse provides all the care to a specific client or group of clients
problem oriented medical record (POMR). a chart organized according to a client's problems
prodromal phase. the early stage of a disease
progesterone. hormone secreted by the corpus luteum that maintains the lining of the uterus for pregnancy
prognosis. the predicted outcome of the course of disease
prolapse. a dropping of an organ from its original place or position
prophylactic. anything used to prevent infection or disease
prospective payment systems (PPS). reimbursement for a specific diagnosis-related group is predetermined and paid regardless of the actual costs incurred
prostate specific antigen (PSA). substance found in both normal and cancerous prostatic cells; used as a tumor marker for prostate cancer
prostatectomy. excision of the prostate gland
prosthesis. (pl., prostheses) an artificial substitute for a part
prosthetist. a person who makes and fits artificial limbs
proteinuria. protein (usually albumin) in the urine
protozoa. microorganisms that are members of the animal kingdom, usually one celled
proxemics. the use and relationship of space to communication
proximal. nearest to a point of reference; opposite of distal
pruritus. itching
pseudocysts. fibrous capsules filled with fluid rather than solid tissue
psoriasis. a skin disorder with dull red lesions surrounded by silver scales
psyche. the mind, both conscious and unconscious
psychobiologic disorders. disorders in which biologic abnormalities in the brain result in altered cognition, thinking, perception, emotion, behavior, and socialization
psychomotor learner. an individual who learns best by doing
psychoneuroimmunology. the field of science that studies the connections among the emotions, the central nervous system, the neuroendocrine system, and the immunologic system
psychosexual developmental stages. developmental stages based on sexual drive as described by Sigmund Freud
psychosocial stages. developmental stages based on social relationships as outlined by Eric Erikson
psychosomatic symptoms. physical changes from stimulation of the autonomic nervous system
psychotherapy. treatment of mental disorders using support, insight, reeducation, and other techniques
ptosis. drooping
puberty. the time when secondary sex characteristics appear and reproductive capacity occurs
public space. the area that begins 12 feet away from an individual
pulmonary edema. fluid in the lungs
pulmonary embolus. a blood clot in the pulmonary circulation
pulmonary hypertension. excess fluid pressure in the pulmonary blood vessels
pulse deficit. the numerical difference between the radial and apical pulse rates
pulse pressure. the numerical difference between the systolic and diastolic blood pressures
pulsus paradoxus. variation in systolic pressure at expiration and inspiration
purge. eliminate nutrients with self-induced vomiting, laxatives, enemas, or diuretics
purines. end products of the digestion of certain proteins
purpura. hemorrhage into the skin and mucous membrane

purulent. containing pus
pustule. a small elevation on the skin that contains pus or lymph
pyuria. presence of pus in the urine

Q

quadriplegia. paralysis of all four extremities; synonym: quadriplegia
quiescent. inactive, dormant

R

race. any of the various populations of humans distinguished by genetically determined biologic variations
radiation. the emission of alpha, beta, or gamma rays
radiation therapy. the use of high-energy ionizing radiation to destroy cancer cells
radioactive isotope. an isotope capable of giving off gamma rays; used for therapeutic or diagnostic purposes
radioactivity. the ability of a substance to emit alpha, beta, and gamma rays
radiograph. x-ray
radioimmunoassay. method for determining the concentration of a substance in blood plasma
radioisotope. an isotope that is radioactive
radionuclide imaging. injection or ingestion of a radioactive substance to examine a body organ by passing a scanner over the structure
radiopaque. cannot be penetrated by x-rays; dye appears white or light on radiographs
radiosensitive. sensitive to radiation; easily affected by radiation
rale. abnormal crackling breath sound heard in chest caused by air passing over secretions or exudate in the airways; synonym: crackles
reality orientation. techniques for promoting awareness of the present
rebound tenderness. pain that increases after releasing pressure
receptor. binding site on the surface of cells
rectocele. protrusion of the rectum against the posterior wall of the vagina
red bone marrow. bone marrow found primarily in the sternum, ileum, vertebrae, and ribs that manufactures blood cells and hemoglobin
reduction mammoplasty. cosmetic breast procedure to reduce extremely large breasts
Reed-Sternberg cells. cells present in Hodgkin's lymphoma
refraction. bending of light rays to focus a visual image on the retina
refractory. resistant to treatment; in the cardiac cycle, resistant to electrical stimulation
regeneration. identical replacement of damaged cells
regurgitation. to flow in the opposite direction of normal
reminiscence therapy. increasing feelings of self-worth and connectedness by encouraging older adults to discuss their personal histories
renin-angiotensin-aldosterone mechanism. complex series of chemical events involving the kidneys, lungs, and adrenal glands that result in a rise in blood pressure
repolarization. realignment of ions after depolarization
reservoir. the environment in which an infectious agent is able to survive and reproduce; may be human, animal, or nonliving, such as food and water
residual urine. urine remaining after voiding
resolution. damaged cell recovery without replacement
resorption. loss of a substance either by a normal physiologic or by a pathologic process
respiration. the exchange of carbon dioxide and oxygen
respirator. a mechanical device that substitutes for or assists with breathing
respite care. care provided by another to give the primary caregiver relief
retrograde ejaculation. ejaculate is expelled backward into the urinary bladder
retrovirus. an RNA-containing tumor virus
reuptake. a process by which neurochemicals are recaptured by the releasing neuron
rheumatic disorder. diseases marked by inflammation and degeneration of connective tissue
rhinitis. inflammatory reaction of the nasal mucosa to various allergens
rhinorrhea. discharge of nasal mucus
rhonchus. (pl., rhonchi) a noise resembling snoring coming from the throat; synonym: gurgle
rhythmicity. rhythmic activity; the heart's ability to repeat each cycle with regularity
rickettsia. parasitic microorganisms between the size of bacteria and viruses that require living cells for growth
right. that to which one is legally and morally entitled
right-sided heart failure. ineffective pumping by the right ventricle
risk management. the process of identifying and reducing the incidence of unwanted events
roentgenography. the obtaining of a film by use of roentgen rays (x-rays)
role confusion. failure to develop self-identity; a negative characteristic acquired during the developmental stage of young adulthood according to Erikson
rubella. German measles
Rule of One Hundreds. method for assessing impending alcohol withdrawal based on vital sign elevation

S

salicylism. a set of symptoms resulting from excessive ingestion of a salicylate
salpingo-oophorectomy. removal of the ovaries and fallopian tubes
sandwich generation. middle-aged adults with responsibilities for children and aging parents
sanguineous. drainage containing blood
sarcoma. a malignant tumor that arises from connective tissue
satiety. a feeling of comfortable fullness after eating
scar formation. replacement of damaged cells with fibrinous connective tissue
schizophrenia. a thought disorder characterized by deterioration in mental functioning, altered sensory perception, and changes in affect
sclerosed. narrowed or occluded
sebum. oily substance secreted by sebaceous glands of the skin
second-intention healing. healing from widely separated wound edges inward
secondary care. referrals for testing, diagnosis, or consultation
secondary condition. one that develops as a result of another condition
secondary gain. indirect benefit of being ill
secondary hypertension. elevated blood pressure due to some other disease process
sedative. an agent that exerts a calming effect
seizure. another term for a convulsion or an epileptic attack
senescence. the last stage in the life cycle

sensitivity. in microbiology, inhibition of bacterial growth with a specific antibiotic
sepsis. the presence of pathogens in the blood
septicemia. the presence of infective microorganisms in the bloodstream
sequela. following and resulting from a disease
sequestrum. pocket of necrotic bone
serosanguineous drainage. containing blood cells and serum
serotonin. a neurotransmitter that regulates mood and sleep
serous drainage. containing serum
shame. a feeling of disgrace or loss of self-respect (or the respect of others); a negative characteristic acquired during the developmental stage of early childhood according to Erikson
shearing. a physical force that separates layers of tissue in opposite directions; often occurs when clients are pulled up in bed
shock. life-threatening condition that occurs when there is inadequate arterial blood flow and oxygen delivery to cells and tissues
short-term goals. outcomes expected during a brief hospitalization
sign. objective data
signing. method for communicating by spelling the alphabet or creating word symbols with the hands
simple mastectomy. surgical treatment of breast cancer in which all breast tissue is removed but no lymph node dissection is performed
sinus bradycardia. regular heart rhythm and rate <60 beats/min
sinus tachycardia. regular heart rhythm but at a rate between 100 and 150 beats/min
sinusitis. inflammation of the sinuses
skeletal traction. mechanical pull applied directly to one or more bones
skin traction. mechanical pull applied to skin and indirectly to the skeletal system
sleep apnea. periodic cessation of breathing while asleep
social space. the area around an individual that extends from 4 to 12 feet
soma. the physical body as distinguished from the mind
somatization. converting unconscious emotional distress into physical symptoms
somatoform disorders. disorders in which physical symptoms are due to underlying and unconscious psychological factors
source oriented record. a chart in which each caregiver documents information on a separate form
specific gravity. weight of a substance compared with water, which has a specific gravity of 1.000, measured with a hydrometer
spermatogenesis. sperm production
sphincter. a circular muscle around an opening
sphygmomanometer. apparatus used to measure blood pressure
spider angiomata. tiny blood vessels that radiate from a central area
spinal shock. loss of sympathetic reflex activity below the level of spinal injury
spondylitis. inflammation of the vertebrae
splenomegaly. enlargement of the spleen
sprain. injury to the ligaments surrounding a joint
sputum. fluid raised from the respiratory passage
stagnation. lack of motion; a negative characteristic acquired during the developmental stage of middle adulthood according to Erikson
Standard Precautions. techniques used to reduce the potential for transmitting pathogens in blood or other body fluids when a person's infectious status is unknown
Starling's law of the heart. the physiologic principle that the length of myocardial stretch influences the force of its contraction
stasis. stagnation; stoppage of normal flow of fluids
status epilepticus. a state of sustained seizure activity
statute of limitations. the designated amount of time within which one may file a lawsuit
statutory law. laws enacted by legislatures or regulations established by governmental agencies
steatorrhea. stools containing undigested fat
stem cell. undifferentiated blood cell
stenosis. constriction, narrowing
stent. a device used to support tubular structures
stereotype. a fixed attitude about all people who share a common characteristic such as age, gender, race, or culture
stertorous. noisy, labored breathing
stoma. opening; mouth; artificially created opening
stomatitis. inflammation of the mouth
stool softener. a drug that softens the stool, thereby easing passage
strain. injury to a muscle when it is stretched or pulled beyond its capacity
streptokinase. a streptococcal enzyme that breaks down the fibrin in clots
stress. a physiologic response to biologic, psychological, or sociologic stressors
stress incontinence. incontinence of urine when sneezing, coughing, or laughing
stress management. techniques for reducing stress including relaxation and other coping strategies
stress-related disorders. disorders that are exacerbated by stress
stress ulcer. erosion of stomach mucous membrane due to ischemic damage to mucosal cells
stressor. an incident or condition capable of causing stress
stricture. a narrowing of a lumen
stridor. a high-pitched harsh sound during respiration; indicative of airway obstruction
stroke volume. the amount of blood pumped per contraction of the heart
subculture. a unique cultural group that exists within a dominant culture
subcutaneous. below or beneath the skin
subcutaneous emphysema. the presence of air in subcutaneous tissue
subcutaneous mastectomy. surgical treatment for breast cancer in which all breast tissue is removed but the skin and nipple are left intact
subjective data. information only the client can reveal
subluxation. partial dislocation
substance abuse. use of legal or illegal drugs for other than their intended purpose
substance P. a neurotransmitter that transmits pain impulses along nerve pathways to the brain
subtotal gastrectomy. removal of part of the stomach
sump tube. vented gastric suction tube
supine. lying on the back
suprapubic. above the pubic bone
susceptibility. prone to disease
sympathectomy. excision of a portion of the sympathetic nervous system, usually of a nerve, ganglion, or plexus
symptom. subjective data
syncope. fainting
syndrome. a group of signs and symptoms
synovial fluid. lubricating liquid within a movable joint

synovial membrane. the membrane lining the capsule of a joint
syphilis. a sexually transmitted disease caused by *Treponema pallidum*
systems method. an approach to the physical assessment that examines each body system separately
systole. contraction of the atria and ventricles (adj., systolic)
systolic blood pressure. pressure within the vascular system at the time of ventricular contraction

T

tabes dorsalis. a sequelae of syphilis characterized by degeneration of the central nervous system, resulting in loss of peripheral reflexes and vibratory and position senses
tachycardia. heart rate that exceeds 100 beats/min
tachyarrhythmia. rapid abnormal heart rhythm
tachypnea. rapid respiratory rate
task-oriented touch. personal contact that occurs as a result of performing nursing procedures
teaching plan. a formal plan for teaching new information; includes times frames and goals
team nursing. a method for delivering nursing care in which nurses with various levels of education are assigned specific aspects of client care; uses the team conference as a way to plan care
telemetry. monitoring from a distance
tenacious. clinging, adhesive
tenesmus. spasms of the rectum or bladder
tepid. lukewarm
terminating phase. the stage of the nurse–client relationship when the relationship ends
tertiary care. care provided by specialists, using complex technology
testicular self-examination. technique of self-assessment of the testes for signs of cancer
testosterone. male sex hormone produced by the testes
tetany. tonic spasms
tetraplegia. paralysis of all extremities; synonym: quadriplegia
therapeutic communication. using techniques that facilitate communication to improve the client's sense of well-being or ability to cope with problems
third-intention healing. delayed form of healing after exudate is removed
third-spacing. the translation of fluid to tissue compartments
thoracentesis. puncture of the chest wall to drain fluid from the thorax
thoracotomy. an opening into the thorax
thrill. palpable vibration
thrombectomy. surgical removal of a thrombus
thrombocytopenia. decreased number of platelets
thrombolytic. an agent capable of breaking up a thrombus
thrombophlebitis. vein inflammation with the formation of blood clots
thrombosis. development of a thrombus
thrombus. a stationary clot within the lumen of a blood vessel
thyroid-stimulating hormone (TSH). hormone produced by the anterior pituitary that stimulates thyroid gland hormone production
tinnitus. ringing in the ears
tolerance. needing a higher drug dosage to achieve the same effect as originally experienced with a lower dose
tonic. characterized by rigid contraction of the muscles
tophi. (sing., tophus) subcutaneous nodules of urate crystals
torts. violations of civil law
total parenteral nutrition (TPN). all essential nutrients including fats and proteins administered through intravenous infusion
toxic shock syndrome. severe, sudden illness caused by *Staphylococcus aureus* and associated with tampon use
toxigenicity. microbial ability to produce a toxin
toxin. a poisonous substance
toxoid. a weakened toxin
tracheostomy. the creation of a tracheal opening
tracheotomy. an incision of the trachea
traction. mechanical pull applied to the body to relieve muscle spasm and align fractures
tranquilizer. a drug that calms and reduces tension without interfering with normal mental activity
transcultural nursing. nursing care that demonstrates respect for people with diverse cultural values and beliefs
transcutaneous. through the skin
transillumination. passing a light through body tissues to observe for densities
transmission-based precautions. infection control techniques specific to the manner in which a particular pathogen is spread
transvenous. through the vein
Trichomonas. a parasitic protozoa
trochanter roll. a device placed parallel to the upper thigh to prevent external rotation of the hip
Trousseau's sign. muscle spasm of the arm and hand induced by exceeding systolic blood pressure; evidence of hypocalcemia
trust. a belief in the integrity and reliability of someone or something; a positive characteristic acquired during the developmental stage of infancy according to Erikson
tumor markers. substances synthesized by tumors and released into the circulation in excessive amounts
Turner's sign. a bluish gray discoloration on the flanks indicating pancreatic bleeding

U

ulcer. craterlike lesion in skin or mucous membranes
ultrasonography. diagnostic study using sound waves
ultraviolet light. light beyond the violet end of the visible spectrum
unilateral. on one side
unintentional torts. lawsuit involving harm to a person or property even though no harm was intended
urea. end product of protein metabolism
uremia. accumulation of nitrogenous substances in the blood (adj., uremic)
uremic frost. a precipitate that forms on the skin when the kidneys fail
urethritis. inflammation of the urethra
urinalysis. laboratory examination of the urine
urinary diversion. surgical procedure in which urine is redirected from its normal route
urticaria. hives
utilitarianism. ethical theory holding that an act is judged to be right or wrong depending on the consequences

V

vaccine. dead or weakened form of an infectious agent given to establish immunity to an infectious disease
vaginitis. inflammation of the vagina
vagotomy. surgical interruption of the vagus nerve to terminate the transmission of impulses along the nerve pathway

validation therapy. affirming the feelings that may underlie inappropriate behavior in the cognitively impaired older adult
Valsalva's maneuver. forced expiration against closed glottis
valvuloplasty. dilation of a stenosed cardiac valve with a balloon-tipped catheter
varicella. chickenpox
varices. (sing., varix) dilated, engorged veins
varicosities. tortuous veins in legs or lower trunk
vascular compartment. inside blood vessels
vasectomy. ligation of the vas deferens
vasoconstriction. constriction or narrowing of the diameter of a blood vessel
vasodilatation. dilatation or enlargement of the diameter of a blood vessel
vasodilator. a drug that increases the lumen of blood vessels
vasomotor nerves. nerves that control the size of blood vessels
vasopressor. a drug capable of constricting blood vessels, particularly arteries and arterioles
vector. an insect or animal that transfers an infectious agent from one host to another
vegetations. clumps of abnormal tissue on the cardiac valves, caused by bacteria
veins. blood vessels that carry unoxygenated blood
venereal diseases. any of the diseases contracted and spread by sexual activity
venereal warts. a sexually transmitted disease caused by the human papillomavirus
venipuncture. puncture of a vein
venography. radiograph of the veins using contrast dye
venostasis. the trapping of blood in an arm or leg by compression of a vein; interruption in the normal flow of venous blood; stagnation of venous blood
ventilation. the movement of air in and out of the lungs
ventricular assist device (VAD). a device that reroutes oxygenated blood in the left atrium directly to the aorta
ventricular fibrillation. quivering of the ventricle
venules. the smallest veins
verbal communication. communication using words
vertigo. sensation of moving or sensing that stationary objects are moving; may be used as a synonym for dizziness
vesicants. capable of causing blisters and necrosis of tissue
vesicle. a small sac that contains fluid
virulence. ability to cause disease
virus. a microorganism that lives in and is dependent on living cells for nutrition, growth, and reproduction
viscous. thick
visual acuity. ability to see clearly
visual field examination. assessment of ability to see in the periphery
vital capacity. a measure of the amount of air a person can expire after maximal inspiration

W

water loading. deliberate intake of large amounts of fluids before weight measurement; a method used by anorectics to suggest weight gain
wellness–illness continuum. the range of health from highest level to impending death
Western blot test. the confirming test for infection with human immunodeficiency virus (HIV)
wheal. a raised lesion often accompanied by severe itching; a hive
whole blood. blood cells and plasma
withdrawal. the physical symptoms and craving that occur when an abused substance is abruptly stopped
working phase. the stage of the nurse–client relationship when mutual care planning and implementation occur

X

xanthelasma. raised yellow plaques in the skin about the eyelids
xerostomia. dry mouth

Y

yeast. a member of the fungus family
yellow bone marrow. bone marrow found in long bones consisting primarily of fat cells and connective tissue

Index

Page numbers in *italics* indicate illustrations; those followed by *t* indicate tables; those followed by *b* indicate boxed and display text.

G

H

J

K

M

P

Q

R

S

Art was used from the following Lippincott Williams & Wilkins sources:

Becker, K.L. (1995). *Principles and practice of endocrinology and metabolism.* Philadelphia: JB Lippincott.
Figure 56-1, Figure 56-4, Figure 56-10

Beyers, M. & Dudas, S. (1984). *Clinical practice of medical-surgical nursing.* Boston: Little, Brown
Figure 56-9

Bullock, B. (1996). *Pathophysiology: Adaptations and alterations in function* (4th ed.). Philadelphia: Lippincott-Raven.
Figure 21-5, Figure 21-6, Figure 21-7, Figure 21-8, Figure 28-2, Figure 28-8, Figure 28-9, Figure 28-12, Figure 28-13, Figure 55-10, Figure 56-2, Figure 56-8, Figure 58-10, Figure 60-5, Figure 60-10, Figure 61-1, Figure 61-2, Figure 61-3

Carpenito, L.J. (1997). *Nursing diagnosis: Application to clinical practice* (7th ed.). Philadelphia: Lippincott-Raven.
Figure 19-8

Ellis, J.R., Nowlis, E.A., & Bentz, P.M. (1996). *Modules for basic nursing skills* (6th ed.). Philadelphia: Lippincott-Raven.
Figure in Clinical Procedure 18-1, Figure 23-9

Fuller, J. & Schaller-Ayers, J. (1994). *Health assessment: A nursing approach* (2nd ed.). Philadelphia: JB Lippincott.
Figure 21-4, Figure 55-11

Harrington, N., Smith, N., & Spratt, W.E. (1996). *LPN to RN transitions.* Philadelphia: Lippincott-Raven.
Box 5-1, Box 5-5

Haviley, C. et al. (1992). Pharmacologic management of cancer pain: A guide for the health care professional. *Cancer Nursing, 15*(5), 331–346.
Table 19-7

Huff, J. (1997). *ECG workout: Exercises in arrhythmia interpretation* (3rd ed.). Philadelphia: Lippincott-Raven.
Figure 33-1, Figure 33-12, Figure 33-13

Hunt, R. & Zurich, E.L. (1997). *Introduction to community nursing.* Philadelphia: Lippincott-Raven.
Figure 2-2

Judge, R.D., Suidema, G.D., et al (1982). *Clinical diagnosis* (4th ed.). Boston: Little, Brown.
Figure 56-5

May, K.A. & Mahlmeister, L.R. (1994). *Maternal and neonatal nursing: Family centered care* (3rd ed.). Philadelphia: JB Lippincott.
Figure 58-3

Memmler, R.L., Cohen, B.J., & Wood, D.L. (1996). *The human body in health and disease.* Philadelphia: Lippincott-Raven.
Figure 52-2, Figure 55-4, Figure 60-1

Metheny, N.M. (1996) *Fluid and electrolyte balance: Nursing considerations.* Philadelphia: Lippincott-Raven.
Figure 56-7

Nettina, S. (1996). *The Lippincott manual of nursing practice* (6th ed.). Philadelphia: Lippincott-Raven.
Figure 41-3

Porth, C. M. (1998). *Pathophysiology: Concepts of altered health states* (5th ed.). Philadelphia: Lippincott-Raven.
Figure 28-1, Figure 28-3, Figure 28-5, Figure 30-3

Rosedahl, C. (1995) *Textbook of basic nursing* (6th ed.). Philadelphia: JB Lippincott.
Figure 18-1

Rubin, E. & Farber, J.L. (1994). *Pathology* (2nd ed.). Philadelphia: JB Lippincott.
Figure 56-3

Smeltzer, S. & Bare, B. (1996). *Brunner and Suddarth's textbook of medical-surgical nursing* (8th ed.). Philadelphia: Lippincott-Raven.
Table 19-11, Table 19-12, Table-26-1, Figure 27-1, Table 28-2, Figure 30-4, Figure 30-5, Figure 38-1, Figure 41-4, Figure 44-7, Figure 54-1, Figure in Clinical Procedure 54-1, Figure 60-3

Taylor, C., Lillis, C., & LeMone, P. (1997). *Fundamentals of nursing: The art and science of nursing care* (3rd ed.). Philadelphia: Lippincott-Raven.
Figure 8-2

Timby, B.K. & Harrison, L.O. (1996). *Fundamental skills and concepts in patient care* (6th ed.). Philadelphia: Lippincott-Raven.
Figure 3-1, Figure 4-1, Figure 4-2, Figure 9-2, Figure 9-1, Figure 9-3, Figure 9-4, Figure 10-1, Table 11-3, Figure 18-3, Figure 20-1, Figure 20-2, Figure 21-1, Figure 21-2, Figure 21-3, Table 21-2, Table 21-3, Table 21-4, Figure 23-2, Figure 23-3, Figure 23-4, Figure 23-5, Figure 23-7, Figures in Clinical Procedure 23-1, Figure in Clinical Procedure 26-1, Figure in Clinical Procedure 28-1, Figure in Nursing Guidelines 28-2, Figure in Nursing Guidelines 28-3, Figure 1 in Clinical Procedure 34-1, Figures in Clinical Procedure 38-1, Figure 46-7, Figure 48-3, Figure 48-4, Figure in Box 49-1, Figure in Clinical Procedure 51-1, Figures in Nursing Guidelines 51-2, Figures in Nursing Guidelines 53-1, Figures 57-2, Figures in Nursing Guidelines 57-2, Figures in Clinical Procedure 57-1, Unnumbered figures in Chapter 58